NUTRITION

For Living

Fourth Edition

Janet L. Christian

Janet L. Greger

University of Wisconsin-Madison

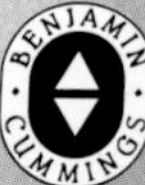

The Benjamin/Cummings Publishing Company, Inc.
Redwood City, California • Menlo Park, California • Reading, Massachusetts • New York
Don Mills, Ontario • Wokingham, U.K. • Amsterdam • Bonn • Sydney • Singapore • Tokyo • Madrid • Sa

To Jack and Jeff with love.
Janet L. Christian

To all my students over the years; and, of course, to my parents and sister.
Janet L. Greger

Executive Editor: Patricia L. Cleary
Project and Production Editor: Wendy Earl
Developmental Editor: Elizabeth Maynard Schaefer
Text and Cover Design, Art Director: Jeanne Calabrese
Electronic Artist: Robert Voigts
Art and Photo Coordinator: Frank Edward Vaughn
Photo Researcher: Sarah Bendersky
Food Photographer: Richard Tauber
Food Stylist: Barbara Tauber
Copy Editor: Sally Peyrefitte
Proofreader: Eleanor Renner Brown
Indexer: Elinor Lindheimer
Compositor and Prepress Supplier: GTS Graphics
Printer and Binder: Von Hoffmann Press, Inc.
Cover Source: Comstock, Inc.

Library of Congress Cataloging-in-Publication Data

Christian, Janet L.
Nutrition for living / Janet L. Christian, Janet L. Greger.
p. cm.
Includes bibliographical references and index.
ISBN 0-8053-1570-5
1. Nutrition. I. Greger, Janet L. II. Title
QP141, C548 1994
613--dc20 93-34107
CIP

ISBN 0-8053-1570-5

2 3 4 5 6 7 8 9 10 -VH - 97 96 95 94

The Benjamin/Cummings Publishing Company, Inc.
390 Bridge Parkway
Redwood City, California 94065

Preface

We hear a great deal about nutrition from a variety of sources today. Increasingly, television newscasts, talk shows, and advertisements all focus on nutrition. Popular magazines and newspapers feature articles on nutrition. At the food market, shelves and freezers bulge with new products claiming to be nutritionally superior to their competitors. Best-seller lists often boast a title or two about nutrition.

With all of this information already available to you, why should you read *Nutrition for Living*? Can't you learn what you need to know just by paying attention to the TV, magazine, and food product promotions?

Not really. It's hard to get a good nutrition education by picking up scattered bits and pieces of information. Without first seeing the big picture, it's difficult to understand where the details fit in. Furthermore, some of what you see around you may sizzle and pop with excitement, but it may not be valid.

By contrast, our goal in writing *Nutrition for Living* is to provide college nonmajors with a comprehensive overview of the science of nutrition, highlighting many intriguing and useful facts along the way. What you read here stems from scientific research, which continues to uncover new findings every day. Altogether, such information is the basis for our advice about how to eat healthfully.

What's New in the Fourth Edition?

In the process of updating the research findings to provide a solid foundation and responding to the expanding needs of nutrition curricula, we have modified much of the text narrative. And although we have continued many of the popular features of previous editions, we have renamed some of them. *Slice of Life* boxes provide real-life examples of principles discussed in the text. *Act on Fact* exercises encourage you to analyze your diet and compare it with recommended standards. *Consider This* boxes suggest dietary changes that are in line with current nutrition goals. But the Fourth Edition provides much more than this.

The Food Guide Pyramid and New Food Labels

The United States government has taken two important initiatives to promote better nutrition among U.S. citizens. First, the Department of Agriculture has developed the Food Guide Pyramid, a new graphic for helping people choose a varied, moderate, and balanced diet. Second, Congress mandated a new food label format that is required on most packaged foods as of the summer of 1994. You will see examples of both of these new developments throughout the Fourth Edition.

Focus on Controversial Issues

Because some of the effects of nutrition on health occur over several years, and because many factors other than nutrition affect health, the effects of nutrition are not always clear-cut. We meet these issues, along with the controversies they have spawned, head on. You will have a chance to meet prominent experts through personal interviews on selected cutting-edge topics—lipids and heart disease, weight control, folic acid supplementation, biotechnology, and nutrition and AIDS.

Expanded Emphasis on Critical Thinking

Throughout the text, special sections called "Thinking for Yourself" present controversial topics and invite you to use critical thinking techniques to develop an informed opinion. You have the opportunity to assess the accuracy of the information presented, consider other factors, and decide on an action plan that makes sense to you.

Greater Emphasis on Fitness

Surely, good nutrition alone cannot ensure good health; adequate exercise is also important. Throughout this edition, we discuss more thoroughly the importance of exercise in a healthy lifestyle. A small icon of a runner appears in the margin at the beginning of sections about exercise and fitness. Look for expanded coverage of exercise and fitness in the chapters on water, carbohydrates, proteins, energy, body weight, and minerals.

More Global Coverage

In this edition, the last chapter of the book is devoted to "Expanding Your Concerns." It provides a perspective on nourishing all the world's people, a matter that is intertwined with the health of the environment. This chapter ends with ideas that outline how the efforts of even one person can help.

More Accessible and Interactive Writing Style

In keeping with the popularity of user-friendly educational materials, this edition is more conversational and accessible than ever before. Scan a few pages for a sample of our modified style. Also, read one of the "You Tell Me" boxes located throughout the text. These new features ask questions that help you apply the material just covered.

Supplementary Materials

A complete package of supplementary materials accompanies this text.

The Student Study Guide

Written by Dr. Susan Nitzke of the University of Wisconsin-Madison, this helpful guide follows the organization of the textbook. Each chapter provides an overview of the equivalent text chapter, a suggested study plan, learning objectives, a detailed chapter outline, a section on memory aids, including suggestions for constructing one or more concept maps, self-testing exercises, and application exercises. The last section of the Study Guide contains perforated self-assessment forms that are keyed to the Act on Fact diet assessments in the text.

Diet Analysis and Fitness Evaluator Software

The Diet Simple and Fitness Evaluator software package, created by N-Squared Computing, contains an interactive graphics diet analysis program that calculates nutritive analyses of single foods or combinations of foods in your diet. Its fitness component allows you to determine energy requirements consistent with weight gain/loss goals, and generate activity schedules to achieve those goals. The Diet Simple/Fitness Evaluator software runs on the IBM PC, AT, and XT, as well as the Macintosh computers.

The Instructor's Guide

This guide, by Dr. Marsha Read of the University of Nevada-Reno, includes chapter learning objectives, a brief outline of each chapter in the text, critical thinking activities, a list of additional classroom resources, and a testbank of multiple choice and short answer questions. Testbank questions are correlated with the learning objectives and are classified according to level of difficulty. The last section of the Instructor's Guide contains self-assessment forms that are keyed to the Act on Fact diet assessments in the text. These forms may be reproduced for student use.

Color Transparencies

A set of 45 full-color transparency acetates and 30 black and white transparency masters of key illustrations in the text is available to qualified adopters of the text.

Computerized Testing Software

The test questions in the Instructor's Guide are also available on The Benjamin/Cummings Microcomputer Testing Software, available for the IBM PC, AT, and XT, and the Macintosh computers. Qualified adopters of *Nutrition for Living* may obtain this software by contacting the publisher or your local representative.

Acknowledgments

Many committed and talented people have helped prepare this book.

At Benjamin/Cummings, we thank our executive editor, Patti Cleary, for providing all the resources that made this edition possible.

In our developmental editor, Beth Schaefer, we found an experienced science writer with exceptional insight, sensibility, and professionalism. We also appreciate the innovative interviews she conducted with five nutrition experts.

We thank Wendy Earl, our project and production editor, for her diplomatic coordination of all the people and tasks necessary to move words and illustrations onto the printed page expediently.

Jeanne Calabrese, the book's designer and art director, brought to her work an uncommon blend of creativity and the ability to incorporate others' ideas. We also thank electronic artist Robert Voigts for his computerized transformation of this edition's artwork.

Sarah Bendersky, photo researcher, found many handsome new images that eloquently make their points, and our thanks go to Rich Tauber for his mouth-watering food photographs.

We also appreciate the authors of this edition's Study Guide, Dr. Susan Nitzke, and the Instructor's Guide, Dr. Marsha Read. They took our newly revised textbook chapters, added their expertise, and created suggestions that will help teachers and students use the textbook to its best advantage.

Finally, we appreciate the many careful reviewers and consultants who advised us on various portions of this book, and we are indebted to all of the instructors who shared their experiences using previous editions. Their insights and suggestions have helped refine the pages of this edition.

We warmly thank you all.

Janet L. Christian
Janet L. Greger

Reviewers and Consultants[a]

Paul Addis,
University of Minnesota

Andrea Arguitt,
Oklahoma State University

Rebecca A. Benedict,
St. Olaf College

Joan Benson,
University of Utah

Nancy Betts,
University of Nebraska

Laurel Jean Branen,
Washington State University

Wen Chiu,
Shoreline Community College

Maxine Cochran,
William Penn College

Dorothy Coltrin,
DeAnza College

Marie Cross,
University of Kansas

Lael Cutler,
Northeastern University

Marjorie Dibble,
Syracuse University

Susan Dougherty,
Monroe Community College

Joan Downham,
Normandale Community College

Bessie Fick,
Auburn University

B.L. Frye,
University of Texas

Sylvia Gartung,
Michigan State University

Nancy Green,
Florida State University

Yolanda Gutierrez,
University of San Francisco

Ed Hart,
Bridgewater State College

Wendy T. Hunt,
American River College

Amy Ireson,
College of San Mateo

Debra K. W. Jahner,
California State University, Long Beach

Charlotte Juntunen,
University of Minnesota, Duluth

Joan Karkeck,
University of Washington

Janet King,
University of California, Berkeley

Sondra King,
Northern Illinois University

Judith Listman,
Purdue University

Bo Lonnerdal,
University of California, Davis

Sharleen Matter,
University of Louisville

Sally McGill,
Canada College

Glen McNeil,
Arizona State University

Barbara Mitchell,
University of Houston

Diane C. Mitchell,
Pennsylvania State University

Elizabeth Mills,
Central Michigan University

Susan Nitzke,
University of Wisconsin-Madison

Earl Nolenberger,
Shippensburg University

Mary Ann Page,
Dixie College

Ellen Parham,
Northern Illinois University

Marsha Read,
University of Nevada, Reno

Ellyn Satter,
Jackson Clinic, Madison

Barbara Schneeman,
University of California, Davis

Charles Seiger,
Atlantic Community College

Jean Skinner,
University of Tennessee ▸

[a] For one or more of the four editions

Joanne Slavin,
University of Minnesota

Anne Smith,
University of Utah

Diana Marie Spillman,
Miami University

Katherine Staples,
North Dakota State University

Bernice Stewart,
Prince George's Community College

Katherine Stewart
University of Nevada, Reno

Jon Story,
Purdue University

Susan Strahs,
California State University, Long Beach

Kathryn Sucher,
San Jose State University

Barry Swanson,
Washington State University

Steve Taylor,
University of Wisconsin-Madison

Mary Ann Thompson,
Waubonsee Community College

Linda Vaughan,
Arizona State University

Jane Voichick,
University of Wisconsin

Rosemary C. Wander,
Oregon State University

Kathy Watson,
Arizona Western College

Margaret West,
Chicago State University

Loyanne Wilson,
Eastern Kentucky University

Billie Wood,
Daytona Beach Community College

Kathy Yadrick,
University of Southern Mississippi

Margaret Younathan,
Louisiana State University

Brief Contents

Detailed Contents

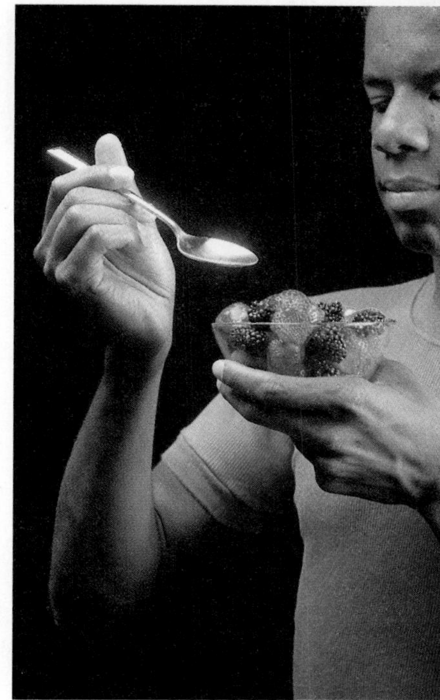

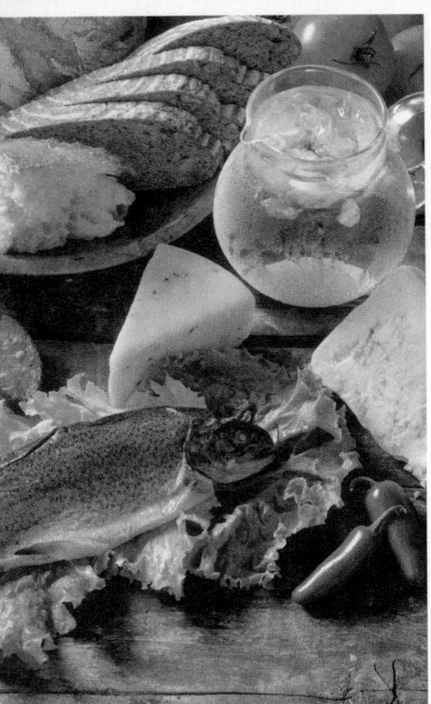

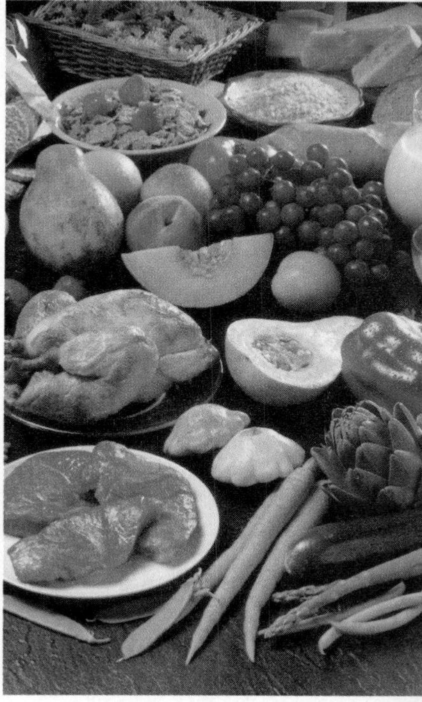

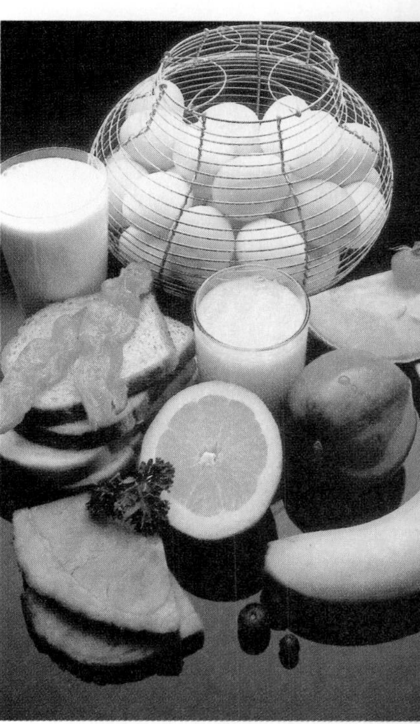

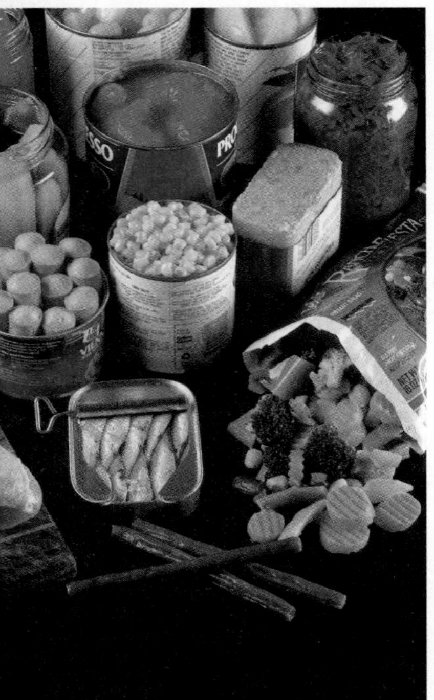

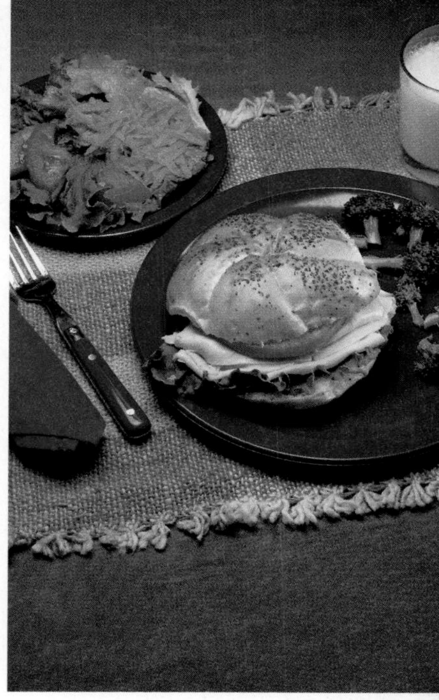

Special Features

Thinking for Yourself

Interviews

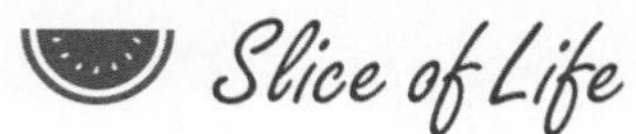

Act on Fact

Consider This

This icon is used throughout the text to highlight material pertaining to fitness and nutrition.

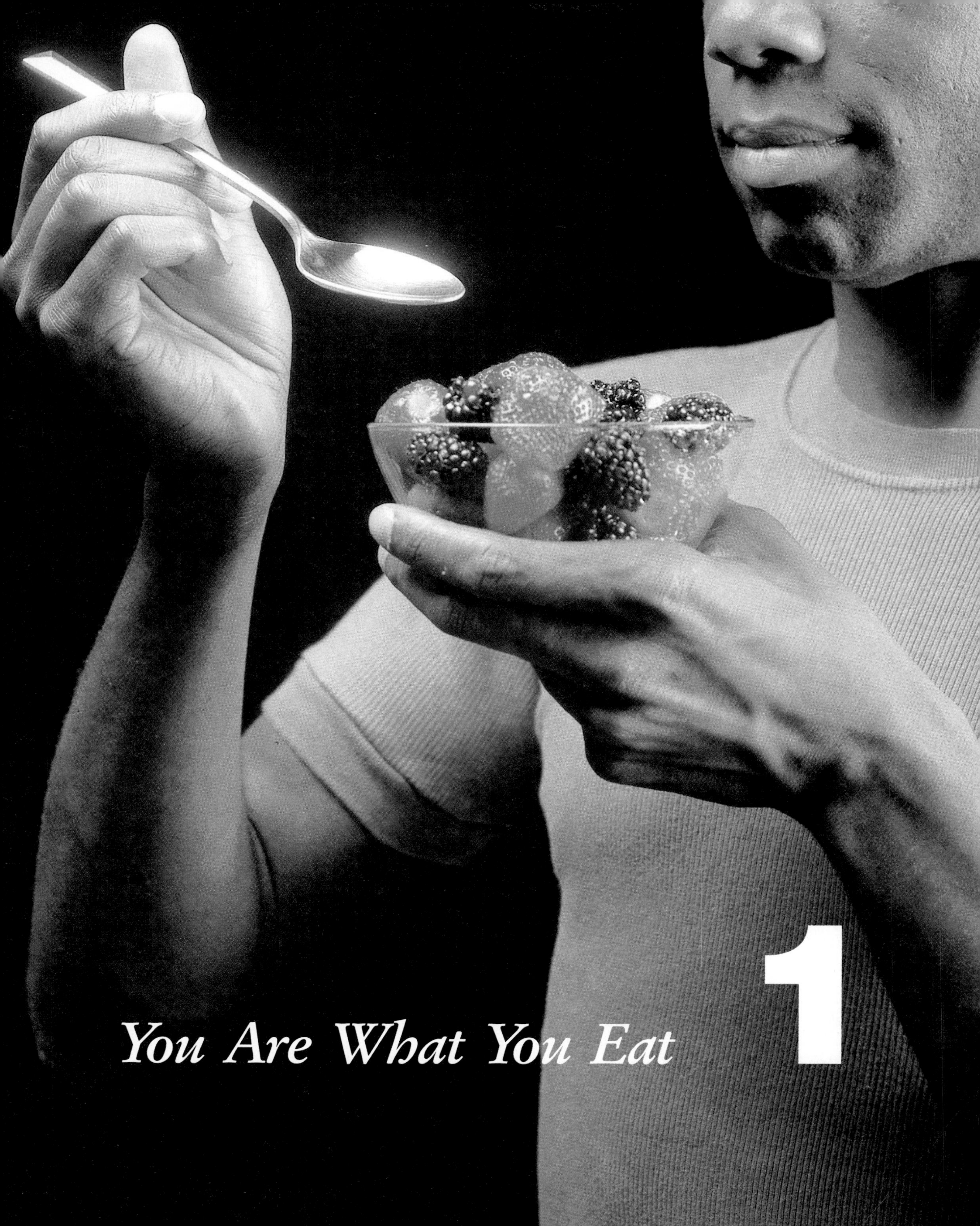

1

You Are What You Eat

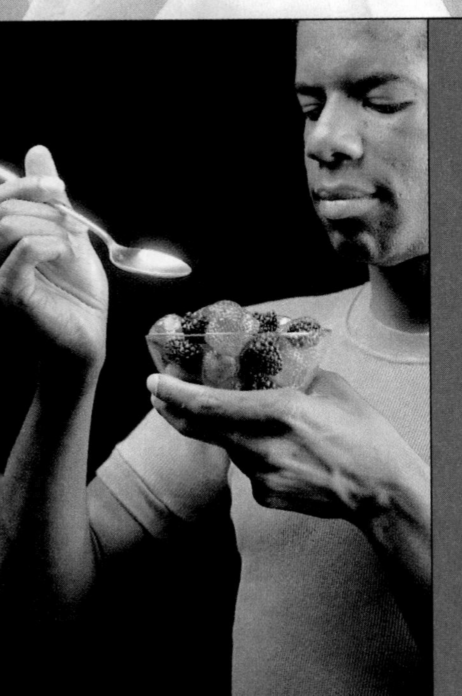

IN THIS CHAPTER

Why You Eat What You Do

The Science of Nutrition

Chapter 1

How Food Affects You

If you could have whatever you wanted to eat for your next meal, what would it be? Pizza, salad, and a can of soda? Lomi salmon and poi bread? Tacos or a burrito? Fried chicken, cornbread, black-eyed peas? Vegetable stir-fry? Hummus and pita bread?

You may be surprised to start a course in **nutrition** by thinking about your food preferences, but it's an excellent way to begin. Foods are the carriers of **nutrients,** so the factors that affect your food choices have major effects on how well-nourished you are.

nutrition—the interactions between a living organism and its food

nutrient—a specific substance that must be taken into the body preformed and in sufficient quantity to meet the body's needs for growth, reproduction, and maintenance of health

It's important to recognize up front—right in the first part of the first chapter—how influential these factors are, so that you can appreciate the great benefits of your good eating habits. And if, as you progress through this course, you decide that you would like to improve some of your habits, your understanding of what affects food choice can help you learn how to make changes.

Your food choices reflect a personal blend of many diverse, overlapping influences. Choosing what to eat involves such factors as which tastes you like, what your mood is at the moment, and how much money you have in your wallet. Your preferences can reach way back to what you were fed as a young child and how you reacted to those foods, and you are probably also influenced by ethnic factors that you may not even recognize until you get away from home territory. Many people try to eat in a way that will make them healthier—but their good intentions sometimes actually backfire, if their information about nutrition is not accurate.

Instead of using a hit-or-miss approach, you can develop healthier eating habits by learning about the science of nutrition. In the second part of this chapter, we present the basics of nutritional science—clarifying what nutrients are, explaining what they do, and considering what happens if you take in either too few or too many nutrients. You'll find out how scientists acquire nutrition knowledge and how you can use this information to evaluate claims you read here and elsewhere about nutrition. Then you'll be ready for more in-depth study in the chapters that follow.

Let's begin!

Why You Eat What You Do

Out of tens of thousands of types of food items available in the United States, one expert has estimated that only about 100 foods account for 75% of the total amount of food we consume (Molitor, 1980). How do we narrow down our choices from such an incredible array of possibilities?

At times, it may seem obvious to you why you eat what you do. ("I like it." "It was there." "I saw it advertised on TV.") However, what you eat arises from a complex, interwoven background of genetic and environmental factors that you do not consciously think about every time you put something in your mouth (Figure 1.1).

Inborn Factors

You may think that a newborn arrives with no food preferences. That is not the case, as you'll see in the following section.

Inborn Taste Preferences All babies and young children like sweet foods; infants who are tested in their first few days of life all respond happily when they are given sweetened water. Water with a bitter taste, by contrast, will bring scowls or crying (Rozin, 1988). Although appreciation for sweetness may decline as people age, the predilection for some degree of sweetness

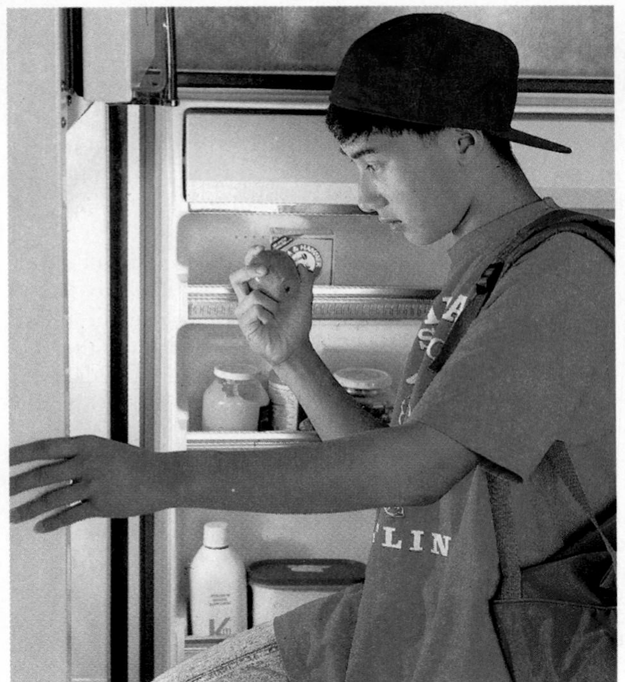

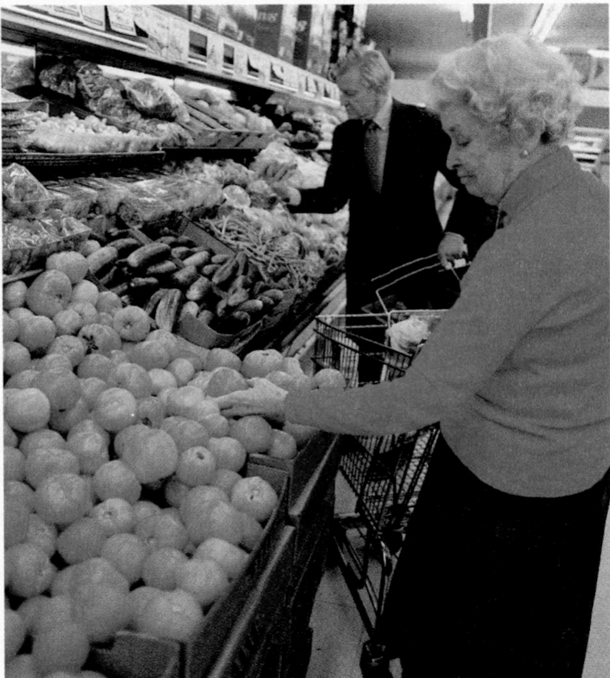

FIGURE 1.1
Influences on food choices.

Although it may seem at times that choosing what to eat is a purely impulsive act, your food preferences are influenced by an underlying complex of innate, cultural, and individual factors. These factors come into play whenever and wherever you make food choices.

persists throughout life. Psychologists suggest that this has been important to our survival, because the naturally sweet (sugar-containing) foods that early humans encountered, such as fruits and honey, were a source of life-sustaining energy.

In recent years, sugar-sweetened foods have been cast in a dim light because of people's belief that these foods cause undesirable weight gain. How do people cope with this, given their liking for sweet things? You have seen the solution: a whole industry—the sugar substitute industry—has developed to resolve the conflict.

Infants reject the bitter taste, however (Rozin, 1988). Psychologists suggest that this may stem from the fact that many bitter substances in nature are toxic; those people who avoided toxic substances survived long enough to become our ancestors.

Some inborn biases can be modified, and they often are, by experience and conditioning. For example, some people *acquire* a taste for foods that are decidedly bitter. Others come to like foods so spicy that their mouths burn and eyes water when they eat them. One psychologist dubbed this behavior of eating foods that produce somewhat unpleasant sensations "benign masochism," because it provides the thrill of apparent danger although it is really harmless (Rozin and Vollmecke, 1986).

You Tell Me

Culture can change your taste preferences. Although all infants like sweetness, in some people the appreciation of the sweet taste gradually declines; and although as newborns we instinctively dislike bitterness, we can learn to like it.

Do you still like foods as sweet as you did when you were younger? Do you like some bitter or spicy foods? Do you remember at what age you started to find such foods appealing?

Cautious Interest in New Foods By nature, we all are interested in new foods; at the same time, we tend to be cautious about trying them. This inborn trait allowed early humans to expand their dietary variety gradually in relative safety. This interest in new foods is not limited to early humans in the distant past, though; we are still experimenting. The great popularity of ethnic restaurants, even among people whose own ethnic background is different than the restaurant's culture, testifies to our interest in trying something new.

This attraction to novelty is also expressed in the use of such exotic items as flower blossoms in salads or as condiments, and in some people's recently renewed interest in foraging for wild foods. If these sound appealing, trust your instinct to be cautious, and learn first which varieties of flowers or wild foods are safe to eat. Check with your county's agricultural expert for information about plants not traditionally used as human food.

Cultural Factors

Wherever we are, the people and culture around us influence our food choices. Anthropologists point out that in all societies, eating is an important way of initiating and maintaining human relationships: eating and socializing experiences are tightly intertwined.

Family and Caregivers Infants learn to associate food and feelings from the first feeding. Caregivers usually give food and affection at the same time; this reinforces the baby's interest in eating. As the child grows and begins to eat a variety of foods at home, an association between these foods and feelings of security develops (Figure 1.2). Even years later, many people find that eating favorite foods of childhood can provide a sense of comfort.

At the other end of the spectrum, unhappy childhood associations with food can also linger, as the Slice of Life on page 6, about Native American Ron Paquin, sadly demonstrates.

National Origin Ethnicity is a strong predictor of food preference. Ethnic groups and nationalities develop their unique cuisines through a combination of environmental and social factors. Each ethnic group encourages the

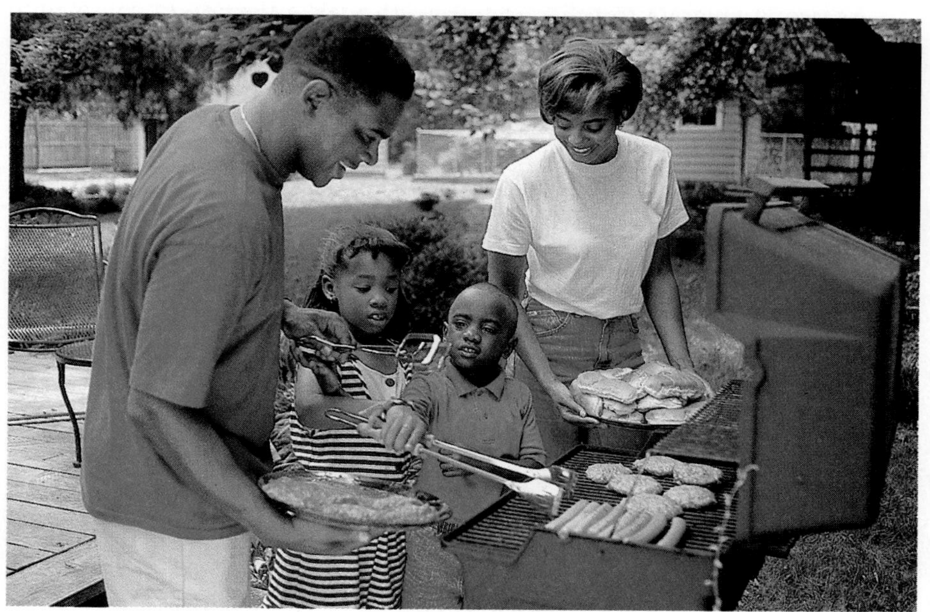

FIGURE 1.2
Happy childhood associations with food can carry through into later years.

If some of the foods you like today are things you remember eating at happy family events when you were a child, you are experiencing a typical cultural effect on food choice.

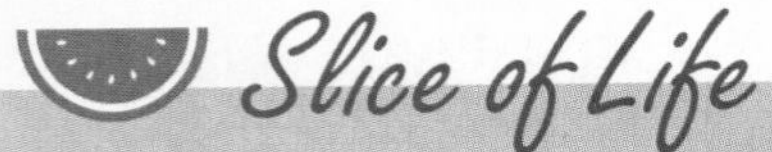

Bad Childhood Memories Can Affect Food Choices, Too

Just as *happy* past associations with food can affect present food choices, *unhappy* connections between food and childhood can also persist. This recollection from the beginning of *Not First in Nobody's Heart* by Ron Paquin and Robert Doherty provides an example.

> *Well, here goes.* My name is Ronald Joseph Paquin. I was born September 4, 1942, behind Al Wright's Bar in a little cabin, to Alec and Theresa Paquin of St. Ignace, Michigan. My twin brother, Donny, and I was delivered by the doctor there. We stayed with our parents for just lacking two years, I think, and my mother took sick, so my aunt went and got us to live with her.
>
> We wasn't happy at my aunt and uncle's, the Hartwicks. They showed us some affection for a while, but then we got to be probably a burden to them, maybe. I don't know. There was a lot of beating that went on too. My aunt had quite a time with that razor strop.
>
> My uncle ate like a pig. He'd hog the good food, the lean meat. He'd grab the lean, most of it, and give us the fatty parts. To this day I can't eat fat. (Paquin and Doherty, 1992.)

use of only some of the foods available to it while discouraging the use of others, even to the extent of designating them "taboo" (Bryant, 1985).

Some indigenous groups of people believe that the characteristics of what is eaten can be acquired by the eater (a rather literal interpretation of "You are what you eat"). For example, some people believe that eating part of an animal known for its ferocity will make them brave. Certain Eskimos believe that if a lactating mother eats duck's wings, her child will grow up to be a good paddler. Such mystical thinking is an attempt to explain and gain control over an environment that is often unpredictable and hostile (Harper, 1988).

Many cultures have a staple food around which the rest of the cuisine has developed and which may have been the key to the people's survival over the ages; the rice of Asia and the wheat bread of Europe are examples. These foods are so important that in some cases cultures have assigned supernatural attributes to them. For example, the Mayan word for corn, *ixim*, literally means "the grace of God."

As people migrate to other countries, they take their food habits with them. Because the population of the United States represents an ethnic mosaic, the foods eaten here reflect our cultural diversity (Figure 1.3). Currently, the predominant racial and ethnic groups in the United States are

FIGURE 1.3
No wonder ethnic restaurants are popular!

Ethnic foods can appeal to you for a variety of reasons. They might be part of your own culture of origin, or you may just enjoy their flavors. Some may be real bargains or have a reputation for being healthy. You may be attracted to exotic foods because they appeal to your sense of adventure—or because your friends are trying them. In another area of the world, a meal of a hamburger and fries would be regarded as ethnic: American!

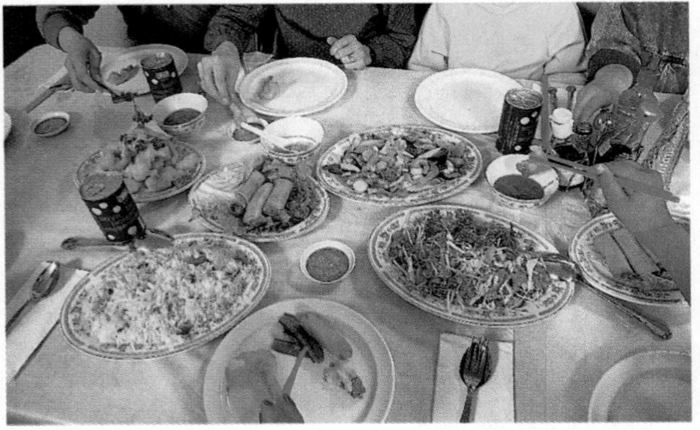

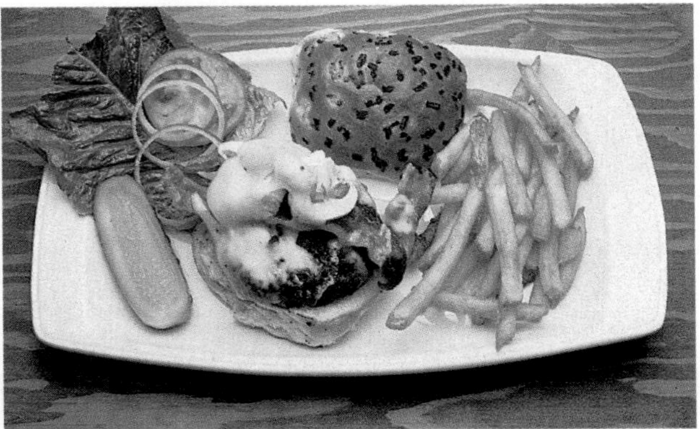

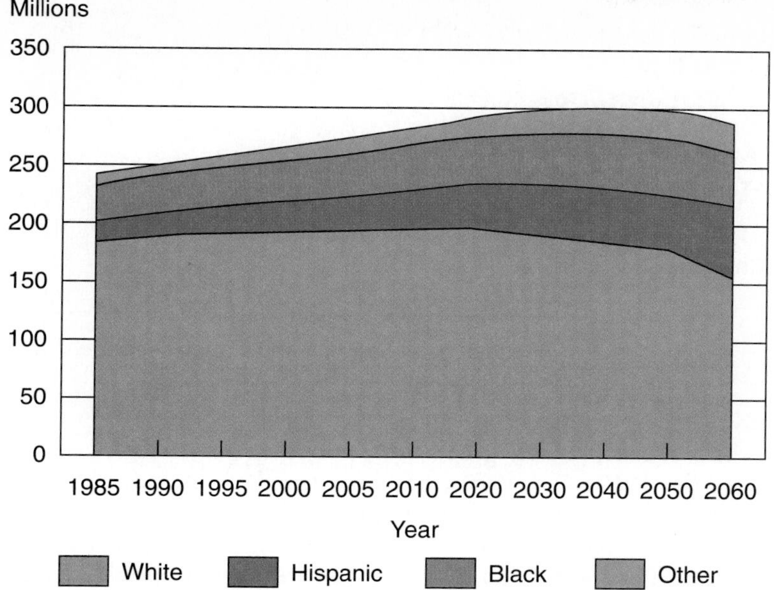

FIGURE 1.4
Projected total U.S. population by ethnic group.

As people of different ethnic backgrounds come to the United States to live, they bring their food preferences with them, providing more food choices for all of us.

(Adapted from Senauer, Asp, and Kinsey, 1991)

white, black, and Hispanic (Figure 1.4); the greatest numbers of new immigrants are currently Asian and Latin American (Senauer et al., 1991).

The changing population mix is expected to have increasing impact on what foods will be available in restaurants, schools, and food stores; this may affect your food choices. Beyond the popular nachos, tacos, pastas, and stir-fried dishes that are already widely available, we will also see the growing popularity of such ethnic cuisines as Cajun, Thai, Afghani, and South American, which were formerly found only in limited regions.

Although many Americans enjoy the variety and richness of ethnic flavors, they are not necessarily concerned about authenticity; ethnic hybrids can also gain acceptance (Owen, 1990). Consider that pizza and chow mein are U.S. creations, fashioned from ingredients characteristic of other cultures. More recently, chizza (pizza crust topped with Chinese vegetables and sauces) and buritskis (a burrito stuffed with Polish sausage) have been test marketed (Owen, 1990).

Religious Affiliation Some religions have developed dietary practices that are so elaborate and important to their followers that they refer to these practices as "laws." The Jewish kosher dietary laws (Regenstein and Regenstein, 1988) and Islamic dietary laws (Twaigery and Spillman, 1989) are examples.

Because many religious food practices stem from ancient traditions, the original motivations for these practices are often not known. There are likely possibilities, though, such as ethical considerations, food safety, health maintenance, and symbolic values. Whatever their origins, these practices give a sense of unity and identity to the groups that maintain them.

Ethical Stances Ethical as well as religious considerations can affect a person's food choices. You or your friends, for example, may be concerned about eating behaviors that cause unnecessary stress on the **ecosystem**; these issues have produced a movement called *green consumerism,* which is expected to have a major impact on the food industry in the 1990s (Wittwer, 1992).

ecosystem—a system formed by the interaction of a community of plants and animals with their environment

FIGURE 1.5
Efficiency of converting grain to other forms of food.

Animals that produce food for human consumption sometimes eat plants that could have been consumed directly by humans. This illustration shows how many pounds of grain (or grain and soy) an animal consumes in producing one pound of the stated product.

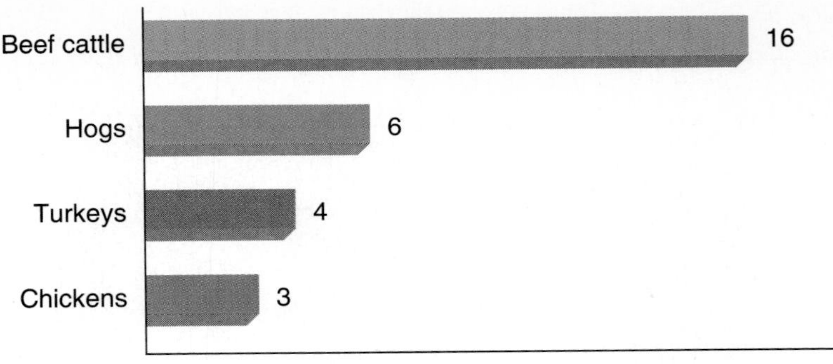

This movement, which grew from concerns raised by world hunger activists of the 1960s and 1970s, has broadened to include environmental concerns. Activists point out that the production of grain-fed beef cattle is wasteful, because to produce one pound of muscle (meat) requires 16 pounds of grain and soy (Lappe, 1982) (Figure 1.5). If people ate the plant products themselves instead of using them to feed animals, less acreage would need to be cultivated, and the soil would be less depleted of nutrients. These considerations have led some people to avoid grain-fed beef. Range-fed cattle, by contrast, are often grazed on domestic land that is unusable for other forms of agriculture; they therefore *add* to the food supply.

Some environmentalists also view with disfavor eating beef that has been imported from tropical regions. Some of that beef comes from cattle grazed on land that has been cleared by cutting down sections of rainforest, a practice that increases the destruction of the endangered rainforest ecosystem (Nations and Komer, 1986). This destruction leads to the extinction of many species of plants and animals as their habitat disappears.

Excessive depletion of energy for food processing is another ethical issue. The food industry uses a large amount of fossil fuel for moving ingredients and products into and out of processing plants and distribution centers and for elaborate packaging of products. This suggests that if we used fewer convenience foods, considerable energy could be saved. However, there are exceptions. For example, the shipping of dried milk powder for reconstitution—instead of fluid milk—can save on energy consumption (Jesse and Cropp, 1987).

Solid waste enters into the ethical picture as well. Space for disposal of solid waste is becoming scarce in most heavily populated areas of the world, especially in the developed countries. Some people concerned with this issue are rallying around a new version of the 3 R's: reduce, reuse, and recycle (Wittwer, 1992) (Figure 1.6). Some trash collection departments now require citizens to separate their refuse according to its recycling potential.

You Tell Me

Many colleges and universities have taken the lead in their communities by establishing campus recycling programs.

Does your campus have a recycling program in place? What materials are collected? Is there evidence that students and staff cooperate in this effort?

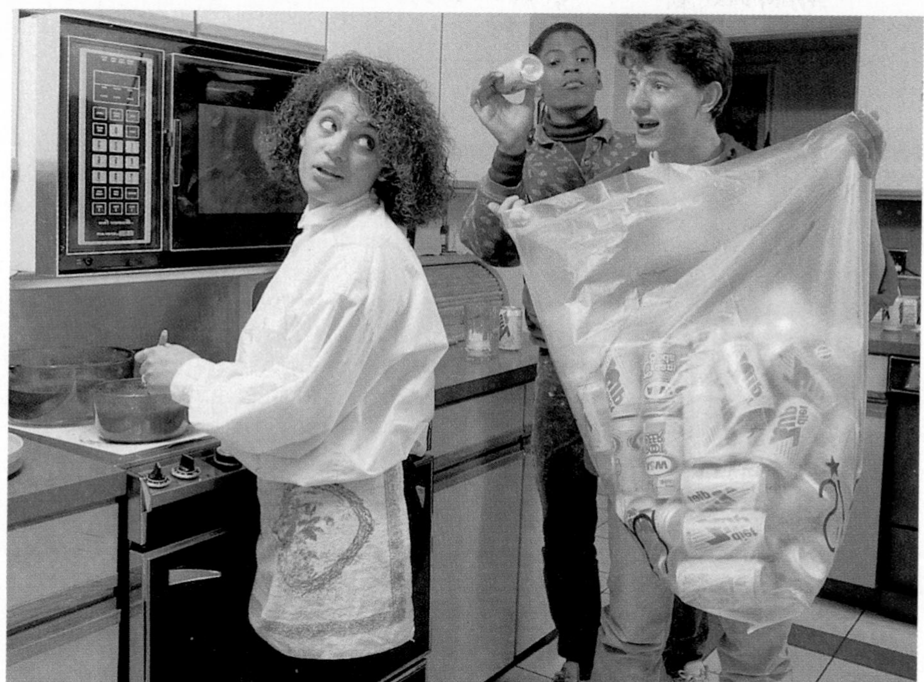

FIGURE 1.6
Recycling starts at home.

In some communities, mandatory separation of trash into plastic, paper, metal, and glass enables once-used materials to be used again repeatedly.

Public Health Information and Nutrition Education Campaigns During the last decade, Americans have received an ever-increasing amount of information about how the foods they eat (or don't eat) may affect their health. These messages address four major health concerns: heart disease, cancer, high blood pressure, and osteoporosis.

Much of this educational outpouring has originated in federal agencies and health organizations, such as the Food and Drug Administration, the National Institutes of Health, and the Surgeon General's Office. To get their messages across, these agencies rely heavily on the mass media; word is spread through press reports and public service announcements.

In the fall of 1984, the National Cancer Institute (one of the National Institutes of Health) allowed one of its health messages to be delivered in a new way—through product labeling and advertising. The Kellogg Company stated in its cereal ads that the National Cancer Institute recommended eating a high-fiber diet to reduce the risk of some types of cancer. The effectiveness of this campaign was evident: in a follow-up survey asking which foods are good sources of fiber, over two-thirds of those asked cited breakfast cereals (Lecos, 1988).

Although this ad delivered information very effectively to the American public, it created a regulatory nightmare. Other food producers wanted to make health claims for their products as well. Developing policies about what claims may say—so that they inform and not mislead—is difficult, because the unique nature of each food makes it impossible for a generic policy to cover all cases easily. Furthermore, experts question how much credit any one food should be given for being nutritious or for reducing risk of disease. As we'll discuss throughout this book, your *health and nutritional status are affected by the total of what you have eaten over a long period of time, not just by one food you have consumed for a few weeks or months.*

Nonetheless, the Food and Drug Administration has decided to allow certain standardized health messages to be used on product labels for appro-

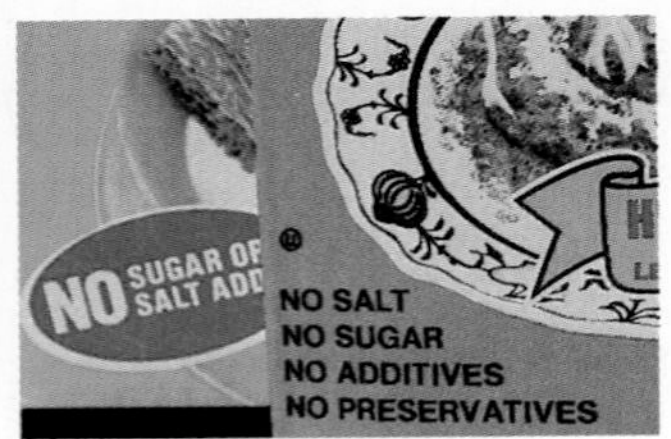

FIGURE 1.7
Nutrition sells.

A large proportion of new food products are promoted on the basis of beneficial nutritional qualities.

priate foods. Seven different label messages may be used to indicate the relationships between various dietary constituents and osteoporosis, cancer, coronary heart disease, and high blood pressure.

Food Product Advertising and Promotion Food ads represent more than 20% of all direct consumer advertising in the United States, making the food industry the largest advertiser in the country. In 1988, the food industry spent $11.5 billion on advertisements (Senauer et al., 1991).

Food advertising is designed to shift people's consumption from one item within a product class to another: most promotions attempt to develop loyalty to a specific brand of product. Basic food items have traditionally received little advertising attention. Recently, though, agricultural commodity groups that produce such foods as dairy products, eggs, beef, pork, and turkey have sponsored national television and print advertising campaigns.

Another type of change has occurred. A decade or two ago, many of the most heavily promoted items, such as alcoholic beverages, frozen baked goods, dessert mixes, mayonnaise, and sweeteners, were foods that had little to recommend them nutritionally. More recently, good nutrition has become an effective selling point. Increasingly, advertisers are marketing products as "bundles of attributes," promoting healthful characteristics such as being low in fat or having less salt (Figure 1.7). This trend is very apparent in the ad campaigns that launch new products and is likely to continue.

Peer Influences Do you and your friends have a favorite restaurant or club where you meet after classes or work? Have you ever been persuaded by your friends or family to try a new food or drink because they liked it? Peer influence can lead you to make food choices that are different from those you might have made on your own (Figure 1.8).

FIGURE 1.8
Peer groups can have a strong influence on food choice.

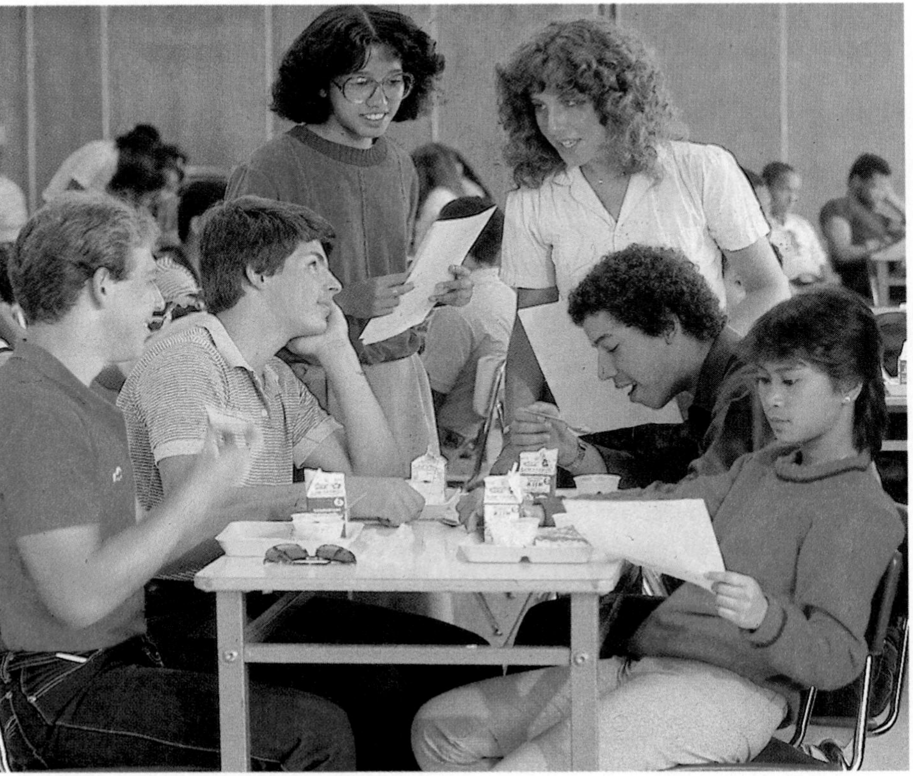

Sometimes you might depart from your usual choices and select foods to make a calculated impression on others. You might, for example, show a sense of adventure by ordering something unfamiliar on the menu, or affluence and sophistication by ordering an expensive wine.

Unique Personal Factors

Along with the various inborn and cultural influences that affect all of us, factors *unique to you* govern what foods you eat. These are the ultimate determinants of your food choices.

Taste and Other Sensory Characteristics The way food appeals to your senses heavily influences your food choices. In almost every survey in which consumers are asked why they chose a particular meal or the items in their shopping cart, *taste* repeatedly has come up as the strongest determinant.

Technically, there are just four basic tastes—sweet, sour, bitter, and salty—and our inclinations regarding them are affected by individual preference as well as by inborn and cultural influences. We also respond to certain food smells. The sensation of flavor is the combination of tastes and smells; this is what many people really mean when they use the term *taste*. Texture also figures into the total picture of what we like: you may respond differently to foods that have crisp, soft, tender, chewy, granular, or smooth textures, for example. Other sensory characteristics that can affect preferences are temperature, moisture, color, and the shape and size of food pieces.

You Tell Me

We appreciate a variety of sensory characteristics in food. Scientists who do research in this area have found that a meal is more satisfying when it includes many of the sensory characteristics a person likes (Rolls, 1991).

Thinking of the various properties of food (taste, texture, and so on), identify what specific characteristics you enjoy (e.g., sweet taste, smooth texture). Describe a meal including foods that provide as many of these characteristics as possible. If you ate this meal, would you feel satisfied?

Available Time and Money The amount of time and money you have available for food can also affect your food choices (Figure 1.9). Fast food restaurants and carry-out foods represent one extreme; make-it-from-scratch items, the other. Many people fall in between, buying some prepared items and assembling other meal components. Two-income families and some self-supporting singles may be time-poor and money-rich and therefore consume more convenience foods.

Although there are wide variations in the amounts that individuals and families in the United States spend on food, the averages suggest some important points. In 1989, families and individuals spent 11.7% of their disposable personal income on food. Food expenditures at home accounted for 7.3%, and 4.3% was spent on food eaten away from home. These figures mean that in the United States, food is an incredible bargain. In some countries of Europe—Spain, Italy, Sweden—consumables on average eat up

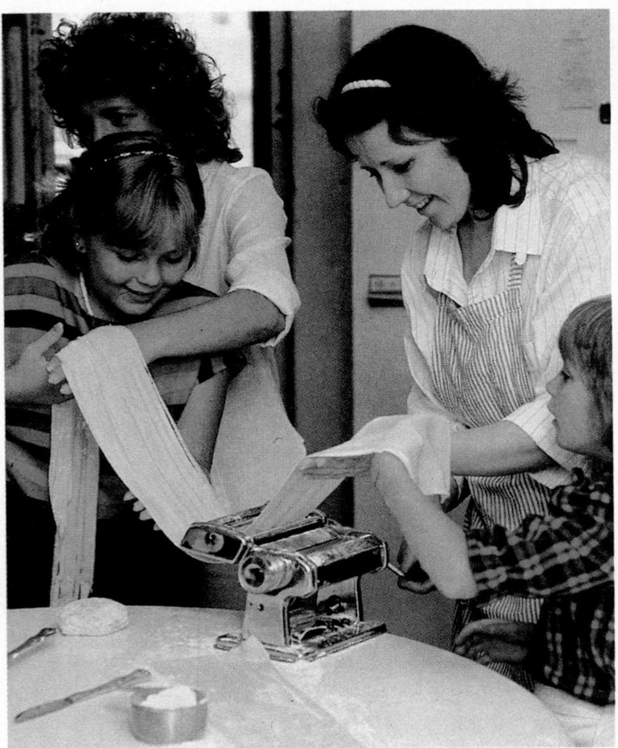

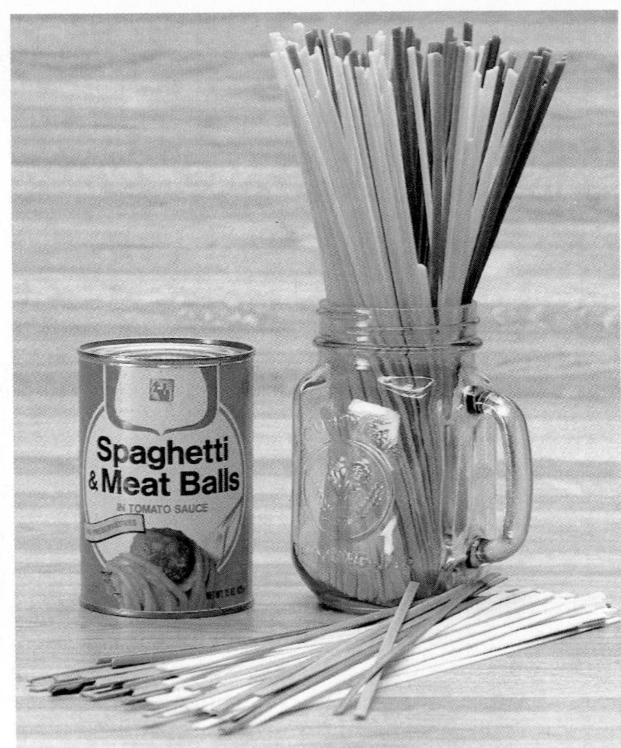

FIGURE 1.9
Which pasta meal is "you"?

Your lifestyle, the amount of time you have available to spend on food preparation, and your financial status can influence which form of food you choose.

20–25% of income; in many less developed countries—such as India and Sri Lanka—food purchases account for 50–55% of a household's income (*Food Review,* 1992).

No matter what the averages are, your own financial situation is a critical factor for you. If your income is less than average, you will spend a larger proportion on food (Figure 1.10). In 1988, those in the United States earning $5,000 to $9,999 spent 28.2% of disposable income for food, whereas households earning $40,000 to $49,999 spent only 11.9% for food (Putnam, 1990).

Emotions Food is part of celebrating: in every culture, food is a part of happy occasions. This is probably the most universal association of food and mood. Food can also be associated with negative emotions. Have you ever had the impulse to eat when you've had a bad day? Psychologists point out that when some people feel insecure or lonely, they want to eat foods associated with a more secure, earlier time of life. If during childhood you were rewarded for good behavior with certain "treat" foods, years later you may still feel you *deserve* that ice cream cone or candy bar after a demanding study session or a busy day at work. On the other hand, you might respond to such stresses by losing your appetite; it's a very individual matter.

Emotions can drive to extremes the *amount* of food people consume. People who regularly overeat for security and comfort are practicing maladaptive behaviors, because the weight gain that inevitably results may compound the original problems. As Chapter 9 (on body weight) and Chapter 10 (on eating disorders) show, some people's psychologic state suppresses their eating, sometimes to a life-threatening degree.

Lower Income
($5,000 - 9,999 annual household income after taxes)

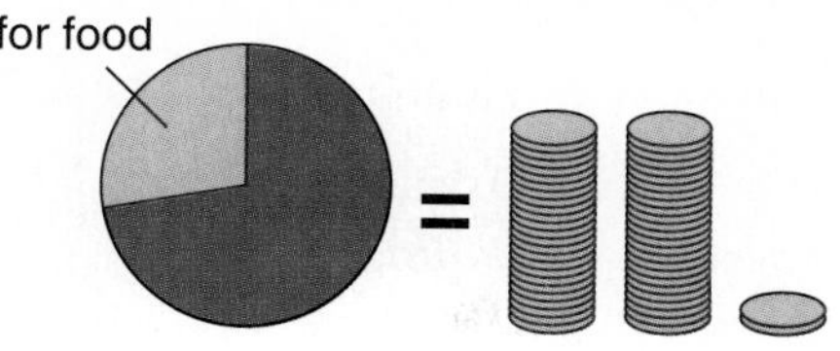

28% of $7,500 = $2,100 spent for food per year

Higher Income
($40,000 - 49,999 annual household income after taxes)

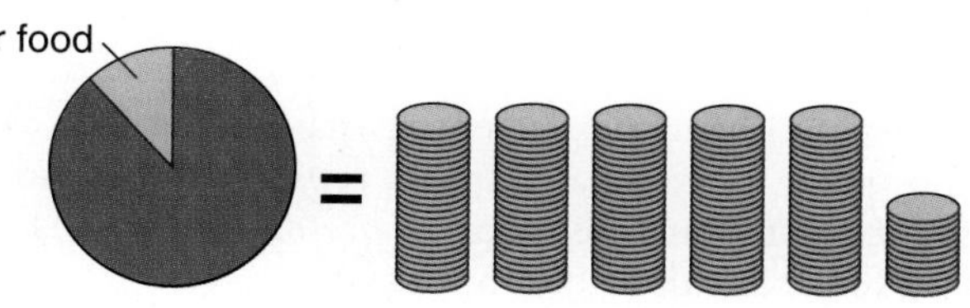

12% of $45,000 = $5,400 spent for food per year

FIGURE 1.10
As you earn more, do you spend more for food? Yes and no.

Higher-income households spend more *dollars* for food than do lower-income households, but the *proportion* of income they spend is far smaller than that spent by lower-income families.

Food, Nutrition, and Your Beliefs about Health Beliefs about the *long-term* effects of food on health also affect people's food choices: 96% of consumers surveyed about their grocery-shopping habits said that nutrition was a somewhat or very important factor in their decisions (Food Marketing Institute, 1992).

Your age has a lot to do with your willingness to make dietary changes. As people get older and more vulnerable to diet-related chronic diseases, they tend to become increasingly willing to modify their diets. In fact, data show that there is a closer relationship between health practices and age than between health practices and gender, race, income, or occupation (Owen, 1990).

However, concerns about nutrition do not necessarily affect all food choices in the same way. People tend to be more attentive to nutrition when they are choosing main-course items than when selecting sweets or snack foods (Schutz et al., 1986). At times, beneficial changes may actually be canceled out when accompanied by other, less healthy, dietary changes. For example, if you select the leanest of meats and switch to low-fat salad dressings in an attempt to lower your fat intake, but then treat yourself to cheesecake or premium ice cream, you may not have lowered your total fat intake.

Therefore, even if you are intent on changing your diet to improve your health, you may not derive any benefit unless you are acting on accurate information about nutrition. To help you start acquiring that knowledge, let's shift our focus now to the basics of the science of nutrition.

The Science of Nutrition

In the first section of this chapter, we recognized the many diverse, overlapping factors that help us select our food from among a banquet of possibilities. Having reflected on both the overt and the more subtle influences that cause you to choose one food instead of another, now you need to step back from these factors and appreciate the most important point of all: it is good that we are attracted—by whatever means—to food, because food is the source of nutrients that keep us alive.

TABLE 1.1 Classes of Essential Nutrients and Their Elemental Components

Water	Carbohydrates	Lipids	Proteins	Vitamins	Minerals
Oxygen	Oxygen	Oxygen	Oxygen	Oxygen	22 separate mineral elements, including calcium, sodium, iron, iodine, phosphorus (see Chapter 12 for complete list)
Hydrogen	Hydrogen	Hydrogen	Hydrogen	Hydrogen	
	Carbon	Carbon	Carbon	Carbon	
			Nitrogen	Nitrogen[a]	
			Sulfur[a]	Sulfur[a]	
				Cobalt[a]	

[a]Found in some but not all members of the class.

Over the last two centuries, scientists have identified close to 50 nutrients our bodies need for normal growth, reproduction, and maintenance of health. These nutrients must be taken in *preformed*; that is, your body cannot assemble them from their components.

The nutrients are grouped into six classes: *water, carbohydrates, lipids* (commonly called fats), *proteins*, *vitamins*, and *minerals*. Table 1.1 identifies the **elements** of which they are composed. Although many nutrients have similar constituents—note how often oxygen, hydrogen, and carbon appear on the lists—the nutrients themselves are different substances and generally cannot substitute for each other.

elements—the more than 100 basic chemical substances of which the earth is composed

macronutrients—the nutrients you need in larger amounts: water, carbohydrates, lipids, and proteins

micronutrients—the nutrients you need in smaller amounts: vitamins, minerals

liter—the basic unit of volume in the metric system; approximately 1.06 quarts

gram—the basic unit of mass in the metric system; approximately 1/30 of an ounce

The classes of nutrients you need in the largest amounts are water, carbohydrates, lipids, and proteins; for this reason, they are called **macronutrients**. Vitamins and minerals, which you need in only very small amounts, are **micronutrients**.

Scientists generally use the metric system of measures rather than the English system, on which common U.S. measures are based. The basic unit of fluid volume is the **liter**, and the basic unit of mass is the **gram**. The values most often used in nutrition, and their equivalents in common U.S. measures, are inside the front cover of this book for your convenience. It may help to keep in mind that there are approximately 30 grams in an ounce, and that a liter is slightly larger than a quart.

Carbohydrates, lipids, and proteins are measured in grams. Typical daily intakes of carbohydrates are in the range of 200–400 grams, and you probably consume 50–100 grams each of protein and fat daily. The micronutrients are measured in *milligrams* (thousandths of a gram) or *micrograms* (millionths of a gram). The prefix *kilo-* means 1,000 of something, as in *kilogram*; a kilogram is approximately 2.2 pounds. A liter of water has a mass of 1 kilogram.

You Tell Me

In scientific discussions, body weights are expressed in kilograms.

What is your weight in kilograms? You will use this value often as you apply to yourself what you learn in this book.

General Functions of Nutrients

Together, the nutrients perform three basic functions for your body (or for any other living organism): they provide structural material; they yield energy; and they serve as regulators of **biochemical** processes. Let's take a closer look at these functions.

biochemical—pertaining to all of the chemical reactions that take place within a living organism

Structure The cliché "You are what you eat" states the truth: your body consists of materials that were created from nutrients that you—or your mother when she was pregnant with you—consumed. Many of those materials have been biochemically rearranged to form the building blocks of your unique body structures.

This is not to say that your food choices can completely determine what you become. Each of us has genetic limits to our physical potential, but nutrition substantially influences the degree to which you achieve that potential. For example, if your genes (the materials that determine hereditary characteristics) contain instructions for developing unusually long bones, you have a chance of being taller than others whose genes do not carry that information. But if you receive far less than the level of nutrients you should have as you grow, your chances for basketball stardom may be limited.

Similarly, if a baby is very seriously deprived of adequate nutrients during periods of rapid brain growth both before and after birth, brain size may be smaller than normal. For the body to be able to generate the full extent of well-organized tissues, organs, and systems for which it has the potential, it must have the appropriate level of raw materials.

The nutrient classes that contribute in a major way to body structure are water, lipids, proteins, and minerals.

Energy Another vital function of nutrients is to provide energy. Without energy production, life ceases.

Energy is measured in a unit of heat called the **kilocalorie**, which will be abbreviated in this book as **kcalorie** or **kcal**. (The term *calorie* is in popular use, although this use is not technically correct, since a calorie is only 1/1000 as large as a kcalorie.) Most adults use between 1500 and 3000 kcalories in a day.

kilocalorie (kcalorie, kcal)—the amount of heat needed to raise the temperature of 1 kilogram of water 1 degree Celsius; a measure of energy

Carbohydrates, lipids, and proteins are nutrients that provide energy. These nutrients are available both from food and from your own body stores of these substances, as we explain more thoroughly in upcoming chapters.

Equal masses of the various energy nutrients do not provide equal numbers of kcalories. Carbohydrates and proteins each have the potential to produce 4 kcalories per gram, and fat produces 9. Alcohol, not usually classified as a nutrient, furnishes 7 kcalories per gram.

Your body generally functions better if it derives energy from more than one source. As we discuss in Chapter 6, the body utilizes fat better if some carbohydrate is available simultaneously. This does not mean that it is best to take in equal amounts of carbohydrates, lipids, and proteins. Some distance athletes think that ingesting a higher proportion of carbohydrate (for example, getting 70% of their kcalories from carbohydrate) gives them greater endurance (Figure 1.11). This is discussed more thoroughly in Chapter 5.

Regulation The third important function that nutrients perform is regulation of body processes. The biochemical reactions that take place in a living system, which are cumulatively called **metabolism**, do not occur in random fashion; they are intricately controlled. Water, proteins, vitamins, and minerals are the chief regulators.

metabolism—the biochemical reactions that take place in a living entity

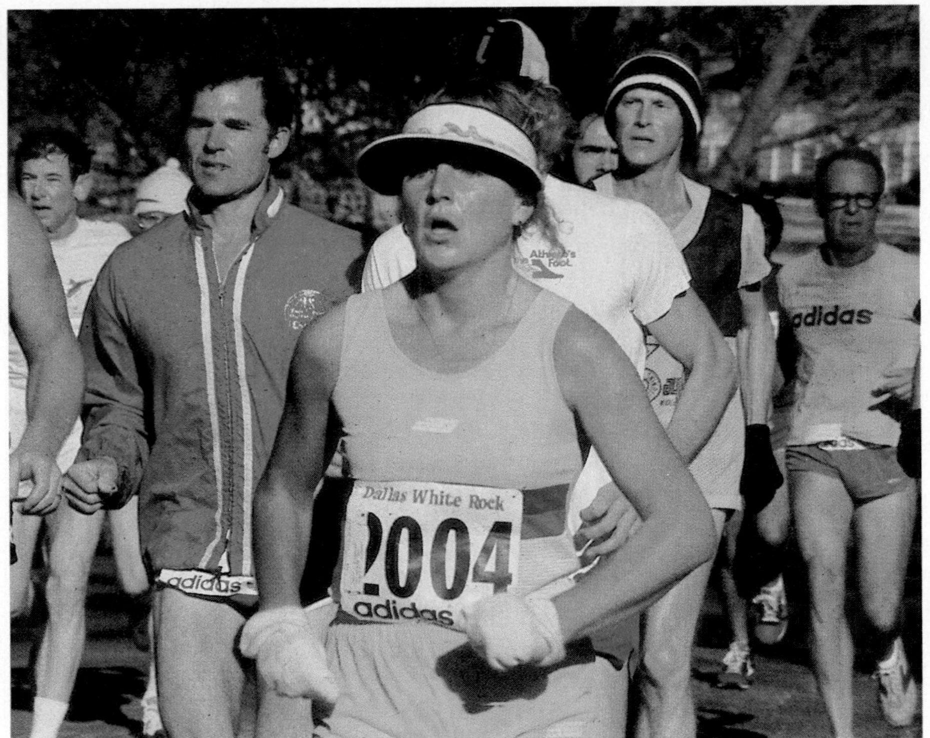

FIGURE 1.11
Endurance and nutrition.

Some athletes in continuous events that last more than an hour find that a high carbohydrate intake helps them go farther.

For example, many of the vitamins and minerals participate in the series of chemical reactions that are needed to generate energy, although they themselves are not energy sources. If some of these nutrients are missing or inadequate, one of the effects will be that the body will not be as efficient a producer of energy and will therefore have poor work capacity and limited growth.

Certain essential minerals such as sodium and potassium help regulate how water is distributed in the body; protein also performs this function.

Phosphorus and chloride influence the acidity or alkalinity (the opposite of acidity) of various body substances. This function is critical because a balance between acidity and alkalinity must be maintained in most of the body; departure from this balance in the blood can result in death. Normally, however, these mechanisms work so well that even though we take in foods and produce body substances of widely varying acidity and alkalinity, the balance in the blood is maintained.

Malnutrition—Too Little or Too Much

For any nutrient, there is a beneficial range of intake; an intake either below or above that range is usually undesirable, as shown in Figure 1.12. Both *undernutrition* and *overnutrition* are forms of **malnutrition**.

malnutrition—poor nutritional status resulting from intakes either above or below the beneficial range

What Happens in Undernutrition If all or some of the nutrients are totally missing, a person will stop growing, fail to thrive, be more susceptible to infection, be incapable of reproduction, and eventually die. If a person does consume all of the nutrients, but in inadequate amounts, the consequences will be less severe: in children, the likely results are stunted growth (Schelp et al., 1986) and increased susceptibility to infection; in adults the likely effects are low body weight, poor work capacity, and increased susceptibility to infection.

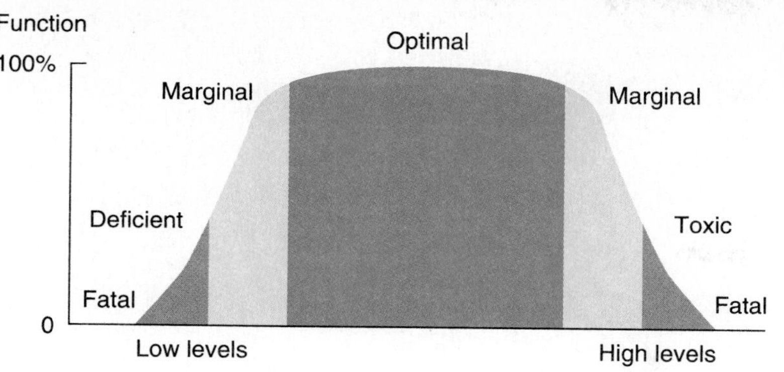

FIGURE 1.12
Effect of the level of intake of a nutrient.

Either too little or too much of a nutrient can interfere with growth and health. (Adapted from Mertz, 1983.)

If just one nutrient in your diet is restricted to low levels while the others are adequate, you are likely to experience more specific effects. For example, if your body does not get enough vitamin A over a period of years, your visual acuity at night may decrease (a condition known as night blindness). Worse than that, eye damage serious enough to cause permanent blindness could eventually result in some situations. Although such a severe vitamin A deficiency is unusual in people in the developed countries, in the developing countries thousands of children become blind each year from this cause.

How quickly could you develop an obvious deficiency if your intake of a particular nutrient were extremely low? For most nutrients, it would take at least a couple of months. For example, if you took in no vitamin C from foods, beverages, or supplements, in a month or two you would probably find that your gums bleed somewhat when you brush your teeth. Bleeding of the gums is not the only effect of vitamin C deficiency, of course, but it is likely to be the first obvious, visible symptom.

Upcoming chapters will point out the consequences of severe, prolonged inadequate intake for each nutrient.

What Happens in Overnutrition Just as an inadequate intake of a nutrient has damaging effects, a consistent and substantial overdose of a nutrient will also cause health problems. For example, if you consume vitamin A for a period of many months in amounts that are much higher than recommended, you may develop toxicity symptoms, including headache, nausea, and vomiting. These high doses could result in elevated pressure of the fluid surrounding your brain, causing a condition that can be mistaken for a brain tumor.

The dangers of excess nutrient intake have become more apparent in recent years. Because concentrated nutrients can be formulated inexpensively in the laboratory as pills, powders, or liquids, overdosing is possible if people use such products inappropriately (Figure 1.13). Although nutrient toxicities have resulted once in a great while from eating too much *food* that is high in a particular nutrient, nutrient overdoses are caused much more often by the indiscriminate use of nutritional *supplements.*

Another example of the danger of supplement overdose involves vitamin B-6, a nutrient formerly thought to be safe at high levels of intake. Now we know that when vitamin B-6 is consumed for long periods of time in amounts that are hundreds or more times the recommended intake, nerve problems that interfere with muscle coordination can occur. Reports describe office workers whose typing abilities were impaired and people who were no longer able to walk unassisted.

FIGURE 1.13
Nutritional supplements: boon or bane?

Although concentrated nutritional supplements are useful in some circumstances, they also carry the potential for harm.

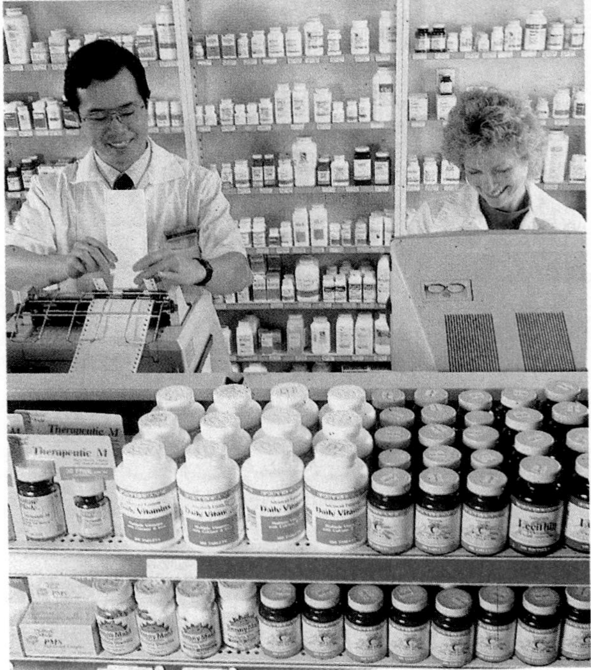

This is not to say that using vitamin supplements is always dangerous: in some situations (e.g., in infancy), they are very beneficial if used properly. In Chapter 11, we discuss situations in which supplementation is recommended.

As the examples above demonstrate, the symptoms of excessive intake usually take months or even years to show up, but there are exceptions. If a child took a whole bottle of potent supplements at once, for example, toxicity symptoms and even death could occur in as little as a couple of hours.

How Important Is Nutrition to Overall Health?

As you start to learn about how severe the effects of malnutrition can be, you might get the impression that nutrition is the only factor that determines health; this is not the case, however. Important as it is, there are limits to what good nutrition can accomplish. Other factors influencing your health are how much exercise and sleep you get, whether you smoke, whether you protect yourself from excessive environmental and psychologic stresses, and whether you get good medical help when you need it. Genetics also plays an important role. We have already noted that genetics limits body structure, no matter what your diet; genetics also affects your likelihood of developing certain diseases.

In fact, your chances of developing some diseases are *totally* determined by genetic inheritance; for certain other conditions, genetics *and* nutrition (and often other factors) interact to varying degrees (Figure 1.14). Some of the major health problems that bedevil Americans—heart disease, cancer, and obesity—are linked to a combination of factors; that is, they are **multifactorial**. Any circumstance statistically associated with a particular disease is referred to as one of its **risk factors**.

multifactorial—having many contributing factors or causes

risk factor—a circumstance statistically associated with a particular disease

If nutrition is only partly responsible for a condition, then nutrition can play only a limited role in prevention. For example, if your genetic makeup predisposes hypertension (high blood pressure), you probably will eventu-

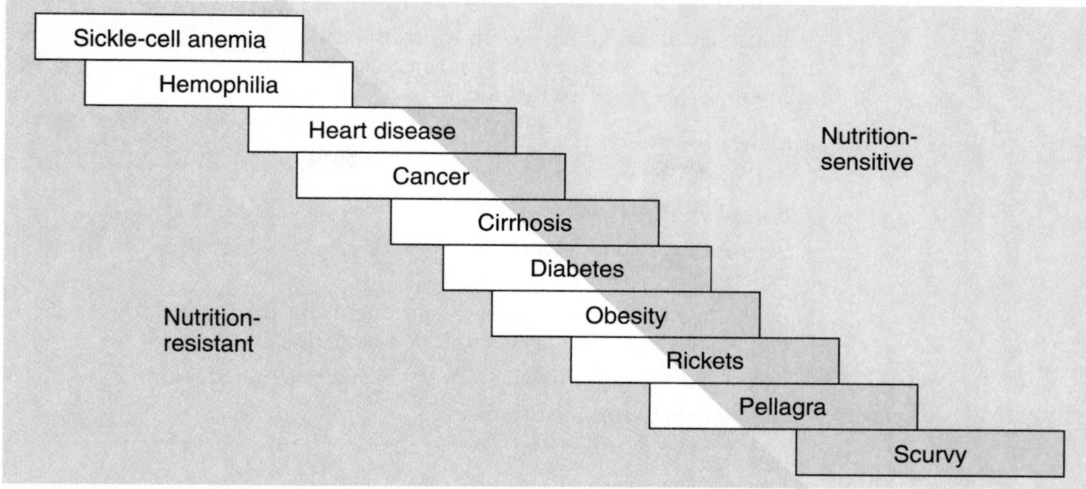

FIGURE 1.14
The influence of nutrition on some health conditions.

Health conditions vary in the extent to which nutrition can influence them. You can estimate the relative effectiveness of nutrition in modifying these diseases if they already exist by noting how much of the bar is in color. (Adapted from Olson, 1978.)

ally develop hypertension even if you take all the right dietary steps to try to prevent the disease. In the meantime, however, you may at least delay its onset through your choice of diet. Similarly, if a person develops a multifactorial condition, diet can serve as only part of its treatment or control.

However, if you are *not* genetically predisposed to a certain disease, there is probably little need to concern yourself about risk factors for that disease; you're not likely to get it anyway. To extend the example above, if you have not inherited the tendency for your blood pressure to rise when you consume salt, you can use salt as you like and not worry about hypertension.

The problem with this approach is that scientists currently don't know how to test for genetic predisposition for most diseases. It would be ideal if researchers could find easy-to-evaluate *biologic markers* (such as a substance in blood or urine) that could serve as a reliable indicator of disease risk. Some scientists expect to be able to "read" an individual's genetic code, or **genome**, in the next 20 years or later in the 21st century. This has exciting implications for predicting and treating inheritable diseases.

genome—the complete set of hereditary factors contained in a sperm or egg

Unless and until such methods are accessible to most of the population, the best strategy to take in the meantime is to try to reduce risk factors by modifying lifestyle factors, including diet. The possible benefits from reducing risk factors for heart disease and cancer are substantial: deaths from these causes represent about two-thirds of all deaths in the United States.

Ways Scientists Learn about Nutrition

Because nutrition often acts along with other factors to influence health and because some consequences may not be apparent for years, distinguishing and describing the effects of nutrition can be challenging for scientists. Nutritional scientists, like all scientists, use the scientific method (Table 1.2) to do research.

After raising questions about something he or she has observed, a scientist forms **hypotheses**—possible explanations—for what was observed.

hypothesis—a supposition that attempts to explain certain phenomena and is used as a basis for experiments

TABLE 1.2 The Scientific Method

Scientists in all disciplines search for truths about the world by making observations and testing them. Although no list can adequately describe the process, the following steps are often included:

1. Make observations.
2. Ask questions.
3. Form hypotheses.
4. Perform experiments to test the hypotheses. (See discussion of various experimental methods in text.)
5. From the hypotheses that survive testing, make predictions about what will happen in similar (but as yet untested) situations.
6. Perform more experiments to verify or refute the predictions.
7. Use all data to formulate a theory.

Then the scientist develops experiments to test the hypotheses. Although performing experiments is listed as just one step, a single experiment can take many years, and many studies may be needed to test a hypothesis. A hypothesis that holds up to testing is then used to predict what would happen in various situations, which calls for more experiments. Only after additional studies verify the hypothesis does it become an accepted theory.

To develop a perspective on new scientific findings, you need to understand this process. Each experiment is just one part of a lengthier process; therefore, not every research finding you hear on the news calls for an immediate change in your diet. Furthermore, a conflict in the results of scientific studies is not a sign that you should distrust science. Rather, it means that scientists are still testing the hypothesis.

General Ways of Conducting Research Now we need to focus on the experimental phase of the scientific method. Generally, research is conducted in one of two ways. In one method, investigators strictly *observe* situations but do not intervene in them. In the other, scientists *intervene* and deliberately change conditions and measure the results. Intervention studies are effective for establishing a cause-and-effect relationship, whereas observational studies usually are not.

Various types of nutrition studies are conducted in these two general ways. In the following sections, we will discuss those most commonly used for nutrition research. They are the basis for the information in this book.

epidemiologic studies—assessments of the health status of a large, defined group (or groups) of people

statistical correlation—the mathematical relationship between the measurements of two (or more) factors based on the same group of subjects

positive correlation—a statistically based statement indicating that when the amount of one factor goes up, the other goes up proportionately; when one measurement goes down, so does the other

negative correlation—a statistically based statement indicating that when one measurement goes up, the other goes down

Epidemiologic Studies Epidemiology is the study of disease as it occurs within populations. **Epidemiologic studies** (also known as *ecologic* or *correlation studies*) are observational; scientists assess the health status of a large, defined group of people, such as all the residents of Framingham, Massachusetts, or all members of a particular professional organization in the United States. At the same time, the researchers observe the dietary patterns and other lifestyle features of the population. The people are not asked to change their diets in any way: the scientists simply record what they normally consume. The researchers then observe other populations that have different diets, recording their health status as well. They note which health factors and diets exist together (Figure 1.15), or show a **statistical correlation**. Statistical correlations are either **positive** or **negative**.

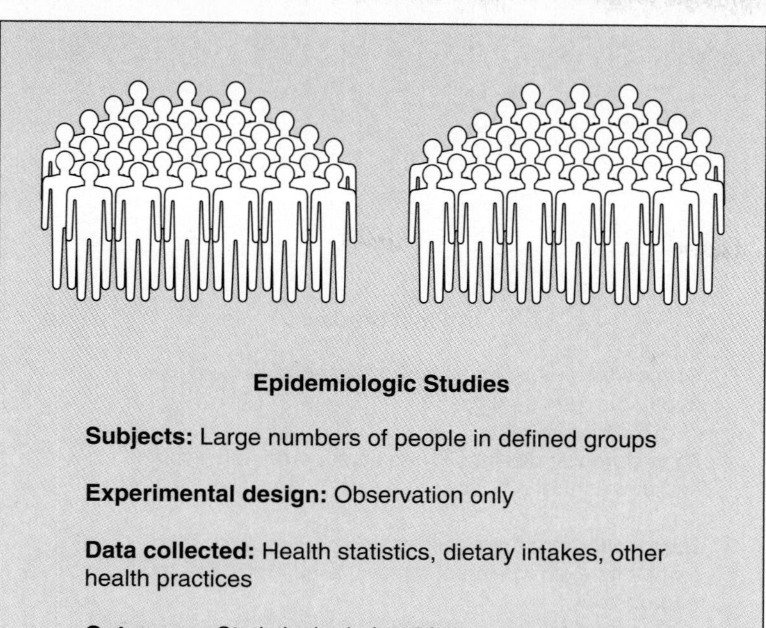

FIGURE 1.15
Epidemiologic studies.

For example, several decades ago, physicians practicing in Africa noticed that natives who ate high-fiber diets rarely developed appendicitis, bowel cancer, or heart disease but frequently contracted infectious diseases; that is, there was a negative correlation between the high-fiber diet and the first three conditions, and a positive correlation between the high-fiber diet and infectious diseases. Europeans living there, by contrast, had a different experience: they developed appendicitis, bowel cancer, and heart disease more freqently than the natives did but had much lower rates of infectious diseases. Their diets were different, too: they contained less fiber than those of the Africans.

It is tempting to conclude that the level of fiber in the diets was responsible for the type of health problems these two groups of people experienced. However, *the correlation of two conditions* (here, the high-fiber diet and the incidence of infectious diseases) *does not prove that either causes the other.* Although it is possible, it is just as likely that the two conditions are present together by coincidence or that a third factor causes both. Therefore, **one cannot assume that there is a cause-and-effect relationship simply because two conditions coexist. It is a common mistake to believe that statistical correlations prove causation. They do not.**

Even when there is a cause-and-effect relationship, other factors are also usually involved in the disease process. In this example, the diets of the two groups varied not only in levels of fiber but also in levels of fat, protein, and other substances—and the activity levels and overall lifestyles of the two groups differed markedly.

Even though the findings of the epidemiologic studies involving fiber intake and various diseases did not establish a cause-and-effect relationship, they did spark other types of studies that were designed to demonstrate such a relationship. One of these types is animal studies, described in the following section.

FIGURE 1.16
Animal studies.

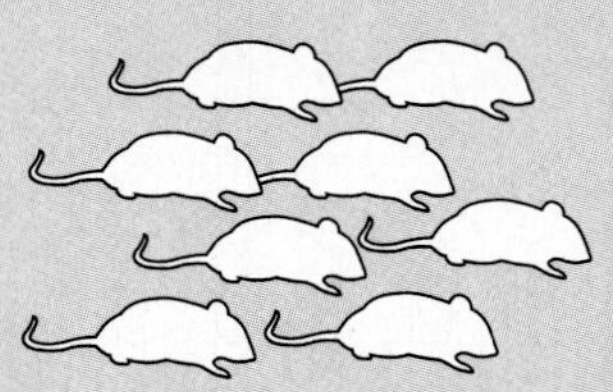
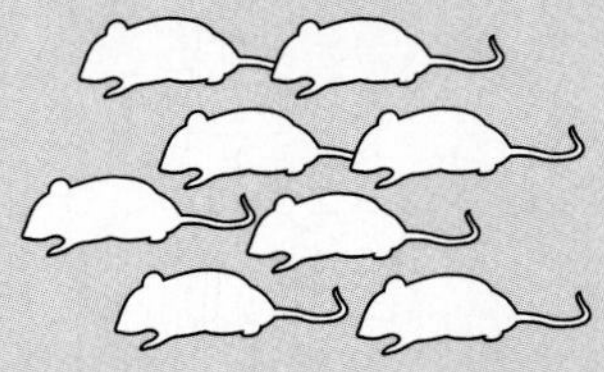

Animal Studies

Subjects: Usually small laboratory animals, such as mice, rats, guinea pigs

Experimental design: Preselected, randomly assigned test and control groups

Data collected: Metabolic changes associated with test diets; examination of internal tissue changes at end of study

Outcomes: Evidence about the effects of various levels of nutrients on tested species and on how nutrients function

control—a normal group of animals or humans against which effects in test subjects can be compared

feces—solid waste from a human or animal

Animal Studies Animal studies involve intervention. In these studies, researchers design a set of diets for groups of animals; the levels of the nutrient(s) or other food substances being studied are varied among groups while all other nutrient levels are kept constant.

Usually, an additional group of the same type of animals is used as a **control** for the experiment. These animals are fed a diet that is exactly like the test diet(s), except for the variable being tested. That way, the researchers can compare differences in the test and control animals. These differences may be detected by such methods as weighing the animals, examining and analyzing body tissues, and measuring substances excreted in urine or **feces** (Figure 1.16). The differences between the test animals and the control animals are the result of the test substance.

Animal studies offer several advantages over similar studies using human subjects. The normal life span of a small laboratory animal such as a mouse, rat, or rabbit is just a fraction of a human's; therefore, an animal study that encompasses the whole life cycle can be done in a few years.

The fact that the animals are caged is another advantage because there is no possibility that they will consume other than the designated diet. In addition, it might be possible to feed the animals more extreme levels of nutrients than would be ethical to feed humans; seeing these effects may help scientists to forecast what might happen in people. Finally, because animals are usually killed at the end of a study, a great deal of detailed information can be gained from postmortem examinations and chemical analyses of tissues and organs.

The major drawback of animal studies is that although they yield a wealth of detailed information about the nutritional needs of laboratory animals, it is not always clear how much information they yield on human nutrition. If the objective of an animal study is to yield information that could eventually contribute to knowledge of human nutrition, it is important to select a type of animal for the study that uses the test nutrient(s) in

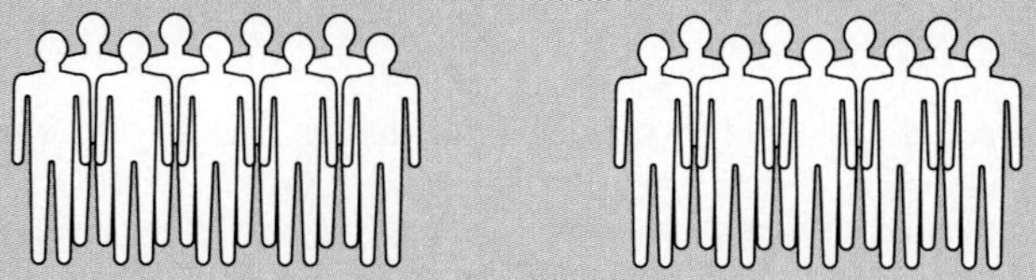

Human Metabolic (Clinical) Studies

Subjects: Large or small numbers of individuals

Experimental design: Preselected test and experimental groups

Data collected: Metabolic changes in blood, urine, and feces associated with test diets; various chemical and physical measures

Outcomes: Conclusions about the effects of various levels of nutrients on humans and on how nutrients function

FIGURE 1.17
Human metabolic (clinical) studies.

a way similar to the way people do. For example, vitamin C is an essential nutrient for humans, but rats do not need it in their diets because their own bodies produce it. Therefore, the guinea pig, which does require vitamin C, is a better choice for vitamin C research.

Human Metabolic Studies Studies using human subjects may be called *human metabolic, clinical,* or *human* studies. In these studies, as in experiments with laboratory animals, careful chemical analyses are done. A major difference, however, is that usually only substances in blood, urine, and feces are analyzed. Physical measurements such as body weight and blood pressure may be collected as well.

The scope of human metabolic studies can vary considerably, depending on the objectives of the study (Figure 1.17). Some involve up to thousands of subjects studied over many years. Generally, fewer types of data are collected in such studies, and the assessments are often done at widely spaced intervals, for example, every other year.

However, most human metabolic studies involve fewer subjects and shorter data-collection periods. For example, as few as 8–12 subjects may be studied for a month or two. Every bite of their food intake would probably be rigidly controlled, and they would be monitored often for various biochemical changes. Researchers sometimes use such studies to establish levels of nutrient requirement by finding out how much of a nutrient the subject must consume to stay **"in balance"**—that is, to have an intake of the nutrient equal to excretion of the nutrient.

in balance—condition in which intake equals excretion

If you were a subject in this type of study, you would have to be able to tolerate food restrictions for weeks at a time. But, as the Slice of Life on page 24 points out, you would receive some encouragement to comply: subjects are usually paid for their cooperation. Other benefits of participating may include gaining information about your health indicators, such as blood chemistry values and blood pressure, as well as a sense of satisfaction from contributing to scientific research.

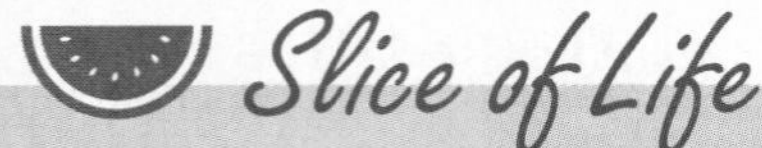

Being a Subject in a Human Metabolic Study

As the alarm rings, Tom awakens with the realization that this is going to be an unusual day: it is *day one* of a human metabolic study regarding the mineral zinc, for which he has agreed to be a subject. He recalls the recent chain of events that led to his signing up: seeing the ad for subjects on a campus bulletin board, interviewing with the major professor and the graduate students who make up the research team, and being examined by the project's physician.

He shuts off the alarm and stretches, thinking about the ways in which his life will be different for the 51 days of the study. He will still live in his apartment, but he will get everything he eats and drinks from the kitchen of the research unit: 51 identical-looking and -tasting breakfasts, 51 identical lunches, and 51 identical dinners. Even the water he drinks must be from the study, because it must be distilled to get rid of the naturally occurring traces of minerals that would interfere with the study result.

He steps into the bathroom, realizing that even this activity will be different during the study. He will have to collect all body wastes in the containers given to the subjects.

During the weeks of study, Tom learns a great deal about himself, including his relationship to food. At first he doesn't mind the repetitious menus and being restricted from eating other foods, but after about two weeks he realizes that he has the "blahs." He's tired of eating the same three meals a day—every day of the week—in the same place, and he'd like to leave town for a weekend. But the research team is depending on him to complete the study, and he wants to earn the full payment. Besides, he has come to enjoy the company of the other subjects and the "TLC" he gets from the researchers.

Finally, with just days to go, everybody is counting down the last meals and anticipating the party that will be held at the end of the study . . . with different food! And in the weeks to come, a gradual return to normalcy.

Tom's story demonstrates how totally accountable a subject in a human metabolic study needs to be regarding intake and output and provides an indication of the attention to detail that is characteristic of a properly planned and conducted study. Protocols for buying, preparing, portioning, and serving food are no less precise; the subsequent laboratory analysis, statistical handling, and writing of the papers for publication must be done with equal care.

Such efforts stand in sharp contrast to untested (or inadequately tested) nutrition claims.

placebo—a food or pill superficially identical to a substance being tested, but without its effect

blind studies—experiments in which the subjects (or the subjects and the researchers) do not know who is receiving the test substance; the first type of study is a **single-blind study**, and the second is a **double-blind study**

Sometimes it is important to keep those involved in nutrition research from knowing who is receiving the test substance or during which phase of the study it is being administered. To accomplish this, the researchers give the subjects a **placebo** (a food or pill made to look, taste, and smell like the test substance but without its effect) when the experimental treatment is withheld. Such studies are called **blind studies**.

In **single-blind studies**, only the subjects are kept unaware of whether they are receiving the test substance. This is done for studies in which the subjects' expectations might influence test results. For example, if a study is being done to test the effect of caffeine on blood pressure, subjects should not know whether they received the caffeine or not, because psychologic factors can modify blood pressure. The subjects' expectations may cause their blood pressure to rise or fall, which would be different from the effects of the caffeine alone.

In **double-blind studies**, neither the subjects nor the researchers working directly with the subjects know who is receiving the test substance; this eliminates the likelihood of bias on the part of the researchers as well. For example, if a test were being done to see whether vitamin E supplements ease respiratory problems, and the person on the listening end of the stethoscope knew which subjects had received the vitamin, she might "hear" the person's breathing a little differently, depending on her expectation. (Of course, somebody in charge of the study has to know who got what—but the information is not revealed until the study is over.)

When researchers who conduct human metabolic studies publish their results, they are careful to explain under what circumstances they obtained the findings. The results might have been different if a different test diet or other conditions had been used.

Molecular Biology Techniques Scientists are always developing more sophisticated methods of discovery. One expanding group of technologies being applied to both observational and interventional studies is molecular biology techniques.

Molecular biology involves the study of basic biologic processes at the cellular and subcellular levels. Scientists in this rapidly growing field might, for example, study the differences between the ways normal human cells and cancerous cells metabolize nutrients, or they might even learn the ways nutrients gain entry into cells or affect the genetic material within cells.

molecular biology—area of science in which inheritance and protein synthesis are studied at a molecular level

These techniques, which are generally carried out in a test tube or other laboratory systems, are referred to as **in vitro studies** (contrasted with **in vivo studies**, which involve studying effects within a living organism). The new techniques of molecular biology allow a precision greater than that attainable in in vivo studies. Therefore, molecular biology has much to offer to the nutritional sciences; it will help scientists complete the picture of how nutrition affects us.

in vitro studies—experiments conducted in a test tube or otherwise outside living organisms

in vivo studies—experiments conducted in living animals or other organisms

Hallmarks of Good Studies

As you were reading about the experimental methods described in the previous sections, did you find yourself wondering about some of the nutrition claims in popular magazines? Are these claims the result of such thorough testing? Often, popular press articles do not mention how the studies were conducted, so you have to look for other clues about the likely validity of the experiments.

The next sections describe other characteristics of good studies, which you may be able to apply to what you read.

Time Line Considerable time and effort are required to develop, fund, operate, analyze, and publish a well-designed study. Even one of the smaller, shorter studies can take anywhere from 2 to 5 years from the time a researcher conceives the idea until the findings have been published. Studies in which the test period itself runs for several years, of course, take much more total time. The fact that a study took a long time to do, though, does not necessarily mean that it is well done or particularly meaningful.

Qualifications of Researchers Ideally, researchers working in human nutrition should have earned *advanced degrees (MS, PhD, MD) in human nutrition, medicine, or biochemistry from universities of good reputation.* Unfortunately, some "PhD" diplomas in nutrition are available by mail order from unscrupulous groups for a price and do not denote authentic scientific training. Some individuals with a PhD in literature, music, or some unrelated field claim to be nutrition experts also. You should not automatically trust a person who claims to hold an advanced degree: first find out what academic discipline the diploma represents and where it was earned.

You Tell Me

Harvey and Marilyn Diamond, authors of the bestseller *Fit for Life*, earned "nutrition certificates" from a correspondence school, The American College of Life Sciences, located in the Austin, Texas, area. According to the Texas Board of Higher Education, this school is not accredited.

There are no prerequisites for entering the program, which usually consists of about 100 lessons (each of a few pages), after which enrollees must take a 25- to 50-question test (Milner, 1992).

Does this program sound as rigorous as the training involved in earning a masters or PhD degree? Should you question the quality of education from an institution that cannot gain accreditation? Is *Fit for Life* likely to be a source of reliable nutrition information?

Reputation of Journals A careful scientist will also be particular about having his or her research published in respected journals. Journals that are *refereed* are more likely to contain accurate information, because articles submitted to them are carefully critiqued by other experts in the field before they can be published. A list of refereed publications that carry nutrition research and review articles is given in Appendix A. Journals that do not use a rigorous review process are more likely to contain errors in study procedures and/or conclusions.

Reproducibility of Results Even after publication, nutrition research is not immediately accepted as truth by other nutritionists. Only after thorough discussion by fellow scientists, and replication (repeating) of the same study elsewhere with similar results, does the new information become part of mainstream thinking within the nutrition community. Of course, the time, expertise, equipment, and effort involved in conducting research cost money. Depending on where they do their work, scientists may have to obtain funds from a variety of sources to pay for their projects. Researchers at a public university, for example, may receive some support from their institution; but they also may have to compete for grants from government agencies, industry, and/or private foundations to hire help, buy equipment and supplies, or even secure part of their own salaries. For this reason, it often takes years for the scientific community to prove or disprove new theories and recommendations about nutrition. (In our opinion there should be a balance of public and private funding sources, because the funding agency determines which projects it will support. Private funds have supported much worthwhile research that would otherwise have required tax dollars or perhaps might not have been done at all. However, sufficient public funding is also critical for maintaining research programs that respond to broad general public interests.)

anecdotal report—a superficial description of an isolated case

Inadequacy of Individual Reports One type of "evidence" that is not reliable is the **anecdotal report**. An anecdotal report is someone's personal testimony that leads to a nutritional claim. For example, somebody might say, "I had a red, itchy rash on one leg for a couple of weeks, but after I took these nutritional supplements for a few days, it cleared up. This is wonderful stuff." Such personal experience can be interesting and dramatic, but it cannot prove anything about the relationship between the condition and nutrition. The rash may have cleared up because the person changed soaps or avoided walking through the woods in shorts again, or for any of a variety of other reasons.

Product advertising, which sometimes features celebrity testimonials, provides many other examples.

You Tell Me

A recognized track-and-field star credits his success to his use of a particular breakfast cereal, which he endorses on television and in print advertisements.

Does his endorsement of the product prove its effectiveness?

Another type of individual report is the **case study** or *case report*, which is often used in the medical literature to illustrate a particular condition and its treatment. In a case study, the researcher offers extensive scientific evidence regarding a particular patient's initial condition and the consequences of efforts to modify it. Well-documented though it may be, even the case study is not in itself sufficient evidence of a nutrition cause-and-effect relationship, because it does not employ enough subjects or have adequate controls.

case study—well-documented description of a patient's medical condition and the result of efforts to treat it

Now that you are familiar with types of nutrition studies and characteristics of quality work, build your critical thinking skill by evaluating the situation in Thinking for Yourself below.

Nutrition Spokespersons to Trust

There are likely to be people in your own community who could give reliable opinions on the validity of a particular claim. They include nutritionists employed by governmental agencies; dietitians (preferably registered dietitians, or RDs) in hospitals, clinics, or nursing homes; cooperative extension agents in county extension offices; and home economists in business.

A number of companies that sell or represent food products also produce nutrition education materials that attempt to interpret nutritional science findings for the general public. Such materials run the gamut from scientifically misleading, thinly veiled "infomercials" for products to thoroughly responsible, accurate applications of the scientific literature.

Here, again, you may be confused about what is valid and what is not. Read such materials carefully, and apply your critical thinking skill to them as well.

Thinking for Yourself

Is This Study Valid?

The Situation

You are scanning the array of vitamin preparations in the nutritional supplement section of your grocery store, and you notice a stack of brochures titled, "Vitamin X—An Aid to Physical Performance." You pick up a copy and drop it in your shopping cart.

At home, you sit down to read the brochure. It states that an independent testing lab studied the effects of "vitamin X" on healthy young men who ran the same two-mile course every day for three weeks. There were two groups of 10 men; the experimental group received the vitamin at the daily recommended level in a single dose every day, and the control group received a placebo. The study was double blind.

Every day, after each man had completed his run, he was asked for a *rating of perceived exertion (RPE)* on a scale from 6 to 20, with 6 representing no effort and 20 indicating maximal effort. When the results were analyzed, 8 of 10 of the men who had received the vitamin supplement perceived their effort to be 3 points less at the end of a three-week study than it had been at the beginning, indicating that it felt easier to run the course.

Is this study likely to be valid?

Is Your Information Accurate and Relevant?

- You can only assume that the data supplied by researchers was accurately reported; all research depends on this trust. (When an occasional scientist is found to have fabricated or falsified data, it makes big news in the scientific community, and the person's career is summarily over.)
- Rating of perceived exertion (RPE) is a self-awareness tool developed by sports psychologists and exercise physiologists (Morgan, 1981). When these subjective ratings are used in research, physiologic measurements also usually are taken to provide objective data (Wilmore et al., 1986). In this brochure, however, only RPEs were reported.

What Else Should You Consider?

An individual's RPE at a given moment is affected by complex physiologic and psychologic factors (Morgan, 1981). Certainly, such factors mutually *affect* physical performance, but RPE does not *measure* performance. There *are* tests that effectively measure performance; a simple one is to time the subjects' two-mile runs every day, after instructing them to run as fast as they could but still complete the course. Perhaps such a test was done, but if so, the brochure neglected to mention it.

Another important consideration: to evaluate the effect of any variable (in this case, "vitamin X") on physical performance, you need to separate the effect of the variable from other factors in the study. Here, you need to control for the fact that running daily will improve running performance over time and that it will improve performance to the greatest extent in previously untrained individuals. Therefore, the two groups of men need to be matched carefully so that their initial *training states* are similar.

Focusing next on the nutrient, the brochure says only that the experimental group received a daily supplement containing the daily recommended intake for "nutrient X," but you do not know their intake of this substance from foods and beverages. Depending on their diets, it is possible that some of the men *not taking the supplement* could have consumed as much or more "nutrient X" as the men *receiving the supplement;* another possibility is that some of those not receiving the supplement and not getting much of it in their diets may have had a marginal deficiency of the nutrient. The levels of other nutrients could also have been important, because nutrients can substantially affect one another. None of these considerations were addressed.

The report of results was also lacking in information: how did the control group fare? We are told nothing about their results; they may have done worse, better, or the same as the experimental group.

On the back of the brochure is a statement that the complete study is available on request. The brochure was published by a manufacturer of nutritional supplements.

Now What Do You Think?

How useful is the information in the brochure?

- Option 1 Trust the information as presented. Give the benefit of the doubt that all appropriate tests were done—but not reported in this brief brochure—and that the data support the stated outcome of better performance.
- Option 2 Trust the information that seems well documented (which do you think is valid?) but not the rest.
- Option 3 Reserve judgment. Send for the complete study and evaluate it on the basis of all available information.
- Option 4 Be skeptical of this study, but consult trustworthy sources such as this nutrition text; or ask your instructor or a registered dietitian (RD) at a sports medicine clinic or hospital whether this nutrient is known to enhance physical performance.
- Option 5 Disregard the study totally. No amount of additional information could validate this study.

Can you think of additional options or combinations of options? Which do you think are appropriate?

Summary

- A complex of inborn, cultural, and personal factors influences food choices. Because foods are the carriers of nutrients, all of these factors, in turn, affect your nutrition.
- Food preferences are affected, first of all, by inborn factors. We all have an innate liking for sweet foods and a dislike of bitter tastes. We are interested in trying new foods, but we're also cautious.
- Cultural influences on our food choices include the people who take care of us as children; our ethnic or religious heritage; ethical considerations, which may include concerns about our **ecosystem**; health information; advertising; and our peers.
- Unique personal factors influencing our food choices include sensory preferences, emotional factors, available time and money, and beliefs about the effects of food on our health.
- **Nutrition** is the sum of all the interactions between an organism and the food it consumes. Foods contain approximately 50 **nutrients**, which must be taken in preformed, because the body cannot make them from their **elemental** constituents. Nutrients can be grouped into six classes: water, carbohydrates, lipids, proteins, vitamins, and minerals. The first four classes are **macronutrients**; vitamins and minerals are **micronutrients**.
- Nutrients are used for three basic purposes: (1) to form body structures; (2) to provide energy, which is measured in **kilocalories**; and (3) to help regulate the body's **biochemical** reactions, collectively called **metabolism**.
- Both inadequate and excessive intakes of nutrients are unhealthy, and both result in **malnutrition**. The effects of malnutrition can be general or specific, depending on which nutrients and what levels of deficiency or excess are involved.
- Genetics influences many aspects of our bodies and health. In the future, it may be possible to read the entire genetic code, or **genome**, of human beings. Nutrition is believed to be one factor involved in diseases of **multifactorial** origin, that is, diseases for which there are multiple **risk factors.**
- Nutritional scientists test **hypotheses** by performing experiments of various types to uncover the truths about nutrition. **Epidemiologic studies** address the health status of large groups of people, identifying **positive** and **negative statistical correlations**. Animal and human metabolic studies usually involve more detailed assessments of the effects that occur when controlled levels of nutrients are given. **Single-** and **double-blind studies** and the use of **placebos** and **controls** help remove some of the possible sources of bias created by human expectations. Experiments using animals must be designed and interpreted with care if they are to yield any meaningful information about human nutrition. Research in **molecular biology**, which generally uses **in vitro** rather than **in vivo** studies, can clarify the effects of nutrition at the cellular and molecular levels. Individual experiences, including **anecdotal reports** and **case studies**, do *not* provide valid evidence of nutritional effects.
- Knowing the hallmarks of good studies can help you identify which nutrition claims are likely to be valid. Good studies are carefully designed, conducted by qualified researchers, published in refereed journals, and replicated by other scientists before the conclusions become generally accepted. Good studies often take years to complete.

References

Bryant, C.A., A. Courtney, B.A. Markesbery, and K.M. DeWalt. 1985. *The cultural feast.* St. Paul: West Publishing Company.

Food Marketing Institute. 1992. *Trends—consumer attitudes and the supermarket, 1992.* Washington, DC: Food Marketing Institute.

Food Review, 1992. Changes in World Markets. *Food Review,* vol. 15, (no. 1), 18–22.

Harper, A.E. 1988. Nutrition: From myth and magic to science. *Nutrition Today* 23:8–17.

Jesse, E. and B. Cropp. 1987. Fluid milk reconstitution: Issues and impacts. *Marketing and Policy Briefing Paper,* Department of Agricultural Economics, University of Wisconsin-Madison.

Lappe, F.M. 1982. *Diet for a small planet.* New York: Ballantine Books.

Lecos, C. 1988. We're getting the message about diet–disease links. *FDA Consumer* May, 1988:6–9.

Leonard, R.E. 1982. Nutrition profiles: Diet in the 80's. *Community Nutrition* 1(5):12–17.

McBean, L.D. 1990. Genetics and nutrition. *Dairy Council Digest* 61(1):1–5.

Mertz, W. 1983. The significance of trace elements for health. *Nutrition Today* 18(5):27.

Milner, I. 1992. Diploma mills grind out self-styled nutritionists dispensing bad advice. *Environmental Nutrition* 15(no. 1):1, 6–7.

Molitor, G.T. 1980. The food system in the 1980s. *Journal of Nutrition Education* 12(no. 2)supplement: 103–111.

Morgan, W.P. 1981. The 1980 C.H. McCloy research lecture: Psychophysiology of self-awareness during vigorous physical activity. *Research Quarterly for Exercise and Sport* 52:385–427.

National Research Council. 1989. *Diet and health.* Washington, DC: National Academy Press.

Nations, J.D. and D.I. Komer. 1986. Rainforests and the hamburger society. In *The nutrition debate: Sorting out some answers*, ed. J.D. Gussow and P.R. Thomas. Palo Alto, CA: The Bull Publishing Company.

Olson, R.E. 1978. Clinical nutrition—where human ecology and internal medicine meet. *Nutrition Today* 13(4):18–28.

Owen, A.L. 1990. The impact of future foods on nutrition and health. *Journal of the American Dietetic Association* 90(9):1217–1222.

Paquin, R. and R. Doherty. 1992. *Not first in nobody's heart: The life story of a contemporary Chippewa.* Ames, IA: Iowa State University Press.

Putnam, J.J. 1990. Food consumption, prices, and expenditures, 1967–1988. *Statistical Bulletin 804.* Washington, DC: USDA Economic Research Service.

Regenstein, J.M. and C.E. Regenstein. 1988. The kosher dietary laws and their implementation in the food industry. *Food Technology* 42:86–94.

Rolls, B.J. 1991. Determinants of food intake and selection. In *Nutrition in the 90's: Current controversies and analysis*, ed. G.E. Gaull, F.N. Kotsonis, and M.A. Mackey. New York: Marcel Dekker, Inc.

Rozin, P. 1988. Cultural approaches to human food preferences. In *Nutritional modulation of neural function*, ed. J.E. Morley, M.B. Sterman, J.H. Walsh. San Diego: Academic Press, Inc.

Rozin, P. and T.A. Vollmecke. 1986. Food likes and dislikes. *Annual Reviews of Nutrition* 6:433–456.

Schelp, F.P., P. Pongpaew, N. Vudhivai, and S. Sornmani. 1986. Relationship of "weight for height" to "height for age"—a longitudinal study. *Nutrition Research* 6:369–373.

Schutz, H.G., D.S. Judge, and J. Gentry. 1986. The importance of nutrition, brand, cost, and sensory attributes to food purchase and consumption. *Food Technology* 40:79–82.

Senauer, B., E. Asp, and J. Kinsey. 1991. *Food trends and the changing consumer.* St. Paul: Eagan Press.

Twaigery, S. and D. Spillman. 1989. An introduction to Moslem dietary laws. *Food Technology* 43:88–90.

Wilmore, J.H., F.B. Roby, P.R. Stanforth, M.J. Buono, S.H. Constable, Y. Tsao, and B.J. Lowdon. 1986. Ratings of perceived exertion, heart rate, and power output in predicting maximal oxygen uptake during submaximal cycle ergometry. *The Physician and Sports Medicine* 14:133–143.

Wittwer, S.H. 1992. The "greening effect": Implications for consumer food choices. *Food and Nutrition News* 64(3):1–3.

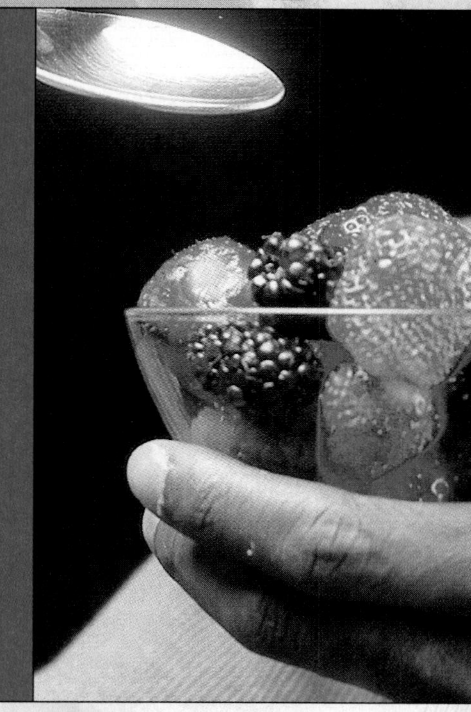

IN THIS CHAPTER

Chapter 2

How Do You Rate Nutritionally?

Do you think you're well nourished?

It wouldn't be surprising if you were uncertain about this. Perhaps one of the reasons you're studying nutrition is to answer that question for yourself.

nutritional status—the extent to which your needs for nutrients are being met

The mixed messages we get may contribute to your confusion about your **nutritional status.** On the one hand, we hear that Americans eat too much; it seems logical to suppose, then, that we must get fairly high levels—wouldn't you presume adequate amounts?—of nutrients. On the other hand, various messages cast doubt on Americans' nutritional well-being. For example, a nutritional supplement ad suggests that if you've felt sluggish (and who hasn't, at one time or another?), your diet is clearly to blame; an article claims that if you miss drinking your orange juice for a few mornings, you've started the slippery slide toward vitamin deficiency.

Relying on such sources of information gets you nowhere: you can't learn much about *yourself* from information about *averages,* or from insinuations or blatant misinformation sometimes offered by those who have products to sell.

nutritional assessment techniques—methods of rating nutritional status

There are, fortunately, many **nutritional assessment techniques** for finding out about your nutritional status, and they are described in this chapter. There are two general types of methods: one is based on evaluating various aspects of your body; the other involves analyzing your diet (Figure 2.1). All of these techniques have some appropriate uses, but all also have limitations.

In this book, we primarily use diet analysis to determine nutritional status. You can follow the step-by-step instructions for evaluating your diet not just today, but whenever you want to check on how well you're nourishing yourself. This chapter provides two methods for looking at the overall quality of your diet. Later chapters provide many other techniques for assessing more specific aspects of your diet.

Once you have analyzed your diet, the results may prompt you to think about making some changes. Your current eating habits have developed over many years and are well entrenched. Even if you want to change, you may also resist the idea of eating differently. To help you find ways to overcome such resistance, we have devoted the last part of this chapter to the principles of behavior modification, which you can use to shape new dietary habits that can provide benefits throughout your life.

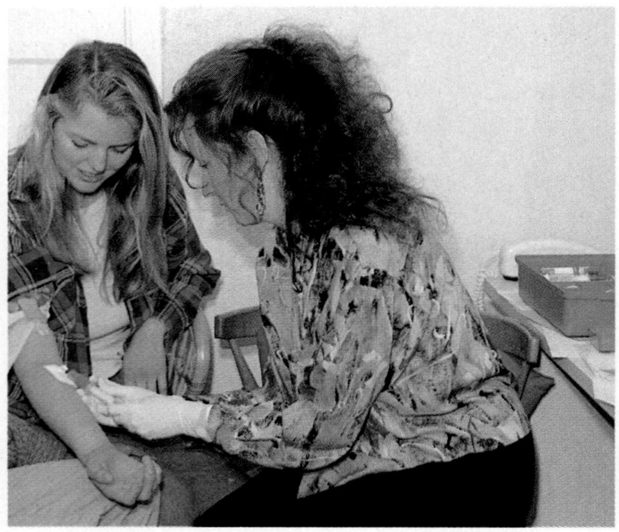

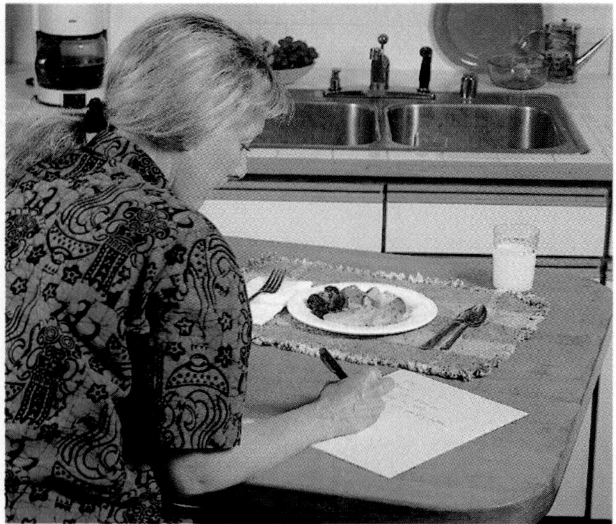

FIGURE 2.1
Methods of nutritional assessment.

There are two general approaches to finding out how well-nourished you are: evaluating your body in various ways and analyzing your diet. You will have many opportunities to evaluate your diet throughout this book.

Body Indicators of Nutritional Status

Before we plunge into the methods of nutritional assessment, it is useful to consider what happens when good nutrition goes awry. Here are a couple of extreme scenarios.

If usually you were well nourished, but you suddenly and dramatically *reduced your intake of a particular nutrient for a few months,* what would happen?

Initially, in the first several weeks, you probably would not notice anything different about the way you felt or looked; however, the amount of the nutrient and related chemicals in your blood might start to decrease. In response, your body would mobilize the nutrient from storage sites to try to normalize the blood level. If your intake continued to be deficient, the level of the nutrient and related compounds in your blood, other body tissues, and/or urine would progressively decline. (This sequence of events is typical but does not apply strictly to all nutrients.)

If the deficiency went on for an extended period of time—a couple of months or more—some of your body's functions and structures could begin to change. You could start to feel and look unhealthy. Eventually, death could result from severe, prolonged deficiency of some nutrients.

Fortunately, death directly attributable to severe undernutrition is quite rare in the United States; marginal undernutrition is much more common. However, severe undernutrition *is* a common cause of death in the developing countries, where an estimated 38,000 children under the age of 5 died each day from hunger and related causes in the late 1980s (UNICEF, 1988). (These numbers were undoubtedly higher in the early 1990s, but accurate numbers are impossible to obtain.) In these cases, usually the children were deficient in many nutrients for a long period of time.

If you *overconsumed a nutrient for an extended period,* the level of the nutrient or its related compounds in your blood, other tissues, and/or urine initially might increase. If you continued to take in more than you needed, your body might be unable to handle the excessive level of the nutrient. You might notice toxic effects in the way you felt, looked, and functioned.

Some substances, most notably the fat-soluble vitamins A and D, can accumulate to toxic levels. Serious permanent effects—even death—have occurred from such overdosing.

It's also important to realize that an excessive intake of *one* nutrient can sometimes interfere with your body's handling of *other* nutrients. This is one way in which people who take large doses of nutritional supplements—believing them to be beneficial—can actually create problems.

These are, of course, extreme examples. It is unlikely that you ever have or ever will experience such situations. Nevertheless, none of us gets exactly the amounts of nutrients that we need each day. Usually, we alternate between brief periods (a couple of days or a week) of moderate underconsumption and overconsumption of nutrients, with the intakes averaging out to an adequate level. This is normal and not considered damaging to health. Chances are, this describes your nutritional status.

But *what if it doesn't?* How could a nutritional problem be detected? Several techniques can be used to uncover information about your body's possible nutritional problems. Some need to be done by medical personnel, and some anyone can do.

Biochemical Tests

Biochemical tests use chemical analysis to evaluate substances from the body. Blood and urine are the materials most often analyzed. Although

biochemical tests—chemical analyses of body substances, such as blood or urine

these tests are not perfect, they are the most accurate means of evaluation we currently have.

metabolites—products of biochemical reactions

Blood Tests A sample of your blood can be analyzed to determine whether certain nutrients and/or the **metabolites** they produce are within normal ranges. When you know what level of a nutrient is *circulating in your blood,* it does not necessarily indicate how much is *present elsewhere* in the body. For example, one way to find out whether your body contains an adequate amount of iron is simply to measure the quantity of iron *in your blood.* A more accurate way, however, is to perform several different analyses, some of which indicate the likely amount of iron stored in your liver.

Of course, abnormal levels of nutrients in the blood could be present for reasons other than poor diet: in some illnesses, even normal levels of nutrients are used in an abnormal way. For example, a high level of sugar in the blood could mean that the person's body is unable to handle even a moderate sugar intake in a normal way. Such a disorder may be due to a disease such as diabetes mellitus.

Because blood tests are also very helpful in diagnosing and monitoring disease conditions, they have become a routine part of general health checkups and hospitalizations, as well as nutritional status surveys.

Urine Tests Chemical analysis of urine also involves skilled laboratory procedures. Like blood tests, urine tests can reveal whether the levels of some nutrients and/or their metabolites are within normal ranges, giving clues to nutritional status or the presence of disease. This technique is commonly used in general health checkups, hospitalizations, and nutritional status surveys to measure levels of certain vitamins.

Anthropometric Tests

anthropometric tests—external measurements of the body, such as height, weight, and skinfold thickness

Anthropometric tests involve taking various external measurements and comparing them with population standards; such assessments provide information about overall nutritional status and are less specific than biochemical tests. The most commonly used anthropometric tests are described here.

Height and Weight Because nutrition helps determine how far you grow toward your genetically determined size limits, measurements of height and weight have some value for nutritional assessment.

In children, both height and weight measurements can provide a rough evaluation of general nutritional status, particularly of energy intake and output. In adults, weight changes usually testify either to *fluctuation in body water, body fat, muscle mass,* or even *bone mass* (Frisancho, 1988).

Height and weight tables are one standard to which a person's measurements can be compared. Because these tables are based on averages and are expressed as broad ranges, they cannot tell you or anybody else specifically what you should weigh. In Chapter 9 we discuss other concerns about such tables and describe many other factors that you should take into account in determining your healthy body weight.

skinfold calipers—device for measuring thickness of skin and underlying fat

Skinfold Thickness An experienced professional can make judgments about a person's past energy intake and expenditure by measuring the thickness of the skin and underlying fat layer at various body sites using special **skinfold calipers** (Figure 2.2). If many more kcalories have been eaten than expended over a period of time, the fat layer will be thicker than before. Conversely, if a person used more energy than was consumed during past

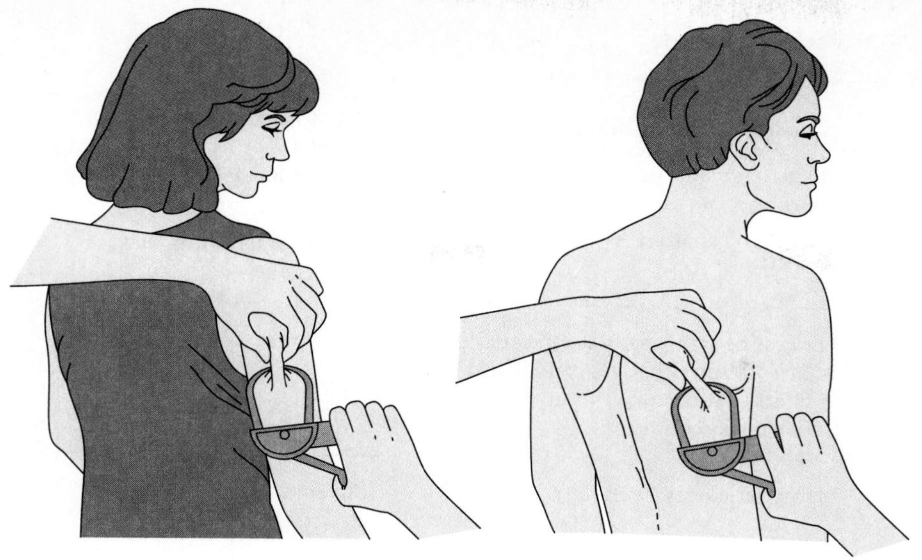

FIGURE 2.2
Using skinfold calipers to measure body fatness.

One way of determining how much body fat a person has is to measure the fat that has accumulated under the skin in various locations on the body. Among the many other possible locations at which the skinfold can be measured are the biceps, chest, abdomen, thigh, and calf.

weeks or months, the fat layer will be measurably thinner. Some fitness programs use changes in skinfold thickness to help measure a person's progress in losing fat.

Tables based on large numbers of people have been developed to show typical fat thicknesses at various body sites. Any individual's measurements can be compared to the tables to determine body fatness relative to the reference group. Like the use of height and weight tables, this method of assessment is not very precise. Chapter 9 provides a more extensive discussion of this method and its shortfalls.

Appearance and Sense of Well-Being

Of the methods of nutritional assessment, evaluating one's appearance and sense of well-being is the least specific. Nonetheless, changes in appearance and loss of well-being can indicate that a problem exists and provide useful clues to further testing.

Appearance Changes in appearance are sometimes used as a rough means of assessing nutritional status. Table 2.1 shows some typical outward signs that often accompany severe, long-term malnutrition.

Because looking for these changes requires no special equipment, you might think that this would be a good method of assessment to use for yourself. However, because even trained health professionals do not always correctly identify malnutrition or its cause when using this method, it is not in itself reliable. Furthermore, few people in the developed countries, especially in the young adult population, experience *undernutrition* severe enough to result in obvious external changes. If you have one of the signs, your nutritional status is probably not the cause. Note that Table 2.1 offers alternative explanations for some external symptoms.

The few Americans and Canadians who might be undernourished enough to show such signs usually are the elderly and the chronically (persistently) ill, including alcoholics. The vast majority of cases of obvious undernutrition are found in developing countries.

TABLE 2.1 A Few Signs of Nutritional Problems . . . or Something Else?[a]

Noticeable Sign	Possible Nutrient Involvement(s)	Possible Other Explanation(s)
Dry, scaling skin	Deficiency of vitamin A, zinc, protein, or essential fatty acid Excess of vitamin A	Chapping from cold or wind Sunburn Chemical irritation, e.g., detergents
Increased yellow pigmentation of skin	Excess of carotene, a compound in carrots and other vegetables and fruits that becomes vitamin A (harmless condition)	Liver disease
Fingernails or toenails that separate from nail bed	Iron deficiency anemia	Physical injury Psoriasis Fungal infection Use of nail hardeners
Swollen, bleeding gums	Deficiency of vitamin C	Poor dental hygiene Medication side effect
Swelling of feet and ankles due to fluid retention (edema)	Deficiency of thiamin or protein	Pregnancy Hot weather Standing for long periods Medication side effect Cardiovascular problems Kidney disease
Cracks in lips and at corners of mouth (cheilosis)	Deficiency of riboflavin, multiple B vitamins, or protein	Cold, windy weather Repeated wetting or rubbing of lips Viral infections
Obesity	Excessive kcalorie intake in relation to energy output	Possible hormone imbalance in rare cases

[a]References: McLaren, 1988; Heymsfield and Williams, 1988; Weinsier and Butterworth, 1981; "Your fingernails: What do they reveal about your health?" 1991.

One type of obvious *overnutrition* that is commonly seen in North America is obesity. Cases of overnutrition of specific nutrients are more unusual but do occur.

Sense of Well-Being Sometimes, but not always, you may be aware of changes in the way you feel or function. Like changes in appearance, these self-reports are of limited value because they are very subjective and are not necessarily the result of nutritional problems. For example, although tiredness can result from prolonged inadequate iron or kcalorie intake, it can also be caused by such nonnutritional factors as too little sleep, mental depression, or other illness. (However, malnutrition is not always accompanied by

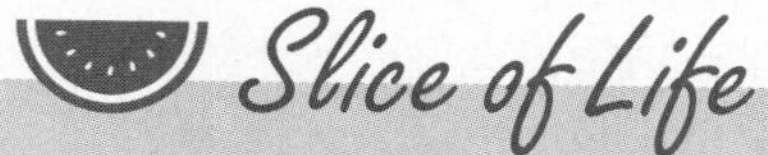

The Unreliability of Hair Analysis

Stephen Barrett, a physician who helped found the National Council Against Health Fraud, put to the test some laboratories that chemically analyze hair samples.

He took hair samples from two healthy 17-year-old girls and sent cuttings from each of them to 13 labs for mineral analysis. The reports he received back from them varied widely: several laboratories reported values for most minerals that were at least ten times those stated by others. One lab reported 2200 times more of a certain mineral than another!

Six labs included supplement advice in their reports, and the types and amounts suggested varied widely from lab to lab for each girl. Some reports noted "trends or tendencies" to diseases: among the conditions suggested for these two girls were goiter, uremia (toxic metabolites in the blood), and "depression of central nervous system" (Barrett, 1985).

Because the girls were known to be healthy, the most charitable statement that can be made about the lab reports is that many of them seem to have been in error. Of course, people who receive reports from such laboratories are likely to take them seriously, because they trusted the service enough to seek it out. Unfortunately, what they may actually be receiving for their money is needless worry about their health. When they receive advice to purchase nutritional supplements to correct the supposed "nutritional deficits," people spend even more money on products that are probably unnecessary or may even be dangerous.

a feeling of being under par: some people are surprised when, on the basis of blood tests, they are diagnosed with severe health or nutritional problems; they may claim that they feel fine or they may have attached no importance to their symptoms.)

No matter what the cause may be, you should report such observations to your doctor so that a professional can provide an evaluation, diagnosis, and plans for appropriate care.

Tests of Limited or Very Questionable Value

Several types of tests do *not* provide useful information about your nutritional status. Some of these tests, in addition, can be very expensive.

Hair analysis has very few valid uses. It can sometimes help in identifying mineral poisoning (arsenic poisoning, for example) and in comparing the status of various population groups in regard to certain minerals. But that's all.

In recent years, some enterprising pseudoscientists have marketed the service of analyzing hair samples to determine chemical content, and reporting their findings as evidence of nutritional status. This is not a reliable means of nutritional assessment.

Why? Biochemistry experts say that although it certainly is possible to analyze the amounts of various minerals present in hair, there are currently few standards as to what values are normal. Furthermore, the composition of hair is not likely to reflect the current composition of other body tissues. In addition, products that come in contact with hair can change its chemical composition: shampoos, bleaches, dyes, solutions used for permanents, and even the water supply can remove or add chemicals. For these reasons, hair analysis currently has little value for nutritional assessment or for diagnosis and treatment of diseases (Klevay, et al., 1987).

On top of all those problems, there is evidence that laboratories that market hair analysis to the general public may not do consistent work. The Slice of Life above explains.

Some tests have even less validity. One of these, according to William Jarvis, PhD (1989), a staff member of the Loma Linda School of Medicine and former president of the National Council Against Health Fraud, is the *cytotoxic* (or *leucocytoxicity*) *test.* In this test, which supposedly identifies allergies, a blood sample is mixed with food extracts and the reactions of the white blood cells are then observed under a microscope. Another technique of questionable value is *applied kinesiology.* Practitioners using this test press down on a client's extended arm or leg, claiming that any perceived weakness can be strengthened with nutritional supplements. Applied kinesiology was invented by a chiropractor using his psychic abilities (Jarvis, 1989).

Estimating Your Nutritional Status from Your Diet

A thorough nutritional assessment includes not only the techniques that focus on your body, but also others that focus on your diet. Dietary assessment involves analyzing your intake and comparing it to a predetermined standard or set of recommendations.

Dietary recommendations have changed considerably, especially in the last two decades. The history of these changes can help you understand why the current advice differs from what you may have learned in the past about planning and evaluating your diet.

A Brief History of U.S. Dietary Recommendations

dietary recommendations (guides, guidelines)—advice for the general public about what types and amounts of foods constitute a healthy daily diet

Dietary recommendations, guides, or **guidelines** are tools for choosing a healthy diet. Based on scientific findings, they translate technical information into practical suggestions for selecting your food. Such guidelines have been used in the United States since the early 1900s.

Food Group Guides in the First Half of This Century The first dietary recommendations in the United States were designed to help people avoid nutritional deficiencies, which were significant problems at that time. The early recommendations divided foods into groups—sometimes as many as 12 different groups—and advised people to eat, at minimum, a specific number of servings from each group every day. Some of the early recommendations were issued by governmental groups, and others were circulated by special trade groups that highlighted their own products.

Although these recommendations were based on much less nutrition knowledge than we have today, and although some may have seemed questionable because they promoted specific commercial products, the principle on which they were based was valid then—and still is today. Foods of the same general type (such as wheat, rice, and oats, all of which are grains) usually have similar nutrient values, although their specific levels are not identical. By recommending that people consume given numbers of servings from various food groups, these guides helped people consume the full spectrum of nutrients at adequate levels of intake.

***The Basic Four Food Guide*—Important for a Quarter Century** In 1958, the United States Department of Agriculture (USDA) released a food group plan, *Food For Fitness—A Daily Food Guide.* More commonly known as the *Basic Four,* it would prove to be an important nutrition education tool for more than two decades. Its most significant difference from its predecessors was that it consisted of only four food groups, a number easier to remember and use. The guide advised people to eat at least the number of

Pieces of the Pyramid

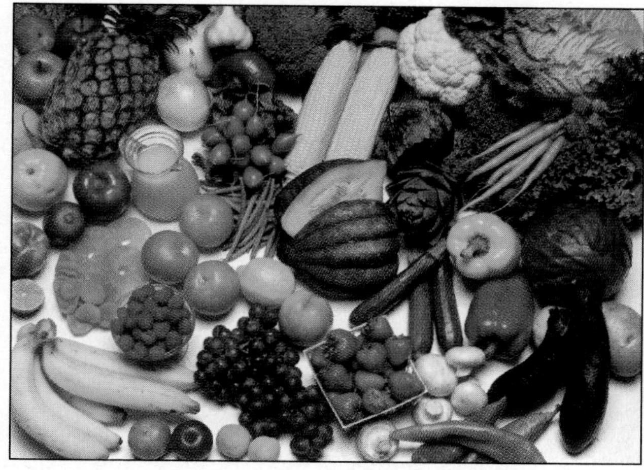

The Pyramid is a tool you can use to quickly evaluate or plan your food intake. It recommends what kinds and amounts of foods you should eat to get enough nutrients; it also tells you the levels of fat, sodium, and added sugar in representative foods.

You will find a page for each of the five basic groups of foods. In the box on each page is the daily recommended intake range for adults. Below the intake recommendations, you will find other important information, including examples of serving sizes.

Within the **bread, cereal, rice, and pasta group,** you are encouraged to use several whole grain items each day.

When considering the **meat, poultry, fish, dry beans, eggs, and nuts group,** you are advised to think in terms of amounts equivalent to meat, because the quantities of the various alternatives are so different.

For the **milk, yogurt, and cheese group,** note that different intakes are recommended for various groups of people.

In addition to the pages for the basic food groups, you will find a page each for **combination foods** and for **fats, oils, and sweets** to help provide a sense of their contributions.

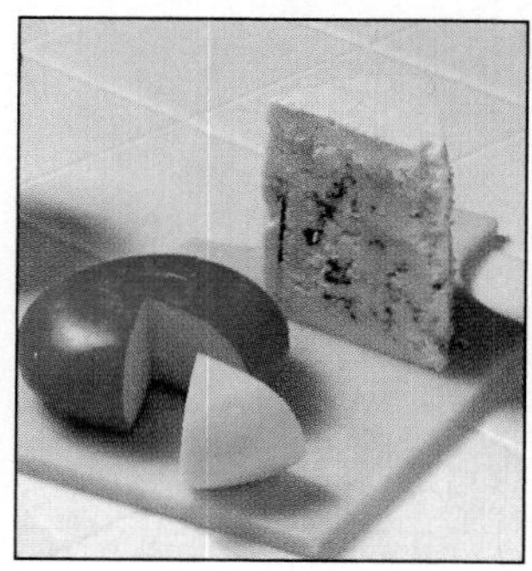

Bread, Cereal, Rice, and Pasta

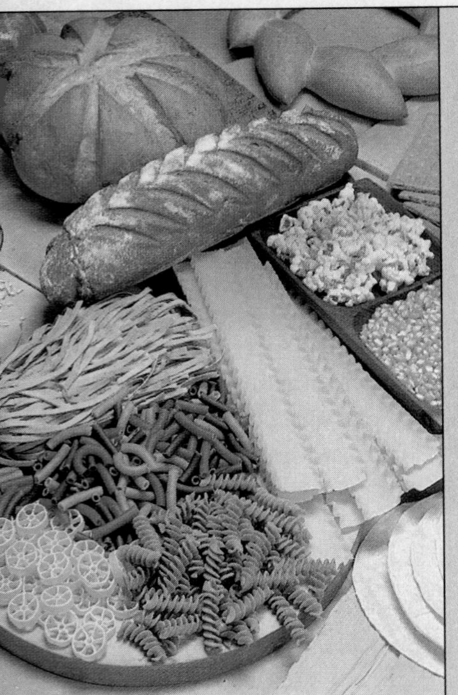

6–11 SERVINGS DAILY

Include several whole-grain products

EACH OF THESE IS A SERVING:

1 slice of bread or medium dinner roll
½ hamburger bun, hot dog bun, bagel, or English muffin
1 ounce ready-to-eat cereal
½ cup cooked cereal
3 cups popped popcorn
1 tortilla, pancake, or waffle square
½ cup cooked pasta, rice, or other grains
6 saltines, snack crackers, or 3-ring pretzels
3 graham cracker squares or small unfrosted cookies

HOW MUCH FAT, SODIUM, AND ADDED SUGAR ARE LIKELY TO BE FOUND IN GRAIN PRODUCTS?

(When no serving size is specified, assume that the serving size stated above applies.)

Grams of Fat

- 35–
- 30–
- 25–
- 20–
- 15–1 large (2 oz.) croissant
- 10–1 oz. fried snack foods
  - –4 small oatmeal raisin cookies
- 5– Compare with 1 t. fat; Quick breads, baking powder biscuit, 2 medium cookies
- 0– Plain bread, saltines; Rice, pasta, most cereals

Milligrams of Sodium

- 1400–
- 1200–
- 1000–
- 800–
- 600–Compare with ¼ t. salt
- 400–Cornflakes
- 200–Saltines, 1 oz. corn chips
  - –Plain bread
- 0–Corn tortilla

Grams of Added Sugar

- 35–
- 30–
- 25–
- 20– 4 small oatmeal raisin cookies
- 15–Sugar Smacks
- 10–Frosted Mini-Wheats
- 5–Compare with 1 t. sugar
  - Medium muffin
- 0– Plain bread, tortilla, saltines, pasta, Cheerios

Vegetables

3–5 SERVINGS DAILY

EACH OF THESE IS A SERVING:

1 cup raw leafy vegetable
½ cup other fresh, frozen or canned vegetable
¾ cup fresh, frozen, or canned juice
¼ cup dried vegetable

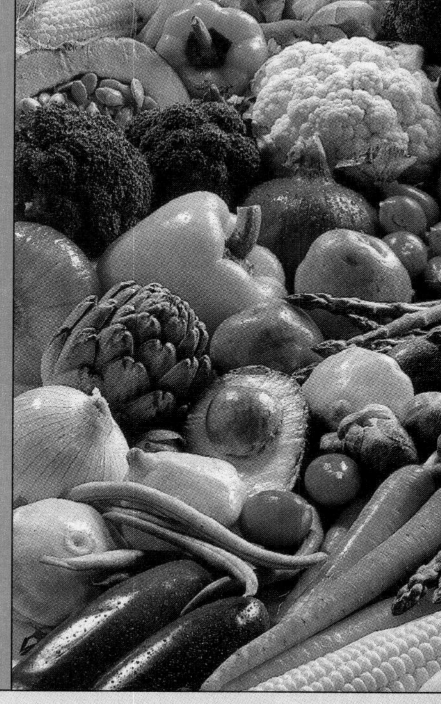

HOW MUCH FAT, SODIUM, AND ADDED SUGAR ARE LIKELY TO BE FOUND IN VEGETABLES AND VEGETABLE PRODUCTS?

(When no serving size is specified, assume that the serving size stated above applies.)

Grams of Fat

Grams	Food
35	
30	
25	
20	
(between 20 and 15)	1/6 of 9-inch sweet potato pie
15	
10	1 oz. potato chips
5	Compare with 1 t. fat
0	Plain fresh, frozen, or canned vegetables or juice

Milligrams of Sodium

Milligrams	Food
1400	
1200	
1000	
(between 1000 and 800)	1 c. canned vegetable soup
800	½ c. sauerkraut
(between 800 and 600)	1 3¾ inch dill pickle
600	Compare with ¼ t. salt
400	Vegetables frozen in sauce
200	Many canned vegetables
0	Most plain fresh or frozen vegetables

Grams of Added Sugar

Grams	Food
35	
30	
25	
20	
15	
10	
5	Compare with 1 t. sugar
0	Plain fresh, frozen, or canned vegetables or juice

Fruits

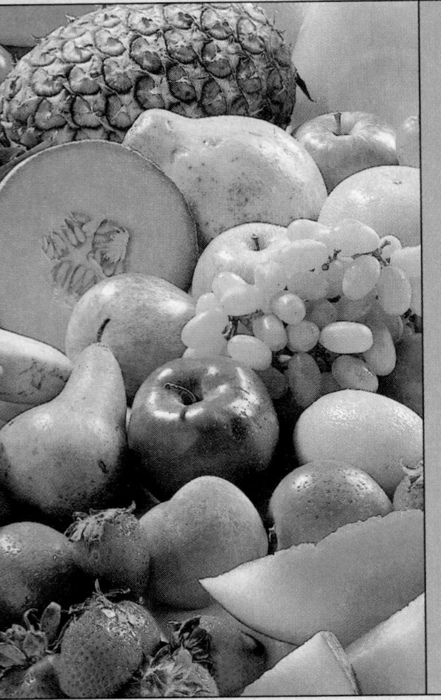

2–4 SERVINGS DAILY

EACH OF THESE IS A SERVING:

1 medium apple, banana, orange
½ cup of raw, cooked, or canned fruit
¾ cup of fruit juice
¼ cup of dried fruit

HOW MUCH FAT, SODIUM, AND ADDED SUGAR ARE LIKELY TO BE FOUND IN FRUIT AND FRUIT PRODUCTS?

(When no serving size is specified, assume that the serving size stated above applies.)

Grams of Fat

35–
30–
25–
20–
–⅙ of 9-inch apple pie
15–
10–
5–Compare with 1 t. fat
0–{Plain fresh, frozen, or canned fruit or juice

Milligrams of Sodium

1400–
1200–
1000–
800–
600–Compare with ¼ t. salt
400–
200–
0–{Plain fresh, frozen, or canned fruit or juice

Grams of Added Sugar

35–
30–⅙ of 9-inch apple pie
25–
20–
15–
10–Fruits frozen or canned with sugar
5–Compare with 1 teasp. sugar
0–Fresh fruit; fruit or juice frozen or canned without sugar

Milk, Yogurt, and Cheese

2–3 SERVINGS DAILY

2 servings (most people)
3 servings (teenagers, young adults through age 24, women who are pregnant or breast-feeding)

EACH OF THESE IS A SERVING:

1 cup milk or yogurt
1½ ounces natural cheese
2 ounces processed cheese food
2 cups cottage cheese
1 cup sauces or puddings made with milk
1½ cups ice cream, ice milk, or frozen yogurt

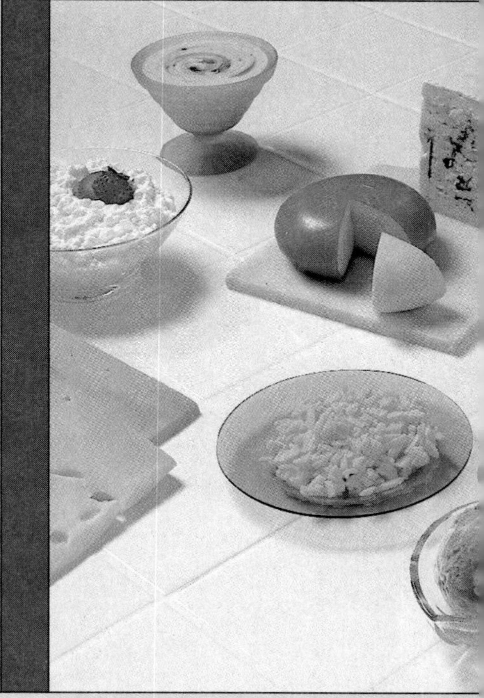

HOW MUCH FAT, SODIUM, AND ADDED SUGAR ARE LIKELY TO BE FOUND IN MILK AND MILK PRODUCTS?

(When no serving size is specified, assume that the serving size stated above applies.)

Grams of Fat

35–
30–
25–
20–Ice cream
15–Processed cheese
–Cheddar cheese
10 Ice milk
Whole milk
5–Compare with 1 t. fat
–2% milk
–1 cup low-fat yogurt
–low-fat cottage cheese
0–Skim milk

Milligrams of Sodium

1400–
1200–
1000–1 cup low-fat cottage cheese
Instant pudding
800–Processed cheese food
600–Compare with ¼ t. salt
400–
Regular pudding from mix
200–Cheddar cheese
–Milk
0–

Grams of Added Sugar

35–
–Pudding
30–Ice cream
–Fruited yogurt
25–
20–
15–
10–
5–Compare with 1 t. sugar
0–Milk, cheese, plain yogurt

Meat, Poultry, Fish, Dry Beans, Eggs, and Nuts

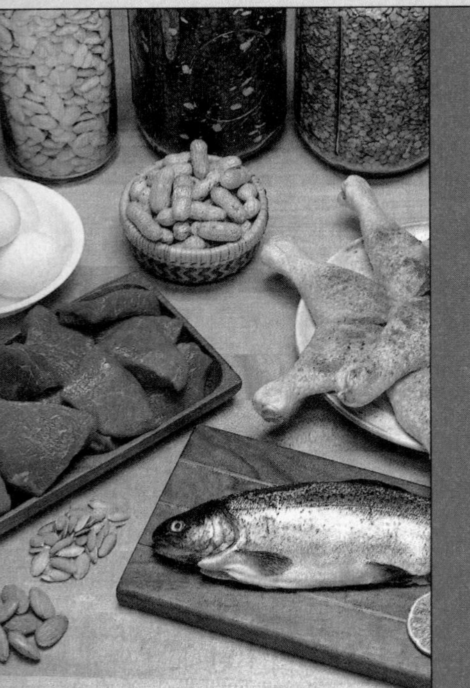

2–3 SERVINGS DAILY

Totaling an equivalent of 5–7 ounces of meat per day

EACH OF THESE IS A SERVING:

2–3 ounces lean, cooked meat, fish, or poultry (no bone)
(a piece about the size of a deck of cards)

The following can substitute for 1 ounce of meat:

1 egg
½ cup cooked legumes (e.g., black, garbanzo, kidney, lima, navy, pinto, soybeans; lentils; split peas)
3 ounces tofu
1 ounce (approximately ¼ cup) nuts or seeds
1 ounce (approximately 2 tablespoons) nut or seed butters

HOW MUCH FAT, SODIUM, AND ADDED SUGAR ARE LIKELY TO BE FOUND IN MEAT AND MEAT ALTERNATES?

(When no serving size is specified, assume that the serving size stated above applies.)

Grams of Fat

35
30
25
20
–1 oz. nuts
–2 oz. bologna
15–2 oz. ham
–2 oz. ground beef
–2 oz. fried chicken
10–2 oz. fried perch
–3 oz. tofu, 1 egg
5–Compare with 1 t. fat
–2 oz. broiled chicken (no skin)
0–Cooked legumes

Milligrams of Sodium

1400
1200
1000
800–2 oz. ham
600–Compare with ¼ t. salt
–½ cup baked beans
400–2 oz. bologna
200
–1 oz. salted peanuts
–2 oz. fried perch
0– 2 oz. meats, poultry, cooked legumes, tofu, nuts (all unsalted)

Grams of Added Sugar

35
30
25
20
15
10
5–Compare with 1 t. sugar
–½ c. canned baked beans
–Some processed lunch meats
0– Plain cooked legumes, meat, fish, poultry, nuts

Combination Foods

You can use the Pyramid to evaluate a combination food by mentally separating it into its ingredients and estimating the amounts of basic foods present. The following examples of different types of combination dishes can be used as guidelines when you estimate similar dishes.

1 cup canned beef noodle soup
1/2 oz. meat = 1/4 serving meat
1/4 c. noodles = 1/2 serving grain

1/8 of 15-inch cheese pizza
1 1/3 oz. cheese = 1 serving milk
pizza dough = 2 servings grain
1/4 c. vegetables = 1/2 serving vegetables

1 cup canned macaroni and cheese
1 oz. processed cheese food = 1/2 serving milk
1 c. macaroni = 2 servings grain
2 oz. milk = 1/4 serving milk

1 cup cream of asparagus or mushroom soup, made with milk
1/2 c. milk = 1/2 serving milk
1 1/4 T. flour = 1/2 serving grain
2 T. vegetable = 1/4 serving vegetable

1 cup chicken chow mein
3 oz. meat = 1 serving meat
1/2 c. vegetables = 1 serving vegetables

1 6-oz. bean burrito
1/2 c. beans = 1/2 serving meat alternate
1 tortilla = 1 serving grain

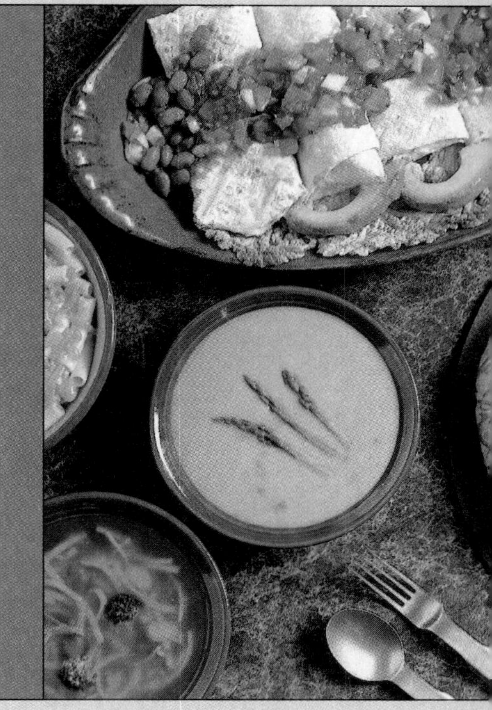

HOW MUCH FAT, SODIUM, AND ADDED SUGAR ARE LIKELY TO BE FOUND IN COMBINATION FOODS?

(When no serving size is specified, assume that the serving size stated above applies.)

Grams of Fat

35–
30–
25–
20–
–Canned cream of mushroom
15–soup
Bean burrito
10–Canned spaghetti and meatballs
–Canned macaroni and cheese–
–1/8 of 15" cheese pizza
5–Compare with 1 t. fat
–Canned beef noodle soup
0–

Milligrams of Sodium

1400–
1200–
1000– { Canned cream of mushroom soup; Bean burrito; Canned spaghetti with meatballs; Canned beef noodle soup }
800–
–Chicken chow mein
600–Compare with 1/4 t. salt
–1/8 of 15" cheese pizza
400–
200–
0–

Grams of Added Sugar

35–
30–
25–
20–
15–
10–
5–Compare with 1 t. sugar
–Many items with tomato sauce
–Many canned soups
0–

Fats, Oils, & Sweets

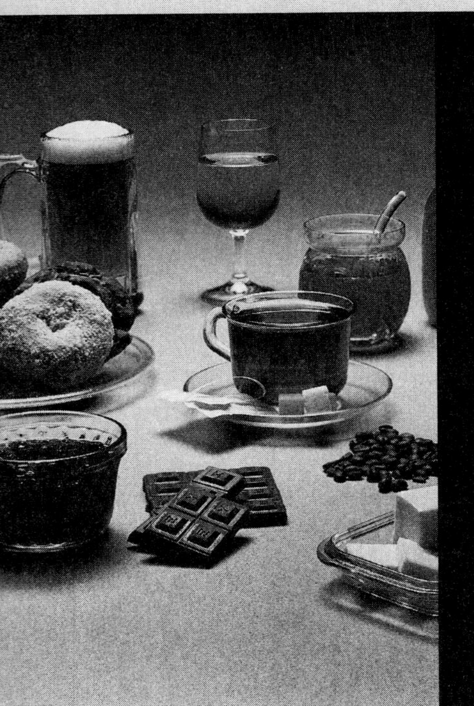

These foods are not needed for good nutrition. These foods don't contain significant amounts of nutrients. They should be used only as limited supplements rather than as mainstays of the diet.

Many of these foods have kcalories that add up quickly. If you are overweight, you can cut kcalories by eating fewer of these foods. If you are at your best weight, it is reasonable to use some of these foods daily, provided that you have included all the recommended foods as the basis of your diet.

Some items on this list have both low kcalories and low nutrient levels, such as tea, coffee, broth, low-kcalorie soft drinks, and diet gelatin desserts. Although low in most essential nutrients, they do contribute water. You can decide how much seems reasonable to consume after you have read the material on caffeine (Chapter 14), sodium (Chapter 12), and additives (Chapter 14).

Grams of Sugar in Sugary Foods

40–12 oz. cola beverage
35
30–½ c. sherbet
25
20–½ c. gelatin dessert, 1 T. honey
15–1 T. syrup, ½ oz. hard candy
–1 oz. chocolate candy
10
–1 t. jam, jelly
5–Compare with 1 t. sugar
0

Grams of Fat in Fatty Foods

20–1 oz. Italian salad dressing
–1 oz. French salad dressing
15–1⅓ oz. cream cheese
10–3 slices bacon, 1 oz. chocolate
5–Compare with 1 t. fat
5–{1 t. oil, 2 T. sour cream; 1 t. butter, margarine, lard, shortening, mayonnaise}

Milligrams of Sodium in Salty Foods

1400
1200
1000–1 T. soy sauce
800–1 c. canned broth
–1 T. teriyaki sauce
–1 oz. low-kcal French dressing
600–Compare with ¼ t. salt
400–1 oz. regular French dressing
–4 green olives
200–3 slices bacon
–1 T. catsup
–1 oz. Italian dressing
0

Grams of Alcohol in Alcoholic Beverages

35
30 Compare with 1 oz. pure alcohol
25
20
–5 oz. wine
15–1 oz. liquor
10–12 oz. beer
5
0

Evaluating Your Diet Using the Pyramid

Familiarize yourself with the Pieces of the Pyramid, and then follow these steps:

1. On a form similar to that used in the accompanying sample, record all the foods and beverages you consume in a day and the amounts of each. For combination foods, estimate the components and list them separately.
2. Using the information in Pieces of the Pyramid, decide which group each food belongs to and how many servings (or what part of a serving) each represents. Enter the numbers in the appropriate columns. For items that belong in the last column—fats, oils, and sweets—simply put an *x* in the column.
3. Add the figures in each column, and total the *x*'s.
4. On the small chart below, check the group you belong in based on your sex, age, and estimated activity level. Take the recommended serving numbers from this chart, and on the diet record chart, fill in your standards for the five food groups. If you are a vegetarian or a person who needs to eat as inexpensively as possible, check Table 2.3 for standards modified for your situation.
5. Compare your intake to the standards. Record any *shortages* on the bottom line. If your intake of foods from certain groups is consistently low, you are probably getting less than you need of that group's major nutrients.

What if you have consumed more than the recommended number of servings? If you are at a weight that is healthy for you, eating more than the recommendations is probably not a problem. If you are overweight or obese, however, the numbers can suggest where your intake is excessive. First look at how many fatty and sugary items you consumed; cutting down on your intake of these foods is the best way of cutting kcalories without sacrificing the nutrients you need. Then check the basic foods columns. If your intake is much above the standards, you can reduce kcalories by gradually bringing your intake down closer to the standards; don't drop below them, though, or you will shortchange yourself on nutrients. You can also replace some of the foods in each group that are higher in fat and/or sugar with other group members whose levels are lower. In Chapter 9, we describe further strategies for reducing fats and sugars in your diet.

Check Your Group		Recommended Servings				Ounces
		Bread Group	Veg. Group	Fruit Group	Milk Group	Meat Group
✓	Many sedentary women; some older adults	6	3	2	2–3[a]	5
	Most children, teenage girls, active women, many sedentary men	9	4	3	2–3[a]	6
	Teenage boys, many very active men, some very active women	11	5	4	2–3[a]	7

[a]Women who are pregnant or breast-feeding, teenagers, and young adults to age 24 need 3 servings.

Sample Act on Fact 2.1

This is the food record of a college woman who, like many of her classmates, is not very active; other than walking from class to class, she gets little activity. Therefore, the sedentary standard applies.

Food or Beverage	Amount Eaten	Number of Servings (Oz. for Meat)					Fats, Oils, and Sweets
		Bread	Veg.	Fruit	Milk	Meat	
Cornflakes	1 oz.	1					
2% milk	1 c.				1		
Sugar	2 t.						X
Orange juice	3/4 c.			1			
Hot dog:							
Bun	1	2					
Frankfurter	1					1	
Catsup	1 T.						X
Relish	1 T.						X
French fries	10 pieces		1				
Diet 7-up	12 oz.						X
Red beans and rice							
Beans	3/4 c.					1 1/2	
Rice	3/4 c.	1 1/2					
Boiled greens	1/2 c.		1				
Biscuits	1	1					
Jam	1 T.						X
2% milk	1 c.				1		
Popcorn	3 c.	1					
Diet cola	12 oz.						X
Group Totals		6 1/2	2	1	2	2 1/2	6
Standards		6	3	2	2	5	
Shortages		—	1	1	—	2 1/2	

TABLE 2.4 Exchange Lists for Meal Planning

The six exchange lists below can be used for meal planning and evaluating food intake. Foods are grouped together on a list because they are similar in composition of energy-containing nutrients. Every food on a list has about the same amount of carbohydrate (CHO), protein (Pro), fat, and kcalories (kcal), except as noted. Any serving of food on a list can be exchanged or traded for any other serving of food on the same list.

Starch/Bread
Each of these equals one starch/bread serving.
(15 g CHO, 3 g Pro, trace fat, 80 kcal)

½ cup pasta or barley

⅓ cup rice or cooked dried beans and peas

1 small potato (or ½ cup mashed)

½ cup starchy vegetables (corn, peas, or winter squash)

1 slice bread or 1 roll

½ English muffin, bagel, or hamburger/hot dog bun

½ cup cooked cereal

¾ cup dry cereal, unsweetened

4–6 crackers

3 cups popcorn, unbuttered, not cooked in oil

Milk
Each of these equals one milk serving.
The calories vary for each choice.
(12 g CHO, 8 g Pro, variable fat and kcal)

1 cup skim milk (90 calories)

1 cup low-fat milk (120 calories)

8-oz. carton plain low fat yogurt (120 calories)

Fruit
Each of these equals one fruit serving.
(15 g CHO, 60 kcal)

1 fresh medium fruit

1 cup berries or melon

½ cup canned in juice or without sugar

½ cup fruit juice

¼ cup dried fruit

Vegetables
Each of these equals one vegetable serving.
(5 g CHO, 2 g Pro, 25 kcal)

½ cup cooked vegetables

1 cup raw vegetables

½ cup tomato/vegetable juice

Meat and Substitutes
Each of these equals one meat choice.
(7 g Pro, variable fat, 55–100 kcal)

1 oz. cooked poultry, fish, or meat

¼ cup cottage cheese

¼ cup salmon or tuna, water packed

1 T. peanut butter

1 egg (limit to 3 per week)

1 oz. low-fat cheese, such as mozzarella, ricotta

Each of these equals 2 meat choices.

1 small chicken leg or thigh

½ cup cottage cheese or tuna

Each of these equals 3 meat choices.

1 small pork chop

1 small hamburger

cooked meat, about the size of a deck of cards

½ of a whole chicken breast

1 medium fish fillet

Fat
Each of these equals one fat serving.
(5 g fat, 45 kcal)

1 t. margarine, oil, mayonnaise

2 t. diet margarine or diet mayonnaise

1 T. salad dressing

2 T. reduced-calorie salad dressing

The Exchange Lists are the basis of a meal-planning system designed by a committee of The American Diabetes Association and The American Dietetic Association. While designed primarily for people with diabetes and others who must follow special diets, the Exchange Lists are based on principles of good nutrition that apply to everyone.

Nutritional Standards

As you read about the food group guides, you may have wondered how the people who developed these guides for *food intake* knew what levels of *nutrient intake* were needed.

Recommended Dietary Allowances (RDAs)—document identifying daily nutrient intake recommendations established by the National Academy of Sciences of the United States

For over 50 years, a document called the **Recommended Dietary Allowances (RDAs)** has been the standard for nutrient intake in the United States. The RDAs have been the basis for the food guides you learned about earlier. You can also use RDAs directly to evaluate your diet, a process we will encourage you to do at the end of this chapter.

The Recommended Dietary Allowances (RDAs)

The *Recommended Dietary Allowances (RDAs)* is the title of the document that identifies the levels of nutrients, usually expressed in grams, milligrams, or micrograms, that satisfy or exceed the needs of practically all healthy people in the United States.

The RDAs were first established by a group of nutritional scientists in 1941. Approximately every five years since then, the National Academy of Sciences (NAS) has appointed a new committee to review recent research on nutrient needs. At the end of the evaluation, the committee prepares a report, which is then thoroughly reviewed by other scientists. Following the reviewers' input, the NAS issues a new set of RDAs. The most recent RDA was published in 1989. A table summarizing its main points is located on the inside back cover of this textbook.

The United States is not the only country to establish nutritional standards: many of the developed countries produce their own. For example, Canada's Department of National Health and Welfare prepares *Nutrition Recommendations*; its summary table from the 1990 edition is located in Appendix B. The World Health Organization of the United Nations has also developed nutritional standards for nations that do not have their own.

The RDAs reflect the fact that a person's actual level of need for any given nutrient can be influenced by sex, body size, growth, and reproductive status. Therefore, various subgroups, defined by sex, age, pregnancy, and lactation, receive their own distinct recommendations.

Of course, levels of need also vary among individuals within any given subgroup. *A recommended nutrient level established by the NAS is usually high enough to include the needs of practically all (98%) healthy people in that group.* In addition, the recommendations are generous enough to allow for some loss of the nutrient as it makes its way through the body. For example, the RDAs allow for losses that occur during the absorption or conversion from one chemical form to another, when some of the nutrient's activity may decrease.

In addition to the nutrients for which RDAs have been established, recent editions of the report have included a number of Estimated Safe and Adequate Daily Dietary Intakes (ESADDI) of selected vitamins and minerals. These are nutrients for which fewer data exist. The ESADDI values are expressed in ranges and are summarized in the table opposite the RDA table inside the back cover of this book.

There is, however, one set of values in the RDA that the NAS does *not* set high enough to meet the needs of almost all of the people in the specified category: kcalorie recommendations. Instead, to discourage overconsumption, the NAS has based its kcalorie recommendations on an *average* level of need for each age group. See Table 8.2.

The RDAs do not take into account the effects of illness or injury, which raise the body's need for nutrients. People who are recovering from infection, surgery, and wounds (including burns) or taking certain medications may need higher levels of nutrients. The RDAs apply to healthy people only.

Taking all the above factors into account, you can see that *almost every healthy person whose diet contains RDA levels of nutrients will actually be getting a greater quantity of nutrients than his or her body needs and can use.* For most healthy people, there would be no benefit to take in more.

In fact, *at much higher levels of intake,* there is risk of toxicity. Because taking excessive amounts of concentrated supplements is the most common cause of nutrient toxicity, the American Medical Association in 1989 advised that people not take supplements that exceed 150% of RDA levels (Council on Scientific Affairs, 1987). Then, in 1989, the National Research Council recommended that people avoid taking dietary supplements in excess of 100% of the RDA in any one day (National Research Council, 1989a). Although it is not dangerous to have *total* nutrient intakes (from your diet and supplements together) somewhat above the RDA, scientists know of no benefits to most healthy people of consuming more than the RDA. For this reason, most nutritional scientists discourage healthy people from using supplements.

You Tell Me

A vitamin supplement ad promotes a product that provides between 200% and 1000% of the RDA per unit dose (that is, per tablet or per capsule) for all vitamins present.

Is this product more likely to offer benefit or risk to a healthy person?

Using the RDA to Evaluate Your Diet

You have just made your way through some pretty intense material, which you will soon use to evaluate your diet. But first you need to consider an issue that can affect the accuracy of your diet analysis: how you collect your information about what you eat.

We could have discussed this issue before you used the Food Guide Pyramid to analyze your diet, but it is even more relevant here: an understanding of how you collected your information will allow you to make more precise comparisons between your intake and your RDA than the rougher approximations you got earlier using the Pyramid.

Three methods are described below. They are valid only if you accurately list everything you eat and drink. This can be a challenge, especially when it comes to including such details as the mayonnaise on a sandwich or the butter in which an egg is fried. It also may be difficult to estimate correctly the *amounts* you consumed.

Using a Twenty-Four-Hour Recall As the name implies, a 24-hour recall consists of remembering and recording everything you consumed during an entire day (usually the preceding day). You have to include all eating situations—whether they were meals, snacks, or just having something to drink. Many people get 10–20% of their daily intake at times other than during meals.

Do you think it would be easy to do a 24-hour recall? Many people find it difficult to remember every food and beverage (and how much of each) they consumed in a day. That can be a problem if you choose the food recall method.

However, if you do have an excellent memory for the items and quantities you consume, this method can provide a reasonable snapshot of *that day's intake*—but it may not effectively represent your average, overall intake. People's diets vary considerably from day to day. Think of your own experience: you probably don't eat the same way on weekends as on weekdays; or you may eat unusual items or amounts on a given day or change your eating habits from one season to another. Therefore, any technique that is limited to getting information about just one day's intake is of limited value for indicating your overall intake; however, such techniques are used for surveying a large group of people, where they may be carried out in combination with other methods.

Using a Food Record To avoid forgetting what you've eaten (a big problem with the food recall method), you can record your intake as the day goes on, carrying your record with you throughout the day so that you won't miss a thing. Food records are generally thought to provide the most accurate self-supplied information regarding diet. For this reason, we will encourage you to keep and analyze food records at many junctures throughout this book.

This method offers another advantage: you can keep food records over many days and average the results for a more accurate picture of your overall nutritional intake. Experts in diet analysis suggest various minimal time periods (e.g., 3 days or a week) for achieving reasonable accuracy. Longer recording periods and/or multiple recording periods generally provide a better (although not completely accurate) picture of typical nutrient intake.

Other potential problems regarding the food record's accuracy can also surface. Because you are writing down your intake, you may be tempted to change your eating habits during the recording period to *what you think you ought to eat* instead of *the way you usually do eat.* The more typically you eat when you are recording your intake, the more useful will be the information you get from your diet analysis.

Knowing how much food you eat is critical to determining what levels of nutrients you consume. Another possible pitfall of all of these methods is the difficulty of accurately estimating food quantities. The Slice of Life on page 59 and Figure 2.4 below suggest how to improve your skill in estimating amounts of foods and beverages.

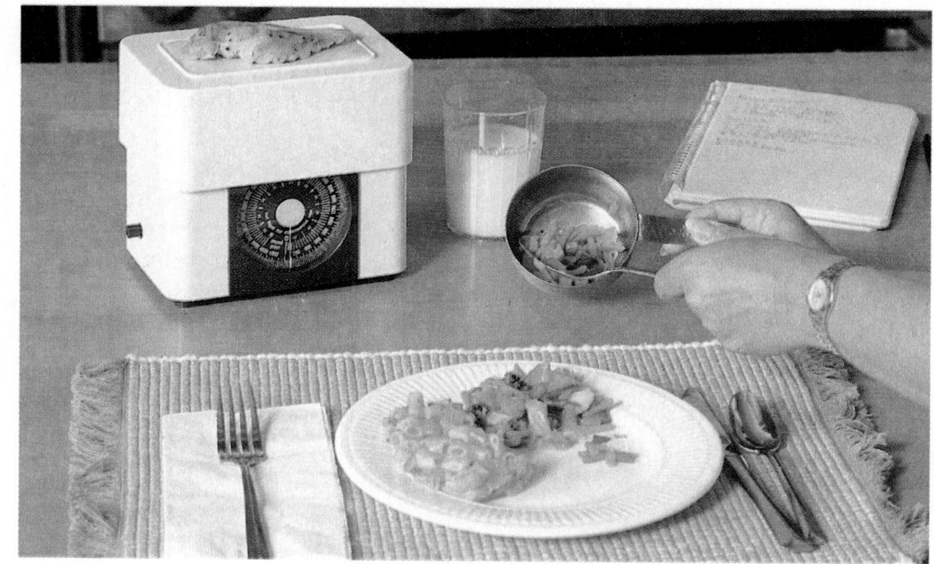

FIGURE 2.4
Estimating your intake: how good are you?

If your estimates are not accurate, your diet analysis won't be either. You can improve your ability to estimate by measuring the portions you usually eat and noticing what that amount looks like on the plate or in the bowl. Measure the capacity of the cups and glasses you usually use to help estimate beverage quantities.

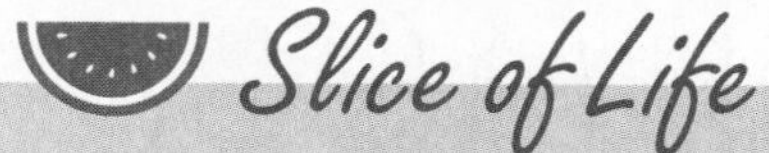

What Did You Eat? Guess Again!

It's not as easy to do a 24-hour recall or a food record as you might think. The point came home to Jane when she tried it herself.

Jane started jotting down what she had eaten the day before. *Let's see . . . I had a bagel with cream cheese just before I left for my 9:55 Econ class . . . a bowl of chili and a carton of yogurt when I met Ted at the cafeteria for lunch . . . didn't eat again until I got home after work. . . .*

As she looked over the list she made, she realized that she had forgotten to list the beverages she had drunk, both with her meals and in between. When she tried to recall them, she remembered that she had taken a vitamin pill with orange juice when she first got up; she added it to her list. *Oh, yes, somebody made popcorn at work . . . and I'd better write down the oil it's popped in, too.*

Estimating amounts was another challenge. *How much popcorn did I eat? Maybe five handfuls, but how much is a handful? And how much chili do you get at the cafeteria?* She couldn't exactly recall the size of the bowls.

Jane decided that she would do a food record the next day and try to improve her accuracy by actually measuring the things she ate at home.

She was on the right track with this idea. Training your eye by looking at a known quantity of food can improve subsequent estimates. At Ohio University at Athens, it was found that students who were given a 10-minute training session using food models made better estimates than untrained students made (Yuhas et al., 1989). In an earlier study at Penn State University, Helen Guthrie, PhD, RD (Registered Dietitian), also found that people tend to be poor judges of the amounts they consume. She offered a free breakfast or lunch to 147 young adults and asked them to write down what and how much they had taken from the buffet table. Among the most common errors were overestimating use of butter and forgetting to mention salad dressing, and four out of ten were more than 50% off in judging the amount of milk they poured on their cereal (Guthrie, 1985). In the Ohio University study, solids (meatloaf and fish) were better estimated than liquids (soup and milk), which were better estimated than amorphous items (spaghetti and applesauce).

Studies such as these show that to prepare yourself for estimating food quantities, it might be worth taking the time to measure your typical portion sizes to develop an eye for food quantities.

Food Frequency Questionnaires A more general method of estimating food intake is the **food frequency questionnaire.** It lists common foods or categories of foods and asks you to indicate how many times a day (or some other time period) you are likely to consume these foods. You can use this method for overall nutritional assessment or for estimating your intake of specific nutrients. In Chapter 6, you will have an opportunity to use food frequency data to assess your fat intake.

food frequency questionnaire—tool for ascertaining intakes of food or groups of foods in a specific time period; used for estimating intake of one or more nutrients

The results of food frequency questionnaires are likely to be less accurate than the results of food records (Krall and Dwyer, 1987). Generally, people overestimate their intake when using this technique (Bergman, et al., 1990). Nutritionists are therefore trying to fine-tune such questionnaires to help elicit more accurate information (Block, et al., 1992). Food frequency questionnaires are easy and inexpensive to administer—real advantages both for individual counseling and for some large studies (Connor, et al., 1992) and results can even be obtained by telephone (Fox, et al., 1992) and by mail (Zulkifli and Yu, 1992).

Assessing Levels of Nutrients in Your Diet

Your next step is to find out what levels of nutrients were in the foods you ate. Tables of food composition data provide you with this information.

Thousands of foods have been analyzed by government, university, and industry laboratories to discover what levels of nutrients they contain. This is a costly and slow process because of the substantial time, skill, and special equipment that are involved.

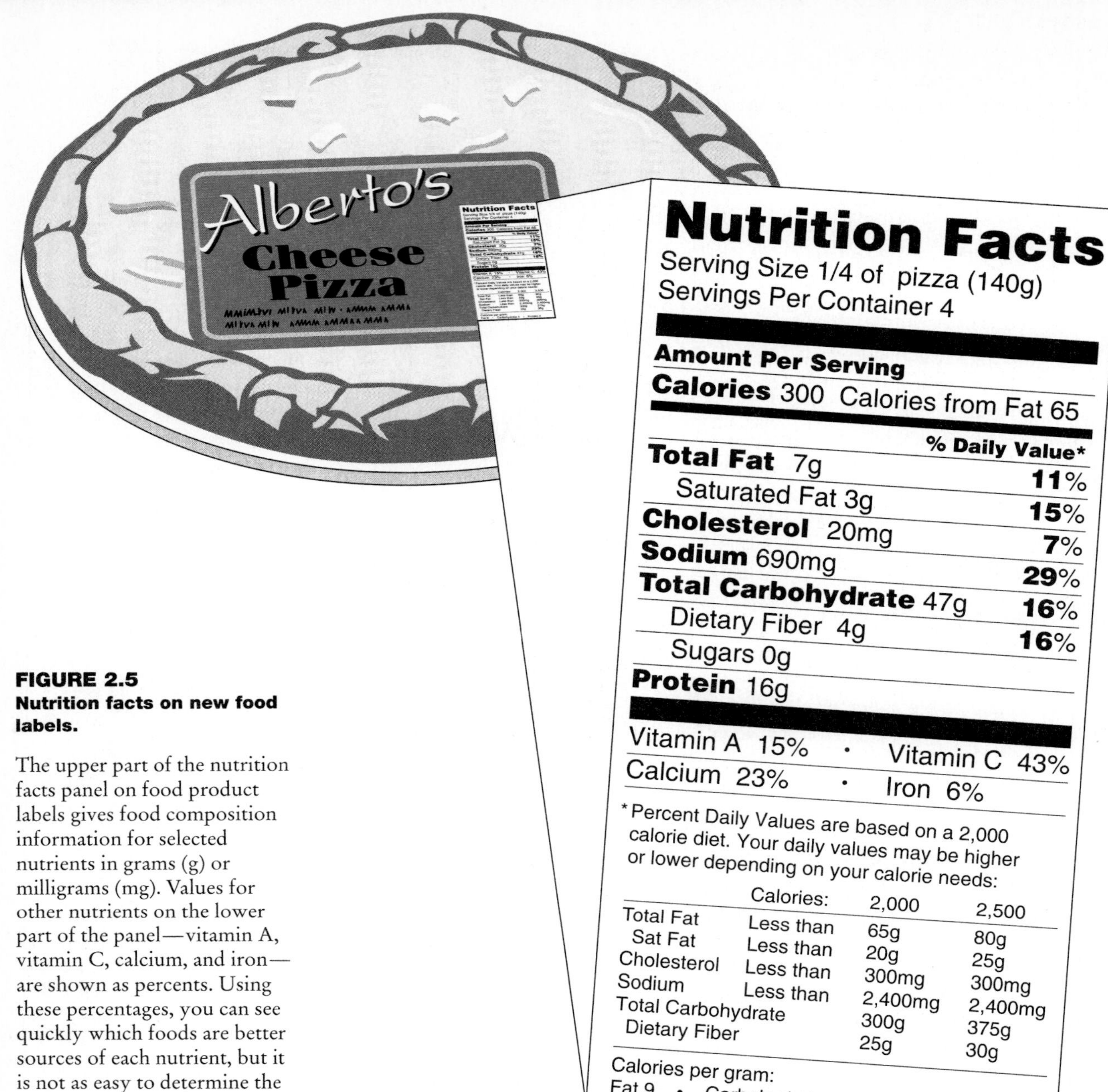

FIGURE 2.5
Nutrition facts on new food labels.

The upper part of the nutrition facts panel on food product labels gives food composition information for selected nutrients in grams (g) or milligrams (mg). Values for other nutrients on the lower part of the panel—vitamin A, vitamin C, calcium, and iron—are shown as percents. Using these percentages, you can see quickly which foods are better sources of each nutrient, but it is not as easy to determine the true amount of the nutrient (see text).

The USDA has been the leader in the United States in analyzing food and assembling and publishing information about food composition; USDA's *Agricultural Handbook 8* contains more than 4000 items. Other authors have also pulled together food composition data from USDA and other sources. In Appendix C, you will find over 2,000 items from one such compilation. Do not be surprised if after consulting several food composition tables you find that the values for a particular food do not agree exactly (Hollman and Katan, 1988); different laboratory methods by which data can be derived are likely to yield somewhat different results. Furthermore, different samples of food contain varying levels of nutrients.

You can also get food composition information from the *Nutrition Facts* panel on most commercially packaged food products. The top part of the label provides grams per serving of fats, carbohydrates, and protein, and milligrams per serving of cholesterol and sodium (Figure 2.5).

It is more difficult to determine the absolute values of the micronutrients given on the lower part of the label—that is, vitamin A, vitamin C, calcium, and iron. The amounts of these nutrients are expressed in percentages, which must be applied to a set of absolute values giving a recommended daily intake for each nutrient. The original set of reference values for labels, called the *United States Recommended Daily Allowances (U.S. RDAs),* was developed in 1968 and needs updating.

The reference values are scheduled for revision as early as 1994, but until they have been revised and implemented on all food product labels, the 1968 standards will be used. Meanwhile, if you want to estimate how much vitamin A, vitamin C, calcium, and iron are in a particular food, check a food composition table. For a very rough estimate you may apply the percentages to your own RDA.

Comparing Your Nutrient Intake with Your RDA Act on Fact 2.2 on page 63 takes you step-by-step through the process of determining your nutrient intake using food composition data. It also provides a sample chart showing how one person compared his intake of various nutrients with his RDA. You can use this method to find out how close your intake comes to your RDA on a given day—or, better yet, on several typical days.

As you may be thinking, this method lends itself very well to computerization. Nutrient data bases and diet analysis software are increasingly being used in research, health care settings, and nutrition education, saving much time that would otherwise have been spent in hand calculation.

We need to sound some notes of caution about computerized diet analysis. Many programs are available, and the quality of the data in different software varies considerably. In some computerized data banks, for example, foods for which some nutrient values have not been entered are included in the data set. When intake values are compiled for the day, nutrients for which some values were missing will be artificially low. This is particularly apt to occur in analyses of dietary fiber, copper, selenium, and vitamin B-6. In addition, various diet analysis programs may produce very different kinds of output. For example, some programs provide only totals of nutrients consumed, whereas others give itemized lists of the foods eaten and their nutrient contents.

If you are ever in the market for such software, be sure to identify the features you want first and to find out what features the various packages include.

Changing Your Eating Habits for Good

Now that you have analyzed your diet, how do you feel? Inspired? Overwhelmed? Perhaps you have analyzed your diet using one or both of the methods described in this chapter, decided that some changes are in order, and committed yourself to making them. Or maybe you're more skeptical about improving your diet—particularly if you're aware that people who have tried to suddenly overturn their long-standing eating habits have usually failed.

That's true, but it doesn't mean that deliberate dietary change is impossible. What it takes is having good reasons for changing, strong motivation, attainable goals, and procedures to help you gradually form new habits. Therefore, you can see that you need to do quite a bit of *thinking* about your diet before you start *doing* anything about it.

The first step is to *assess whether you really need to make any changes.* What have the Act on Fact exercises in this chapter told you about your eating habits? Does your diet generally meet the standards for good nutrition and health, or does it fall short (or is it excessive) in some way? Do you have nutrition-related disease risk factors that call for a change in your diet?

Second, are you *sufficiently motivated*? It takes energy to change habits, and a strong commitment can help. Experts recommend that people who are not highly motivated should not even try to make changes, because they won't be able to carry these changes through. Repeated failures can have negative mental and physical consequences (Kayman, 1989) and may even damage your health.

behavior modification—process used to bring about gradual, sustainable changes in behavior

If you are convinced that you need to change your diet and are motivated to do it, your next step is to consider a process known to be helpful in achieving dietary change: **behavior modification.** This method was developed by psychologists to help people change many different kinds of behaviors, including eating habits. Dietitians and nutritionists often teach clients to use such techniques (Holli, 1988), but you can implement them yourself.

As you read about the process, note the importance of setting reasonable goals. Another important principle for success is to think positively throughout the program. Also consider whether you might benefit from social support; some of us do, some don't. You can enlist support by telling your family and friends about what you are trying to do, asking them to praise you as they see you doing it, and urging them not to tempt you to deviate from your program. Some people make a written contract with a friend who will provide encouragement along the way. You have to know yourself in order to decide whether such measures would be helpful to you.

Even if you employ all the methods suggested below, don't expect perfection; there will be times when you'll slip back into your old behaviors. But don't despair or give up. When you experience an occasional lapse, renew your determination and "get back on the horse." Be proud of the successes you *have* achieved, and learn from your mistakes.

Techniques for Behavior Modification

A behavior modification program can help you make a success of dietary change. Below you will find techniques that can help you *make and maintain* the changes that you want in your eating habits. Design a program for yourself using these techniques, but do not regard this list as ironclad; while you are using your program, feel free to go back and make adjustments in various features as needed.

What follows is an outline and explanation of each step of behavior modification. You should follow these steps regardless of the habit(s) you are attempting to change. To show you how the process works, let's create a scenario. Suppose that, after analyzing your diet using the Pyramid, you decide that you need to eat more fruits and vegetables. The sections that follow include examples of what might happen during each step of your behavior modification program.

Record Your Current Food Intake Find out what you are eating by keeping a record of your intake and your thoughts about eating for several days. Make note of the time of day; the amount of each food and beverage you

Analyzing a Day's Intake Using Food Composition Data and Your RDA

1. Record the items and amounts you consumed throughout a day on a form similar to that used in the sample.
2. Find the nutrient content of each item on a food composition table such as Appendix C, and adjust the values to your serving sizes. For example, if you drank 1/2 cup of milk but the table gives values for 1 cup, you need to divide all values in half before you record them.
3. After entering all nutrient values, calculate the sum for each nutrient.
4. Enter the RDA (see inside back cover) for your sex, age, and reproductive status on the line below the sums. (Note: there are no RDAs for total fat, saturated fat, cholesterol, and carbohydrate.) Above the chart, indicate your characteristics.
5. Compare the sums to your RDAs: divide the sum for each nutrient by your RDA for the nutrient. Multiply your answer by 100 to get the percentage. If you took in less than your RDA for a nutrient, the percentage will be less than 100; if you took in more, the percentage will be more than 100.

To appreciate their significance, you have to think back to how the RDAs are derived. What do the percentages mean? Because most healthy people's nutrient needs are actually below the levels recommended by the RDAs, you might very well be able to meet your need for a particular nutrient with an intake of less than 100% of the RDA. Some experts in nutritional assessment judge a diet to be acceptable if it contains at least 70% of the RDA values for all nutrients, although other experts disagree. (Remember, we're talking only about healthy people here; people who are ill may have higher nutritional needs.)

Sample Act on Fact 2.2

Characteristics: Sex M Age 20 Pregnant? — Lactating? —

Food or Beverage	Approximate Measure	Food Energy kcal	Protein g	Total Fat g	Saturated Fat g	Cholesterol mg	Carbohydrate g
Egg bagel	1	163	6	1	—	8	31
Jelly	1 T.	50	0	0	0	0	13
Lemon lime soda	12 oz.	148	0	0	0	0	38
McDonald's Cheeseburgers	2	620	30	28	10	106	62
French fries	regular	220	3	12	5	9	26
Caramel ice cream sundae	1	323	8	10	5	26	53
Cola drink	12 oz.	151	0	0	0	0	38
Pork chop, lean, broiled	2 oz.	169	18	10	3	63	0
Baked potato with skin	1 medium	220	5	—	—	0	51
Frozen peas	1/2 c.	63	4	—	—	0	12
Butter	2 t.	72	—	8	6	22	—
Iceberg lettuce	2 c.	14	2	—	—	0	2
French Dressing	3 T.	201	—	18	6	6	9
2% milk	1 c.	125	9	5	3	18	12
Graham crackers	4 squares	112	4	4	—	0	20
Totals		2651	89	96	38	258	367
Your RDA			58				
% of Your RDA			153				

Calcium mg	Phosphorus mg	Sodium mg	Potassium mg	Iron mg	Zinc mg	Vitamin A RE	Thiamin mg	Riboflavin mg	Niacin mg	Vitamin B-6 mg	Vitamin B-12 µg	Folic Acid µg	Vitamin C mg
23	37	198	41	1.46	.29	24	.21	.16	1.94	.02	.05	13	0
4	1	3	14	.3	—	0	0	.01	0	—	—	—	1
7	0	41	4	.25	.18	0	0	0	.06	0	0	0	0
398	354	1500	446	4.6	4.18	236	.58	.42	7.72	.24	1.88	36	4
10	91	110	484	.52	.35	0	.14	0	1.84	.18	.08	22	8
201	231	208	338	.23	.88	56	.07	.31	1.01	.05	.64	13	4
11	44	15	4	.11	.04	0	0	0	0	0	0	0	0
5	184	50	276	.61	1.93	2	.64	.28	3.93	.30	.71	3	—
20	115	16	844	2.75	.65	—	.22	.07	3.32	.70	0	22	26
19	72	70	135	1.26	.75	54	.23	.08	1.19	.09	0	47	8
2	2	82	2	.02	—	16	0	—	—	0	.02	—	0
22	22	10	174	.56	.24	36	.06	.04	.20	.04	0	62	4
6	6	642	36	.3	.03	9	—	—	0	—	.06	3	0
313	245	128	397	.12	.98	150	.10	.42	.22	.11	.94	13	2
12	44	132	112	1.00	.20	0	.04	.16	1.00	.04	0	4	0
1053	1448	3205	3307	14.09	10.7	583	2.29	1.95	22.43	1.77	4.38	238	57
1200	1200	500–2400[a]	2000–3500[a]	10	15	1000	1.5	1.7	19	2.0	2.0	200	60
88	121	134	OK	141	71	58	153	115	118	89	219	119	95

[a]These values are not on the RDA summary table; they are given within the text of *Recommended Dietary Allowances*, 10th ed., (Washington, DC: National Academy Press, 1989).

Time	Food or Beverage	Amount Consumed	Location of Eating	Thoughts about eating before and during eating	Thoughts about eating after eating
8:30 a.m.	Wheat cereal	2 c.	Kitchen	I'm hungry &	
	2% milk	1 c.		late. This is	Satisfied
	Coffee	1 c.		fast.	
11:00 a.m.	Sweet roll	1 medium	outside	Bored & have	
			classroom	time to kill.	
12:30 p.m.	Beef macaroni	1 c.	Union		
	tomato casserole		cafeteria	Chose stuff I	At least
	Bread	2 slices		like. The veg.	there was
	Butter	3 pats		salads & fresh	tomato & onion
	Cola	12 oz.		fruit didn't	in the casserole.
	Chocolate pie	1 piece		appeal to me.	
6:15 p.m.	Fried fish	5 oz.	Kitchen		
	Tartar sauce	2 T.		Because I didn't	Good job -
	Hash browned potatoes	1 c.		do so well earlier,	2 vegetables
	Lettuce salad	1 c.		I made myself	here!
	2% milk	½ c.		fix the lettuce.	
	Frosted white cake	1 piece			
9:30 p.m.	Corn snacks	3 oz.	living room	I'm tired. I deserve	Fruit just
	Cherry pop	12 oz. can		something I like.	wouldn't have
					done it.

FIGURE 2.6
Diet record and log of thoughts.

If you want to make changes in your eating habits, it is useful to keep diet records of what you were thinking about before, during, and after you ate.

consumed; where you were at the time; and the thoughts you had before, during, and after eating (Figure 2.6). This not only documents your current eating pattern and establishes a baseline against which you can compare your behavior as you change it, but also gives you the chance to see whether your patterns are helping or hurting your efforts.

Example: For several days, you complete diet records. This day, you find that you ate several servings of fruits and vegetables. On other days, you ate none or just one serving.

Set Realistic Goals Decide exactly what you want your eating habits to be. You have a general idea already—after all, you had something in mind when you decided dietary changes were in order—but now you need to get more specific. Are you trying to eat *more* of a certain kind of food? If so, how many servings do you eventually want to eat per day? Are you trying to eat *less* of something? What's consistent with eating guidelines for good health? Do you think you can achieve those levels? We can't overemphasize the importance of setting reasonable goals; evidence shows that they can be the most useful feature of a lifestyle change program (Berry, et al., 1989).

Make sure you write your goals in terms of *behaviors* and not particular health *outcomes,* such as a drop in blood pressure or lower body weight. *It is important to deal with behaviors here because they are under your control, whereas the rate at which your body responds is not within your control.* Surely, at some point you will want to find out whether you are achieving positive results from your changed behaviors, but there is no point in paying much attention to that at first.

Example: You decide you eventually want to consume two servings of fruit and three servings of vegetables per day, as recommended by the Pyramid.

Evaluate Why You Practice Unwanted Behaviors Psychologists point out that most eating behaviors, like many other types of behavior, consist of a chain of events: a *cue* brings you to think about the behavior, you *do it,* and then there is a *consequence.* If you understand what cue causes an unwanted behavior again and again, you can think of a way to interrupt that chain of events and have more control over the behavior and its consequence.

Consequences are of two types: either a *reinforcement that encourages* or a *punishment that discourages* that behavior in the future. Generally, reinforcement has a stronger effect on future behavior than punishment. Reinforcers may either be *positive* (a good thing happens as a result of the behavior) or *negative* (a bad thing goes away as a result of the behavior).

Example: You realize that one reason you don't eat many fruits and vegetables is that you think it's a nuisance to fix them for yourself. Furthermore, on several previous occasions when you bought fresh vegetables and put them into your refrigerator drawer, you forgot about them, and they spoiled. Since you quit buying fresh produce, you have been glad not to have any more of those disgusting surprises and were thereby reinforced not to purchase fresh vegetables.

Plan for Gradual Change and Then Do It Decide which of your goals you would like to work toward first. If it represents a large departure from your current habits, plan to take it in stages. In other words, as you begin, plan to get only partway there. Once you become fairly comfortable with the new habit, set your sights a little higher.

Keep in mind what cues commonly trigger your unwanted behavior. Are there features of your environment that you can change to avoid or eliminate the cues? Change those features. Are there places or certain situations you should avoid? Stay away from them, at least until you form new habits. Are there situations you can set up for yourself to cue your intended behaviors? Create those situations for yourself.

Example: To begin with, you decide to eat at least one serving of fruit and one serving of vegetable per day. You decide to buy types of produce that keep better, to store them properly, and to keep them more visible in the refrigerator so that you will be reminded to use them. You realize that when you and your apartment-mate fix meals together, you don't mind fixing salads and cooked vegetables; you agree that you will make three dinners together each week.

Reward Yourself for Success Plan some rewards that will give you additional reinforcement. One reward to use regularly is *positive self-talk*; that is, congratulate yourself every time you do as you intended. This can be surprisingly empowering, because it calls attention to your increasing mastery of your behavior, which further increases your likelihood of success (Holli and Calabrese, 1991).

If you have asked people close to you for their support, they can add more reinforcement. Plan other rewards, such as buying something you have wanted or taking time to do something you enjoy. Rewarding yourself as promptly as possible provides the best reinforcement.

Example: Immediately tell yourself that you did the job right. Further reward yourself for meeting your dietary goals by calling a friend and arranging to go to a movie you have been eager to see.

Once You Have Begun Your Program, Think Positively Positive thinking supports new behaviors. Check your diet record and log of thoughts, and credit yourself for positive thoughts. When you have negative thoughts, practice "thought stopping" (Holli, 1988). Whenever you catch yourself with a pessimistic or self-defeating thought, simply say to yourself, "Stop," and deliberately replace that thought with a more positive idea. A great deal of negative thinking is predictive of impending relapse (Holli and Calabrese, 1991).

Example: At some points, you catch yourself thinking that, in the whole scheme of things, eating enough fruits and vegetables isn't all that important. STOP. Change your thoughts to something like this: "I know that there is nutritional benefit from doing this. I know that soon it will be a habit, and I won't even have to think about it."

Practice Relapse Prevention Some of the cues that trigger your unwanted behavior, such as stress and certain social situations, may be hard to avoid. Think about those situations before they occur, and rehearse how you will handle them successfully. This practice is called **relapse prevention.** Of course, this doesn't guarantee you will avoid all pitfalls, but it does help. Even if you have a *lapse* (a single slip) in your behavior, it doesn't need to result in total *collapse* (complete loss of control) of your program. Focus on your successes, and go on.

relapse prevention—planning how to cope successfully with situations that might cause you to fall back into old behaviors you now want to avoid

Example: To practice relapse prevention, think about the fact that you don't want to fix vegetables at the end of an especially stressful day. Think about how you could carry through on meeting your goal. If you can afford it, you might go out for dinner and include a salad and/or cooked vegetable in the meal. Alternatively, you might pick items that don't require much preparation (fruit that only needs to be washed, a can of vegetables that only need to be heated).

Monitor Your Progress and Fine-Tune Your Program Check up on yourself as you go along. Periodically keep another series of diet records, and compare them with your earlier records. Are you making progress? If so, keep up the program, or even step it up a bit. If it is not successful enough, analyze what is causing your lapses, and modify your program.

Example: Two weeks after you begin your behavior modification effort, you record your diet for a few days. You find that you're pretty consistently getting one fruit and two vegetables per day, but sometimes less. You decide to continue using the same technique, but you advance to a goal of two fruits and two vegetables per day.

As you can see, it takes considerable effort to dislodge an old habit and replace it, even if you are fully aware of the benefits of the new behavior. Using the techniques of behavior modification can ease the process and contribute to your chances of success.

As you reevaluate your diet in various ways throughout this course, you may find that you would like to make some changes. Using these ideas could make the difference between success and failure.

Summary

- Most of us alternate between overconsuming and underconsuming moderate amounts of the nutrients we need. This is normal and does not negatively affect your **nutritional status** or damage your health. However, long-term over- or underconsumption, which can be documented with various **nutritional assessment techniques,** can have many negative effects.

- There are several body-based means of measuring nutritional status. **Biochemical tests** involving the chemical analysis of blood or urine require special techniques and equipment but yield relatively specific information about levels of circulating nutrients and their **metabolites. Anthropometric tests** of height and weight or estimates of fatness using **skinfold calipers** are easier to do but provide less specific information about nutritional status. Changes in appearance or sense of well-being may be related to nutritional status, or they may have another cause entirely.

- For most healthy people, diet analysis is more useful and practical than body-based measurements for estimating nutritional status. Various **dietary recommendations** have been used in the United States since the early 1900s; two important current guides are the **Dietary Guidelines** and the **Food Guide Pyramid.** These emphasize foods of high **nutrient density** and discourage the intake of too much fat, cholesterol, sodium, sugar and alcohol, which are related to the development of many diseases that affect people in the United States and other developed countries.

- In the United States, the standard of nutritional adequacy is the *Recommended Dietary Allowances;* in Canada, *Nutrition Recommendations.* Both are periodically updated to take new scientific findings into account. You can analyze your diet by determining the nutrient content of the foods you eat in one day, summing these values, and then comparing the totals with your RDA.

- You can describe your diet by using a 24-hour recall, a diet record, or a **food frequency questionnaire.** None of these methods is entirely accurate, but the diet record is generally thought to come closest to your actual intake.

- **Behavior modification** can help people who want to make changes in the way they eat. Self-monitoring can help you determine whether your habits are what you think they are. If you decide to make changes, it is important to be realistic in your goals. Evaluate why you practice the unwanted behaviors, and plan carefully for gradual change. Think positively, and reward yourself regularly for success in behavior change. However, it is also wise to practice **relapse prevention** for the expectedly difficult times. Periodic monitoring will tell you how you are doing and give you insights about how to fine-tune your program.

References

American Diabetes Association, Inc. and the American Dietetic Association. 1986. *Exchange lists for meal planning.* Alexandria, VA: The American Diabetes Association. Chicago, IL: The American Dietetic Association.

Barrett, S. 1985. Commercial hair analysis: Science or scam? *Journal of the American Medical Association* 254:1041–1045.

Bergman, E.A., J.C. Boyungs, and M.L. Erickson. 1990. Comparison of a food frequency questionnaire and a 3-day diet record. *Journal of the American Dietetic Association* 90:1431–1434.

Berry, M.W., S.J. Danish, W.J. Rinke, and H. Smicilas-Wright. 1989. Work-site health promotion: The effects of a goal-setting program on nutrition-related behaviors. *Journal of the American Dietetic Association* 89:914–920, 923.

Block, G., F.E. Thompson, A.M. Hartman, R.A. Larkin, and K.E. Guire. 1992. Comparison of two dietary questionnaires validated against multiple dietary records collected during a 1-year period. *Journal of the American Dietetic Association* 92:686–693.

Connor, S.L., J.R. Gustafson, G. Sexton, N. Becker, S. Artaud-Wild, and W. Connor. 1992. The diet habit survey: A new method of dietary assessment that relates to plasma cholesterol changes. *Journal of the American Dietetic Association* 92:41–47.

Council on Scientific Affairs, American Medical Association. 1987. Vitamin preparations as dietary supplements and as therapeutic agents. *Journal of the American Medical Association* 257:1929–1936.

Fox, T.A., J. Heimendinger, and G. Block. 1992. Telephone surveys as a method for obtaining dietary information: A review. *Journal of the American Dietetic Association* 92:729–732.

Frisancho, A.R. 1988. Nutritional anthropometry. *Journal of the American Dietetic Association* 88:553–555.

Guthrie, H.A. 1985. Selection and quantification of typical food portions by young adults. *Journal of the American Dietetic Association* 84:1440–1444.

Heymsfield, S.B. and P.J. Williams. 1988. Nutritional assessment by clinical and biochemical methods. In *Modern Nutrition in Health and Disease,* ed. M.E. Shils and V.R. Young. Philadelphia: Lea & Febiger.

Holli, B.B. 1988. Using behavior modification in nutrition counseling. *Journal of the American Dietetic Association* 88:1530–1536.

Holli, B.B. and R.J. Calabrese. 1991. *Communication and education skills: The dietitian's guide.* Philadelphia: Lea & Febiger.

Hollman, P.C. and M.B. Katan. 1988. Bias and error in the determination of common macronutrients in foods: Interlaboratory trial. *Journal of the American Dietetic Association* 88:556–563.

Jarvis, W. 1989. Dubious health assessments. *Nutrition & the M.D.* 15(no.2):1–3.

Kayman, S. 1989. Applying theory from social psychology and cognitive behavioral psychology to dietary behavior change and assessment. *Journal of the American Dietetic Association* 89:191–202.

Klevay, L.M., B. R. Bistrian, C.R. Fleming, and C.G. Neumann. 1987. Hair analysis in clinical and experimental medicine. *American Journal of Clinical Nutrition* 46:233–236.

Krall, E.A. and J.T. Dwyer. 1987. Validity of a food frequency questionnaire and a food diary in a short-term recall situation. *Journal of the American Dietetic Association* 87:1374–1377.

McLaren, D.S. 1988. Clinical manifestations of nutritional disorders. In *Modern Nutrition in Health and Disease,* ed. M.E. Shils and V.R. Young, Philadelphia: Lea & Febiger.

National Research Council. 1989a. *Diet and health.* Washington, DC: National Academy Press.

National Research Council. 1989b. *Recommended dietary allowances,* 10th ed. Washington, DC: National Academy Press.

UNICEF. 1988. UNICEF annual report 1988. New York: UNICEF Headquarters.

U.S. Department of Agriculture, Consumer Nutrition Division. 1983. *The thrifty food plan, 1983.* Hyattsville, MD: Human Nutrition Information Service, U.S. Department of Agriculture.

U.S. Department of Agriculture and U.S. Department of Health and Human Services. 1980, 1985, 1990. *Nutrition and your health: Dietary guidelines for Americans.* Home and Garden Bulletin No. 232; U.S. Government Printing Office.

Weinsier, R.L. and C.E. Butterworth. 1981. *Handbook of clinical nutrition.* St. Louis: The C.V. Mosby Company.

Your fingernails: What do they reveal about your health? *Mayo Clinic Health Letter* October 1991.

Yuhas, J.A., J.E. Bolland, and T.W. Bolland. 1989. The impact of training, food type, gender, and container size on the estimation of food portion sizes. *Journal of the American Dietetic Association* 89:1473–1477.

Zeman, T. and D.M. Ney, 1988. *Applications of clinical nutrition.* Englewood Cliffs, NJ: Prentice-Hall.

Zulkifli, S.N. and S.M. Yu. 1992. The food frequency method for dietary assessment. *Journal of the American Dietetic Association* 92:681–685.

IN THIS CHAPTER

Digestion: Preparing Nutrients for Absorption

The Cell: Where Nutrients Are Used

Circulation: Delivering Nutrients Where They Are Needed

Excretion: Getting Rid of Waste

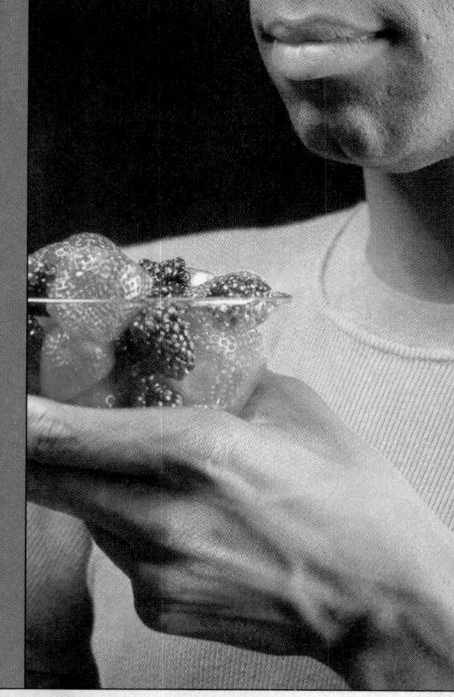

Chapter 3

Physiology for Nutrition

What happens to the food you swallow? And what happens to the nutrients it contains?

You might think that just *eating* food should guarantee that all of its nutrients will be used by your body. Before the nutrients can be used, though, your body must first break food apart and then move the nutrients through physical and chemical screening devices.

Because the healthy body is so efficient at doing this, we tend to take these functions for granted. An appreciation of the ingenious design and normally smooth operation of the systems that accomplish this is crucial to your understanding of nutrition. Such background will equip you in upcoming chapters to understand what nutrients can do for you and to understand certain abnormalities that can occur in the way your body handles nutrients.

We will discuss several processes involved in the food-using activity: digestion, which prepares food to move through the screening devices; absorption, which moves nutrients into your body's interior tissues; circulation, which carries nutrients and oxygen to the **cells** and waste products from them; metabolism, during which nutrients are used in a variety of chemical reactions; and excretion, which transports the waste products out of your body. We will also look at your body's cells, the ultimate users of nutrients.

cell—the fundamental structural and functional unit of living organisms

Along the way, you will become acquainted with the basic **anatomy** and **physiology** of several body systems: the digestive, circulatory, and excretory systems. In this way, you'll be prepared for later chapters, where we will take a more detailed look at how the body handles each of the six classes of nutrients.

anatomy—study of the structure of the body

physiology—study of the function of the body

Digestion: Preparing Nutrients for Absorption

Digestion is the process of breaking food down into substances that can be absorbed. **Absorption** is the uptake of these substances into the body's interior tissues. Both occur in the **alimentary canal,** or **gastrointestinal (GI) tract.** The GI tract absorbs the digested fragments through its lining into the blood as it breaks food down into the nutrients that will eventually be used at the cellular level.

digestion—the process of breaking food down into substances small enough to be absorbed

absorption—the process of taking digested substances into the body's interior

alimentary canal, gastrointestinal (GI) tract—the main part of the digestive system: a hollow tube beginning at the mouth and ending at the anus

General Characteristics of the Digestive System

Many digestive organs—your mouth, salivary glands, stomach, intestines and liver, to name a few—contribute to the work of disassembling the food you have eaten into its various subunits. There are many special features of this system that enable it to carry out its unique tasks.

Shape The main part of your digestive system consists of a hollow tube called the GI tract. The tube begins at your mouth and takes a turning and twisting route before it ends at your anus. Its entire length, if straightened out, would be several times your height. As you look at the structure of this tract (Figure 3.1), you can see that its various specialized sections have different diameters, from the considerable width of the stomach to the relatively narrow tubes of the esophagus and small intestine.

Lining The entire tract has a lining that can be thought of as an internal skin separating the contents of the tract from the body's *interior* tissues

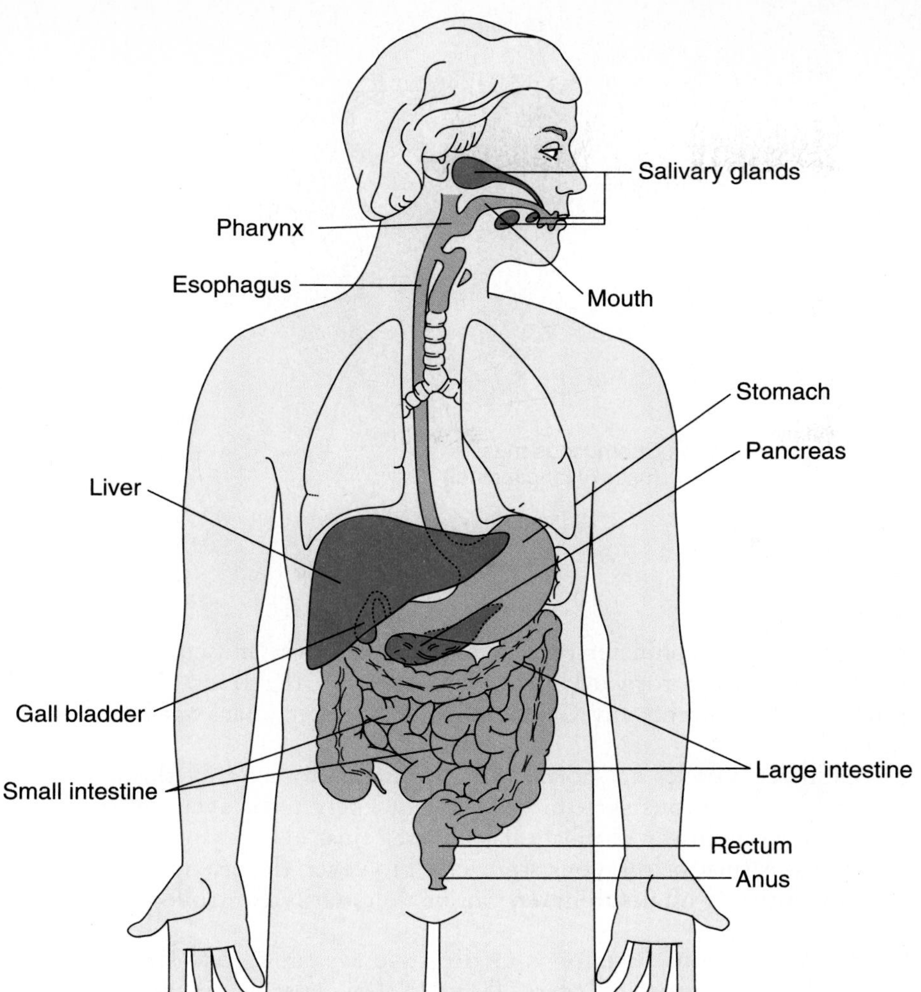

FIGURE 3.1
The anatomy of the digestive system.

Organs of the alimentary canal are shown in red. The organs in purple release their digestive secretions into the GI tract.

(Figure 3.2). Food that is moving through the central space within the tract, called the **lumen,** is still technically "outside" your body. The lining of the tract is called the **mucosa;** it selectively allows certain types of substances to be absorbed. An important criterion in this screening process is that the materials be particles small enough to pass through the lining.

lumen—the central space within which food passes through the GI tract

mucosa—the internal lining of the GI tract

Substances that are too large to be absorbed will simply pass through the entire length of the GI tract and exit the system. For example, if a toddler swallows a small plastic button, the button will be prevented from entering the child's body and will simply pass through and exit the system within a few days. Similarly food fiber, the plant constituents that the human body is unable to digest, will not pass through the mucosa but will travel through the tract and leave the body as solid waste.

Muscles The GI tract has many layers besides the mucosa; several of these are composed of muscles that control the progress of the contents through the tract. Longitudinal muscles run the length of the system, and others encircle it (Figure 3.2).

The enlarged special circular muscles that are found between different areas of the tract and at the end of it are called **sphincters.** When a sphincter is relaxed, that part of the tube is open, and the contents can pass

sphincters—circular muscles between different sections of the GI tract that help regulate the passage of materials

FIGURE 3.2
The layers in the GI tract.

Different regions of the GI tract have many similarities in structure, even though they vary considerably in the size of the lumen (central space through which food passes) and in some other characteristics. This cross-sectional drawing shows the features the regions have in common.

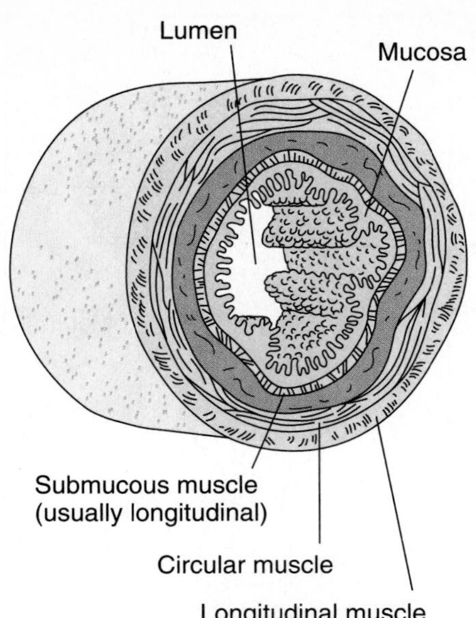

through. When a sphincter contracts (constricts), the muscular ring closes tightly, preventing forward movement through the tract. A contracted sphincter also prevents any GI contents from moving backward (up) in the tract.

Sphincter muscles are normally controlled automatically through stimulation by the nervous system. You are not likely to be aware of the functioning of your lower esophageal sphincter (just above your stomach) or your pylorus (just below your stomach). However, the last sphincter in the tract, the **anus** or **anal sphincter,** can be voluntarily controlled.

anus, anal sphincter—the last sphincter in the GI tract; can be voluntarily controlled

Secretions Various parts of your digestive system secrete large amounts of fluids—approximately 8 liters (about 2 gallons) per day in most people—that contain the following types of substances that assist in digestion:

mucus—slimy material produced by the mucosa

1. **Mucus** is a slimy material produced by certain cells in the mucosa; it lubricates the tract, keeping the lining moist and allowing food to move more readily through the system, as well as coating the lining to protect it from some of the tract's harsher secretions.
2. **Acids** and **alkalies** are chemical compounds that are needed for digestion; they are produced in various regions of the tract.
3. **Enzymes** are proteins that speed up the rate of biochemical reactions in the body. Enzymes are produced in various parts of the digestive system to help break down food. Names of enzymes can often be recognized by their "-ase" endings—for example, prote*ase,* an enzyme that acts on protein; lip*ase,* an enzyme that acts on lipid (fat); and amyl*ase,* an enzyme that acts on starch.
4. **Hormones** are chemical messengers produced in one region of the body and targeted to affect a process at some other body site. Hormones influence many aspects of digestion. Names of hormones often end in "-in" or "-ine"—for example, epinephr*ine,* gastr*in,* secret*in.*

enzymes—proteins that speed up biochemical reactions; usually have names ending in *-ase*

hormones—chemical messengers produced in one region of the body that affect a process in another region

transit time—the time that elapses between ingestion of food and elimination from the body of the solid waste from the food

Transit Time The amount of time it takes from ingestion of a food until its solid waste leaves the system is called the **transit time.** Transit time is often from 24 to 72 hours in a healthy individual, although remnants of a given meal may remain in the system for a week or more. In the United

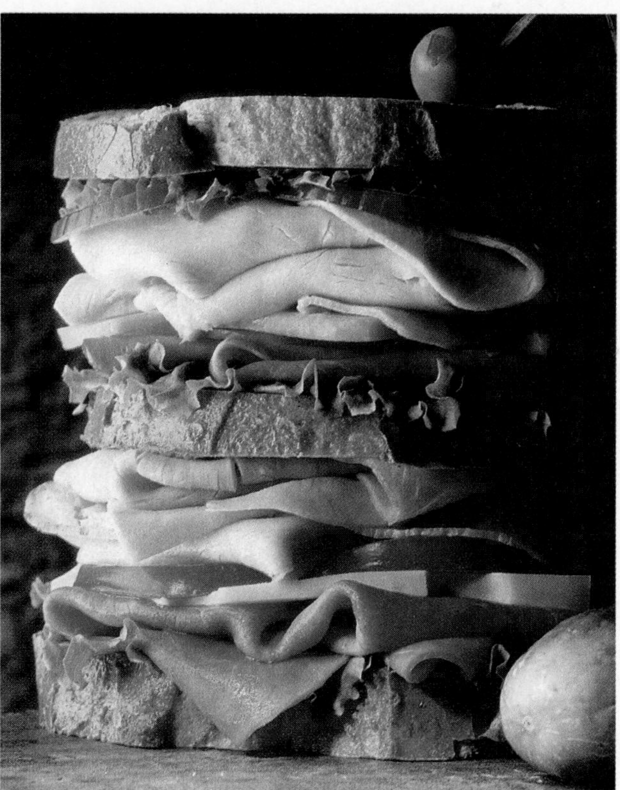

FIGURE 3.3
Does this photo start the cephalic phase of digestion for you?

Digestive processes can begin even without your putting food into your mouth.

States, **defecation** rates that range anywhere from three times a week to three times a day are considered normal.

defecation—elimination of waste from the GI tract

Factors that can influence the rate of transit in your body, either speeding it up or slowing it down, include the content of your diet, medications, emotions, physical activity, and various illnesses. If transit time is much faster than normal, diarrhea results; if it is much slower, constipation occurs.

Maintenance The innermost lining of your GI tract, which directly contacts food, renews itself every 2–3 days. This replacement is necessary because even though there are mechanisms to protect the mucosa from damage, the digestive secretions and the moving of food through the tract cause wear and tear.

Phases of Digestion and Absorption

Just as the different sections of the GI tract vary in structure, they also vary in function. Digestion and absorption represent a series of coordinated activities and responses that work together. Let's look at these steps.

Cephalic Phase: Sometimes the First Step in the Process *Cephalic* means "pertaining to the head"; just thinking about food can initiate digestive processes. If you see food, smell it, or even hear sounds associated with it, you might sense your digestive processes beginning, even though you have not eaten anything. Your stomach might growl, and your saliva and other digestive juices might flow more copiously in anticipation. In some instances, the responses of the GI tract can be as active as if you had actually eaten the food (Mattes and Mela, 1988).

These sensations may make you *want* to eat, but your body does not necessarily *need* food when you experience them (Figure 3.3).

FIGURE 3.4
"Hot" doesn't necessarily mean "irritating."

Peppers that feel like they are burning your mouth are not likely to damage your stomach.

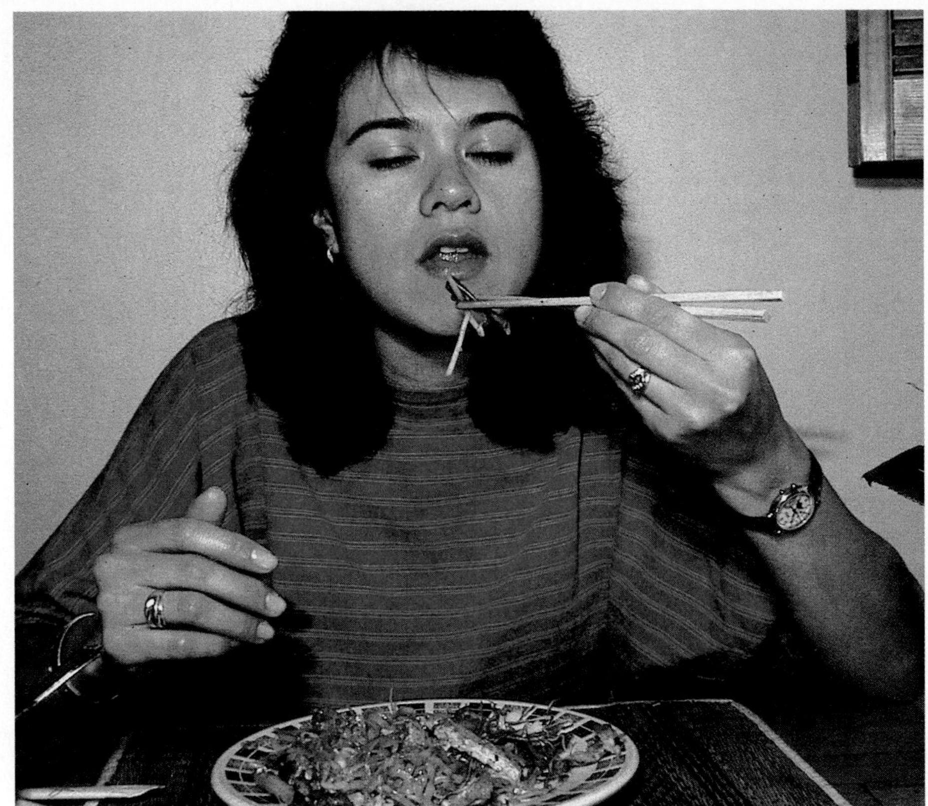

The Mouth: Point of Entry When food enters your mouth, digestive processes begin if they haven't already. With your teeth, you cut, grind, and mash food, making it easier to swallow and more accessible to the various digestive substances it will encounter along the way.

In addition, the presence of food stimulates the flow of saliva, the watery mucus produced in the mouth. Saliva not only lubricates the upper part of the GI tract, but also moistens dry foods and turns them into a cohesive wad. Furthermore, saliva contains the first of many enzymes involved in digestion: *amylase.* Amylase begins the breakdown of starch, a form of carbohydrate. Saliva plays an important role even after you have swallowed your food: it rinses the surface of your teeth, helping to prevent their decay. The amount of saliva you produce and swallow throughout the day probably totals 1 to 1½ liters (Marieb, 1991).

The tissues of your mouth can tolerate nearly all of the tastes, temperatures, and textures of the foods you eat and can help you appreciate them. Hot peppers, however, are known for their irritation of the mouth. They cause a burning sensation because they contain the chemical *capsaicin,* which binds to the tissues of the mouth. If you enjoy "hot" cuisine, you probably relish this sensation to some degree, but at times you may find that the burn gets out of control. One way to cool your mouth is to reach for a glass of milk: *casein,* the main protein in cow's milk, is thought to displace the capsaicin from its binding sites on mouth tissues (Henkin, 1991).

pharynx—section of the GI tract just beyond the mouth

The Pharynx: Origin of the Swallow The **pharynx,** located just beyond the mouth, is a common pathway for both the digestive and respiratory systems. It is part of the GI tract for food and part of the airway for breathing. When it is being used for food, openings to the other portions of the airway are normally closed by muscles controlled automatically by the nervous system.

Because it contains the muscles for swallowing, the pharynx's special function in digestion is to move food along to the next region of the tract, the esophagus.

The Esophagus: The Stomach Connection The **esophagus** is a conduit between the pharynx and the stomach. Once food arrives in the esophagus, it is moved along by rhythmic waves of muscular contraction that are automatically controlled by the nervous system. This involuntary digestive muscular activity is called **peristalsis;** it occurs in every region of the GI tract from the pharynx to the rectum. Usually gravity, too, plays a role in helping move foods down the esophagus, but peristalsis can accomplish the task by itself if you are not in an upright position.

esophagus—passageway that conducts food from the pharynx to the stomach

peristalsis—rhythmic waves of involuntary muscular contraction that move food in the proper direction through the GI tract

At the bottom of the esophagus is a sphincter that relaxes to allow food to pass into the stomach but then closes to prevent digestive juices and food from moving back into the esophagus. Sometimes this sphincter does not stay tightly closed while food is being mixed with digestive juices in the stomach, and part of the stomach contents wash back up into the lower part of the esophagus. Because the stomach juices contain chemicals that are irritating to the lining of the esophagus, repeated contact causes pain that is referred to as **"heartburn,"** although it has nothing to do with the heart. This sphincter is also open during vomiting.

"heartburn"—waves of warmth or burning sensation occurring behind the breastbone; generally caused by stomach acid in the lower part of the esophagus

The Stomach: Mixer and Reservoir Your stomach is a pouchlike enlargement in your GI tract. It has the elasticity to accommodate from 1 to 2 liters of food and fluid. Although one of its important functions is simply to hold what you have eaten until the lower portions of your tract are ready to receive and process its contents, it also has several unique roles.

Mixing Activity Peristaltic contractions in the stomach are very strong. The muscles squeeze and churn the contents, mixing digestive juices with the food particles. The slushy blend that results is called **chyme.**

chyme—slushy mixture of food and digestive juices produced in the stomach

Secretions The stomach produces digestive juices that contain strong hydrochloric acid and enzymes that begin the process of digesting protein. The presence of food in the stomach stimulates the production of these juices. Emotions can either increase or decrease these secretions: when people feel aggressive, resentful, angry, hostile, sad, afraid, or depressed, the rate at which these substances are produced may either speed up or slow down.

Because the tissues of the stomach are composed of protein, you might think that they would be vulnerable to digestion by their own gastric (stomach) juices. However, under normal circumstances the tough material and tight construction of the stomach lining prevent self-digestion. Furthermore, the mucus produced there sets up a protective barrier. In most cases, these features of the stomach also protect it against damage from acids in food (which are generally weaker than stomach acid anyway) and from spices in foods. A study done in Texas showed that two spicy Mexican-style meals consumed one day by 12 normally healthy people left no significant stomach irritation in 11 of them, as observed the next day (Graham et al., 1988).

However, these fail-safe mechanisms can break down if the stomach frequently produces excessive amounts of acid, and/or the stomach is unusually vulnerable to its acid (Guyton, 1992). Known irritants such as alcohol, caffeine, and tobacco can provoke or worsen the situation, as, it seems, can certain bacterial infections (Alper, 1993). Drugs can also be powerful irri-

FIGURE 3.5
Peptic ulcers can affect the lining of the esophagus, the stomach, or the small intestine.

The most common sites are indicated.

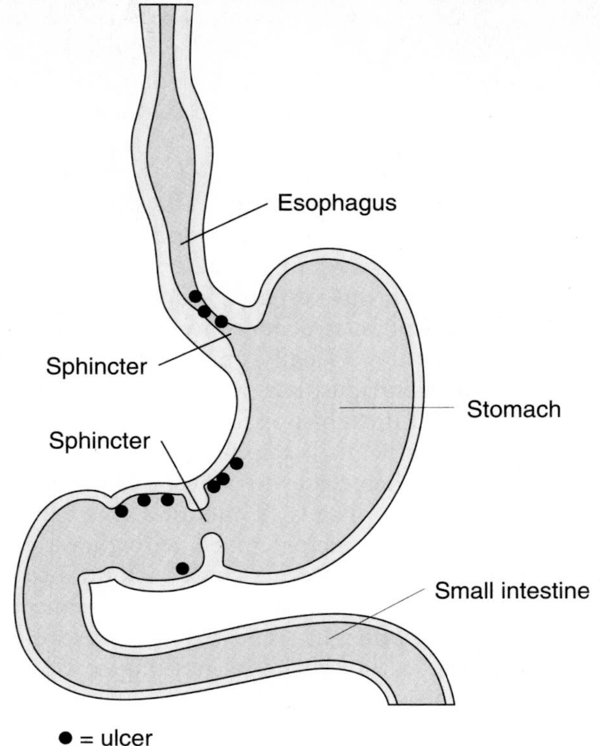

tants. In another part of the Texas study cited above, 11 of 12 people showed significant damage the next day from having taken a total of six aspirin tablets with bland (nonirritating) meals the previous day. If irritation eventually wears deep into the lining, a **peptic ulcer** results (Figure 3.5). (This term is often used for ulcerations that occur in the lower part of the esophagus or in the upper part of the small intestine as well as in the stomach; this is discussed further later in the chapter.)

peptic ulcer—open sore in the lining of the esophagus, stomach, or small intestine; irritated by acidic digestive juices and/or other substances

Absorption Little absorption takes place through the stomach. Two common substances can be absorbed without being digested first—water and alcohol—and they are absorbed from this site in only small amounts. (Some drugs can also be absorbed through the stomach.)

Emptying Chyme is emptied from the stomach over a period of several hours; it is released from the stomach into the small intestine at intervals when the sphincter between them is relaxed. The rate at which the stomach empties depends on a number of factors. Consistency of the material influences emptying: liquids leave the stomach more rapidly than solids do. The macronutrient composition also makes a difference: if you were to eat a meal consisting exclusively of carbohydrate, protein, or fat, the carbohydrate meal would empty the fastest, the protein meal more slowly, and the fat meal the most slowly. But because most consumables are *mixtures* of macronutrients, their emptying time depends on the relative nutrient content of each. Not surprisingly, the volume of what has been eaten is also a factor: a huge meal takes longer to empty entirely than a smaller one.

Stomach (or gastric) emptying is regulated more by the small intestine than by the stomach itself, although both are involved. When chyme contacts the intestinal mucosa, hormonal messages based on the composition of the chyme are sent back to the sphincter at the lower end of the stomach; this controls when and how much chyme will be released. The nervous system can also prompt the opening or closing of the sphincter, depending on how distended the small intestine is, and on various chemical factors.

Emotions may affect emptying as well, either slowing or hastening it. A physician who x-rayed the stomachs of college football players found that meals the players ate before the game took 2–4 hours longer to empty from their stomachs, presumably because of stress (Mirkin and Hoffman, 1978). •

The Small Intestine: Scene of the Major Action In a length of ten to twenty feet, your **small intestine** accomplishes the major work of digestion. It divides most of the carbohydrates, proteins, and fats into small units and then absorbs them. It also absorbs the substances that are small enough to pass through the lining without digestion: water, vitamins, minerals, and alcohol.

small intestine—longest section of the GI tract, performing the major work of digestion and absorption

Secretions In addition to the enzyme-containing digestive juices produced by the intestinal mucosa, secretions from two organs connected to the tract also enter the intestinal lumen. The **liver** is a large multifunction organ that filters blood and processes and stores various body substances. It produces **bile,** a solution that is stored in the **gallbladder** until it is needed. Bile is necessary for the digestion of fat. Because fat is not soluble in water, it would be likely to form a glob in the midst of the watery material; but bile acts to keep fat **emulsified** (divided into small droplets) after intestinal muscular activity mechanically breaks it apart. This makes the fat more accessible to enzymes for digestion and absorption.

The **pancreas** also has several functions, one of which is to produce secretions that contain alkali, which neutralizes the hydrochloric acid in the chyme. (If this process fails, or if the amount of stomach acid is excessive, a peptic ulcer can develop in the small intestine. The region in which ulceration is most often seen is the part immediately below the stomach called the *duodenum;* therefore an ulcer here is more specifically called a *duodenal ulcer.*) In addition, the pancreas produces various amylases, proteases, and lipases.

liver—organ that produces bile; performs many metabolic functions

bile—liquid produced in the liver and stored in the **gallbladder** until needed for fat digestion in the small intestine

emulsified—dispersed in small droplets through another substance with which the dispersed material ordinarily does not mix

pancreas—organ producing secretions that neutralize the acidity of the chyme and enzymes that help digest macronutrients

Mechanical Activity Two kinds of muscular activity take place in the small intestine to mix and move the contents. Peristalsis, as in other areas, is evident here. In addition, circular muscles constrict at intervals to produce a "sausage-link" effect. After the contents between the contracted muscles have been mixed for a time, the muscles relax, and then other muscles constrict to form a new series of "links"; these are called *segmentation contractions.*

Absorption The structure of the lining of the small intestine equips it perfectly for its additional critical role of absorbing the end-products of digestion. Millions of thin, flexible fingerlike projections extend from the lining, giving the effect of a terrycloth-lined tube. Called **villi** (singular: *villus*), these projections waft about in the intestine, ready to absorb digested macronutrient particles, water, vitamins, and minerals.

Projecting from the villi are even smaller strands called **microvilli,** which enlarge surface area further (Figure 3.6). It is estimated that this convoluted construction multiplies the intestinal surface area by 600 times what it would have been if the intestine were smooth. If the absorptive surface could be flattened out, it would measure approximately 200 square meters

villi—thin, fingerlike projections of the intestinal mucosa that extend into the lumen, greatly increasing the surface area for absorbing nutrients

microvilli—microscopic projections from the villi that increase the intestine's absorptive surface area even further

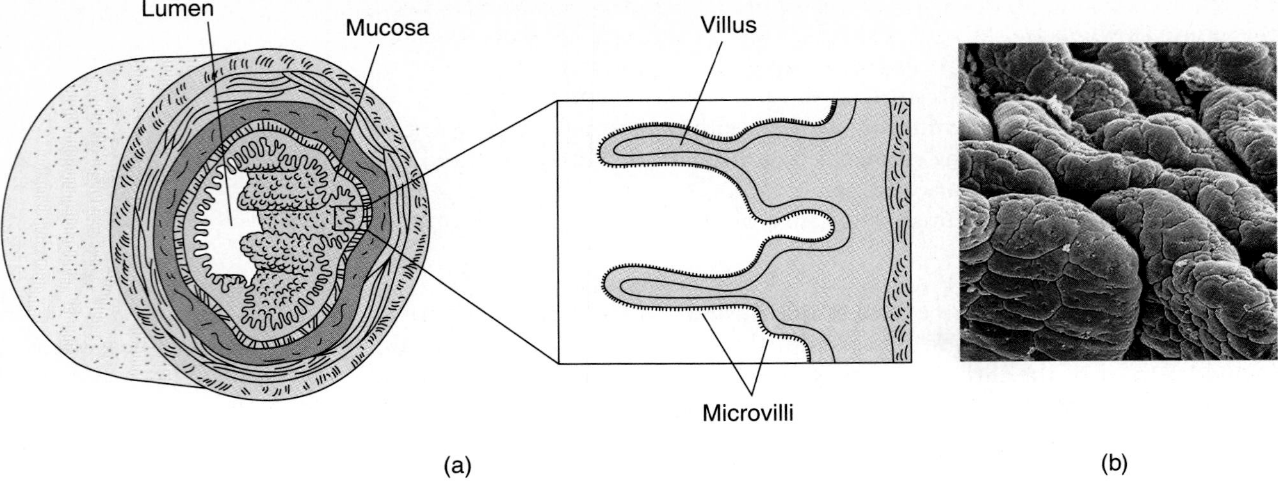

FIGURE 3.6
The villi of the small intestine.

(a) The left side of this illustration represents a cross section of the small intestine, showing how the villi project into the lumen. The right side is a magnification of two villi, showing their microvilli. These projections greatly enlarge the absorptive surface beyond what it would be if the lining were smooth. (b) This photograph taken through an electron microscope shows the microvilli on a single villus.

(Ganong, 1991), an area equivalent to the size of a tennis court. (The estimates of other physiologists vary.) After the nutrients have been absorbed, they are distributed to the body's cells via circulation, which is described later in this chapter.

The small intestine of a healthy person does a thorough job; it is here that 90% or more of the carbohydrate, fat, and protein that were consumed are digested and absorbed. The absorption of vitamins and minerals from the small intestine is less predictable, because the presence of other food constituents influences the absorption of these nutrients. Water is also absorbed here, as well as in the large intestine.

large intestine, colon, bowel—last major section of the GI tract, serving as a collection chamber for solid waste, a home for bacteria, and an absorption site for water and certain minerals

The Large Intestine: Absorber and Reservoir You may think that there is nothing left for the **large intestine** (**colon** or **bowel**) to do after the small intestine has played its major role. However, this section of your digestive tract performs several important functions.

Collection The large intestine serves as a collecting chamber for solid waste, which it holds until the feces are excreted. Of all the regions of the digestive system, food spends the longest time here, often 24 hours or more.

Holding and Harboring of Bacteria Because peristalsis and segmentation contractions move contents more slowly through the colon, bacteria have an opportunity to become established and to flourish. Their population is impressive: the number of bacteria in the GI tract is estimated to be more than ten times the number of cells in the human body (Savage, 1987).

Bacteria nourish themselves with portions of food that have not yet been digested and absorbed by your system. Some of the chemical products of bacterial metabolism are able to be absorbed from your colon: research suggests that up to 10% of the kcalories a person absorbs may come via this route (McNeil, 1984).

These bacteria also produce some vitamins during the course of their own metabolism that seem to be partially absorbed by the body. Small amounts of the B vitamins and vitamin K are thought to be obtained by this absorption.

As bacteria metabolize food, they produce gas as one of their waste products. If the amount is small, it causes no symptoms; however, if a great deal of gas accumulates, it is emitted through the anus.

Absorption The colon offers the body its last chance to absorb much of the remaining water and the nutrients sodium and chloride. If the colon fails to do this, diarrhea results. Normally, however, much of these materials is reclaimed before the solid waste is excreted.

Defecation The solid waste, called feces or fecal material, is excreted when the anal (rectal) sphincter at the end of the colon is relaxed; this process is called defecation or laxation. In babies, it is automatic and uncontrolled; as children mature, they learn to recognize the sense of fullness in their rectum and temporarily delay defecation.

What is considered a comfortable and convenient frequency of laxation varies from person to person. Even cultural patterns influence expectations; the "once a day" standard that many Americans think is best is not the only healthy pattern. But when an unusually long time passes between one defecation and the next, the feces may become hard and difficult to eliminate. This condition is called **constipation.** People sometimes use a **laxative** to relieve the situation.

One of the common causes of constipation is **irritable bowel syndrome,** also known as *spastic colon* or *nervous bowel;* this condition usually develops in late adolescence or early adulthood, and affects twice as many women as men. If you have irritable bowel syndrome, you might have bouts of constipation that alternate with episodes of cramping and **diarrhea** or with normal GI function. Physicians have not been able to identify a structural cause of irritable bowel syndrome, but because stress often precedes it, psychologic factors are thought to play a role (West, 1991). Other researchers have suggested that allergies might be involved (Mullin, 1991).

Because there are some causes of constipation that have very serious consequences, you should seek a physician's evaluation if you experience the condition frequently or persistently.

You have now taken a tour through the GI tract. Figure 3.7 summarizes the processes that occur there by reviewing the regions of the canal in which the mixing, moving, and absorbing activities occur. Table 3.1 on page 83 summarizes the digestive secretions that act on carbohydrate, fat, and protein and indicates the organs in which these actions take place. We next focus on the microscopic unit of your body that *needs* the nutrients: the cell.

constipation—infrequent or difficult evacuation of feces

laxative—a medication that promotes defecation

irritable bowel syndrome—periodic bouts of constipation and/or diarrhea, with no obvious physiologic explanation

diarrhea—condition characterized by watery fecal material and usually more-frequent-than-normal defecation

The Cell: Where Nutrients Are Used

Although it may look smooth, your skin is actually made up of millions of individual cells that work together to create a protective barrier. Other body materials—bones, muscles, fat—are composed of a multitude of tiny cells that work together to accomplish a particular function. It is within the cell that the most basic life processes take place, including the release of chemical energy from nutrients.

All living animals—from spiders to humans—have certain structural and functional similarities in their cells. Figure 3.8 on page 83 illustrates these similarities.

FIGURE 3.7
Schematic summary of gastrointestinal tract activities.

Most products of digestion are absorbed through the villi of the small intestine into the blood vessels; however, many fat fragments are absorbed into the lympahtic vessels. Some water and other nutrients are absorbed from the large intestine.

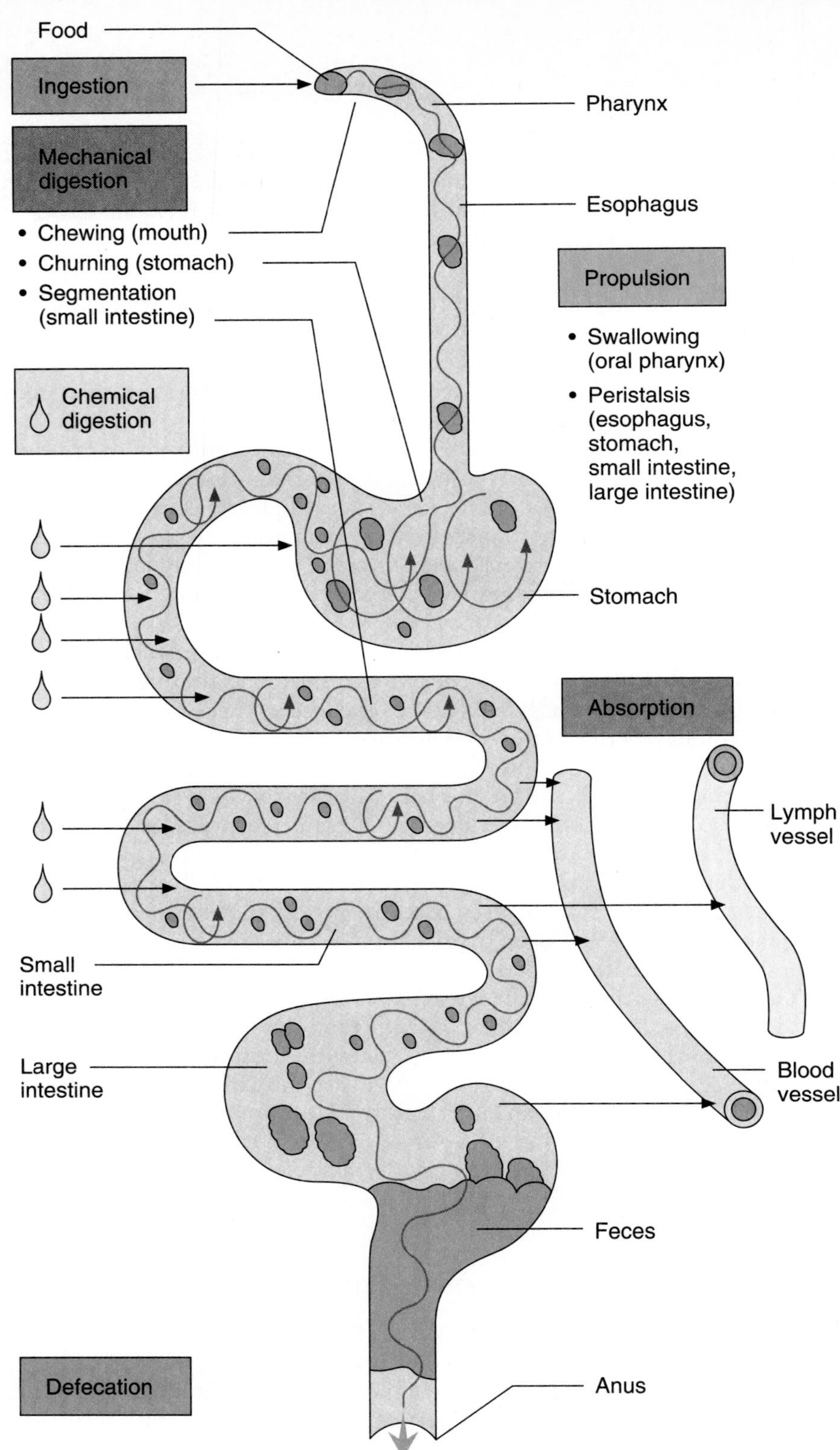

TABLE 3.1 Summary of Major Secreted Agents That Help Break the Macronutrients Apart in the GI Tract

Location	Agents Acting on Carbohydrate	Agents Acting on Fat	Agents Acting on Protein
Mouth	Amylase in saliva		
Stomach			Hydrochloric acid Protease
Small intestine	Amylase from pancreas Enzymes from mucosa that complete carbohydrate digestion	Bile produced by liver Lipase from pancreas	Proteases from pancreas Enzymes from mucosa that complete protein digestion
Large intestine	(Here bacteria carry out their own chemical processes on remaining nutrients.)		

- A thin, selectively permeable **cell membrane** that encloses and protects the contents by controlling what substances come into and go out of the cell.
- **Cytosol,** the fluid that fills the cell and in which all the cell bodies are suspended. The cytosol and its suspended bodies together are called the *cytoplasm.*
- A **nucleus,** which contains genetic information that enables new cells of the same type to form by division from the original.
- **Mitochondria,** small bodies within the cell in which most energy production takes place.
- An **endoplasmic reticulum,** a network of membranous channels involved in synthesis of protein and fatty materials.
- Various other types of small bodies that make or store protein or fat, or destroy materials for which there is no further need.

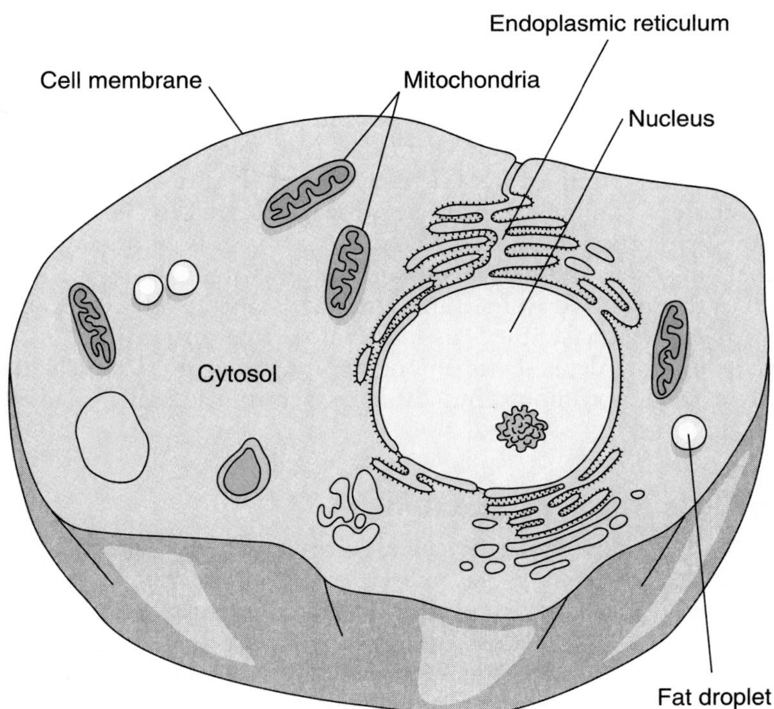

FIGURE 3.8
The cell.

Animal cells have certain structural similarities, which are pictured.

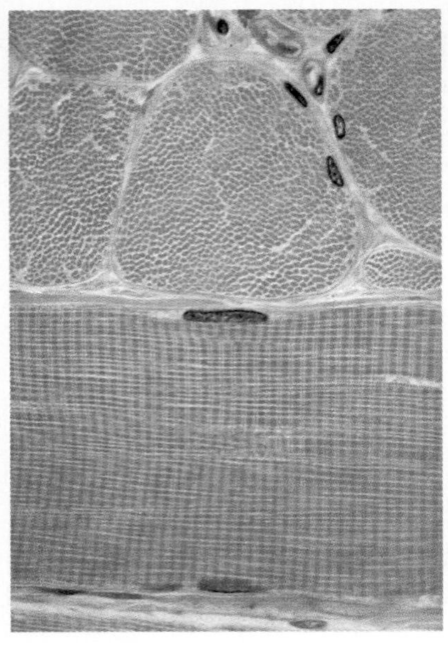

(a)

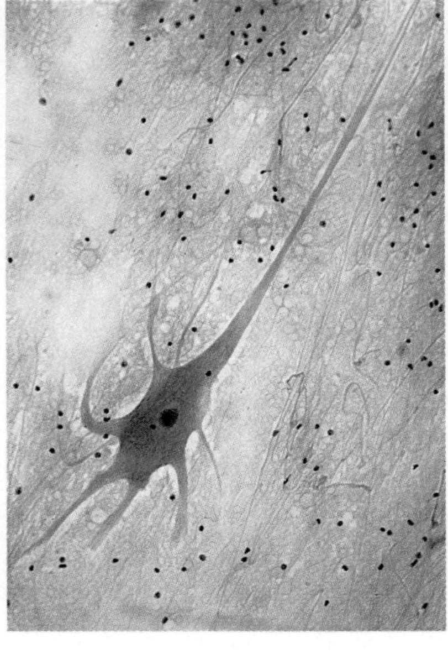

(b)

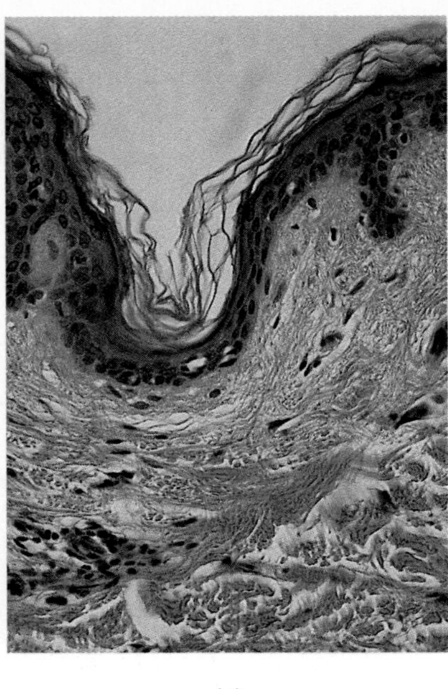

(c)

FIGURE 3.9
Specific types of cells look different from each other but have similar structural features.

These photographs show (a) skeletal muscle cells; (b) nerve cells; (c) epithelial cells.

Although a cell is microscopic, its importance cannot be overestimated. Some single cells are able to function independently; bacteria and yeasts are examples. When cells are grouped together in a more complex life form, they are seldom so tightly packed that their membranes touch each other. Rather, there are spaces between the cells called *interstitial spaces,* which are filled with **interstitial fluid.** You have seen interstitial fluid when it has oozed from a minor abrasion or a scrape in your skin that was not deep enough to cause bleeding. This same fluid has a role to play in nutrition that will be described soon.

Building a Body from Cells

When many cells of the same type are grouped together within an organism to perform a similar function, they are collectively referred to as a **tissue.** Your body includes *muscular, nervous, connective* (for binding together and supporting body structures), and *epithelial* (for coverings and linings, such as the skin or the lining of the GI tract) tissues (Figure 3.9).

Several tissues can combine to form **organs,** which are capable of more complex physiologic processes; the stomach, for example, is an organ made up of epithelial, muscular, and nervous tissues. Several organs combine into **systems,** such as the digestive system, and function cooperatively to accomplish a major physiologic task. Systems unite into a total **organism.**

This variety and interdependence among the functions of cells make the body not only extremely complex, but also very versatile and able to adapt to different conditions.

interstitial fluid—fluid that fills the spaces between cells

tissue—similar cells united to perform a particular function

organ—a specialized body part composed of various types of tissues that work together to perform a particular function or functions

system—a set of interdependent organs that together perform a function that none could do alone

organism—any individual living thing, whether plant, microbe, or animal; the most complex forms consist of a set of interdependent systems that together sustain life

Sustaining Cells Through Metabolism

As mentioned early in this book, the chemical processes that take place in the living cell are referred to by the umbrella term *metabolism.* A regular supply of nutrients is needed to support your body's ongoing metabolism.

Metabolic reactions occur all the time in every living cell. Synthesis reactions build up new substances that will become part of the body's structure or will be used to help it function. These metabolic processes are collectively referred to as **anabolism.** Simultaneously, breakdown reactions dismantle other materials into smaller units, a process called **catabolism.**

Although both are occurring in all cells at the same time, anabolism and catabolism may take place at different rates at different times or in different cells. During periods of growth—such as childhood, pregnancy, muscle building, and healing—more synthesis than breakdown occurs. At other times, such as during illness or injury, breakdown predominates.

anabolism—the combining of simpler substances into more complex substances by a living system

catabolism—the breakdown of complex substances into simpler substances by a living system

Circulation: Delivering Nutrients Where They Are Needed

Every cell of your body continuously needs nutrients. How do the nutrients reach the cells? This task is accomplished by the **circulatory system,** which has two parts. The part more familiar to most people is the cardiovascular system, which contains blood as its transport medium. The less familiar part is the lymphatic system, which carries substances in a fluid known as lymph.

circulatory system—cumulatively, the structures that move materials to and from body cells; includes both the cardiovascular and lymphatic systems

General Characteristics of the Cardiovascular System

The **cardiovascular system** is a closed, continuous network of elastic blood vessels in which the body's 4–6 liters of blood cycle repeatedly. The heart provides the power that keeps this vital fluid pulsing throughout the body nonstop from before birth until death.

cardiovascular system—the closed, continuous network of vessels in which blood cycles repeatedly throughout the body

The Heart The heart is a cone-shaped organ about the size of your fist, located in the middle to upper part of your chest behind your lungs. It is composed of strong muscles forming two pumps that cooperate to keep blood moving through your body. The muscles of the heart normally contract and relax 50–90 times per minute when the body is at rest.

The vessels that enter and leave the heart are few in number but large in size. The body's entire blood supply is channeled through them.

Two Loops There are two loops through which the blood in your body is routed: one that circles between the heart and the lungs (the *pulmonary circuit*), and one that connects the heart to all the other parts of the body (the *systemic circuit*). Each circuit is powered by a different side of the heart, as shown in Figure 3.10.

Here's what happens in the pulmonary circuit:

1. Blood is pumped from the right side of the heart to the lungs through a network of branching blood vessels.
2. In the lungs, where the vessels are especially small and permeable, the blood releases carbon dioxide (a waste product of cellular activity) to be exhaled and takes in oxygen from the newly inhaled air.
3. The blood returns to the left side of the heart.

The following takes place in the systemic circuit:

1. Blood is pumped from the left side of the heart to all areas of the body through a network of branching blood vessels.
2. Where the vessels are very small and permeable, oxygen and nutrients move out through the vessel walls, and carbon dioxide and other cellular metabolic products pass into the blood.
3. The blood returns to the right side of the heart.

This sequence is repeated continuously throughout your life.

FIGURE 3.10
Schematic diagram of circulation.

This drawing represents the route blood takes through the two circuits that begin and end at the heart. (Note that in anatomic drawings, the right and left sides are pictured as though you were looking at the body from the front.) Red indicates blood that is richer in oxygen; blue is for blood carrying more carbon dioxide.

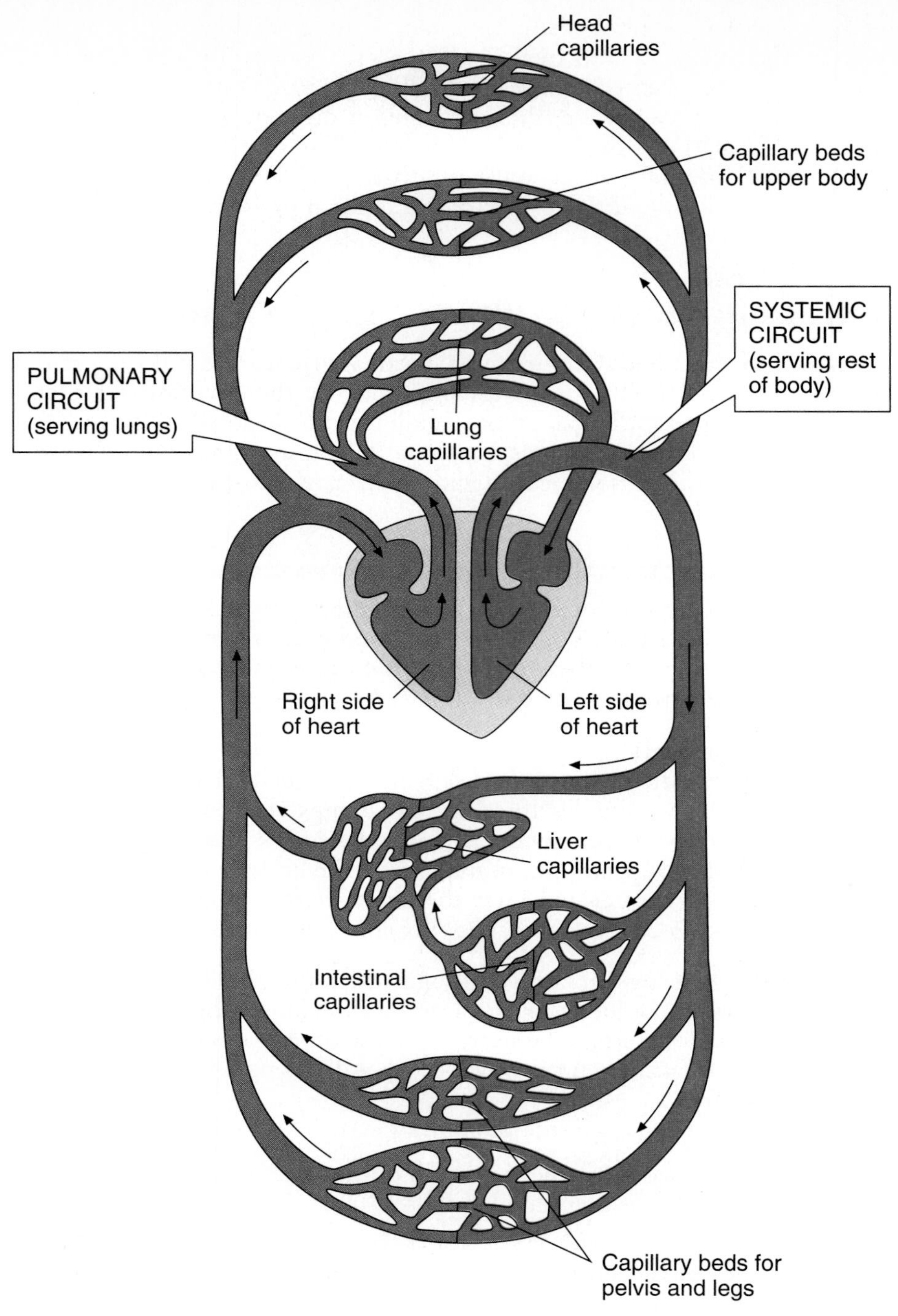

Names of Vessels Although the blood vessels form a continuous system, they are called by different names, depending on where they are in the circuit. The large vessels that carry blood away from the heart are called **arteries.** They divide into many branches in order to distribute blood to different areas of the body.

arteries—vessels that carry blood away from the heart

After each branching, they are more numerous and smaller in diameter. Small arteries are called *arterioles,* and the very smallest versions, through which the exchange of nutrients from the blood supply and wastes from body cells finally occurs, are called **capillaries.** The network of tiny blood vessels that serves a given region of the body is its *capillary bed.*

capillaries—smallest blood vessels, through which exchange of nutrients from the blood supply and wastes from body cells occurs

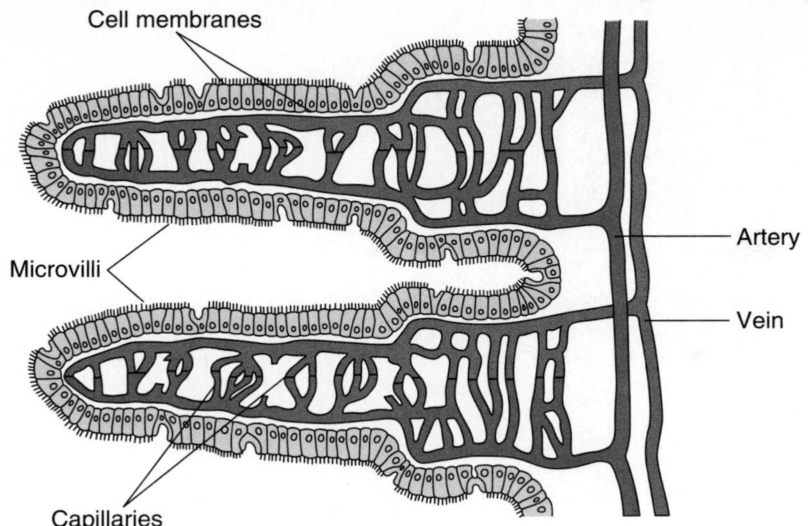

FIGURE 3.11
The villi and their blood vessels.

Each villus is laced with a network of capillaries that take in nutrients absorbed during digestion.

You can imagine how numerous the blood vessels need to be to have a capillary close to every body cell—every cell of skin, bone, nerve, muscle, and so on. You have approximately 60,000 miles of blood vessels within you to accomplish this!

To complete the circuit, blood returns toward the heart through *venules.* These merge to form **veins,** large vessels that funnel blood back into the heart.

veins—vessels that carry blood to the heart

Although the description of these routes may seem involved, your cardiovascular system repeatedly and reliably does the job for you. Next, let's consider how nutrients make their entry into this system.

The Route Taken by Nutrients Entering the Bloodstream

Recall that nutrients are absorbed into the villi in the small intestine. There are capillaries in each villus (Figure 3.11), which are ready to take up nutrients that are absorbed.

Capillaries take in mostly water-soluble nutrients. Many of the digested nutrients that are absorbed into the cardiovascular system need more modification before they can be used by the body's cells. For this reason, the venous blood leaving the small intestine goes to the liver, where such changes can be made.

The liver is the body's major metabolic clearinghouse. In the liver, many nutrients are made more suitable for circulation, energy production, or storage. Some nutrients remain in the liver; others resume their journey via the veins back to the heart.

As these veins merge with those returning from other body areas, the blood they are carrying mixes, and the nutrients are distributed through it. The dissolved nutrients keep recycling in the blood as described here and as shown in Figure 3.10: from the heart to the lungs, then back to the left side of the heart, which pumps them to all regions of the body.

Getting the Nutrients into Cells

When nutrients are distributed via the circulation to all of your capillary beds, they are able to move through the thin selectively permeable capillary

FIGURE 3.12
The route taken by nutrients from the capillaries to the cells.

Nutrients are carried by the circulation to all regions of the body. They pass through the selectively permeable capillary walls into the interstitial fluid, and from there into the cells.

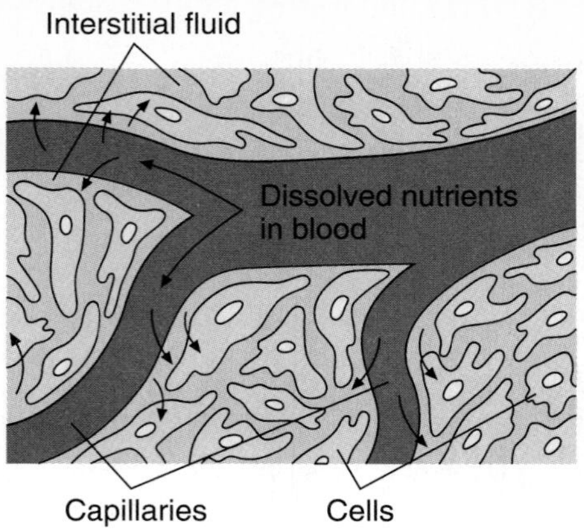

membranes into the interstitial fluid (Figure 3.12). From the interstitial fluid, the nutrients are absorbed through the individual selectively permeable cell membranes into the interior of the cells.

While they are taking in nutrients, the cells are simultaneously releasing wastes and other products of their metabolism into the interstitial fluid. Many of these products are then absorbed back into the capillaries and thereby into the general circulation. In a later section, we will describe how the body gets rid of wastes.

Distributing Blood to Various Body Regions

The volume of blood that is channeled to each of the body's various regions is determined largely by the amount of blood that is *needed* there at any given time. When there is increased demand in particular tissues, the muscles in the walls of arterioles in that region relax to allow more blood to flow to those tissues.

When your body is at rest, your heart typically directs to your abdomen about half of the total amount of blood it pumps; approximately one-sixth goes to skeletal muscle (muscle that is attached to bone); and the rest is shared by your heart, brain, skin, and other organs (Ganong, 1991). This distribution is adequate to meet resting needs. However, when a person is engaged in strenuous physical activity, as much as seven-eighths of the blood supply may be directed to the active skeletal muscles, which are in immediate need of oxygen and nutrients for energy production.

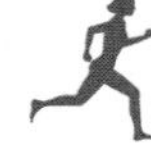

If you have recently eaten a large meal, a greater-than-normal portion of your blood supply will be committed to your intestines in order to pick up the nutrients that are absorbed. If you eat a large meal shortly before strenuous exercise, your skeletal muscles and GI tract will both need a greater blood supply at the same time. These increased demands cannot both be met fully and simultaneously. It is possible, therefore, that physical performance and digestion may be temporarily impaired. (Eating just a *small* amount is not likely to interfere with physical performance, though.) For this reason it is not a good idea to eat a large meal within 3 hours of intense physical activity. ●

lymphatic system—one-way system of vessels; one function is to absorb and transport certain nutrients; eventually empties into the cardiovascular system

lymph—fluid, derived from interstitial fluid, found in lymphatic vessels

A Sidekick for the Cardiovascular System: The Lymphatic System

The **lymphatic system** is a second system of vessels that provide circulating fluids to the body. It carries **lymph,** the clear fluid filtered from inter-

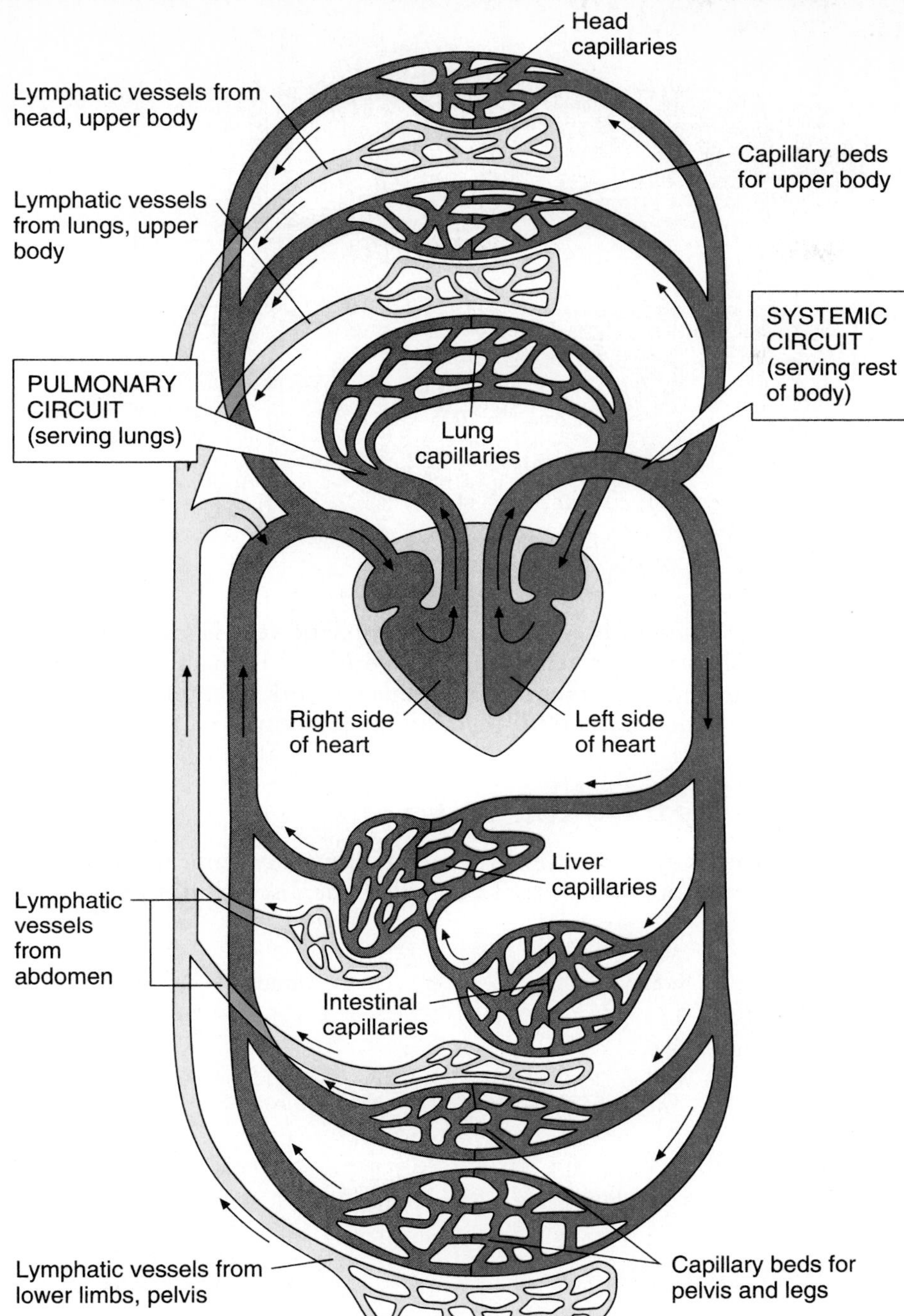

FIGURE 3.13
Schematic drawing of the lymphatic system.

This system carries lymph (which has been filtered from interstitial fluid) and nutrients (which have been picked up in the small intestine). Both enter the bloodstream where the lymphatic system connects with major veins near the heart.

stitial fluid, which flows into tiny lymphatic vessels. These vessels constitute a one-way network that eventually funnels lymph from all over the body into two large lymphatic vessels that empty into major veins returning to the heart (Figure 3.13). This system drains surplus fluid away from the tissues, which would otherwise become swollen.

It is the lymphatic vessels that serve the small intestine that have an important role in nutrition. Besides collecting lymph, they also absorb and transport some of the nutrients that the blood capillaries in the villi do not

FIGURE 3.14
Lacteals.

Each villus in the small intestine, besides housing capillaries, contains a lacteal. The lymphatic system absorbs the fatty products of digestion.

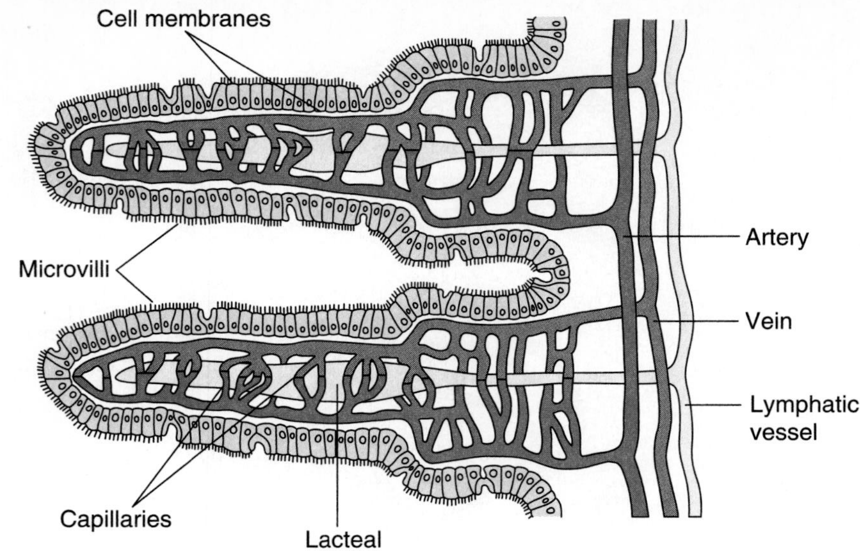

lacteals—small lymphatic vessels in the villi

carry. Figure 3.14 shows how these small lymphatic vessels, called **lacteals,** fit into the total absorption scheme. The lacteals take in mainly fatty products of digestion and carry them through this network, merging with larger and larger lymphatic vessels until they join major veins.

Excretion: Getting Rid of Waste

You have learned a great deal in this chapter about how your body digests, absorbs, and transports nutrients. To complete the discussion, let's consider

FIGURE 3.15
The urinary system and some neighboring structures.

The two kidneys are the body's chief organs for cleansing its internal fluids of soluble waste and excreting surplus water and nutrients. Ureters carry the urine to the bladder for storage until it is excreted through the urethra.

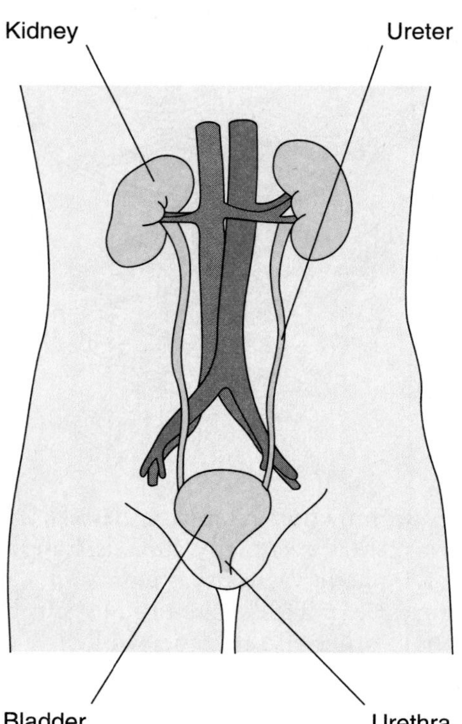

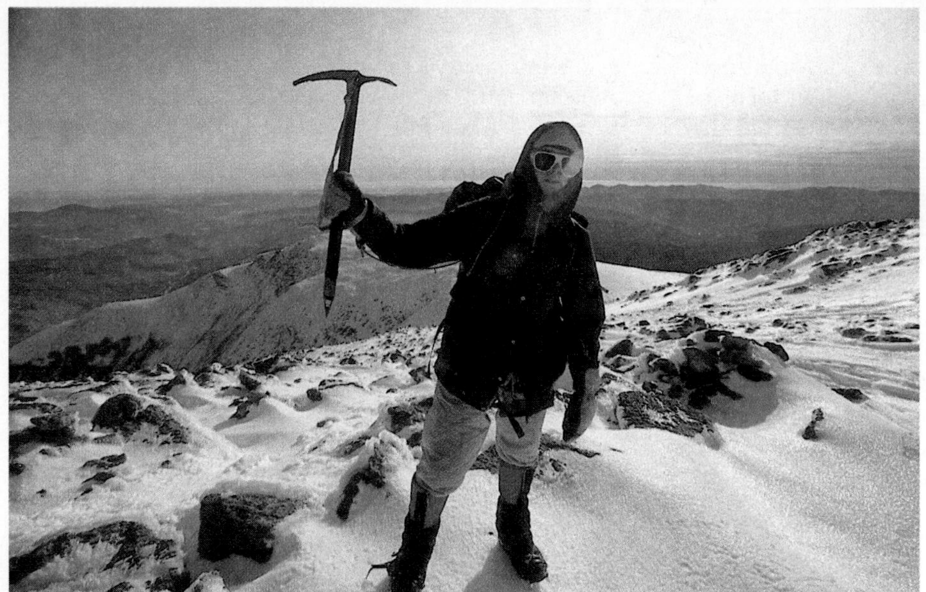

FIGURE 3.16
Hooray for you!

Whatever physical feats you may accomplish, your body's internal processes keep pace, with the help of the adaptable systems described in this chapter. They deserve credit as well!

how you dispose of the substances for which you have no further use. When solid waste is excreted from the body as feces, some water is also lost, because plant fiber and bacteria in the feces hold a certain amount of water and take it out with them.

Several other routes exist by which water and soluble substances leave the body. The greatest amount of water exits the body via the **urinary system.** As the body's blood supply continuously flows through the capillaries of the kidneys, much of the water and many of the dissolved substances (solutes) in the blood pass from the capillaries into the functional units of the kidneys, which are called *nephrons.* The role of the nephrons is to filter waste products out of the blood. Most of the water and solutes are reabsorbed back into the bloodstream from the nephrons; those that are not reabsorbed become urine. This process is under strict hormonal control to ensure that the body keeps adequate water and other substances to support its life processes. The urine is collected and held in the urinary bladder until it is excreted (Figure 3.15).

urinary system—system that filters wastes out of the blood and excretes them in the urine

Perspiration, body water loss due to sweating or surface evaporation, is another route by which water and some minerals leave the body. Although everybody loses some moisture through the skin every day, the amounts lost in this way by different people and on different days are extremely variable. This is discussed further in Chapter 4 (on water).

perspiration—loss of water due to sweating or evaporation from body surfaces

Along with the carbon dioxide they exhale, people also lose some water vapor through the capillaries of the lungs. The amounts lost in this way are proportional to the rate at which a person breathes. For example, when you are exercising hard, you lose much more carbon dioxide and water by this route than you would if you were at rest. You will also lose more via the lungs when you first arrive at a high altitude, because you need to breathe more often to get enough oxygen into your body.

Summary

• **Digestion** is the process of breaking food down into substances small enough to be taken into the body's interior. This intake process is called **absorption.**

• The main part of the digestive system consists of a hollow tube called the **alimentary canal** or **gastrointestinal (GI) tract.** Its many specialized sections vary in diameter, but all sections have a **lumen** (space through which food passes) and a **mucosa** (inner lining). Longitudinal and circular muscles—some of the latter called **sphincters**—control the passage of material from one section of the tract to the next. **Mucus, enzymes,** and **hormones** are secreted at various points along the way to assist in digestion.

• The amount of time food spends in the tract **(transit time)** is affected by diet, drugs, emotions, physical activity, and state of health.

• Digestion and absorption have several phases, and each section of the tract has its own functions to perform. (1) Food is ground in the mouth. (2) The **pharynx** moves food into the **esophagus,** where involuntary muscular contractions called **peristalsis** transport the food to the stomach. (3) The stomach is very active in digestion, attacking food both mechanically and chemically to produce a slushy blend called **chyme.** (4) Digestion continues in the **small intestine** with the aid of secretions from other organs. The **liver** produces **bile,** which **emulsifies** fats (divides them into small droplets), and the **pancreas** produces digestive enzymes and substances that help to neutralize the acid in the chyme. Most of the absorption process also occurs in the small intestine, whose **villi** and **microvilli** project into and expose an enormous surface area to the chyme. (5) The **large intestine** collects solid waste, provides a home for bacteria, and absorbs water and some minerals.

• Feces are retained until the **anus,** or **anal sphincter,** is relaxed, allowing for **defecation.** If this occurs too infrequently, **constipation** occurs; if feces are excreted before the usual amount of water is absorbed, **diarrhea** results.

• Some people experience problems with the structure and/or function of these systems. **"Heartburn"** occurs when stomach acid irritates the lower portion of the esophagus. **Peptic ulcer** occurs in the stomach, esophagus, or small intestine when acid causes damage deep into the linings of these organs. **Irritable bowel syndrome,** of uncertain origin, involves intermittent constipation and diarrhea.

• The chemical processes of metabolism take place continuously in every living cell. The process of building more complex substances from simpler materials is **anabolism;** that of breaking complex into simpler substances is **catabolism.** Synthesis and breakdown reactions can take place at different rates at different times.

• The **circulatory system,** which moves materials to and from the body's cells, actually consists of two systems. The **cardiovascular system** delivers nutrients and oxygen to all the body's cells. It is powered by the heart, which moves blood through a closed system of vessels. The section of the system that loops between the heart and the lungs is the pulmonary circuit, and that which circles between the heart and all other parts of the body is the systemic circuit. **Arteries** carry blood away from the heart; **veins** carry blood back to it; and the exchange of nutrients and wastes takes place across the walls of the smallest vessels, called **capillaries.** Most nutrients enter the bloodstream through the capillaries of the small intestine.

• The **lymphatic system** is a one-way network of vessels that carry **lymph** as well as some of the products of fat digestion. The nutrients are picked up at the intestinal villi by small vessels called **lacteals.**

• Waste products are excreted via several routes. Solid waste is excreted from the body as feces. Most water leaves the body by way of the **urinary system,** which also has the job of filtering waste products out of the blood. Additional water is lost by **perspiration** and by exhalation of water vapor from the lungs.

References

Alper, J. 1993. Ulcers as an infectious disease. *Science* 260:159–160.

Ganong, W.F. 1991. *Review of medical physiology,* 15th edition. Norwalk, CT: Appleton & Lange.

Graham, D.Y., J.L. Smith, and A.R. Opekun. 1988. Spicy food and the stomach. *Journal of the American Medical Association* 260:3473–3475.

Guyton, A.C. 1992. *Human physiology and mechanisms of disease,* sixth edition. Philadelphia: W.B. Saunders.

Henkin, R. 1991. Cooling the burn from hot peppers. *Journal of the American Medical Association* 266:2766.

McNeil, N.I. 1984. The contribution of the large intestine to energy supplies in man. *American Journal of Clinical Nutrition* 39:338–342.

Marieb, E.N. 1991. *Human anatomy and physiology,* 2nd edition. Redwood City, CA: The Benjamin/Cummings Publishing Company.

Mattes, R.D. and D.J. Mela. 1988. The chemical senses and nutrition: Part II. *Nutrition Today* 23:19–25.

Mirkin, G. and M. Hoffman. 1978. *The sportsmedicine book.* Boston: Little, Brown and Company.

Mullin, G.E. 1991. Food allergy and irritable bowel syndrome. *Journal of the American Medical Association* 265:1736.

Savage, D.C. 1987. Factors influencing biocontrol of bacterial pathogens in the intestine. *Food Technology* 41:82–86.

West, J.B., ed. 1991. *Best and Taylor's physiological basis of medical practice.* Baltimore: Williams and Wilkins.w

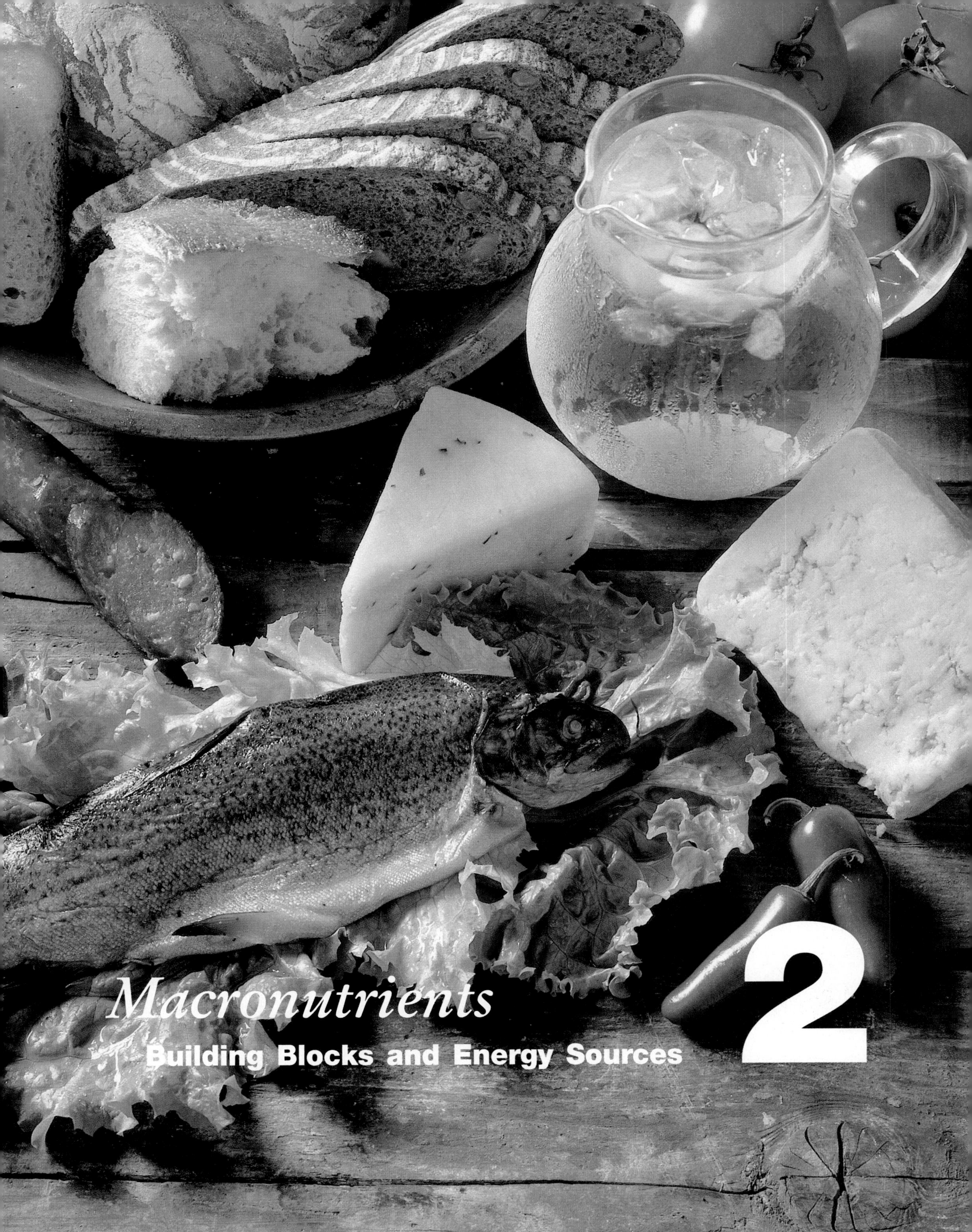

2 *Macronutrients*

Building Blocks and Energy Sources

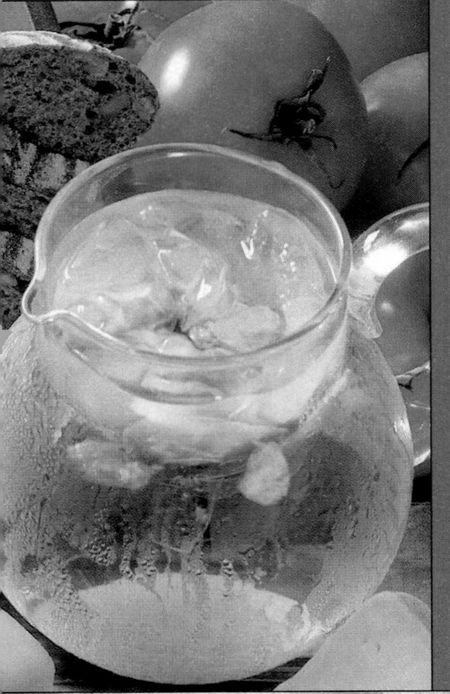

IN THIS CHAPTER

Chapter 4

Water: Not to Be Taken for Granted

Have you ever become light-headed while out hiking for the day or playing volleyball at the beach? Have you ever found yourself almost unbearably thirsty after rushing off to class from an hour of aerobics? Perhaps part of the reason you felt this way was that you were experiencing **dehydration.**

There's a reason why we have a strong drive to drink fluids: we would die if we had to go without water for more than a few days, whereas we can last for weeks without other nutrients. If you were stranded in a desolate area, finding water would be much more pressing than finding food.

Most of the time, though, we easily get enough water by drinking plain water or beverages such as coffee, tea, juices, milk, and soda. We can get a lot of water even from the foods we eat, especially fruits and vegetables. To restore a healthy state of **hydration,** we must replace the amount of water we lose every day.

hydration (dehydration)—the adequacy (or inadequacy) of water in the body

In this chapter, we consider why water is so important and how our bodies deal with the water we take in from the various beverages and foods we consume. We also discuss strategies for maintaining adequate water intake. This is particularly important for athletes, for whom thirst may not be an adequate prompt to restore lost water. People who are physically active need to be especially attentive to meeting their needs for water, or they will not be able to perform as well as they have been trained to do.

Much Water, Many Functions

You get a sense of why this substance is so important when you consider how much of the body is water: water accounts for 60% of the body weight for the typical young adult male and 50% for the young adult female (Randall, 1988).

Water is found throughout the body. Fluids such as **blood plasma** and interstitial fluid are over 90% water. Because the cytosol within cells is also primarily water, every kind of tissue in your body contains water. Muscle tissue is almost 72% water by weight, bones are about 25% water, teeth are about 10% water, and fat tissue varies from 20% to 35% water (Figure 4.1).

blood plasma—the watery portion of the blood, from which the red blood cells and other cells have been removed

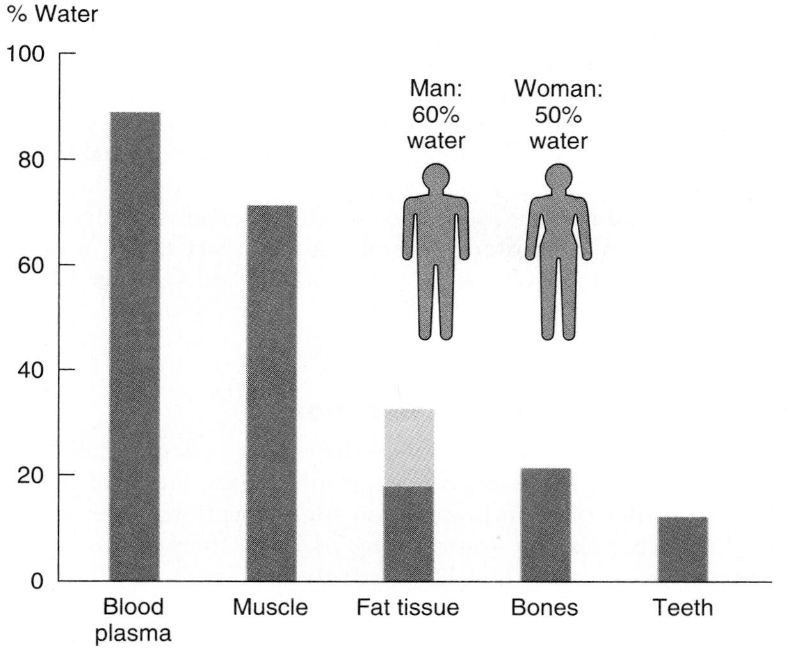

FIGURE 4.1
Percentage of water in various body tissues.

The percentage of water in most body tissues is fairly predictable, although the proportion of water in fat tissue varies within a range, as shown. Because men have a higher proportion of lean body mass, they also have a higher percentage of water.

From the information depicted on the graph, you can see that the exact percentage of body water can vary from person to person, according to the percentage of fat in the person's body. If you have a higher-than-average proportion of body fat, which contains relatively little water, you are likely to have a lower percentage of body water than a thinner person of the same age. Similarly, the average woman, who has a higher proportion of body fat than the average man, has a lower percentage of body water.

Age makes a difference too: a newborn infant may consist of as much as 75% water. By the time a child is a year old, water content in the body is close to 60%.

But what does water actually *do* in the body?

solvent—a substance that dissolves another to form a solution

solute—substance dissolved in water or another solvent

ions, electrolytes—particles that carry an electrical charge in solution

acidic solution—solution containing an excess of positively charged hydrogen ions (H^+), also known as protons

basic (alkaline) solution—solution containing an excess of negatively charged ions that can bind H^+

neutral solution—one containing equal numbers of H^+ and negatively charged ions that can bind H^+

pH scale—a measure of the concentration of hydrogen ions (H^+) in solution

buffer—chemical substance or system that minimizes changes in pH by releasing or binding hydrogen ions

hydrolysis—chemical breakdown process in which water is one of the reacting substances

Medium in Which Reactions Happen

Many biochemical reactions can take place only if the reacting compounds are dissolved in water: water is the critical biochemical **solvent.** In fact, almost all water in the body contains **solutes;** no body fluid is 100% water.

Many chemicals, when they are dissolved in water, dissociate (break apart) into electrically charged particles called **ions** or **electrolytes.** Certain electrolytes such as sodium and potassium have a great deal of influence on how water is distributed in the body. This is discussed more thoroughly later in the chapter.

When a solution has an excess of positively charged hydrogen ions (H^+), also known as protons, the solution is **acidic.** When a solution has an excess of negatively charged ions that are capable of uniting (binding) with hydrogen ions, the solution is **basic** or **alkaline.** For example, a solution that contains an excess of negatively charged hydroxyl ions (OH^-)—which are capable of binding H^+—is basic. If H^+ ions outnumber the negatively charged ions, the solution is acidic. When there are equal numbers of H^+ and negative ions that can bind with H^+, the solution is **neutral.** Water itself (H_2O or HOH) is an example of a neutral substance, because a small portion of its molecules dissociate into equal numbers of H^+ and OH^- ions.

The **pH scale** is a measure of the concentration of hydrogen ions in solution. Figure 4.2 shows a pH scale; 7 is the neutral value, with values below 7 being acidic and values above 7 being alkaline. The strongest acid has a pH of 1; the strongest base has a pH of 14.

The body is very sensitive to changes in pH. Blood and lymph are normally maintained within a very narrow range around 7.4, just slightly basic. If the pH varies by only a few tenths of a pH unit, the normal functioning of many body systems can be interrupted. It is not surprising, then, that your body has a number of mechanisms that help maintain a constant pH; some of these are called **buffers.** Several nutrients participate in buffer systems; we discuss them in Chapter 7 (on proteins) and Chapter 12 (on minerals).

Participant in Biochemical Reactions

In some situations, water itself is one of the reacting compounds. For example, in the process of digestion, when carbohydrates, fats, and proteins are broken into smaller units in preparation for absorption, water participates in the splitting process by contributing its own components to the new compounds. This reaction is called **hydrolysis.** Figure 4.3 illustrates how this process occurs.

Medium of Transport

Some body fluids outside of cells have as their major function the task of carrying substances throughout the body. Blood is the prime example of a nutrient- and waste-transporting body fluid (as discussed in Chapter 3 and shown in Figure 3.9); interstitial fluid and lymph (Figure 3.12) are other examples. In addition, water-based secretions of your gastrointestinal (GI) tract carry digestive enzymes to where they are needed.

Lubricant and Cushion

Some body fluids serve as lubricants that enable solid materials to slide against each other. Your saliva, for example, promotes easier movement of food through the upper part of the digestive tract; tears allow the eyeballs to rotate smoothly in their sockets. Synovial fluid, a thick liquid encapsulated within many of your joints, provides a protective cushion for the tissues of these joints.

Temperature Regulator

Another key function of water is to help control body temperature. This is important because there is a rather narrow range of internal temperatures in which human life processes can continue. If your temperature, which is normally about 37°C (98.6°F), were to fall below about 27°C (80°F) or rise above 42°C (108°F), you would not be likely to survive. These values are for oral temperatures; the actual internal (or core) temperatures are approximately 0.6°C (1°F) higher.

Water is involved in temperature control in several ways. One important property of water is that it does not change temperature as readily as some other substances do in response to environmental temperature changes. Therefore, the body maintains its normal temperature more easily than it would if it were filled with other fluids. Your blood and interstitial fluid, because of their high water content and wide distribution throughout the body, are very important in keeping your core temperature stable.

Sometimes, though, either internal factors (such as an increasing body temperature resulting from vigorous physical activity) or external factors (such as very hot or very cold environmental temperatures) may threaten the consistent internal temperature of the body. In these cases, various mechanisms help body fluids moderate the changes in body temperature or even bring it back toward normal. For example, if you are in a very cold environment without adequate clothing and your body temperature is beginning to fall, your body conserves heat by constricting (narrowing) the blood vessels near the skin surface. This causes less blood to be circulated near the surface, thereby slowing the loss of heat from your blood. Conversely, if you are overheated, blood vessels of the skin dilate, bringing a larger volume of blood near the surface, where it loses some heat to the environment. At the same time, you may exude fluid from the skin—*perspiration*—the evaporation of which reduces your temperature further.

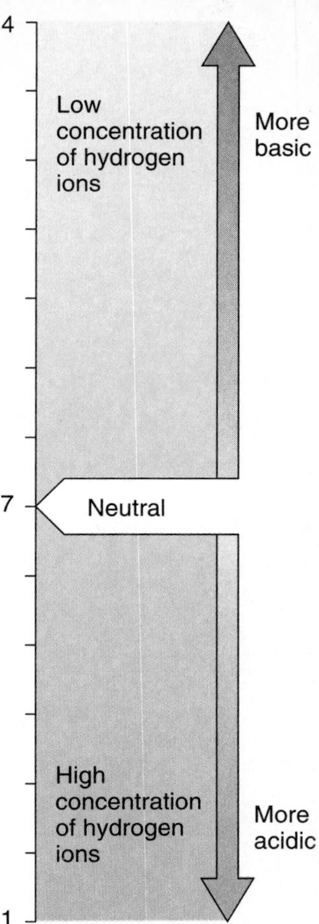

FIGURE 4.2
The pH scale.

The measure of strength of acids and bases.

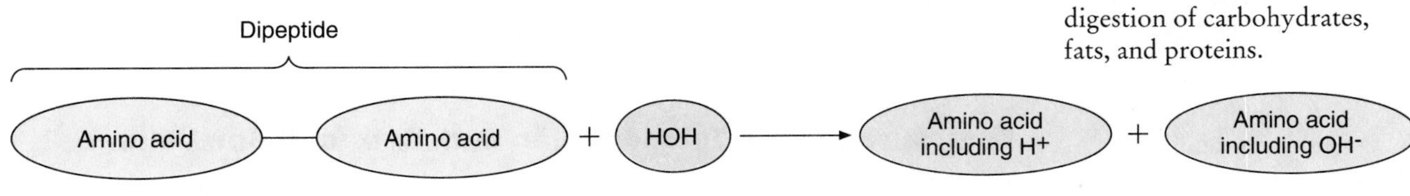

FIGURE 4.3
Hydrolysis: an important biologic function of water.

In this example, a dipeptide containing two amino acids (the units that compose proteins) is split, and the water itself is divided between the two new units. This type of reaction is involved in the digestion of carbohydrates, fats, and proteins.

Mechanisms That Aid in Maintaining the Body's Water Balance

For water to carry out the functions described above, there needs to be enough water in your body, and it needs to be distributed properly. A number of mechanisms help accomplish these two tasks.

Thirst

Your sense of thirst plays an important role: it prompts you to take in water when it is needed—in fact, before you have lost 1% of your body weight as water. Thirst occurs when receptors in the brain (in the region called the *hypothalamus,* which controls many basic body functions) are stimulated in response to certain physiologic changes. If the volume of your body fluids decreases, or if the concentration of substances dissolved in the blood increases, or if the mucosa of your mouth and pharynx become dry, then these receptors are stimulated and you become thirsty (Ganong, 1991; Marieb, 1991).

There is also a mechanism that signals when you have had enough water and should stop drinking, but it is not very well understood. It appears to be located in the GI tract, because our sense of thirst is inhibited before ingested water has reached the bloodstream (Marieb, 1991). It is apparent that social factors also play a role. For example, we sometimes drink when there is no physiologic stimulus to do so, and we sometimes stop drinking before we have restored all lost fluids (Greenleaf, 1992).

Nonetheless, physiologic mechanisms work quite well to help healthy people maintain body water balance, with a few exceptions. During illness, for example, you might not drink enough to meet your needs for water; maybe you feel too uncomfortable to notice your thirst, or perhaps your illness causes you to feel satisfied after drinking only a little. Similarly, if you have been exercising hard and sweating heavily for a long period of time, you are unlikely to drink enough to restore your losses if you count only on thirst. Also, studies have shown that some elderly people have a blunted sense of thirst (RDA Subcommittee, 1989; Hoffman, 1991). We will consider these situations again later in the chapter, when we discuss deliberate steps you can take to make sure you meet your fluid needs.

Absorption of Water from the Gastrointestinal Tract

Water that has been consumed needs to be absorbed before it can do its work in your body.

Water does not need to be broken down into smaller units prior to absorption. The first site in the GI tract at which it can be absorbed is the stomach. Actually, only a minute amount is absorbed here, but this is notable nonetheless because so few substances can be absorbed at all from this organ.

Over 80% of the water you take in is absorbed by the villi of the small intestine (Ganong, 1991). The remainder goes through to the large intestine, where much of what remains is reclaimed. Ninety-eight percent of the water contained in all of the fluids that enter the GI tract, including both dietary sources and fluids secreted into the tract from the body, is eventually absorbed (Ganong, 1991).

Distribution into Intracellular and Extracellular Volumes

Once absorbed, water is distributed between two general locations: inside and outside body cells. The water inside all body cells is collectively referred

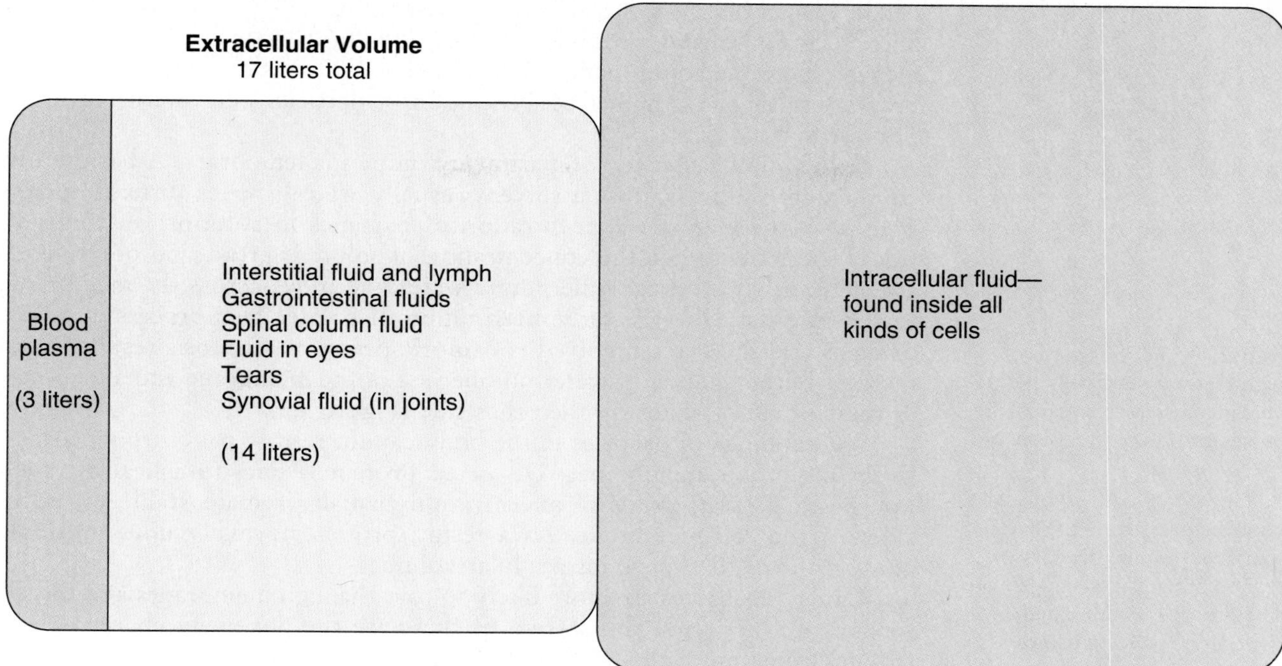

FIGURE 4.4
Body fluids.

Intracellular and extracellular volumes in an average 70-kg (154-pound) male. (Note: total body fluid varies with body size and composition.)

to as the **intracellular volume** or **compartment;** the water outside cells is called **extracellular.**

Extracellular water, the smaller volume, includes blood plasma, interstitial fluid and lymph, gastrointestinal fluids, fluids contained within the spinal column and eyes, tears, and the synovial fluid that cushions the joints.

In a typical 70-kg (154-pound) man, there are approximately 42 liters of total body water. The intracellular volume represents approximately 60% (25 liters) of the total (Figure 4.4).

intracellular volume (compartment)—water contained within all the cells of the body

extracellular volume (compartment)—body water not contained within cells

Implications of Changing Volumes Now that you know what water does for you, what do you suppose would happen if you lost a lot of fluid from one of these volumes?

If your intracellular fluid volume decreases, cellular metabolism, including energy production, may not take place efficiently. If your extracellular fluid volume decreases, blood volume drops; this means that less oxygen can be delivered to body cells. In addition, body temperature rises because the heat produced by metabolic processes is being absorbed by a smaller volume of fluid, which is less able to get rid of the surplus heat. This jeopardizes the functioning of the brain, the circulatory system, the skeletal muscles, and every other body system. What causes such changes in fluid volume?

Factors Involved in Internal Fluid Movement Let's focus on cell membranes to understand what can cause changes in compartment volumes.

In Chapter 3, we mention that water can pass easily through the selectively permeable membranes that enclose body cells. When equal volumes of water move through these membranes in both directions, there is no change in compartment volumes.

Sometimes, however, more water passes through in one direction than the other, resulting in changes in the volumes. To understand why this can occur, remember that the selectively permeable cell membranes will not allow certain substances dissolved in body fluids to pass through. This means that some solute particles accumulate on one side of the cell membrane, resulting in a higher concentration of particles per volume of solution on that side.

Such an imbalance in compartment volumes is temporary. A basic principle of physiology is that a solvent (usually water) moves through membranes to equalize the concentration of particles in solution on the two sides. Therefore, when the concentration of solute is greater on one side of a membrane than on the other, more water will move across the membrane to the side with the greater concentration of solute. This process is called **osmosis** and the force involved is **osmotic pressure.** Osmosis results in an increase in the volume of water on one side of the membrane and a decrease in the volume of water on the other side (Figure 4.5).

osmosis—movement of solvent across a selectively permeable membrane to equalize the concentration of the solute on the two sides

osmotic pressure—the force that occurs when the concentration of particles is higher on one side of a membrane than the other; results in osmosis

Several kinds of particles in the body cannot readily pass through selectively permeable membranes. Dissolved protein is one. In a healthy, well nourished person, protein concentrations usually remain stable on both sides of the cell membrane. As a result, protein normally does more to *maintain* than to *change* intracellular volumes.

Other substances are more likely to pass through membranes and therefore to produce fluid shifts. Two of these are the positively charged electrolytes potassium and sodium. However, the great majority of your body's potassium ions are located inside body cells, whereas your sodium ions are found mostly outside cells. A mechanism in the cell membrane, called the sodium–potassium pump, actively transports potassium through the cell membrane into the cell but ejects sodium, segregating it to the extracellular fluid. If the concentration of positive ions like potassium inside the cell dif-

FIGURE 4.5
How osmosis affects fluid volumes in a simple model.

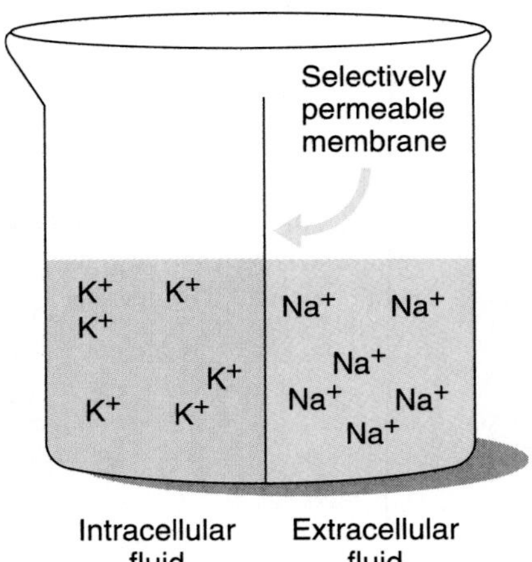

When ions (represented here by potassium [K^+] and sodium [Na^+]) are equally concentrated in the intracellular and extracellular fluid, the volumes of water are equal on both sides of the selectively permeable membrane.

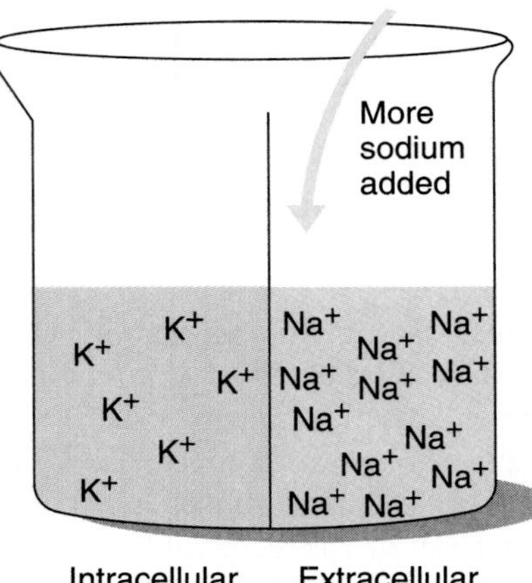

When more sodium is added to the extracellular fluid, the concentration of ions becomes higher in that compartment.

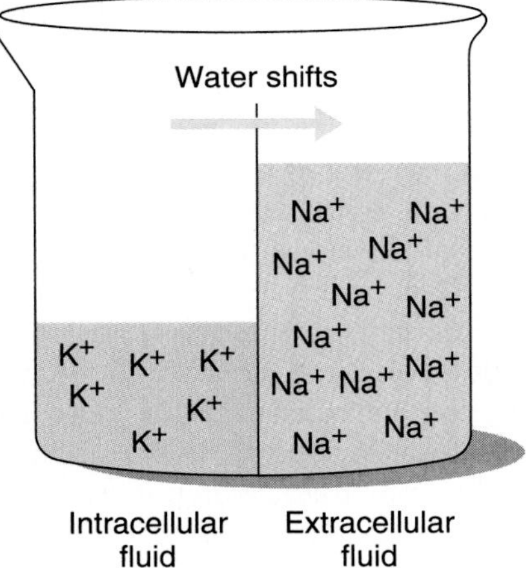

To equalize the concentrations, water moves through the selectively permeable membrane by osmosis from the compartment where ions are less concentrated to the compartment where they are more concentrated. The volumes of both compartments change in the process.

fers from the concentration of positive ions like sodium outside the cell, there will be a water shift in the direction of the greater concentration of ions.

Many other dissolved materials are also segregated largely to one side of the cellular membrane or the other. For example, negatively charged chloride and bicarbonate ions are mainly outside the cell and, along with sodium, influence extracellular volume. On the other hand, positively charged magnesium and negatively charged sulfur- and phosphorus-containing complexes help maintain the intracellular volume.

Excretion of Water

Water leaves your body by four routes: via the kidneys as urine; via the GI tract in the feces; via the skin as perspiration; and via the skin and lungs as **insensible losses,** which occur as water evaporates from body cells that are in contact with dryer surrounding air. As water losses occur by the latter three routes, and as fluid intake fluctuates, your kidneys adjust the amount of urine produced to maintain a healthy hydration status.

insensible loss—a loss that occurs without its being perceived

Typically, the healthy body loses 2–3 liters of fluid per day by all routes combined. Figure 4.6 indicates what proportions are lost by each of the four routes, but these values vary greatly from person to person, and from day to day. Even environmental factors can have a big impact on water losses. If you are in the mountains, for example, insensible losses are much higher than at sea level. This is due to the low humidity of the atmosphere at high altitude and your increased rate of respiration resulting from the air's lower oxygen content (Askew, 1989).

In addition to their role in water excretion, the kidneys also regulate the body's electrolyte status to maintain **homeostasis** in regard to body fluids. The kidneys can produce urine ranging from dilute (with only low levels of electrolytes present) to quite concentrated (with much higher levels of one or more electrolytes). A number of hormones are involved in regulating these processes.

homeostasis—maintenance of the body's normal internal environment, accomplished by biochemical control mechanisms

For example, when electrolytes are becoming too concentrated in the blood, the hormone *antidiuretic hormone (ADH)* causes the kidneys to

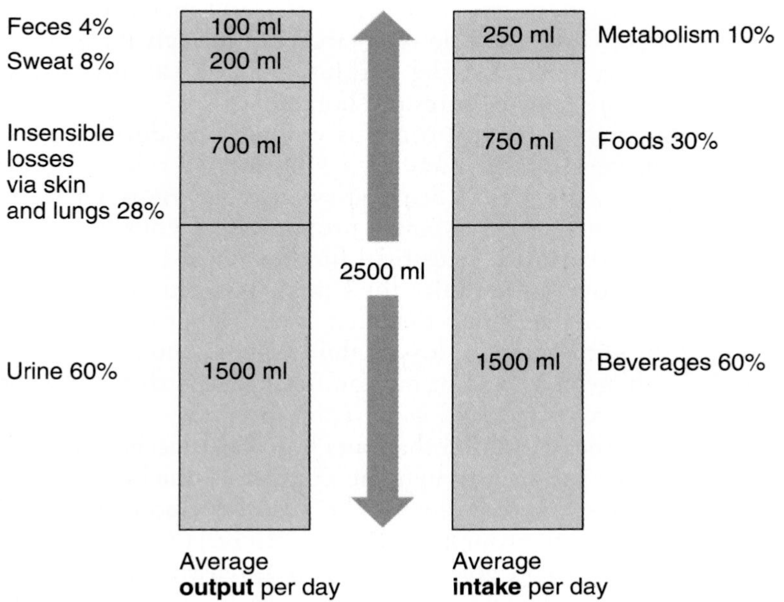

FIGURE 4.6
Major routes of water output and intake.

When total output and intake are in balance, the body is adequately hydrated. The volumes shown are typical for the moderately (not extremely) active adult.

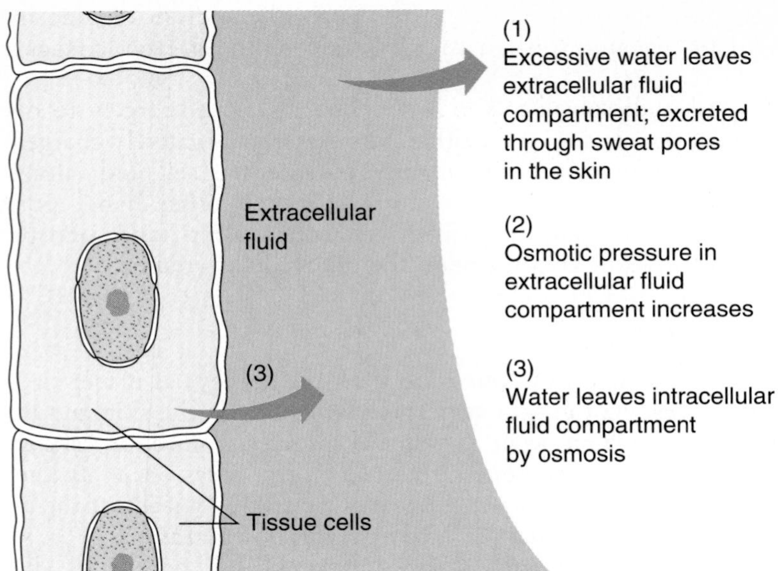

FIGURE 4.7
What happens when you perspire?

Sweat is produced primarily from extracellular fluid. As the dissolved materials in the extracellular fluid become more concentrated because of the loss of water, osmotic pressure increases and causes fluid to move from within cells into the extracellular fluid.

excrete proportionately less water and more electrolytes. On the other hand, when sodium ions in body fluids are beginning to fall (or potassium is relatively in excess), a complex set of hormonal mechanisms involving the hormone *aldosterone* causes the kidneys to hold back sodium that would ordinarily have been excreted in the urine (Marieb, 1991). Let's take a look at some examples of how these mechanisms work in your daily life.

Examples of Fluid Regulation

If you eat a bag of salty pretzels, the salt (which is a compound made of sodium and chloride) will be absorbed and will appear in your blood and interstitial fluid as sodium and chloride ions. Because the concentration of the sodium ions in the interstitial fluid and blood is likely to be higher than that of the positive ions like potassium inside the cell, water will move by osmosis from inside the cells to the interstitial fluid until the concentrations of the ions in the water on both sides of the membrane are equalized. As a result, you will become thirsty, and your body will produce ADH. Soon after this, as sodium and chloride ions circulate through the kidneys, the kidneys will gradually discard the surplus ions via the urine. Working together, these mechanisms help restore homeostasis.

The physiologic changes that occur as you perspire during heavy exercise—such as during a soccer game or a long bicycle ride—also demonstrate fluid shifts (Figure 4.7). When you sweat, you lose water from your interstitial fluid, as well as a very small proportion of your body's sodium and chloride. Your remaining interstitial fluid contains a higher concentration of ions than your intracellular fluid does; this causes water to move mainly from your body cells into the interstitial spaces to equalize the concentration. At the same time, the loss of fluid volume causes you to become thirsty and simultaneously sets in motion mechanisms that cause the kidneys to withhold electrolytes and water from the urine.

Diarrhea is another condition that puts hormonal mechanisms to work. When fecal material moves through the colon too quickly for the usual amount of electrolytes (and water) to be absorbed, body sodium levels decrease, and aldosterone prompts the kidneys to reclaim sodium and, consequently, water that would otherwise have been released in the urine. This mechanism is usually sufficient to correct for fluid and electrolyte losses if

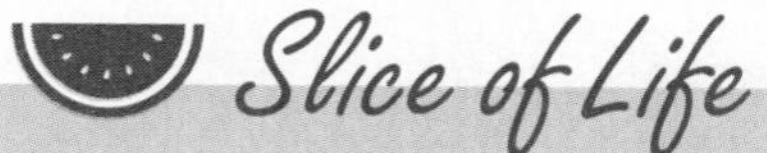

Fluid Losses During Physical Activity

People who exercise for extended periods can experience substantial fluid losses. Here are some examples of amounts of body water lost by people in particular situations:

- Enrico likes on pleasant weekend afternoons to head out of the city on his bicycle to "open up" on the rolling country roads. In a ride of several hours, he commonly loses 3–5 pounds, even though he drinks the contents of his water bottle (and sometimes several refills) along the way.
- Min, an enthusiastic volleyball player, easily loses 2 pounds of body fluids during a couple of hours of vigorous play with friends.
- Cornelius, a 235-pound university football linebacker, lost 9 pounds playing in the spring game. The temperature rose into the 80s that afternoon; other factors promoting fluid loss were the heavy pads and clothing that he wore. Nate, a 290-pound defensive tackle, lost 15 pounds in the same game.
- Gary, a lean and fit man in his thirties, lost 3 pounds while playing 1½ hours of nonstop recreational basketball on an indoor court where the temperature was maintained at approximately 65°F.
- Karen, a woman in her fifties, ran a 20-mile race one morning when the temperature was over 70°F. Although she drank fluids at every water stop along the course, downed a couple of cups of juice at the finish, and sipped on a huge root beer during the ride home, she weighed 6 pounds less when she got home than she had weighed before the race.

If you were to engage in these activities under similar conditions, your fluid losses would not necessarily match those in the examples above; individual variability plays a big role in fluid loss.

Remember: you will—and *should*—regain such body water losses quickly by drinking generous amounts of fluids. Do not confuse water loss with fat loss; the vast majority of weight that you lose during a bout of exercise is due to water loss.

the diarrhea is not severe or prolonged and if the person is able to drink and eat. However, as the next section points out, the body's attempts to correct for these losses are not always successful.

The Serious Consequences of Dehydration

Sometimes a person's fluid intake can be so low or his losses so high that mechanisms designed to maintain hydration are not equal to the task. In such cases, the person becomes dehydrated, and body functions are impaired. At worst, death occurs.

For example, many infants and young children in the developing countries get diseases that cause diarrhea. (Many of these diseases are caused by drinking water that came from supplies contaminated with disease-causing microorganisms.) As fluid and electrolyte losses continue, the child is often unwilling or unable to consume sufficient fluids or food, and dehydration proceeds rapidly. At losses of 10–20% of body water, death results; millions of infants and young children die annually from such diseases. Drinking simple solutions that replace water, electrolytes, and other substances can change the outcome: in 1987, it was estimated that at least half a million children were saved by such *oral rehydration therapy* (UNICEF, 1988).

Even in healthy people, various degrees of dehydration can occur; this is a common problem for the endurance athlete. With moderate sweating, individuals generally produce 1 to 2 liters of sweat per hour (Pivarnik, 1989), but in warm weather some athletes have been found to produce more than 2 liters (4 pounds) of sweat per hour (Costill, 1986). When you consider that the stomach can accommodate only about 1 liter per hour, you can see that even when a person drinks as much fluid as possible along the way, a fluid deficit is likely to occur. The Slice of Life above gives examples of net

TABLE 4.1 Adverse Effects of Dehydration

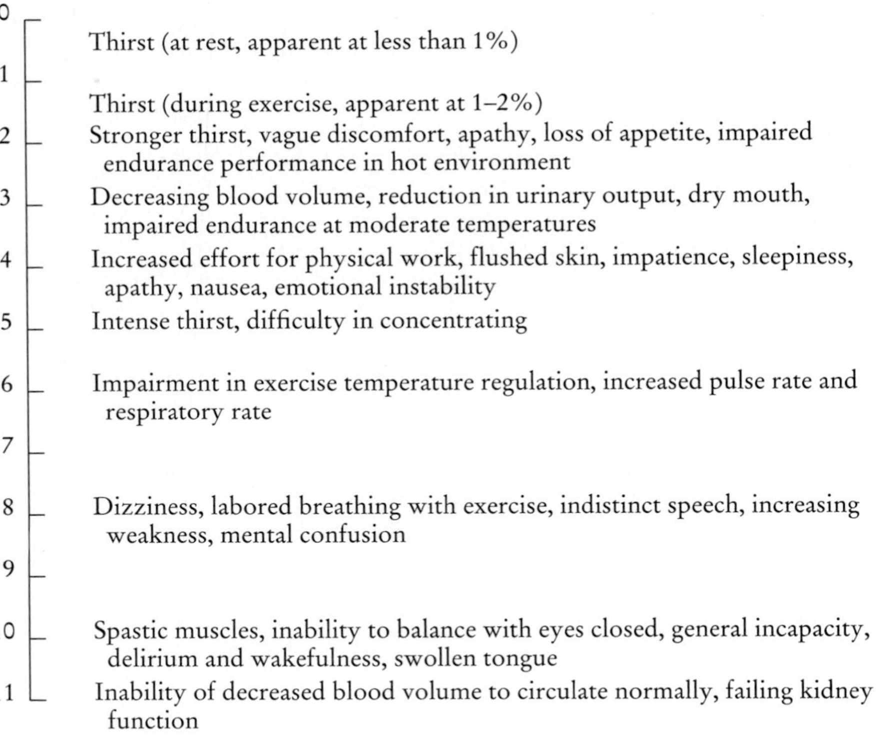

% Body Weight Loss	
0	
	Thirst (at rest, apparent at less than 1%)
1	
	Thirst (during exercise, apparent at 1–2%)
2	Stronger thirst, vague discomfort, apathy, loss of appetite, impaired endurance performance in hot environment
3	Decreasing blood volume, reduction in urinary output, dry mouth, impaired endurance at moderate temperatures
4	Increased effort for physical work, flushed skin, impatience, sleepiness, apathy, nausea, emotional instability
5	Intense thirst, difficulty in concentrating
6	Impairment in exercise temperature regulation, increased pulse rate and respiratory rate
7	
8	Dizziness, labored breathing with exercise, indistinct speech, increasing weakness, mental confusion
9	
10	Spastic muscles, inability to balance with eyes closed, general incapacity, delirium and wakefulness, swollen tongue
11	Inability of decreased blood volume to circulate normally, failing kidney function

Reference: Greenleaf, 1982

losses of weight due to losses of water that people have experienced during extended physical activity.

Loss of water-weight is a problem if you compete in distance activities. At moderate temperatures, losing as little as 3% of your normally hydrated body weight will impair your speed and endurance. In hot weather, a 2% loss of weight due to dehydration will bring about these punishing effects (Sawka, 1992).

One study quantified the effects of a 4% loss of water-weight in young men who had sweated in a sauna: their muscular endurance decreased by about 30% (Torranin et al., 1979). Even 4 hours after they had drunk enough water to restore their body weight, their muscular endurance was not back to normal; it takes time for ingested water to make its way to all the body cells that need it. This fact has sobering implications for wrestlers, who sometimes deliberately dehydrate themselves to make their weight classes, and then expect to be at top strength within a couple of hours after drinking some water. ●

Table 4.1 identifies consequences of various levels of fluid deficit.

You Tell Me

Thirst by itself does not prompt us to drink enough water during heavy sweating; nevertheless, a recent survey of aerobic dance instructors

found that over half the instructors believed thirst to be an *adequate* indicator of needs for fluid during exercise (Soper et al., 1992).

If an instructor leading a 45-minute workout waited until the participants became thirsty before breaking for water, how serious a risk would this be?

Sources of Water

Your body functions best if its fluid losses are replaced promptly. You can rightly assume that beverages are a major source of water (see Figure 4.6). What may be less obvious is that almost all solid foods contribute water as well. In fact, some "solid" foods have a higher percentage of water by weight than do some liquids. Table 4.2 demonstrates this.

When average dietary intakes are evaluated in large surveys, it is found that beverages usually account for more than half of the 2–3 liters that are taken in daily, and foods account for less than half. However, these values can vary considerably with food and beverage choices. An additional but smaller amount comes from within the body itself: when carbohydrates, fats, and proteins are metabolized to produce energy, they also yield carbon dioxide and water. Figure 4.6, earlier, shows typical volumes of water supplied daily from the three sources.

Depending on your dietary habits, it may be best for you to consume more than the usually recommended amount of water. Consider This on page 109 points out some of the ways food and beverage intakes can influence your body's water balance.

Are some fluids better for you than others? Water itself is an excellent choice; but if you prefer other beverages, there are a couple of things to consider. If you are primarily thinking about what *volume of water* you can get from various beverages, there is not much difference among them: most beverages are approximately 90% water by weight. However, some beverages contain **diuretics**—substances that increase urine production and consequent body water loss. Caffeine (found primarily in coffee, tea, and some carbonated beverages) and alcohol (in beer, wine, whiskey, and others) have a diuretic effect. Consequently, beverages with high concentrations of these chemicals are less desirable water sources than beverages that don't contain such chemicals or have only low concentrations of them. (Caffeine and alcohol have other effects on the body that you may want to limit or avoid; these are discussed in Chapters 14 and 17.)

diuretics—substances that cause increased urine production

Another consideration when you choose a beverage is what nutrients it contains besides water. For example, fruit juices contain carbohydrates and possibly vitamins A and/or C; milk beverages contain protein, carbohydrates, calcium, phosphorus, riboflavin, and other nutrients; and sugared carbonated beverages and fruit-flavored drinks contain considerable levels of carbohydrates. Therefore, beverages can make a substantial nutritional contribution to the day's intake; you need to consider their energy and nutrient values as well as their water content.

In recent years, Americans have been buying more beverages overall, particularly soft drinks, fruit juices, and fruit drinks; meanwhile the consumption of coffee, tea and milk has declined. In the 1980s, the per capita consumption of soft drinks surpassed that of milk; in fact, it exceeded the consumption of milk and fruit juices combined.

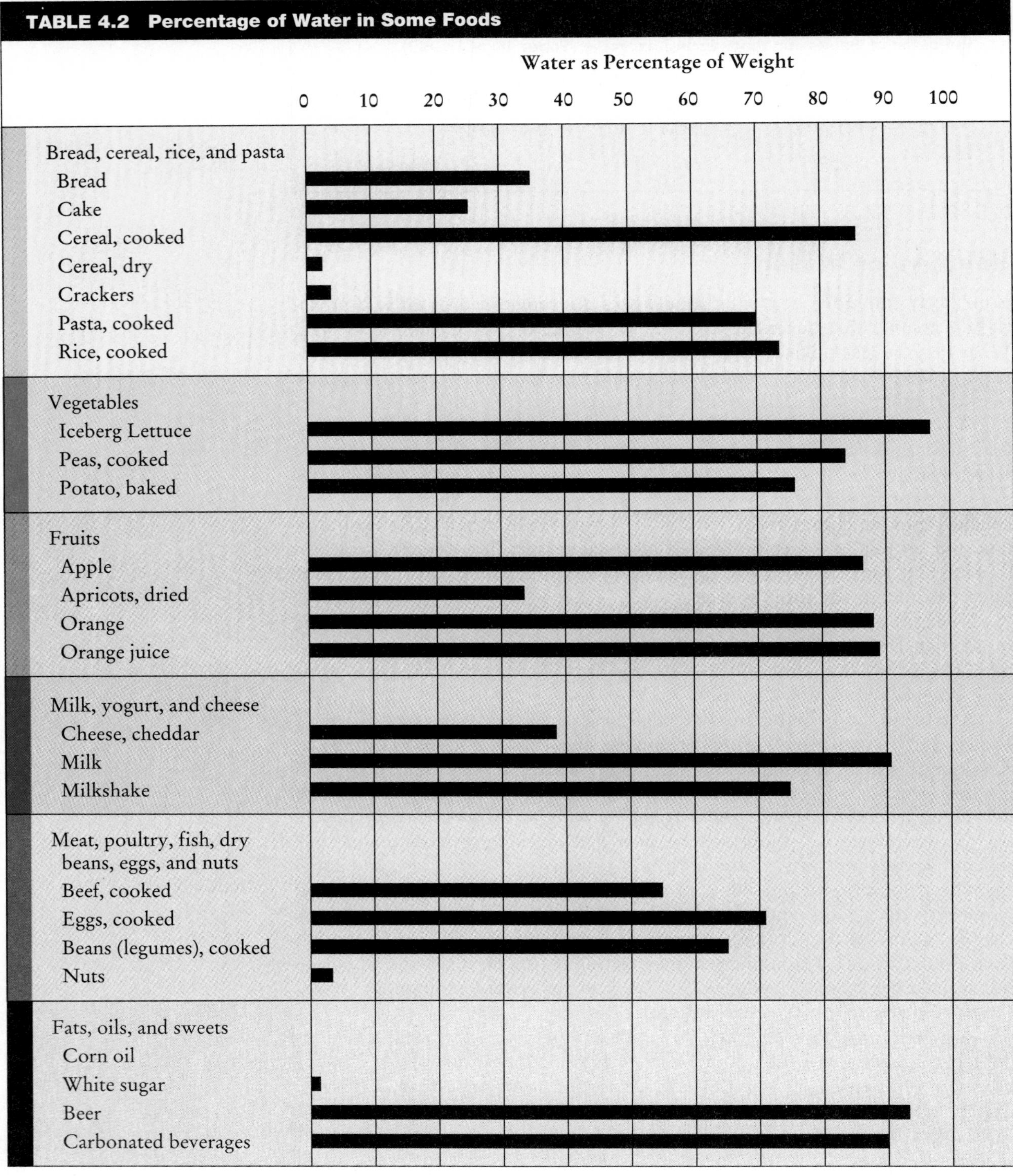

The popularity of bottled water has increased significantly. The reason seems to have less to do with nutrition than with the general public's concerns about possible contamination of public and private water supplies. Thinking for Yourself on page 110 addresses this issue.

To improve your water balance, if you eat or drink

This	*. Consider this*
Many whole-grain products; any fiber-added items	**Drink extra fluids. Fiber absorbs and holds water in your GI tract until it is excreted, so you need to make up for these losses.**
Salty foods	**Drink extra fluids. You need more water to carry the surplus sodium out of your body.**
Alcoholic beverages	**Drink less alcohol, more of other fluids. Alcohol causes increased fluid losses. A dry mouth "the morning after" reflects your dehydrated condition.**
Caffeine-containing beverages	**Substitute some caffeine-free fluids. Caffeine has a mild dehydrating effect. In large amounts, caffeine can also make you jittery or upset your GI tract.**

Recommendations for Fluid Intake

Sometimes your sense of thirst is not enough to keep you aware of your body's need for water. This section offers several recommended strategies to help you maintain hydration.

Consume Water in Proportion to Kcaloric Expenditure

The 1989 RDA recommends that moderately active, healthy people (including the elderly) consume from 1 milliliter (ml) to 1.5 ml of water per kcalorie expended (RDA Subcommittee, 1989). This amounts to at least 1 liter (approximately 1 quart) of fluid from all sources per 1000 kcalories used. (If you don't know approximately how many kcalories you expend per day, see Table 8.3 for a quick way to estimate your use.) People on low-kcalorie diets should note that this standard applies to kcalories *expended,* not to kcalories taken in; therefore, *you should drink at least as much fluid while on a weight reduction diet as you did before.*

Infants routinely need 1.5 ml of water per kcalorie. Not only do their cells have a higher water content, but their immature kidneys also require more fluid for removing metabolic wastes.

These standards based on energy usage are not likely to meet your needs if you are extremely physically active; in this case, the following two guidelines are more appropriate.

Replace Weight of Water Lost

This guideline is useful for physically active people. Rehydration is especially important for athletes because the sense of thirst alone is not likely to prompt a person to rehydrate adequately during exercise and after hours

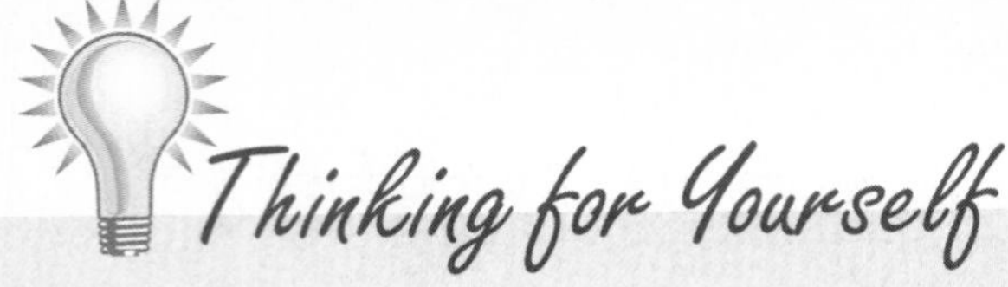

Is Bottled Water Better?

The Situation

The radio is playing as you are getting dressed. "Is your drinking water pure?" the advertisement asks. "Join the thousands who are now using Brady's Bottled Water. . . ." Although you have heard the ad many times before, this time you pause. You recall a TV news item you saw a few nights ago, in which residents of a local community questioned the safety of their water supply. At the grocery store the next day, you noticed how much shelf space is devoted to bottled water. You had regarded the recent interest in bottled water as a fad, but now you are beginning to wonder: is bottled water better?

Is Your Information Accurate and Relevant?

- The ad insinuates that water, to be drinkable, should be *pure.* Absolutely pure water is almost nonexistent, although if water is distilled and deionized, it comes close. In fact, many of the dissolved and suspended substances in natural water do not affect its safety, and some even give it sought-after flavors. It is important, however, for water to be *safe;* that is, the levels of potentially harmful dissolved and suspended substances it contains need to be lower than levels that are known to cause harm.
- Although the vast majority of public water supplies in the United States meet the standards established by the Safe Drinking Water Act of 1974 (amended in 1986), the concern about water quality *is* increasing. The Environmental Protection Agency (EPA) is charged with testing water supplies, and Congress has given the EPA a timetable through 1994 for setting limits on additional chemicals not dealt with in the earlier legislation.
- It is true that the use of bottled water has grown considerably in recent years. In 1990, Americans consumed 8 gallons per person (Putnam, 1992), and sales are expected to grow by 10% per year.

What Else Should You Consider?

In the United States, approximately half the population uses public water supplies that come from *surface water*—that is, from rivers, streams, reservoirs, and lakes. The other half uses water that comes from underground sources, called *groundwater,* which is obtained from either a public water supply or a private well.

It is possible for either surface water or groundwater to become contaminated. In developing countries, where many people do not have access to clean public water and adequate sewer systems, *pathogenic (disease-carrying) organisms* from contaminated water cause millions of deaths per year.

In developed countries, 98% of citizens have access to clean water (Myers, 1984). In the United States, the EPA sets standards for public water supplies, which define allowable levels of microbial contaminants and other pollutants. Substances believed to be carcinogenic are permitted at a level that would allow a one-in-a-million cancer risk over a 70-year life span. When public water supplies do not meet the standards, contaminants are filtered out, or chemicals are added to make them settle out. Then chlorine is added to kill any microorganisms that might be present.

For people who have their own wells, public health officials recommend testing at least yearly for microbial safety and for other likely contaminants, based on the source of supply. Some local and state public health departments will do such tests, or they can recommend reputable laboratories (Baumeister, 1990).

What Substances Are Considered Contaminants, and Where Do They Come From?

Substances used in *agriculture* can run off into surface water or seep into groundwater, potentially reaching levels that are unacceptable. The substances of major concern are nitrates (nitrogen-containing compounds from both natural and chemical fertilizers), herbicides, and insecticides (National Research Council, 1989). Pollutants from *petrochemical industries, mining, and manufacturing* can also be a problem. These include such substances as hydrocarbons (e.g., crude oil, gasoline, and creosote) and heavy metals.

Lead is another substance of concern. Although it is possible for lead to be present in surface or groundwater supplies, the cause of excessive lead in drinking water is likely to be closer to home. If lead is present in household water pipes or solder or in the service lines from public water mains, small amounts can dissolve into water moving through those pipes. It is more likely that lead will leach into water if the water is hot, if it is acidic, and if it stands in the pipes for several hours (e.g., overnight or all day). The only way to determine if there is a problem is to have your water tested. Until you have such testing done, here's a way to reduce the (possible) lead content of water: whenever water has been standing in the pipes for 5 or 6 hours, open the tap, and let the water run for 2–3 minutes before consuming any.

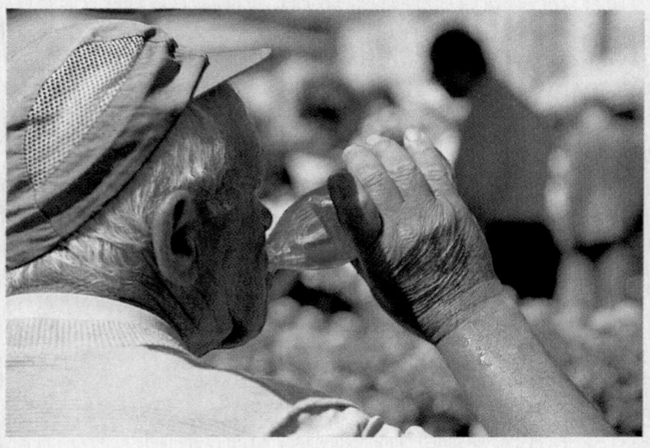

Increasing popularity of bottled water.

Bottled water is not necessarily purer or safer than tap water, but it may offer advantages to some.

Some states now require that the plumbing and solder in new construction be lead-free and that the pH of public water supplies be adjusted to at least 8 (mildly alkaline) (Raloff, 1989).

How do all of these standards compare to those for bottled water?

The U.S. Food and Drug Administration is responsible for setting the standards for bottled water. For many years, the FDA standards for bottled water were identical to the EPA standards for public water supplies, with an additional proviso that the bottling conditions be sanitary. Under these regulations, water could be bottled from ordinary public supplies and then filtered, flavored, deionized, or carbonated to change the taste. Now the FDA is writing definitions for the various types of bottled waters available today. In January, 1993, the FDA proposed new standards and labeling regulations, but the previous rules apply until the new standards take effect.

Tests have shown that bottled waters are not always in compliance with standards; in a test of 37 brands of domestic and imported mineral waters bought off the shelves in Chicago and Pittsburgh, 24 had one or more substances that were not in compliance with the drinking water standards in the United States (Allen et al., 1989). And the Massachusetts Department of Public Health, in testing 15 brands of bottled water, found that 13 of them exceeded one or more guidelines for limits on pollutants.

It is equally possible that bottled water might be missing something you want: fluoride. An important mineral for reducing the risk of tooth decay, fluoride is added to most public water supplies in the amount of one part per million; many bottled waters, however, do not contain this amount.

Although you might assume that *mineral water* includes fluoride, there is no guarantee. California and Florida, two states that have already defined mineral water, specify only that it must contain 500 parts per million of dissolved solids. New federal standards and labeling regulations are under development, but the content of mineral waters will continue to vary greatly.

Now What Do You Think?

So, should you use bottled water instead of tap water? As you think through these options, consider whether your choice would be different if your tap water came from a public supply or from a private well.

- Option 1 Without having your tap water tested, you use bottled water as a precaution for all drinking and cooking purposes.
- Option 2 You have your tap water tested. If it meets water safety standards, you decide to use it and to enjoy flavored or carbonated bottled waters on occasion.
- Option 3 You have your water tested for substances for which you think there may be some risk; if the water exceeds standards for safety, you use bottled water or choose one of the following options.
- Option 4 If tests indicate that lead is a problem after water has been standing in pipes but not after several minutes of running the water, you do the following: you "flush" the pipes by leaving the tap open for 2–3 minutes after water has been standing for several hours; you use bottled water after long periods of disuse but not at other times; you install an approved treatment device or have your plumbing replaced.
- Option 5 If tests indicate that other chemicals are a problem, you ask the testing agency whether there are filtering systems that will reduce the levels to acceptable limits, and you install such recommended systems.
- Option 6 You forget the issue if there are no reports of problems regarding water quality in your area.

Do you see other options, or reasonable combinations of options, that would be acceptable to you?

of heavy sweating. When you are exercising hard, you probably won't feel thirsty until you have lost 1–2% of your weight through dehydration (Williams, 1992). By that time, dehydration could already be starting to impair your performance.

Moreover, you can sweat fluid faster than you can absorb it through your small intestine. Some people sweat 3 liters of fluid per hour during activity but can absorb only about half that amount per hour through the small intestine. If you are perspiring heavily, therefore, the best you can usually accomplish, even when following sound recommendations, is to *minimize* your losses during activity.

Here is the guideline for restoring fluid losses: weigh yourself (without clothing) before the activity and again afterward. For every pound lost, drink 2 cups of fluid. Pace the drinking at whatever rate is comfortable for you, such as 1 cup every 15 minutes or so, until you have restored the entire amount.

If you rely only on thirst to tell you how much fluid you need for rehydration, you will probably take in only about half the needed amount in the first 24 hours (Saltin, 1978). It may take as long as three days to replace the fluid lost in one day of heavy sweating, unless you drink more than thirst prompts you to consume.

Successive days of vigorous activity without deliberate replacement of water can lead to progressive dehydration, which has resulted in the tragic, easily preventable deaths of some athletes. Mistakenly, some athletes and coaches believe that players can be "trained" not to need much water, and some believe that withholding water will make players "tougher." The fact is that a dehydrated athlete, like any dehydrated person, becomes impaired (see Table 4.1). Because players might not pay attention to their own hydration status, coaches or trainers should weigh their players daily.

You Tell Me

In the United States, overheating with severe dehydration during exercise is the third most prevalent cause of death among high school athletes (Hubbard, 1990). (Head and neck injuries are first; heart failure is second.)

What can coaches and trainers do to prevent deaths from dehydration?

During this discussion, you may have been mentally protesting that body weight losses also reflect the loss of fat resulting from strenuous activity, and that therefore it should not be necessary to drink so much that the person's original weight is restored. Although it is true that fat is lost, the weight of the fat lost during any vigorous activity of a few hours' duration is usually very small compared to the weight of the water lost. As an extreme example, most runners of average size lose *less than a pound of body fat during a marathon* (26 miles, or several hours of running) but can easily perspire between 10 and 20 pounds of fluid (4½–9 liters) during that experience. Therefore, weight loss is indeed a suitable approximate measure of water loss.

Hydrate Before, During, and After Heavy Perspiration

If you are going to exercise hard, you can minimize dehydration if you drink water before and during heavy activity, as well as replacing water afterward. Table 4.3 suggests a schedule.

TABLE 4.3 Amounts of Water Needed for Extended Physical Activity

When to Drink	Approximate Amount to Drink
Before activity	
2 hours before	½–¾ liter (2–3 cups) of water
10–15 minutes before	½ liter (2 cups) of cold (40–50°F) water
During activity	
Every 10–15 minutes	~¼ liter (½–1 cup) of cold water
After activity	
Every 15 minutes, or at comfortable intervals	¼ liter (1 cup of fluid); continue until 2 cups have been consumed for every pound lost

Endurance athletes help themselves by consuming extra fluids *before* they start exercising. This leads to a condition called *hyperhydration* or *superhydration;* it helps ensure that hydration is adequate to begin with (Williams, 1992). Then, *during* activity, it is important to drink small amounts frequently. Nonetheless, if you exercise for a long time, you cannot keep up with your losses. Recommendations for maintaining hydration during physical endurance activities, then, are compromise measures that will allow you to achieve only partial rehydration; you must complete the rehydration process after the activity.

Some aspects of the recommendations in Table 4.3 deserve explanation. Drinking *cold* water (4–10°C, or 40–50°F) is suggested because cold water increases the motility of the stomach and leaves the stomach faster than warmer water. This hastens the water's absorption and its beneficial effects

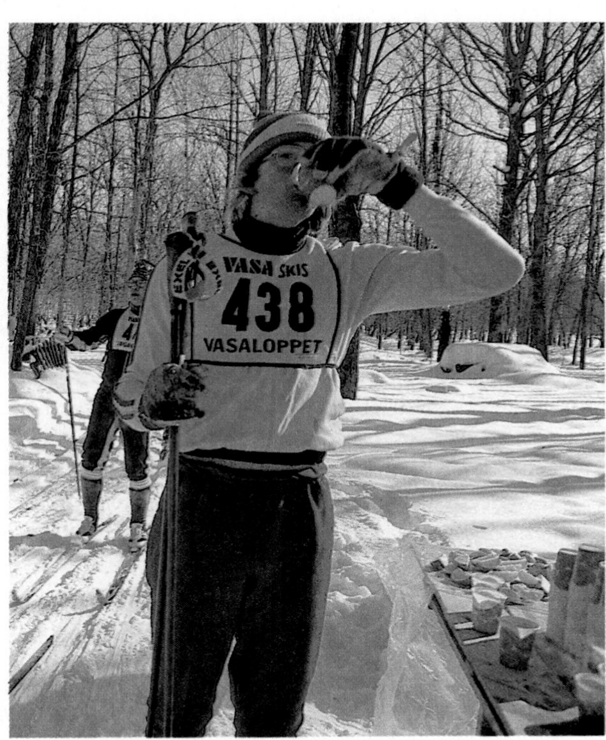

FIGURE 4.8
Replacing lost body fluids.

This skier is attempting to restore water she has lost through perspiration and respiration.

(Fink, 1982). Water at the temperatures and volumes suggested in Table 4.3 does not appear to cause stomach cramps. Such distress is more likely to occur when larger volumes are consumed (Costill, 1986).

Replenish Carbohydrates and Electrolytes

Notice that in Table 4.3 we recommend you drink *water* rather than other fluids. When you are involved in short-term activities—up to about an hour of continuous performance—water is the only substance you need to worry about replacing. Because most of us are not continuously active for longer than an hour at a time, plain, cool water usually is adequate; moreover, it is absorbed more quickly than many other drinks.

However, if you are continuously active for more than an hour at a time, you need to replace carbohydrate as well. The amount of carbohydrate you have in your muscles limits the amount of time you can continue the activity; therefore, consuming a beverage that contains some carbohydrate can extend your endurance. The carbohydrate can be in the form of sucrose or glucose (all simple forms of sugar) or glucose polymers (a somewhat more complex, manufactured carbohydrate). These are discussed more thoroughly in Chapter 5.

Be careful, though: if the drink is too concentrated in carbohydrate, it will interfere with the absorption of the water. The upper limit of carbohydrate that can help without significantly hindering hydration is a 10% solution (Davis et al., 1990); that is, there should be no more than 100 grams (g) of carbohydrate in 1 liter (or no more than 24 grams in an 8-oz serving) of the beverage. Check the content of whatever you consider using; most unsweetened fruit juices and many commercially prepared sports drinks fall within the limit, but carbonated beverages may not. Another alternative is to make your own solution by adding 20–24g (5–6 teaspoons) of sugar to each 240ml (8 ounces) of water. (Carbohydrate and endurance are discussed further in Chapter 5.)

Some endurance athletes wonder about the need for drinks that also contain the electrolytes sodium, chloride, and potassium. Actually, your body does not lose much potassium during exercise. Sodium and chloride are lost in sweat, but they are exuded in lesser concentrations than are present in body fluids. Because the *relative* concentration of sodium and chloride in body fluids actually *increases* while you perspire, you ordinarily don't need to be concerned about replacing these substances during exercise. Of course, the *absolute* amount of sodium in your body decreases somewhat, but this is of no consequence with short-term exercise.

However, if you are a *superendurance athlete* who competes for more than 4 hours at a time and rehydrates with plain water, your absolute levels of sodium could eventually drop dangerously low. This drop could result in epileptic-type seizures or even death (Williams, 1992). You can prevent this problem, however. If you lose 6–8 pounds or more in a day of activity or are going to be exercising continuously for more than 4 hours—especially in hot weather—consider sodium replacement. We offer specific guidelines for sodium replacement in Chapter 12 (on minerals). Generally, though, by salting food a little more liberally and using a sport drink that contains 50–100 milligrams (mg) of sodium per 240 ml (1 cup), you will get enough sodium. (One hundred mg of sodium is the amount in about 1/25 of a teaspoon of salt, a very small amount.) These beverages supply another benefit to the superendurance athlete: the presence of sugar and sodium together enhances the absorption of water (Williams, 1992). ●

Can You Get Too Much Water?

Throughout this chapter we have stressed the importance of taking in enough water. But you might be asking yourself, is it possible to consume *too much* water?

The answer is that it is possible, but very unlikely. Experts estimate that the healthy human body can cope with an intake of approximately 20 liters (about 5 gallons) of water per day. (Barr and Costill, 1989). Beyond that level, the kidneys probably can't produce urine fast enough to remove the excess water.

It is extremely rare for anyone to consume this much fluid. The only cases of which we are aware involved two psychotic individuals who, in misguided efforts at self-purification, drank so much water that they eventually overwhelmed their bodies' ability to cope with the fluid and died (Rendell et al., 1978). Nonetheless, these rare examples demonstrate the principle that even substances as critical to our well-being as water can be toxic if consumed in excessive quantities.

Summary

- Although the average person devotes little thought to his or her hydration, water is crucial to survival. Water is the largest body constituent, is found in every body tissue, and normally accounts for at least half of body weight.
- One of water's most important roles is as a biochemical **solvent.** Many types of **solutes,** including charged particles called **ions** or **electrolytes,** are dissolved in body water. An **acidic solution** contains an excess of positively charged hydrogen ions, or **protons** (H^+), and a **basic solution** contains an excess of negatively charged ions that can bind H^+. A solution containing equal numbers of H^+ and negative ions is **neutral.** The **pH** of a solution is a measure of its H^+ ion concentration, which is given on a scale from 1 (very acidic) to 14 (very basic). The body is extremely sensitive to changes in pH, and several nutrients participate in **buffer** systems that help maintain it at the proper level.
- Water also participates in certain metabolic reactions, such as **hydrolysis** of lipids, proteins, and carbohydrates; acts as a transport medium and lubricant; and helps to regulate body temperature.
- Water must be present in the right places in the body as well as in the right amounts. Water enters the body through the digestive system (mainly via the small intestine) and, once absorbed, becomes part of either the **intracellular** or **extracellular compartment.** Water moves between the two compartments across cell membranes. The process of movement, which results in an equal concentration of solutes in water on both sides of the membrane, is called **osmosis.** Given sufficient time, the body of a healthy individual can compensate for the effects on water balance of eating an unusually salty food or losing a great deal of water in perspiration—provided that the person consumes enough water to make up for the losses. The kidneys play a major role in maintaining the body's **homeostasis.**
- Like all other nutrients, water has a beneficial range of intake. Thirst is an important, but not infallible, indicator of need; other guidelines, such as those for athletes, focus on replacing losses. Although it would be difficult to consume too much water under ordinary circumstances, overconsumption is possible.
- Water is available from three sources: (1) beverages, (2) foods, and, in much smaller amounts, (3) the body's own metabolic processes.
- Water is lost by four routes: (1) urine excretion, (2) **insensible loss** and perspiration (both involving evaporation of water from the skin), (3) exhalation of water vapor, and (4) excretion in the feces. The amounts of water lost by these routes can vary considerably; for example, prolonged strenuous exercise increases water loss through perspiration as well as respiration.
- If body water losses exceed intake, progressive dehydration occurs with accompanying penalties. If your normal body weight decreases by as little as 3% (or 2% in a hot environment) because of water loss, your physical performance will be impaired. Greater losses have even more serious consequences and when water loss reaches 10–12% of body weight, death can result.

References

Allen, H.E., M.A. Halley-Henderson, and C.N. Hass. 1989. Chemical composition of bottled mineral water. *Archives of Environmental Health* 44(no.2):102–116.

American Dietetic Association. 1987. Position of the American Dietetic Association: Nutrition for physical fitness and athletic performance for adults. *Journal of the American Dietetic Association* 87:933–939.

Applegate, L. 1991. *Power foods.* Emmaus, PA: Rodale Press.

Applegate, E. 1991. Nutritional considerations for ultraendurance performance. *International Journal of Sport Nutrition* 1:118–126.

Askew, E.W. 1989. Nutrition and performance under adverse environmental conditions. In *Nutrition in exercise and sport,* ed. J.F. Hickson and I. Wolinsky. Boca Raton, FL: CRC Press, Inc.

Barr, S.I. and D.L. Costill. 1989. Water: Can the endurance athlete get too much of a good thing? *Journal of the American Dietetic Association* 89:1629–1635.

Baumeister, R. 1990. Personal communication. Madison, WI: Chief, Public Water Supply Section, Wisconsin Department of Natural Resources.

Coleman, E. 1988. *Eating for endurance.* Palo Alto, CA: The Bull Publishing Company.

Costill, D.L. 1986. *Inside running.* Indianapolis, IN: Benchmark Press, Inc.

Davis, J.M., W.A. Burgess, C.A. Slentz, and W.P. Bartoli. 1990. Fluid availability of sports drinks differing in carbohydrate type and concentration. *American Journal of Clincal Nutrition* 51:1054–1057.

Environmental Nutrition. 1988. Bottled waters making big splash with more than 700 varieties on market. *Environmental Nutrition* 11(no.5):4–5.

Fink, W.J. 1982. Fluid intake for maximizing athletic performance. In *Nutrition and athletic performance: Proceedings of the conference on nutritional determinants in athletic performance,* ed. W. Haskell, J. Scala, and J. Whittam. Palo Alto, CA: The Bull Publishing Company.

Frizzell, R.T., G.H. Lang, D.C. Lowance, and S.R. Lathan. 1986. Hyponatremia and ultramarathon running. *Journal of the American Medical Association* 255:772–774.

Ganong, W.F. 1991. *Review of medical physiology,* 15th edition. Norwalk, CT: Lang.

Greenleaf, J.E. 1982. The body's need for fluids. In *Nutrition and athletic performance: Proceedings of the conference on nutritional determinants in athletic performance,* ed. W. Haskell, J. Scala, and J. Whittam. Palo Alto, CA: The Bull Publishing Company.

Greenleaf, J.E. 1992. Problem: Thirst, drinking behavior, and involuntary dehydration. *Medicine and Science in Sports and Exercise* 24:645–656.

Hoffman, N.B. 1991. Dehydration in the elderly: Insidious and manageable. *Geriatrics* 46:35–38.

Hubbard, R.W. 1990. An introduction: The role of exercise in the etiology of exertional heatstroke. *Medicine and Science in Sports and Exercise* 22:2–5.

Knox, C.E. 1988. What's going on down there? *Science News* 134:362.

Marieb, E.N. 1991. *Human anatomy and physiology,* 2nd edition. Redwood City, CA: The Benjamin/Cummings Publishing Company.

Myers, N. 1984. *GAIA: An atlas of planet management.* New York: Doubleday.

National Research Council. 1989. *Alternative agriculture.* Washington, DC: National Academy Press.

Pivarnik, J.M. 1989. Water and electrolytes during exercise. In *Nutrition in exercise and sport,* ed. J.F. Hickson and I. Wolinsky. Boca Raton, FL: CRC Press, Inc.

Putnam, J. 1992. Personal communication. USDA, Economics Research Service.

Raloff, J. 1989. EPA proposes new rules to get the lead out. *Science News* 134:118.

Randall, H.T. 1988. Water, electrolytes, and acid-base balance. In *Modern nutrition in health and disease,* ed. M.E. Shils and V.R. Young. Philadelphia: Lea & Febiger.

RDA Subcommittee. 1989. *Recommended dietary allowances.* Washington, DC: National Academy Press.

Rendell, M., D. McGrane, and M. Cuesta. 1978. Fatal compulsive water drinking. *Journal of the American Medical Association* 240(no.23):2557–2559.

Saltin, B. 1978. Fluid, electrolyte, and energy losses and their replenishment in prolonged exercise. In *Nutrition, physical fitness, and health.* International series on sports sciences, volume 7, ed. J. Parizkova and V.A. Rogozkin. Baltimore: University Park Press.

Saltin, B. and D. Costill. 1988, Fluid and electrolyte balance during prolonged exercise. In *Exercise, nutrition, and energy metabolism,* ed. E.S. Horton and R.L. Terjung. New York: Macmillan Publishing Company.

Sawka, M.N. 1992. Physiological consequences of hypohydration: Exercise performance and thermoregulation. *Medicine and Science in Sports and Exercise* 24:657–670.

Soper, J., R.A. Carpenter, and B.M. Shannon. 1992. Nutrition knowledge of aerobic dance instructors. *Journal of Nutrition Education* 24:59–66.

Torranin, C., D.P. Smith, and R.J. Byrd. 1979. The effect of acute thermal dehydration and rapid rehydration on isometric and isotonic endurance. *The Journal of Sports Medicine and Physical Fitness* 19:1–9.

UNICEF. 1988. Oral rehydration therapy. *UNICEF annual report 1988.* NY: UNICEF Headquarters.

Williams, M.H. 1992. Nutrition for fitness and sport. Dubuque, IA: William C. Brown, Publishers.

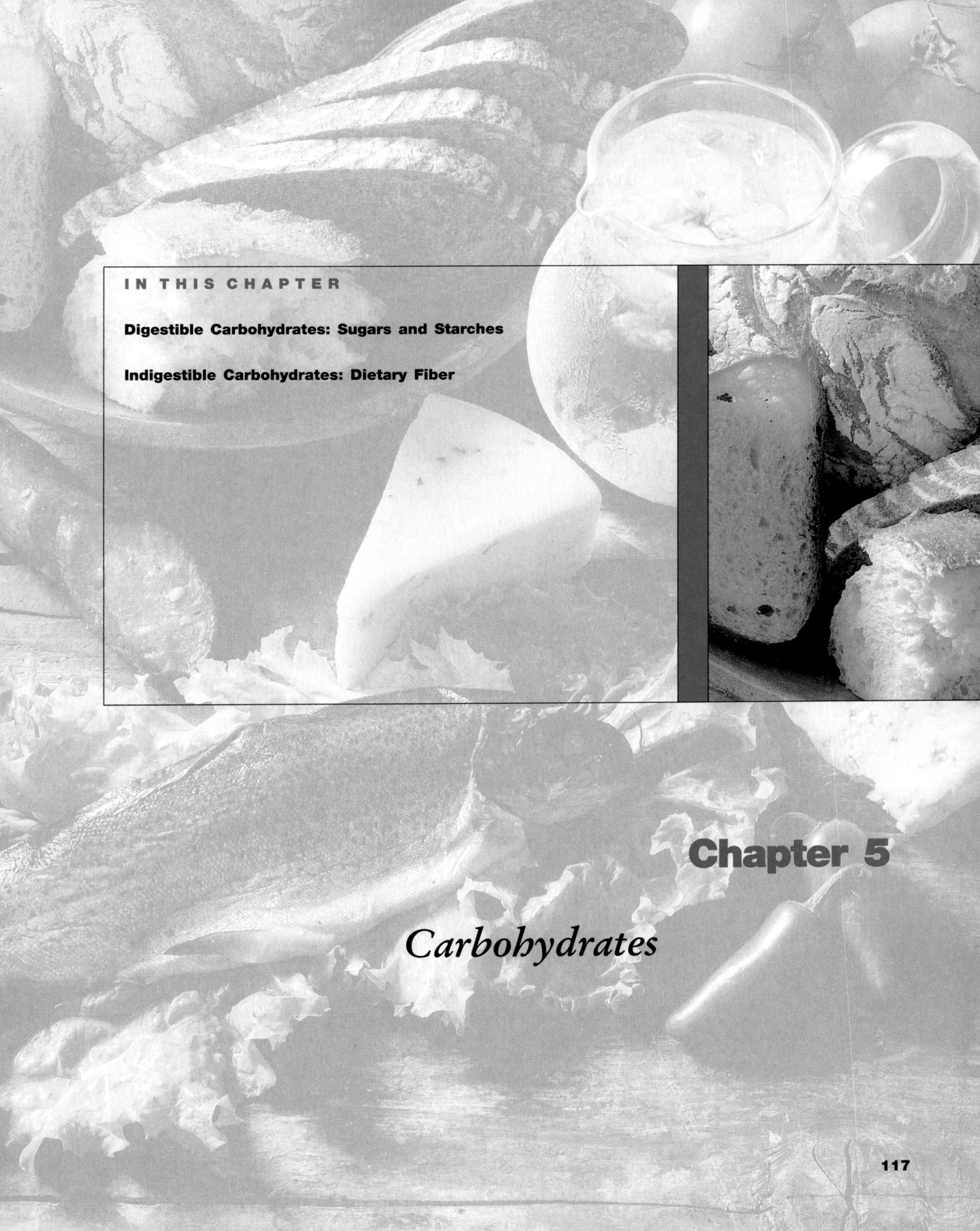

IN THIS CHAPTER

Digestible Carbohydrates: Sugars and Starches

Indigestible Carbohydrates: Dietary Fiber

Chapter 5

Carbohydrates

What do the following foods have in common: heaps of steaming pasta, a candy bar, carrot sticks, a bowl of cereal, a plate of baked beans, a can of cola, and dried apricots?

carbohydrates—compounds consisting of one or more basic units composed of 5- or 6-carbon skeletons with only hydrogens and oxygens attached

You're right if you said they are all high in **carbohydrate**. There are many different forms of carbohydrate—you probably know them as sugars, starches, and fiber—and these foods contain the whole gamut. All forms of carbohydrate are composed of carbon, hydrogen, and oxygen atoms arranged into similar chemical units.

Nonetheless, there are marked differences among the different types of carbohydrates in food. Carbohydrates can be classified into two major categories, based on a quirk of their structure and of our biology. One major type, called **digestible carbohydrates,** can readily be broken into smaller units by our bodies, absorbed, and used to generate energy. Digestible carbohydrates include *sugars* and *starches.* **Indigestible carbohydrates,** or *dietary fiber,* make up the other category. Our bodies are unable to uncouple the connecting links between the units of these carbohydrates, so the large molecules move through the gastrointestinal (GI) tract relatively unchanged.

digestible carbohydrates—sugars and starches that can be hydrolyzed by human gastrointestinal processes

indigestible carbohydrates—carbohydrates linked together in such a way that they cannot be separated by human digestive secretions; dietary fiber

A seemingly small structural variation, then, results in major differences in how these two categories of carbohydrate function in our bodies. As a result, each type offers different health risks and benefits, and we should consume different amounts of each. Most Americans don't get enough of either type to receive the greatest possible benefits, so during our discussion we will urge you to consider eating more of the foods that contain carbohydrates. Even so, remember that, as with all nutrients, it is possible to consume too much.

Let's start by considering the digestible carbohydrates.

Digestible Carbohydrates: Sugars and Starches

The vast majority of digestible carbohydrates are produced by plants. All foods of plant origin—whether fruits, vegetables, or grains—contain them, and typically several different kinds are found in the same food. The only significant animal sources are milk and some products made from milk.

In this section you'll learn what digestible carbohydrates do for you and in what forms they occur in foods, both naturally and as the result of processing.

The Function of Digestible Carbohydrates

Digestible carbohydrates are the fundamental human fuel. Sugars and starches furnish 4 kcalories per gram and are metabolized by your body to help meet its energy needs. All of your cells readily utilize **glucose,** the major breakdown product of digestible carbohydrate, but red blood cells and the cells of the central nervous system have a particular preference for it. In fact, inadequate intake of dietary carbohydrate can result in impaired functioning of the higher centers of the brain (Macdonald, 1987).

glucose—a simple carbohydrate that is found both in animals and plants; it is a readily available source of energy and a building block for more complex forms of carbohydrate

Digestible carbohydrate not only is itself a major source of energy but also plays a role in metabolizing fat for energy. A small amount of carbohydrate is needed for the series of reactions involved in fat metabolism; therefore, even when you derive a high proportion of your energy from fat, a small amount of carbohydrate *must* be involved.

If sufficient carbohydrate is not available for your body's energy needs, your metabolism will shift gears and begin to break down *protein* to use for energy instead. This, of course, is not desirable, because protein is needed for other functions only it can accomplish. When a person consumes at least the recommended level of digestible carbohydrate, therefore, protein that is needed for other purposes is spared from being used for energy.

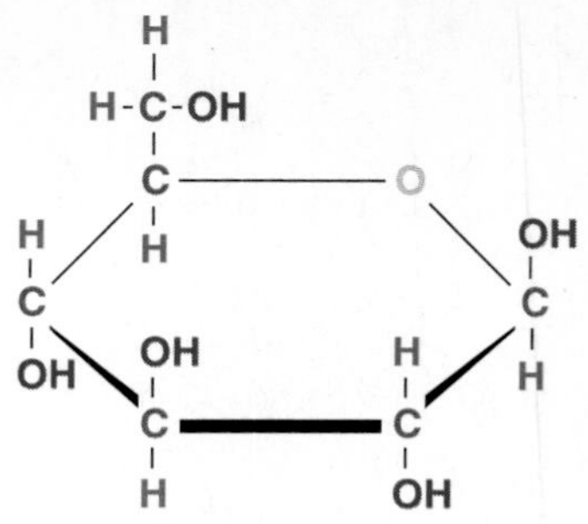

FIGURE 5.1
The structure of glucose.

This structural model of a single molecule of glucose exemplifies the organization of carbohydrates: their units have a carbon skeleton, with oxygen, hydrogen, and hydroxyl groups attached to the carbon.
Key: C = carbon, H = hydrogen, O = oxygen, and OH = hydroxyl group.

Sugars in Nature

Sugars are the smallest and least complicated of the carbohydrates; they are of varying sweetness and are soluble in water. Their solubility allows them to move readily through the watery systems of plants and animals. Names of sugars are easy to recognize by their *-ose* endings: gluc*ose,* fruct*ose,* sucr*ose.*

Green plants produce **sugar** by *photosynthesis,* a sunlight-requiring process in which carbon dioxide and water are combined to yield the simple sugar glucose and oxygen. Plants use the glucose they produce for energy.

The structure of this basic carbohydrate, as the biochemist depicts it, is shown in Figure 5.1. Although you will not see many chemical structures in this book, an occasional one gives you an idea of the composition and relative complexity of various substances. This one illustrates that six carbon (C) atoms form the skeleton of glucose. Hydrogen (H), oxygen (O), and OH groups, called *hydroxyl groups,* are attached to the carbons in an arrangement that is specific for glucose.

Glucose is one of many sugars found in nature. Others are formed with similar 6-carbon frameworks (or sometimes 5-carbon frameworks), with the H, O, and OH units in different arrangements. These types of sugars are called **monosaccharides.** *Fructose* is another example of a monosaccharide.

Glucose, fructose, and other monosaccharide molecules can be combined into **disaccharides,** which consist of two monosaccharide units linked together. Two molecules of glucose can unite to form a molecule of *maltose* (Figure 5.2), or a molecule of glucose can join a molecule of fructose to form *sucrose.* Several types of sugar usually exist simultaneously in a food of plant origin.

Sugars—in fact, all carbohydrates—contain the equivalent of one water molecule for each carbon in the structure. The term *carbohydrate* reflects the carbon, hydrogen, and oxygen contained in all carbohydrates. Scientists refer to substances that contain carbon—such as carbohydrates, fats, pro-

sugars—simple forms of carbohydrate that are sweet and soluble in water; names end with suffix *-ose*

monosaccharides—sugars consisting of a single 5- or 6-carbon unit

disaccharides—sugars consisting of two 5- or 6-carbon units

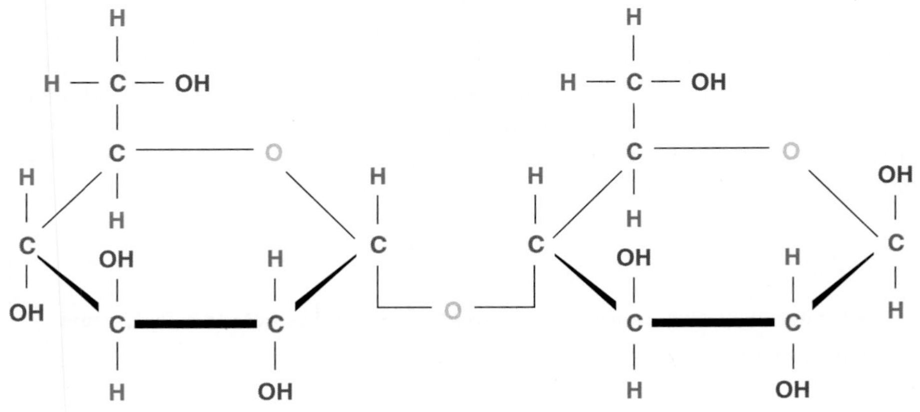

FIGURE 5.2
The structure of a disaccharide.

This model shows how two monosaccharide units (here, two units of glucose) are joined in a disaccharide (here, maltose). In more complex forms of carbohydrates, similar bonds join many monosaccharide units together in either long chains or branched structures. Starches, for example, are composed of many units of glucose.

TABLE 5.1 Most Common Sugars in Nature

Source	Monosaccharides	Disaccharides
Plants	Glucose	Sucrose = 1 glucose + 1 fructose
	Fructose	Maltose = 2 glucose
Animal milks		Lactose = 1 glucose + 1 galactose

organic—scientific definition: carbon-containing substances that originate either in nature or in the laboratory

teins, and vitamins—as **organic** substances. All living organisms, both plant and animal, use and/or produce organic materials. (*Note:* in recent decades, the term *organic* has also been used to suggest that a food has been produced without manufactured chemicals. This use of the term is discussed more thoroughly in the Slice of Life in Chapter 11 and the Thinking for Yourself in Chapter 13. Unless otherwise specified, however, the scientists' use of the term applies in this textbook.)

In which plants are sugars found? Actually, all plants contain some sugar in their juices, although the amounts vary from one part of the plant to another. Fruits usually contain more liberal amounts of sugar; most roots, leaves, stems, and tubers contain less; and seeds have varying amounts. There are a few unusually rich nonfruit sources of sugar, though, such as sugar cane (stem) and sugar beet (root).

A major sugar that occurs naturally in animal foods is the disaccharide *lactose,* which is found in animal milks. Lactose consists of a unit of glucose joined to a unit of *galactose,* another 6-carbon sugar molecule.

Table 5.1 summarizes the most common sugars in nature.

Sugars and Processing

concentrated sugars—solid or liquid substances consisting largely of sugar; added to other foods as sweeteners (examples: cane sugar, beet sugar, maple syrup, honey, corn syrup)

As you've just learned, nature produces sugars in many foods. However, many foods also contain sugar that people—not nature—have put there. Everyone is born with a preference for the sweet taste, and although this preference tends to diminish to some degree after childhood, sweetness continues to influence many people's food choices. Therefore, we extract **concentrated sugars** such as maple syrup, molasses, brown sugar, white sugar (pure sucrose), and honey from naturally sweet sources and add them to our food.

Food scientists have also found ways to produce sweeteners from the starches in grains such as corn, rice, and barley. These are the sources of many of the sweet syrups and much of the glucose (sometimes called *dextrose*) and fructose (sometimes called *levulose*) currently used in processed foods. They are major ingredients in such products as sherbet, ice cream, gelatin desserts, sweet baked goods, and some cereals. *High fructose corn syrup* is a common sweetener in soft drinks. Lactose, another sugar commonly added to foods, is obtained from whey, the watery by-product of cheesemaking. Other carbohydrate terms you may see are *turbinado sugar* (a steam-cleaned, partially refined sugar) and *total invert sugar* (a modified, liquefied form of sucrose that is used commercially).

You Tell Me

An advertisement claims that a food contains "sweeteners only from natural sources."

Which sweeteners could these be? Which would be excluded? What do you think the advertiser wants you to believe about these sugars?

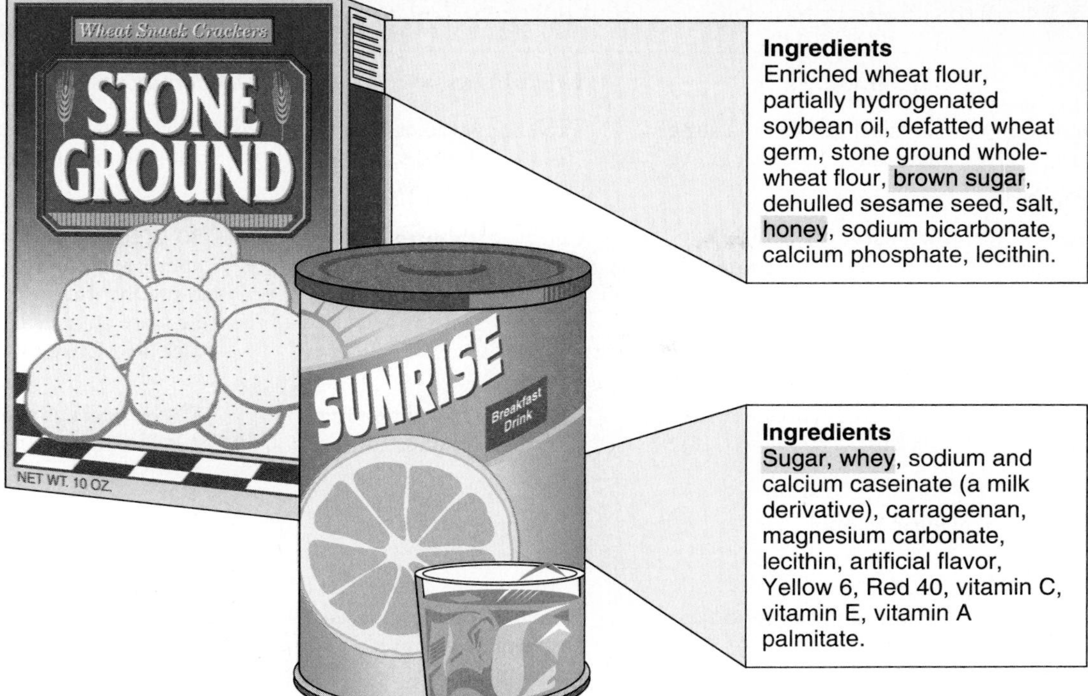

FIGURE 5.3
Examples of sugars in two processed foods.

You can find out which sugary components your foods contain by checking their ingredient lists. Ingredients must be listed in order from the most to the least amount in the product.

Read the ingredient list on the labels of foods you eat, and see how many sugar sources you can identify. Figure 5.3 shows two examples. You can get a rough idea of how much added sugar a food contains by noting the position of the sugars on the list, because ingredients must be ranked according to their weights in the product, from the largest to the smallest.

Data collected by the United States Department of Agriculture indicate that in recent years, approximately 127 pounds per person per year of all types of concentrated sugars together "disappeared" from the U.S. marketplace. However, it is not accurate to assume that per capita consumption is actually this high. Such *disappearance data* do not take into account waste that occurs during production, distribution, storage, and usage of foods, nor do they account for the sugar that goes into such products as pet food and alcoholic beverages. It is difficult to estimate how much less than 127 pounds the actual average consumption is.

Some people, maybe including you, want to enjoy the sweetness of sugar without experiencing the negative consequences of sugar ingestion, such as weight gain and tooth decay. To meet this demand, the food industry has developed a number of **sugar substitutes** for use in food products. Some sugar substitutes are chemical derivatives of naturally occurring carbohydrates or other natural components of food, and others are completely new additions to the food supply.

sugar substitutes—substances that are sweet but chemically different from ordinary natural sugars; may or may not have kcaloric value

To circumvent the problem of tooth decay, derivatives of sugars and starches called **sugar alcohols,** which are sweet but do not promote tooth decay, are used in some foods. The sugar alcohols are *maltitol, mannitol, sorbitol,* and *xylitol.* In fact, xylitol has been shown in a number of studies actually to *inhibit* tooth decay (Pepper and Olinger, 1988). But here's a fact that may surprise you: the sugar alcohols have the same energy value as carbohydrates; that is, because of their close structural relationship to carbohydrates, they provide 4 kcalories per gram.

sugar alcohols—compounds structurally related to sugars and used as sweeteners

TABLE 5.2 Sugar Substitutes

Substance	Description	Typical Uses	Comments
Acesulfame-K Sunette® Sweet One®	Chemical not in food supply naturally	Table top sweetener, dry foods and mixes, chewing gum, soft drinks	200 times as sweet as sucrose; no kcalories
Aspartame Nutrasweet® Equal®	Two naturally occurring components of protein linked together	Candy, carbonated beverages, chewing gum, gelatin dessert, puddings	180–200 times as sweet as sucrose; has 4 kcal/gram, but contributes few kcal because so little is needed (see also Chapter 7)
Maltitol Lycasin® Almalty®	Sugar alcohol made from starch	Candy; approval pending for more applications	75% as sweet as sucrose; has 4 kcal/g; does not cause tooth decay
Mannitol	Sugar alcohol	Chewing gum	65% as sweet as sucrose; has 4 kcal/g; does not cause tooth decay
Saccharine	Chemical not in food supply naturally	Primarily being replaced by aspartame but used in some chewing gums	300–400 times as sweet as sucrose; has no kcalories (see also Chapter 14)
Sorbitol	Sugar alcohol made from glucose	Candy, chewing gum, cough drops, breath mints	50% as sweet as sucrose; causes bloating and diarrhea in some people; has 4 kcal/g; does not cause tooth decay
Thaumatin Talin®	Protein	Chewing gum	400–2000 times as sweet as sucrose; few kcalories because so little is needed
Xylitol	Sugar alcohol made from substances high in hemicellulose; naturally present in many fruits and vegetables	Special diet candies and chewing gums	Same sweetness as sucrose; has 4 kcal/g; helps prevent tooth decay

References: Institute of Food Technologists (IFT), 1989b; IFT, 1987; Jain et al., 1987.

You Tell Me

A package of "sugar-free" chewing gum that contains sugar alcohols for sweetening is labeled "NOT NONCALORIC."

What does this mean?

Because some people want to avoid the kcalories in sugar and sugar alcohols, sugar substitutes that have few, if any, kcalories are used in many products. Table 5.2 summarizes information about many sugar substitutes. Some, such as *aspartame* and *thaumatin,* consist of chemicals similar to those that occur naturally in the food supply, though not as sugars. Others are very different from substances commonly found in the food supply; examples of such artificial sweeteners are *acesulfame-K* and *saccharine.*

Because sugar substitutes vary considerably in their characteristics and effects, you need to be selective to get the feature(s) you want. The safety of some sugar substitutes has been questioned; this issue is discussed in the appropriate chapters. Aspartame is discussed in Chapter 7 (on proteins); more information on other artificial sweeteners is found in Chapter 14 (on food safety issues).

Starches in Nature

Some of the glucose produced in plants is converted into **starches,** the insoluble, nonsweet forms of carbohydrate in which plants store energy. Because a single starch molecule can consist of hundreds of units of glucose linked together, they are also referred to as *polysaccharides* or *complex carbohydrates.*

starches—nonsweet, complex forms of carbohydrate consisting of sugar units linked together

Starches usually concentrate in plant seeds, roots, and tubers. Grains, nuts, legumes, root vegetables, and potatoes are particularly good sources. Fruits have much less of these complex carbohydrates.

Starches and Processing

Various processing methods are used to alter the nature of starches. When starch is exposed to dry heat, as it is in the production of cold cereals or in the baking of bread, some of the large starch molecules are broken down into somewhat smaller units called *dextrins.*

For use in the brewing industry, grain (especially barley) is *malted* (sprouted) and then dried. The enzymes produced in the malting process split starch within the sprouted grain into dextrins and maltose. These products, in turn, nourish the growth of the yeast that produces alcohol. Various malted grains are also used as ingredients in some ready-to-eat breakfast cereals.

Modified starch, which you find in some processed foods such as puddings, is starch that has been treated to enhance its ability to thicken or gel.

Amounts of Digestible Carbohydrates in Foods

Table 5.3 shows how the total amounts of digestible carbohydrates compare among the foods of the Pyramid's groups. The solid parts of the bars represent naturally occurring sugars and starches; the broken parts of the bars indicate added concentrated sugars.

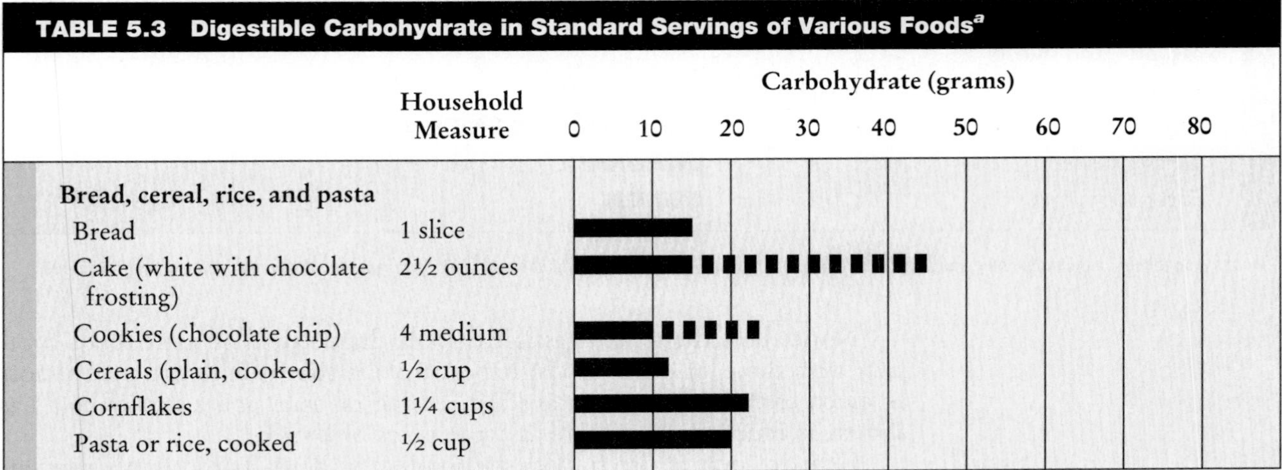

TABLE 5.3 Digestible Carbohydrate in Standard Servings of Various Foods[a]

	Household Measure	Carbohydrate (grams): 0 10 20 30 40 50 60 70 80
Bread, cereal, rice, and pasta		
Bread	1 slice	
Cake (white with chocolate frosting)	2½ ounces	
Cookies (chocolate chip)	4 medium	
Cereals (plain, cooked)	½ cup	
Cornflakes	1¼ cups	
Pasta or rice, cooked	½ cup	

[a]Broken sections of bars represent added concentrated sugars. Data sources: Matthews, 1987; Pennington, 1989; calculation from recipes.

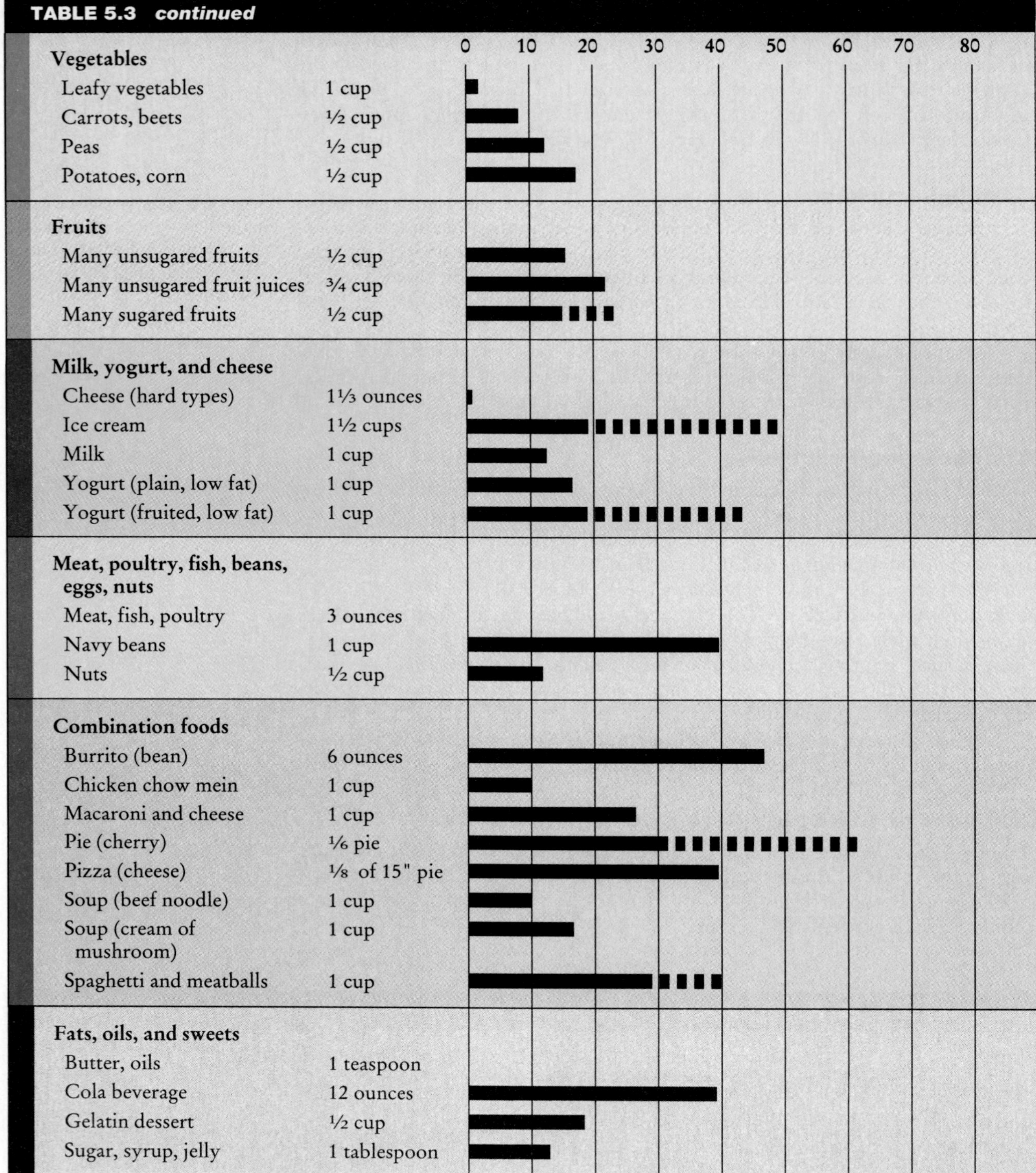

[a]Broken sections of bars represent added concentrated sugars. Data sources: Matthews, 1987; Pennington, 1989; calculation from recipes.

Notice how the total digestible carbohydrate values of some foods compare with those of other foods: for example, a cup of milk contains almost as much carbohydrate as an average serving of fruit, and a can of cola has almost as much carbohydrate as three slices of bread.

Other resources also provide carbohydrate values. For example, Appendix C gives digestible carbohydrate values for hundreds of foods, and as of

protein in milk. A protein allergy is distinctly different from lactose intolerance. (Allergies are discussed in Chapter 7.) Protein allergy is most likely to occur in very young infants, but fewer than 1% of babies have this condition (Scrimshaw and Murray, 1988). People allergic to milk protein will not be helped by avoiding lactose.

Ingestion of Sugar Alcohols Sugar alcohols, which do not require digestion, are absorbed relatively slowly because of a special mechanism by which they are transported through the villi of the small intestine. Therefore, a portion of ingested sugar alcohols usually fails to be absorbed and moves on to the colon. Some people may experience symptoms similar to those of lactose intolerance when they consume large amounts of sugar alcohols. The amount that is present in a single stick of chewing gum is not usually large enough to cause this effect, but chewing several sticks of gum or eating a number of pieces of candy sweetened with sugar alcohol causes symptoms in some people. The sugar alcohol sorbitol also occurs naturally in many fruits; prunes have the most.

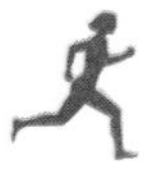

Concentrated Sugar Plus Athletic Activity Sometimes athletes consume concentrated sugary foods or drinks before or during athletic activity, thinking that the sugars will provide extra energy. Generally they do, but in some situations this practice may be counterproductive.

One possible problem involves the GI tract. If your intestines react to activity (or the nervousness that may accompany competition) by moving material through the small intestine more rapidly than usual, undigested disaccharides and/or unabsorbed monosaccharides will reach the colon, which can result in a very inopportune bout of diarrhea, appropriately nicknamed "runner's trots."

Consuming large amounts of sugar during exercise can also have a negative effect on hydration. A high concentration of sugar delays stomach emptying and hence absorption of water; concentrations higher than 10% (that is, 100 grams of fructose and/or glucose per liter of beverage, or 24 grams per 8 ounces) cause some interference (American Dietetic Association, 1987). Some fruit juices, fruit drinks, and other sugar-sweetened beverages have more than this amount. If the sugar content of the beverage you want to use exceeds 24 grams per 8 ounces of beverage, you should dilute it. Table 5.6 gives the sugar content in various sports beverages and some ordinary beverages. •

You Tell Me

After a person has had a severe gastrointestinal infection with diarrhea, the levels of enzymes that are normally present in the GI tract to digest carbohydrates may be reduced for an additional couple of days.

What would be the likely consequence of this? Does a brief continuation of the diarrhea necessarily indicate that the infection is still in process?

What Happens to Glucose Inside the Body

After you've eaten potatoes, bread, or some other carbohydrate-containing food and the carbohydrate has been digested and absorbed into your villi, most of the sugars travel via the bloodstream to your liver. There, the major-

TABLE 5.6 Sugar Content of Various Beverages

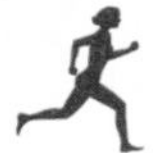

Many experts recommend that during endurance exercise it is best to drink beverages with a carbohydrate concentration of 12–24 grams per 8 ounces (5–10%). If the beverage that you want to use is more concentrated than that, you can add water to bring it into the right range.

Beverage	Carbohydrate (g) per 8 oz.	% Carbohydrate (by volume)
Fruit Juices		
Apple	29	12
Cranberry	36	15
Grape	32	13
Grapefruit	24	10
Orange	27	11
Carbonated Beverages		
Coca Cola	26	11
Sprite	24	10
Commercial sport drinks		
Bodyfuel 450	10	4
Carbo Energizer	59	25
Exceed Fluid Replacement	17	7
Exceed High Carb.	59	25
Gatorade	14	6
Isostar	18	7
Sqwincher	16	7
Ultra Fuel	50	21
Other		
Kool Aid	20	8
Lemonade from frozen concentrate	28	12

ity are converted to glucose. What happens to the glucose after this? Ultimately, of course, your body's cells use it for energy production, but not all of it is needed at once. In fact, only a small amount of glucose is metabolized for energy right away. Another small portion stays conveniently available in your bloodstream and interstitial fluids. The largest amounts are converted to energy-storage materials.

Several factors work together to determine how and when the glucose is handled. These factors include the activity of your liver and its enzymes, several hormones, and your muscles.

The Liver and Its Enzymes After every meal, your body puts most of the glucose you have absorbed into energy-storage forms: enzymes in your liver convert much of it into materials that will later make up **glycogen** and fat molecules. This helps keep the level of glucose in your blood within a normal range, even after a substantial carbohydrate intake. (A condition in which the body does not respond normally to carbohydrate intake—called reactive hypoglycemia—will be discussed shortly.)

glycogen—complex carbohydrate produced in animals that is somewhat similar to the starch produced by plants

Conversely, if you don't eat anything for several hours, your blood glucose gradually drifts to a low level within the normal range. This prompts other enzymes in your liver to break glycogen apart into glucose and release

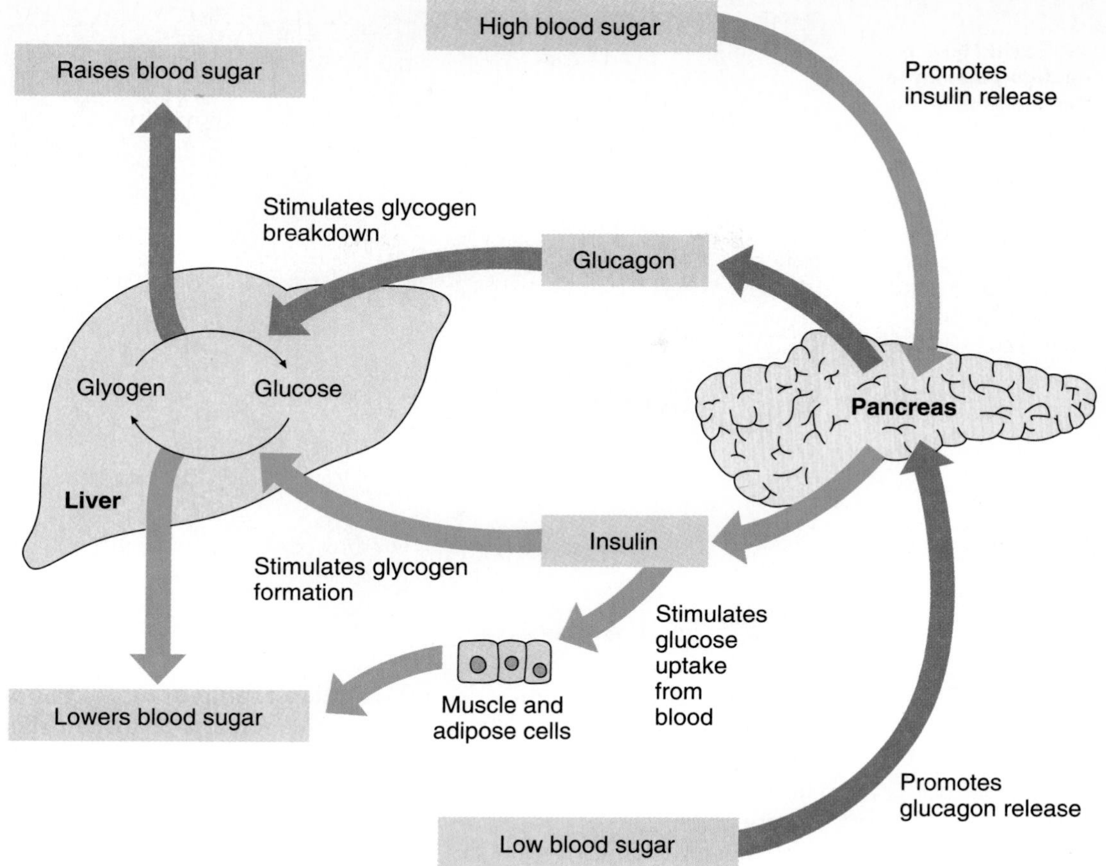

FIGURE 5.5
Regulation of blood sugar levels by insulin and glucagon.

When blood sugar levels are high, the pancreas releases insulin. Insulin stimulates sugar uptake by cells and glycogen formation in the liver, which lowers blood sugar levels. Glucagon, released when blood sugar levels are low, stimulates glycogen breakdown and thereby raises blood sugar.

it into the blood, raising the glucose level back up. You can often sense when these events are occurring. When your blood glucose drops to low-normal, you initially feel hungry and possibly tired; after a while, however, even if you still don't eat anything, the hunger and tiredness seem less pronounced as glycogen is converted into blood glucose. This sequence of events is totally normal and desirable.

Hormones Several hormones also cooperate in regulating your blood sugar level. **Insulin,** a hormone produced by the pancreas, has a major influence. Part of its function is to help glucose get into various body cells.

When your blood glucose level rises, your pancreas produces more than the maintenance level of insulin and releases it into the bloodstream. The insulin causes body cells to remove the excess glucose from your blood. Then in both liver and skeletal muscle cells, the insulin promotes the production of glycogen; in both liver and fat cells, it promotes the formation of fat. At the same time, insulin discourages the breakdown of fat for energy, causing the body to rely more heavily on the recently ingested carbohydrate for energy production.

When your blood sugar level falls, your pancreas increases its production of a different hormone, **glucagon,** which has the opposite effect of insulin. Glucagon encourages the liver to break glycogen back down into glucose. Glucagon also promotes the utilization of fat. Some other hormones have this same effect, particularly *epinephrine,* which is produced by the adrenal glands when the body has a sudden, high demand for energy. Figure 5.5 shows the effects of various levels of blood glucose on the production of insulin and glucagon.

insulin—hormone produced by the pancreas; helps to regulate the blood sugar level by promoting glucose utilization, protein synthesis, and formation and storage of lipids

glucagon—hormone produced by the pancreas; has the opposite effect of insulin, helping to regulate the blood sugar level by promoting the breakdown of glycogen and fat

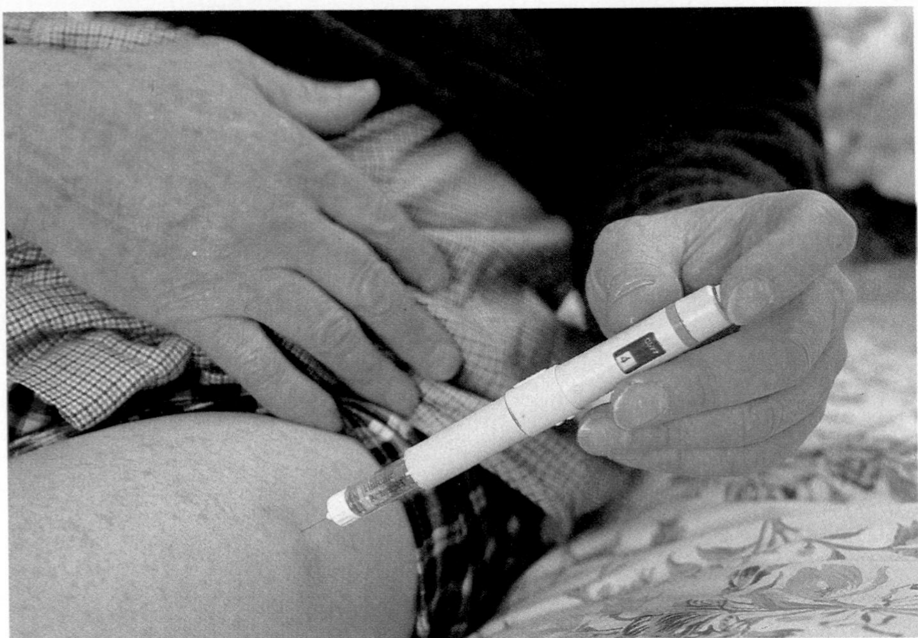

FIGURE 5.6
Insulin-dependent (Type I) diabetic injecting insulin to supply what the body does not produce.

If you were a Type 1 diabetic, your health care professionals would recommend the type, amount, and timing of your insulin injections, taking into account your weight, your diet, and your exercise habits.

Some people's bodies do not handle carbohydrate in the ways just described because of an abnormality in the amount of insulin their bodies produce or in the way their cells react to the insulin. Approximately 11 million Americans are estimated to have these conditions (Surgeon General's Report, 1988).

In some people, the pancreas does not produce enough insulin to accomplish its usual tasks. In such instances, sugar builds up in the blood; without sufficient insulin, sugar cannot be taken into body cells for energy production or converted to glycogen or fat. This condition is called **insulin-dependent (Type I) diabetes:** people with this disease need to inject insulin to make up for their lack of it (Figure 5.6). Note that eating sugars and starches is not the cause of diabetes; rather, researchers theorize that diabetes may result from a hereditary tendency of a person's body to destroy insulin-producing cells and/or from a viral infection.

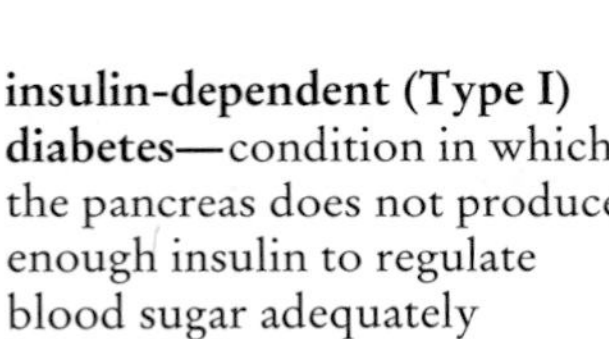

insulin-dependent (Type I) diabetes—condition in which the pancreas does not produce enough insulin to regulate blood sugar adequately

In the past, insulin-dependent diabetics have been advised to restrict their carbohydrate intake rigidly. But in recent years, studies of insulin-dependent diabetics have shown that blood sugar levels are influenced not only by the total amount of carbohydrate eaten but also by the type of carbohydrate and/or the food(s) in which it was consumed. Some researchers have attempted to identify the rate and extent to which various foods influence blood sugar concentration, representing these values on a scale called the *glycemic index* (Anderson, 1988). However, it is difficult to apply these glycemic index values in practical situations. In general, diabetics can achieve good blood sugar control on diets that are high in complex carbohydrates and soluble fiber (Anderson et al., 1987). (Soluble fiber is discussed later in this chapter.)

Some people (usually adults) produce plenty of insulin, but for some reason the insulin cannot perform its role of carrying glucose into body cells. This is a form of diabetes quite different from and approximately ten times more prevalent than the one just mentioned; it is called **non-insulin-dependent (Type II) diabetes.** Because people who get it are often overweight, it is primarily treated with a weight-reduction program, which may in itself bring the condition under control. Sometimes, a diet that is high in

non-insulin-dependent (Type II) diabetes—condition in which adequate amounts of insulin are produced but not used normally

soluble fiber or an oral drug that helps lower blood glucose is also part of the treatment. There is probably a hereditary influence on this condition.

A much more unusual metabolic dysfunction is the *overproduction* of insulin in response to carbohydrate ingestion. In this case, a small rise in blood glucose from a normal diet causes an abnormally large outpouring of insulin from the pancreas, and blood sugar drops sharply below the normal range 2–4 hours after a meal. At the same time, sweating, tremulousness, palpitations, headaches, hunger, weakness, and anxiety occur. The condition is called *reactive hypoglycemia* (Kanarek and Marks-Kaufman, 1991). **Hypoglycemia** simply refers to blood sugar that has fallen below the normal range for any of a number of reasons. The adjective *reactive* specifies that the hypoglycemia occurs *in reaction to* normal amounts of ingested carbohydrate.

hypoglycemia—general term for condition in which blood sugar falls below the normal range; can occur for any of a number of reasons

Many people who superficially appear to have reactive hypoglycemia really don't have it; they are actually experiencing reactions to stress and anxiety. Stress causes the release of the hormone *epinephrine,* which ultimately brings about some of the same symptoms as does excessive insulin. Only carefully conducted laboratory tests and accompanying reports of the patient's symptoms can provide an accurate diagnosis.

For those few who do have it, reactive hypoglycemia can be controlled (but not cured) by limiting the amount of carbohydrate consumed at each eating occasion. It helps to eat small, frequent meals throughout the day.

Muscles Your muscles also affect what happens to glucose within your body. Exercise depresses insulin production. You might think that this would interfere with your cells' uptake of glucose and therefore interfere with energy production; however, exercise also prompts skeletal muscle cells to take in more glucose from the bloodstream than usual. With more glucose in your muscle cells, you can produce more energy so that your muscles can continue their work.

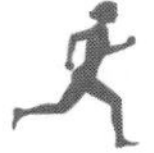

For Endurance Athletes: Using Carbohydrate to Advantage

Athletes who begin endurance activities (sports in which they are continuously active for more than an hour) with the largest possible amount of glycogen in their liver and muscles can perform longer. Classic studies have demonstrated that the amount of glycogen in muscles at the start of a bout of exercise is directly proportional to the amount of time an athlete can perform before exhaustion sets in (Figure 5.7).

If you exercise hard day after day, you need to consume a high-carbohydrate diet to deposit glycogen before exercise and restore it afterward. Whereas the average nonathlete is advised to get at least half his or her kcalories from carbohydrate, the endurance athlete is often advised to get 60–70% of kcalories from carbohydrate (Applegate, 1991a; Sherman and Wright, 1989). Sports nutritionist and triathlete Liz Applegate gives an example of how you can change a high-fat diet into a high-carbohydrate one (Table 5.7). Later, in the Act on Fact on page 142, you will learn how to assess your own intake of carbohydrate.

Some athletes preparing for an endurance event attempt to achieve the highest possible muscle and liver glycogen through a process called **glycogen loading** or **carbohydrate loading.** The process begins about a week before the event and involves modifying the nature of both your workouts and your diet. Early in the week, you train hard; but as the week progresses, you taper off, just resting or doing an easy warm-up a day or two before

glycogen loading, carbohydrate loading—maximizing body stores of glycogen by controlling both exercise and food consumption

FIGURE 5.7
The relationship between diet, muscle glycogen, and endurance.

When subjects were fed high-fat/high-protein diets for several days, leg muscle glycogen was low, and endurance for pedaling an exercise bicycle was lower than normal. When fed a high-carbohydrate diet (approximately 80% of kcalories) for several days, both muscle glycogen and work increased automatically. (From McArdle, et al., 1991. Adapted from Bergstrom, 1967.)

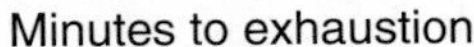

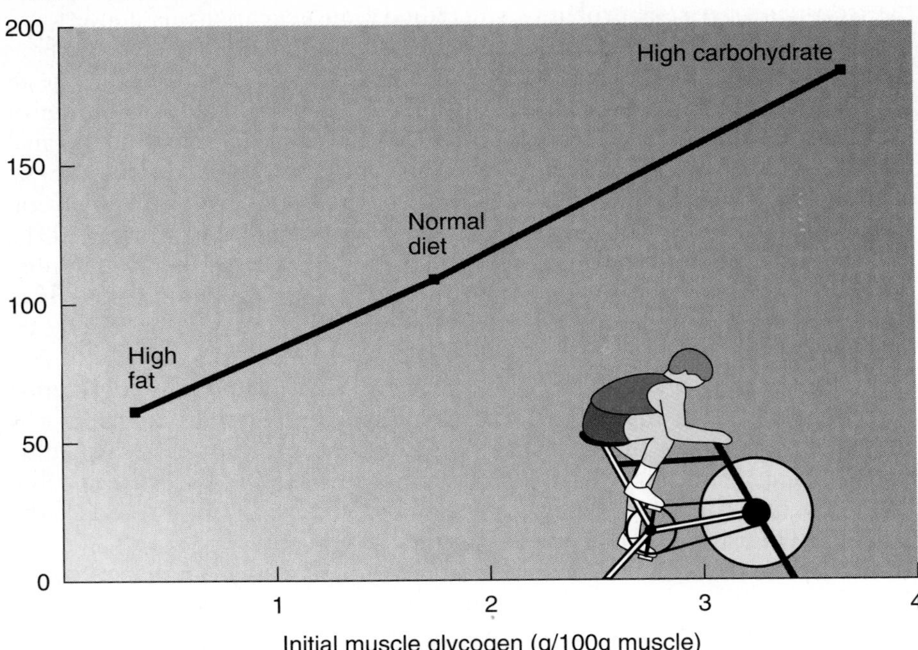

TABLE 5.7 Meal Makeovers: Moving from a High-Fat to a High-Carbohydrate Diet

High-Fat (Before)	High-Carbohydrate (After)
Breakfast	
At fast-food restaurant	
1 croissant breakfast sandwich	2 bagels and fruit spread
6 ounces orange juice	1 cup low-fat yogurt with ¾ cup strawberries
Coffee with cream	Coffee with low-fat milk
Lunch	
At restaurant	
2 cups pasta with seafood and cream sauce	2 cups bean chili
Tossed green salad with house dressing	Salad with vinegar or lemon juice dressing
1 slice French bread with butter	2 slices French bread
	¾ cup fruit sorbet
Dinner	
From take-out restaurant	
2 egg rolls	Stir-fry vegetables
1 cup fried rice	1 cup steamed rice
1 cup chow mein	1 cup beef and broccoli stir-fry
1 ice cream cone	5 fig bars
Analysis	
Total calories: 2420	Total calories: 2220
42% carbohydrate	60% carbohydrate
40% fat	24% fat

Source: Applegate, 1991b.

the event. (This has led some athletes to refer to the training regimen as "loaf loading.")

Meanwhile, at the beginning of the week, you should eat whatever you usually do. In the last few days before the event, however, eat very high amounts of carbohydrate—in the range of 500 to 600 grams per day. Some research suggests that this high absolute amount of carbohydrate, rather than a particular percentage, may be what is important. Scientists discovered in one study that a group of competitive college swimmers who consumed 500 grams of carbohydrate per day, which—because of their very high total energy intakes—represented only 43% of their kcaloric intake, achieved times that were as good as those of team members who consumed a higher percentage of kcalories from carbohydrate (Lamb et al., 1990).

People vary markedly in their reaction to glycogen loading. Those who like it say that it allows them to continue farther and/or faster at the end of an endurance activity (such as the last several miles of a marathon) than they could otherwise have done. Glycogen loading does not, however, provide any benefit in the earlier stages of the event (Williams, 1992).

Other athletes have not felt any benefit at all; in fact, they have been bothered by the extra water-weight they carried as a result of glycogen loading: for every gram of glycogen stored, 2.7 grams of water are also retained.

You Tell Me

The typical amount of glycogen stored in the muscles of a 150-pound man is approximately 400 grams. Glycogen loading can double or triple this amount.

If a 150-pound man loaded carbohydrate and increased his muscle glycogen to twice the usual amount, what would be the weight of the extra water in these muscles? How do you think your muscles would feel if they contained this amount of extra fluid? Do you think you should try carbohydrate loading for the first time before an event that is important to you?

What about the *last meal eaten before an event?* The advice from some exercise physiologists: "A carbohydrate meal or beverage can be consumed from 4 hours before exercise up to minutes before exercise without a detrimental effect on performance in most athletes" (Sherman and Wright, 1989). However, Applegate, the nutritionist/triathlete, takes into account the possibility that pre-event nervousness could cause stomach upset if the athlete eats too close to competition; therefore, she recommends that athletes eat a light meal of 300–600 kcalories, mostly as carbohydrate, about 3 hours before exercise. The ultraendurance athlete probably needs an even higher energy intake at that time (Applegate, 1991a).

It also helps to take in some carbohydrate *during endurance exercise* (Figure 5.8). The recommended intake is 15–20 grams of carbohydrate every 15–20 minutes. As with carbohydrate loading before an event, consuming carbohydrate during an event does not improve your performance at the *beginning* of activity but can extend endurance at the *end* of a very long event. If you are consuming carbohydrate as a fluid, a 5–10% solution (that is, 12–24 grams of carbohydrate per 8 ounces of fluid) is recommended (Williams, 1992).

FIGURE 5.8
Fueling on course.

If you are vigorously and continuously active for more than an hour, you would probably benefit from taking in some carbohydrate along the way.

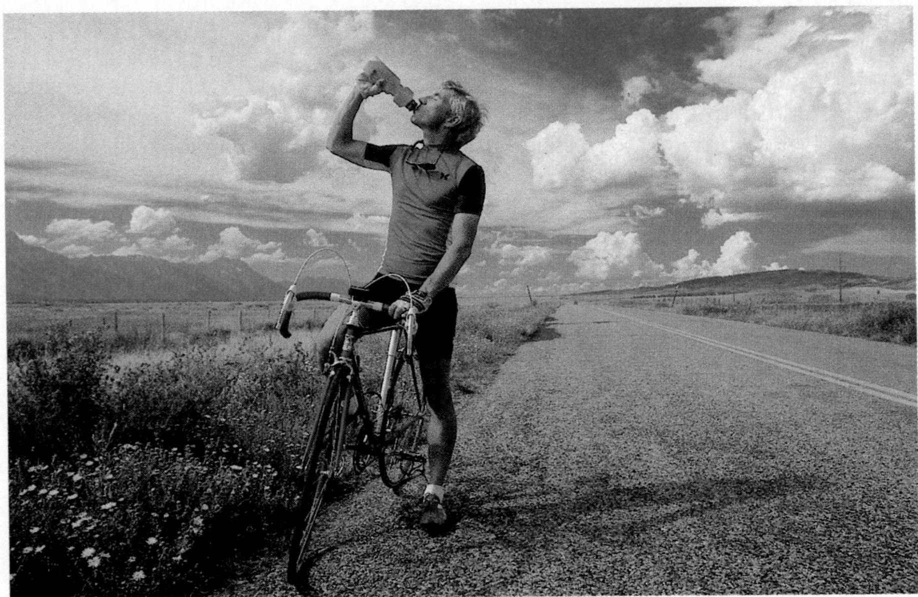

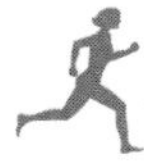

Research shows that it doesn't matter what form of carbohydrate you take in: about 99% of the carbohydrate—whether glucose, fructose, sucrose, *maltodextrins,* or *glucose polymers*—is converted by your body to glucose and starts to appear in the bloodstream about 5 minutes after ingestion (Costill, 1990). (Maltodextrins and glucose polymers are synthetically produced; their molecules are larger and less sweet than disaccharides but smaller than dextrins.)

Carbohydrate consumption *after exercise* is also important, especially if you want to exercise again within a day or two after an exhausting competition or workout. Glycogen restoration in your liver and muscles is influenced by when and how much carbohydrate you consume. Applegate (1991b) recommends small carbohydrate meals or snacks starting right after competition and every 2 hours after that; Gisolfi and Duchman (1992) recommend at least 50 grams of carbohydrate *per hour* during the first 2 hours. If you can't tolerate solid food right after exercising, high-carbohydrate beverages might help; those that contain the less-sweet forms of carbohydrate, such as maltodextrins and glucose polymers, might be more palatable and therefore more successful (Ivy, 1989). •

Digestible Carbohydrates and Health Problems

Sugars and starches have been accused, most often unjustly, of damaging health. Now let's take a look at the various accusations, both warranted and unwarranted, that have been fired at carbohydrates.

Unfair Accusation: Sugars and Starches Make People Fat Digestible carbohydrates are not inherently fattening. What makes people overly fat is an excess intake of kcalories from *all energy sources combined.* The kcalories from sugars and starches are no more fattening than surplus kcalories from proteins, fats, or alcohol; in fact, there is some evidence that they are less so. (This issue is discussed further in Chapter 8.) Further, a recent study of food intakes of over 30,000 people in the United States revealed that high consumers of added sugar had body weights similar to those of moderate consumers (Lewis et al., 1992).

Unfair Accusation: Sugars Cause Hyperactivity Studies done in the last decade show that sugars do *not* cause hyperactivity (Kanarek and Marks-Kaufman, 1991). In well-controlled dietary challenge studies, consumption of sugar has not been shown to have negative effects on motor activity, spontaneous behavior, performance in psychologic tests, learning, memory, attention span, or problem-solving abilities.

Why, then, do many people associate sugar with hyperactivity? The results of a small correlational study published in 1980 were widely misreported in the popular media, and despite much research to refute it, the myth persists. Many educators, parents, and even physicians are misinformed on this matter (Kanarek and Marks-Kaufman, 1991). (For more information, see Chapter 16.)

Justifiable Concern: Digestible Carbohydrates Promote Dental Caries Sugars and cooked starches bear some guilt in the matter of tooth decay. In essence, **dental caries,** or **cavities,** occur when susceptible teeth are exposed over time to acids, which are produced when bacteria metabolize any fermentable carbohydrates in the mouth.

dental caries, cavities—destruction of tooth enamel and decay of interior tooth materials; caused by acids that dissolve mineral out of enamel

Let's look first at factors that promote acid production and tooth decay. Then we'll discuss ways you can prevent tooth decay.

Some people's teeth are more prone to decay than others'. *Susceptibility* can be inherited, but diet can also be involved. A child who has had access to a sufficient amount of the mineral fluoride during the tooth-forming years has a denser tooth surface (enamel) that is less likely to decay throughout life than does the child who has not. As a result, susceptibility is individually variable.

A factor that almost everybody is subject to is *mouth bacteria.* The organism most often implicated is *Streptococcus mutans,* a common mouth resident that metabolizes fermentable carbohydrates. The bacteria produce acid by-products that slowly dissolve the minerals from the enamel on the outside of the tooth, making the softer structures inside the tooth more vulnerable to decay. Other bacteria are thought to play a less important role.

The common sugars sucrose, glucose, fructose, maltose, and lactose are all highly fermentable and are almost equally likely to cause decay on a gram-for-gram basis. This is true whether the sugars occur naturally in the food or are added to it. Cooked starches—that is, starches that have been processed with heat—also support the growth of mouth bacteria; cooked starches are found in such foods as breads, cereals, pasta, and popped corn. Sugar alcohols, by contrast, are not as easily metabolized by mouth bacteria. For this reason, they are commonly used in "sugarless" chewing gum and candy.

Another factor in dental caries is a food's *stickiness.* Sticky foods cling to tooth surfaces, making food available to mouth bacteria for an extended period. Which foods are most likely to leave small particles around your teeth? Although the classic villains, such as caramels, rank as moderately sticky, dried fruits are worse, and foods most likely to cling are cereals, crackers, and cookies.

Frequency of eating is important as well, because acid production continues for approximately 30 minutes after the last mouthful is swallowed (National Research Council, 1989). That means, for example, that it is less damaging to eat a popsicle, which is eaten quickly, than to eat hard candy with an equivalent amount of sugar at intervals throughout the day. Even apples, once thought of as "nature's toothbrush," can contribute to tooth decay if consumed very frequently: farm workers who ate at least 8 apples per day during the harvest season had substantially more decayed, missing, and filled teeth than controls (Grobler and Blignaut, 1989).

FIGURE 5.9
Factors that together promote tooth decay.

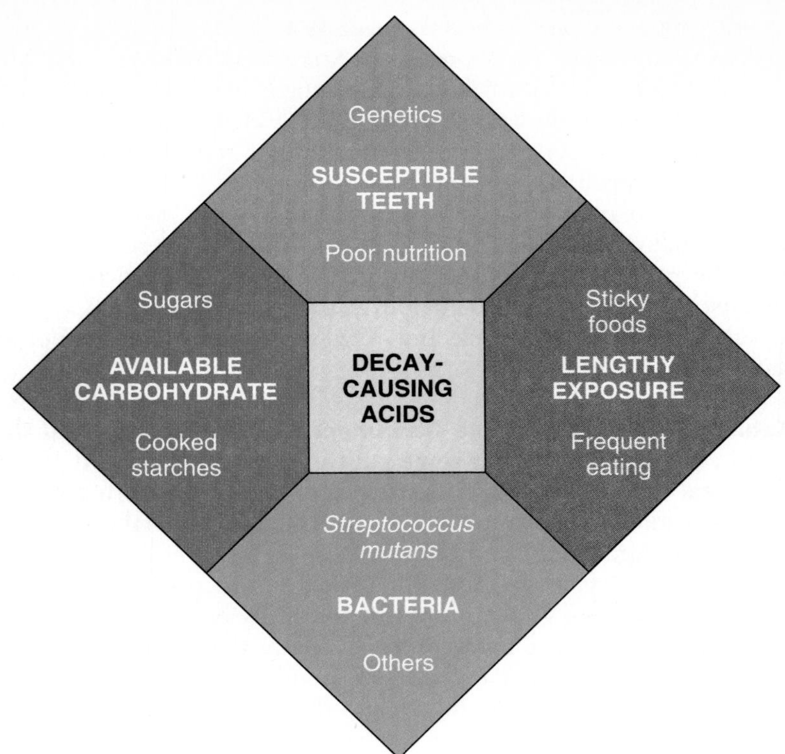

Timing of eating also plays a role: fermentable carbohydrates consumed *between meals rather than with meals* are more likely to result in tooth decay. For example, researchers found that drinking soft drinks *with* meals was not associated with high incidence of decay; drinking sodas three times or more *between* meals daily, however, was associated with almost twice the incidence of decay (Nutrition Reviews, 1987).

Figure 5.9 summarizes the factors that increase the risk of decay.

There are positive things you can do to discourage decay. *Saliva* helps deter decay in a number of ways: it washes sugars away from teeth, and it contains materials that actually promote remineralization of eroded tooth enamel to a certain extent (Featherstone, 1987). As a result, any practice that stimulates saliva production is helpful. For example, eating fibrous foods stimulates saliva flow, and eating sugary foods with meals (when saliva flow is more copious) results in fewer cavities than does eating sugary foods between meals.

Some scientists think that *certain food components* are protective. Fats may provide a coating for teeth, and high phosphorus foods may be protective as well. These experts suggest that ending a meal with cheese or nuts may help prevent dental caries.

Xylitol, as mentioned earlier, has been found to discourage the formation of dental caries. In a study funded by the World Health Organization, xylitol was substituted for some of the sugar in the diets of children living on two islands, while the children on another island (with dietary habits originally similar to the other two) continued their usual diets. After almost 3 years, the children who were ingesting xylitol as part of their diet had significantly fewer dental caries than those who were not (Kandelman and Hefti, 1988). A number of other studies have produced similar findings (Pepper and Olinger, 1988).

Of course, *good dental hygiene* immediately after eating reduces the amount of time that sugars are in the mouth and therefore helps prevent dental caries. The American Dental Association incorporates these suggestions into its decay-prevention program: it recommends a nutritious diet, limited snacking (especially on sweets), careful hygiene, and regular dental checkups.

Possible Concern: Concentrated Sugars "Dilute Nutrients" White sugar is pure carbohydrate; other high-sugar sweeteners such as brown sugar, maple syrup, honey, and molasses, contain only tiny amounts of micronutrients. Therefore, if such substances constitute much of your intake, the other items in your diet have to provide practically all the vitamins and minerals you need. For this reason, the Pyramid Food Guide recommends that you eat no more than about 1 ounce of concentrated sugars if your kcalorie intake is 1600 per day, and no more than about 2½ ounces if you consume about 2800 kcalories per day (Human Nutrition Information Service, 1992). In either example, sugars are limited to no more than 10% of your total energy intake. These limits apply to the total amount of sugar added by you and by commercial food processors together.

So what's the bottom line for those of us who enjoy an occasional chocolate chip cookie? Will our consumption of added sugars put us at serious risk of falling far short of our RDA intakes of nutrients? In general, it doesn't appear that way. In the study cited earlier of the relationship between U.S. sugar consumption and body weight, the researchers also evaluated the micronutrient intake of the one-fourth of the population that had the highest intake of added sugars. Even these people, on average, took in at least 100% of their RDA for most nutrients; for remaining nutrients, intakes were 70% of the RDA or better (Lewis et al., 1992). Nonetheless, if your food choices are very poor, it is possible that added sugar might dilute dietary quality substantially.

How Much Digestible Carbohydrate Should You Get?

Even though carbohydrate is a basic source of energy, there is no RDA for it, because as we mentioned earlier, people can survive without it by producing it from protein. Of course, if body proteins were used heavily for carbohydrate production, physiologic damage would eventually result. Therefore, experts have estimated how much carbohydrate is needed to protect body protein.

Experts in the United States recommend that, *at the very least,* you take in 50–100 grams of carbohydrate daily (RDA Subcommittee, 1989). The United Nations and the World Health Organization suggest a more generous *minimum* of 180 grams daily. If you add up the carbohydrate in the minimum amounts of foods recommended by the Pyramid Food Guide, you will find that it ranges anywhere from about 160 to 240 grams, depending on which foods are selected—especially on whether legumes are used as meat alternatives.

Interestingly, the traditional diets of many of the world's cultures emphasize high-carbohydrate foods. For example, rice is a staple food in much of China, Japan, and southeast Asia; for many people in Ireland and in the Andes Mountains, potatoes are a very important food; and bread is basic to many Europeans. People who follow such dietary practices will probably take in these recommended amounts of carbohydrate with no difficulty.

Carbohydrate recommendations are sometimes expressed in another way: as a proportion of kcalories. The 1989 RDA recommends that more than 50% of a person's energy requirement be provided by carbohydrates. Endurance athletes who train daily are advised to consume even more to prevent becoming progressively glycogen-depleted. People consuming 50% or more of their kcalories as carbohydrate will get far more carbohydrate than the minimums suggested above.

How can you determine whether you meet the recommendations? Act on Fact 5.1 on page 142 gives you instructions for comparing your digestible carbohydrate intake with these two standards. Then, if you find that your intake is less than what is recommended, Consider This on page 141 offers ways to increase it.

Indigestible Carbohydrates: Dietary Fiber

Fiber is the second major category of carbohydrate found in our food. Chances are that fiber is no stranger to you, because it has been the focus of much recent scientific research that has caught the attention of the popular media. It has also been featured—often with much fanfare—as an ingredient in new food products.

Of course, fiber is a natural constituent of all plants and therefore has always been part of the food supply. Prominent in cell walls, fiber gives plants the strength to stand upright. Fiber is most concentrated in the outer layers that protect seeds, fruits, and vegetables.

Fiber, whether it is a natural constituent of a food or has been added during processing, is called **dietary fiber.**

dietary fiber—plant components made of linked carbohydrate units that cannot be separated by human digestive secretions

The Function of Dietary Fiber

Dietary fiber resists being hydrolyzed by your digestive processes. Much of it remains as solid material in your large intestine after other components of food have been absorbed. The bulk fiber provides (and the water it holds) dilutes the other materials in the colon and gives intestinal muscles the opportunity for healthy muscular work, moving solid waste through the colon more rapidly.

Fiber also serves as a food source for bacteria in the gut. Although human digestive processes cannot break fiber apart, bacteria can partially use it. These organisms thrive, multiply, and are eventually excreted, thereby making a major contribution to the mass of solid waste.

In addition, fiber in the gut can have an effect beyond the GI tract itself: some types of fiber are believed to lower blood *cholesterol,* a substance that, in excessive amounts, can increase a person's risk of heart disease. Although the mechanism is not well understood, it appears that certain types of fiber reduce the absorption of cholesterol from the GI tract.

Chapter 6 provides much more information about cholesterol and the risk of heart disease.

Fiber in Nature

There are two major types of fiber, and both can be present in the same food. One type is **insoluble fiber,** the rigid material that gives structure to plants and does not dissolve in water. *Cellulose,* which is found in the cell walls of fruits, vegetables, grains, nuts, and seeds, is an example of insoluble fiber. It is also concentrated in the protective outer layers of whole grains, called the *bran layers,* and in seeds and edible skins and peels. Insol-

insoluble fiber—indigestible carbohydrate that does not dissolve in water; an example is cellulose, a major component of wheat bran

To improve your carbohydrate intake, instead of

This	*Consider this*
Fewer than 5 fruits and vegetables daily	**At least 2 fruits and 3 vegetables every day**
Fewer than 6 servings of bread, rice, cereal, and pasta daily	**6–11 servings every day; choose from bread, pita, rolls, rice, cereal, crackers, popcorn, pasta, couscous, tortillas, chapatis, matzo**
Exclusively wheat products	**More variety of grains: try products made from oats, rye, rice, corn, barley, millet, triticale**
Very few starchy beans and peas	**More of these: in soups (lentil, black bean); in salads (kidney beans, garbanzo beans); in sandwiches (hummus made from chickpeas); in entrees (lima bean and ham casserole, chili con carne)**

Remember: Gradual changes are more likely to last, and they give your body time to adjust.

uble fiber represents two-thirds to three-fourths of the total fiber ingested in a mixed diet (Marlett, 1990).

The other major type of fiber is **soluble fiber**. *Pectins, gums,* and *mucilages* are all types of soluble fiber. Apples are a notable source of pectin; other fruits have less. Gums and mucilages are generally found in only small amounts in common plant foods. Soluble fiber is likely to be metabolized by colonic bacteria to a greater extent than is insoluble fiber.

soluble fiber—indigestible carbohydrate that dissolves in water; an example is pectin, found in apples

Fiber and Food Processing

Food processing can change the fiber content of foods. On the one hand, the most fibrous parts of a food are sometimes removed and discarded during processing; apple skins are peeled away during the making of applesauce, and the bran layers of wheat are removed in the production of white flour (Figure 5.10 on page 144).

On the other hand, fiber is sometimes added to food by processors in response to the positive public image fiber currently enjoys. For example, the bran of various grains is being added to an increasing number of breakfast cereals. Bran is also marketed by itself so that consumers can add it to other foods. Cellulose that has been refined from wood is added to some breads, both to raise the fiber content and to lower the kcalories by substituting it for some of the available carbohydrates.

Assessing Your Digestible Carbohydrate (and Fat and Protein) Intake

Use this worksheet to compare your intake of digestible carbohydrate with the standards for absolute intake (in grams) and proportion of kcalories (in percent).

As you calculate the percentage of kcalories from carbohydrate, you can easily do the same for protein and fat. It will be convenient to have this information when you study these nutrients in the next two chapters.

1. Keep a 24-hour food record on as typical a day as possible, using a form similar to that shown in the sample. List all foods and beverages consumed. (Add a column if you also consumed alcohol.)
2. Use Appendix C to find the protein, fat, and carbohydrate contents of those foods. Adjust the values to correspond to the amounts of food you consumed, and enter the values in the appropriate columns. For example, if you drank 2 cups of milk and the appendix gives values for 1 cup, you will have to double all values as you record them.
3. Figure the sum for each column.

> Did you achieve at least the bare-bones minimum of 50 grams of digestible carbohydrate? __√__ yes ____ no

4. Multiply the sum for each column by the energy value per gram of each nutrient: 4 kcal/g (protein); 9 kcal/g (fat); 4 kcal/g (carbohydrate); and 7 kcal/g (alcohol) if you consumed any.
5. Total the kcalories from all nutrients. If you consumed an alcoholic beverage, you can determine how many kcalories the alcohol provided by subtracting the kcalories provided by the beverage's protein, fat, and carbohydrate from the total kcalories in the beverage.
6. Divide the kcalories from each energy substrate by the total kcalories consumed; this yields a decimal fraction.
7. Multiply each decimal fraction by 100 to get the percentages; round each to the nearest percent.

> Did you get at least 50% of your kcalories from carbohydrate? ____ yes __√__ no

Sample Act on Fact 5.1

Calculating the percentage of kcalories from protein, fat, and carbohydrate in a day's menu.

Food or Beverage	Amount Eaten	Protein (g)	Fat (g)	Carbohydrate (g)
Pork sausage, 2 small links	1 ounce	6	8	0
Fried egg	1 large	6	7	1
Hash browned potatoes	½ cup	3	9	22
Toast, wheat	2 slices	6	2	26
Butter	2 t.	0	8	0
Coffee	2 cups	0	0	0
Cola	12 oz. can	0	0	37
Swiss cheese sandwich				
Rye bread	2 slices	4	2	24
Swiss cheese	2 ounces	16	16	2
Mayonnaise	1 T.	0	11	0
Lettuce	1 leaf	0	0	0
Potato chips	1 oz. (~15)	2	10	15
Dill pickle	½ medium	0	0	1
Coffee	2 cups	0	0	0
Cola	12 oz. can	0	0	37
Roast beef	3 ounces	19	30	0
Mashed potatoes	1 cup	4	1	37
Gravy, canned	¼ cup	2	1	3
Peas	½ cup	4	0	12
Bread, Italian	2 slices	6	0	34
Butter	2 t.	0	8	0
2% milk	1 cup	9	5	12
Totals		87	118	263
Multiply by kcal/g of nutrient		×4	×9	×4
to get kcal from each nutrient		348	1062	1052
Total the kcal		348 +	1062 +	1052 = 2462
Divide nutrient kcal by total kcal		÷ 2462	÷ 2462	÷ 2462
which yields a decimal fraction		.14	.43	.43
Multiply by 100 to get percent		14%	43%	43%

FIGURE 5.10
A kernel of wheat.

The three parts of a wheat kernel have different nutrient characteristics. The endosperm contains most of the starch and protein; the bran and germ contain most of the fiber and micronutrients. When wheat is milled and made into white flour, much of the bran and germ are removed.

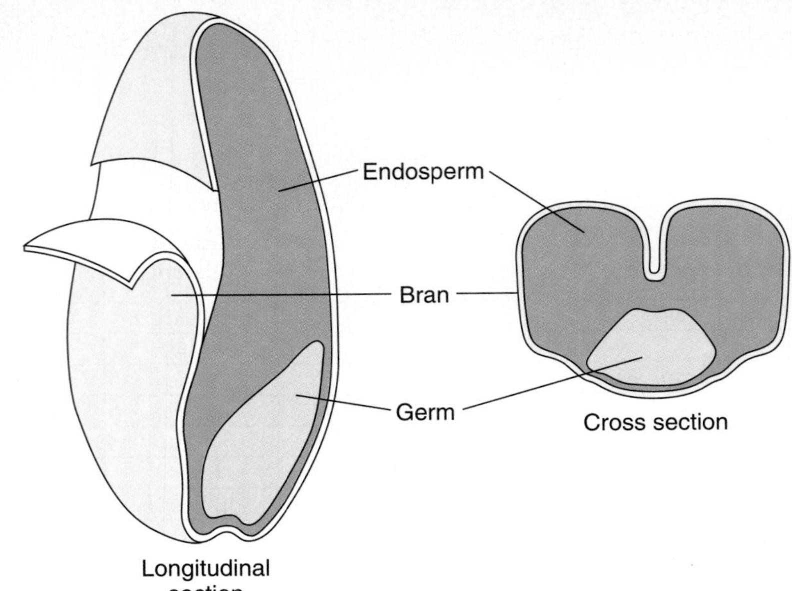

Sometimes pectins and gums are refined and used as additives to thicken, gel, or stabilize foods or to emulsify foods so that their different components do not separate. Commercially, pectin is usually refined from citrus peel and apples and is added to jams, jellies, and candies. Gums are extracted from less familiar sources; certain African and Asian shrubs, trees, and seed pods are their natural origins. Gums are used in ice cream, fruit drinks, and canned meats, to name just a few. You have seen gums listed on labels as *guar gum, locust bean gum, gum tragacanth, gum arabic,* and *xanthan gum. Agar, carrageenan,* and *alginates* are extracts of seaweed that are also widely used as stabilizers and thickeners.

In recent years, a new fiberlike substance, *polydextrose,* has been developed primarily for use as a bulking and moisture-retaining agent and a texturizer in reduced-kcalorie processed foods. Although this substance does not yield to *human* digestive processes, it nonetheless provides approximately 1 kcalorie/gram to humans from by-products of colonic *bacterial* metabolism.

Amounts of Fiber in Foods

Although most of us have been inundated with ads and reports about fiber, there are gaps in our knowledge about the amount of it in food. In a recent large survey of American adults, 4 out of 5 people knew that bran flakes are a good source of fiber; only 1 in 5, however, knew that baked beans are (Cremer and Kessler, 1992).

Those people weren't alone in their ignorance: even scientists have trouble determining exactly how much fiber is in food. To measure fiber content, they have had to develop special laboratory analyses to approximate human GI processes; there are no simple, universally accepted procedures (Institute of Food Technologists [IFT] Expert Panel, 1989a). Table 5.8 provides data thought to be among the most accurate (Marlett, 1992). The solid parts of the bars represent insoluble fiber, and the open sections represent soluble fiber. A more extensive table is found in Appendix D.

Unfortunately, the fiber values published thus far by Marlett do not include any pairs of refined and whole-grain products (e.g., white bread and

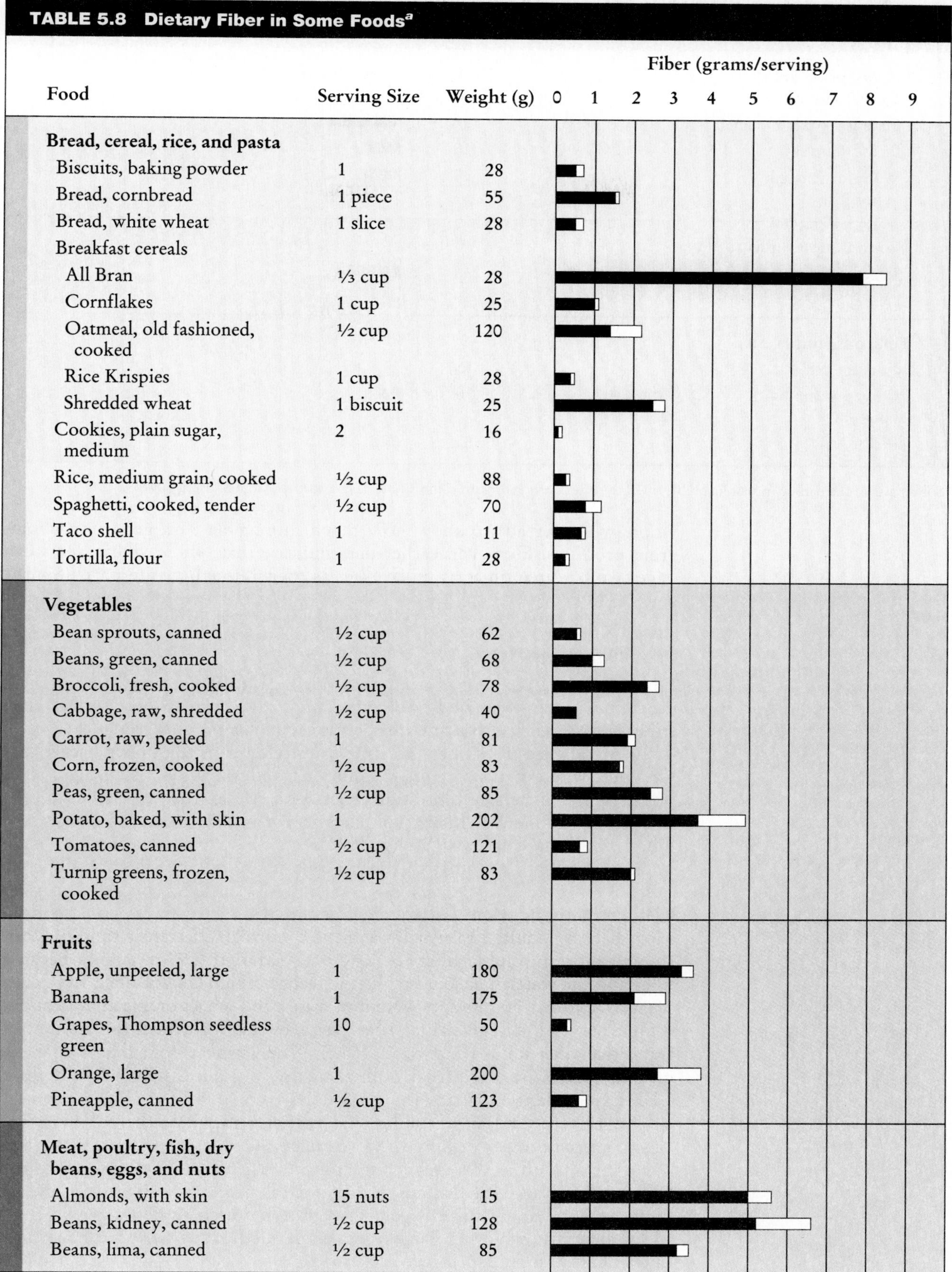

TABLE 5.8 Dietary Fiber in Some Foods[a]

Food	Serving Size	Weight (g)
Bread, cereal, rice, and pasta		
Biscuits, baking powder	1	28
Bread, cornbread	1 piece	55
Bread, white wheat	1 slice	28
Breakfast cereals		
All Bran	⅓ cup	28
Cornflakes	1 cup	25
Oatmeal, old fashioned, cooked	½ cup	120
Rice Krispies	1 cup	28
Shredded wheat	1 biscuit	25
Cookies, plain sugar, medium	2	16
Rice, medium grain, cooked	½ cup	88
Spaghetti, cooked, tender	½ cup	70
Taco shell	1	11
Tortilla, flour	1	28
Vegetables		
Bean sprouts, canned	½ cup	62
Beans, green, canned	½ cup	68
Broccoli, fresh, cooked	½ cup	78
Cabbage, raw, shredded	½ cup	40
Carrot, raw, peeled	1	81
Corn, frozen, cooked	½ cup	83
Peas, green, canned	½ cup	85
Potato, baked, with skin	1	202
Tomatoes, canned	½ cup	121
Turnip greens, frozen, cooked	½ cup	83
Fruits		
Apple, unpeeled, large	1	180
Banana	1	175
Grapes, Thompson seedless green	10	50
Orange, large	1	200
Pineapple, canned	½ cup	123
Meat, poultry, fish, dry beans, eggs, and nuts		
Almonds, with skin	15 nuts	15
Beans, kidney, canned	½ cup	128
Beans, lima, canned	½ cup	85

[a]Solid parts of the bars represent insoluble fiber; the open parts represent soluble fiber. Data adapted from Marlett, 1992.

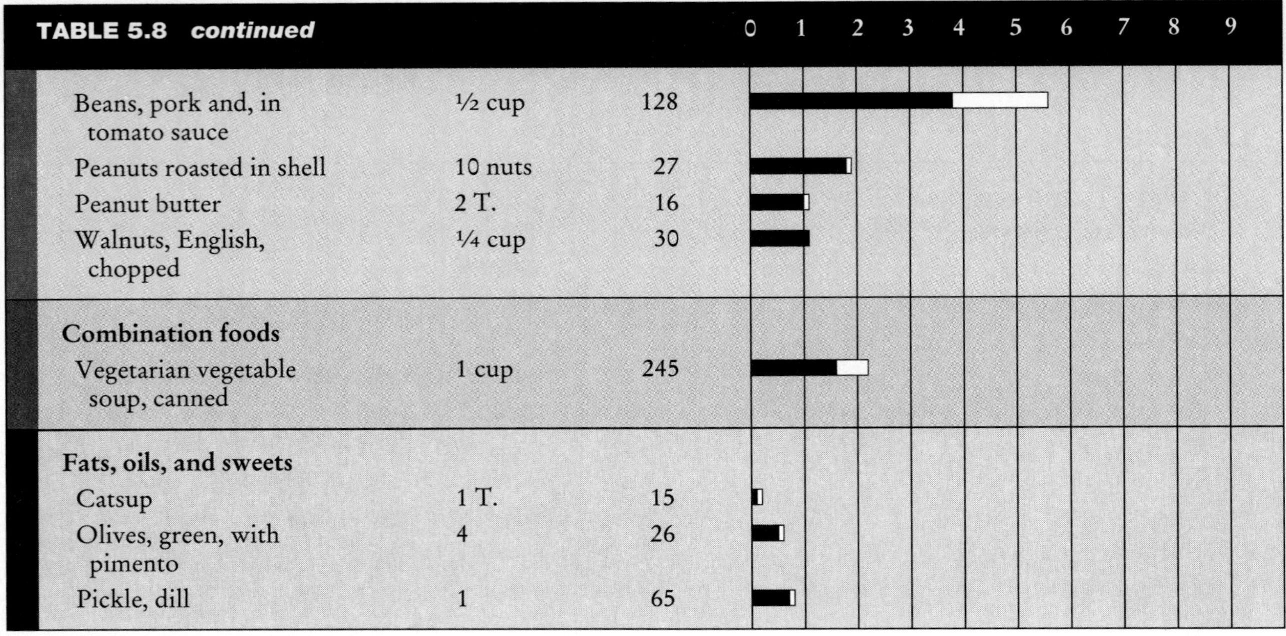

TABLE 5.8 continued

Food	Serving	Weight	0 1 2 3 4 5 6 7 8 9
Beans, pork and, in tomato sauce	½ cup	128	
Peanuts roasted in shell	10 nuts	27	
Peanut butter	2 T.	16	
Walnuts, English, chopped	¼ cup	30	
Combination foods			
Vegetarian vegetable soup, canned	1 cup	245	
Fats, oils, and sweets			
Catsup	1 T.	15	
Olives, green, with pimento	4	26	
Pickle, dill	1	65	

[a]Solid parts of the bars represent insoluble fiber; the open parts represent soluble fiber. Data adapted from Marlett, 1992.

whole-wheat bread) to show how much more fiber you get from whole-grain products. However, earlier data indicate that whole-wheat items can have two to three times as much fiber as their refined counterparts (Southgate, 1986).

Fiber and Health

Fiber is unique in the way it affects your health. Whereas most substances do their work in your body only after they have been absorbed, fiber contributes to your health primarily because you *cannot* absorb it.

Generally, soluble fiber has its greatest effects in the upper part of the GI tract, where it delays gastric emptying and slows down absorption of nutrients from the small intestine (Eastwood, 1992). Insoluble fiber is typically more influential in the colon, where it speeds intestinal transit and dilutes intestinal contents (Slavin, 1990).

Let's look at how fiber can play a role in various health conditions.

Relieves Constipation Adequate fiber in the diet relieves constipation. Most healthy adults can usually achieve a normal GI transit time by consuming more insoluble fiber for 2–4 days (Marlett, 1990), largely because fiber and the water it absorbs make the feces bulkier. Carrot fiber, for example, can hold 20–30 times its weight in water, and wheat bran can hold about 5 times its weight. The size of fiber particles also influences the amount of water that fiber holds (Eastwood, 1992). Whole-wheat flour that is coarsely ground results in more fecal bulk than finely ground whole-wheat flour (IFT Expert Panel, 1989a).

Bulky feces and larger undigested particles stimulate the colonic muscles to exercise more, making them stronger and able to function better and move the fecal mass through the tract more easily. If your diet contains the recommended amount of fiber, transit time is typically between 24 and 72 hours; if your fiber intake is very low, transit time may be longer.

Vegetarians who rely largely on plant foods and therefore have high fiber intakes rarely experience constipation.

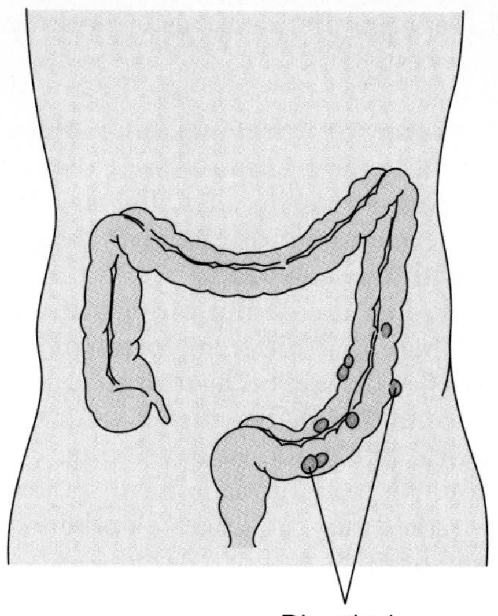

FIGURE 5.11
Diverticular disease.

In diverticular disease, a common condition in the elderly, outpouchings form in the wall of the colon.

Relieves Diverticular Disease **Diverticular disease** is a condition in which pressure in the lumen of the colon causes outpouchings (diverticula) to occur in its wall (Figure 5.11). An estimated 30–40% of people aged 50 and over in the United States are thought to have this condition, although they may not be aware of it (National Research Council, 1989). Diverticula will not cause any pain unless waste collects in them and causes irritation, resulting in *diverticulitis.* (The suffix *-itis* means "inflammation.")

diverticular disease—condition in which pressure in the lumen of the colon causes outpouchings called diverticula to occur in its walls

A diet generous in fiber has been found to help relieve the symptoms of uncomplicated diverticular disease. Some epidemiologists further believe that a high-fiber diet may help prevent the condition, because increased fecal bulk and decreased transit time also decrease colonic pressure.

May Decrease Colon Cancer Cancer is a disease in which body cells multiply out of control. Research over the past several decades suggests that there may be over 100 different clinical conditions with such runaway cell division; all are called cancer. Because certain components in the diet have been linked to cancer, this topic is on the leading edge of nutrition research.

One of the sites in which cancer commonly develops is the colon. Epidemiologic studies suggest that dietary fiber may provide protection against colon cancer: populations that consume a high-fiber diet tend to have less colon cancer than populations that eat low-fiber diets (Thun et al., 1992). Note, however, that high-fiber diets are often also lower in fat and kcalories than are low-fiber diets. Consequently, it may be just as valid to suggest that the low-fat and/or low-energy features of the diet are protective—it may even be that none of the three factors is involved. Other possibilities are that some types of fiber may be protective whereas others are not or that another substance associated with fiber in food is a helpful factor (Kritchevsky, 1991a). Animal studies have been done to try to clarify the relationship between fiber and colon cancer, but they have not produced consistent results (National Research Council, 1989).

Despite these uncertainties, the National Cancer Institute and many other health organizations recommend that Americans eat both types of fiber in a large number of fiber-containing foods. It is possible that fiber may help; in any event, it won't hurt. The fiber intakes of many populations are double or more those of average Americans and have not caused detrimental effects (Greenwald and Lanza, 1986).

The possible link between diet and cancer is further discussed in later chapters where it is relevant.

Helps Reduce a Risk Factor for Cardiovascular Disease The effect of diet on cardiovascular (heart and blood vessel) disease is a topic that has been on the nutrition frontier for decades. Dietary fats are believed to be more influential in the development of cardiovascular (CV) disease than are carbohydrates, so we will devote a major section in Chapter 6 (on fat) to this health concern, including the definition of many important terms.

It is enough to say here that different forms of carbohydrates seem to have different effects on CV disease because of their influence on blood cholesterol, a fatty substance in blood. The higher your total blood cholesterol, the greater your statistical likelihood of developing CV disease.

Studies of both animals and humans have indicated that the bran of grains such as oats, corn, and rice can lower blood cholesterol levels in some people, whereas wheat bran does not (Anderson, Gilinsky, et al., 1991; Whyte et al., 1992). Some researchers suggest that this may be a consequence of lower fat intake rather than higher fiber intake, but several recent studies show that decreasing fat and increasing fiber have independent cholesterol-lowering effects (Kritchevsky, 1991b).

Legumes and some fruits and vegetables also lower blood lipid levels. These effects are generally also attributed to the soluble fibers present (Anderson and Gustafson, 1988; National Research Council, 1989). In addition, a water-soluble fiber found in psyllium seed, originally marketed as a bulking agent, has also been found to reduce blood cholesterol (Abraham and Mehta, 1988; Anderson, Zettwoch, et al., 1988).

Of course, reality is rarely simple. Now it has been found that some types of soluble fiber do *not* lower blood cholesterol (Haskell et al., 1992). Never mind: because several different types of soluble fiber are usually present in a given food, most foods with significant soluble fiber will have some cholesterol-lowering effect. Nonetheless, this is a good illustration of why nutritional scientists are very wary of making "always" or "never" claims.

If you're trying to decrease your blood cholesterol level, you may not need to consume dramatic levels of fiber to achieve some benefit. Moderately increasing your intake of fibrous foods may lead to small, persistent decreases in blood cholesterol levels that may significantly lessen risk over a long period. The debate about the benefits of fiber in reducing the incidence of CV disease continues.

You Tell Me

Epidemiologic studies of Seventh Day Adventists, who are vegetarians—and are therefore likely to consume large amounts of starch and fiber—document that they have considerably less heart disease than the general population. Seventh Day Adventists are also less likely to smoke and consume alcohol than the general population.

Do such studies prove that fiber is responsible for the decrease in heart disease? Do they prove that it is not? Do they prove that all vegetarians are at lower risk of heart disease?

May Interfere with Absorption of Nutrients Studies of both animals and humans have shown that consuming high levels of fiber can decrease the absorption of certain vitamins and minerals. This occurs because fiber can bind some minerals in inabsorbable complexes as well as speed up the activities of the gut. (Other compounds in the food may be involved as well.)

For example, when approximately 7 tablespoons of wheat bran were added to the test meals of subjects in a metabolic study, the absorption of calcium from milk at that meal was reduced by about 25% (Knox et al., 1991). But because most metabolic studies are of short duration, scientists do not know whether some people would adjust to higher levels of fiber with time, allowing mineral absorption to return to normal. This seems possible, because some of the world's people appear to have adequate mineral status although they customarily consume very high levels of dietary fiber.

Recommended Intake for Fiber

So how much fiber do you need? Despite remaining uncertainties about fiber, some scientific and health organizations have issued recommendations about how much fiber is optimal in light of current knowledge. Their guidelines pertain to total fiber intake rather than addressing soluble and insoluble fiber separately.

In the mid-1980s, the National Institutes of Health suggested that Americans should eat foods that provide a total of 25–35 grams of fiber per day. Later, a panel convened by the Life Sciences Research Office of the Federation of American Societies for Experimental Biology recommended an intake range of 20–35 grams per day for the healthy adult population. The American Dietetic Association followed suit with a similar recommendation. The upper limit reflects scientists' concern that higher levels of fiber might reduce absorption of some vitamins and minerals.

How do these recommendations compare with current American intakes? The typical range of intake in the United States is 10–20 grams per day, so these recommendations suggest that most Americans should try to increase their intakes. However, some vegetarians in our own population already consume 40–50 grams of dietary fiber daily without apparent ill effect (Slavin, 1987). In countries such as China, intakes average around 75 grams with no noticeable problems from the fiber.

As far as recommended sources of fiber are concerned, the *Dietary Guidelines, 1990* (USDA and USDHHS), states it well: "Dietary fiber—a part of plant foods—is in whole-grain breads and cereals, dry beans and peas, vegetables, and fruits. It is best to eat a variety of these fiber-rich foods because they differ in the kinds of fiber they contain. It's best to get fiber from foods rather than from supplements."

Act on Fact 5.2 on page 150 shows how you can assess your fiber intake. If you find that increasing your fiber intake is warranted, the Thinking for Yourself on page 152 and Consider This on page 154 offer suggestions.

Estimating Your Fiber Intake for One Day

1. Keep a record of your food intake for 24 hours on a form similar to the one in Sample Act on Fact 5.2.
2. For each food that contains fiber, check Table 5.8 or Appendix D to determine the content of soluble, insoluble, and total fiber. If you have eaten a high-fiber cereal that is not on either table, check the label for specific data for that product. There can be considerable differences among products.

Did your intake include both insoluble and soluble fiber?
_√_ yes   ____ no

3. Total the fiber columns.

How does your total fiber intake compare with the recommended intake of 20–35 grams per day? Check whether it is:
_√_ less than recommended
____ within the recommended range
____ above the recommended range

4. If your intake for this day was outside the recommended range, suggest in the space below some changes you could have made to bring it in range.

Changes for improvement:

- Substitute a higher fiber cereal
- Eat fresh fruit as snacks
- Eat more vegetables
- ____
- ____

Sample Act on Fact 5.2

Estimating your fiber intake for one day.

Food or Beverage	Amount Eaten	Fiber (grams/serving) Insoluble	Soluble	Total
Orange juice	1 cup	tr	(est.) tr	tr
Special K	1 1/3 cup	0.7	0.1	0.8
2% milk	3/4 cup	0	0	0
Sugar	1 t.	0	0	0
Submarine sandwich				
Roll—est. equiv. to	3 sl. white bread	1.5	0.6	2.1
Meat	2 oz.	0	0	0
Cheese	2 oz.	0	0	0
Lettuce, chopped	1/2 cup	0.5	(est.) tr	0.5
Tomato, fresh	3 thin slices	0.3	(est.) 0.1	0.4
Cola	12 oz.	0	0	0
Quarter pound hamburger				
Bun	1	0.7	0.3	1.0
Ground beef	1 patty	0	0	0
French fries	~ 15 pieces	1.3	0.3	1.6
Milkshake	16 oz.	0	(est.) tr	tr
Side salad:				
Lettuce	1 cup	1.0	(est.) tr	1.0
Tomato	2 wedges	0.3	(est.) 0.1	0.4
Shredded carrot	2 T.	0.5	tr	0.5
French dressing	2 T.	0	(est.) tr	tr
Ice cream	1 cup	0	(est.) tr	tr
Cone	1 cone	0.3	0.1	0.4
Fiber Totals		7.1	1.6	8.7

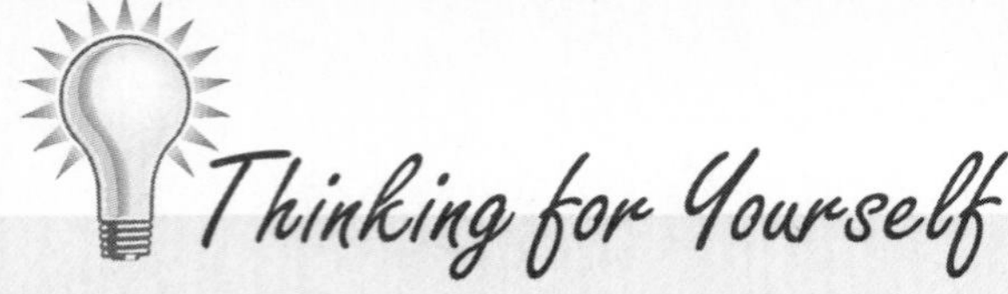

Fiber, Fiber Everywhere—So What?

The Situation

You are watching your favorite TV morning news show as you eat breakfast, and another breakfast cereal commercial appears. The last one was for a cereal that had oat bran added to it—the ad said it may keep your blood cholesterol down. This one is for a wheat bran cereal, and they're claiming it may reduce your risk of colon cancer.

You take a bite of your English muffin, and you eye it somewhat critically. No bran here, from the looks of things. You wonder whether you ought to start eating a fiber-enriched cereal for breakfast, as everybody seems to be recommending, instead of your usual muffin or bagel.

Is Your Information Accurate and Relevant?

- It is true that a diet including oat bran has been found to lower blood cholesterol somewhat. In one metabolic study, patients with elevated blood cholesterol who ate two servings of instant oats per day experienced almost a 6% drop in cholesterol after 8 weeks (Van Horn et al., 1991).
- Studies show that diets higher in whole grains correlate with lower risk of colon cancer. Animal studies using grain fiber have yielded mixed results, but wheat bran has had the most consistent beneficial effect in this regard (National Research Council, 1989).
- The recommendation to include sources of fiber in the diet has been one of the most consistent pieces of dietary advice given to Americans since the early part of this century.

What Else Should You Consider?

Fiber and its relationship to health is a hot research topic now, and that means there is much yet to be learned.

Although in general it appears that diets higher in fiber offer some protection against heart disease and cancer, it is not always clear whether it is the *presence of the fiber per se,* or *the presence of a particular type or amount of fiber,* or *either the presence or absence of something else in high-fiber diets* that has the beneficial effect. For example, when oatmeal is added to the diet and blood cholesterol goes down, scientists do not know whether soluble fiber is responsible for the reduction, or whether it may be—at least in part—that the oatmeal has displaced some high-fat, high-kcalorie foods from the diet, thereby helping to lower blood cholesterol. More research on both laboratory animals and humans is needed.

For these reasons, many scientists and scientific groups are hesitant to make very specific recommendations for fiber intake. Most do not recommend fiber supplements but do recommend that we eat a variety of foods that are naturally high in fiber.

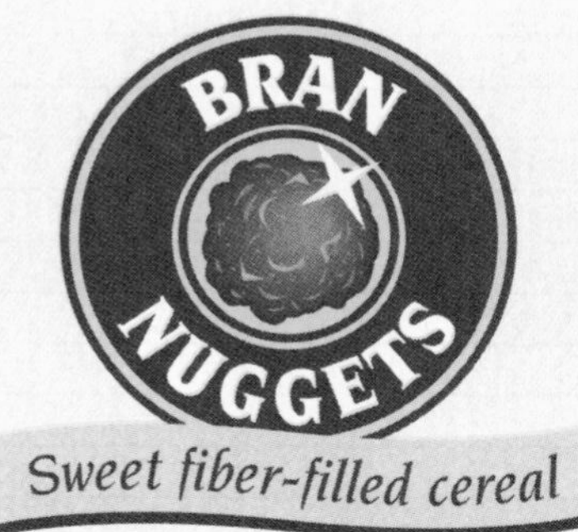

Ingredients: Oat bran, wheat bran, brown sugar, partially hydrogenated soybean oil, sugar, corn syrup, walnuts, wheat starch, salt.

There are some possible negative effects of high fiber intake. A few individuals who have taken fiber supplements without adequate fluid have produced compacted feces that were difficult to eliminate. Of more general concern is that at some level of intake, certain types of fiber may reduce absorption of minerals such as calcium and iron—which are already in short supply in the diets of many Americans.

Many products now being promoted as fiber-enriched vary not only in the types of fiber they contain but also in the amounts included. By May, 1994, the labels on processed foods will indicate how many grams of fiber are present in each product.

Now What Do You Think?

So, should you increase your fiber intake, and, if so, what's the best way to get the benefits of fiber without the possible penalties?

Here are some options to consider:

- Option 1 You decide that because quite a bit is unknown about fiber, there's no point in changing your fiber intake.
- Option 2 You decide not to worry about fiber intake at present but to increase your overall carbohydrate intake and lower your fat intake. You'll ask your physician's advice at your next checkup.
- Option 3 Using Act on Fact 5.2, you evaluate your diet for its current fiber content on a typical day. If you find that you usually consume over 20 grams of dietary fiber per day, you decide there is no need to increase your fiber intake at this time. If you find your fiber intake is less than 20 grams, you consider options 4 and 5.
- Option 4 You decide to use more foods with their natural fiber intact: more whole-grain products instead of refined products, and more fruits and vegetables with edible peels.
- Option 5 You decide to try one of the fiber-enriched cereals.

Do you see other options? Which approach makes most sense to you, and why?

OAT BRAN ADDED!
HEARTLAND
English Muffins
Ingredients: Enriched flour, malted barley flour, water, whole blueberries, sugar, yeast, oat bran, salt, corn meal, baking powder, lactic acid.

BACK-FORTY
Whole Grain Cereal
Ingredients: Cracked wheat, cracked rye, whole flax.

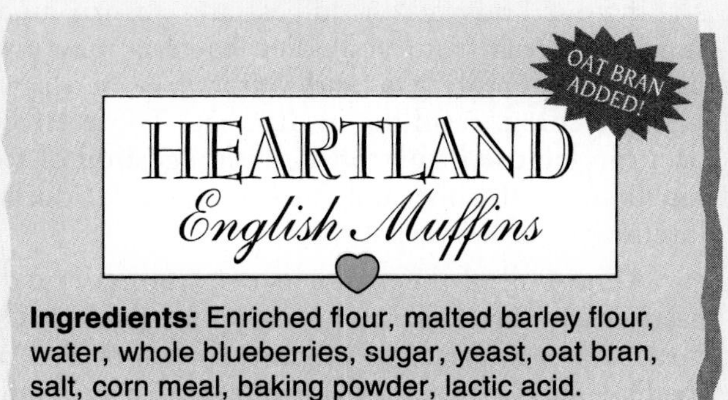

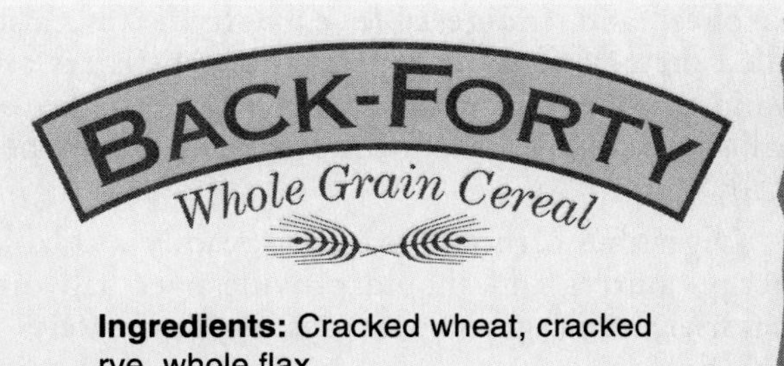

To increase your fiber intake, instead of

This	*Consider this*
Many servings of juices	**More whole fruits and vegetables**
Peeled friuts and vegetables	**Fruits and vegetables with edible peels, such as apples, pears, potatoes**
White breads, pastas, rice	**Several whole-grain items each day, such as whole-grain bread, crackers, or pasta; brown rice**
Very few starchy peas and beans	**More of these; they are high in fiber as well as digestible carbohydrates**

Remember: Gradual changes are more likely to last, and they give your body time to adjust.

Summary

- There are two types of **carbohydrate: digestible carbohydrates,** consisting of **sugars** and **starches;** and **indigestible carbohydrates,** also called **dietary fiber.** These **organic** substances are found primarily in plants, where many forms of carbohydrate are likely to be present simultaneously.

- Digestible carbohydrates are readily available energy sources and should provide over half our kcalories; each gram provides approximately 4 kcalories.

- Sugars such as **glucose** and fructose are **monosaccharides,** which your body can absorb as they are; sucrose and lactose are **disaccharides,** which are normally readily digested and absorbed. **Sugar alcohols** are closely related to sugars. All of these substances occur in nature and can be concentrated or even produced by technologic processes. Now many **sugar substitutes** are also available.

- Starches are polysaccharides that are readily hydrolyzed by **amylases** in your digestive system and absorbed. During food processing, starches may be converted to dextrins, malted, or modified to enhance thickening.

- If your body fails to digest and absorb much sugar or starch from your diet, bacteria may produce considerable gas, and water may be drawn into the colon, resulting in diarrhea. Those effects occur in **lactose intolerance,** with ingestion of too much sugar alcohol, and (in some people) during intense physical activity.

- Almost all of the products of carbohydrate digestion are converted by the body into glucose. The distribution and fate of glucose are controlled by the liver and its enzymes, hormones such as **insulin** and **glucagon,** and muscular activity. Abnormal insulin production or responses result in **insulin-dependent (Type I) diabetes** and **non-insulin-dependent (Type II) diabetes.** Epinephrine can also affect blood glucose levels and cause **hypoglycemia.** Distance athletes can extend their endurance by consuming high levels of carbohydrate, either by occasional **glycogen loading (carbohydrate loading)** or by routinely high carbohydrate intakes.

- Sugars and starches are unfairly accused of causing various health problems. However, the major justifiable concerns are that sugars promote

dental caries (cavities) and that a diet high in concentrated sugars reduces the nutrient density of the diet. In general, Americans should consume more carbohydrate, especially starches.

• There are two major types of dietary fiber: **soluble fiber,** which is not visually obvious in foods; and **insoluble fiber,** which is most concentrated in the outer layers of grains, fruits, and vegetables. Food processing may either remove or add fiber to foods.

• In general, soluble fiber encourages the growth of colonic bacteria and may bind cholesterol in the gut. Insoluble fiber provides bulk in the colon, speeds intestinal transit, and may bind some vitamins and minerals. These effects account for the ability of dietary fiber to relieve constipation, relieve (or even prevent) **diverticular disease,** reduce blood cholesterol levels, and possibly reduce the risk of colon cancer. On the down side, too much fiber may bind certain vitamins and minerals, making them unavailable to the body.

• Most Americans should increase their consumption of fiber-containing foods.

References

Abraham, Z.D. and T. Mehta. 1988. Three-week psyllium-husk supplementation: Effect on plasma cholesterol concentrations, fecal steroid excretion, and carbohydrate absorption in men. *American Journal of Clinical Nutrition* 47:67–74.

American Dietetic Association, House of Delegates. 1987. Position of the American Dietetic Association: Nutrition for physical fitness and athletic performance in adults. *Journal of the American Dietetic Association* 87:933–939.

Anderson, J.W. 1988. Nutrition management of diabetes mellitus. In *Modern nutrition in health and disease,* ed. M.E. Shils and V.R. Young. Philadelphia: Lea & Febiger.

Anderson, J.W., N.H. Gilinsky, D.A. Deakins, S.F. Smith, D.S. O'Neal, D.W. Dillon, and P.R. Oeltgen. 1991. Lipid responses of hypercholesterolemic men to oat-bran and wheat-bran intake. *The American Journal of Clinical Nutrition* 54:678–683.

Anderson, J.W. and N.J. Gustafson. 1988. Hypocholesterolemic effects of oat and bean products. *American Journal of Clinical Nutrition* 48:749–753.

Anderson, J.W., N.J. Gustafson, C.A. Bryant, and J. Tietyen-Clark. 1987. Dietary fiber and diabetes: A comprehensive review and practical application. *Journal of the American Dietetic Association* 87:1189–1197.

Anderson, J.W., N. Zettwoch, T. Feldman, J. Tietyen-Clark, P. Oeltgen, and C.W. Bishop. 1988. Cholesterol-lowering effects of psyllium hydrophilic mucilloid for hypercholesterolemic men. *Archives of Internal Medicine* 148:292–296.

Applegate, E.A. 1991a. Nutritional considerations for ultra-endurance performance. *International Journal of Sport Nutrition* 1:118–126.

Applegate, E.A. 1991b. *Power foods.* Emmaus, PA: Rodale Press.

Bergstrom, J. et al. 1967. Diet, muscle glycogen and physical performance. *Acta Physiologica Scandinavica* 71:140.

Costill, E.L. 1990. Carbohydrate for athletic training and performance. *Contemporary Nutrition* 15(no. 9). Minneapolis, MN: General Mills.

Cremer, S.A. and L.G. Kessler. 1992. The fat and fiber content of foods: What Americans know. *Journal of Nutrition Education* 24:149–152.

Eastwood, M.A. 1992. The physiological effect of dietary fiber: An update. *Annual Review of Nutrition* 1992:19–35.

Featherstone, J.D. 1987. The mechanism of dental decay. *Nutrition Today* May/June, 1987:10–16.

Gisolfi, C.V. and S.M. Duchman. 1992. Guidelines for optimal replacement beverages for different athletic events. *Medicine and Science in Sports and Exercise* 24:679–687.

Gray, G.M. 1992. Starch digestion and absorption in non-ruminants. *Journal of Nutrition* 122:172–177.

Greenwald, P. and E. Lanza. 1986. Dietary fiber and colon cancer. *Contemporary Nutrition* 11(no.1). Minneapolis, MN: General Mills.

Grobler, S.R. and J.B. Blignaut. 1989. The effect of a high consumption of apples or grapes on dental caries and periodontal disease in humans. *Clinical Preventive Dentistry* 11:8–12.

Haskell, W.L., G.A. Spiller, C.D. Jensen, B.K. Ellis, and J.E. Gates. 1992. Role of water-soluble dietary fiber in the management of elevated plasma cholesterol in healthy subjects. *The American Journal of Cardiology* 69:433–439.

Houts, S.S. 1988. Lactose intolerance. *Food Technology* 42:110–113.

Human Nutrition Information Service. 1992. *USDA's eating right pyramid.* Home and Garden Bulletin Number 249. Washington, DC: United States Department of Agriculture.

Institute of Food Technologists (IFT). 1987. Sweeteners: Nutritive and non-nutritive. *Contemporary Nutrition* 12 (no. 9).

Institute of Food Technologists (IFT), Expert Panel on Food Safety and Nutrition. 1989a. Dietary fiber. *Food Technology* 43:133–139.

Institute of Food Technologists (IFT). 1989b. Ingredients for sweet success. *Food Technology* 43:94–116.

Ivy, J.L. 1989. Carbohydrate supplementation for rapid muscle glycogen storage in the hours immediately after exercise. In *The theory and practice of athletic nutrition: Bridging the gap*, ed. A.M. Cameron. Columbus, OH: Ross Laboratories.

Jain, N.K., V.P. Patel, and C.S. Pitchumone. 1987. Sorbitol intolerance in adults. *Journal of Clinical Gastroenterology* 9:317–319.

Kanarek, R.B. and R. Marks-Kaufman. 1991. *Nutrition and behavior.* New York: Van Nostrand Reinhold.

Kandelman, A.B. and A. Hefti. 1988. Collaborative WHO xylitol field study in French Polynesia. *Caries Research* 22:55–62.

Knox, T.A., Z. Kassarjian, B. Dawson-Hughes, B.B. Golner, G.E. Dallal, S. Arora, and R.M. Russell. 1991. Calcium absorption in elderly subjects on high- and low-fiber diets: Effect of gastric acidity. *American Journal of Clinical Nutrition* 53:1480–1486.

Kolars, J.C., M.D. Levitt, M. Aouji, and D.A. Savaiano. 1984. Yogurt—an autodigesting source of lactose. *New England Journal of Medicine* 310:1–3.

Kritchevsky, D. 1991a. Evaluation of publicly available scientific evidence regarding certain nutrient-disease relationships. 5. Dietary fiber and cancer. Bethesda, MD: Life Sciences Research Office.

Kritchevsky, D. 1991b. Evaluation of publicly available scientific evidence regarding certain nutrient-disease relationships. 6. Dietary fiber and cardiovascular disease. Bethesda, MD: Life Sciences Research Office.

Lamb, D.R., K.F. Rinehardt, R.L. Bartels, W.M. Sherman, and J.T. Snook. 1990. Dietary carbohydrate and intensity of interval swim training. *American Journal of Clinical Nutrition* 52:1058–1063.

Lewis, C.J., Y.K. Park, P.B. Dexter, and E.A. Yetley. 1992. Nutrient intakes and body weights of persons consuming high and moderate levels of added sugars. *Journal of the American Dietetic Association* 92:708–713.

Macdonald, I. 1987. Metabolic requirements for dietary carbohydrate. *American Journal of Clinical Nutrition* 45:1193–1196.

Marlett, J.A. 1990. Dietary fiber. *Nutrition and the M.D.* 16(no.8):1–2.

Marlett, J.A. 1992. Content and composition of dietary fiber in 117 frequently consumed foods. *Journal of the American Dietetic Association* 92:175–186.

Martini, M.C., D. Kukielka, and D.A. Savaiano. 1991. Lactose digestion from yogurt: Influence of a meal and additional lactose. *American Journal of Clinical Nutrition* 53:1253–1258.

Matthews, R.H., P.R. Pehrsson, and M. Farhat-Sabet. 1987. Sugar content of selected foods. Washington, DC: United States Department of Agriculture.

McArdle, W.D., F.I. Katch, and V.L. Katch. *Exercise physiology: Energy, nutrition and human performance.* Philadelphia: Lea & Febiger.

National Dairy Council. 1989. Food sensitivity and dairy products. *Dairy Council Digest* 60:25–30.

National Research Council. 1989. *Diet and health: Implications for reducing chronic disease risk.* Washington, DC: National Academy Press.

Nutrition Reviews. 1987. Diet and dental health as measured by NHANES I data. *Nutrition Reviews* 45:302–304.

Pennington, J.A. 1989. *Food values of portions commonly used.* New York: Harper & Row.

Pepper, R. and P.M. Olinger. 1988. Xylitol in sugar-free confections. *Food Technology* 42:98–106.

RDA Subcommittee. 1989. *Recommended dietary allowances.* Washington, DC: National Academy Press.

Savaiano, D.A. and C. Kotz. 1988. Recent advances in the management of lactose intolerance. *Contemporary Nutrition* 13(no. 9, 10). Minneapolis, MN: General Mills.

Scrimshaw, N.S. and E.B. Murray. 1988. Lactose tolerance and milk consumption. *American Journal of Clinical Nutrition* 48:1059–1083.

Sherman, W.M. and D.A. Wright. 1989. Preevent nutrition for prolonged exercise. In *The theory and practice of athletic nutrition: Bridging the gap,* ed. A.M. Cameron, Columbus, OH: Ross Laboratories.

Sinden, A.A. and J.L. Sutphen. 1991. Dietary treatment of lactose intolerance in infants and children. *Journal of the American Dietetic Association* 91:1567–1571.

Slavin, J.L. 1987. Dietary fiber: Classification, chemical analysis, and food sources. *Journal of the American Dietetic Association* 87:1164–1171.

Slavin, J.L. 1990. Dietary fiber: Mechanisms or magic on disease prevention? *Nutrition Today* 25:6–10.

Southgate, D.A. 1986. Dietary fiber content of selected foods by the Southgate methods. In *CRC handbook of dietary fiber in human nutrition,* ed. G.A. Spiller. Boca Raton, FL: CRC Press, Inc.

Southgate, D.A. and I.T. Johnson. 1987. New thoughts on carbohydrate digestion. *Contemporary Nutrition* 12(no.10).

Surgeon General. 1988. *Surgeon General's report on nutrition and health.* Washington, DC: United States Department of Health and Human Services.

Thun, M.J., E.E. Calle, M.M. Namboodiri, W.D. Flanders, R.J. Coates, T. Byers, P. Boffetta, L. Garfinkel, and C.W. Heath, Jr. 1992. Risk factors for fatal colon cancer in a large prospective study. *Journal of the National Cancer Institute* 84(no.19):1491–1500.

USDA and USDHHS. 1990. *Nutrition and your health: Dietary guidelines for Americans.* Home and Garden Bulletin No. 232; U.S. Government Printing Office.

Van Horn, L., A. Moag-Stahlberg, K. Liu, C. Ballew, K. Ruth, R. Hughes, and J. Stamler. 1991. Effects on serum lipids of adding instant oats to usual American diets. *American Journal of Public Health* 81:183–188.

Whyte, J.L., R. McArthur, D. Topping, and P. Nestel. 1992. Oat bran lowers plasma cholesterol levels in mildly hypercholesterolemic men. *Journal of the American Dietetic Association* 92:446–449.

Williams, M.H. 1992. *Nutrition for fitness and sport.* Dubuque, IA: William C. Brown, Publishers.

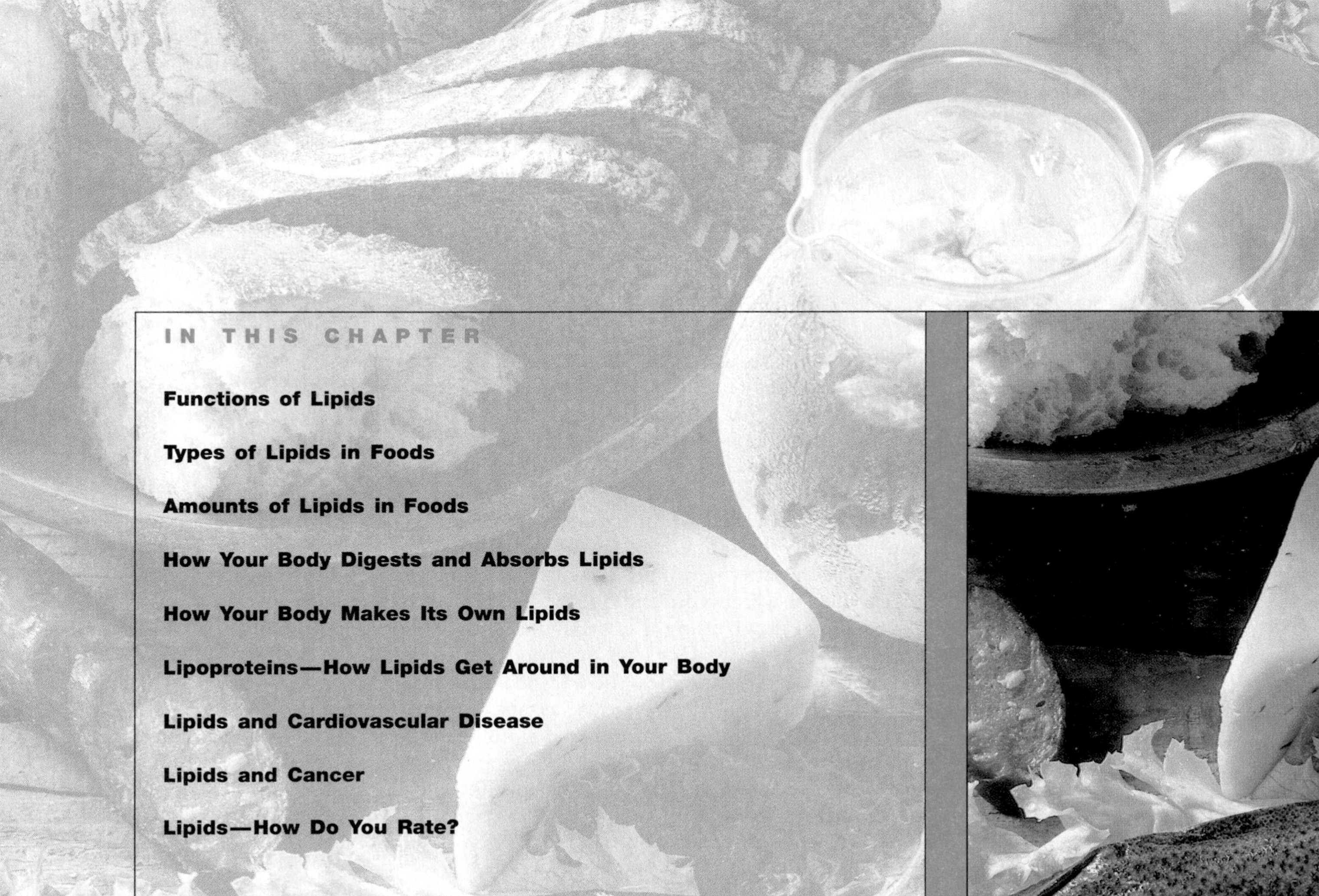

IN THIS CHAPTER

Chapter 6

Lipids

What's *canola oil?* What are the *monoglycerides, diglycerides,* and *lecithin* you see on food product ingredient lists? Have you ever had a laboratory test done to determine the level of your *blood cholesterol?* These substances are all examples of lipids.

lipids—fatty substances that usually do not dissolve in water because of their chemical structure

fats—lipids that are solid at room temperature

oils—lipids that are liquid at room temperature

Lipids are fatty substances that usually do not dissolve in water but that do dissolve in the common organic solvent ether. Two closely related terms are *fats* and *oils:* **fats** are lipids that are solid at room temperature, and **oils** are pourable at room temperature. (In ordinary usage, people often say "fats" when they intend the broader meaning of *lipids;* we'll do that ourselves in this chapter when it isn't likely to cause confusion. In the next paragraph, for example, we'll refer to a "high-fat diet," although it would be more accurate to say "high-lipid diet.")

Fats, oils, and their chemical relatives have developed a bad reputation in recent years. One reason is cosmetic; our society, at this time, regards obvious body fat as ugly—and eating a high-fat diet can lead to increased body fat. Other reasons are health related. Over the years, we have heard time and again that eating too much fat increases risk of heart disease, cancer, and an assortment of other ills, none of which you'd want to write into your life plan.

So we've learned to *think* negatively about lipids. Nonetheless, we do like *eating* them, and we find ourselves repeatedly attracted to them. Lipids contribute to the tantalizing aromas of foods; they also largely account for the sense of satiety (hunger satisfaction) you get from eating rich foods. Magazines in which you find buttery recipes coexisting with a feature about how to slim down using a low-fat diet show that we have conflicting attitudes toward fat: we like it in our foods, but not on our bodies.

This chapter examines these aspects of lipids, starting with a little-recognized fact: all of us *need* a certain amount of fat in our diets. We'll describe the forms and amounts of lipids found in foods, both as nature produces them and as food technology modifies them. We'll also discuss how your body handles them, and you'll look at the evidence on how your health can be affected by the lipids you consume. You will then learn what levels are recommended and how to help yourself achieve these levels.

Functions of Lipids

Despite the bad press lipids have faced in recent years, a certain amount always has been and always will be an important contributor to our health and well-being. As dietary constituents, lipids perform all three of the general functions of nutrients: providing energy, supplying materials for body structures, and serving as regulators of physiologic processes. Although excess body fat is a real problem for some people, a certain amount of fat serves us well.

Lipids are the most potent providers of energy. At 9 kcalories per gram, they provide more than twice as much energy as the 4 kcalories per gram that carbohydrates and proteins furnish. Because fat is such a concentrated source of energy, high-fat diets are more likely to result in high energy intakes and body fat gain than are low-fat diets.

adipose tissue—an aggregation of cells specialized for fat storage

A large share of the body's lipids is stored in **adipose tissue** (body fat) (Figure 6.1). It is fortunate that we can store energy in such a compact form: we would be very much larger and heavier if the kcalories carried as fat were stored as glycogen instead (Leibel, 1992). For example, if the energy contained in 25 pounds of fat were stored in your body as glycogen, the glycogen would weigh about 55 pounds, and the water associated with it

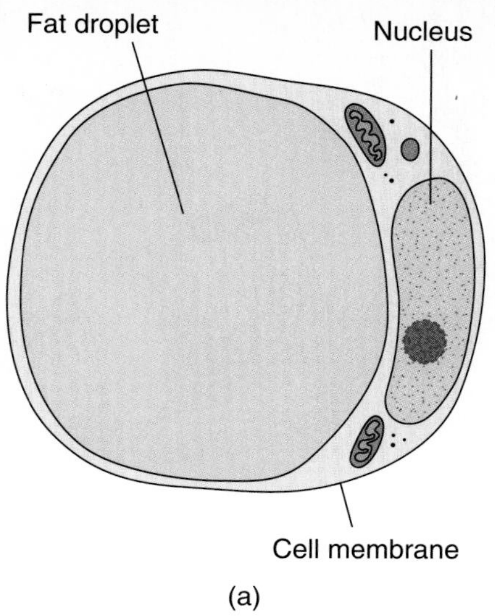

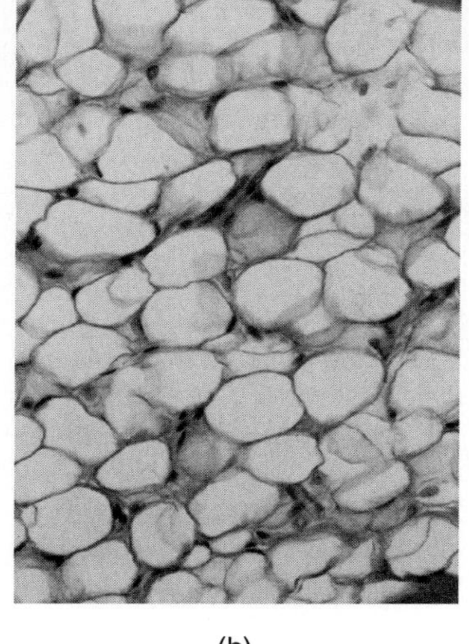

FIGURE 6.1
An adipose cell.

(a) Although every call can hold some fat, cells of adipose tissues are designed for storage of large amounts of fat. Other normal cell components—the nucleus and other bodies—are compressed into a small portion of the cell. (b) Pictured here are adipose cells. Note the large droplets of lipid in each.

would weigh over 150 pounds, making you more than 180 pounds heavier than the 25 pounds of fat would!

Besides serving as a depot for energy, adipose tissue has other uses. About half of your adipose tissue is located just under your skin. Called *subcutaneous fat,* it serves as an internal blanket to hold in your body heat. The rest of your adipose tissue surrounds your internal organs, where it cushions them from shocks and bruises.

Your body fat is also important because lipids contain essential nutrients: two are **linoleic acid** and **linolenic acid.** There probably are others (Connor et al., 1992; Simopoulos, 1991). Both linoleic and linolenic acid are abundant in plant oils.

linoleic acid and **linolenic acid**—essential fat components present in lipids

A deficiency of linoleic acid, although rarely seen in humans, results in scaly, rough skin, a tendency to bleed, abnormal kidney function, and diminished reproductive capacity (Kinsella, 1988). If a child does not get enough linoleic acid, growth is impaired. Fortunately, linoleic acid is widespread enough in the food supply that most people who eat a varied diet are likely to fulfill their need for this nutrient. Deficiency of linolenic acid is even more unlikely.

Further, fats help us by carrying fat-soluble vitamins into the body. Some vitamins—A, D, E, and K—are absorbed into the body much more easily if they are dissolved in fat. This is a good example of how nutrients influence each other in your body.

Once they are absorbed, fats serve as components for many body materials. Besides being the stuff of which adipose tissue is largely made, lipids constitute over half of the structural materials of the brain's communication network (Crawford, 1992). They are prominent in the retina of the eye, some hormones and **prostaglandins** (hormonelike substances), nerve coverings, vitamin D, and some digestive secretions. Lipids known as *phospholipids* are necessary components of the membrane of every type of cell (Figure 6.2).

prostaglandins—certain naturally occurring lipid substances with hormonelike activity; they have important effects on various body systems and functions

Cholesterol is one lipid that performs many of these functions. It is important for you to know that cholesterol, which has had so much bad press, is a necessary body substance. In fact, it is so important that people's bodies actually *produce* it, usually in larger amounts than people consume in their diets.

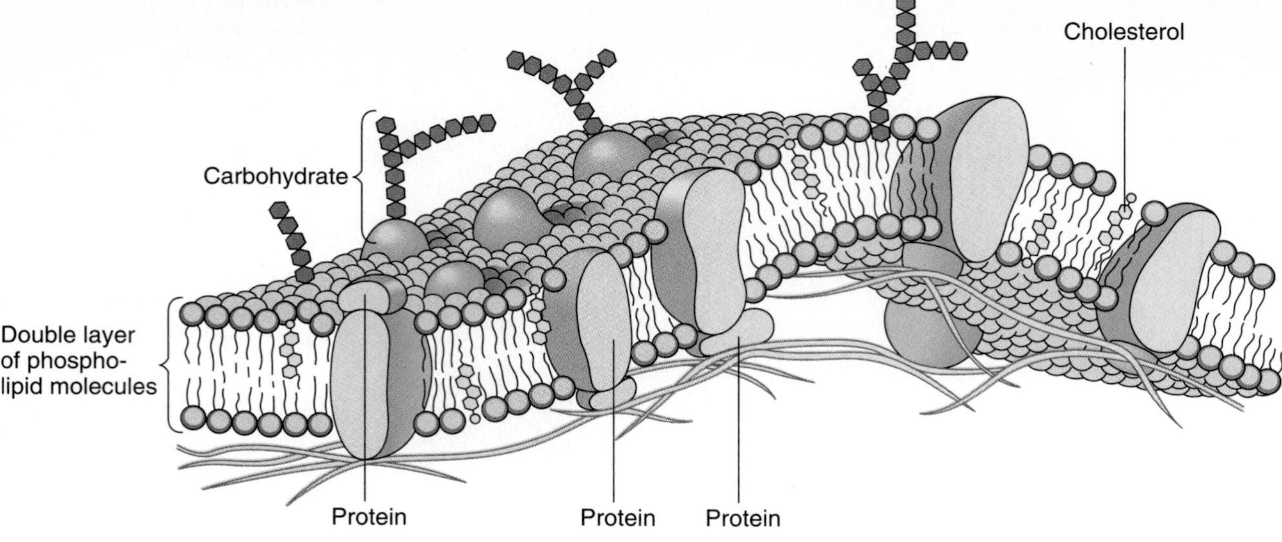

FIGURE 6.2
All your cell membranes are made largely of lipids.

As the cross-sectional diagram shows, the bulk of the material in cell membranes is two layers of phospholipid, shown here in lavender. Cholesterol, another lipid, is shown in yellow. Proteins and carbohydrate components make up the rest of the membrane.

Types of Lipids in Foods

Lipids are categorized according to their structural characteristics. We will deal here with glycerides, phospholipids, and sterols. These groups are of major importance because of their prevalence in your diet and your body and because of their implications for health. We will discuss lipids that occur in nature as well as various technologic modifications developed for using lipids in food.

Glycerides in Nature

Glycerides are the most common forms of lipids. They consist of a molecule of the 3-carbon compound **glycerol** to which one, two, or three **fatty acids** are attached *(mono-, di-,* or *triglycerides).* Figure 6.3 shows how these components fit together to form glycerides.

Triglycerides (called *triacylglycerides* by some biochemists) account for about 90% of the weight of lipids in foods; fats and oils are both largely triglycerides. Mono- and diglycerides also occur in nature, as do some unattached or "free" fatty acids.

Even though the name of these compounds draws attention to the glycerol portion of the lipid molecule, the attached fatty acids are the components responsible for the characteristics of different glycerides. Fatty acids differ from each other in several ways.

glycerides—the most common lipids, consisting of one, two, or three fatty acids attached to a molecule of glycerol; triglycerides have three fatty acids

glycerol—the 3-carbon compound that is the backbone of glycerides

fatty acids—units mainly composed of carbon chains and hydrogen; attached to glycerol in glycerides

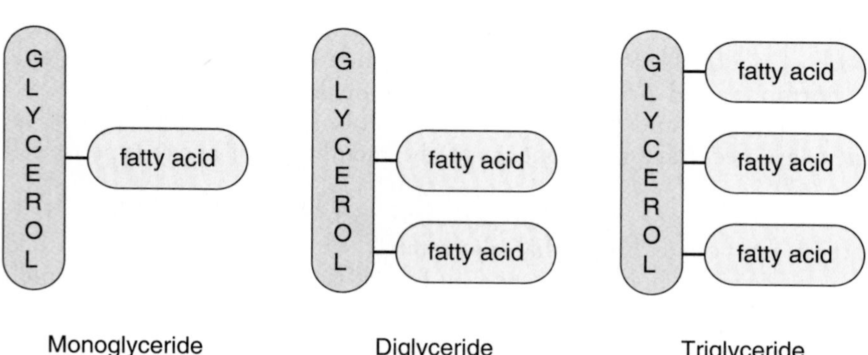

FIGURE 6.3
Glycerides.

Glycerides consist of glycerol with one, two, or three chains of fatty acids attached. Triglycerides are the most common form: they account for over 90% of all the lipids in food and in the human body.

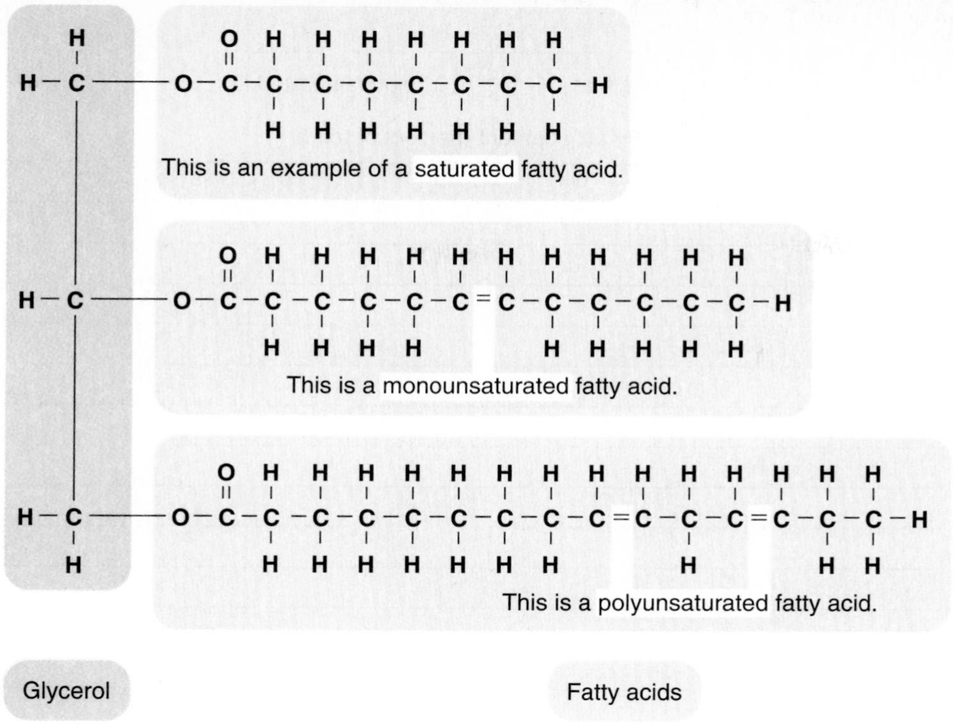

This is an example of a saturated fatty acid.

This is a monounsaturated fatty acid.

This is a polyunsaturated fatty acid.

Glycerol

Fatty acids

FIGURE 6.4
Theoretical example of a triglyceride.

Triglycerides consist of a molecule of glycerol with three fatty acids attached. Fatty acids can be saturated (no double bonds between carbon atoms); monounsaturated (one double bond); or polyunsaturated (two or more double bonds). Fatty acids can also differ in the position of their double bonds and the length of their carbon chains.

One such difference is their *chain length,* the number of linked carbon atoms in the fatty acid skeleton. Chain length is significant because, generally, the shorter its fatty acid chains, the more likely a glyceride is liquid at room temperature. (Milk fat has many short-chain fatty acids.) Triglycerides with long fatty acids, such as those found in red meats, tend to be solid at room temperature. Fatty acids may have anywhere from 4 to 22 carbons; oleic acid, the most common fatty acid in nature, has 18 carbons in its chain.

Another important characteristic of a fatty acid is its *degree of saturation.* **Saturation** refers to the number of hydrogen atoms attached to the carbons in the fatty acid skeletons. If the fatty acid chain can accommodate more hydrogen than it currently does, the fatty acid is said to be *unsaturated.* The unsaturated carbons are connected by double bonds.

A fatty acid with no double bonds between carbons is a *saturated fatty acid (SFA).* A fatty acid with one double bond is a *monounsaturated fatty acid (MUFA).* A fatty acid with two or more double bonds is a *polyunsaturated fatty acid (PUFA).*

saturation—the degree to which hydrogen atoms fill all available positions along the fatty acid skeleton; a saturated fatty acid is holding as many hydrogens as it has room for, whereas an unsaturated fatty acid is not

Figure 6.4 shows a theoretical example of a triglyceride containing fatty acids of different chain lengths and degrees of saturation. Although this much variation among fatty acids within a single triglyceride is not typical of what you would find in nature, the figure illustrates the types of fatty acids you find in lipids overall. Nevertheless, the fatty acids within a triglyceride are not likely to be identical.

You often hear the lipids in food referred to as "saturated fat" (or "unsaturated fat"). This does not mean that all the food's fatty acids are saturated (or unsaturated), but that the majority are.

Triglycerides containing large amounts of SFAs are usually solid at room temperature and are generally found in animal products, such as beef fat and butter. Triglycerides containing mostly MUFAs are usually liquid at room temperature and are generally found in plant products, such as olive oil and

TABLE 6.1 Comparison of Dietary Fats

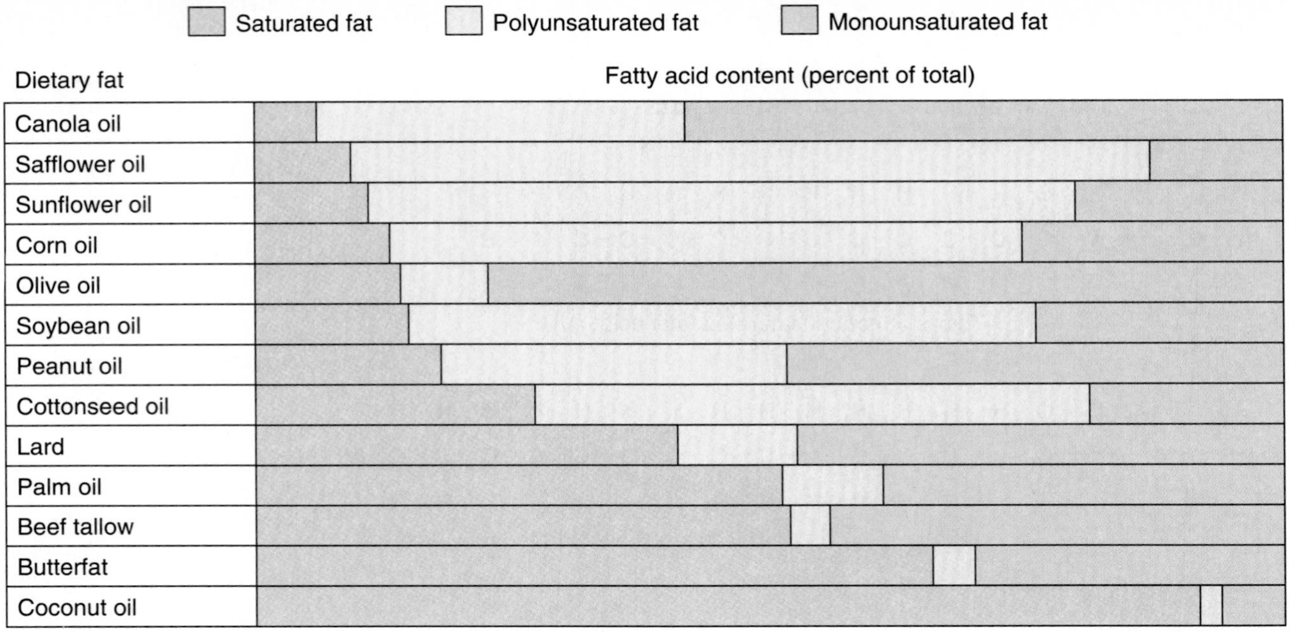

Saturated fat | Polyunsaturated fat | Monounsaturated fat

Dietary fat	Fatty acid content (percent of total)
Canola oil	
Safflower oil	
Sunflower oil	
Corn oil	
Olive oil	
Soybean oil	
Peanut oil	
Cottonseed oil	
Lard	
Palm oil	
Beef tallow	
Butterfat	
Coconut oil	

nuts. Triglycerides containing mostly PUFAs are also usually liquid at room temperature and are generally found in plant products, such as cottonseed oil and corn oil.

There are some notable exceptions to these general rules. Coconut, palm, and palm kernel oils contain lipids called *tropical oils;* because they are from plant sources, you would expect them to be more unsaturated than saturated. However, the opposite is true. Another exception is fish oils, which might be expected to contain primarily SFAs, but, in fact, contain many PUFAs. Table 6.1 shows the proportions of saturated, monounsaturated, and polyunsaturated fatty acids in various lipids.

There is another important variable in unsaturated fatty acids: the *position* of the last unsaturated bond. This, along with the other distinguishing characteristics of fatty acids, is discussed further in the section on lipids and health.

phospholipids—compounds that are similar to triglycerides but have a phosphorus-containing unit in place of one of the fatty acids

lecithin—type of phospholipid that mixes well with both watery and oily substances

emulsifiers—substances that mix with both fat-soluble and water-soluble materials to help create and maintain suspensions

Phospholipids in Nature

Phospholipids are compounds that resemble triglycerides, except that a phosphorus-containing unit takes the place of one of the fatty acids. Phospholipids in the body primarily function in cell membranes. **Lecithins** are the most prevalent phospholipids.

Phospholipids, including lecithin, have the biologically useful characteristic of mixing well with both watery and oily substances; the phosphorus-containing part of the molecule attracts water, and the fatty acids attract fat. This property classifies phospholipids as **emulsifiers** and enables your cell membranes to allow both water-soluble and fat-soluble materials to pass through the membrane into your cells.

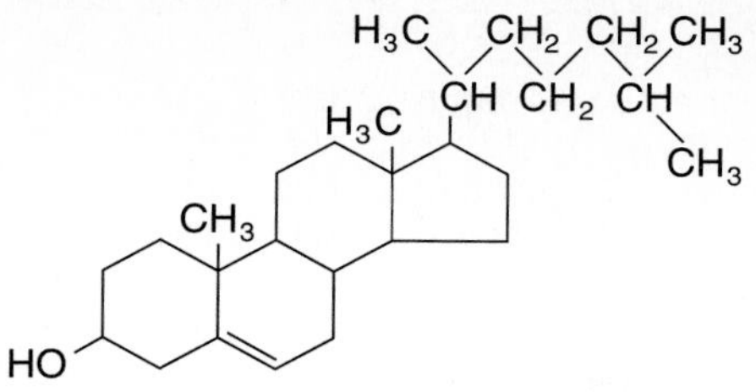

H_3C CH_2 CH_2 CH_3
CH CH_2 CH
H_3C
CH_3
CH_3
HO
Cholesterol

FIGURE 6.5
Cholesterol.

Cholesterol is constructed of connected ring structures (shown here as hexagons) rather than the chains seen in glycerides. In chemical shorthand, the six points of a hexagon represent carbon atoms, each with 2 hydrogen atoms attached.

Sterols in Nature

Sterols are unlike triglycerides in the organization of their carbon, hydrogen, and oxygen components. Sterols consist of rings of carbon chains attached to each other, sometimes with fatty acids attached. Nonetheless, sterols qualify as lipids because they are organic substances that are insoluble in water and soluble in ether.

sterols—class of lipids that includes certain hormones and vitamin D

Undoubtedly the best-known sterol is **cholesterol,** a compound produced by animals, including humans (Figure 6.5). Cholesterol is particularly abundant in egg yolks and organ meats, such as liver. Although cholesterol and saturated fats are both lipids typically found in animal products, they are distinctly different from each other. Other sterols in food include vitamin D and **precursors** of vitamin D; they are discussed in Chapter 11 (on vitamins).

cholesterol—important sterol that is produced by the body and ingested in foods of animal origin

precursor—a substance from which another substance is formed

Lipids and Processing

Food scientists have developed ways to modify food fats, just as they have modified carbohydrates. For example, it is possible to separate fats (such as butter and lard) and oils (such as soybean, peanut, and safflower oils) from their natural sources so that they can be used as ingredients or as frying agents. Food technology can also prolong the shelf life and sensory appeal of fats and oils through such techniques as refining, bleaching, and deodorizing.

The food industry has also used other properties of some of the naturally occurring lipids. Mono- and diglycerides are good emulsifiers, for example, so they are often used as additives to prevent the separation of watery and fatty fractions of salad dressings, margarines, baking batters, and other products. Lecithin, a phospholipid discussed above, can also serve that purpose.

Another application of food science to lipid modification is the **hydrogenation** of oils. This process forces hydrogen into oils with a high PUFA content, thereby increasing their degree of saturation, firming them, and lengthening their shelf life. Hydrogenation can be partial or complete. A whole range of margarines and shortenings on the market have been hydrogenated to varying degrees; to some extent, you can judge the level of hydrogenation by how firm or soft they are. Figure 6.6 shows examples of lipids listed on food labels.

hydrogenation—the forcing of hydrogen into unsaturated oils to make them firmer and to prolong shelf life

In recent years, other fat-related innovations have appeared on the market, and interest in them is growing. We're talking about **fat substitutes.** These products have some of the sensory characteristics (such as look, taste, and/or mouth feel) of common dietary fats without the same high kcaloric value. When fat substitutes are used as ingredients, foods have a lower

fat substitutes—substances that have the sensory properties of fat without the high kcalorie value of fat

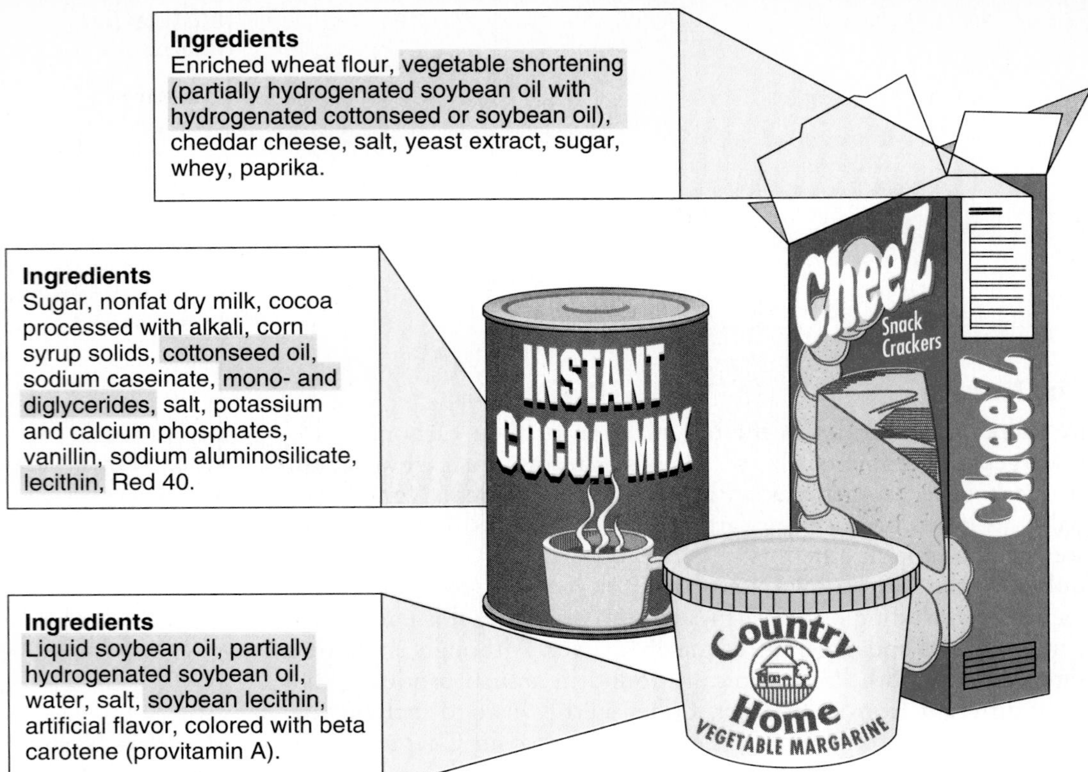

FIGURE 6.6
Examples of lipids in three processed foods.

kcalorie value than their traditional counterparts. Each type of fat substitute has physical and chemical characteristics that restrict its use; Table 6.2 lists several of them and describes their applications.

Fat substitutes are made from a variety of materials. Carbohydrate-derived products, such as *maltodextrin* and *polydextrose,* have been used as partial fat replacements for more than a decade. Proteins from egg white and/or milk are used to produce *Simplesse®*, a recent addition to the "fake fat" roster. Because these substances are made from energy nutrients, they are not kcalorie-free, but they are lower in kcalories than the fat they replace. Because they are made from materials present in the natural food supply, they more easily gain the approval of the Food and Drug Administration (FDA) for inclusion in the food supply.

sucrose polyester—a laboratory-produced fat substitute made from the union of carbohydrate and lipid components

Other types of fat substitutes are waiting in the wings for approval. **Sucrose polyester** (proposed brand name: *Olestra*) is an example. Not present in nature, it is an indigestible compound of sucrose units and fat components. Because it cannot be broken apart and absorbed in the gastrointestinal (GI) tract, it will provide no kcalories. Before a new fat substitute of such unusual molecules can be put onto the market, research on its safety must undergo careful FDA evaluation.

The maker of the proposed product must pay for extensive testing regarding its safety and effects on other food components. The producer must deliver the test data to the FDA, where the data are interpreted and a decision is reached. The testing, evaluation, and approval for one product usually take many years, if approval is obtained at all. (Chapter 14 provides more details about the approval process for substances which are new to the food supply.)

TABLE 6.2 Fat Substitutes

Substance	Description	Typical Uses	Comments
Maltodextrin Maltrin®	Hydrolyzed corn-starch; water can be added	Used commercially in salad dressings, table spreads, frozen desserts	1–4 kcal/g, depending on water content; can partially replace fat
Nutrifat C®	Hydrolyzed dextrins from wheat, potato, corn, tapioca	Used commercially in cakes, ice cream, mayonnaise, salad dressings	1.2 kcal/g; can partially replace fat
Polydextrose	Water-soluble fiber made from dextrose	Used commercially in baked goods, frostings, frozen desserts, puddings, dry cake and cookie mixes	1 kcal/g due to partial metabolism; serves as a bulking agent and partial replacement for fat and sugar
Shortening replacer N-Flate®	Mixture of emulsifiers, modified food starch, guar gum, nonfat dry milk	Used commercially in baked goods	Can reduce kcal content of cakes by one-third
Simplesse®	Physically modified milk protein and/or egg white protein; water added	Original version used in frozen desserts, suitable only for unheated foods; second version suitable for baked products	1–2 kcal/g, depending on formulation; original version breaks down if heated; second version withstands cooking and baking
Sucrose polyester Olestra®	Chemical union of sucrose and lipid components	Pending approval; suitable for frying; potentially wide variety of uses	0 kcalories; indigestible; will only partially replace fat
Tapioca dextrin N-Oil®	Hydrolyzed tapioca starch; water can be added	Used commercially in salad dressings, table spreads, frozen desserts	1–4 kcal/g, depending on water content
Trailblazer®	Similar to Simplesse® but by different manufacturer	Pending approval	See comments for Simplesse®

References: "Fats, oils and fat substitutes," 1989; "Fat substitute update," 1990; Waring, 1988; "Nutrifat," 1988; The Nutrasweet Company, Consumer Affairs Division (personal communication), 1992.

While the various proposed products are awaiting approval, there is speculation on matters besides their possible toxicity. Will people be likely to use products containing a new generation of fat substitutes? It looks that way: a survey of 2000 households showed that approximately half of consumers wanted to try fat-reduced spreads (butter, salad dressings, mayonnaise, and cheese), and over 70% were interested in purchasing a fried or baked product in which some of the fat is replaced with a fat substitute (Bruhn et al., 1992).

How much of a reduction in fat could you achieve by using fat-reduced products instead of what you usually eat? Researchers have calculated the effect of substituting all available types of fat-reduced products for current comparable food choices and found that average total daily fat intakes would decline by 10 grams, saturated fat by 3 grams, and cholesterol by 13 mg (Lyle et al., 1992).

Of course, that's just a forecast; questions remain about what will happen once such products come into more widespread use (Mela, 1992). For example, if we decrease our intake of fat by using a fat-free salad dressing instead of a traditional oily dressing, will we tend to compensate by eating more butter on our dinner rolls? Only time will tell, but public education about these products could help people learn to use them to best advantage (American Dietetic Association, 1991).

Amounts of Lipids in Foods

Although you can sometimes see how much lipid is in a food simply by looking at it (such as the fat on meat, or the butter on bread), fats are often hidden in food (such as the shortening in pie crust or the fat in an avocado). Therefore, it is hard for most people to estimate their fat intake. In the United States, people consume a higher proportion of "hidden" fats than visible ones (National Research Council, 1989). Table 6.3 compares the approximate amounts of saturated and unsaturated fats that are present in various foods and food groups, and Appendix C provides values for more than 2000 additional foods.

Glycerides

Fruits, vegetables, and grains, as found in nature, have little fat. Fats added during processing or home cooking, however, can substantially raise the lipid level of a product. Look at what happens when plain, fresh vegetables such as potatoes are processed into potato chips, and note that although flour has very little fat, the fat content of some baked goods is higher.

The foods that are naturally high in fat include some dairy products, many meats, and nuts. In the case of dairy products, food technology has developed ways of removing fat to provide some lower fat options: skim milk is almost devoid of fat, for example, as are products made from it, such as yogurt cultured from skim milk. Several cheeses that can be made from partly skimmed milk, such as mozzarella, ricotta, and low-fat cottage cheese,

TABLE 6.3 Amounts of Saturated Fat[a] and Unsaturated Fat[b] in Standard Servings of Various Foods

Food	Household Measure	Lipids (g) 0 5 10 15 20 25 30 35 40 45
Bread, rice, cereal, pasta		
Plain bread, white	1 slice	
Cake, frosted chocolate	2 ounces	
Cookies, oatmeal	4 small	
Corn chips	1 ounce	
Plain rice, pasta, most cereal	½ cup	
Vegetables		
Most plain, fresh, frozen, canned vegetables	½ cup	tr[c]
Potato chips	1 ounce	

[a]Solid parts of bars denote total saturated fatty acids. In the future, dietary recommendations may limit some (rather than all) saturated fatty acids.
[b]Open parts of bars denote total monounsaturated and polyunsaturated fatty acids.
[c]Trace

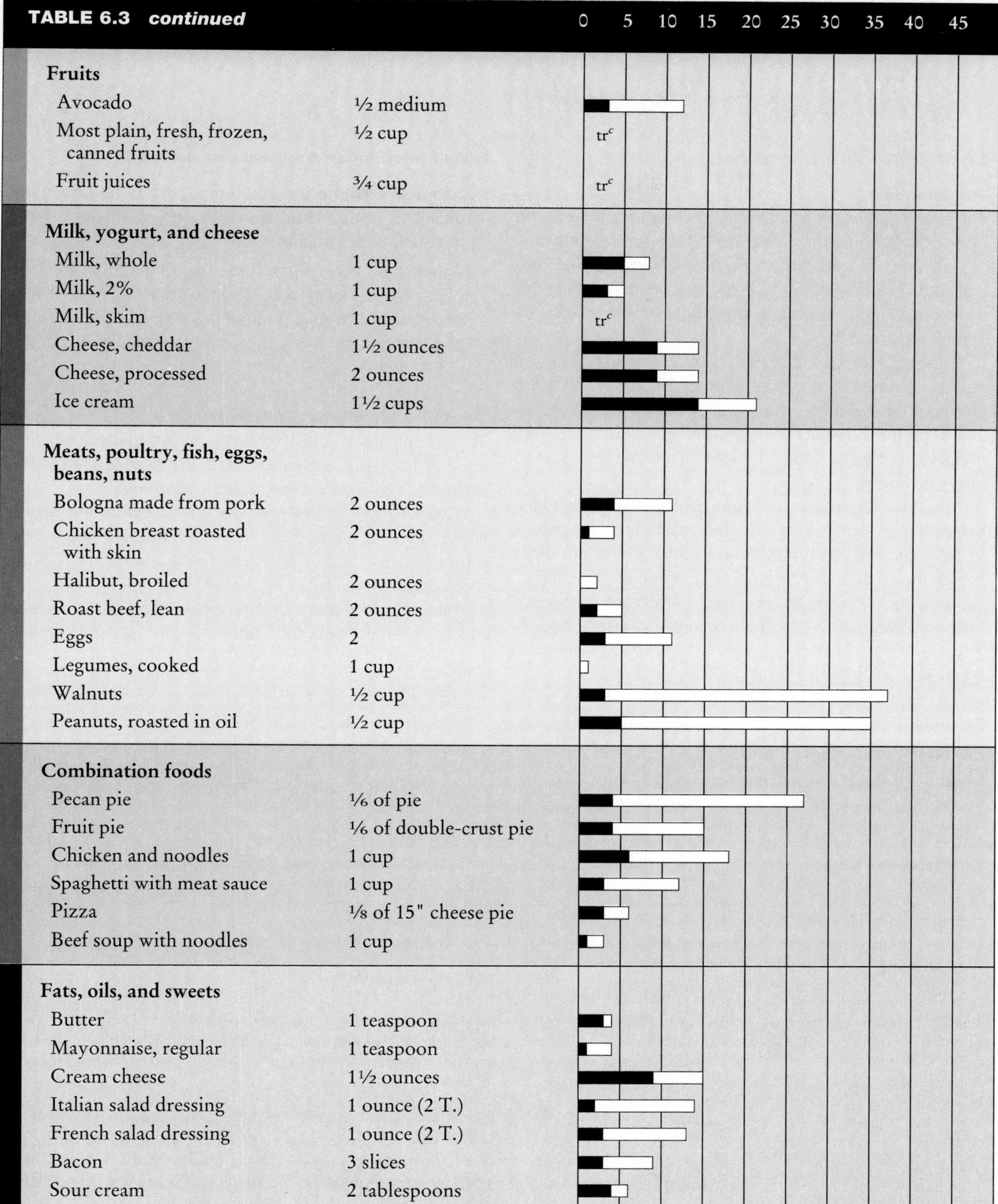

TABLE 6.3 *continued*

Food	Serving	0 5 10 15 20 25 30 35 40 45
Fruits		
Avocado	½ medium	
Most plain, fresh, frozen, canned fruits	½ cup	tr[c]
Fruit juices	¾ cup	tr[c]
Milk, yogurt, and cheese		
Milk, whole	1 cup	
Milk, 2%	1 cup	
Milk, skim	1 cup	tr[c]
Cheese, cheddar	1½ ounces	
Cheese, processed	2 ounces	
Ice cream	1½ cups	
Meats, poultry, fish, eggs, beans, nuts		
Bologna made from pork	2 ounces	
Chicken breast roasted with skin	2 ounces	
Halibut, broiled	2 ounces	
Roast beef, lean	2 ounces	
Eggs	2	
Legumes, cooked	1 cup	
Walnuts	½ cup	
Peanuts, roasted in oil	½ cup	
Combination foods		
Pecan pie	⅙ of pie	
Fruit pie	⅙ of double-crust pie	
Chicken and noodles	1 cup	
Spaghetti with meat sauce	1 cup	
Pizza	⅛ of 15" cheese pie	
Beef soup with noodles	1 cup	
Fats, oils, and sweets		
Butter	1 teaspoon	
Mayonnaise, regular	1 teaspoon	
Cream cheese	1½ ounces	
Italian salad dressing	1 ounce (2 T.)	
French salad dressing	1 ounce (2 T.)	
Bacon	3 slices	
Sour cream	2 tablespoons	

[a]Solid parts of bars denote total saturated fatty acids. In the future, dietary recommendations may limit some (rather than all) saturated fatty acids.
[b]Open parts of bars denote total monounsaturated and polyunsaturated fatty acids.
[c]Trace

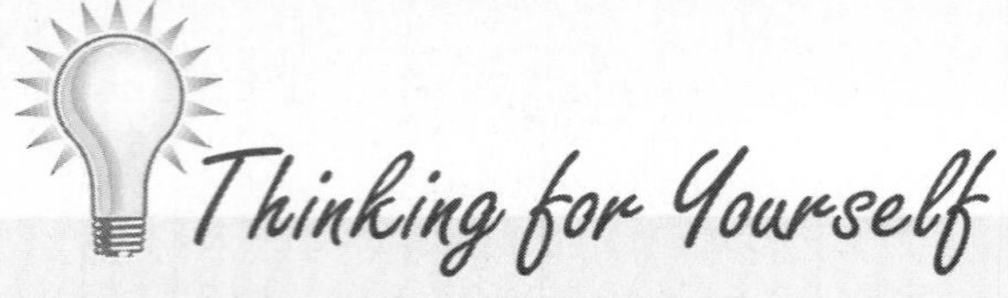

Using Fat Claims and Facts

The Situation

You are shopping for food, trying to find products lower in fat than your usual fare. You know (from having analyzed several days' diet records using Act on Fact 5.1) that your typical daily intake of fat exceeds the recommended 30% of kcalories, and you have decided that it's time to do something about it.

Pushing your cart through the supermarket, you see various products with label claims suggesting that the products don't contain much fat. A box of muffins is labeled "fat free." A lunchmeat product is called "lean," and a frozen entree is labeled "light." A salad dressing is marked "low fat."

You have heard that the word *light* has no legal definition and that some processors use it simply to get people to buy their products. However, you think that the other terms are legitimate. As you pick up a few of these items, you wonder: What do these terms really mean? How can I use this information to reduce my fat intake?

Is Your Information Accurate and Relevant?

- Although it is true that the term *light* has had no legal definition for use on labels in the past, now it does have meaning (more on this later).
- The terms *fat free, lean, and low fat* each specify an upper limit for fat in food. New food labeling regulations stipulate that by mid-summer of 1994, these terms can be used only on foods that meet the published criteria (CFR, 1993).

What Else Should You Consider?

Terms that describe fat contents on food labels are defined in Table 6.A. Note that there are more terms on the table than appeared in the situation above.

Two terms—*fat free* and *low fat*—describe the upper limit of total fat allowed per serving of food. Although the amounts of fat defined for these terms are different, both are modest amounts.

Two other descriptors—*lean* and *extra lean*—express allowable amounts of total fat, saturated fat, and choles-

TABLE 6.A Label Language: Fat

By mid-summer, 1994, these terms are allowed on products that match the definitions below:

Fat free: Contains less than 0.5 grams of total fat per serving

Low fat: Contains no more than 3 grams of total fat per serving

Low in saturated fat: Contains no more than 1 gram of saturated fat per serving

Cholesterol free: Contains less than 2 mg of cholesterol and 2 grams of saturated fat per serving

Low in cholesterol: Contains no more than 20 mg of cholesterol and 2 grams of saturated fat per serving

Extra lean: Contains less than 5 grams of total fat, 2 grams of saturated fat, and 95 mg of cholesterol per 100-gram (approximately 3-ounce) serving of meat or poultry product

Lean: Contains less than 10 grams of total fat, 4 grams of saturated fat, and 95 mg of cholesterol per 100-gram (approximately 3-ounce) serving of meat or poultry product

Reduced fat, less fat, lower in fat, lower fat: Contains at least 25% less total fat than the regular product

Light: Contains at least one-third fewer kcalories and/or 50% less fat than the regular product

have less fat than their full-fat counterparts. Read the label to be sure. Now, thanks to food processing techniques, cheeses that taste like traditional Swiss and cheddar are also produced with reduced fat content.

Many meats and meat products are also being trimmed of their traditionally higher fat values. Both the methods of raising the animals and of processing the meat contribute to this decrease in fat (see Chapter 13).

Commercially prepared convenience foods are also on the low-fat bandwagon. In product categories such as single-serving frozen entrees and

terol per 100 grams of meat and poultry products. For example, *lean ham* can have up to 10 grams of fat per 100 grams of ham, which is the same as saying that it can be as much as 10% fat by weight. Don't think this means that only 10% of the kcalories are from fat, though. If a 100-gram portion (approximately 3 ounces) of ham has 10 grams of fat, the fat provides 90 kcalories (10 g fat x 9 kcal/g). The same serving of ham has approximately 23 grams of protein, which provides 92 kcalories (23 g protein x 4 kcal/g). Note that practically half—49%—of the kcalories in the lean ham comes from fat.

Other terms—*reduced, less, fewer, lower in, lower, and light*—are relative terms. Although the definition of these terms do not give the grams or mg of lipids per serving, such information is close by on the nutrition facts panel (see right), where the product's contents of total fat, saturated fat, and cholesterol are shown (a). These values are also expressed as a percentage of the Daily Value (b), which is the recommended daily upper limit for a person who consumes about 2000 kcalories per day.

A final point: Although the new labels give you tools for carefully controlling the amount of fat in your diet, remember that *you need some fat.* You cannot be healthy without adequate amounts of the essential fatty acids, so don't use this information to cut your fat intake too drastically.

Nutrition Facts

Serving Size ½ cup (90g)
Servings Per Container 8

Amount Per Serving

Calories 110 Calories from Fat 20 (c)

	% Daily Value*
Total Fat 2g	**20%**
(a) Saturated Fat 1g	**25%**
Cholesterol 7mg	**10%** (b)
Sodium 80mg	**28%**
Total Carbohydrate 19g	**11%**
Dietary Fiber 0g	**0%**
Sugars 19g	
Protein 4g	

Vitamin A 2% • Vitamin C 0% • Calcium 14% • Iron 1%

*Percent Daily Values are based on a 2,000 calorie diet. Your daily values may be higher or lower depending on your calorie needs:

	Calories:	2,000	2,500
Total Fat	Less than	65g	80g
Sat Fat	Less than	20g	25g
Cholesterol	Less than	300mg	300mg
Sodium	Less than	2,400mg	2,400mg
Total Carbohydrate		300g	375g
Dietary Fiber		25g	30g

Calories per gram:
Fat 9 • Carbohydrate 4 • Protein 4

Now What Do You Think?

- Option 1 You decide that it is too much work to deal with all this information; you would rather eat high-fat foods less often or in smaller servings than you currently do—and increase your intake of other types of food that are generally lower in fat, such as pasta, plain breads, fruits, and vegetables.
- Option 2 You decide that as a first step, you will try the *lower in fat* and *light* products, find out whether you like them, and evaluate your diet afterward to see whether the percentage of fat in your diet comes within recommendations.
- Option 3 You decide first to determine what your recommended limit is for fat per day (Act on Fact 6.1 helps with this) and then to control your intake using the absolute amounts of fat listed on nutrition facts panels.
- Option 4 You decide to take guidance from the % Daily Values on the label, setting a limit for how high you can go for any single food item.
- Option 5 You decide to set a limit on what proportion of kcalories in the food you eat can come from fat, such as one-third. For an individual food, you will divide Calories from fat by Calories (see above[c]) to see whether the food is within the limit.

Which of these options—or any other you can think of—will work best for you?

desserts, you can now find many items produced with greatly reduced fat contents, as compared with their traditional counterparts.

But how can you know when you shop for food which items really net you a significant fat saving? Information on food labels can be a great help. By May, 1994, a new format for food labels will be required on processed products which specifies not only total fat but also saturated fat per serving. The Thinking for Yourself above acquaints you with the meanings of the fat-related terms the new labels will carry and invites you to use the information the new labels provide.

TABLE 6.4 Cholesterol in Some Foods

Food	Household Measure	Cholesterol (mg) 0 100 200 300 400 500 600
Bread, cereal, rice, pasta		
Bread, plain	1 slice	
Cake (most plain mix or commercial)	1 piece	tr
Cereal, pasta, grains	½ cup	
Vegetables		
All types	½ cup	
Fruits		
All types	½ cup	
Milk, yogurt, and cheese		
Milk, whole	1 cup	
Milk, 2%	1 cup	
Milk, skim	1 cup	
Cheese, cheddar	1⅓ ounces	
Ice cream	1½ cups	
Meat, poultry, fish, eggs, beans, nuts		
Beef, ground, baked	2 ounces	
Chicken, baked, with skin	2 ounces	
Chorizo	2 ounces	
Fish (cod), baked	2 ounces	
Shrimp, boiled	2 ounces	
Eggs	2 large	
Legumes; nuts	½ cup	
Liver, beef	2 ounces	
Fats, oils, and sweets		
Alcoholic beverages	1 serving	
Butter	1 tablespoon	
Cream cheese	1½ ounces	
Mayonnaise	1 tablespoon	
Vegetable oils	1 tablespoon	

Cholesterol

Compared to glycerides, cholesterol occurs in only minute amounts in foods. An average serving of food may contain many *grams* of triglycerides, but will contain only *milligrams* of cholesterol. Your own body produces more cholesterol than your diet provides. Cholesterol and diet are discussed in more detail later in this chapter, in the section on heart disease.

As we mentioned earlier, cholesterol is found only in products of animal origin. Table 6.4 compares the amounts of cholesterol in standard serving sizes of certain foods, and Appendix C gives the values for many more. Notice that there are not many concentrated sources of cholesterol; egg yolk is the only commonly eaten food that stands out.

TABLE 6.5 Phases of Digestion and Absorption of Two Types of Lipids

	Triglycerides	Cholesterol and Cholesterol Esters
Mouth	—	—
Stomach	—	—
Small intestine	Emulsification by bile acids; enzymatic hydrolysis to glycerol, fatty acids, and monoglycerides by pancreatic and intestinal enzymes; ferrying by micelles to intestinal wall cells; absorption	Enzymatic hydrolysis of cholesterol esters to free cholesterol and fatty acids; secretion of bile acids (containing cholesterol); ferrying by micelles to intestinal wall cells; absorption
Large intestine	—	—

You may wonder why we have not discussed the amount of phospholipids in foods. Scientists do not believe that the low levels in food are significant to health, so extensive analysis has not been warranted. For the same reason, the remainder of this chapter focuses on glycerides and cholesterol.

How Your Body Digests and Absorbs Lipids

Now that you have an idea of where the most important lipids are in your diet, let's consider their digestion and absorption. In this section, we discuss triglycerides, which represent the overwhelming majority of lipids we consume, and cholesterol, which not only is an important structural material but also is associated with heart disease.

Digestion and Absorption of Triglycerides

Most lipid digestion takes place in your small intestine. There, two substances—*bile* and *lipases*—play vital roles in preparing lipids for absorption.

Bile is a greenish liquid that is synthesized in the liver and released into your small intestine when fat is present. It contains cholesterol, lecithin, and **bile acids,** which are emulsifiers. Bile salts help keep the triglycerides in small droplets, making them more available to digestive enzymes.

bile—substance produced by the liver that maintains emulsions in the small intestine

bile acids—derivatives of cholesterol that are components of bile

Lipases, the enzymes that digest lipids, are produced primarily in the pancreas and in the small intestine. Lipases break down triglycerides into monoglycerides, glycerol, and fatty acids, all of which are then incorporated along with bile salts into conglomerations called *micelles.* Micelles ferry the lipid fragments to the intestinal wall cells for absorption, after which most of the remaining components are recycled to continue the process.

lipases—enzymes that digest lipids

Normally, this system works very effectively. If an abundance of bile salts is present, a healthy small intestine usually digests and absorbs over 95% of all fats (RDA Subcommittee, 1989).

Digestion and Absorption of Cholesterol

Cholesterol in food often has a fatty acid attached to it, a compound called a **cholesterol ester.** The fatty acid must be removed before you can absorb cholesterol. Enzymes in the small intestine accomplish this task. Cholesterol is best absorbed when micelles are available to ferry it to the intestinal wall cells. You don't absorb all of the cholesterol you consume; estimates range from 25% to 75% (Kantor, 1989), with the average at about 55% (McNamara, 1987). Table 6.5 summarizes the phases of digestion and absorption of both triglycerides and cholesterol esters.

cholesterol ester—chemical combination of cholesterol and fatty acid(s)

How Your Body Makes Its Own Lipids

The absorbed products of lipid digestion—glycerol, fatty acids, cholesterol—do not stay in these smaller particles for long. Right in the cells lining your small intestine, they mix and mingle with each other and with similar substances previously in your body to form your body lipids.

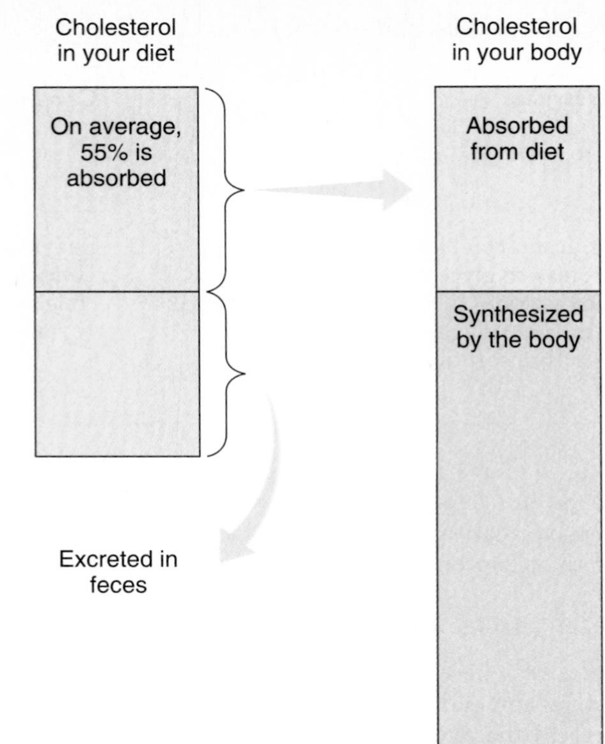

FIGURE 6.7
Where the cholesterol in your body comes from.

Only part of the cholesterol in your body is absorbed from food. On average, we absorb 55% of the cholesterol present in the small intestine; therefore, the typical North American 70-kg man, who consumes approximately 450 mg of cholesterol per day, absorbs approximately 250 mg of it. The body of that same man synthesizes approximately 840 mg of cholesterol per day, largely in his liver. (From McNamara, 1987.)

Triglycerides

Your triglycerides, just like triglycerides in foods, are formed from glycerol and fatty acids. Your body may absorb some of these components but others may have been synthesized from surplus carbohydrate, protein, or alcohol; your body can make fat components from all these sources. This metabolic thriftiness has been an important survival mechanism in times of scarcity through the ages. But if food supplies are abundant and you consistently eat more than you need, you will gradually accumulate an excessive amount of body fat.

Cholesterol

The cholesterol you absorb from food is not the only cholesterol in your body; your body, especially your liver, readily produces cholesterol so that there is always enough for its many important functions.

Your liver can produce cholesterol from fragments of any of the energy nutrients. In most people, the liver adjusts the amount of cholesterol it produces according to the amount absorbed from the diet. In general, the more cholesterol in the diet, the less the liver produces; the less the diet contains, the more the body produces. For most people, this *feedback mechanism* works effectively to keep the total amount of cholesterol in their blood quite stable under ordinary circumstances (McNamara et al., 1987). Some people's bodies, however, do not compensate as successfully for the cholesterol absorbed from the diet. At least one-third of the population experiences an increase in blood cholesterol when they consume dietary cholesterol (National Research Council, 1989). Nevertheless, for most people, the amount of cholesterol produced by the body (primarily in the liver) is substantially larger than the amount absorbed from the diet (Figure 6.7).

You Tell Me

> **The March 28, 1991, edition of the *New England Journal of Medicine* published a case study of an 88-year-old man who claimed he had eaten *25 eggs per day for at least 15 years;* yet, his blood cholesterol was normal (Kern, 1991).**
>
> **Which of the physiologic factors that determine how the body handles cholesterol could explain this? Would eating this many eggs have the same effect on everyone?**

Why is it that the body is so intent on making sure it has enough cholesterol? As we have mentioned, cholesterol is a very important biologic substance. The major function of cholesterol in the body is to help form bile acids. Additionally, cholesterol is an important structural element in cell membranes, forms the protective covering on nerves, and is the material from which steroid hormones, vitamin D, and various other body substances are derived. Unfortunately, cholesterol can also accumulate in blood vessel walls; this is the one characteristic that is not healthy, because it can cause narrowing of the affected vessels and could ultimately result in blockage. This is how the most common form of cardiovascular disease develops.

We'll say much more about this later in the chapter. In preparation, let's become familiar with how lipids are transported in the body.

Lipoproteins—How Lipids Get Around in Your Body

As you have read, many of the absorbed lipid breakdown products are quickly reassembled inside the cells of the small intestine into glycerides and cholesterol esters. Other components are not; for example, short- and medium-chain fatty acids, which are water-soluble, can be absorbed directly into the bloodstream and are transported via the portal vein to the liver. But the reassembled triglycerides and cholesterol esters are not soluble in water. They must be put into a water-soluble form, because otherwise they would clump together and possibly clog up your vessels. Your body makes them soluble by combining them into conglomerates with phospholipids and encasing them in a surface coat that includes protein. The resulting soluble compounds are called **lipoproteins** (Figure 6.8). Lipoproteins can be made not only in the cells of your small intestine but also in your liver. The various types of lipoproteins differ from one another in the amounts of triglyceride, phospholipid, and cholesterol they contain. They also differ in the amounts and types of protein they contain.

lipoprotein—water-soluble aggregates of triglycerides, phospholipids, cholesterol, and protein that can be transported in the bloodstream

Lipoprotein Formed in the Intestine

The principal type of lipoprotein formed in the intestinal wall cell is the **chylomicron.** It contains more triglyceride than any other type of lipoprotein. Chylomicrons move from the intestinal wall cells into the lacteals of the lymphatic system and eventually join the bloodstream. As these and other lipoproteins move through the body, many of them give up their triglycerides to muscle and fat cells along the way.

chylomicron—principal type of lipoprotein formed in the intestinal wall cells after a meal; consists mostly of triglyceride

Chylomicrons are short-lived: by several hours after an average meal, chylomicrons have been broken apart and their components used for energy

FIGURE 6.8
General structure of lipoproteins.

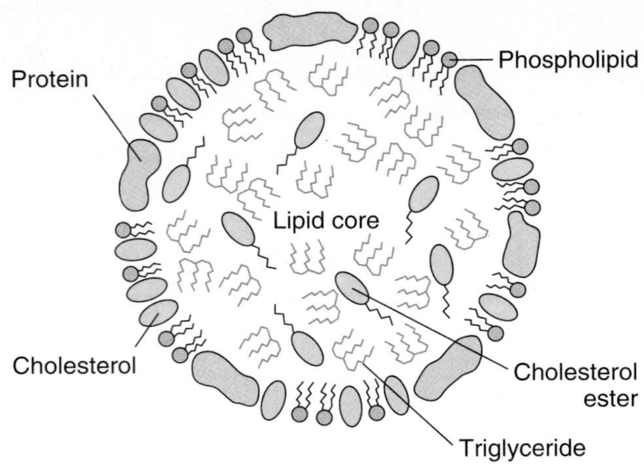

and for making other lipids. If you have a blood sample drawn an hour or two after a meal, it will reveal a much higher level of chylomicrons than a sample drawn after many hours without food (Linscheer and Vergroesen, 1988).

The levels of lipoproteins that are synthesized by the liver, by contrast, tend to be present in the blood at more consistent levels throughout the day, because they are regulated by the feedback mechanism that was described earlier.

Lipoproteins Formed in the Liver

high density lipoprotein (HDL)—lipoprotein containing a high proportion of protein

low density lipoprotein (LDL)—lipoprotein containing a high proportion of cholesterol

very low density lipoprotein (VLDL)—lipoprotein containing about half its substance as triglyceride

The lipoproteins formed by the liver are named according to their relative *density* (mass per unit volume). The substances within lipoproteins that are the most dense are the proteins; therefore, the lipoproteins containing the most protein are called **high density lipoproteins (HDL).** Other lipoproteins produced by the liver are **low density lipoproteins (LDL)** and **very low density lipoproteins (VLDL).** All of these lipoproteins are released from the liver into the bloodstream, where they undergo considerable change: components of various lipoproteins are plucked off and traded back and forth, a process that sometimes even changes the lipoproteins into different types. For example, much of the VLDL eventually is converted into LDL. Table 6.6 indicates the relative size of these lipoproteins and proportions of various components they contain.

From here on, we will deal primarily with HDL and LDL, the two types of lipoproteins that assume particular importance in the upcoming discussion of cardiovascular disease.

In all people, there is much more LDL than HDL present in the blood; this is normal. But there is considerable individual variation in the absolute amounts of LDL and HDL. Statistics show that people who have elevated total cholesterol or elevated LDL cholesterol are statistically at greater risk of coronary heart disease (CHD). High blood HDL levels, however, are *inversely* correlated to CHD; that is, *the higher your HDL, the less your risk.* This is why the popular press often refers to LDL as "bad cholesterol" and to HDL as "good cholesterol."

But what is it that *makes* "bad cholesterol" bad and "good cholesterol" good? Scientists are trying to find the answer. It appears that HDL is likely to take cholesterol *away* from the tissues (i.e., from the linings of blood vessels) and carry it back to the liver, where it does no harm, at least for a while.

TABLE 6.6 Some Important Lipoproteins in the Bloodstream

Type of Lipoprotein	Major Site of Synthesis	Relative Size and Composition	Comments
Chylomicrons	Small intestine	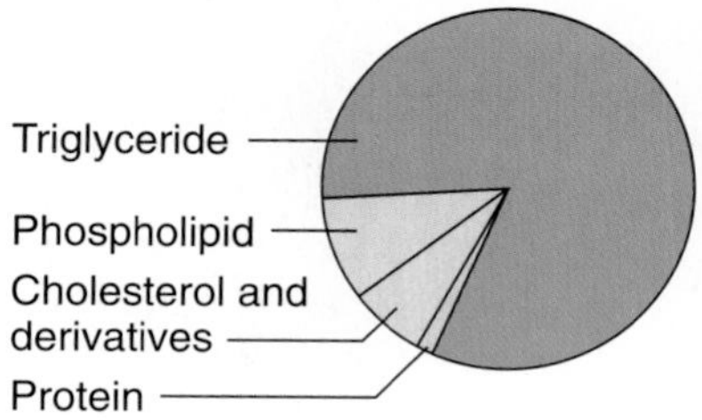 Triglyceride; Phospholipid; Cholesterol and derivatives; Protein	Present in blood for a few hours after meals; are processed into other forms
Very low density lipoproteins (VLDL)	Small intestine Liver	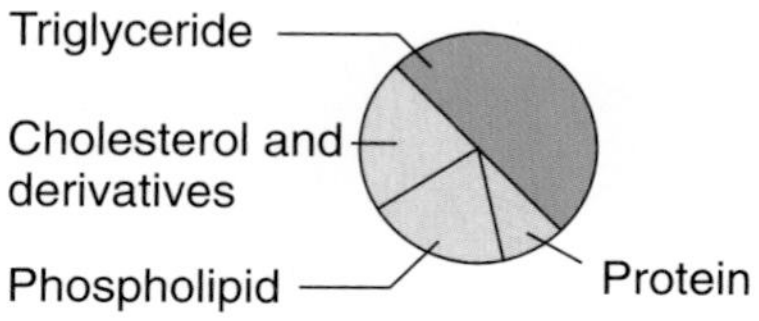 Triglyceride; Cholesterol and derivatives; Phospholipid; Protein	Most gets converted to LDL
Low density lipoproteins (LDL)	Liver	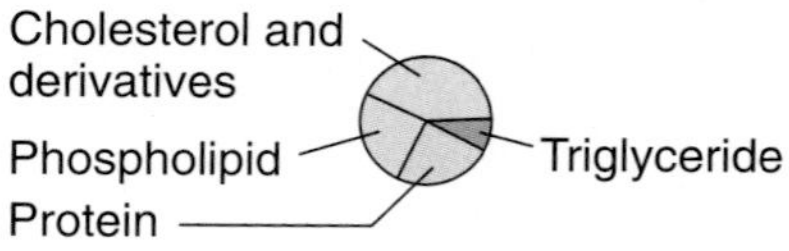 Cholesterol and derivatives; Phospholipid; Protein; Triglyceride	Some used for bile production; the rest circulates in blood for use in other body materials. Some may accumulate in the walls of blood vessels
High density lipoproteins (HDL)	Liver	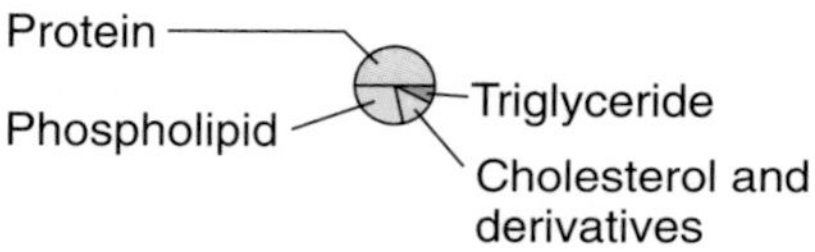 Protein; Phospholipid; Triglyceride; Cholesterol and derivatives	Some used for bile production; the rest circulates in blood for other uses

Data source: Linscheer and Vergroesen, 1988.

Researchers Michael Brown and Joseph Goldstein (1986) shed light on another factor that can affect levels of blood cholesterol. They discovered that there are special structures, *lipoprotein receptors,* on the membranes of liver cells that enable the cells to take in lipoprotein cholesterol, thereby removing cholesterol from the blood and inhibiting cholesterol synthesis by liver cells. If a person's liver cells have fewer of these receptors than normal, or if they are less responsive than normal, the level of cholesterol in the blood is likely to be higher. The relative number of cholesterol receptors a person has appears to be an inherited trait. This discovery was deemed so important that Brown and Goldstein received a Nobel Prize for their work.

Additional research suggests that the receptors recognize lipoproteins based in part on the type of *protein* they contain (Linscheer and Vergroesen, 1988). This is an important topic of current research.

Cholesterol that enters liver cells can be used in various ways. It may be recycled into different lipoproteins or used to make bile acids. As we mentioned earlier, cholesterol is more likely to become a part of bile than to be used for anything else. Approximately 1000 mg of biliary cholesterol enters a person's intestinal tract each day. Of that, about half is reabsorbed and the other half excreted (McNamara, 1987). This is the major way in

FIGURE 6.9
Where the cholesterol in your body goes.

Your body needs cholesterol—many important body substances contain it. More goes into bile than into anything else, and about half of the cholesterol from bile is reabsorbed (McNamara, 1987). The one negative characteristic of cholesterol is that sometimes it is deposited in the linings of blood vessels, where it may eventually interfere with blood flow.

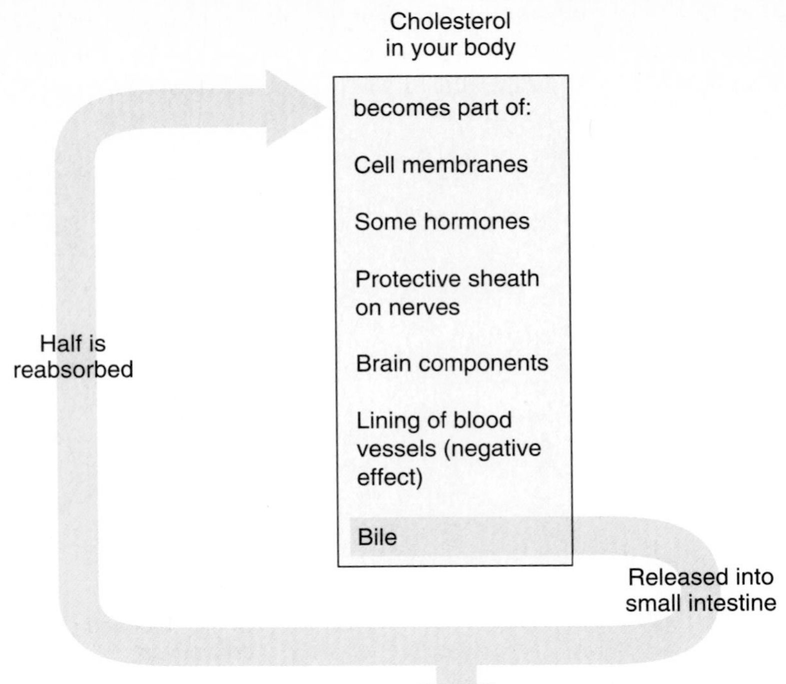

which the body rids itself of cholesterol. Figure 6.9 summarizes the various ways in which the body uses cholesterol and recaptures part of what is in bile.

Lipids and Cardiovascular Disease

Up to now, we have focused on how food lipids are digested and rebuilt into body lipids and how they contribute to your body's healthy functioning. Now we have to take a look at the darker side of lipids—the health problems they may contribute to in some people. In this section, you'll have a chance to look critically for yourself at the evidence for and against the roles of lipids in cardiovascular disease. First, we'll discuss an all-too-common disease of the cardiovascular system.

atherosclerosis—disease in which certain materials gradually accumulate in the lining of blood vessels, interfering with their function

Atherosclerosis is the major disease affecting the heart and blood vessels. Heart and blood vessel diseases are the leading causes of death in the United States and other developed countries. Although the number of these deaths has been declining steadily in the United States since the 1960s, heart and blood vessel diseases still account for almost half the deaths in this country.

Although atherosclerosis has been the subject of thousands of studies of various kinds, *there is still no absolute proof as to what causes it.* There are two major theories, however (Addis and Park, 1989). One theory proposes that a minor injury to a blood vessel lining—caused by high blood pressure, for instance—prompts certain blood cells, lipoproteins, and other substances in the blood to attach to the injured site, which in turn stimulates the blood vessel to produce more cells to cover over the area. Another theory suggests that the presence of high levels of blood cholesterol or cholesterol metabolites initiate the process by unusually close contact with the

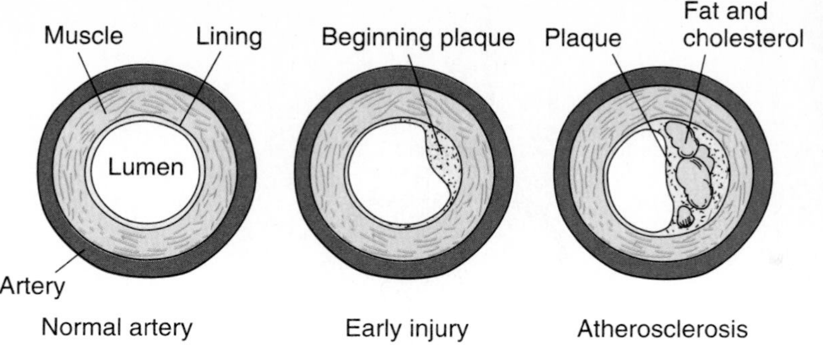

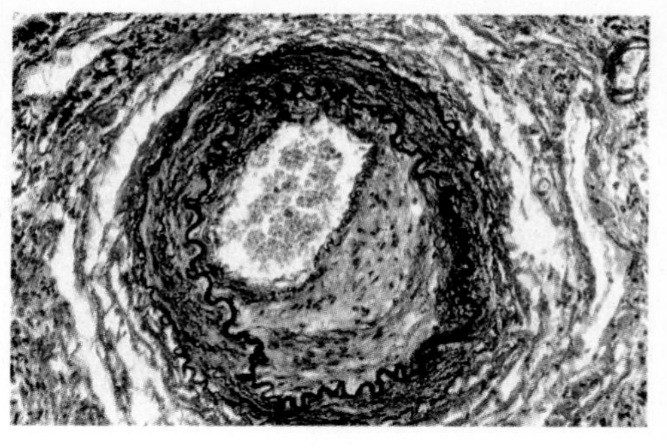

FIGURE 6.10 The development of atherosclerosis.

(a) This figure shows the progression of atherosclerosis in the cross section of an artery. The lumen of the vessel becomes progressively smaller as the disease advances, restricting blood flow. (b) This micrograph shows a human artery that is almost completely blocked.

blood vessel linings. Some recent investigation focuses on whether the oxidized form of cholesterol might be more damaging than the unoxidized form (Salonen et al., 1992; Regnstrom et al., 1992). Cholesterol can be converted to the oxidized form during food processing or even in blood vessels. In any event, the material that accumulates inside the blood vessel, which is called **plaque,** progressively narrows the opening (lumen) of the blood vessel and causes it to lose its flexibility (Figure 6.10).

As plaque builds up in a blood vessel, the chances for damage increase: a bit of loose plaque or blood clot (called a *thrombus*) could clog the narrowed vessel, a spasm could block the vessel, or a rise in blood pressure could become severe enough to cause the vessel to rupture. Any of these occurrences interrupts the delivery of oxygen and nutrients to the body cells served by the vessel, causing these cells to die within a couple of hours. If the group of cells that die is very important and/or very extensive, the person dies. With less damage, varying degrees of recovery are possible.

Although atherosclerosis can occur in various regions of the body (Figure 6.11), two areas in which the effects of atherosclerosis are most critical are the brain and heart. If atherosclerosis interrupts blood flow to the brain, a **stroke** or **cerebrovascular accident (CVA)** occurs. If atherosclerosis causes interference with blood flow to the heart muscle, a **heart attack, myocardial infarction (MI),** or **coronary occlusion** results. The development of atherosclerosis in any of the body's blood vessels, including those of the heart, is known as **cardiovascular disease (CVD);** when atherosclerosis occurs in the heart, it is usually called **coronary heart disease (CHD).**

Although both heart attacks and strokes can result in death, they are not always fatal; important determining factors are the extent of damage and the promptness and quality of care. One-third of heart attack victims die within hours of the attack. Here we will look mainly at what is known about CHD, a common type of atherosclerosis that has been the subject of much research.

plaque—patches of material that form in the lining of blood vessels in a person with atherosclerosis; consists of cells of the blood vessel lining, cholesterol, calcium, blood cells, and various other materials.

stroke, cerebrovascular accident (CVA)—result of interruption of blood flow to the brain

heart attack, myocardial infarction (MI), coronary occlusion—result of interruption of blood flow to the heart

cardiovascular disease (CVD)—impairment of the *body's* blood vessel function

coronary heart disease (CHD)—impairment of the *heart's* blood vessel function

Risk Factors for CHD

You probably know someone who has heart disease, and you may have pondered *why* this person happens to be affected. Although scientists are not certain of the direct cause(s) of CHD, epidemiologic and animal studies have shown that it occurs with greater frequency in association with certain risk factors. One epidemiologic study that has provided much data began in the late 1940s in the town of Framingham, Massachusetts; data are still being collected and analyzed today on the more than 5000 original participants.

FIGURE 6.11
More common locations of atherosclerosis.

Typical sites of atherosclerosis are shown in green in this diagram of the major arteries. Plaque tends to collect at points where an artery branches.

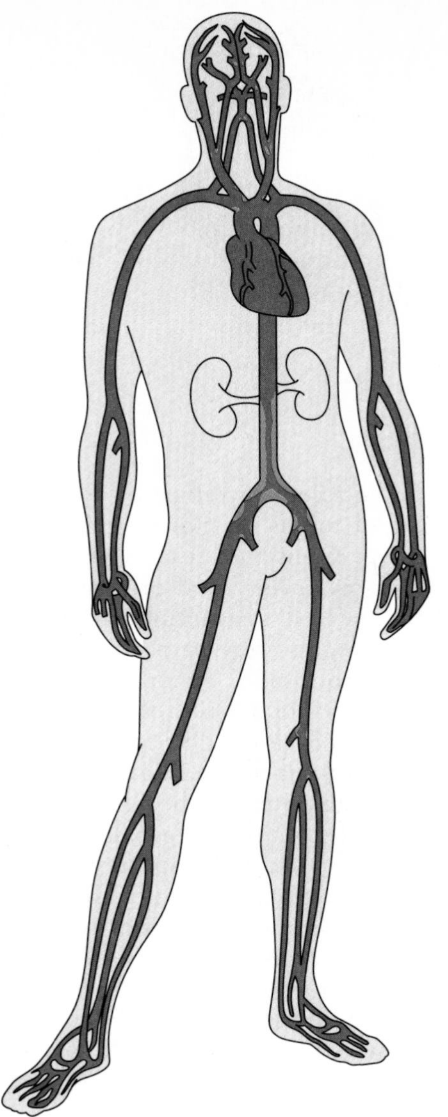

Another long-term study involves the community of Tecumseh, Michigan, and the Seven Countries study makes a broad geographical sweep. Cardiovascular risk factors in children are being evaluated in Bogalusa, Louisiana, and Muscatine, Iowa. These and thousands of other studies have identified over 20 risk factors for CHD.

There are various types of risk factors. Some cannot be changed; being male, growing older, and having a family history of atherosclerosis are *uncontrollable risk factors.* Certain *clinical measurements* indicate other risks, including such factors as high blood pressure (hypertension), obesity, high blood cholesterol, abnormal electrocardiogram (test of electrical activity of the heart), and diabetes. In addition, particular *lifestyle habits,* such as smoking, consuming too many kcalories and/or fats, being physically inactive, and taking certain medications, correlate with risk. Figure 6.12 shows many of these factors and some of their relationships. Notice that your *diet* can affect several of these risk factors.

Of the risk factors you can do something about, smoking, high blood pressure, and high blood cholesterol emerge as the most important: they

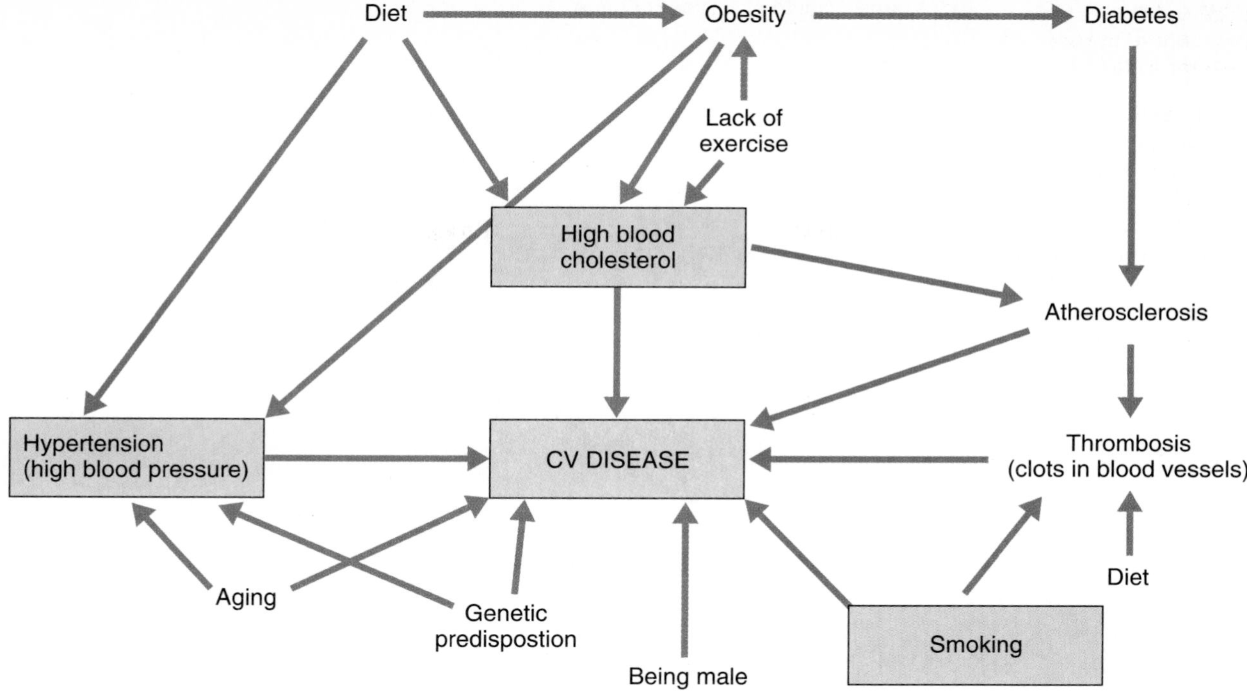

FIGURE 6.12
Some known contributors to cardiovascular disease (CVD).

This model represents some of the risk factors for CV disease that have been identified and some ways they are interrelated. The three most influential *modifiable* risk factors are smoking, hypertension, and high blood cholesterol. Diet influences several risk factors. (Modified from Zilversmit and Stark, 1984.)

have the strongest statistical association with heart attacks in white American males, the most studied population segment for connection of risk factors and CHD. Figure 6.13 shows how these factors affected the occurrence of first heart attacks during a ten-year period. Notice several important points: (1) the more of these risk factors the men had, the more likely they

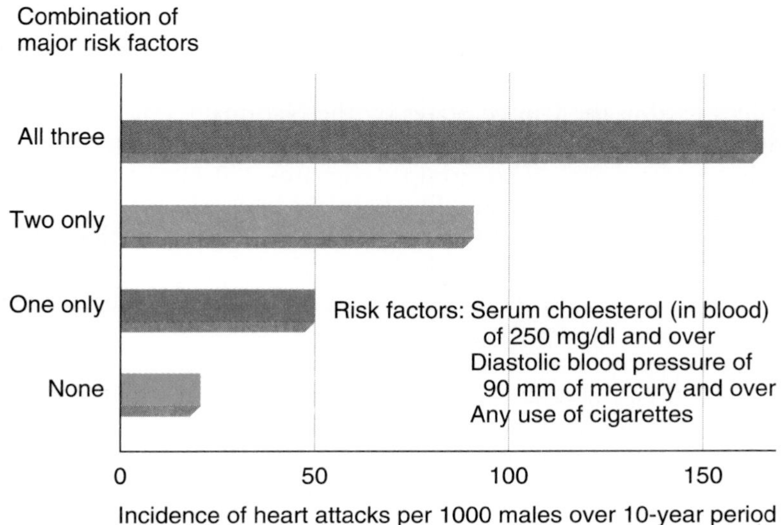

FIGURE 6.13
The effect of three major risk factors on the incidence of heart attacks in white American males.

When the data from many studies were assembled in the National Cooperative Pooling Project, the impact of having one, two, or all three of the risk factors was evaluated. Each additional risk factor almost doubled the risk. (Adapted from Farrand and Mojonnier, 1980.) Diastolic blood pressure is the lower number in a blood pressure value, such as 125/72. The 72 indicates the pressure in the arteries when the heart is relaxing. The upper number is the systolic pressure, the pressure in arteries when the heart is contracting.

FIGURE 6.14
Relationship of serum cholesterol to CHD death.

These data were collected on over 350,000 men ages 35 to 37 who were followed for an average of 6 years. Each point represents the median for 5% of the men. (From National Research Council, 1989.)

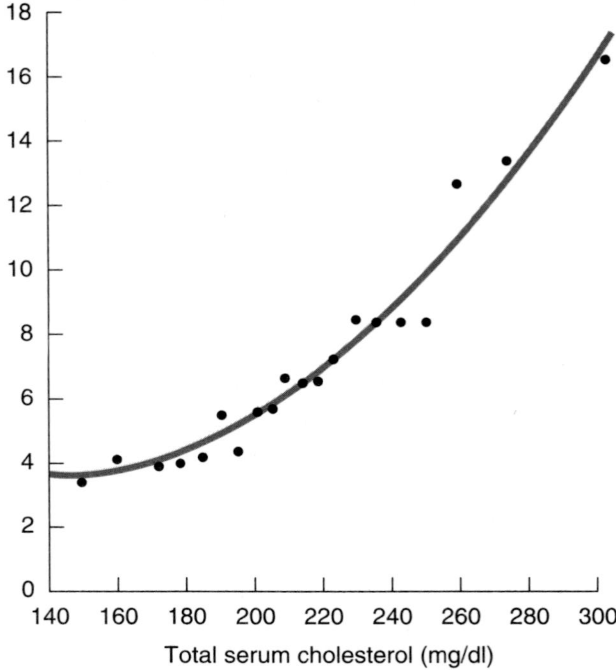

were to have a heart attack; (2) even if they had none of these three risk factors, 20 out of 1000 had heart attacks anyway; and (3) even if they had *all three* of these risk factors, 830 out of 1000 did not have heart attacks during the ten years. It is obvious, then, that although these factors are influential, they do not explain all occurrences of heart disease. Nonetheless, their relative importance has made them the target of major efforts to reduce the incidence of heart disease.

Blood Cholesterol as a Risk Factor for CHD

What about blood cholesterol by itself? How great a risk factor is it? Figure 6.14 gives data from a study involving 350,000 men, showing the relationship between serum cholesterol levels and men who died of CHD.

Based on such data, scientists have estimated the levels of risk associated with various concentrations of total blood cholesterol. Table 6.7 indicates the values used in the United States by the National Cholesterol Education Program (NCEP, a public health education campaign involving 20 major health organizations). This group designates 200 mg of cholesterol per deciliter of blood as the dividing line between low risk and borderline-high risk; 240 mg/dl marks the beginning of high risk. (A deciliter [dl] is equal to one-tenth of a liter.) Although the cutoffs are somewhat arbitrary, many doctors use test results as indications to begin cholesterol-reduction therapy.

Recently, however, researchers have identified more sensitive predictors of CHD than total cholesterol: the types of lipoproteins in which the cholesterol is found. Studies have now shown that risk of CHD increases *when LDL (which accounts for most of a person's cholesterol) is unusually high* or *when HDL (normally a much smaller amount) is abnormally low.*

TABLE 6.7 Blood Cholesterol Values (mg/dl) That Define Different Levels of Cardiovascular Risk

	Desirable	Borderline-high	High
Based on total cholesterol[a]	<200	200–239[b]	>240
Based on LDL cholesterol[a]	<130	130–159	>160

[a]National Cholesterol Education Program, 1988. Treatment of High Blood Cholesterol in Adults. *Archives of Internal Medicine* 148:36-69.
[b]Patients in this range are at high risk if two or more of the following apply: male sex, family history of premature coronary heart disease, cigarette smoking, hypertension, HDL concentration <35 mg/dl, diabetes mellitus, personal history of vascular disease, >30% overweight.

If you've had a cholesterol test and you received a result indicating only your total cholesterol level, you might wonder why HDL and LDL determinations aren't done automatically. Traditionally, total cholesterol has been regarded as a reasonable starting point. If the test for total cholesterol indicates risk, then the more expensive tests for HDL and calculations for LDL are called for. More recently, however, some experts have advocated that HDL levels be determined *routinely,* because they believe that this value contributes significantly to risk assessment.

Blood cholesterol tests lack precision in another way: values vary, depending on several factors: the time of day, how much time has passed since you ate your last meal, the season of the year, your anxiety level, the body position you assumed when the blood was drawn, and even the laboratory method used (Koch et al., 1988). Shopping mall samples, for instance, are notoriously inaccurate. Ideally, the test should be done on several different occasions at a medical facility before a diagnosis is made or treatment is initiated.

An approach commonly used is to *consider blood cholesterol along with other risk factors.* The NCEP considers that if your total blood cholesterol level is in the "borderline-high" range (201–239 mg/dl) and you have two or more of certain other risk factors, you are at high risk, just as though your blood cholesterol level had been over 240. The other risk factors include being male, having a personal or family history of CHD, having hypertension, having diabetes, smoking cigarettes, and being more than 30% overweight.

You Tell Me

Your friend had a "finger stick" blood cholesterol test at a shopping mall and learned that his blood cholesterol value was 201 mg/dl.

Can you say what degree of risk this represents? How likely is it that if your friend had another test, the results would be the same?

Despite all of this research, there are some differences of opinion among both scientists and health care professionals about how much blood cholesterol influences cardiovascular health. At the extremes, some have staked their careers on the belief that the influence is great, whereas others believe cholesterol's importance has been seriously overblown. Some researchers are looking for additional factors that may be involved, such as the nature of

FIGURE 6.15
To help your heart, go take a walk.

Many studies have shown that people who exercise frequently have healthier cardiovascular systems. Although vigorous activity seems to be better, even moderate activity such as walking is clearly better than warming the couch.

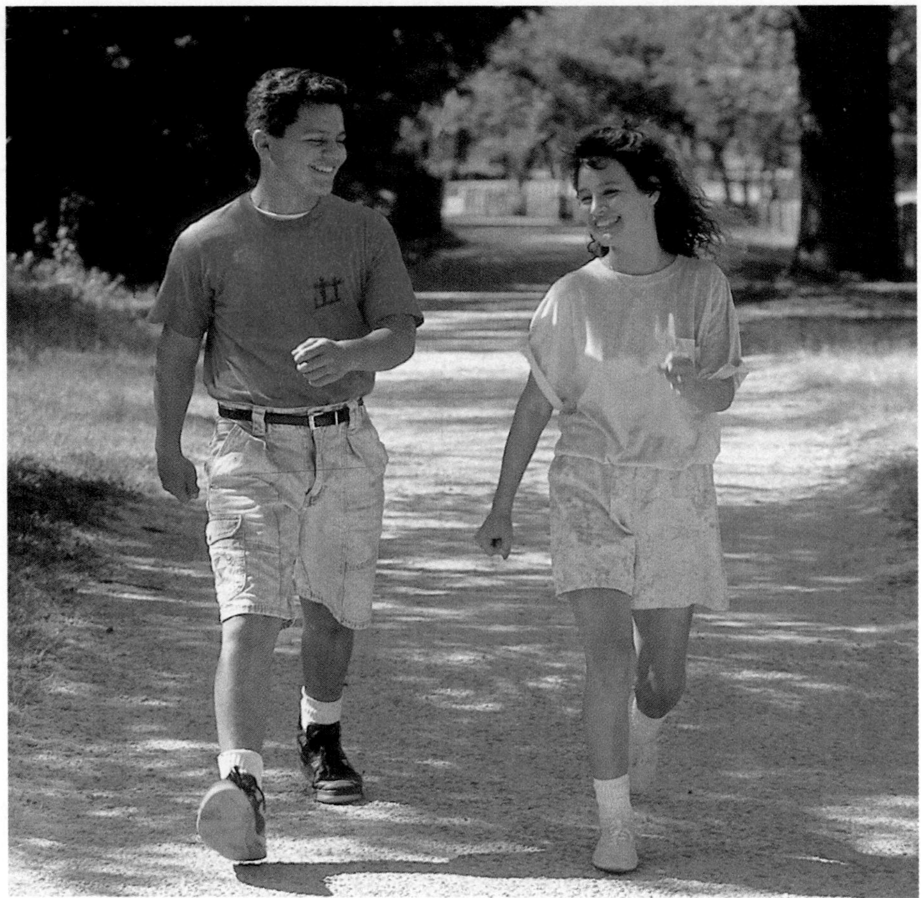

the *proteins* in the lipoproteins. Most experts and clinicians believe that concern about elevated blood cholesterol has at least some validity, but that it doesn't deserve to be the focus of a patient's entire diagnosis and treatment program.

Ways to Control Blood Cholesterol

A great deal of research has been targeted at identifying what factors affect blood cholesterol levels. These studies have provided various recommendations for keeping your blood cholesterol level in the desirable range or bringing it down if it's too high.

For those who smoke, quitting smoking is critical: it lowers cholesterol, improves circulation, and reduces the likelihood of clots forming in the blood vessels, among other things. Exercise helps, too, primarily by raising HDL levels and helping control body weight (Figure 6.15). There are medications that reduce blood cholesterol—from ordinary aspirin to high-tech lovastatin—but all have undesirable side effects, and many are expensive. Then, of course, there is diet.

A variety of dietary factors has been shown to affect blood cholesterol levels. In Chapter 5, you learned about one that has a modest effect—soluble fiber. In Chapter 11, you will learn about the effect of certain vitamins; in Chapter 17, about the effect of alcohol. Here, we focus on lipids in the diet, which may have the greatest impact of all.

But before we begin, we have to warn you that reducing dietary lipids will not be a panacea, either. **People vary tremendously in how much they**

can change their blood cholesterol levels through dietary modifications. At best, a person can reduce blood cholesterol by around 20%. Most people, however, can decrease it by only 10–15% (Kwiterovich, 1989), and some people see even less change—or no change at all. Generally, the people who have the greatest success are those who have a very high blood cholesterol level to begin with, who are younger, who lose weight in the process, who implement more restrictive diets, and who are blessed with a genetic background that allows it. Even with the best of success, changes in diet may not lower blood cholesterol levels enough, and additional measures such as drug therapy may be necessary.

Nevertheless, it's important to realize that most people can bring about at least *some* effect by modifying their diets. In the remainder of this discussion, we'll describe the factors involved. In each section, we'll tell you what the NCEP and the American Heart Association (AHA) have recommended to the general public to help keep blood cholesterol within the low-risk range. If you have an elevated blood cholesterol level, it may take greater restrictions to lower it significantly.

Body Fat People who are obese are likely to have higher levels of blood lipids in general. Losing excess fat and keeping it off often help reduce the damaging forms of blood cholesterol and other lipids.

Total Amount of Dietary Fat How much dietary fat is acceptable? There is considerable debate about this point. On the one hand, the NCEP and the AHA recommend that we all *limit our total fat intake to 30% of kcalories,* which is lower than the average U.S. consumption of 35–40%. If people reduce their fat intake (and don't greatly increase their intake of other energy nutrients at the same time), they will lose weight, which can lower blood lipids. Cutting down on fat, then, certainly could be beneficial to those who are overweight and have high blood cholesterol.

Furthermore, when you reduce your overall intake of fat, you probably also consume less saturated fat, and saturated fatty acids are known to raise blood cholesterol. (The next section discusses this further.)

On the other hand, there is no evidence to prove that restricting fat to 30% of kcalories will help if you don't also decrease your overall kcalorie intake and your saturated fat intake (Barr et al., 1992). Previous studies have shown that although total blood cholesterol can drop when fat is restricted to 30% of kcalories, both LDL *and HDL* can be lowered in the process. Furthermore, some populations, such as those of the Mediterranean region, consume more than 30% of kcalories as lipids but have relatively little heart disease.

Nonetheless, on the strength of the first two arguments, the NCEP and AHA stand behind their recommendation to limit fat intake to 30% of total kcalories.

Saturated Fatty Acids (SFAs) in the Diet Saturated fatty acids (SFAs) are known to be strong promoters of higher LDL levels. Why? Scientists aren't sure, but one theory is that SFAs reduce your liver's ability to take cholesterol out of your blood (Ney, 1990). This means that less cholesterol goes into bile, some of which would ultimately have been excreted. SFAs, by interfering with your mechanisms for disposing of cholesterol, cause your blood cholesterol to rise.

One of the most emphasized pieces of heart-smart advice for the public is to *limit your intake of saturated fat to no more than 10% of kcalories;* some experts would like the percentage to be even lower. Because SFAs are

TABLE 6.8 Omega-3 Fatty Acids in Selected Seafoods

A number of fatty acids can be classified as omega-3. Two of the most common[a] are very long (20 or 22 carbons) and very unsaturated (5 or 6 unsaturated bonds). This table lists the amount of these two fatty acids that are thought to lower the risk of CVD. In general, the best sources (in bold type) are fatty fish that live in extremely cold water.

Food Item	Mg of certain omega-3 fatty acids[a] 2 oz. of fish
Finfish	
Anchovy, European	**0.8**
Bass, striped	**0.5**
Bluefish	**0.7**
Catfish	0.2
Dogfish, spiny	**1.1**
Halibut, Greenland	**0.5**
Herring	**1.0**
Mackerel, Atlantic	**1.5**
Pike, walleye	0.2
Pompano, Florida	0.4
Salmon, different varieties	**0.5–0.8**
Trout, lake	**1.0**
Tuna	0.3
Whitefish, lake	**0.8**
Crustaceans and mollusks	
Clams, softshell	0.2
Shrimp, different varieties	0.2–0.3
Oysters	0.2–0.4
Squid	0.2

[a]Omega-3 fatty acids are considered here to be equal to the content of eicosapentaenoic acid (EPA) and docosahexaenoic acid (DHA).
Data source: Hepburn et al., 1986.

found primarily in animal products (meats and full-fat dairy products) and tropical oils (coconut, palm, palm kernel oil, and cocoa butter), these would seem to be the foods that you should restrict.

But even this advice might not hold. Recent research indicates that all SFAs are not equal in their cholesterol-raising potential (Denke and Grundy, 1991). The effect seems to vary according to *the length of the chain of the SFA.* For example, one study showed that when subjects consumed a liquid diet high in a 16-carbon SFA (palmitic acid) and then were switched to a diet high in an 18-carbon SFA (stearic acid), blood cholesterol went down (Bonanome and Grundy, 1988). Other studies also see differences according to the length of the SFA chains.

More research on this topic is in progress. It is important, because the results could affect dietary advice considerably. If it is true that 18-carbon SFAs do not elevate blood cholesterol, then it is not appropriate to steer people away from the SFAs in meat and in chocolate, because many of the

SFAs in these foods are of the 18-carbon variety. Obviously, it's a complicated business scientifically, and it could have major ramifications in the food marketplace.

Polyunsaturated Fatty Acids (PUFAs) in the Diet Various studies have shown that some PUFAs—particularly linoleic acid, an essential fatty acid that is prevalent in vegetable oils—can lower LDL and HDL somewhat (Grundy, 1991). However, in some (but not all) studies on laboratory animals, certain PUFAs have increased the incidence of cancer. Therefore, to get the LDL-lowering benefit but avoid increased risk of cancer, the NCEP and AHA recommend that we *consume up to (but not more than) 10% of our kcalories from PUFAs.* This recommendation applies primarily to linoleic acid (Grundy, 1991). Currently, Americans get approximately 7% of their kcalories from linoleic acid.

Not all types of PUFAs in foods act in the same way, a fact that is related to the structure of the fatty acid. (This is getting to be a familiar story, isn't it?) In this case, the critical structural feature is *the location of the last double bond in the fatty acid chain.* An *omega-6 fatty acid,* for example, is a PUFA whose last double bond is 6 carbons from the last carbon (the omega carbon) of the chain. Linoleic acid, the focus of the discussion above, is an omega-6 fatty acid.

Omega-3 fatty acids represent another important group of PUFAs. Omega-3 fatty acids are most prevalent in the oil of cold-water fish (Table 6.8). Although these substances don't necessarily lower cholesterol levels, a number of epidemiologic studies show that people who regularly eat fish high in omega-3 fatty acids are less likely to die of CVD than those who do not eat fish (Connor, 1991). In a study done in the Netherlands, only half as many cardiac deaths occurred among men who ate at least 1 ounce of fish per day as among those who ate none (Kromhout et al., 1985). A study involving almost 19,000 U.S. men treated for CVD also showed benefits of omega-3 fatty acids (Dolecek, 1992). Because of such studies, we are urged to *eat one or two meals including fish per week* (Figure 6.16). The fish should be baked, poached, or broiled (not fried), so that the beneficial effects of the fish oil are not negated by adding other fats.

omega-3 fatty acids—highly unsaturated fatty acids found primarily in cold-water fish

You Tell Me

Some people, on learning about the benefits of fish oil, have presumed it would be better to eat canned tuna fish packed in oil, rather than packed in water. However, oil-packed tuna is packed in vegetable oil, not fish oil, and any type of oil adds 9 kcalories per gram.

In light of this, which form of canned tuna would you choose?

The beneficial effects of eating fish are not necessarily due to changes in blood cholesterol. When you eat fish, your blood cholesterol levels can either increase or decrease, depending on such factors as your intake of omega-3 fatty acids and saturated fat. What omega-3 fatty acids do, though, is reduce the levels of other blood lipids that may be involved in atherosclerosis, and they promote the production of certain *prostaglandins* (hormonelike substances) that improve the flexibility and reduce the stickiness of red blood cells. This means that clots are less likely to form in blood vessels, and a heart attack is less likely (Ney, 1990).

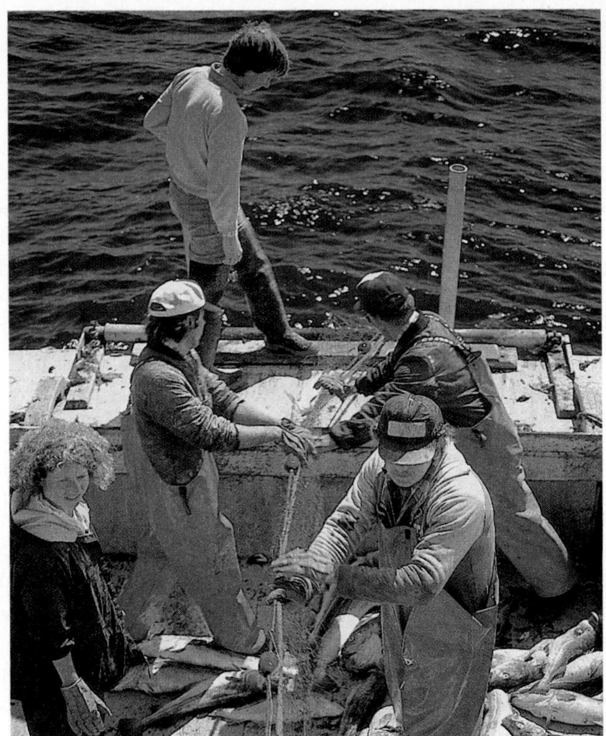

FIGURE 6.16
Net yourself lower risk for heart disease.

Studies show that people who eat cold-water fish a couple of times each week are less likely to die of heart disease.

Unfortunately, the very biologic activities of omega-3 fatty acids that help reduce atherosclerosis can have a negative effect if these PUFAs are consumed to excess. At very high levels of intake, omega-3 fatty acids make bruising, bleeding, and strokes more likely. For this reason, experts are concerned about fish oil supplements that have come onto the over-the-counter market; *researchers and health care professionals are unanimous and emphatic in advising against their self-prescribed use.*

Another strike against these products is that they may not have been purified to remove toxins from the ocean's food chain that became concentrated in the fish and its oil. In human studies and for selected patients, however, highly purified fish oils are sometimes used as appropriate treatment.

Monounsaturated Fatty Acids (MUFAs) in the Diet MUFAs are most prominent in olive oil, canola oil, nuts, and avocado. Table 6.1 shows their occurrence in some other common fats and oils.

Scientists used to think that MUFAs were neutral in their effect on blood cholesterol. Not anymore. Scientists now think that MUFAs lower LDL by about the same amount as do PUFAs from plant sources, but, fortunately, they do not lower HDL at the same time (Grundy, 1991). This characteristic actually gives a risk-reducing advantage to the diets with MUFAs over those with PUFAs, a finding supported by an increasing number of studies (Mata et al., 1992; Valsta, et al., 1992).

Epidemiologic studies have also found MUFAs associated with good health. People in the Mediterranean countries, where monounsaturated olive oil is liberally used in food, have a low incidence of heart disease, even though their intake of fat (based on percentage of kcalories) is as high as that of people in the United States. There's more good news about MUFAs: they are not associated with an increased risk of cancer.

As far as recommendations for intake are concerned, the NCEP advises that *MUFAs can make up whatever part of the 30% fat allowance is not taken up by saturated and polyunsaturated fat.* Research continues.

You Tell Me

Some popular writers have called MUFAs "no fault fat" because they reduce the risk of heart disease and cancer, compared with other lipids.

But is it smart to consume unlimited amounts?

Trans Fatty Acids Trans fatty acids are another form of fatty acids. They occur naturally in food in very small amounts, and they occur in some processed foods, such as hydrogenated margarines, in larger amounts. (The term *trans* indicates that the hydrogen atoms are positioned around the double bond in a certain way.)

Unfortunately, trans fatty acids seem to have a troublesome effect on blood cholesterol. One study showed that when high levels of intake of trans fatty acids and SFA were compared, LDL rose with both test diets, but with the trans fatty acid diet, HDL dropped in addition (Zock and Katan, 1992). In another study when subjects consumed trans fatty acids, their blood cholesterol values changed so as to increase their risk of heart attack (Troisi et al., 1992). It is not yet clear whether the extent of the effect of trans fatty acids is the same or different from that of saturated fatty acids.

Does this mean than you should totally avoid margarine, or, as some newspaper stories have suggested, that it's better to eat butter? No, even the experts do not say that; they point out that the amounts of trans fatty acids present in the test diets were more than three times the average intake by margarine-consuming Americans (Grundy, 1991). Furthermore, margarines contain no cholesterol (Katan and Mensink, 1992).

Cholesterol in the Diet Reducing cholesterol in your diet can lower total blood cholesterol, but, as you have learned, the extent of the change varies greatly among individuals. In fact, for most people, reducing the intake of dietary cholesterol appears to be the least important influence on their level of blood cholesterol (Kris-Etherton, 1988). In a recent seven-page review of the effects of diet on risk of heart disease, the authors dismiss dietary cholesterol with this single statement: "Some readers would doubtless wish dietary cholesterol to be included although the evidence for its importance seems weak" (Ulbricht and Southgate, 1991).

Even so, others think that dietary cholesterol should not be ignored (Grundy, 1991). The NCEP and the AHA both *recommend limiting daily intake of dietary cholesterol to 300 mg.*

You Tell Me

In recent years, foods of plant origin—from bananas to margarine to salad dressings—have been promoted on the basis that they contain no cholesterol.

From what you know of these foods, is the claim for these products accurate? Is it misleading? Are there other substances in these foods that could affect risk of CHD?

Obviously, lipid researchers vary in their beliefs about the effects of the various lipids discussed above on heart disease. For the opinions of one scientist who has explored these ideas for several decades, read the interview with David Kritchevsky on the next page.

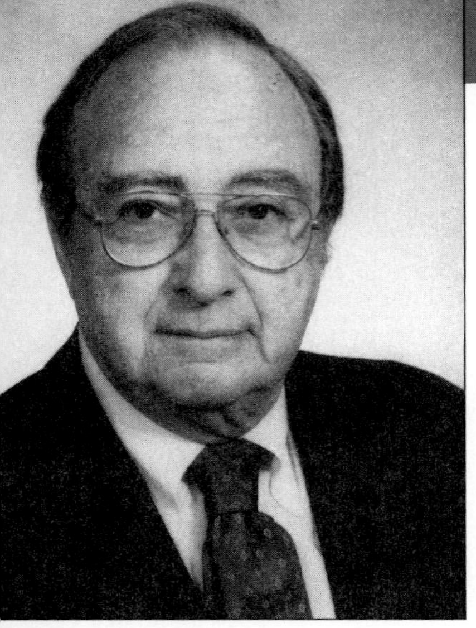

Interview with David Kritchevsky, PhD
Lipids and Heart Disease

How important are the lipids in your diet in determining whether you'll develop heart disease? And which kinds of lipids are of greatest concern? Dr. David Kritchevsky is a scientist who has devoted his career to answering such questions. Dr. Kritchevsky is a professor at the Wistar Institute of Anatomy and Biology in Philadelphia, and at the University of Pennsylvania. In addition to generating an extensive list of research publications, he has been the author or editor of numerous books on lipid research and nutrition, and has written songs and poems on these topics as well.

What kind of scientific training did you have, and how did it lead to your study of lipids and heart disease?

After I got my PhD in 1950, I went to Switzerland on a post-doctoral fellowship, where I worked on steroids. Then they needed a cholesterol expert at the University of California at Berkeley. They were just discovering the lipoproteins and they wanted to trace their pathway through the cell with radioactive cholesterol. So, I made the cholesterol and we did some experiments. In fact I wrote the first book on cholesterol; that was in 1958.

What I became primarily interested in was the nutritional aspect of cholesterol. I spent the next 5 years working in industry, and while I was there we did the very first studies showing that unsaturated fat decreased atherosclerosis in rabbits. We published a lot of papers on the effects of different fats, fatty acids, and cholesterol on rabbits, and on atherosclerosis in rabbits. That led me to study other aspects of the diet; we did a lot of work on fiber. Actually in 1964, I wrote a letter to the *Journal of Atherosclerosis* suggesting that the fiber in the diet played a role in atherosclerosis. So, I've been at this work for quite a few years.

We read a lot in the news these days about fat and heart disease. Do you think that fat is related to heart disease? And if so, what specifically do you think is the real cause for concern—fat per se, the kcalories it contains, saturated fat, cholesterol?

This is a very complex area. One of the problems is that we don't have a simple diagnosis for the impending coronary event. Even if serum cholesterol *is* a risk factor, a risk factor is a statistical diagnosis, not a medical diagnosis. If you are worried about, let's say, tuberculosis, you go to the doctor and he does a simple test, and he says "yes" or "no". But if you run a cholesterol test he says, "This is the percentile you're in". Now that is better than nothing, but it is not as good as a diagnosis, because we don't know exactly what will precipitate heart disease.

The fat plays a role. The real question is: Is the role of fat due to the fat itself, something in the fat, or the calories from the fat? Which aspect of fat contributes? In the U.S. we have this real "lipo-hysteria"—all you hear about is cholesterol. I think you should know your cholesterol level, primarily because we don't know what else to measure.

You also have to realize that cholesterol tends to vary diurnally (daily) and seasonally, so a single reading is meaningless. A lot of things affect cholesterolemia (high blood cholesterol levels) that have nothing to do with diet. A paper published last year looked at 160,000 Britons and over 40,000 Japanese and found that their cholesterol levels vary during the year. Stress raises cholesterol, too. There are studies that have been done on medical students in which you take a blood sample on Monday morning of every week, give the samples to a technician to run, and don't look at the results until the end of the semester. Then when you plot cholesterol levels versus time you get a peak the week of every examination. There is a lot of data like this and only now is it being appreciated. The lesson in this is that you have to do more than one reading.

How about diet? Most of the diet studies show that cholesterol in the diet does not have a huge impact on blood cholesterol levels. Several years ago William

Dawber, who used to be the director of the Framingham project, showed that whether people ate one egg a week or nine eggs a week made little difference to their cholesterol levels.

The biggest dietary impact is from the saturation of the fat—a number of studies show that. The difficulty is that a high cholesterol level doesn't automatically mean a coronary; it means risk for a coronary. Cholesterol is important, but it is just one part of this dietary complex.

Some researchers are very concerned about *trans* fatty acids. What are they? And are they worth the concern?

First of all, a double bond can be in either what is called the *cis* or the *trans* configuration. If it is in the *cis* configuration, it means that the two hydrogens are on the same side of the molecule. When it's in the *trans* configuration though, hydrogens are on opposite sides of the molecule. This changes the geometry of the molecule. Now, *trans* fatty acids are not unknown in nature—they occur at low levels in dairy foods, and some plants have a lot of them. But in our diets the major source of *trans* fatty acids is the hydrogenated fat in shortening, margarines, things like that.

Now the question is, are they good or bad for you? They do raise cholesterol levels. If you feed them to rabbits, as we and other people have done, in either a cholesterol-containing or a cholesterol-free diet, they raise cholesterol. But they do not increase atherosclerosis significantly.

This has been a topic of interest in the literature since the 50s. Most recently, a U.S. Department of Agriculture study had people on a rotating diet, starting with a diet in which they used olive oil or some other fat that was not hydrogenated, and rotating through diets with two levels of *trans* fat. They found that as the *trans* fat increased there was a slight increase in cholesterol level—an increase that normally isn't considered very high, but which might make a difference when translated to population levels. So my feelings about the *trans* fat is that it is only dangerous in that it raises cholesterol levels. There are a few recent studies suggesting that dietary *trans* fat raises levels of the lipoprotein "Lp(a)," which may be the link between atherosclerosis and thrombosis (blood clot formation). If this becomes a general observation, we'll have to take a much closer look at *trans* fat.

Some researchers are now advocating a Mediterranean diet as a means of decreasing the risk of heart disease. Why are some people promoting it? Is it worthwhile?

It's sort of worthwhile because it tastes good. But while Mediterraneans have a different diet, they also have a different lifestyle. A lot of things are different. It's interesting that in Greece they eat more fat than we do, but they still have less heart disease. Look at the French, who eat more fat and cholesterol and more red meat than anybody else in Europe, and have the lowest incidence of heart disease. They also use red wine.

What we have to decide, I think, is do we want people to have lower cholesterol? Lower weight? What is it you're going for? What we have to do is look at the total diet and its interactions, instead of everybody jumping at their favorite nutrient. We have done studies, for instance, on animal versus vegetable protein in animals. Rabbits fed casein (an animal protein) have a higher cholesterol level than rabbits fed soy protein. But if we feed them casein and alfalfa, they have the same cholesterol levels as rabbits fed soy protein and cellulose. So all of these things interact and we really don't have a lot of information on how they do that. Every time, you get back to the importance of moderation in the diet.

What other factors might influence heart disease? How important do you think soluble and insoluble fiber might be?

Soluble and insoluble fiber influence cholesterol readings. Nobody has studied fiber intake in humans long enough to say, "These people have more or fewer coronaries than a control group." But heart disease is such a complex thing, and everybody is trying to reduce it to a simple prescription, usually a prescription that only includes one thing. I think that one of the reasons for that is that watching your diet, watching your weight, is not what people want; they want a quick fix.

Is it true that you have written songs and poems about the biochemistry of cholesterol?

Oh, I have many. Over the years, I've taught this way. Probably the most popular thing I wrote, originally published in the *New England Journal of Medicine* in 1960, goes like this:

Cholesterol is poisonous,
 so never, never eat it
And fatty food will do you in,
 there is no way to beat it
Sugar too is bad for you
 be certain to avoid it
Some food was rich in vitamins
 but processing destroyed it
So let your life be ordered
 by each document and fact
Die of malnutrition
 but with arteries intact.

Should You Change Your Diet? Nutrition and health experts are divided about who should be encouraged to make dietary changes in an attempt to avoid or delay CHD. The experts are likely to fall into one of two camps.

One group believes that the entire population should make dietary changes without delay. This is the position of the NCEP, the AHA, and various other health agencies and professional societies in the United States. Groups in many other countries have already made recommendations to their populations as well.

The other camp believes that there is not enough evidence that dietary change of the type described above would accomplish significant reductions in blood cholesterol and CVD. Nine studies were evaluated (involving a total of more than 20,000 subjects) to determine the effects of a diet similar to what the NCEP and the AHA recommend for the U.S. public (Ramsay et al., 1991). The researchers found that the average cholesterol reduction in these studies was only about 2%. Other researchers have assessed that for every 1% reduction in blood cholesterol in a population, incidence of cardiovascular disease goes down by 2½% (Holme, 1990).

Therefore, the whole-population approach seems to yield some results, but are they enough to be worthwhile? One study, using a mathematical model to predict how much longer we would live if the whole population reduced saturated fat and cholesterol intake as recommended, estimated an *average* of 3–4 months; of course, *individuals'* benefits would vary a great deal (Browner et al., 1991). Critics question whether the relatively limited effects of these large-scale programs are worth the resources. Some studies even show that when deaths from CVD go down, deaths from other causes go up, resulting in no net change in the rate of death (Kaplan, 1992; Jacobs et al., 1992).

In light of all these facts and opinions, most experts believe that we should identify and treat people at high risk for CVD. Of course, those with preexisting disease should be treated; they are the most likely to benefit (Silberberg and Henry, 1991). Their dietary restrictions will need to be greater than those described above.

There is evidence that an extremely aggressive program *can actually lessen a patient's atherosclerosis* over time (Ornish et al., 1990; Gould et al., 1992). The program involves adhering to a vegetarian diet with less than 10% of kcalories from fat and less than 5 mg of cholesterol per day, doing daily moderate aerobic exercise, practicing stress management, and stopping smoking. The number of people involved in this program is small, and only time will tell whether this approach is practical. Continued monitoring of these patients over many years will show whether they can maintain the program and whether the regression of atherosclerosis continues.

Many physicians recommend that families of CHD patients adopt the same diet as the patient, because if one person in a family is at risk, other members are likely to be at risk as well. In addition, family members who attend nutrition education programs together comply with the diet more closely and achieve greater risk reduction (McMurray et al., 1991).

As we conclude this section on heart disease, you should bear in mind that if you want to follow the advice of world experts on this matter, you are in a tough spot because they aren't all humming the same tune. For more personalized advice in determining your risk factors, see your physician.

cancer—general term for what are probably many diseases, all characterized by uncontrolled cell growth

Lipids and Cancer

Cancer accounts for the second largest number of deaths per year in the United States. Statistic projections suggest that 1 in 4 of us will develop can-

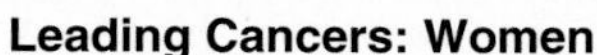

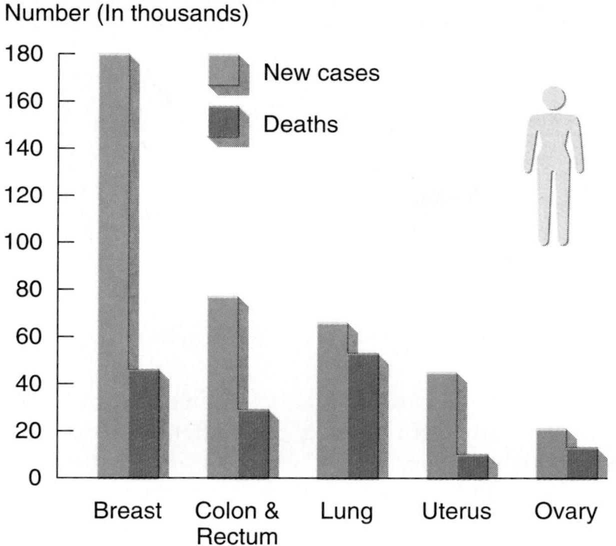

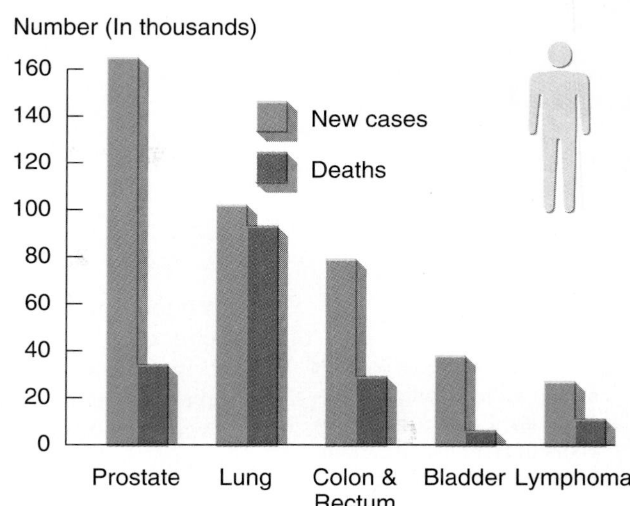

FIGURE 6.17
New cases and deaths due to various cancers in women and men in the United States (1993 estimates).
(Adapted from American Cancer Society, 1993.)

cer during our lifetimes, and 1 in 8–10 will die of the disease. As with atherosclerosis, considerable evidence links cancer with dietary lipids.

Many experts believe that the term *cancer* encompasses over 100 separate diseases that afflict different body organs by different mechanisms. The most common sites affected are the lungs, colon, breast, pancreas, prostate, stomach, and blood. Figure 6.17 shows the rates of new cases and deaths from some major types of cancer in men and women in the United States.

Cancer occurs when normal body cells, whose growth and division are carefully regulated in healthy individuals, undergo genetic changes *(initiation)* that allow them to ignore the usual controls. If the body's processes for recognizing and destroying such cells are not functioning normally, the abnormal cells can compete with healthy ones for oxygen and nutrients. Eventually, the abnormal cells spread throughout the body if conditions encourage their growth (*promotion* and *progression*) (Butterworth and Goldsworthy, 1991). This process often takes place over a period of several decades (although there are exceptions). Figure 6.18 illustrates the stages in cancer development.

In this section, we'll consider the possible causes of cancer, take a hard look at the evidence linking dietary lipids to cancer, and then learn what dietary strategies are suggested for reducing your risk of cancer.

Possible Causes of Cancer

Although there seems to be a genetic aspect to cancer development, epidemiologic data suggest that most human cancers are influenced by one or more environmental factors called **carcinogens.** Certain dietary constituents are among the environmental carcinogens; several leading epidemiologists estimate that about one-third of all cancer deaths may be linked to diet (National Research Council, 1989).

carcinogen—environmental factor thought to initiate or promote the development of cancer

Lipids are thought to be among the most important of the dietary factors related to cancer development; both epidemiologic evidence and animal studies support this contention. Other dietary factors include excessive amounts of alcohol and toxins produced by molds. (Chapter 14 discusses toxins from molds.) Nondietary factors include tobacco, radiation (such as

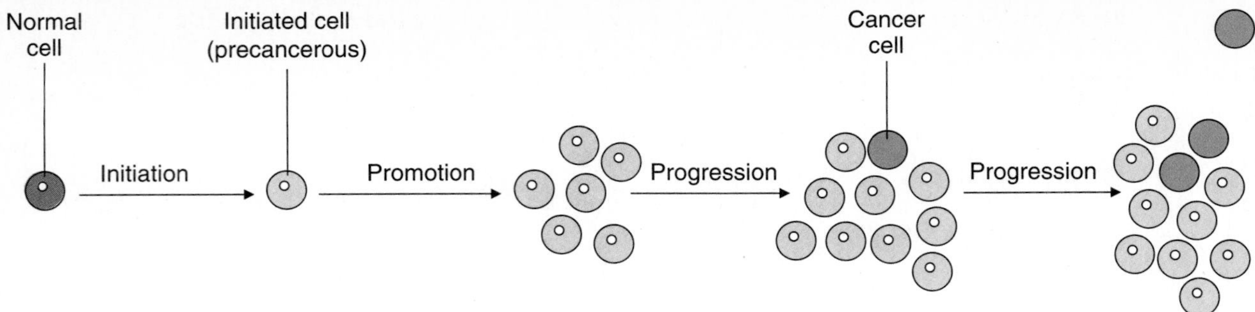

FIGURE 6.18
Stages in cancer development.

Body cells undergo a series of changes in becoming cancerous. Usually, initiation occurs in response to certain environmental conditions, including various dietary factors. It is not inevitable that initiated cells will become cancerous; if levels of cancer-promoting factors are low or if cancer-inhibiting factors are high enough, promotion and progression will not occur. It may take 20 or more years for cancer to develop even when conditions that encourage it exist.

anticarcinogen—environmental factor thought to interfere with the development of cancer

ultraviolet and x-ray radiation), viruses, hormones, and various industrial chemicals.

Just as some substances *encourage* cancer, others—called **anticarcinogens**—*prevent* its development. Fourteen classes of such chemicals occur in common foods from broccoli to whole wheat (Caragay, 1992). Substances thought to be anticarcinogens include nutrients such as carotenoids (precursors of vitamin A), vitamin C, and vitamin E (see Chapter 11), conjugated linoleic acid (see Chapter 14), and non-nutrients in food, such as fiber (see Chapter 5). The important point here is that you should not just view food suspiciously as a potential *cause* of cancer, but recognize that it can also play an important role in cancer *prevention.*

In fact, the National Cancer Institute's Diet and Cancer Branch has recently begun to study how various anticarcinogens in food interfere with cancer. With this information, it may be possible to develop "designer foods"—processed foods to which cancer-preventing ingredients have been added (Caragay, 1992).

Dietary Lipids as a Risk Factor for Cancer

For more than a decade, major reports on the effect of diet on cancer have identified high fat intake as a risk factor for cancer. In 1982, the comprehensive report of the National Academy of Sciences' Committee on Diet, Nutrition, and Cancer stated that lipids seem to be more closely associated with the development of cancer than any other dietary constituent; in 1989, this was still the prevailing opinion of the National Research Council in its report *Diet and Health.*

Although some scientists are not convinced, several kinds of data support the hypothesis that lipids are associated with cancer (Carroll, 1991a). First, epidemiologic data from many countries show a correlation between the average daily dietary fat intake of a population and the incidence of cancer of the colon, breast, and prostate (National Research Council, 1989). Second, the data become more convincing when you see what happens to people who leave their homeland and its diet and adopt a new country and its diet: in a generation or two, the incidence of cancer among those people resembles that in the adopted country rather than that in their country of origin. Of course, other environmental differences between the two countries could also be factors.

Third, certain vegetarian groups have been found to have considerably lower rates of cancer than the general population. Although it may be tempting to attribute this finding to the fact that vegetarian diets are often lower in fat, other aspects of diet and lifestyle could influence the incidence of cancer in these population groups as well. For example, Seventh Day Adventists, approximately 50% of whom avoid meat, experience lower rates of cancer. They generally do not smoke or consume alcohol either—practices that could also lessen their incidence of certain types of cancer. Mortality rates among Seventh Day Adventists are only 50–70% of the general population rates for cancer in body sites *other* than those related to smoking and drinking. Their mortality rates are also lower for sites *unrelated to fat consumption.* More research is obviously needed to explain the reasons—which are likely to be multifactorial—for the impressively lower rates of cancer among Seventh Day Adventists.

Finally, animal tests also strengthen the relationship between dietary fat and cancer (National Research Council, 1989). Animals fed a high-fat diet generally develop more tumors than those fed low-fat diets. This effect may be partially due to the fact that a low-fat diet may also be a low-kcalorie diet, which is known to discourage cancer growth in animals.

Some scientists have been exploring this idea more thoroughly and have become convinced that it is not fat per se that is carcinogenic, but rather *excess kcalories* (Kritchevsky, 1990; Pariza, 1988). They also point to research that supports their theory. For example, a rat study tested the carcinogenic effect of diets that differed in fat and kcalorie values. Surprisingly, the animals receiving the *most fat* had the *lowest* incidence of cancer in their milk-producing glands, but their diet was *lower in total kcalories* by 20% than the other test diets (Boissonneault et al., 1986).

Some human studies have also called into question a link between fat intake and breast cancer in women. One study done in the United States involved almost 90,000 female registered nurses from 34 to 59 years of age. They completed a dietary questionnaire designed to measure consumption of fat as well as other nutrients. During the next 4 years, about 600 cases of breast cancer were diagnosed in these women. When the data were analyzed to determine the relationship between their intake of fat and their incidence of cancer, it was found that *the women consuming the **highest** proportion of their kcalories as fat (44%) had **less** cancer than those consuming the least fat (32%)* (Willett et al., 1987). Other U.S. studies have failed to show a relationship between fat intake and breast cancer.

Given all the other studies we've described that support a connection between dietary lipids and cancer, how can the conflicting results of this breast cancer study be explained? There are many possibilities. First, factors other than diet bear on the incidence of breast cancer. One of these is reproductive history: women who have had a full-term pregnancy early in life or who have had more than one pregnancy have a lower risk of breast cancer (Love, 1988). Genetic differences may also have confounded the dietary effects. In addition, in studies conducted within a country, the intakes of fat among the women studied may not have occupied a broad enough range of fat quantities to show significant effects. Furthermore, even the lowest fat intakes may not have been low enough to affect the incidence. Some experts believe that fat intake earlier in life may be more important than fat intake during adulthood, and studies that assess current diet may not reflect earlier eating habits. Finally, it is possible that total energy intake and body weight, as in the animal study above, were important factors. Until such issues have been addressed, it is impossible to say with absolute certainty whether there is a cause-and-effect relationship between dietary fat and breast cancer.

But what about other cancers? Do they show a clear relationship to dietary lipids? Evidence linking cancer of the colon with dietary fat is stronger (National Research Council, 1989; Henderson et al., 1991). Figure 6.19 shows the relationship using epidemiologic data from around the world. Another study, done in western New York state, substantiated a cor-

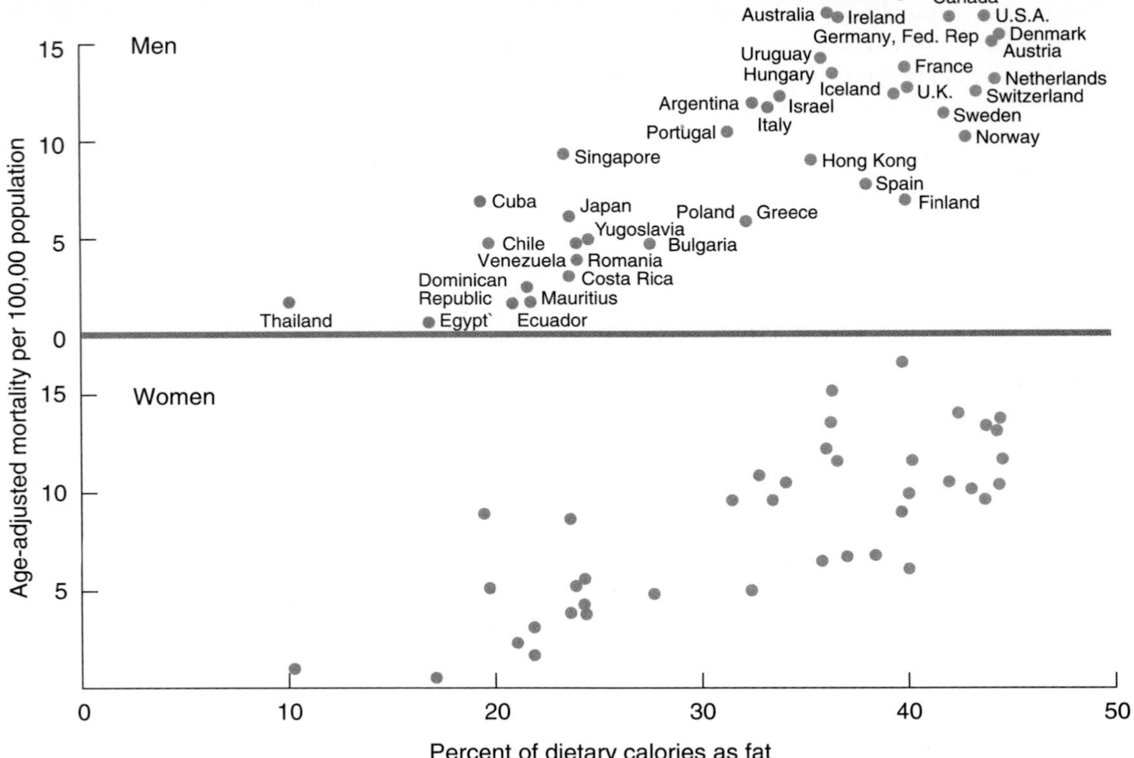

FIGURE 6.19
Relationship between percent of kcalories from fat and deaths from colon cancer.
(Source: Carroll, 1991b.)

relation between high-fat and/or high-kcalorie diets and incidence of colon cancer. Although the influence of other factors, such as obesity and an inherited tendency to colon cancer, was also noted, men with the highest intakes of fat had an incidence of cancer almost three times as high as men with low intakes. For women with high fat intakes, the magnitude of risk was not as dramatic, but data showed the same trend (Freudenheim et al., 1990).

In hopes of pinpointing a specific culprit, other scientists have tried to determine whether certain types of fat—saturated, unsaturated, or the slightly modified *trans fatty acids* that can result from hydrogenation—are more closely associated with cancer development than others. Unfortunately, it appears that the effects are not uniform even within a given type. For example, some animal data suggest that certain polyunsaturated fats (especially those high in linoleic acid) are cancer *promoters,* but epidemiologic data do not provide such evidence. Other studies suggest that saturated fat, especially from red meat, increases risk for colorectal cancers (Henderson et al., 1991).

In a related area of research, there is some evidence that diets containing fish oils may be *protective* against cancer as well as against CHD (National Research Council, 1989; Dolecek, 1992). More studies are needed. In general, the association between total dietary fat and cancer is stronger than the association between any specific type of fat and cancer. But what is known about the relationship between cholesterol and cancer?

Cholesterol as a Risk Factor for Cancer

Although there is a general lack of correlation between intake of *dietary* cholesterol and the incidence of cancer, the link between *blood* cholesterol and cancer incidence may be a different matter. A number of studies involving blood cholesterol levels and incidence of all types of cancer together have suggested that if blood cholesterol is low (e.g., less than 190 mg/dl), the statistical risk of cancer is increased. But (as you are coming to expect!), other studies have not shown this relationship (National Research Council, 1989).

When studies have shown an inverse relationship between blood cholesterol and cancer, there has been much debate about whether the low blood cholesterol levels were the *cause* or the *effect* of the cancer. Some experts believe that because the progression of cancer is often accompanied by falling blood cholesterol levels, some cases of low blood cholesterol in these studies were *a result of* a growing cancer that had not yet been detected. Other researchers seriously consider the possibility that low levels of blood cholesterol *may contribute to the beginning of cancer,* possibly by interfering with the integrity of cell membranes (Isles et al., 1989).

The conflicting information on blood cholesterol and cancer is not yet consistent enough to form the basis for dietary advice. Nevertheless, the relationship between high blood cholesterol and CHD is much more certain; therefore, if your blood cholesterol level is high, you should try to lower it (Kritchevsky and Kritchevsky, 1992).

Fortunately, other suggestions for reducing your risk of cancer through diet are on firmer footing, as the next section describes.

Guidelines for Reducing Your Risk of Cancer Through Diet

In the past decade, many organizations have issued advice to the general public about how to modify your diet to reduce your risk of developing cancer. The Committee on Diet, Nutrition, and Cancer of the National Academy of Sciences issued its advice in 1982, followed by the National Cancer Institute (NCI) of the National Institutes of Health and by the American Cancer Society, both in 1984. In 1988, NCI revised its recommendations (Butrum et al., 1988).

All of these groups have made similar recommendations, as follows:

- Avoid obesity.
- Lower your fat intake to 30% of kcalories or less.
- Increase your intake of whole-grain products. (See Chapter 5.)
- Increase your intake of fruits and vegetables, especially those that are good sources of vitamins A and C and **cruciferous vegetables.** (These are believed to contain various anticarcinogens.)
- Reduce your intake of pickled, salt-cured, smoked, and charred foods. (See Chapter 14.)
- If you consume alcoholic beverages, limit your consumption. (Chronic alcohol consumption increases risk of cancer, especially of the upper GI tract.)

cruciferous vegetables— members of the mustard family; examples are broccoli, Brussels sprouts, cabbage, cauliflower

Of course, there are no guarantees that following these dietary recommendations will protect you from the many forms of cancer, but a large body of epidemiologic, animal, and human evidence suggests that diet can make a difference in reducing the risk of this multifactorial disease within a population.

Some day, it may be possible to determine on an *individual* basis who is most susceptible to cancer. To a very limited extent, that is already happening: scientists have identified certain genes, called *oncogenes,* that are involved in the development of some specific cancers. Perhaps in the future, members of families that experience a high incidence of one of these cancers may be able to have their genes tested and then be given individualized advice about reducing their cancer risk.

As far as we know, oncogenes are not involved in all forms of cancer; for some cancers, repeated exposure to environmental factors (which include dietary factors) is the culprit. Research is in the early stages to determine how people could be tested individually to determine who is at greatest risk from these factors (Marx, 1991)

You Tell Me

Medical ethicists, in anticipation of more advanced technology, are in controversy over whether people should be told what they are likely to die of.

If your family medical history puts you at high risk for a genetically transmitted form of cancer, would you want to be tested? If the test showed you were at risk, would you be able to make constructive use of the information?

Lipids and Body Fat

Excess body fat, as you know, results from surplus kcalories from *any* source, but there are a couple of reasons why, if you eat a lot of dietary fat, you are likely to gain body fat (Dattilo, 1992).

First, the obvious one: lipids, at 9 kcalories/gram, are higher in energy than are proteins or carbohydrates. Because fat is often not visible and does not contribute as much to the bulk of food as various forms of carbohydrate do, even a small serving of some foods can be quite high in fat and kcalories.

But dietary fat may even be more fattening than we have long thought: some research suggests that lipids' kcalorie potential is actually closer to 11 kcalories/gram (Donato and Hegsted, 1985). This is partially due to the fact that your body can very efficiently digest, absorb, and reassemble fat: only 2% of the kcalories in the fat are used up in these processes. If your body is converting surplus carbohydrate to fat, by contrast, an estimated 24% of its kcalories are used up. This metabolic efficiency for fat is a disadvantage for the person who wants to *eat* fat but not *be* fat.

Research is making more progress in finding an association between a high-fat diet and a higher proportion of body fat. More will be said about this in Chapters 8 (on energy) and 9 (on body weight).

Lipids—How Do You Rate?

As you're now well aware, many questions remain about the effects of lipids on health. As a result, you might think it would be difficult to make any recommendations regarding fat intake. However, scientific organizations that are familiar with the literature on both the need for lipids and the risks associated with them have made recommendations that can serve until more is known.

For *linoleic acid,* one of the essential fatty acids, the recommended intake is 1–2% of kcalories (RDA Subcommittee, 1989). Based on USDA data, it is possible that Americans get as much as 5–7% of their kcalories as linoleic acid; therefore, you are at little risk of developing essential fatty acid deficiency and there is little need for you to be deliberate about consuming it. At the other end of the spectrum, it seems unlikely that you are exceeding the recommended limit of 10% of kcalories from this source.

As far as *linolenic acid* (the other essential fatty acid) is concerned, no recommended intake has been set for people in the United States.

Regarding total fat in the diet, the Food and Agriculture Organization/World Health Organization expresses concern that people in developing countries do not get enough fat; these groups recommend that the people increase their fat intake to 15–20% of kcalories. We Americans have more cause to be concerned about too much fat in our diet. In recent years in the United States, estimates of typical consumption of fat range from 36–40% of total kcalories (National Research Council, 1989). However, the 1989 RDA subcommittee and the National Research Council recommend a limit of 30% of kcalories from fat. Guidelines for reducing risk of heart disease and cancer make the same recommendation, as you learned earlier.

In addition to the potential benefits of reducing the risk of disease, lowering fat intake can have a positive effect on overall nutrient content of the diet. In a 100-day study in which people changed their diets from the typical U.S. high-fat diet to a diet containing approximately 25% of energy as fat, subjects increased their consumption of carbohydrates and many vitamins and minerals (Dougherty et al., 1988). This suggests that Americans could benefit in more than one way by lowering their fat consumption.

This study provides encouragement in another way, too: it shows that *it is possible* for people to lower their fat intakes as much as the experts recommend. Other studies support this. In the Women's Health Trial, designed to reduce the risk of breast cancer by lowering fat intake, subjects reduced their intake of fat from 39% of total kcalories to 22% of kcalories; a year later, they had maintained most of their new eating habits (Kristal, et al., 1992). Other studies also show that (depending on the diet you start with), you may be able to get down to the 30% limit by making just a few changes, such as choosing lower fat meat and/or using lower fat dairy products (Smith-Schneider et al., 1992).

With more people eating an increasing number of meals away from home, it is important that restaurants make it possible to choose lower fat foods. In a study of restaurants in six Midwest communities, one-third had changed menu items within the last year to make them lower in fat or had added low-fat options. Two out of five said they were deep-fat frying foods less often, and one in five were broiling meat more often (Weisbrod et al., 1991). These are moves in the right direction.

To help you understand the specifics of your own situation, Act on Fact 6.1 on page 198 shows you how to figure out how much fat you can eat and which foods will help you stay within the recommended 30% limit for total fat and 10% limit for saturated fat. The Consider This box on page 200 shows you some of the general types of changes that can help reduce fat intake.

Determining Your Budgets for Total and Saturated Fat

Guidelines for limiting fat in the diet recommend that you consume no more than 30% of kcalories from total fat and no more than one-third of that total from saturated fat.

We propose that you develop a *daily fat budget in grams* to use as a reference point against which to compare the fat contents (shown in grams on the nutrition label) of particular items you are considering. Use a form similar to the one shown in Sample Act on Fact 6.1, and follow the steps below.

1. Retrieve an estimate of your approximate daily kcaloric intake (e.g., from Act on Fact 2.1 or 5.1) and enter it in (1) below.
2. Calculate 30% of that figure in (2) below.
3. Divide by 9, the number of kcalories in a gram of fat, in (3) below. The answer is your daily total fat budget in grams.
4. Divide your total fat budget by 3 to determine your saturated fat budget in (4) below.
5. Next, you will find it useful to know how much fat you take in routinely (your habitual fat intake). You can estimate this based on the fat content of foods you eat every day: for example, how much (and what kind of) milk are you likely to drink? How much meat do you eat?

   This type of information is called *food frequency data.* Notice that it does not necessarily include everything you eat every day, as the food records in other assessments do. Food frequency questionnaires emphasize foods that contain the nutrient(s) in question; for example, our focus here is on fat. Fried vegetables (a source of fat) are considered, whereas other vegetables (containing little fat) are not. The items that vary in your diet from day to day will be considered in step 6.

   The chart in Sample Act on Fact 6.1 lists commonly consumed sources of fat. Fill it in to reflect your habitual intake. If you consume other fat sources regularly, add those foods to the chart, using fat contents from Appendix C.
6. Now subtract your habitual fat intakes from your fat budgets for the day. These figures give you the number of grams of total and saturated fat available for other things—your *discretionary fat allowances.*

You can spend your discretionary fat allowances as you wish. You may decide to keep your per-item intake of fat to low or moderate levels for all of the foods you eat. Or you may want to eat certain high-fat items occasionally, for which you can compensate by selecting low-fat items for the rest of the day. The person in the sample, for example, might want to have a fast-food quarter-pound hamburger on some days to use her discretionary total saturated fat allowances; on other days, she may want to spend them on more butter or salad dressing.

1. Enter approximate daily kcaloric intake	2700 kcals
2. Calculate 30% of kcaloric intake	× 0.3
Equals kcalories allowed from fat	810 kcals
3. Divide by 9 (kcalories per gram)	÷ 9
Equals total fat budget in grams	90 grams
4. Divide by 3 (⅓ of total fat)	÷ 3
Equals saturated fat budget in grams	30 grams

SAMPLE ACT ON FACT 6.1

Determining your budgets for total and saturated fat

Basic Food	Serving Size	Approximate Fat (grams) Per Serving		Servings You Consume Per Day	Daily Fat (grams) from This Food	
		Total	Sat		Total	Sat
Bread, cereal, rice, and pasta						
Bread, white	1 slice	1	0	3	3	0
Corn chips	1 ounce	9	1			
Muffin, bran	1	5	1			
Popcorn, unbuttered	3 cups	1	0	1	1	0
Snack crackers, many kinds	1 ounce	8–10	3			
Vegetables						
Potatoes, French fried	10 pieces	8	3	1	8	3
Potato chips	1 ounce	10	3			
Milk, yogurt, and cheese						
Milk, whole	1 cup	8	5			
Milk, 2%	1 cup	5	3			
Yogurt, made with 2% milk	1 cup	4	2			
Cheese	1½ ounces	14	9			
Cottage cheese, creamed	2 cups	20	13	¼	5	3
Ice cream, reg.	1½ cups	21	14			
Meat, poultry, fish, eggs, beans, nuts						
Lean meats	2 ounces	5	2	2	10	4
Medium-fat meats	2 ounces	10	4			
Legumes	1 cup	1	0			
Nuts	½ cup	35	5			
Combination foods						
Hamburger sandwich	"quarter-pound"	21	8			
Pizza, cheese	⅛ of 15"	6	3			
Fats, oils, and sweets						
Butter, margarine	1 teaspoon	4	3	3	12	9
Regular salad dressing	1 ounce	14	3	1	14	3
Mayonnaise, regular	1 teaspoon	4	1			
HABITUAL FAT INTAKE (GRAMS)					53	22

5. Calculate your usual daily fat intake
6. Calculate your discretionary fat allowances

	Tot. fat	Sat. fat
Fat budgets	90 grams	30 grams
Minus habitual fat intakes	53 grams	22 grams
Equals discretionary fat allowances	37 grams	8 grams

To decrease the fat in your diet, instead of

This	*. Consider this*
Fried entrees such as fried chicken, fried shrimp, fried fish	**Grilled chicken, boiled shrimp, poached fish**
Meats with obvious fat	**Meat trimmed of fat, smaller portions; leaner cuts of meat, more poultry without skin; more fish**
Whole milk, regular cheese, sour cream, ice cream	**2%, 1%, or skim milk; lower fat cheese; low-fat or nonfat yogurt; ice milk or low-fat frozen yogurt**
Regular mayonnaise, regular salad dressing, butter	**Low-fat mayonnaise or fat-free mayonnaise; low-fat or fat-free salad dressing; diet margarine, less butter**
Potato or corn chips, cheese puffs, nuts, some snack crackers	**Air-popped popcorn, pretzels, lower fat crackers**
Most regular cakes and cookies	**Angel food cake, fig newtons, low-fat cakes and cookies**

Remember: Gradual changes are more likely to last, and they give your body time to adjust.

Summary

• Because of their chemical structure, **lipids** generally do not dissolve in water but do dissolve in such substances as ether. **Fats** and **oils** are common lipids. People think negatively about lipids but enjoy eating them. Evidence of these conflicting attitudes can be found throughout our culture.

• Lipids have many important functions. They provide energy, stored in compact form as **adipose tissue.** They furnish the essential nutrients **linoleic acid** and **linolenic acid.** Along with other components of lipids, these essential fatty acids are building materials for brain tissue, the retina of the eye, cell membranes, and many other body substances. Lipids carry fat-soluble vitamins into your body, insulate you, and protect your internal organs.

• **Glycerides** are the most common forms of lipids. They consist of one, two, or three **fatty acids** attached to the 3-carbon compound **glycerol.** Triglycerides (which have three fatty acids) account for about 90% of the weight of lipids in foods. Fatty acids vary in chain length and in their degree of **saturation** with hydrogen atoms: at room temperature, triglycerides containing long, saturated fatty acids are usually solid (fats), whereas those containing short or unsaturated fatty acids are usually liquid (oils).

- Other lipids common in nature are **phospholipids,** such as the **lecithins** present in cell membranes, and **sterols,** such as **cholesterol** and vitamin D.

- Food science has developed many ways of modifying food fats, such as separating fats and oils from their natural sources and **hydrogenating** unsaturated fatty acids to make them firmer. Many **fat substitutes,** such as **sucrose polyester** and Simplesse®, have been developed for commercial and retail uses. Simplesse® has been approved for use, and sucrose polyester awaits approval.

- The amounts of lipids in different foods vary considerably and are not always obvious on inspection. Foods naturally higher in triglycerides include many dairy products, many meats, and nuts. Cholesterol occurs in variable amounts in food of animal origin and is present in amounts much smaller than triglycerides. Cholesterol is also synthesized by your body.

- Lipids take many forms during digestion, absorption, and transport. Triglycerides in the GI tract are kept in small globules by **bile,** and are subsequently broken down into their components by **lipases.** Then, along with bile salts, triglycerides are incorporated into micelles and transported to the intestinal wall cells. Cholesterol also reaches intestinal cells by this route. Once in the cells, these non-water-soluble substances are packaged along with proteins into water-soluble **lipoproteins,** which can be carried readily in the bloodstream. Lipoproteins are also synthesized in the liver. There are four major categories of lipoproteins: **chylomicrons, very low density lipoprotein (VLDL), low density lipoprotein (LDL),** and **high density lipoprotein (HDL).**

- Lipids concentrate in specific kinds of body substances. Triglycerides are either used immediately for energy or stored as body fat. Phospholipids are found mainly in cell membranes. The fate of cholesterol in the body is currently being studied intensively. Some cholesterol is secreted in the bile; other cholesterol remains in the blood; some remains in body cells; and some is incorporated into **plaque** in the linings of blood vessels. Generally, high levels of LDL cholesterol and/or low levels of HDL cholesterol increase a person's risk of heart and blood vessel disease.

- Lipids are involved or suspected of involvement in the development of several major health problems. **Atherosclerosis** is the major disease affecting the blood vessels and is one of the most common causes of death in North America. Although no clear proof of cause and effect is yet available, a variety of evidence suggests that dietary lipids play a role in its long-term development. **Strokes** and **heart attacks,** caused by interruptions of blood flow to the brain and heart, respectively, are serious consequences of atherosclerosis. Many risk factors have been studied intensively in an attempt to learn more about the cause and prevention of this disease. **Cancer,** a general term for many diseases characterized by uncontrolled cell growth, also may be influenced by dietary lipid consumption. Excess fat intake is also implicated in obesity.

- Many experts recommend limiting overall fat intake to 30% of kcalories and saturated fat intake to 10% of kcalories. Act on Fact 6.1 and this chapter's Consider This give practical advice for modifying fat intake.

References

Addis, P. and S.W. Park. 1989. Role of lipid oxidation products in atherosclerosis. In *Food toxicology: Perspective on the relative risks,* ed. S.L. Taylor and R.A. Scanlon. New York: Dekker.

American Cancer Society. 1992. *Cancer facts and figures—1992.* Atlanta: American Cancer Society.

American Dietetic Association. 1991. Position of the American Dietetic Association: Fat replacements. *Journal of the American Dietetic Association* 91:1285–1288.

Barr, S.L., R. Ramakrishnan, C. Johnson, S. Holleran, R.B. Dell, and H.N. Ginsberg. 1992. Reducing total dietary fat without reducing saturated fatty acids does not significantly lower total plasma cholesterol concentrations normal males. *American Journal of Clinical Nutrition* 55:675–681.

Boissonneault, G.A., C.E. Elson, and M.W. Pariza. 1986. Net energy effects of dietary fat on chemically induced mammary carcinogenesis in F344 rats. *Journal of the National Cancer Institute* 76:335–338.

Bonanome, A. and S.M. Grundy. 1988. Effect of dietary stearic acid on plasma cholesterol and lipoprotein levels. *The New England Journal of Medicine* 318:1244–1248.

Brown, M.S. and J.L. Goldstein. 1986. A receptor-mediated pathway for cholesterol homeostasis. *Science* 232:33–47.

Browner, W.S., J. Westenhouse, and J.A. Tice. 1991. What if Americans ate less fat? *Journal of the American Medical Association* 265:3285–3291.

Bruhn, C.M., A. Cotter, K. Diaz-Knauf, J. Sutherlin, E. West, N. Wightman, E. Williamson, and M. Yaffee. 1992. Consumer attitudes and market potential for foods using fat substitutes. *Food Technology* 46(no.4):81–86.

Butterworth, B.E. and T.L. Goldsworthy. 1991. The role of cell proliferation in multistage carcinogenesis. *Proceedings of the Society for Experimental Biology and Medicine* 198:683–687.

Butrum, R.R., D.K. Clifford, and E. Lanza. 1988. NCI dietary guidelines: Rationale. *American Journal of Clinical Nutrition* 48:888–895.

Caragay, A.B. 1992. Cancer-preventive foods and ingredients. *Food Technology* 46(no.4):65–68.

Carroll, K.K. 1991a. *Evaluation of publicly available scientific evidence regarding certain nutrient-disease relationships: Lipids and cancer.* Bethesda, MD: Life Sciences Research Office.

Carroll, K.K. 1991b. Nutrition and cancer: Fat. In *Nutrition, toxicity, and cancer,* ed. I.R. Rowland. Boca Raton, FL: CRC Press.

CFR, 1993. Food labeling rules. *Congressional Federal Register,* Books 1 and 2, January 6, 1993. Washington DC: Superintendent of Documents.

Committee on Diet, Nutrition, and Cancer. 1982. *Diet, nutrition, and cancer.* Washington, DC: National Academy Press.

Connor, W.E. 1991.*Evaluation of publicly available scientific evidence regarding certain nutrient-disease relationships: Omega-3 fatty acids and heart disease.* Bethesda, MD: Life Sciences Research Office.

Connor, W.E., M. Neuringer, and S. Reisbick. 1992. Essential fatty acids: The importance of Ω-3 fatty acids in the retina and brain. *Nutrition Reviews* 50(no.4):21–29.

Crawford, M.A. 1992. The role of dietary fatty acids in biology: Their place in the evolution of the human brain. *Nutrition Reviews* 50(no.4):3–11.

Dattilo, A.M. 1992. Dietary fat and its relationship to body weight. *Nutrition Today* 27:13–19.

Denke, M.A. and S.M. Grundy. 1991. Effects of fats high in stearic acid on lipid and lipoprotein concentrations in men. *American Journal of Clinical Nutrition* 54:1036–1040.

Dolecek, T.A. 1992. Epidemiological evidence of relationships between dietary polyunsaturated fatty acids and mortality in the multiple risk factor intervention trial. *Proceedings of the Society for Experimental Biology and Medicine* 200:177–181.

Donato, K. and D.M. Hegsted. 1985. Efficiency of utilization of various sources of energy for growth. *Proceedings of the National Academy of Sciences USA* 82:4866–4870.

Dougherty, R.M., A.K. Fong, and J.M. Iacono. 1988. Nutrient content of the diet when the fat is reduced. *American Journal of Clinical Nutrition* 48:970–979.

Farrand, M.E. and L. Mojonnier. 1980. Nutrition in the multiple risk factor intervention trial (MRFIT). *Journal of the American Dietetic Association* 76:347–351.

Fats, oils, and fat substitutes. 1989. *Food Technology* 43:66–74.

Fat substitute update. 1990. *Food Technology* 44:92–97.

Freudenheim, J.L., S. Graham, J.R. Marshall, B.P. Haughey, and G. Wilkinson. 1990. A case-controlled study of diet and rectal cancer in western New York. *American Journal of Epidemiology* 131:612–624.

Gould, K.L., D. Ornish, R. Kirkeeide, S. Brown, Y. Stuart, M. Buchi, J. Billings, W. Armstrong, T. Ports, and L. Scherwitz. 1992. Improved stenosis geometry by quantitative coronary arteriography after vigorous risk factor modification. *American Journal of Cardiology* 69:845–853.

Grundy, S.M. 1991. *Evaluation of publicly available scientific evidence regarding certain nutrient-disease relationships: Lipids and cardiovascular disease.* Bethesda, MD: Life Sciences Research Office.

Henderson, B.E., R.K. Ross, and M.C. Pike. 1991. Toward the primary prevention of cancer. *Science* 254:1131–1137.

Hepburn, R.N., J. Exler, and J.L. Weihrauch. 1986. Provisional tables on the content of omega-3 fatty acids and other fat components of selected foods. *Journal of the American Dietetic Association* 86:788–793.

Holme, I. 1990. An analysis of randomized trials evaluating the effect of cholesterol reduction on total mortality and coronary heart disease incidence. *Circulation* 82:1916–1924.

Isles, C.G., D.J. Hole, C.R. Gillis, V.M. Hawthorne, and A.F. Lever. 1989. Plasma cholesterol, coronary heart disease, and cancer in the Renfrew and Paisley survey. *British Medical Journal* 298:920–924.

Jacobs, D., H. Blackburn, M. Higgins, D. Reed, H. Iso, G. McMillan, J. Neaton, J. Nelson, J. Potter, B. Rifkind, J. Rossouw, R. Shekelle, and S. Yusuf. 1992. Report of the conference on low blood cholesterol: Mortality associations. *Circulation* 86:1046–1060.

Kantor, M.A. 1989. Nutrition, cholesterol and heart disease. Part III: How diet affects blood cholesterol levels. *Nutrition Forum* 6(no.3):17–20.

Kaplan, N.M. 1992. Lipid intervention trials in primary prevention: A critical review. *Clinical and Experimental Hypertension* A14(1&2):109–118.

Katan, M.B. and R.P. Mensink. 1992. Isomeric fatty acids and serum lipoproteins. *Nutrition Reviews* 50 (no.4):46–48.

Kern, F. 1991. Normal plasma cholesterol in an 88-year-old-man who eats 25 eggs a day—mechanisms of adaptation. *New England Journal of Medicine* 324:896–899.

Kinsella, J.E. 1988. Food lipids and fatty acids: Importance in food quality, nutrition, and health. *Food Technology* 42:124–145.

Koch, D.D., D.J. Hassemer, D.A. Wiebe, and R.H. Laessig. 1988. Testing cholesterol accuracy: Performance of several common laboratory instruments. *Journal of the American Medical Association* 260:2552–2557.

Kris-Etherton, P.M., D. Krummel, M.E. Russell, D. Dreon, S. Mackey, J. Borchers, and P.D. Wood. 1988. The effect of diet on plasma lipids, lipoproteins, and coronary heart disease. *Journal of the American Dietetic Association* 88:1373–1400.

Kristal, A.R., E. White, A.L. Shattuck, S. Curry, G.L. Anderson, A. Fowler, and N. Urban. 1992. Long-term maintenance of a low-fat diet: Durability of fat-related dietary habits in the Women's Health Trial. *Journal of the American Dietetic Association* 92:553–559.

Kritchevsky, D. 1990. Nutrition and breast cancer. *Cancer* 66:1321–1325.

Kritchevsky, D. and S.B. Kritchevsky. 1992. Serum cholesterol and cancer risk: An epidemiologic perspective. *Annual Reviews of Nutrition* 12:391–416.

Kromhout, D., E.B. Bosschieter, and C.L. Coulander. 1985. The inverse relation between fish consumption and 20-year mortality from coronary heart disease. *New England Journal of Medicine* 312:1205–1209.

Kwiterovich, P. 1989. *Beyond cholesterol.* Baltimore: The Johns Hopkins University Press.

Leibel, R.L. 1992. Fat as a fuel and metabolic signal. *Nutrition Reviews* 50(no.4):12–16.

Linscheer, W.G. and A.J. Vergroesen. 1988. Lipids. In *Modern nutrition in health and disease,* ed. M.E. Shils and V.R. Young. Philadelphia: Lea & Febiger.

Love, R.R. 1988. Dietary fat and human breast cancer: Epidemiological evidence. *Food and Nutrition News* 60(no. 3):13–15.

Lyle, B.J., K.E. McMahon, and P.A. Kreutler. 1992. Assessing the potential dietary impact of replacing dietary fat with other macronutrients. *Journal of Nutrition* 122:211–216.

Marx, J. 1991. Zeroing in on individual cancer risk. *Science* 253:612–616.

Mata, P., L.A. Alvarez-Sala, M.J. Rubio, J. Nuno, and M. DeOya. 1992. Effects of long-term monounsaturated- vs. polyunsaturated-enriched diets on lipoproteins in healthy men and women. *Journal of Clinical Nutrition* 55:846–850.

McMurry, M.P., P.N. Hopkins, R. Gould, K. Engelbert-Fenton, C. Schumacher, L.L. Wu, and R.R. Williams. 1991. Family-oriented nutrition intervention for a lipid clinic population. *Journal of the American Dietetic Association* 91:57–65.

McNamara, D.J. 1987. Effects of fat-modified diets on cholesterol and lipoprotein metabolism. *Annual Review of Nutrition* 7:273–290.

McNamara, D.J., R. Kolb, T.S. Parker, H. Batwin, P. Samuel, C.D. Brown, and E.H. Ahrens, Jr. 1987. Heterogeneity of cholesterol homeostasis in man. *Journal of Clinical Investigation* 79:1729–1739.

Mela, D.J. 1992. Nutritional implications of fat substitutes. *Journal of the American Dietetic Association* 92:472–476.

Mensink, R.P. and M.B. Katan. 1990. Effect of dietary trans fatty acids on high-density and low-density lipoprotein cholesterol levels in healthy subjects. *New England Journal of Medicine* 323:439–435.

National Cholesterol Education Program. 1988. Report of the expert panel on detection, evaluation, and treatment of high blood cholesterol in adults. *Archives of Internal Medicine* 148:36–69.

National Cholesterol Education Program. 1991. Report of the expert panel on population strategies for blood cholesterol reduction. *Circulation* 83:2154–2232.

National Research Council. 1989. *Diet and health.* Washington, DC: National Academy Press.

Ney, D.M. 1990. The cardiovascular system. In *Clinical nutrition and dietetics,* ed. F.J. Zeman. New York: The MacMillan Publishing Company.

Norum, K.R. 1992. Dietary fat and blood lipids. *Nutrition Reviews* 50(no.4):30–37.

Nutrifat. 1988. *Food Engineering,* November 1988.

Ornish, D., S.E. Brown, L.W. Scherwitz, J.H. Billings, W.T. Armstrong, T.A. Ports, S.M. McLanahan, R.L. Kirkeeide, R.J. Brand, and K.L. Gould. 1990. Can lifestyle changes reverse coronary heart disease? *Lancet* 336:129–133.

Pariza, M.W. 1988. Dietary fat and cancer risk: Evidence and research needs. *Cancer Research* 8:167–183.

Ramsay, L.E., W.W. Yeo, and P.R. Jackson. 1991. Dietary reduction of serum cholesterol concentration: Time to think again. *British Medical Journal* 303:953–957.

RDA Subcommittee. 1989. *Recommended dietary allowances.* Washington, DC: National Academy Press.

Regnstrom, J., J. Nilsson, P. Tornvall, C. Landou, A. Hamsten. 1992. Susceptibility to low-density lipoprotein oxidation and coronary atherosclerosis. *Lancet* 339:1183–1186.

Salonen, J.T., S. Yla-Herttuala, R. Yamamoto, S. Butler, H. Kerpela, R. Salonen, K. Nyssonen, W. Palinski, and J.L. Witztum. 1992. Autoantibody against oxidised LDL and progression of carotid atherosclerosis. *Lancet* 339:883–886.

Silberberg, J.S. and D.A. Henry. 1991. The benefits of reducing cholesterol levels: The need to distinguish primary from secondary prevention. *Medical Journal of Australia* 155:665–670.

Simopoulos, A.P. 1991. Omega-3 fatty acids in health and disease and in growth and development. *American Journal of Clinical Nutrition* 54:438–463.

Smith-Schneider, L.M., M.J. Sigman-Grant, P.M. Kris-Etherton. 1992. Dietary fat reduction strategies. *Journal of the American Dietetic Association* 92:34–38.

Troisi, R., W.C,. Willett, and S.T. Weiss. 1992. Trans-fatty acid intake in relation to serum lipid concentrations in adult men. *American Journal of Clinical Nutrition* 56:1019–1024.

Ulbricht, T.L.V. and D.A.T. Southgate. 1991. Coronary heart disease: Seven dietary factors. *Lancet* 338:985–992.

Valsta, L.M., M. Jauhiainen, A. Aro, M.B. Katan, and M. Mutanen. 1992. Effects of a monounsaturated grape-seed oil and a polyunsaturated sunflower oil diet on lipoprotein levels in humans. *Arteriosclerosis and Thrombosis* 12:50–57.

Waring, S. 1988. Shortening replacement in cakes. *Food Technology* 42:114–117.

Weisbrod, R.R., P.L. Pirie, R.M. Mullis, and P. Snyder. 1991. Healthy menu choices in Midwest restaurants. *Journal of Nutrition Education* 23:303–307.

Willett, W.C., M.J. Stampfer, G.A. Colditz, B.A. Rosner, C.H. Hennekens, and F.E. Speizer. 1987. Dietary fat and the risk of breast cancer. *The New England Journal of Medicine* 316:22–28.

Zilversmit, D.B. and C. Stark. 1984. Diet and cardiovascular disease. *Professional Perspectives,* June 1984. NY: Cornell University Extension.

Zock, P.L. and M.B. Katan. 1992. Hydrogenation alternatives: Effects of *trans* fatty acids and stearic acid versus linoleic acid on serum lipids and lipoproteins in humans. *Journal of Lipid Research* 33:399–410.

IN THIS CHAPTER

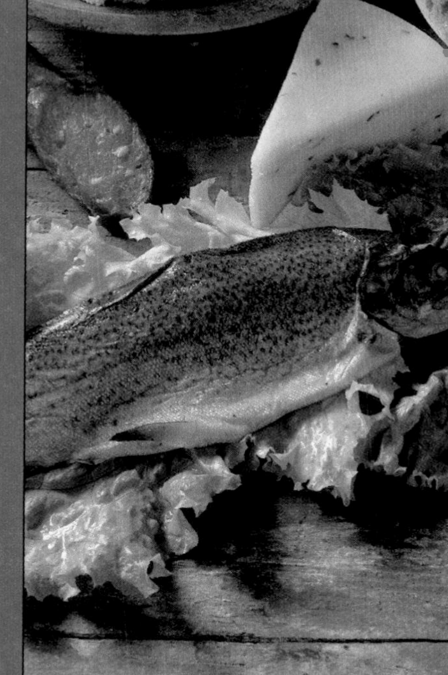

Chapter 7

Proteins

Play the word association game for a few seconds. *Protein.* What words come to mind? *Lean? Lively? Strong, fit,* and *energetic?* Many people associate protein with muscle, vitality, and fitness. It's true that protein is related to life and vitality, because protein is a critical component of every cell. The cells of your body, a bacterium, an apple, a pine tree, a rhinoceros—every living thing contains protein.

Perhaps that's why many people value protein above other classes of nutrients. Just page through a household magazine to see how protein and its most popular sources are treated. Most meals are planned around the primary protein source. People spend hundreds of dollars and devote backyard and kitchen space to grills that are designed primarily to cook meats, and most people spend the largest portion of their food dollars on meats, fish, and poultry, the most popular sources of protein. There is no question about the status protein enjoys in our society. The name itself reinforces the priority we give it: the Greek word *protos,* from which the word *protein* is derived, means "first."

This supervaluing of protein has led to another predictable phenomenon: *we tend to give protein credit for more than it can deliver.* Look at the ads in sports magazines for protein supplements that claim to improve performance, or at articles about diets that imply that protein will melt fat off your body. In light of scientific evidence, it is clear that these claims have *over*rated protein.

In this chapter, you'll cut through the hype and the expectations and take a scientifically realistic look at what protein is, what it does, and what we need to eat to get the healthiest amount of it. Let's start by looking at protein's structure.

Proteins—Built from Amino Acids

protein—thousands of related nitrogen-containing organic substances that have structural, regulatory, and energy-providing functions

amino acids—the approximately 20 "building block" molecules the body uses to construct proteins

Protein is an umbrella term that includes thousands of related substances. In your body, some of them are solids, and others are dissolved within fluids. The unifying feature shared by the thousands of different proteins is that they are all composed of chemical building blocks called **amino acids.**

The Structure of an Amino Acid

An amino acid, being an organic substance, contains carbon, hydrogen, and oxygen. Unlike other organic nutrients, all amino acids also contain nitrogen and sometimes sulfur as well.

Approximately 100 amino acids exist in nature, but only 20 of them are used to build proteins. Human cells can produce certain amino acids needed for protein synthesis, provided that the right ingredients are present: compounds containing carbon, hydrogen, oxygen, and nitrogen. Because carbon, hydrogen, and oxygen are liberally available from various dietary sources, your cells have no trouble coming up with those elements, but to synthesize amino acids, they have a critical need for nitrogen sources. Figure 7.1 shows the general structure of an amino acid and several examples. To form proteins, amino acids are linked together by **peptide bonds.** If two amino acids join, the resulting substance is a *dipeptide;* three amino acids create a *tripeptide.* A larger number of connected amino acids constitutes a *polypeptide.* A protein may be made up of one or more polypeptides.

peptide bonds—the chemical linkages that hold amino acids together

The Structure of a Protein

The structure of a protein is infinitely more complicated: a single protein molecule can contain hundreds of amino acids. These molecules are bent,

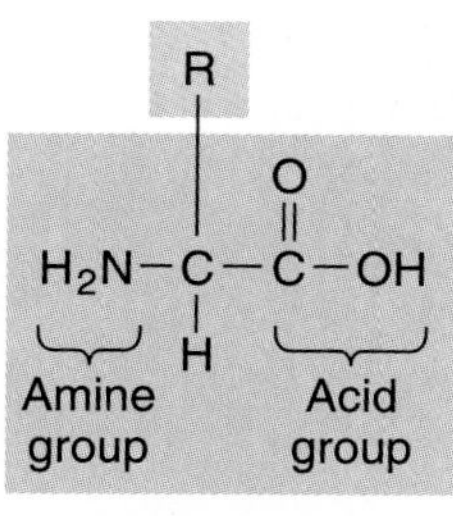

(a) Generalized structure of all amino acids

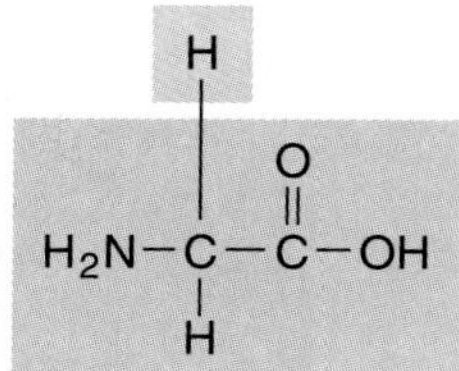

(b) Glycine (the simplest amino acid)

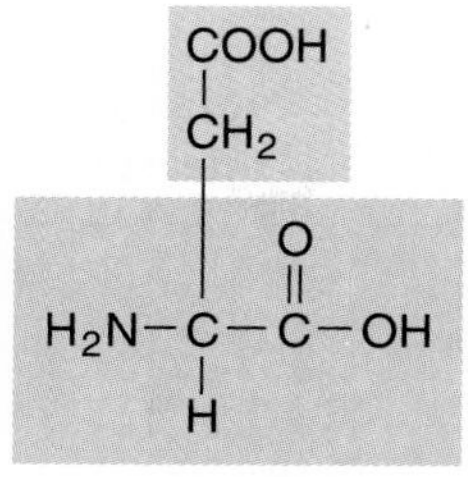

(c) Aspartic acid (an acidic amino acid)

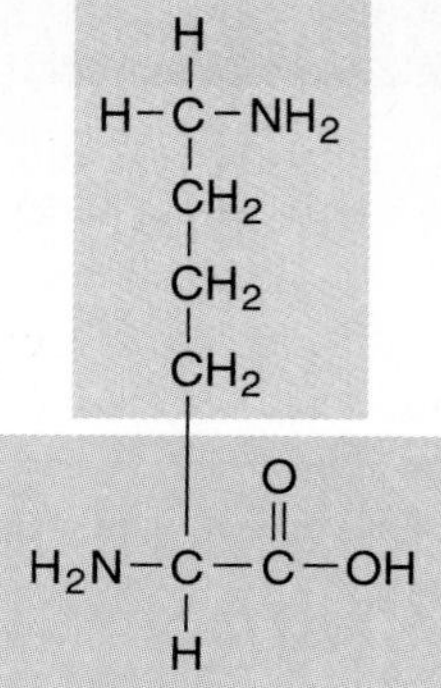

(d) Lysine (a basic amino acid)

FIGURE 7.1
Amino acid structures.

(a) Generalized structure of amino acids. All amino acids have both an amine ($-NH_2$) and an acid ($-COOH$) group; they differ only in the makeup of their R groups (orange). (b)–(d) Specific structures of three amino acids. The simplest (glycine) has an R group consisting of a single hydrogen atom. An acid group in the R group makes the amino acid more acidic. An amine group in the R group makes it more basic.

folded, or coiled into very specific three-dimensional configurations; Figure 7.2 gives examples. The shape of the molecule is provided by the various cross-linkages formed between amino acids at different places in the chain. The same amino acids may appear many times in a single molecule of a protein, and their order is critical: if one is in the wrong place, or if one amino acid substitutes for another, a different protein may result.

An analogy using letters and words demonstrates the point. Let's say that the letters *A, E, M, S,* and *T* each represent a different amino acid. If you combine these "amino acids" in different ways, you can make different "proteins," such as *steam, mates, teams,* and *meats.* If you add other letters, such as an *R* and another *S,* you can then make *masters* and *streams.* Omitting some of the letters, you can make *stem, same, mesas, rate,* and so on. All are distinctly different "proteins," although they were all derived from the same six "amino acids." This analogy breaks down when we consider molecule size: our "proteins" should have hundreds of letters.

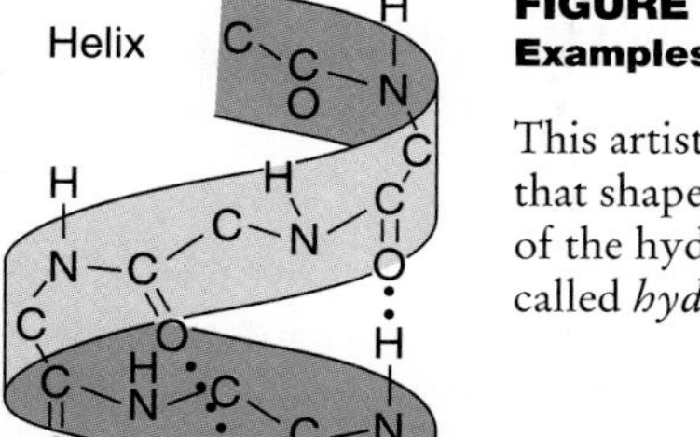
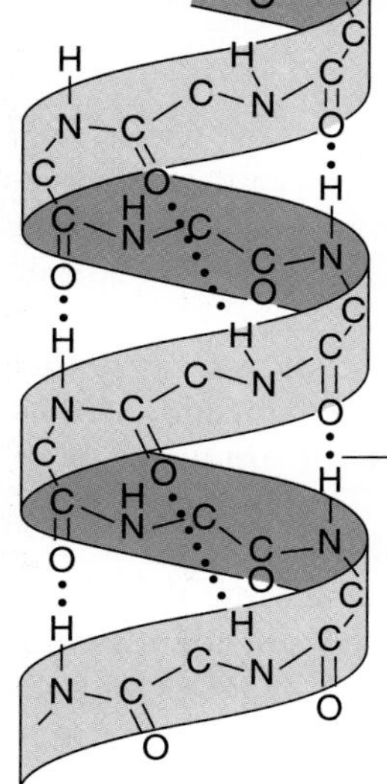

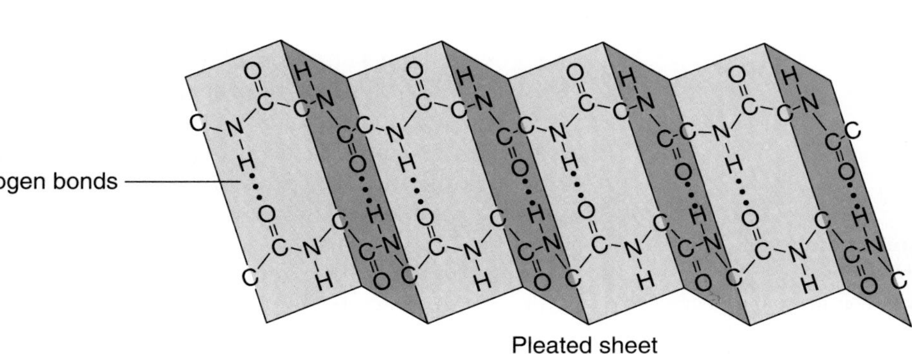

FIGURE 7.2
Examples of protein structures.

This artist's rendering shows two structural patterns—the helix and the pleated sheet—that shape protein molecules. Both patterns depend on weak attractions between some of the hydrogen and oxygen atoms along the polypeptide chain. These attractions are called *hydrogen bonds.*

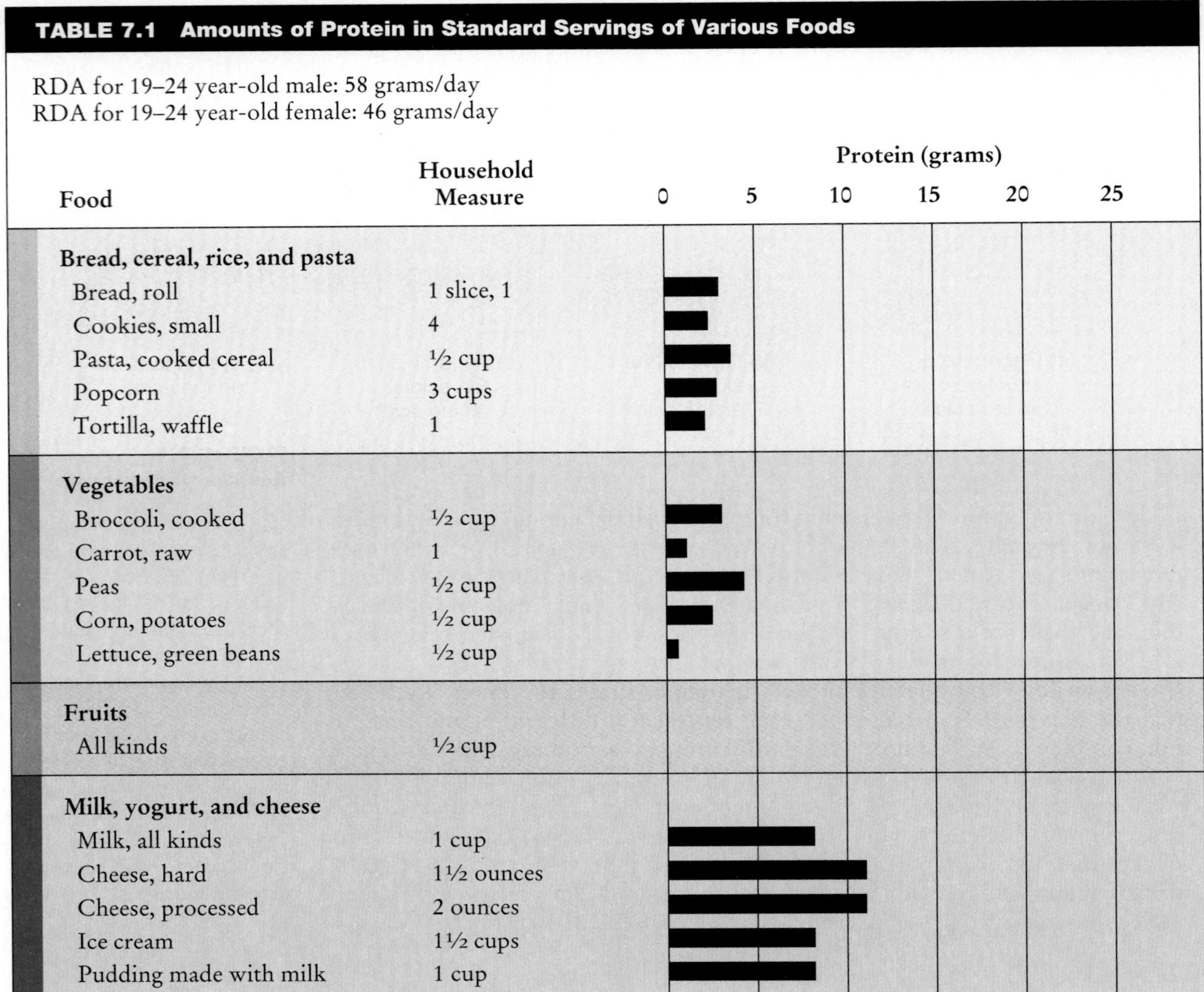

TABLE 7.1 Amounts of Protein in Standard Servings of Various Foods

RDA for 19–24 year-old male: 58 grams/day
RDA for 19–24 year-old female: 46 grams/day

Food	Household Measure
Bread, cereal, rice, and pasta	
Bread, roll	1 slice, 1
Cookies, small	4
Pasta, cooked cereal	½ cup
Popcorn	3 cups
Tortilla, waffle	1
Vegetables	
Broccoli, cooked	½ cup
Carrot, raw	1
Peas	½ cup
Corn, potatoes	½ cup
Lettuce, green beans	½ cup
Fruits	
All kinds	½ cup
Milk, yogurt, and cheese	
Milk, all kinds	1 cup
Cheese, hard	1½ ounces
Cheese, processed	2 ounces
Ice cream	1½ cups
Pudding made with milk	1 cup

The cells of every living organism can synthesize their own proteins, provided the right amino acids are available. All species of plants and animals construct the unique proteins they need to support their own life and growth.

How does your body know how to assemble its different proteins? The answer is found in the nucleus of every cell, where materials called *deoxyribonucleic acid (DNA)* and *ribonucleic acid (RNA)* contain the information that governs the synthesis of each protein. To extend our letter analogy, DNA and RNA dictate the "spelling" of proteins.

limiting amino acid—an amino acid in such short supply that protein synthesis in the body cannot continue

When a cell needs to make a particular protein, it draws from the assortment of amino acids available to it at that time. If a cell needs to continue making a certain protein but runs short of one of the amino acids it needs, it cannot synthesize any more of that protein. The amino acid or acids that are in short supply are called the **limiting amino acid(s).**

The foods we eat contain proteins, but not exactly the same ones that make up our own bodies. The fact that food proteins are not identical to human protein is not a problem: digestion dismantles food proteins so that we can use the components for reassembling our own body proteins (this topic is discussed in more detail later in the chapter).

TABLE 7.1 continued

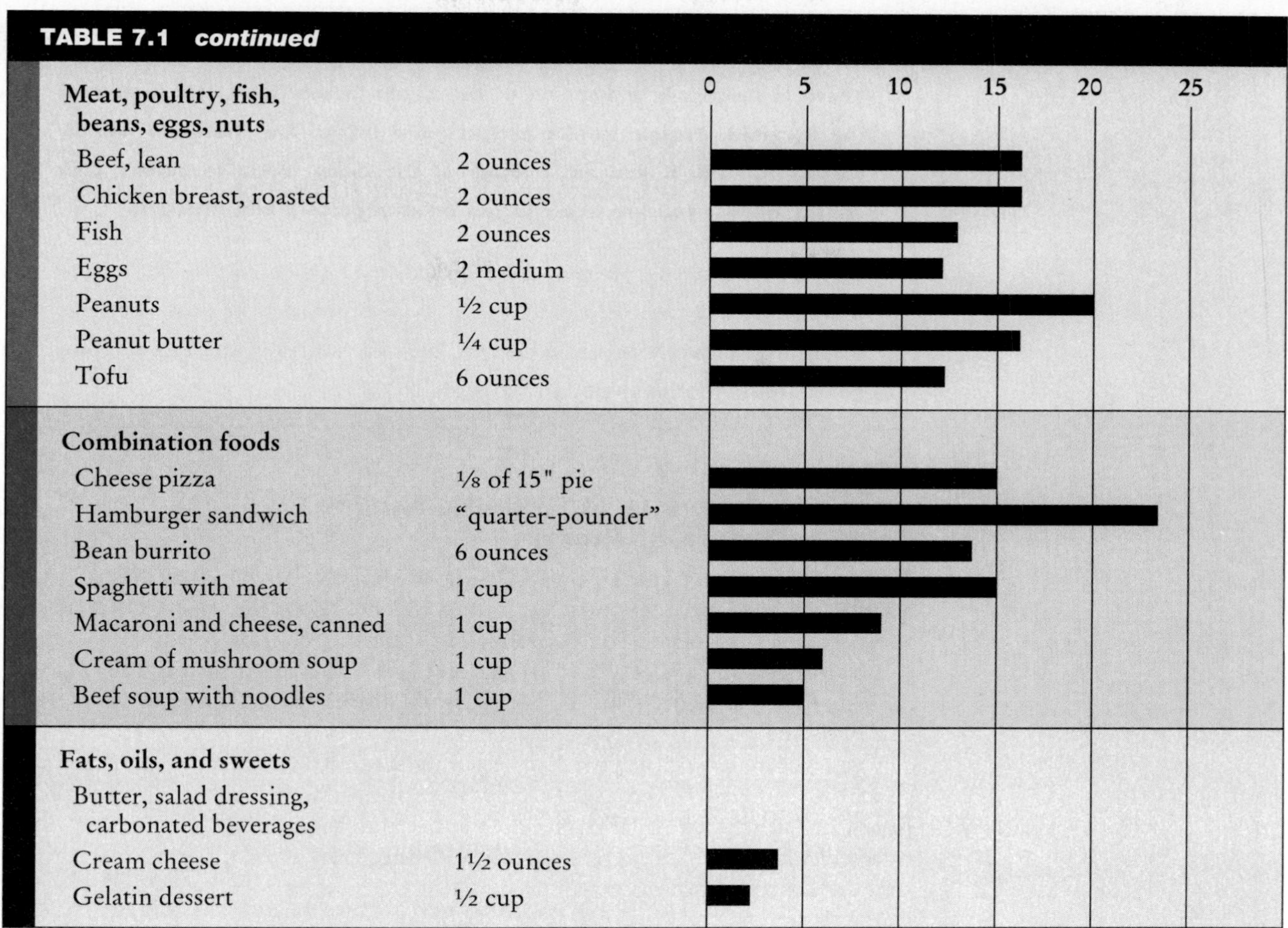

Meat, poultry, fish, beans, eggs, nuts		
Beef, lean	2 ounces	
Chicken breast, roasted	2 ounces	
Fish	2 ounces	
Eggs	2 medium	
Peanuts	½ cup	
Peanut butter	¼ cup	
Tofu	6 ounces	
Combination foods		
Cheese pizza	⅛ of 15" pie	
Hamburger sandwich	"quarter-pounder"	
Bean burrito	6 ounces	
Spaghetti with meat	1 cup	
Macaroni and cheese, canned	1 cup	
Cream of mushroom soup	1 cup	
Beef soup with noodles	1 cup	
Fats, oils, and sweets		
Butter, salad dressing, carbonated beverages		
Cream cheese	1½ ounces	
Gelatin dessert	½ cup	

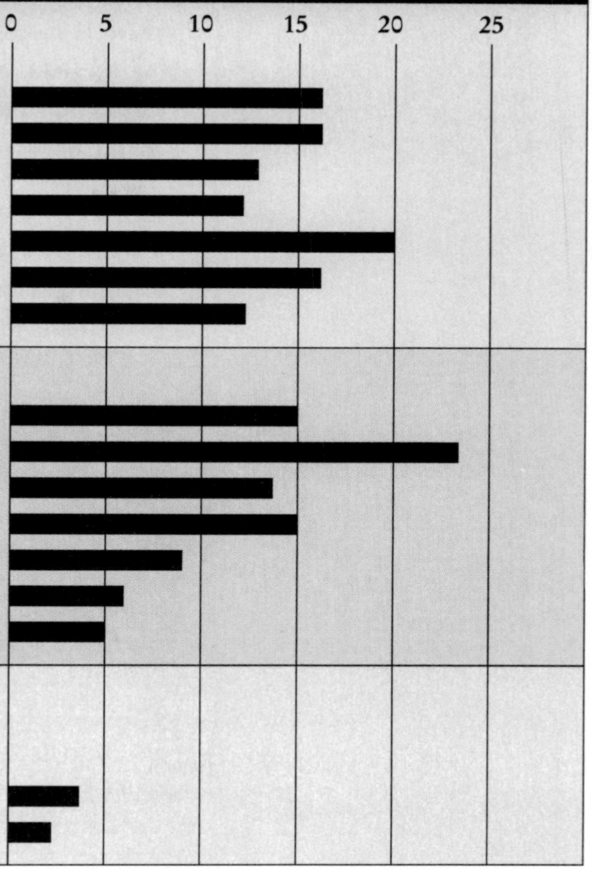

Now let's take a more specific look at exactly what it is that humans need from dietary protein.

The Body's Need for Components of Protein

When nutritionists talk about "protein needs," they are really referring to our need for certain components of protein. First, we need sufficient *nitrogen* from food proteins. Second, we need enough of *certain amino acids* that are necessary for human protein synthesis and that cannot be produced within the body; these are called **essential amino acids.** These two concerns are often referred to as issues of protein *quantity* and *quality.*

essential amino acids—amino acids the body needs for protein synthesis but cannot produce for itself and so must obtain from foods

Adequate Nitrogen = Quantity of Protein

Recall our earlier statement that living cells can synthesize some amino acids if they have a nitrogen source. Once they have the amino acids, the cells synthesize their own unique proteins. In a practical sense, then, the most important protein intake issue is quantity: getting enough protein in the diet to provide the necessary nitrogen for amino acid production.

Table 7.1 shows the protein contents of various foods, grouped according to the categories of the Food Guide Pyramid. You can see that, in general, dairy products, meats, poultry, fish, beans, eggs, and nuts offer the greatest amount of protein per serving. But notice that *most foods offer at least some protein.*

You Tell Me

There is protein in almost all of the foods in the five basic groups of the Pyramid. Protein intake and kcalorie intake are therefore usually closely related. If you eat enough of the basic foods to satisfy your energy needs, you are likely to get enough protein and nitrogen.

If, however, your diet is very low in kcalories, how could this affect your protein intake? Or if you consume a large proportion of your kcalories from foods outside the basic groups, such as fats, oils, and sweets, how could this affect your protein intake?

Adequate Amounts of Essential Amino Acids = Quality of Protein

The second protein intake issue is one of quality. To be considered "good quality," a food protein must contain adequate amounts of essential amino acids your body needs for protein synthesis but cannot produce by itself. Nine amino acids are essential in the diet (RDA Subcommittee, 1989). Table 7.2 lists them, as well as the 11 nonessential amino acids (the ones your body can produce).

Scientists not only have learned that these nine amino acids are indispensable but also have estimated what amounts the human body needs. Research continues on this topic (Young and Bier, 1987). Figure 7.3 illustrates most protein experts' current thinking about our relative needs for specific essential amino acids.

A food protein is considered to be of good quality if it contains the essential amino acids in those approximate proportions. In fact, one way scientists determine protein quality is to calculate a *chemical score,* which reflects the amount of the most limiting amino acids compared with a *ref-*

TABLE 7.2 Essential and Nonessential Amino Acids

Amino Acids Essential in the Diet	Amino Acids Not Essential in the Diet
Histidine	Alanine
Isoleucine	Arginine
Leucine	Asparagine
Lysine	Aspartic Acid
Methionine	Cysteine[a]
Phenylalanine	Glutamic acid
Threonine	Glutamine
Tyryptophan	Glycine
Valine	Proline
	Serine
	Tyrosine[a]

[a] The amino acids cysteine and tyrosine are not essential, but they can substitute in part for methionine and phenylalanine, respectively.

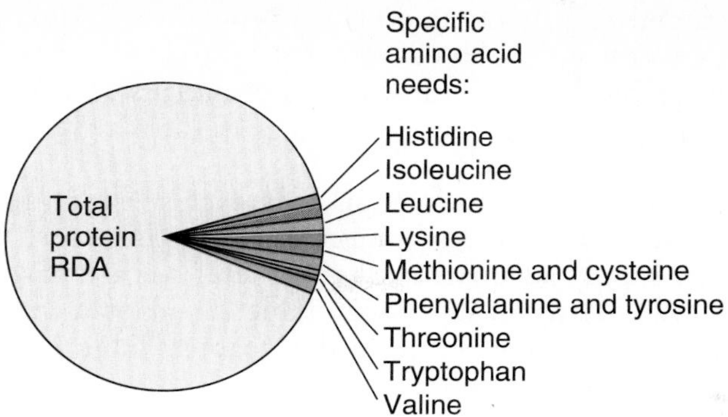

FIGURE 7.3
Relative amounts of essential amino acids and total protein needed by adults.

All together, the essential amino acids represent only a small portion of the recommended total amino acid (protein) intake. Also note that the essential amino acids are not all needed in the same amounts. (RDA Subcommittee, 1989; Young and Bier, 1987.)

erence protein of excellent quality, such as egg or milk protein. In such a system, the proteins with the most desirable proportions of amino acids earn the highest scores.

Other tests involve feeding a particular protein to laboratory animals to assess how much protein was retained or how much it contributed to the animals' growth. The results of all of these tests indicate that food proteins from animal sources are generally of higher quality than proteins from plant sources. Based on an evaluation method that indicates how much protein was retained, here's how various food proteins rated, on a scale of 0 to 100: egg protein, 100; cow's milk, 93; fish, 76; beef, 74; soybeans, 73; whole wheat, 65; peas, 64; peanuts, 55.

The proteins that match human needs best are found in eggs and milk, but meats, fish, poultry, cheese, and soybeans (a notable plant source) also have protein of good quality. The proteins in other legumes, nuts and seeds, most grains, and vegetables get a fair rating. A protein of unquestionably poor quality is gelatin. Note that the poor quality of this animal protein is an exception to the general rule. Gelatin and other proteins at the lower end of the scale are in that position because of their limiting amino acids.

Vegetarian Eating Styles: Few Concerns About Protein Quantity and Quality

Knowing that most animal products provide both a higher quantity and a higher quality of protein, you might think that we would advise against **vegetarian eating styles,** which avoid animal products to one degree or another. Not so, although there are some considerations about protein you need to keep in mind if you are a vegetarian. Before we discuss these issues, let's take a look at some of the variations in vegetarian eating styles.

vegetarian eating styles—eating habits that avoid some or all animal products; common variations include **semivegetarian, lacto-ovo vegetarian, lacto-vegetarian,** and **vegan**

Most vegetarians eat all types of foods of plant origin, and some also eat certain foods of animal origin; therefore, vegetarians are most easily differentiated by which animal foods they include or avoid. The better-known types are as follows:

- **semivegetarian**—avoids only certain kinds of meat, fish, or poultry
- **lacto-ovo vegetarian**—avoids eating animal flesh but does use dairy products and eggs
- **lacto-vegetarian**—avoids eating animal flesh and eggs but does use dairy products
- **vegan**—avoids *all* foods of animal origin, even dairy products and eggs

Note that the first three groups include milk, a protein source of very high quality. When the diets of these vegetarian groups are evaluated, they

omnivores—people who eat all kinds of food

are generally found to contain amounts of protein that are as generous as those in the diets of people who eat all types of food, who are called **omnivores.** Like many North Americans, these vegetarians are likely to take in almost double the protein they need, which gives them a glut of both essential and nonessential amino acids.

The fourth group on the list, vegans, rely exclusively on foods of plant origin. Even most vegans can easily meet their protein needs. Various food group plans that supply adequate intakes for adult vegans have been developed (Mutch, 1988). Early in this book, Table 2.3 adapted the Food Guide Pyramid for the needs of the vegan. In this chapter, Table 7.3 reiterates the guide and shows a sample menu.

TABLE 7.3 Food Guide for the Adult Vegan

The recommended intakes of foods, based on the groups of the Pyramid, are shown below with a sample day's menu. Some vegans will need to eat more to meet their needs for energy.

Summary of Recommendations	Est. Protein per Serving (grams)	Approx. Total (grams)
Bread, rice, cereal, pasta		
Whole-grain yeast bread: 4 slices	2	8
Other grains: 3–7	2	6–14
Vegetables		
4–5 including 2 or more dark leafy greens	2	8–10
Fruits		
2–4 including Vitamin C source	0	0
Beans and Nuts		
Legumes: 2 servings	15	30
Nuts or Seeds: 1 serving	15	15
Total		67–77

Sample Day's Menu

Breakfast

½ cup orange juice
1 cup cooked oatmeal with raisins, dried apples, and cinnamon
2 slices whole-grain toast
2 tablespoons peanut butter

Lunch

1 cup split pea soup
1 whole-wheat English muffin with margarine
1 cup spinach salad with French dressing
2 medium oatmeal cookies

Dinner

Mixed entree of:
1 cup lima beans
½ cup onions, celery, and water chestnuts
½ cup tomato sauce
½ cup broccoli
1 cornmeal muffin with margarine
1 cup apple juice

Snacks

3 cups popcorn
grapes
¼ cup mixed nuts

Remember that humans need essential amino acids in particular proportions. It isn't important that the amino acids present *in any one individual food* match the pattern that represents human needs, as long as the assortment available *from everything eaten during the day* fulfills those needs. The amino acids you consume become part of a general circulating pool from which your body draws amino acids as needed. As long as enough of the essential amino acids enter the pool to restore those used during the day, your body is able to continue normal protein synthesis.

Therefore, even though a given plant protein has one or more limiting amino acids, a more generous amount of that amino acid from another food or foods can make up for the shortfall in the first. This principle is called **complementing** (from the root word *complete*) or **mutual supplementation.** For example, corn is low in the amino acid lysine, whereas many beans have generous amounts of it; by eating both foods in the same day, a person can consume adequate levels of lysine and other essential amino acids. With this in mind, you can see that *getting adequate variety in the diet* is important to the nutritional status of a vegan.

complementing (mutual supplementation)—eating together foods whose amino acids are *collectively* in proportion with human needs, although individually they are not

You Tell Me

Although the proteins in plant foods have their unique limiting amino acids, there are a couple of generalizations about mutual supplementation. One general rule is that the essential amino acids in *legumes* (starchy beans, peas, and lentils) and in *grains* usually mutually supplement each other. *Legumes* and *nuts or seeds* also usually complement each other.

With these generalizations in mind, can you name some combination food items that include complementary ingredients? One example is a soup that includes kidney beans (a legume) and macaroni (a grain product). Another is a snack mix that includes peanuts (actually a legume) plus almonds, pecans, and pumpkin seeds.

If you had trouble answering the You Tell Me above, Figure 7.4 gives other examples of foods whose amino acids substantially complement each other. Note that although it is not necessary to get all the right proportions of essential amino acids within the same meal, these dishes promote healthy variety in protein sources.

Another perspective on the issue becomes clear when you look at Figure 7.3; notice what a small proportion of the total recommended intake for amino acids needs to come from essential amino acids. If you consume your RDA for protein, even from all-plant sources, you are likely to get as much as you need of the essential amino acids. The important principle here is *to eat enough food from the basic food groups* to fulfill your overall needs for energy and protein.

Vegans with Particular Concerns about Meeting Protein Needs

Some groups of vegans find that meeting their needs for optimal amounts and proportions of essential amino acids is a challenge. These are people

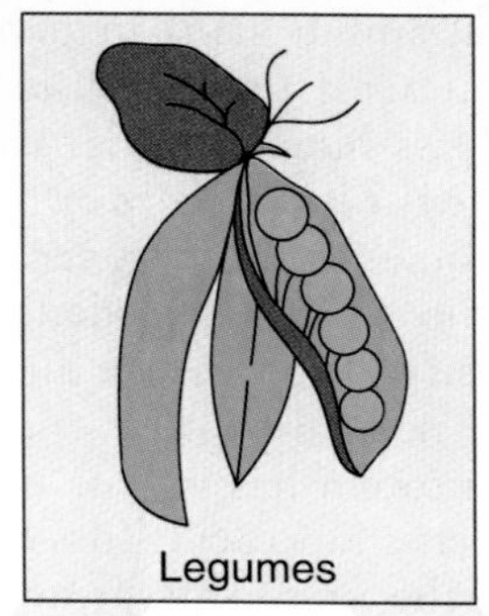

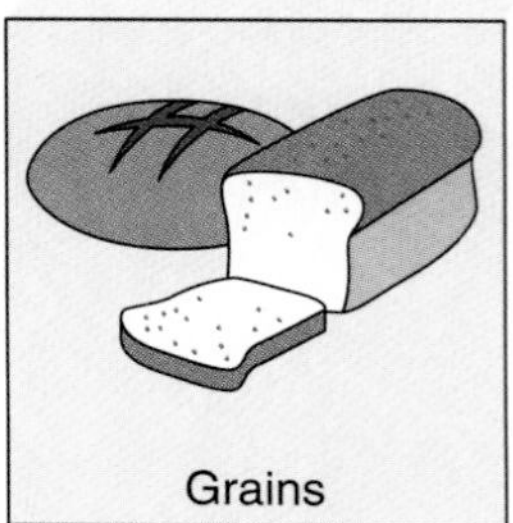

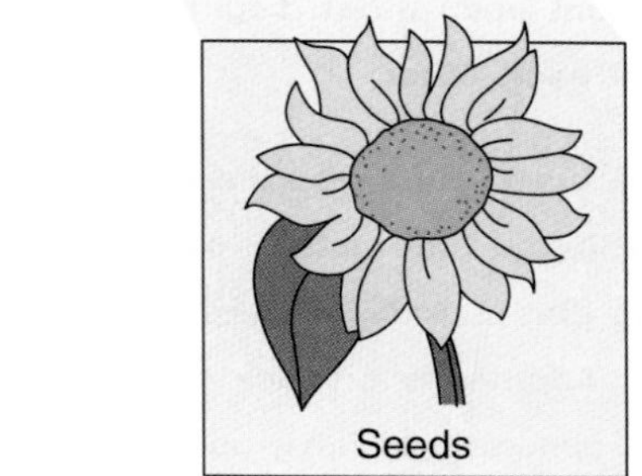

FIGURE 7.4
Improving plant protein quality.

Individual foods of plant origin usually do not have the proportions of essential amino acids that humans need; however, other foods can make up for the lack. Generally, legumes (starchy beans and peas) have complementary relationships with grains and also with nuts and seeds. Each food item listed in the shaded bands is an example of a food that has better protein quality than its individual ingredients have separately.

whose bodies need to make more protein but whose overall food intake may be too low to supply the necessary basic ingredients.

The classic examples are pregnant and lactating vegan women, whose bodies need protein for added maternal tissues, for the fetus, and for milk production. For the pregnant or lactating vegan, it is a wise safeguard to complement protein intakes over the course of the day while generally increasing overall food consumption. This can be accomplished by using a special eating guide (given in Chapter 15) that will help her meet her increased needs for not only protein but also other nutrients.

Vegan children are another concern. Like all children, they need high intakes of energy, protein, and other nutrients to achieve normal growth. They also need more protein of higher quality: almost half their recommended protein intake should be composed of essential amino acids (Young and Bier, 1987). Because the proteins in foods of plant origin tend to be lower in quality and in quantity than those in an equal volume of foods of animal origin, the vegan child may need to eat a larger quantity of food than he or she wants to consume. Other nutrients also are less concentrated in

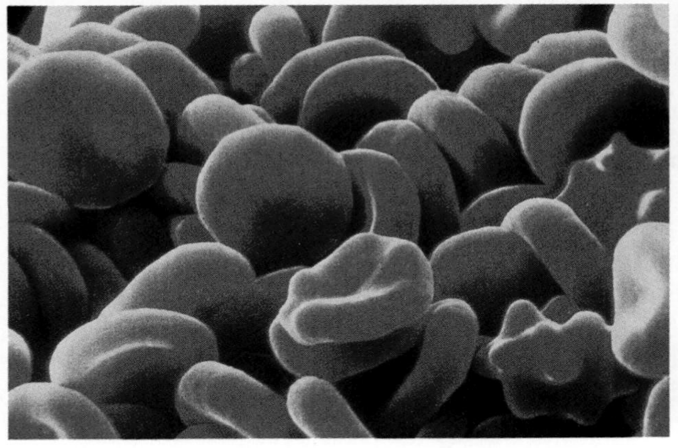

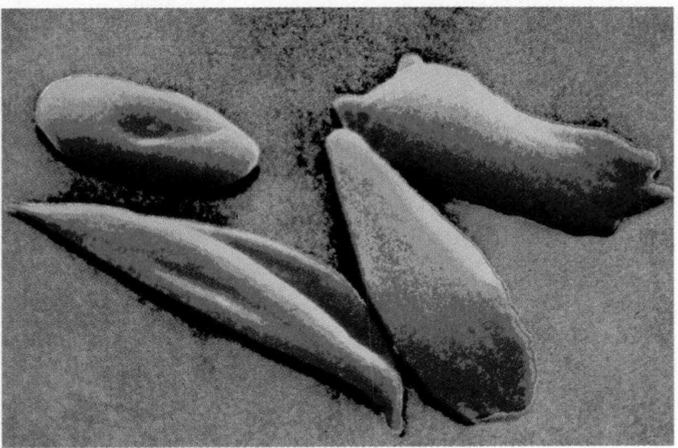

FIGURE 7.5
Serious consequences of an error in protein synthesis: sickle cell anemia.

These scanning electron micrographs show both (a) healthy red blood cells (disk-shaped) and (b) sickle cells (crescent-shaped), which are unable to carry oxygen normally. This drastic difference occurs as a result of one incorrect amino acid in the hemoglobin structure.

foods of plant origin. Unfortunately, some children who consume vegan diets fail to thrive (Williams and Worthington-Roberts, 1988). Therefore, although it is *possible* for vegan children to meet nutritional needs if they eat sufficient quantities of a well-planned plant-based diet, the practicalities suggest that children are likely to be better nourished if they include some animal sources of protein in their diets. Fortunately, vegan parents often see the wisdom of this approach and provide their children with lacto-ovo or lacto-vegetarian diets. Children who consume lacto-ovo vegetarian diets can grow as well as children who eat meat (Sabate et al., 1991).

The Many Functions of Protein

One way of underscoring protein's crucial role in your body is to note its involvement in all three general functions of nutrients. Proteins constitute body structure, regulate various body processes, and are an energy source. In this section we look at examples of how protein performs each of these functions.

Constituting Structure

Protein is a part of every living cell: it is part of the cell membrane (along with phospholipids and cholesterol, as you saw in Figure 6.2), the cytosol, and the small organelles floating in the cytosol, including the nucleus. Protein therefore is a key component in the structure of your body.

Proteins that give structure and definition to your body are prominent in such tissues as skin, muscles of internal organs, skeletal muscle, connective tissue, and the matrix (framework) of bones and teeth. Many different kinds of proteins make up these tissues.

The composition of proteins also varies from one person to another, depending on the DNA code inherited. For example, a slight difference in normal proteins determines whether an individual's blood type is A, B, AB, or O.

Occasionally, an organism is genetically programmed to make a consistent error in protein synthesis. For example, small variations in the amino acid content and arrangement of the blood protein *hemoglobin* can result in serious blood diseases, such as sickle cell anemia (Figure 7.5). In this condition, red blood cells are misshapen and unable to function normally. The course of this disease, which is found predominantly in blacks, is a painful one that often results in early death.

Regulating Processes

Proteins influence a variety of metabolic functions. You have learned about some of these previously; others may be new to you.

Enzymes, Nutrient Carriers, and Hormones You know that enzymes, which are proteins, are critical to the process of digestion. But that is not the only function they perform. There are thousands of different types of enzymes in the human body that accomplish many different tasks. Without enzymes, biochemical reactions would occur so slowly that life as we know it could not exist.

Other proteins in the body serve as carriers for nutrients. Vitamin A, riboflavin, and copper, for example, depend on proteins to transport them around the body.

Hormones, some of which are proteins or peptides, are chemical messengers produced in one part of the body to affect a process in another region. Among the many processes that hormones affect are metabolism and reproduction. Insulin is an example of a protein hormone.

Body Defenses Proteins are also critical to the body's defense network. Because proteins are present in skin, they are part of the body's first line of defense against infection. However, the skin is just one of several protein-dependent defenses.

If disease-causing bacteria attempt to enter the body via any of its various openings, they are likely to be destroyed by bactericidal substances found in mucosal secretions. But if disease-causing bacteria or viruses gain entry anyway, other aspects of the body's immune system take over. The body recognizes that the invading organisms consist of unfamiliar proteins, called **antigens,** and it produces its own proteins, called **antibodies,** to search and destroy the organisms. If your protein intake has been inadequate for an extended period of time, your immune system is not able to function as well, and you are more likely to develop an active case of the disease (Myrvik, 1988).

antigens—foreign substances, such as proteins, that can provoke an immune response

antibodies—proteins that protect the body against antigens by binding to and inactivating them

Mineral and Fluid Regulators Proteins affect mineral balance and fluid balance. The proteins in cell membranes function as gatekeepers that control the access of certain electrolytes to the cell. For example, sodium ions are actively pumped out of the cell by these proteins, whereas potassium ions are pumped in. The appropriate location of these electrolytes is critical to the function of nerves and muscles. Without the right balance of these minerals in intracellular and extracellular fluids, such vital functions as the beating of your heart cannot take place. The location of these minerals also affects distribution of body water, as you learned in Chapter 4.

Protein is involved in fluid balance in a more direct way as well, because soluble proteins hold water. Water readily moves across membranes to equalize the concentration of particles on the two sides, but soluble proteins do not cross these membranes, thereby helping stabilize the fluid in each compartment (see Chapter 4). For example, *albumin,* the most abundant soluble protein in blood, helps maintain the fluid volume within blood vessels. If blood protein levels fall as a result of severely inadequate protein intake for several weeks, some fluid will move from the blood into interstitial spaces. This condition is called *edema.*

pH Regulators Another function of proteins is to help maintain acid–base balance through *protein buffer systems.* A buffer, as you learned in Chapter 4, is a substance that minimizes changes in pH by releasing or binding

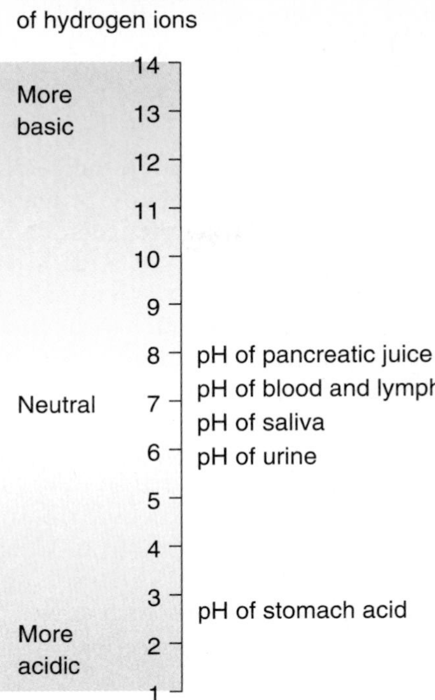

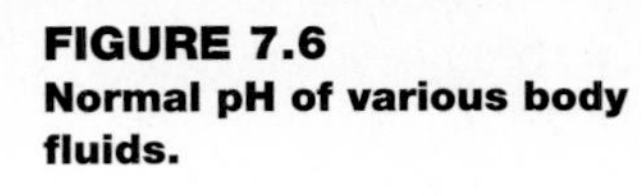

FIGURE 7.6
Normal pH of various body fluids.

hydrogen ions. Soluble proteins, notably those within body cells, are very effective buffers because of the activity of parts of their side groups (see R groups in Figure 7.1). When pH is dropping, the side groups on some amino acids can accept hydrogen, thereby raising the pH. When pH is rising, the side groups on other amino acids can release hydrogen to lower the pH.

pH regulation is important because body systems, to function normally, require that their fluid environments have a specific pH. Figure 7.6 shows the different pH of various fluids in the body. The strong hydrochloric acid produced by the stomach provides the low pH the stomach enzyme *pepsin* needs to begin protein digestion; at any higher pH, the function of pepsin would be compromised. The pH of the bloodstream, by contrast, must be maintained between the narrow range of 7.35 and 7.45, or otherwise essential metabolic processes will cease (Marieb, 1992). In the most severe cases of acid–base imbalance, death results.

Neurotransmitters Some amino acids function as **neurotransmitters**—chemical substances that are released from a nerve cell into the space between it and the adjoining cell(s). These chemicals help nerve impulses get from one cell to the other (Figure 7.7). At least three amino acids, *tryptophan, tyrosine,* and *glutamic acid,* are known to be neurotransmitters or precursors of neurotransmitters. Researchers are working to learn how diet may affect the production of these neurotransmitters and how they in turn may affect behavior and nervous system function within a few hours of consumption.

neurotransmitters—chemicals that aid in the transmission of nerve impulses

The fact that diet can influence these important biochemicals leads people to fantasize about controlling their behavior or mental function by eating certain types of foods. (Wouldn't you like to be assured that your memory and thought processes would be in top form if you ate certain foods before an exam?) However, this area is still highly experimental; it is too early to suggest applications of most of these theories to real-life situations.

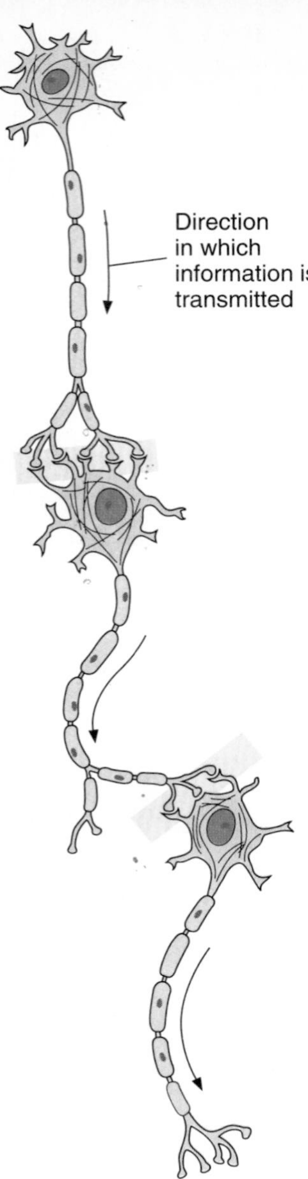

FIGURE 7.7
Some amino acids help your nervous system do its job.

At least three amino acids function as neurotransmitters —chemicals that help nerve impulses travel rapidly through the tiny spaces (synapses) between one cell and another. The highlighted areas show two synapses.

Providing Energy

Like carbohydrates and lipids, proteins can be metabolized for energy. They yield 4 kcalories per gram. However, the body primarily uses available carbohydrates and fats, saving proteins for their unique uses as much as possible. Estimates regarding the proportion of a day's energy use that might ordinarily come from protein range from 1% to 15% (Goodman, 1988).

There are several circumstances in which your body uses more protein for energy. If you don't get enough carbohydrate and fat to meet your body's energy demands—let's say you're running a marathon—some protein will be broken apart, *deaminated* (have its amino groups removed), and then metabolized like carbohydrate. Or, if your body has been totally depleted of carbohydrate—perhaps you haven't consumed any for several days—the same process occurs. (This reemphasizes the protein-sparing function of carbohydrates that you read about in Chapter 5.) Also, during the early weeks of a demanding physical conditioning program, especially in untrained people, more protein is used for energy.

You Tell Me

Some weight loss diets emphasize high-protein foods and severely restrict carbohydrate and fat.

If you were on this type of diet, what would happen to some of the protein?

Your Body's Handling of Protein

Although the structure of protein is complex, your body has no trouble dismantling it. In fact, your body treats proteins pretty harshly, beginning in the stomach. Obviously, the treatment is effective, because 95% or more of the proteins that arrive in the small intestine are absorbed (Ganong, 1991).

Before we discuss the digestion of protein, it is important to point out that food is not our only source of this nutrient; our own bodies provide a substantial amount of protein for internal recycling every day. Both digestive juices and the cells that line the digestive tract (which are sloughed off and replaced every couple of days) contain proteins that are digested and absorbed along with the proteins from food. Some experts estimate that up to 70 grams of protein per day are made available from these sources, compared with 100 grams of protein per day provided by the average American diet (Munro and Crim, 1988). Others estimate that digestive juices and cells sloughed off the lining of the gastrointestinal (GI) tract contribute as much protein as the diet does (Ganong, 1991).

Digestion, Absorption, and Transport of Dietary Proteins

After food is chewed and swallowed, the proteins meet their first chemical challenge in the stomach. Here, hydrochloric acid begins taking apart the large protein molecules. The first step in unfolding the protein structure is

TABLE 7.4 Phases of Protein Digestion and Absorption

	Proteins
Mouth	—
Stomach	Unraveling of protein strands by acid; hydrolysis by enzyme pepsin to polypeptides
Small intestine	Hydrolysis of most proteins by pancreatic enzymes (such as trypsin and chymotrypsin) and enzymes from intestinal wall cells to amino acids, dipeptides, tripeptides; absorption
Large intestine	—

called **denaturation.** (Proteins can be denatured outside the body, too, when they are exposed to heat, alcohol, and certain other chemicals.)

denaturation—unfolding of the three-dimensional structure of a protein

In addition, the stomach enzyme pepsin breaks some of the long protein strands into polypeptide units containing many amino acids. We mentioned earlier that pepsin is specially designed to work in the harsh acid climate of the stomach. Most of the body's other enzymes would themselves be digested by stomach acids, but this one finds the acid environment ideal. In fact, if the stomach juices are not acid enough, pepsin cannot function.

Pepsin has its limits, though; it just begins breaking down proteins so that they are more vulnerable to the battery of enzymes they will face in the small intestine. In the small intestine, other **proteases** from the pancreas and intestinal wall cells take up the task of dividing the long, unraveled protein and polypeptide strands into units suitable for absorption. The enzymes succeed in reducing most proteins to tripeptides, dipeptides, and single amino acids. There is evidence that some large polypeptides, and even intact proteins, escape digestion in the healthy GI tract and are able to be absorbed; however, these are thought to represent a minor proportion of proteinaceous substances absorbed (Gardner, 1988).

proteases—protein-digesting enzymes

After absorption, these substances travel via the portal vein to the liver and then are carried into the general circulation. Table 7.4 summarizes the steps of digestion and absorption.

Food Allergies—An Irregularity in the Body's Handling of Proteins?

For many years, food allergies were presumed to be the consequence of a "leaky" gut that allowed large polypeptides or intact proteins to be absorbed and enter the circulation, where they were recognized as antigens. As a consequence, the immune system produced antibodies, and some sort of allergic reaction ensued.

Now, however, scientists know that at least a small amount of intact protein *normally* enters the bloodstream of a healthy person. It is apparent, then, that had the original explanation been adequate, we would all have allergies (Gardner, 1988). From what we currently know, it is likely that genetic predisposition has something to do with food allergies (allergies tend to cluster in families). Environmental factors—such as foods fed during infancy—probably also have an effect.

Allergies can manifest themselves in surprising ways. An allergy may cause symptoms far removed from the GI tract. A person with a food allergy might experience respiratory symptoms (such as asthma or sneezing); skin symptoms (rash, hives); nervous system symptoms (headache, dizziness); cardiovascular symptoms (rapid heartbeat); urinary symptoms (blood in the urine); or GI symptoms (vomiting, diarrhea). Food allergies can be difficult to diagnose, not only because they can take so many forms, but also because the symptoms may take many hours to develop. Some people, however, react to offending foods within a minute or two.

The American Academy of Allergy and Immunology (AAAI) lists the following foods as the most common causes of allergic reactions in the United States: cow's milk, egg white, peanuts, wheat, and soybeans. Shrimp, tomato, codfish, and crab have also been implicated (Thompson, 1986).

Because food allergies are more likely to occur in infants, the best practice is for the mother to breast-feed her baby and to delay introducing the common allergens into her infant's diet. This is an especially wise tactic for an infant born into a family with a history of allergies. If an infant does develop food allergies, though, they usually subside by about the age of 5. However, it is always possible that other types of substances, such as inhaled pollens or dust, may provoke allergic reactions when the child is older.

We have a few final cautions about food allergies. Because food allergies manifest themselves with such a wide variety of symptoms, some people are tempted to ascribe any puzzling adverse physiologic or behavioral symptoms—such as arthritis or mental or emotional distress—to food allergy, without having an adequate scientific basis for such a connection. If such people severely restrict their diets for a long period of time in an attempt to avoid presumed allergens, they may develop nutritional problems if their "allergy diet" ignores basic nutritional needs. Self-diagnosis and dietary self-treatment can also become a serious problem if such people fail to get an accurate diagnosis of their condition, which should be the basis for treatment.

People who suspect they have food allergies are advised to seek out a physician with specialized training in allergy diagnosis and treatment, such as a member of the AAAI.

The AAAI estimates that fewer than 2% of Americans have true food allergies. An additional small proportion of the population has other food intolerances, which produce symptoms similar to allergies but are not caused by invasion of foreign proteins.

You Tell Me

For the last few weeks, a friend of yours has been having headaches for no apparent reason. He tells you he has just read an article in a popular magazine stating that some people get headaches as an allergic response to wheat products and to milk. He tells you he is going to try avoiding these foods to see whether it helps.

Do you agree with his approach? What problems do his plans pose? What would you do if you were in his place?

Food Technology, Proteins, and Protein Derivatives

Now that you are familiar with how your body handles protein, you have the background to understand technologic modifications of protein and the effects they could have.

New and old processes provide us with a whole range of products that Nature never thought of, from processed proteins shaped into entirely new foods to isolated amino acids. And as with technologic modifications of carbohydrates and fats, there are potential advantages and disadvantages to their use.

Processed Proteins

Soybeans are a high-protein food that is processed in many different ways. For example, soy protein can be separated from most of the other soybean components to yield *soy protein isolates.* These can be spun into strands of texturized vegetable protein and then shaped and flavored into *meat analogues* that resemble such foods as hot dogs, veal cutlets, or meatballs. Sometimes the manufacturer improves on the protein quality of these products by adding limiting amino acids.

Soy protein concentrates, another derivative, are also produced by removing some of the nonprotein components of soybeans, but not as many as are removed to make isolates. Soy protein concentrates are used to provide texture and to aid in emulsification, fat absorption, and water absorption.

The practice of modifying soybeans to produce new forms of food is far from new; Asian cultures have done so since antiquity. *Tofu* is a curd product made from water in which soybeans have been soaked; the soy proteins in the water coagulate and are pressed into a cake, resulting in a product with a texture resembling soft cheese. People who use tofu should realize that a large serving—6 ounces—is needed to provide as much protein as a 2-ounce serving of meat. *Miso,* an Asian soybean paste that is used as a flavoring ingredient or condiment, also contains soy protein. However, miso does not usually contribute much protein to the day's diet, because only small amounts are likely to be used.

Fish is another high-protein food that can be remodeled into new forms. There has been recent commercial interest in an ancient Japanese practice, the production of *surimi,* a slurry made from minced fresh fish. The fish is first washed to remove the fishy taste and then seasoned, flavored, and shaped into look-alikes of lobster, shrimp, or other seafood (Martin, 1988).

Another commercially isolated protein is *casein,* a cow's milk protein. Casein or its derivative, *sodium caseinate,* is used as an ingredient in foods such as frozen dessert toppings and coffee whiteners. *Hydrolyzed vegetable protein* is used as a flavoring component. Figure 7.8 shows some examples of proteins or their derivatives as found in processed foods.

Processed Amino Acids

Food technologists are also able to isolate individual amino acids and combine them to produce dipeptides. The use of these products, however, has met with varying degrees of success. Some amino acids have been added selectively to grain products to enhance their protein quality. The intention was to improve the protein quality in diets of people in developing countries, especially those whose diets are based on one staple grain product. Although this application may seem to have merit, in practice it didn't help much, because the major problem in these countries was an *overall shortage of food.* If sufficient food to supply the energy needed for growth and activity had been available, enough protein would have been present, too. Because the kcalorie intake of these people was inadequate, much of the protein in their diets was metabolized for energy.

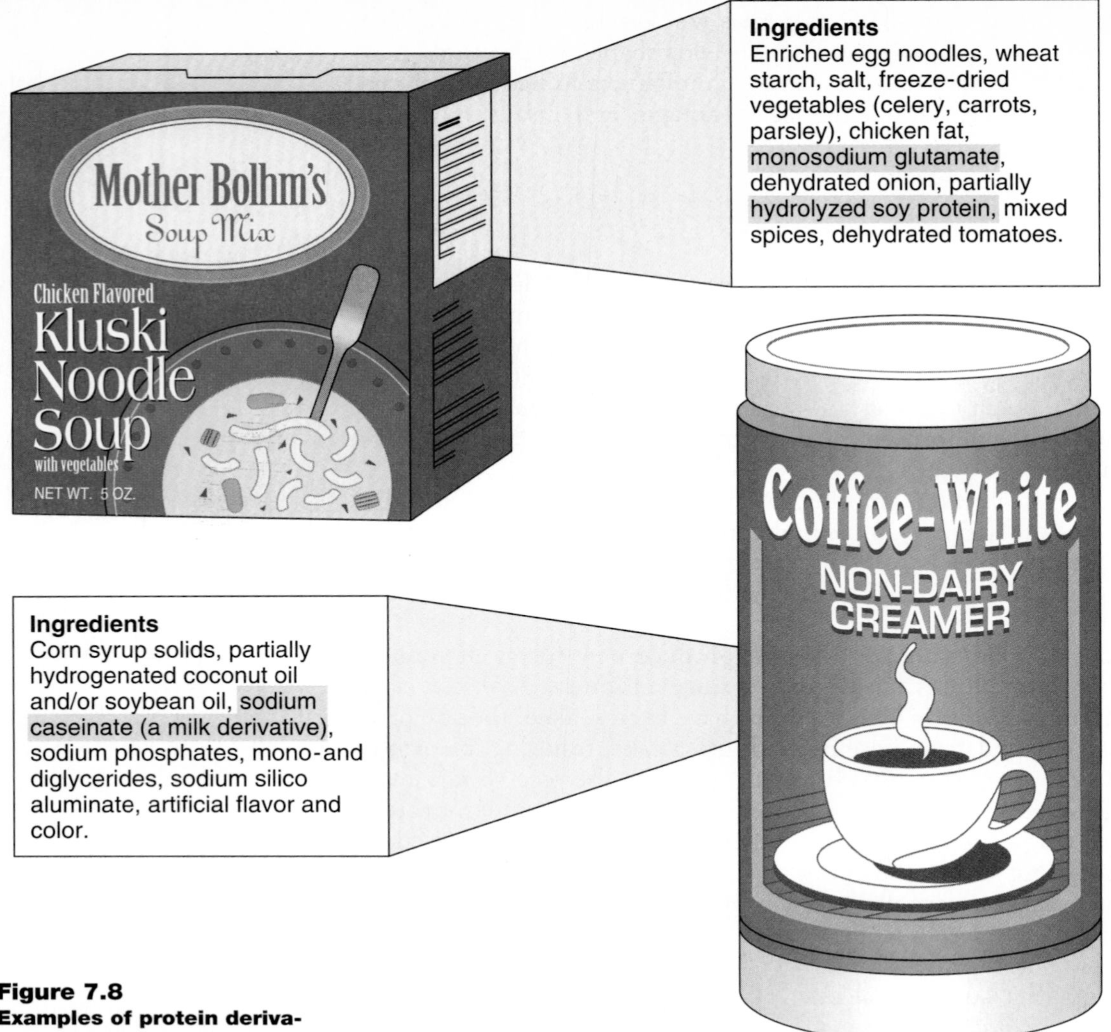

Figure 7.8
Examples of protein derivatives in processed foods.

Monosodium Glutamate (MSG) An amino acid derivative that has been in widespread use for decades is *monosodium glutamate (MSG).* MSG is made from *glutamic acid,* mentioned earlier as a neurotransmitter. MSG, which has been available for decades as the flavor enhancer Accent®, is present in many commercially prepared foods and can be purchased for home use. There has been some question about whether the amounts added to foods might be sufficiently high to approach toxicity in some people, especially young children.

This question was first raised more than 20 years ago, when a researcher demonstrated that a single dose of MSG given orally by itself to rats or monkeys caused damage in one region of the brain, most notably in infant animals. Concerned that the same effects might occur in human babies, he crusaded to have the Food and Drug Administration (FDA) take action preventing the use of MSG. The FDA, armed with test results showing that MSG given to animals *with food* (which dilutes the MSG) does not have the same effect, refused to ban MSG from the food supply—but the baby food industry voluntarily removed the additive. The debate continues today because MSG is present in relatively large amounts in a few products that might be fed to young children, such as instant soups. Other neuroscientists share some concern on this issue, recognizing that when present *in excess,* this neurotransmitter "can actually stimulate nerve cells until they die." However, the exact amount of glutamate or the conditions of use that would cause this to happen in humans have not been determined (Barinaga, 1990).

That has not been the full extent of MSG's troubles: MSG also has been implicated (but not proved to be at fault) in a condition called *Chinese restaurant syndrome (CRS).* CRS is the name given a group of symptoms experienced by a few people when they ingest Chinese or other food that contains large amounts of MSG. For several hours after eating the offending food(s), these people complain of some or all of the following: severe tightness in the chest, asthma, sensations of warmth and tingling, stiffness and/or weakness of the limbs, headache, lightheadedness, heartburn, and gastric discomfort. Although the symptoms of CRS are not life-threatening, they can be unpleasant—and frightening—if mistaken for more serious problems.

Although a considerable amount of circumstantial evidence has been accumulated against MSG in regard to this condition, other studies refute it. For example, in one study six people who claimed to have CRS were given different beverages on two occasions. One beverage contained MSG, the other salt. Four people had *no reaction to either drink,* whereas the other two reacted to *both.* Apparently, then, it takes more than MSG to trigger this syndrome, but it is possible that MSG acts in concert with something else (Kenney, 1986).

In 1992, the Institute of Food Technologists (IFT) issued a scientific perspective on MSG. Although they identified it as "an important flavor enhancer" that is "safe for the vast majority of people" (IFT, Office of Scientific Public Affairs, 1992), they acknowledge that some people may have adverse reactions to it. They advise that if you think you might be sensitive, you should have your physician perform a double-blind test.

To help sensitive people avoid MSG, the FDA requires that food products containing MSG be so labeled. Soon, new labeling regulations may require that MSG be identified when it is a component of other ingredients, such as hydrolyzed vegetable protein.

Aspartame Another use of amino acids involves the dipeptide **aspartame,** which is marketed as a sugar substitute under the names *Nutrasweet®* and *Equal®*. It was accidentally discovered to be a sweet compound when scientists were synthesizing a product for ulcer therapy late in 1965.

aspartame—a sweet dipeptide composed of phenylalanine and aspartic acid; used as a low-kcalorie sweetener

You Tell Me

Aspartame is a dipeptide that is 200 times as sweet as sugar. Composed of the amino acids phenylalanine and aspartic acid, aspartame has the same kcaloric value as protein—4 kcalories per gram—which is also the kcaloric value of sugar.

If aspartame has the same number of kcalories per gram as sugar, what is the advantage in substituting it for sugar? How can its use reduce the kcaloric value of foods?

Aspartame is used in the United States as a tabletop sweetener and in soft drinks, dry beverage mixes, cocoa, instant coffees and teas, milk and shake mixes, cereals, chewing gum, puddings, fillings, gelatin mixes, yogurt, fruit juice beverages, and more. The amino acids in aspartame occur normally in proteins we consume every day: a 4-ounce hamburger has about 12 times more phenylalanine than a can of aspartame-sweetened soda. Despite its natural occurrence in foods, it was necessary to test carefully whether aspartame might have negative effects, based on the concern mentioned earlier that purified amino acids (or in this case, the products of the breakdown of a dipeptide) might cause unwanted effects.

Aspartame was approved in 1981 by the FDA for use up to a level established as the *acceptable daily intake (ADI).* Later, the American Medical Association (AMA) and the Centers for Disease Control (CDC) stated they also thought it was safe. According to the FDA, if aspartame were to replace all the sugar and saccharin (an unrelated artificial sweetener) in the diet, the highest consumption would be far below any level even suspected of causing negative effects (IFT, 1986). A subsequent test with six normal adults who drank the equivalent of two (12-ounce) cans of aspartame-sweetened beverage every hour for 8 hours had no significant effect on blood plasma levels of aspartame or its metabolites (Stegink et al., 1989).

Some experts are more concerned about possible effects on children. The number of aspartame-sweetened beverages and other products that children could consume before they would reach the ADI for their body size has been calculated: for a 6-year-old, the number is 4 beverages and 7 other products, and for an 11-year-old, it is 8 beverages and 10 other products (Thomas-Doberson, 1989). Unfortunately, experts fear that some children in the United States consume close to or more than the ADI for aspartame.

Some adults claim to have experienced problems such as dizziness, panic attacks, hives, swelling of throat tissue, gastrointestinal symptoms, migraines, seizures, and eye damage from aspartame. In response to these claims, the National Institute of Allergy and Infectious Diseases in Bethesda, Maryland, conducted a study. They located people in the area who thought they were aspartame-sensitive to verify whether aspartame was, in fact, the cause of their symptoms. Of the 61 people who were sent by their physicians or came in on their own over a 32-month period, none had reproducible reactions from an aspartame challenge (Garriga et al., 1991). The FDA did a different study, but came to similar conclusions. In evaluating 251 reports of seizures that consumers believed were linked to ingestion of aspartame, FDA staff decided that their analyses did "not indicate any unusual or significant association . . ." (Tollefson and Barnard, 1992).

FIGURE 7.9
Nutrasweet® (aspartame) is not for everybody.

Products containing Nutrasweet are required to carry labels warning people who have phenylketonuria (PKU) not to use the product. In this rare inborn error of metabolism, the body cannot metabolize phenylalanine, one of the components of aspartame.

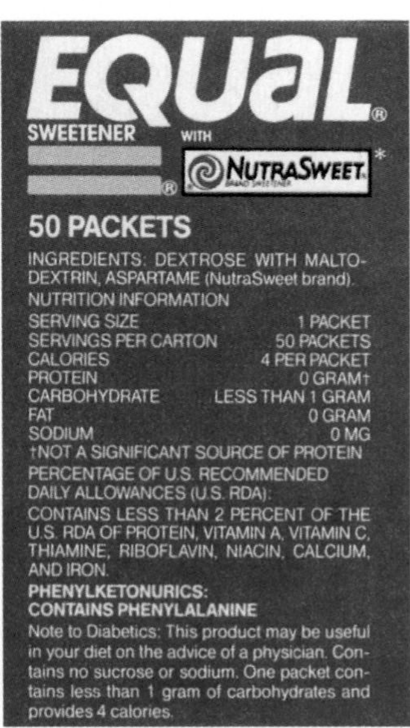

Because these studies have not identified problems from aspartame use, aspartame continues to be widely used in the U.S. food supply. If you want to use it, apply the same guideline for intake as you should for any food component: use it in *moderate* amounts as part of a varied diet.

There is one small group of people who definitely should avoid aspartame, though: people with *phenylketonuria (PKU),* an inborn error of metabolism that results in brain damage if too much phenylalanine is consumed. It is for the benefit of these people (who are usually diagnosed at birth) that all products containing aspartame must be so labeled (Figure 7.9).

Other Amino Acid Products Although MSG and aspartame have been the major amino acid products used in the food supply, many others have appeared on the market. Some formulas designed for weight loss have consisted of amino acids, vitamins, and minerals; Chapter 9 (on body fatness) will deal with the inadvisability of using such products. Products containing amino acids have also been marketed as supplements for athletes. They are discussed in the Thinking for Yourself on page 236.

Amino acids are also sold individually, and most are readily available over the counter. The FDA has classified amino acids as dietary supplements because they are naturally occurring components of food, but that classification may change. Most people who take amino acids do not need them to meet their recommended intake for protein; rather, they are using them—sometimes in very high doses—as drugs. That can be dangerous, because large amounts of individual amino acids that are taken by themselves (not with foods) can act in the body very differently from amino acids that are consumed as part of food.

Animal studies have shown that taking disproportionate amounts of amino acids interferes with growth. This could be due to either direct toxic effects or interference with the function of other amino acids (Munro and Crim, 1988). Animal studies are limited in their application to humans, in part because of species differences and in part because many of the claims made for amino acids relate to how people *feel* rather than to measurable physical effects.

The other source of information about the use of individual amino acids is case reports of human toxicity. Unfortunately, these are only occasionally published. It would be helpful if more were reported so that people could be alerted to the effects of overdoses and the levels of intake at which they occurred. Only people who go to the doctor's office with their problem may become part of the medical literature—provided that the doctor writes up the case study, submits it, and it is published. A cluster of occurrences late in 1989 had important public health implications and the reports about them therefore were widely disseminated in the media. The problem involved supplements of the essential amino acid tryptophan, which have consequently been recalled; it is discussed in the Slice of Life on page 226.

Considering the serious lack of information about the effects of taking purified amino acids, the National Research Council (1989) advises against their use. If you take them, you are experimenting on yourself. If you are taking amino acids—or any other nutritional supplement, for that matter—and experience a health problem, be sure to report your use of the product to your health care professional.

Problems from Too Little or Too Much Protein

As you have very likely recognized, one of the themes of this book is that it is important to get enough of the essential nutrients, but not too much. For every class of nutrients, problems can occur with either underconsumption or overconsumption. Proteins are no exception.

Shortage of Protein

Although we have said that in our society it is usually quite easy to get enough protein, there are places in the world where the common foods are very low in protein or where there is simply not enough food of any kind. In either of these circumstances, concern about inadequate protein is legitimate and very serious.

"Pure" Protein Deficiency Protein deficiency by itself—that is, without accompanying *energy* deficiency—is a rare phenomenon. Protein deficiency is seen in its pure form in just a few places in the world, where the food choice is extremely limited and the staple food is extremely low in protein.

Cassava (a starchy root) and yams are foods that by weight have only about one-third of the protein provided by grains. A study done in Nige-

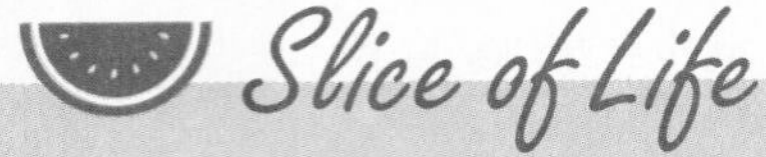

The Tryptophan Mystery

During the bright New Mexico summer, Carol (not her real name) had been sailboarding and winning tennis tournaments. Then she began to experience pain—first in her temples and jaws, then spreading throughout her body until she was completely incapacitated (Steinbrook, 1989).

For several months, her case had doctors completely baffled. Despite extensive testing, there were few clues leading to the cause of her problem. The only abnormal finding was that she had a very high count of *eosinophils,* a type of white blood cell that is usually elevated when a parasitic disease or tumor is present, but she had neither.

While Carol lay in the hospital that fall, three similar cases developed in the area; within 2 more weeks 30 cases had been identified, some outside New Mexico. Physicians, consultants, and public health officials kept in close contact by phone. One of the doctors who had worked with Carol noticed an odd similarity between the histories of the patients: all had been taking the amino acid *tryptophan* before they became ill. Although correlational data do not prove causation, the observation was compelling. The physicians notified federal authorities; in mid-November 1989, the FDA warned the public to stop using tryptophan and asked manufacturers to recall tryptophan supplements and other products in which it was a major ingredient.

Far from being the end of either the problem or the mystery, this was just the beginning. By May 1992 there were 1511 reported cases with 38 deaths among them (Roufs, 1992). In the interim, the condition had acquired a name: *eosinophilia-myalgia syndrome,* referring to the elevated levels of eosinophils in the blood, and the muscle pain that was the principal symptom of the illness. Other symptoms included weakness, fever, joint pain, shortness of breath, rash, and inflammation of the lungs.

But why tryptophan? Why should this amino acid, which had been taken by some people for several years without apparent consequence, be associated with a relatively sudden outbreak of serious—even life-threatening—problems?

One possibility that had to be considered was that tryptophan, in the amounts that were being consumed, might be toxic. However, most people in the United States ordinarily consume between 1 and 5 grams of tryptophan per day as a component of their usual diet, and the patients with eosinophilia-myalgia syndrome had consumed an average of 1.2 grams of purified tryptophan from supplements (with a few as high as 17 grams per day). From a comparison of the average supplemental intakes with the average dietary intakes, toxicity seemed an unlikely explanation. It was still under consideration, however, because consuming an individual amino acid with water gives a different response than consuming the same substance in food. The presence of other amino acids and other compounds in food affects the absorption and utilization of an amino acid.

Another point of consideration was the possibility that some people's bodies are more sensitive to the amino acid in its pure form than others are. Because this product had been available for many years over the counter, however, it would seem that some people would have developed the problem before this latest series of cases.

Others noted that there is a variant of the tryptophan molecule that is known to cause eosinophilia. It is possible that some of this "off-form" developed in the product during processing, shipping, or storage, or it is possible that a highly toxic contaminant found its way into the tryptophan.

The front-running hypothesis is that a contaminant in certain brands of purified tryptophan was responsible (Belongia et al., 1992). Even several years later, the mystery has yet to be solved definitively—if it ever will be. As an additional safeguard, in late March 1990 the FDA expanded its recall to *all products to which tryptophan had been added,* even those including very small dosages. Even so, one expert believes this does not go far enough: he thinks that all amino acid supplements should be removed from the U.S. market (Herbert, 1992).

ria, where these foods are staples, found that only 5–8% of the kcalories in people's diets came from protein (Worthington-Roberts, 1981). Protein deficiency manifested itself in low weight gains during pregnancy, low maternal milk production, high infant mortality (40% in the first 5 years), extremely low weights and heights in children, poor intelligence scores for children, and increased susceptibility to infections.

Protein–Energy Malnutrition (PEM) It is much more common to find long-term protein deficiency associated with severe underconsumption of

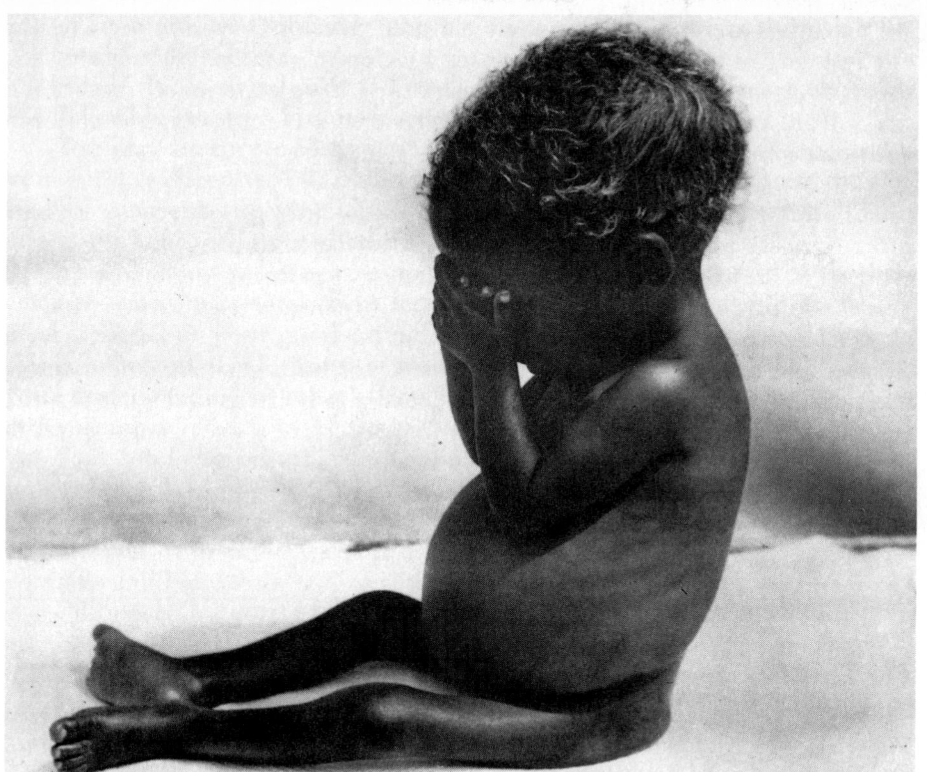

Figure 7.10
A child with kwashiorkor.

Although this child may not appear malnourished to the casual observer, she is. The swelling caused by the fluid in her tissues camouflages her protein–energy malnutrition. The other signs are more obvious—her dark hair has turned reddish, she has a skin condition, and she is feeling miserable.

other energy-producing foods. This condition, called **protein–energy malnutrition (PEM),** is a fairly widespread disorder in the developing countries. Usually, the problem is that the people simply do not have enough food. PEM would be relieved if these people had access to more of what their diet already contained.

protein-energy malnutrition (PEM)—long-term protein deficiency associated with severe energy deficiency; fairly widespread in the less developed countries

PEM affects young children more than others, because their need for protein and other nutrients is greater per unit of body weight. PEM manifests itself in a variety of ways. Two severe conditions are marasmus and kwashiorkor.

Marasmus is a condition in which a person becomes thinner and thinner from a progressive loss of fat and muscle tissue. People with marasmus are extremely weak and listless and have decreased resistance to infection. Many pictures of the people of Somalia, prominent in the media beginning late in 1992, show people with marasmus. **Kwashiorkor** produces quite different physical symptoms; the body becomes swollen with fluid because there is less protein than is normal in the blood, so fluid from the bloodstream migrates into the tissues, causing edema. Sometimes the edema makes the person look healthfully chubby, but other signs quickly disprove this image: dark hair has become red, a dermatitis (skin condition) has developed, and the person obviously feels miserable. Once again, resistance to infection is reduced. Liver damage is characteristic. A child with kwashiorkor is pictured in Figure 7.10.

marasmus—a serious form of PEM characterized by progressive fat and muscle loss

kwashiorkor—a serious form of PEM in which liver damage results and fluid shifts create a swollen appearance

Although kwashiorkor originally was thought to result from protein deficiency alone, more recent thinking is that it also involves inadequate energy intake. PEM experts Benjamin Torun and Fernando Viteri state, "The concept that marasmus or kwashiorkor is the end result of either severe energy or protein deficiency is too simplistic" (1988).

Scientists aren't sure why some children develop kwashiorkor whereas others living in the same circumstances develop marasmus. Perhaps the reason is that many children with kwashiorkor have experienced additional stress from certain infections and parasites that have not plagued children with marasmus.

Susceptibility to Infection In its most severe forms, inadequate dietary protein, as we have said, results in poorer resistance to infection. However, even in milder dietary inadequacies of energy and/or protein, the body's defenses for dealing with invading microorganisms are weaker and/or slower to respond (Myrvik, 1988).

Because infection raises the body's need for both kcalories and protein, it creates an even wider gap between what the body needs and what the diet supplies. For this reason, PEM and infection create a downward spiral in the health of many people in developing countries. Diseases such as measles, which would run a short course in well-nourished populations, become killers among the poorly nourished.

You Tell Me

Mild cases of protein–energy malnutrition (PEM) also occur in people in developed countries, such as the United States. Some people seriously shortchange themselves on kcalories and/or protein because of disease, medication, or deliberate attempts to maintain an unrealistically low body weight. And some people who drink lots of alcohol but who don't want to develop a "beer belly" severely restrict their intake of all other kcalorie and protein sources.

In terms of resistance to disease, what are the likely consequences of any of these actions?

Fatty Liver If a person's liver has inadequate access to protein due to long-term dietary deficiency, fats can accumulate there. (Recall from Chapter 6 [on lipids] that the body needs protein to create lipoproteins, the form in which lipids are transported in the body.) Protein deficiency can also occur among alcoholics in the developed countries if their intake of alcohol replaces a large part of their food intake. However, in alcoholics, the development of fatty liver is also influenced by the fact that alcohol is toxic to the liver, and in alcoholics this damage allows fat to be deposited (Shaw and Lieber, 1988).

Excess of Protein

Americans often consume more than twice the recommended amount of protein, so now let's consider what the consequences of such overindulgence might be.

Excess Kcalories and/or Fat As with any of the macronutrients, an excess of protein can result in the creation of *additional body fat,* if total kcalories consumed exceed the kcalories needed.

Furthermore, many commonly consumed high-protein foods are also high in fat. If your intake of high-protein/high-fat foods is high, the total

TABLE 7.5 Fat Levels That Accompany 7–8 Grams of Protein in Various Kinds of Foods

Food	Protein (grams)	Fat (grams)
Milk and milk products		
Skim milk	8	0
Cheddar cheese	7	9
Animal protein sources		
Haddock, broiled	7	2
Beef ribeye	7	13
Plant protein sources		
Lentils	8	0
Peanuts	8	15

fat content of your diet will be high, making you a candidate for the problems associated with high fat intake. However, you can obviously be deliberate about choosing the lower-fat/high-protein foods. Table 7.5 provides examples of options within dairy, flesh (meat, poultry, fish) protein, and plant protein foods. For a more comprehensive picture of which high-protein foods are high or low in fat, refer back to the Food Guide Pyramid sections on milk products and meats and meat alternatives.

Dehydration If your diet includes too much protein, dehydration is another possible problem. When you consume very high levels of protein, your body dismantles the amino acid surplus. The separated amino groups are metabolized into urea, which is excreted in your urine. These processes demand more work of your liver and kidneys.

Your body needs a sizable volume of water to excrete urea in the urine. To metabolize 100 kcalories of protein, the body uses 350 grams of water, but only 50 grams to metabolize 100 kcalories of carbohydrate or fat (Worthington-Roberts, 1981). So if you consume a great deal of protein but do not also consume a lot of water, dehydration is a possibility. This is why high-protein weight-reduction diets often recommend consuming large volumes of water. It also explains why athletes consuming high-protein diets are in double jeopardy of dehydration, because of both urinary losses and perspiration.

Calcium Loss Some studies show that people who consume protein at levels at least twice as high as the amount recommended by the RDA excrete more calcium in the urine than normal. This may lead to a net loss of calcium from the body if a person consumes less than the RDA for calcium.

In theory, this means that the person who eats a lot of meat but avoids the recommended number of servings of dairy products per day might be slowly but steadily losing bone calcium. It in turn suggests that high protein intakes could contribute to the development of **osteoporosis,** a condition in which gradual loss of bone mass causes weakening of bone and risk of fracture. Surprisingly, though, epidemiologic data do not support that theory. Certainly, it's a complicated issue: many other factors, such as level of dietary phosphorus, gender, age, and activity level can also affect this situation. Chapter 12 (on minerals) discusses this more thoroughly.

osteoporosis—condition in which bone mass decreases, thereby weakening the bone

How Much Protein Do You Need?

Because protein has so many important functions, you surely don't want to shortchange yourself, but you will probably be surprised at how easy it is to get what you need. Generally, your needs will be covered if you eat enough food to match your energy expenditure. People who restrict their energy intake, though, often come up short on protein.

How Scientists Determine Protein Needs

How do scientists know how much protein a healthy adult needs? In essence, they have measured the amount of protein that the body loses in a day's time to find out how much should be replaced. The major losses occur via the urine. Urinary nitrogen is measured, and because protein is 16% nitrogen, it is possible to calculate from this value how much protein has been discarded. Much smaller amounts of protein are lost in the feces, sweat, skin, hair, and nails; collection and analysis of these amounts present their own challenges.

But it is not enough to measure the body's losses; intake of dietary protein is another important part of the equation. Some of the urinary nitrogen may come from excess protein that was in the diet. If a person has eaten more protein than his or her body needs for replacement of worn tissues, the unneeded amino acids are either metabolized for energy or are converted to fat and stored. In either case, the nitrogen from the surplus is excreted in the urine along with whatever nitrogen from worn internal tissues was not recycled.

nitrogen balance study—biochemical test that determines whether protein is being lost, gained, or simply maintained; involves comparing nitrogen intake with loss of nitrogen from all body routes combined

Protein needs, then, are determined using **nitrogen balance studies** that measure both intake and output of nitrogen. If output and intake are equal, the person is said to be *in balance.* If output is greater than intake, the person is losing protein, or is in *negative balance;* this occurs with injury, surgery, illness, and starvation. If intake is greater than output, the body is creating new protein and is in *positive balance;* this occurs during growth, pregnancy, lactation, healing, and muscle building.

Thousands of studies about protein metabolism have shown that people's protein needs vary slightly from one individual to another. This is consistent with the generalization we made in Chapter 1 about people's unique needs for levels of nutrients. The studies also show that there is a strong relationship between the need for protein and the need for kcalories: a person who is losing weight needs more protein to stay in balance than a person who is maintaining body weight (Munro and Crim, 1988), because some of the protein is used for energy.

When experts considered recommendations for the RDA for protein, they took into account as many of these factors as they could. To allow for individual variation, they included a generous margin in the recommendation. They also added a margin to allow for the fact that people's diets are made up of proteins of varying quality. The recommendations do assume, though, that the proteins will come from both animal and plant sources. However, be aware that the protein RDAs are not adequate for a person who is losing weight rapidly or who is ill. During illness and after surgery or serious accidental injury, the appropriate recommendation for protein could be double or more the amount recommended for the healthy person, depending on the nature of the illness and/or the extent of the surgery or injury (Munro and Crim, 1988).

Recommended Protein Intakes for the Healthy Adult

The RDA subcommittee advocates that you calculate your recommended daily protein intake based on body weight. (If you are substantially overweight or underweight at the moment, use your ideal body weight in the calculation; your protein needs are based primarily on lean body tissue and do not change much when your body contains different amounts of fat.) First, convert your weight to kilograms; then multiply it by 0.8 gram per kilogram to get the recommended daily intake. Note that this corresponds to the figures in the RDA table: 58 grams of protein per day for the 72-kilogram man and 46 grams for the 58-kilogram woman.

People who are developing new tissue need more dietary protein. According to the 1989 RDA, the pregnant woman should consume 60 grams each day during pregnancy. During the first 6 months of lactation, she should consume 65 grams per day and thereafter 62 grams per day.

Children's needs vary according to their ages; in the first 6 months after birth, they should take in 2.2 grams of protein per kilogram of body weight. As they get older, the recommendation per unit of body weight gradually decreases until it gets to the adult level of 0.8 gram per kilogram.

Act on Fact 7.1 on page 232 outlines a method for determining the protein intake that is adequate for you.

Recommended Protein Intakes for Athletes

Do athletes need more protein? For many centuries, it was believed that protein was the major fuel required by muscle and, therefore, that a high-protein diet would help a person excel at physical activity. For this reason, some of the original Olympic contenders ate meals primarily of high-protein foods, such as meat, milk, and eggs (Hickson and Wolinsky, 1989).

In 1866, however, two German scientists published the results of experiments proving that protein was *not* the preferred energy source for the working muscle. Many studies have reinforced those early findings. Fat and carbohydrate are undeniably the major energy sources for both athletes and nonathletes.

Nutrition scientists and exercise physiologists in recent years have learned that during strenuous athletic activity, protein may contribute up to 15% of energy (Goodman, 1988), especially when carbohydrate intake is low and/or exercise is prolonged (that is, over 2 hours). In fact, after such a bout of exercise, the body synthesizes more protein. These factors suggest that the serious adult athlete might benefit from more than the 0.8 gram per kilogram recommended for the average adult.

How much is the right amount? There is considerable disagreement on this point. Opinions range all the way from scientists who insist that 0.8 g/kg is adequate for the athlete (they remind us that the RDA has a built-in safety factor) to a few who promote as much as 3 g/kg.

There are many reasons for such disparities. To begin with, some of the studies that people hold up as proof of protein needs lack proper controls. Also, exercise physiologists have learned that protein and amino acid metabolism is affected by the nature and duration of the activity being done (Goodman, 1988). For example, the protein needs of a runner and a weight lifter may be different. Because the vast majority of studies on protein needs during exercise have dealt with endurance activity, such as bicycling or running, these results may not be on target for other kinds of activities.

Determining Protein Intake Adequacy

To find out how your protein intake compares with your needs, follow the steps below.

Calculation of Recommended Daily Intake

1. Convert ideal body weight from pounds to kilograms, using as an example an adult (nonathlete) whose ideal weight is 165 pounds:

$$\text{Body weight in kilograms} = \frac{\text{ideal body weight (lb)}}{2.2\ \text{lb/kg}} = \frac{165\ \text{lb}}{2.2\ \text{lb/kg}} = 75\ \text{kg}$$

2. Circle the basic standard (and extra need) that applies to you:

   Basic standards

Older teen (nonathlete)	0.9 g/kg body weight
Adult (nonathlete)	(0.8 g/kg body weight)
Older teen (athlete)	1.0–1.8 g/kg body weight
Adult (athlete)	1.0–1.6 g/kg body weight

   Extra needs

Pregnant	Add 10 grams to prepregnant recommendation.
Lactating	Add 15 grams to prepregnant recommendation for first six months and 12 grams thereafter.

3. Calculate the amount of protein recommended for you:

$$\begin{aligned}\text{Recommended daily protein intake} &= \left(\text{body weight in kg} \times \text{basic standard}\right) + \text{extra need} \\ &= (75\ \text{kg} \times 0.8\ \text{g/kg}) + 0\ \text{g} \\ &= 60\ \text{g of protein}\end{aligned}$$

Determination of Actual Intake for One Day

1. Keep a record of your intake for 24 hours, as shown in Sample Act on Fact 7.1.
2. Using Appendix C and information from food labels, determine the amount of protein in each item consumed, and enter values on the record.
3. Total the protein column.

Comparison of Recommendation with Intake

1. Calculate what percentage of your recommended intake you actually consumed, using the following formula:

$$\begin{aligned}\text{Percentage of recommendation} &= (\text{intake} \div \text{recommendation}) \times 100 \\ &= (104 \div 60) \times 100 \\ &= 173\%\end{aligned}$$

2. Compare the percent you calculated with guidelines that suggest too little or too much: if your intake is less than 70% or more than 200% of your recommendation (and this is typical for you), you run the health risks described in this chapter.

Food or Beverage	Amount	Protein (grams)
Orange juice	1 cup	2
Scrambled eggs	2 large	14
Bagel	1	6
Margarine	1 T.	tr.
Jelly	1 T.	0
Chili con carne	1 cup	19
Crackers, sesame and wheat	4 squares	1
Sandwich:		
White enriched bread	2 slices	4
Turkey	2 oz.	13
Mayonnaise	2 T.	tr.
Milk, 2%	1 cup	9
Sloppy Joe sandwich		
Bun	1	4
Ground beef	2 oz.	14
Tomato sauce	2 T.	tr.
Green beans	½ cup	2
Mashed potatoes	½ cup	2
Milk, 2%	1 cup	9
Ice milk	1 cup	5
TOTAL		104

Sample Act on Fact 7.1

Determining your protein intake adequacy for one day.

Another issue concerns the selection of subjects for experiments. Exercise physiologists know that when people who are not accustomed to much physical activity start an aerobic training program, they metabolize an increased amount of protein for energy. This causes some body protein to be lost initially, but after a couple of weeks on the program, their metabolism adapts, preventing further losses over time (Hickson and Wolinsky, 1989). The apparent short-term "needs" of people who are unaccustomed to exercise, then, are not representative of the ongoing needs of the regular athlete. At the other end of the activity spectrum, ultraendurance athletes may have somewhat greater needs than endurance athletes with less extreme goals.

The timing of data collection can be important as well. As we mentioned above, *during* endurance exercise, some protein is broken down and used for energy production, but in the hours *after* a bout of exercise, the body gradually begins to synthesize protein. Therefore, the time at which body substances, such as blood or muscle tissue samples, are taken makes a great deal of difference: if you take samples in the midst of an exercise session, you might conclude that activity has a destructive effect, whereas if you take them later, it may seem that exercise promotes formation of protein. It is important not to draw conclusions about overall protein nutrition based on one brief glimpse of protein metabolism at an isolated moment.

Another problem in doing these studies has to do with how the breakdown of body protein is measured. If researchers want to know whether body protein is being lost, they might look for a biochemical "marker" as evidence of muscle tissue destruction. One marker that has been used in many studies, a substance called *3-methylhistidine,* is not a perfect marker for skeletal muscle breakdown (Goodman, 1988). Therefore, there is room for disagreement about the recommendations that come from studies centered around 3-methylhistidine measures.

Other studies of protein utilization during exercise have been done using nitrogen balance studies, which compare nitrogen intake with nitrogen losses. This type of study is difficult to apply to the athlete, because during physical activity a significant amount of nitrogen is lost in sweat, and those losses are very difficult to collect and measure. To recover nitrogen lost by this route, scientists have to rinse the subject with deionized water (containing no dissolved materials) after exercise, rinse the perspiration from the person's clothes, and then analyze all the rinse water for nitrogen. If such care is not taken to determine all losses accurately, studies of nitrogen balance in athletes misrepresent their protein status and needs.

When you consider all of these factors, you can see why recommendations for protein intake for physical activity have covered such a wide range. But which advice is best?

Although some experts continue to believe that the RDA level of 0.8 g/kg of body weight is sufficient for an athlete to maintain muscle tissue, most investigators have concluded from recent studies that more is better. Some recommend approximately 1 g/kg body weight (Tarnopolsky et al., 1988; Meredith et al., 1989), whereas others recommend up to 1.7 g/kg (Lemon, 1991; Williams, 1992). The International Center for Sports Nutrition endorses the range of 1–1.5 g/kg (1990). These upper values all are around the upper limit set by the 1989 RDA Subcommittee, which recommends that protein intake for anybody—athlete or nonathlete—not be more than double the RDA. That means that adults should not consume more than 1.6 g/kg, and older teens should not exceed 1.8 g/kg.

Is it difficult to achieve these levels? Not at all. If you follow the recommendations of the Food Guide Pyramid, you are likely to be within the

protein intake range for athletes. Table 7.6 reiterates the Pyramid's food group ranges, which yield between 69 and 105 grams of protein, depending on how many servings you choose from each group. Larger and very active athletes should consume the number of servings at the upper end of the ranges (or even more, if their energy needs demand it). Smaller athletes and/or those who need to maintain a lower body weight may find the lower end of the ranges more appropriate.

Do athletes in the real world usually get the amount of protein recommended for them? Because athletes vary so much in what they eat, let's look at three patterns that occur. First, many athletes simply select a good, varied diet as described above. If they consume adequate kcalories to maintain normal weight, they get the protein they need automatically.

A second group of athletes, though, may not get enough protein. Those who are restricting kcalories to achieve or maintain a lower body weight for their sport, such as gymnasts and runners, are at greatest risk in this regard. Other athletes, especially endurance athletes, may take in too little protein because they are so focused on getting enough carbohydrate that they largely eliminate the better sources of protein from their diets (Clark, 1990; Applegate, 1991). If carbohydrate replaces necessary levels of other nutrients, both performance and health will suffer.

Finally, there are those athletes who believe that the more protein they consume, the better off they will be. Some take protein supplements in addition to eating high-protein foods (Figure 7.11). If this practice tempts you, the Thinking for Yourself on page 236 can help you decide whether this is in your best interest. ●

if YOU ARE-
TIRED,
FLABBY,
WEAK?
PROTEIN
WILL
STRENGTHEN
YOU THRU THE WEEK
BREAD,
LIFE!

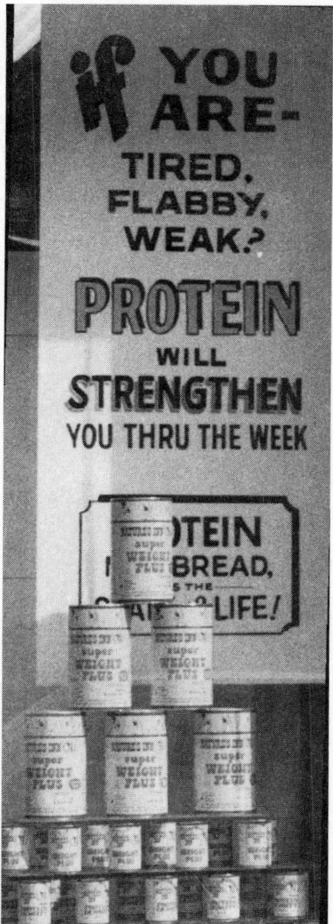

Figure 7.11
Promises that can't be kept.

Protein or amino acid powders are often marketed for muscle building. They are neither necessary nor effective; only a regular, graduated body building program can add muscle mass within genetic limits.

TABLE 7.6 Food Guide for an Athlete

The Pyramid provides plenty of protein . . . even for most young adult athletes. The recommendations of the Food Guide Pyramid are shown below with a sample day's menu. If this is not enough food to meet your energy needs, then eat more, especially from the grain, vegetable, and fruit groups. Eating more will also provide more protein.

Summary of Recommendations	Est. Protein per Serving (grams)	Approx. Total (grams)
Bread, rice, cereal, pasta: 6–11	2	12–22
Vegetables: 3–5	2	6–10
Fruits: 2–4	0	0
Milk, yogurt, cheese: 3 servings through age 24; after that, 2 servings per day	8	16–24
Meat, poultry, fish, beans, eggs, nuts: equivalent to 5–7 ounces of meat	7 per oz.-equiv.	35–49
Total		69–105

Sample Day's Menu

Breakfast

½ cup orange juice
1 oz. breakfast cereal
1 cup 2% milk
1 slice whole wheat toast with butter and jelly

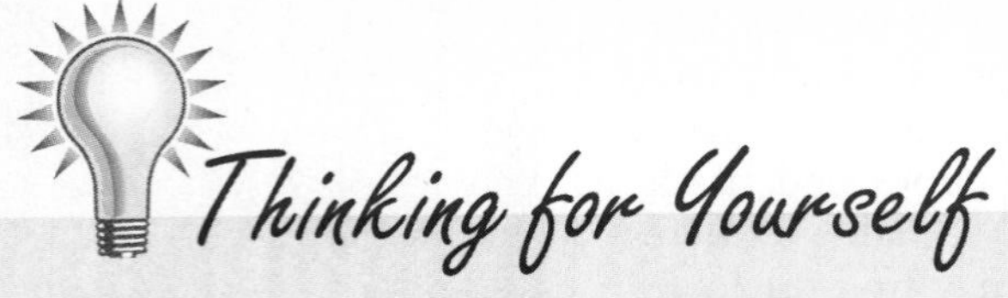

Are Protein Supplements Helpful to an Athlete?

The Situation

You've always been an active person. You use your bicycle for transportation much of the time, and almost every day you participate in some sort of sports activity. Last month, you joined a soccer team that plays two games per week, and recently you've become interested in weight lifting. You've decided you'd really like to excel at these two activities.

Some of the soccer players and weight lifters you've met are very interested in nutrition. Several of them take different types of protein supplements; they are convinced the supplements help their performance, and they're encouraging you to try them. A couple of people have showed you the products they use. One of the packages suggests a daily protein intake of 2 grams of protein per kilogram of body weight; another supplement label recommends 3–3.5 grams of protein per kilogram of body weight. You wonder whether you should give these products a try.

Is the Information Accurate and Relevant?

- Most experts in protein research recommend protein intakes of 1.0–1.6 g/kg for the adult; for the older teenager, the recommended range is 1.0–1.8 g/kg. More is not better; in fact, the 1989 RDA advises against anybody going above these ranges (see text).
- Research has shown no additional beneficial effects on strength, power, enlargement of muscle, or physiologic work capacity from taking protein supplements (Williams, 1989), provided the person has eaten an adequate diet.
- Unless an athlete is consuming a low-kcalorie or extremely high carbohydrate diet, it is unlikely that protein intake will be low.
- If a diet is low in protein nonetheless, a protein supplement may make up the deficit.

What Else Needs to Be Considered?

Essentially, there are three types of protein-based supplements marketed for the athlete: whole (intact) protein supplements, mixtures of amino acids, and individual amino acids.

Whole-protein supplements are generally made from proteins of milk or soybeans. When you use these products, you are getting protein without getting other nutrients the original foods contained. This can be an advantage if you need protein and you want to get it for the fewest

TABLE 7.6 *continued*

Lunch	Dinner
Sandwich of:	Mixed entree of:
2 slices bread	1 cup macaroni
2 oz. sliced turkey	3 oz. lean ground beef
lettuce	¾ oz. cheese
low-fat mayonnaise	½ cup tomato sauce
1 carrot	1 slice French bread
2 plums	½ cup green beans
1½ cups milk	½ cup fruit salad
2 oatmeal cookies	
Afternoon Snack	**Evening Snack**
12 crackers	3 cups popcorn
Carbonated beverage	1 cup fruit-flavored drink

This Menu Contains:

Food Servings	Protein (g)
11 Grains	22
3 Vegetables	6
3 Fruit	0
3 Milk	24
5 (oz.) Meat	35
Total	87grams

possible additional kcalories. A disadvantage to using this type of product is that it is often more expensive than the whole food would be.

Mixtures of amino acids are essentially "predigested proteins." They are promoted as being easier to absorb than whole proteins because they are already in the simplest possible form. However, the normally healthy GI tract easily digests and absorbs over 90% of dietary proteins; in fact, protein experts generally believe that the healthy gut *prefers* dealing with whole proteins. It absorbs the variety of protein particles produced by digestion (amino acids, dipeptides, tripeptides, and even some larger polypeptides and whole proteins) better than it absorbs material reduced entirely to amino acids. (The only circumstance in which such products have valid use are when a person's gut is *not functioning normally:* they are sometimes used in hospitals for patients with severe GI disorders.)

The third category of protein supplements is individual amino acids. Some athletes take certain amino acids hoping they will have anabolic (muscle-building) effects; some pseudoscientific publications have suggested that certain amino acids serve as "growth hormone releasers." But early studies demonstrated that adding amino acids above the requirement level did not promote positive nitrogen balance (Hickson and Wolinsky, 1989). No studies have been done to assess the long-term effects of taking high levels of these individual purified amino acids. Therefore, taking them in high doses is like taking untested drugs (see text). For these reasons, the FDA is considering tightening its regulations regarding the sale of individual amino acids and products containing them.

Now What Do You Think?

- *Option 1* You decide to evaluate your current diet for protein by doing Act on Fact 7.1. If your intake is within the range recommended for athletes your age, you will continue to eat as you have been.
- *Option 2* You decide that if your intake of protein is not high enough, you will eat more high-protein foods to bring it into the range scientists recommend.
- *Option 3* You decide that if your intake is not high enough, you will supplement your diet with a whole-protein type of supplement.

Do you see any other adequate and safe options? Which suits you best?

Summary

- We tend to value **protein** above the other classes of nutrients, to the point of giving it credit for more than it can deliver.
- There are thousands of different proteins that differ widely in complexity and function. However, all consist of **amino acids** joined together by **peptide bonds.** Every amino acid consists of an amine group, an acid group, and a characteristic side group. Approximately 20 amino acids are used to synthesize proteins, and every living cell can produce some of them if it has the necessary raw materials.
- Dietary protein needs are actually needs for nitrogen (to make those amino acids the body can produce itself) and for **essential amino acids** (those the body cannot produce but must obtain in foods). Protein is widespread in our food supply, but not all protein is of the same quality. In general, animal sources are better than plant sources for matching human needs for essential amino acids. **Omnivore** and some **vegetarian** diets (**semivegetarian, lacto-ovo,** and **lacto-**) easily meet essential amino acid needs, but **vegan** diets may do so less well. However, different foods eaten within the same day often contain—*in combination*—acceptable proportions of amino acids, a phenomenon known as **complementing** or **mutual supplementation.**
- Protein's crucial role in the body is evident from its many functions: (1) constituting cell and tissue structure; (2) regulating a wide variety of body processes, including metabolic reactions, hormonal activity, body defenses, mineral and fluid balance, acid–base balance, and nerve impulse transmission; and (3) providing energy (in emergencies, or if present in surplus).
- Proteins can be modified by food technology just as the other macronutrients can. Soy protein isolates and concentrates commonly turn up as meat analogues and texturizers, respectively. Protein supplements of various kinds are marketed for

several purposes, few of which are really legitimate. The amino acid derivative monosodium glutamate (MSG) is a commonly used flavor enhancer, and the dipeptide **aspartame** is an increasingly common sugar substitute.

- The body handles dietary protein very efficiently. **Denaturation** (unfolding) and digestion begin in the stomach with the action of hydrochloric acid and pepsin, and other **proteases** take over the breakdown process in the small intestine. Secreted proteins and proteins from sloughed cells of the GI tract are also digested. Then amino acids, dipeptides, and tripeptides are efficiently absorbed. Occasionally large peptide fragments are absorbed. In some cases these absorbed proteins provoke an immune response, in which case the susceptible individual is said to have a food allergy (the symptoms of which can occur in body sites far removed from the digestive tract). The body is also very efficient at recycling many of its own proteins.

- As for the other nutrients, there is an optimal range of protein intake. Pure protein deficiency is rare, but in the less developed countries **protein–energy malnutrition,** a result of general food shortage, is fairly widespread. Two severe forms of this disorder are **marasmus** and **kwashiorkor.** In addition to its other consequences, inadequate protein intake can lead to increased susceptibility to infection and to fatty liver. Excess protein in the diet can lead to an increase in body fat and in some cases to dehydration.

- A healthy adult can easily meet his or her protein needs by eating a balanced diet. Protein intake guidelines are usually based either on body weight or on the total number of kcalories consumed. Needs vary among individuals; athletes have been shown not to benefit from consuming protein far in excess of the RDA, though people who are recovering from illness or injury may need considerably more than the recommended amount.

References

Applegate, L. 1991. *Power foods.* Emmaus, PA: Rodale Press.

Barinaga, M. 1990. Amino acids: How much excitement is too much? *Science* 247:20–22.

Belongia, E.A., A.N. Mayeno, and M.T. Osterholm. 1992. The eosinophilia-myalgia syndrome and tryptophan. *Annual Review of Nutrition* 12:235–256.

Carroll, P., K.J. Caplinger, and G.L. France. 1992. Guidelines for counseling parents of young children with food sensitivities. *Journal of the American Dietetic Association* 92:602–603.

Clark, N. 1990. *Sports nutrition guidebook.* Champaign, IL: Leisure Press.

Ganong, W.F. 1991. *Review of medical physiology.* Norwalk, CT: Lange Medical Publications.

Gardner, M.L. 1988. Gastrointestinal absorption of intact proteins. *Annual Review of Nutrition* 8:329–350.

Garriga, M.M., C. Berkebile, and D.D. Metcalfe. 1991. A combined single-blind, double-blind, placebo-controlled study to determine the reproducibility of hypersensitivity reactions to aspartame. *Journal of Allergy and Clinical Immunology* 87:821–827.

Goodman, M.N. 1988. Amino acid and protein metabolism. In *Exercise, nutrition, and energy metabolism,* ed. E.S. Horton and R.L. Terjung. New York: The Macmillan Company.

Herbert, V. 1992. L-Tryptophan: A medicolegal case against over-the-counter marketing of supplements of amino acids. *Nutrition Today* 27(no.2):27–30.

Hickson, J.F. and I. Wolinsky. 1989. Human protein intake and metabolism in exercise and sport. In *Nutrition in exercise and sport,* ed. J.F. Hickson and I. Wolinsky. Boca Raton, FL: CRC Press.

Institute of Food Technology (IFT). 1986. Sweeteners—alternatives to cane and beet sugar. *Food Technology* 40 (no.1):116–128.

Institute of Food Technology (IFT), Office of Scientific Public Affairs. 1992. Monosodium glutamate: An Institute of Food Technologists Scientific Perspective. *Food Technology* 46(no. 2):34.

International Center for Sports Nutrition and the United States Olympic Committee Sports Medicine Division. 1990. *Protein implications for athletes.* Omaha, NE: International Center for Sports Nutrition.

Kenney, R.A. 1986. The Chinese restaurant syndrome: An anecdote revisited. *Food and Chemical Toxicology* 24:351–354.

Lemon, P.W.R. 1991. Effect of exercise on protein requirements. *Journal of Sports Sciences* 9:53–70.

Marieb, E.N. 1992. *Human anatomy and physiology.* Redwood City, CA: The Benjamin/Cummings Publishing Company.

Martin, R.E. 1988. Seafood products, technology, and research in the U.S. *Food Technology* 42(no.3):58–62.

Meredith, C.N., M.J. Zackin, W.R. Frontera, and W.J. Evans. 1989. *Journal of Applied Physiology* 66(no.6):2850–2856.

Munro, H.N. and M.C. Crim. 1988. The proteins and amino acids. In *Modern nutrition in health and disease,* ed. M.E. Shils and V.R. Young. Philadelphia: Lea & Febiger.

Mutch, P.B. 1988. Food guides for the vegetarian. *American Journal of Clinical Nutrition* 48:913–919.

Myrvik, Q.N. 1988. Nutrition and immunology. In *Modern nutrition in health and disease,* ed. M.E. Shils and V.R. Young. Philadelphia: Lea & Febiger.

National Research Council. 1989. *Diet and health.* Washington, DC: The National Academy Press.

RDA Subcommittee. 1989. *Recommended dietary allowances.* Washington, DC: The National Academy Press.

Roufs, J.B. 1992. Review of L-tryptophan and eosinophilia-myalgia syndrome. *Journal of the American Dietetic Association* 92:844–850.

Sabate, J., K.D. Lindsted, R.D. Harris, and A. Sanchez. 1991. Attained height of lacto-ovo vegetarian children and adolescents. *European Journal of Clinical Nutrition* 45:51–58.

Shaw, S. and C.S. Lieber. 1988. Nutrition and diet in alcoholism. In *Modern nutrition in health and disease,* ed. M.E. Shils and V.R. Young. Philadelphia: Lea & Febiger.

Smith, E.L., R.L. Hill, I.R. Lehman, R.J. Lefkowitz, P. Handler, and A. White. 1983. *Principles of biochemistry: General aspects,* 7th edition. New York: McGraw-Hill Book Company.

Stegink, L.D., L.J. Filer, Jr., E.F. Bell, E.E. Ziegler, and T.R. Tephley. 1989. Effect of repeated ingestion of aspartame-sweetened beverage on plasma amino acid, blood methanol, and blood formate concentrations in normal adults. *Metabolism* 38:357–363.

Steinbrook, R. 1989. Tracking disease the old way. *The Los Angeles Times,* November 27, 1989.

Tarnopolsky, M.A., J.D. MacDougall, and S.A. Atkinson. 1988. Influence of protein intake and training status on nitrogen balance and lean body mass. *Journal of Applied Physiology* 64(no.1):187–193.

Thomas-Doberson, D. 1989. Calculation of aspartame intake in children. *Journal of the American Dietetic Association* 89:831–833.

Thompson, R.C. 1986. Food allergies: Separating fact from hype. *FDA Consumer* 20:25–27.

Tollefson, L. and R.J. Barnard. 1992. An analysis of RDA passive surveillance reports of seizures associated with consumption of aspartame. *Journal of the American Dietetic Association* 92:598–601.

Torun, B. and F.E. Viteri. 1988. Protein-energy malnutrition. In *Modern nutrition in health and disease,* ed. M.E. Shils and V.R. Young. Philadelphia: Lea & Febiger.

Williams, M.H. 1989. Nutritional ergogenic aids and athletic performance. *Nutrition Today* 24:7–14.

Williams, M.H. 1992. *Nutrition for fitness and sport.* Dubuque, IA: William C. Brown, Publishers.

Williams, S.R. and B.S. Worthington-Roberts. 1988. *Nutrition throughout the life cycle.* St Louis: Times/Mirror-Mosby.

Worthington-Roberts, B.S. 1981. Proteins and amino acids. In *Contemporary developments in nutrition,* ed. B.S. Worthington-Roberts. St Louis: The C.V. Mosby Company.

Young, V.R. and D.M. Bier. 1987. A kinetic approach to the determination of human amino acid requirements. *Nutrition Reviews* 45:289–298.

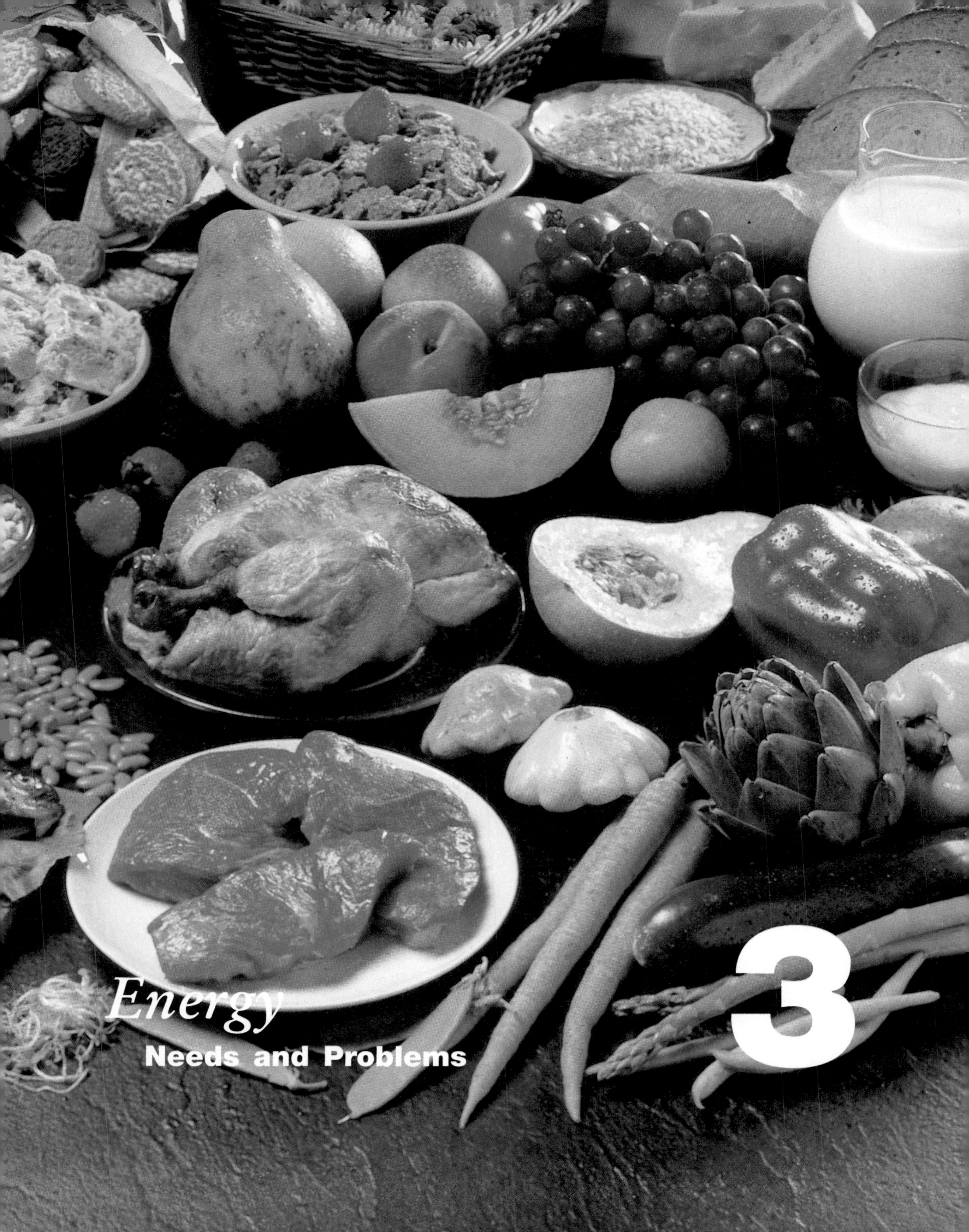

Energy
Needs and Problems

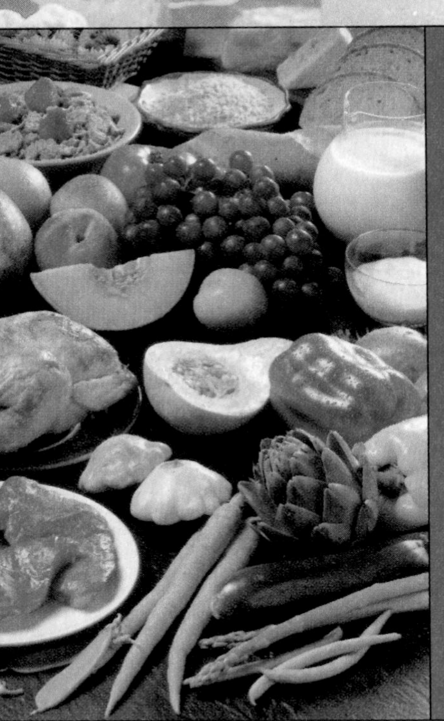

IN THIS CHAPTER

Chapter 8

Energy Sources and Uses

You have just studied the three classes of nutrients that provide energy: carbohydrates, lipids, and proteins. So far, though, we haven't considered why you need energy. That's a major purpose of this chapter.

You might have regarded energy as the commodity you need to be vigorously active—to run with the family dog, dunk a basketball, race a bicycle, swim, bounce on a trampoline. There is no question that such activities use energy, and lots of it. However, you also use energy when you're sitting quietly in a rowboat waiting for the fish to bite, or when you're sleeping in front of the TV: you use energy continuously to carry out the basic processes that keep you alive. The amount of energy you need every day for these processes is approximately the amount of energy you would use to walk 20–25 miles. In an ordinary day, you are likely to use more energy for life-sustaining processes than for physical activity.

Energy takes many forms in the body. Movement demonstrates *mechanical energy.* Energy that powers metabolic reactions is *chemical energy.* The tiny electrical impulses generated by nerve cells represent *electrical energy.* Heat produced by the body is *thermal energy;* most of our energy ultimately takes this form.

energy—the capacity to do work, measured in kcalories; the power to effect physical changes

Whatever form energy takes, it is commonly expressed as *kilocalories* (kcalories, kcal). Energy intake and energy output are both expressed in kcalories: we talk about food providing a certain number of kcalories and about various activities using a particular number of kcalories. (The metric system sometimes quantifies energy in *kilojoules.* There are 4.18 kilojoules in 1 kcalorie. However, because the kcalorie is more familiar, we have used that term throughout this book.)

This chapter describes the functions for which we use energy and gives you several ways of estimating how much energy you use for these tasks each day. Then you'll learn how the macronutrients you eat are sometimes converted to other materials for energy storage. We also discuss what happens at the cellular level to produce energy and what factors influence the proportions of protein, fat, and carbohydrate that are used to generate it.

How Your Body Expends Energy

Scientists know about three general purposes for which your body uses energy: to support life-sustaining functions, to allow physical activity, and to process internally food that has been consumed. Energy also seems to be expended in response to extreme environmental or physiologic stresses. Let's discuss each of these expenditures individually.

Life-Sustaining Functions

Continuously throughout life, your body expends energy for the activities that keep you alive. These activities include breathing, producing heartbeats, maintaining body temperature and muscle tone, and keeping your glands, cells, and nervous system functioning. Collectively, these life-sustaining processes are referred to as **basal metabolism,** and the amount of energy required to maintain them for a specified unit of time is called the **basal metabolic rate (BMR).** To measure a person's BMR takes very specialized equipment and precise conditions. Because the protocol for determining BMR is difficult and inconvenient, it is seldom done except in very specialized research. Basal metabolism usually accounts for 60–70% of the typical North American's daily energy expenditure.

basal metabolism—all the metabolic processes that must take place continuously to sustain the life of an animal

basal metabolic rate (BMR)—the number of kcalories required to maintain life-sustaining activities for a specified amount of time; requires very specific conditions for exact measurement

resting metabolic rate (RMR)—the number of kcalories used during a specified amount of time at rest; usually a slightly higher value than BMR due to measurement under less stringent conditions

Data for research on energy use are now likely to be collected under somewhat less stringent conditions, producing a value called the **resting metabolic rate (RMR)** or resting energy expenditure (REE). If you had your RMR measured, you would need to rest quietly in a comfortable environment for several hours following a meal and physical activity. Under such circumstances, your energy use might be slightly higher than your BMR, because it could include a small amount of energy used for purposes other than basal activities. For most people, RMR usually accounts for 60–75% of total daily energy expenditure (Poehlman and Horton, 1992).

Chances are that you will never have a BMR or RMR test done yourself, but research on others has provided data from which formulas for *estimating* RMR have been derived. One method of calculating RMR is shown in Act on Fact 8.1 (page 252).

A number of individual factors affect your basal or resting energy needs; they are discussed in the paragraphs that follow. As you read, note that several of these factors involve two general variables: how much lean body mass you have (including muscle, which typically represents 35–40% of body weight) and whether the amount of that tissue is changing. Additionally, you should note that certain internal organs are responsible for a disproportionate amount of basal energy usage: your liver and brain, which account for only 4% of body weight, are responsible for 40% of your BMR (Owen, 1988). Therefore, the fairly consistent energy usage of these organs exerts a certain stabilizing effect on your BMR, especially once you have reached adulthood.

Body Size A tall, large person usually has a higher BMR than a short, small person. The different BMRs reflect the different total amounts of lean tissue each body contains. There may not be much difference in BMR between a fat person and a thin person of the same height, though, because fat tissue is not very active metabolically and does not use much energy.

Age Because your mass of lean tissue increases as you progress from infancy through adolescence, the number of kcalories used for basal processes increases during the growth years. The growth process itself increases the BMR further: BMR is high during the growth spurts of the toddler period and adolescence.

After early adulthood (around the mid-20s), lean body mass and BMR decrease gradually by anywhere from 2% to 3% per decade (RDA Subcommittee, 1989).

Sex Males generally have higher BMRs than females of the same age and size, mainly because males usually have proportionately more lean tissue than females have. There may be hormonal influences as well.

Figure 8.1 shows the effects of both sex and age after physical maturity.

Growth When body tissue, whether protein or fat, is added, energy is required to synthesize the tissue—energy that is over and above the energy value of the material itself. The average energy cost is about 5 kcalories per gram of tissue gained (RDA Subcommittee, 1989).

Health Status Fever raises your BMR, as happens when your body is fighting an infection. For every Fahrenheit degree above normal temperature, BMR is about 7% higher; every Celsius degree of fever represents almost a 13% increase in your BMR (Heymsfield and Williams, 1988).

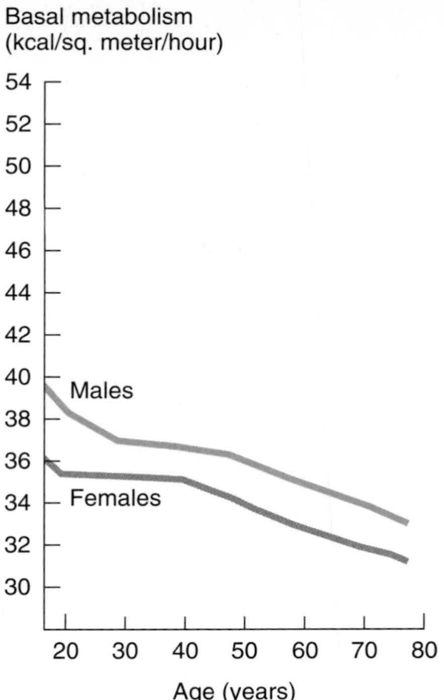

FIGURE 8.1
The effect of sex and age on BMR after maturity.

This graph shows that males usually have a higher BMR than females, even when differences in lean body mass are accounted for (by expressing BMR values per square meter of body surface area). After a person reaches physical maturity (around the mid-20s), the energy used for internal processes gradually declines. (Adapted from Guyton, 1991.)

Injuries and surgery also increase basal needs; extensive burns can double your energy requirement.

Thyroid Hormone Level The thyroid hormone *thyroxin* is a metabolic accelerator. If your body produces less thyroxin than most people's, your metabolic processes are slower, a fact that is reflected in a lower BMR. People who produce an overabundance of thyroxin, by contrast, have higher basal metabolic rates as a result.

If low or high thyroxin production interferes with a person's health, either situation can usually be corrected by medical intervention. Fortunately, both conditions are unusual.

Pregnancy During pregnancy, maternal and fetal growth raises the woman's BMR above its prepregnant level. Energy needs during pregnancy are considered in more detail in Chapter 15.

Individual Variation Some people use more (or less) energy for basal metabolic activities than you would expect from taking into consideration the factors just listed. It is not uncommon for a person's BMR to vary as much as 20% in either direction, and even greater differences have been observed. These variations seem to have a strong genetic component (Poehlman and Horton, 1989).

Physical Activity

The second largest use of energy, typically, is for physical activity. This is the only aspect of energy expenditure over which you have very much control. Because most energy used for physical activity is converted to heat, this component of energy use is referred to as the **thermic effect of exercise (TEE).**

thermic effect of exercise (TEE)—the number of kcalories expended above RMR as a result of physical activity

TABLE 8.1 Energy Cost of Some Activities

Activity	kcal/kg/minute	Activity	kcal/kg/minute
Bicycling (racing)	0.127	Painting outside	0.057
Bicycling (leisurely)	0.042	Playing ping-pong	0.073
Canoeing (leisurely)	0.024	Piano playing	0.018
Carpentry	0.045	Rowing in a race	0.267
Cleaning (light)	0.030	Running (5½ min/mile)	0.269
Cooking	0.015	Running (7 min/mile)	0.208
Dancing (fast)	0.148	Running (9 min/mile)	0.173
Dancing (slowly)	0.050	Sewing (hand or machine)	0.007
Dishwashing	0.017	Singing (loud)	0.013
Dressing, personal care	0.025	Sitting (writing)	0.007
Driving a car	0.015	Skating	0.058
Eating	0.007	Skiing (cross-country, level)	0.099
Field hockey	0.114	Skiing (cross-country, uphill)	0.254
Grocery shopping	0.040	Sleeping	0
Football	0.112	Squash	0.192
Garage work (repairs)	0.046	Standing (relaxed)	0.008
Golf	0.065	Stock clerking	0.034
Gymnastics	0.046	Swimming (2 mph)	0.132
Horseback riding (walk)	0.023	Tennis	0.089
Horseback riding (gallop)	0.112	Violin playing	0.010
Judo	0.175	Volleyball	0.030
Knitting	0.012	Walking (3 mph)	0.039
Laboratory work	0.018	Walking (3 mph, carrying 22 lb)	0.046
Laundry (light)	0.022	Walking (4 mph)	0.057
Lying still, awake	0	Walking downstairs	0.012 kcal/flight
Painting inside	0.014	Walking upstairs	0.036 kcal/flight

Compiled from data published by Taylor and McLeod, 1949; Durnin and Passmore, 1967; Mc Ardle et al., 1981; and Passmore and Durnin, 1955. Values have been modified to eliminate energy expended for BMR and the thermic effect of food (discussed later in the chapter). Because values for the same activity vary from one source to another, these values are unavoidably less precise than they appear.

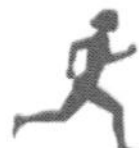

The amount of energy you use for physical activity can vary markedly from one day to the next. This contrasts with BMR, which isn't likely to be much different from day to day. The proportion of energy most people use for physical activity is 15–30% of total kcalories (Poehlman and Horton, 1992). A manual laborer or an athlete training 5 or 6 hours per day might use 50% of the day's energy for activity.

Three factors influence the amount of energy you use for physical activity: the type of activity you engage in, the length of time you do it, and your body weight.

Type of Activity Activities that use a larger amount of muscle mass use more energy. For example, walking requires more energy than sitting and typing because more large muscles are involved in walking. The intensity of an activity also has a direct influence on energy usage: walking, even though it involves some of the same muscles as running, uses less energy per unit

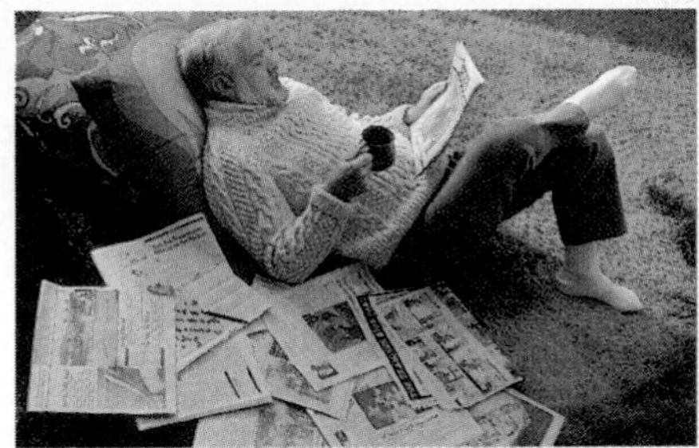

(a)

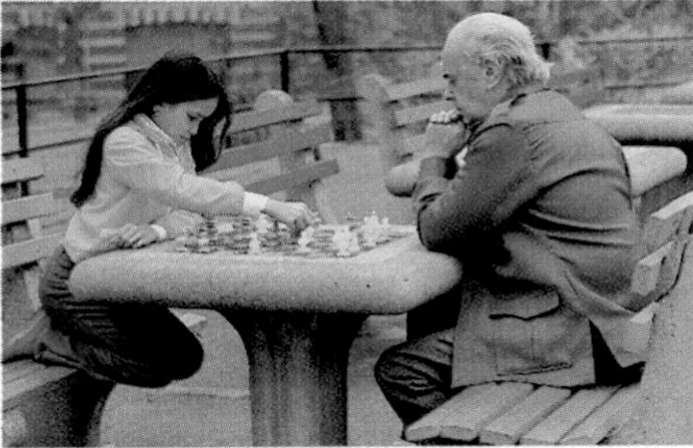

(b)

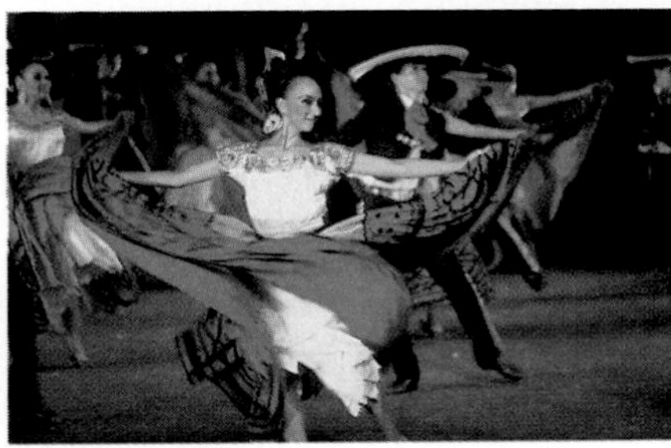

(d)

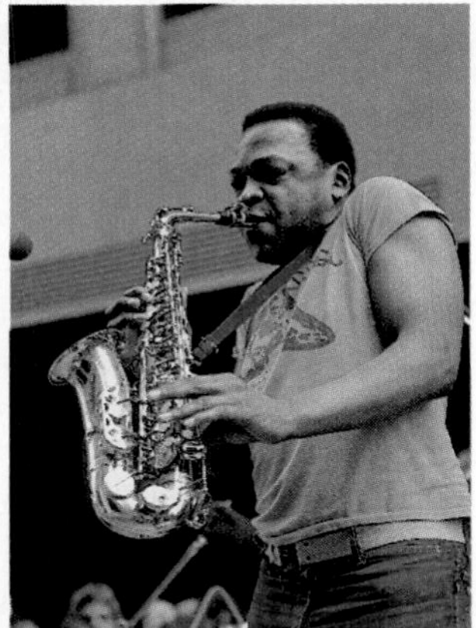

(c)

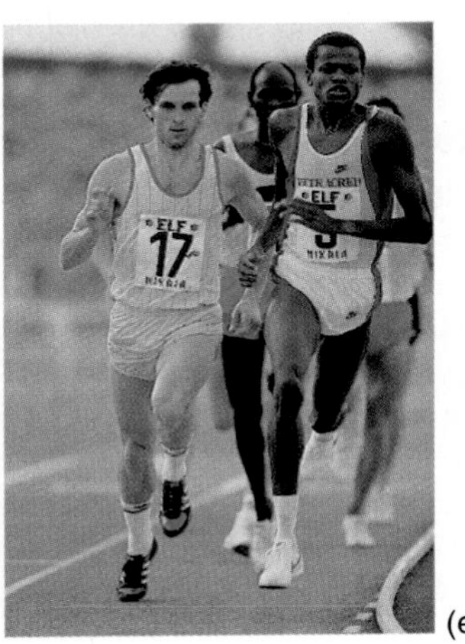

(e)

FIGURE 8.2
Energy cost of various activities.

These activities use different amounts of energy. (a) The person lying still uses very little energy for activity. (b) The chess players use about 30 kcalories per hour for their slight activity. (c) The musician probably uses double that amount, depending on how much he moves as he plays. (d) Folk dancers may use 500 kcalories per hour. (e) The runners use the highest amount of energy: a 154-pound person running 7-minute miles uses almost 900 kcalories per hour for the activity alone.

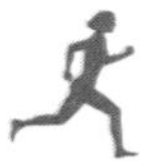

of time because fewer muscle cells are involved, producing a stride that is shorter and less frequent. Table 8.1 and Figure 8.2 give examples of how much energy is expended during various activities. Note that these values are for activity alone and do not include energy that is simultaneously being expended for basal needs.

You Tell Me

Many people think it's possible to burn up hundreds of kcalories in a single bout of exercise. You *can*, but are you *likely to*?

Choose from Table 8.1 one of the more vigorous activities that you do. Taking into account your body weight and the energy cost of the activity, for how many minutes do you have to be active to expend 300 kcalories?

Duration of Activity Time is the second factor to consider when you calculate energy expenditure. As noted above, the longer an activity continues, the more energy will be used.

It is sometimes difficult to estimate how much time is actually involved in an activity if you do it only intermittently. For example, if you spend 8

hours at a downhill ski area, you may spend only a couple of hours skiing, spending the rest of the time in lift lines, on lifts, and in the chalet.

However, small movements, if done repeatedly throughout the day, can expend a significant amount of energy. One researcher has estimated that *fidgeting* can cost 100–800 kcalories per day (Ravussin et al., 1986).

Body Weight Body weight also influences energy expenditure. The heavier you are, the more energy you expend in moving your mass. This means that if you and a friend who is larger exercise together, your friend uses more energy than you while performing the same exercise at the same intensity for the same length of time.

In theory, you could calculate your total day's energy expenditure from physical activity by keeping a careful diary of your activities in 5-minute intervals, multiplying those times by the appropriate figures from Table 8.1, and summing them; such records are very difficult to keep accurately, however. ●

Biologic Processing of Food

For decades, researchers have known that a certain expenditure of energy is required for the physiologic processes of digestion, absorption, and transport and for the storage of food and its nutrients. That is, your body uses a small amount of energy for processing food internally before you have access to the larger amount of energy the food contains, just as it takes an investment of some money to make more money.

thermic effect of food (TEF)—the number of kcalories expended (at rest) above RMR during the several hours following a meal; caused by the energy demands of digestion, absorption, transport, and storage

These processes usually occur within 6 hours following a meal, and the production of heat as a by-product is called the **thermic effect of food (TEF).** Approximately 10% of the energy in the food a person consumes is used for internal processing of food (Poehlman and Horton, 1992).

Responding to Extreme Physiologic and Environmental Stresses

adaptive thermogenesis—energy expended by an animal in response to extreme physiologic or environmental conditions; produces heat but no "work"

In recent years, scientists have been interested in the fact that under certain circumstances, some people seem to expend more (or less) energy than would be expected from the factors discussed above. They refer to this change in energy production as **adaptive thermogenesis** (Van Zant, 1992). There are several situations in which this may occur.

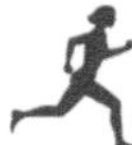

One instance occurs when a person has been in physical training. A person who is physically fit generally has a higher RMR than one who is not in such good shape. Although you might think that this simply reflects that a fit person has a larger muscle mass, there's more to it than that. A given amount of muscle mass in a well-trained man has a higher RMR than the same amount of muscle in an untrained man (Poehlman and Horton, 1992). The same may be true for women, although the data are not as consistent. ●

Other examples of adaptive thermogenesis occur when energy intake changes radically. At one end of the spectrum, the RMR of a person who is losing weight very quickly often decreases; this is one reason why people who are on severe kcalorie-restricted diets lose weight more slowly after they have been dieting for a while. The RMR of a starving person may be as much as 30% lower than that of the same person before deprivation.

At the other end of the spectrum, taking in huge excesses of kcalories may lead to wasting some of the surplus kcalories. A number of studies suggest that some people, when they take in much more energy than they need for RMR, TEE, and TEF, dissipate a portion of those kcalories as more heat (Van Zant, 1992). This occurs particularly when the surplus kcalories come from carbohydrate. Other researchers using more precise methods of measuring energy expenditure doubt that people waste energy in this way (Roberts et al., 1990; Schoeller and Fjeld, 1991). They believe that the technologies used in earlier studies were less accurate and thereby lost track of some of the energy.

Adaptive thermogenesis may also occur in response to environmental cold. It is well known that hibernating animals maintain a steady body temperature in spite of the fact that environmental temperature may vary considerably. Such heat production is called *nonshivering thermogenesis.* It is not known whether this phenomenon also occurs in humans.

brown fat—brown-colored fat tissue found in hibernating animals, newborn humans, and perhaps adults; the color is due to high concentrations of the energy-producing cell structures, mitochondria.

Some scientists theorize that adaptive thermogenesis may occur in animals whose bodies contain, in addition to the usual white fat tissue, a second type of fat called **brown fat** (Kinney, 1988). It is brown because it contains a much larger number of mitochondria, the cellular structures in which much of the body's energy is produced. Although brown fat is known to exist in animals that hibernate and in newborn human infants, it is not yet known whether human adults retain this tissue or how much they might have.

Although some scientists currently refer to adaptive thermogenesis as a separate category of energy use, it is possible that, in the future, kcalories expended in these ways will be described as variations in RMR and/or TEF.

Figure 8.3 summarizes the relative amounts of energy used in a 24-hour period for the functions of resting metabolism, the thermic effect of exercise, and the thermic effect of food. Because of the variable circumstances that cause adaptive thermogenesis, it cannot be represented as a reliable part of daily expenditure.

FIGURE 8.3
Total energy expended in 24 hours.

This represents the proportions of energy used for different types of functions by an adult on a relatively inactive day. Energy expended by adaptive thermogenesis is theoretical (see text). (Adapted from Poehlman, 1989.)

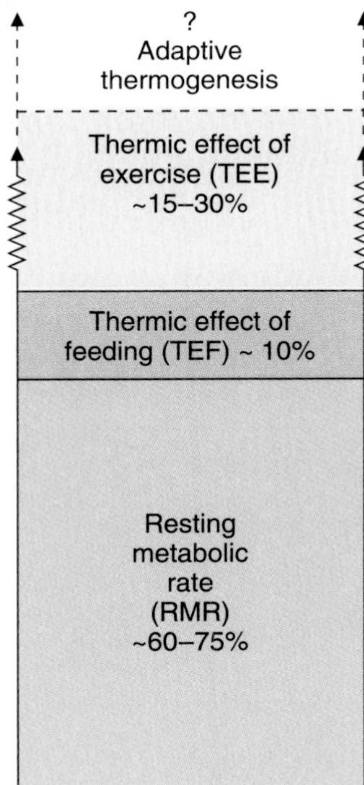

Estimating Your Daily Energy Needs

Authorities have suggested a number of methods for estimating how many kcalories a person uses in a day for all purposes together. The methods we show here vary in their ease of use and in their accuracy.

The RDA Table

The RDA committee has collected data on typical daily kcaloric usage by people of different ages and sexes; these data appear in Table 8.2. The committee usually establishes RDAs as recommendations that meet the needs of most of the population. But for energy, the committee gives *median* values for people with light to moderate activity levels and at body weights indicated in the table for each sex and age. If your body size is substantially different from that stated in the table for your category or if you are much more or less physically active, your energy usage may differ considerably from that suggested. Even if you appear to be similar to the reference person, your energy expenditure might vary by 20% in either direction.

Calculated Estimates of Energy Use

Many formulas, some fairly simple and some more complex, have been developed for estimating kcalories expended in a day. Table 8.3 offers easy formulas that allow you to take into account your sex, weight, and general activity level. These formulas are likely to be more accurate than the RDA table we just discussed, because they use more specific information.

TABLE 8.2 Median Heights and Weights and Recommended Energy Intake[a]

Category	Age (years) or Condition	Weight (kg)	Weight (lb)	Height (in)	Average Energy Allowance (kcal)[b] Per kg	Per day[c]
Infants	0.0–0.5	6	13	24	108	650
	0.5-1.0	9	20	28	98	850
Children	1–3	13	29	35	102	1,300
	4–6	20	44	44	90	1,800
	7–10	28	62	52	70	2,000
Males	11–14	45	99	62	55	2,500
	15–18	66	145	69	45	3,000
	19–24	72	160	70	40	2,900
	25–50	79	174	70	37	2,900
	51+	77	170	68	30	2,300
Females	11–14	46	101	62	47	2,200
	15–18	55	120	64	40	2,200
	19–24	58	128	65	38	2,200
	25–50	63	138	64	36	2,200
	51+	65	143	63	30	1,900
Pregnant	1st trimester					+0
	2nd trimester					+300
	3rd trimester					+300
Lactating	1st 6 months					+500
	2nd 6 months					+500

[a]Adapted from Recommended Dietary Allowances, 10th edition, 1989, with the permission of the National Academy Press, Washington, DC.
[b]In the range of light to moderate activity, the coefficient of variation is ±20%.
[c]Figure is rounded.

You can calculate an even more individualized estimate by using Act on Fact 8.1 on page 252, which was developed from formulas in the 1989 RDA report. Your results will give you a sense of how much energy you use for basal activities, thermic effect of exercise, and thermic effect of food. Of course, all of these are just approximations of your energy use, and there is no way to estimate individual variation or what you might expend in adaptive thermogenesis.

Assessment of Typical Energy Intake

If your weight usually stays quite stable and you are fairly consistent in the amount of exercise you get, there is another way to estimate your daily energy usage: determine your typical daily kcaloric *intake.* Keep diet records for several typical days (such as two weekdays and one weekend day), calculate their energy content, and then average them.

People vary substantially in the amount of energy they use; the values you calculate might be very different from your classmates' estimates. A very small, inactive woman might expend (and therefore need to consume) only about 1200 kcalories per day, whereas a large, active man could use many times that. For example, one recent report of the dietary intakes of male bicycle racers found that they consumed almost 4500 kcalories per day

TABLE 8.3 Simple Method for Calculating Daily Energy Expenditure for Adults

Calculate the number of kcalories you use per day by multiplying your present weight in pounds by the appropriate values (in units of kcalories/pound) below.

For Adults Through Age 55				
	Sedentary	Moderately Active	More Active	Obese adults, All activity levels
Women	10	13	15	10
Men	13	15	17	10
For Adults Age 56 And Above				
	Sedentary	Moderately Active	More Active	
Women and men	10	13	15	

Most values from Kolasa et al., 1991.

to cover their energy needs (Jensen et al., 1992). Such high needs undoubtedly were due partly to a high basal metabolic rate from their large muscle mass and the effect of training. Their energy needs were also due to the energy they expended for physical activity. Adaptive thermogenesis may have played a role as well.

The Energy Value of Food

As you know, the energy value of a food depends on how many grams of protein, fat, carbohydrate, and alcohol it contains. Protein has an approximate energy value of 4 kcalories per gram; fat, 9 kcalories per gram; carbohydrate, 4 kcalories per gram; and alcohol, 7 kcalories per gram. Although these values are not precise, scientists regard them as reasonable averages of the actual energy yielded in the body from various food sources.

Table 8.4 shows the amounts of these substances in a few foods of each food group. Notice that even within some groups, foods can vary considerably in their levels of energy nutrients. For example, vegetables vary widely in their carbohydrate content. Meats, poultry, fish, beans, eggs, and nuts, although they all have high protein levels, have different fat and carbohydrate contents.

In Table 8.4, the energy nutrient that is responsible for the greatest number of kcalories in each food is in bold print. Because fat and alcohol furnish more kcalories per gram than carbohydrate or protein, they can be the largest contributors of energy without being the heaviest components.

Appendix C lists the nutrient contents and kcaloric values for about 2000 foods. Sometimes the number of kcalories shown per serving of food does not exactly match the values you get when you calculate them yourself. The discrepancy is due to the slight differences in conversion factors used to calculate the values in the appendixes. The appendix values are more accurate, but the values you calculate are close, usable estimates.

Estimating Kcalories Used in 24 Hours

Use a form similar to that in Sample Act on Fact 8.1 to do these calculations.

1. **Estimating RMR**
   a. Convert your body weight to kilograms by dividing your weight in pounds by 2.2 lb/kg.
   b. In Table A, below, identify your sex and age range, and copy the adjacent equation for estimating your RMR into the appropriate space of your assessment form.

Table A Equations for Estimating RMR from Body Weight

Sex and Age Range (years)	Equation to Derive RMR in kcal/day
Males	
0–3	$(60.9 \times wt^{a}) - 54$
3–10	$(22.7 \times wt^{a}) + 495$
10–18	$(17.5 \times wt^{a}) + 651$
18–30	$(15.3 \times wt^{a}) + 679$
30–60	$(11.6 \times wt^{a}) + 879$
>60	$(13.5 \times wt^{a}) + 487$
Females	
0–3	$(61.0 \times wt^{a}) - 51$
3–10	$(22.5 \times wt^{a}) + 499$
10–18	$(12.2 \times wt^{a}) + 746$
18–30	$(14.7 \times wt^{a}) + 496$
30–60	$(8.7 \times wt^{a}) + 829$
>60	$(10.5 \times wt^{a}) + 596$

[a]Weight in kilograms
Source: RDA Subcommittee, 1989.

   c. Enter your kg weight into the equation for "wt," and do the calculation; it yields an estimate of the number of kcalories you expend per day for RMR.

2. **Estimating energy expenditure for RMR plus the thermic effect of exercise (TEE)**
   a. Estimate how many hours you spend per day at the various activity levels in Table B in Sample Act on Fact 8.1, and enter the number of hours for each in column 1. The sum of the values in column 1 must be 24 for the hours in a day.
   b. Multiply each number in column 1 by the adjacent value in column 2; figures in column 2 represent how many multiples of a person's

IN THIS CHAPTER

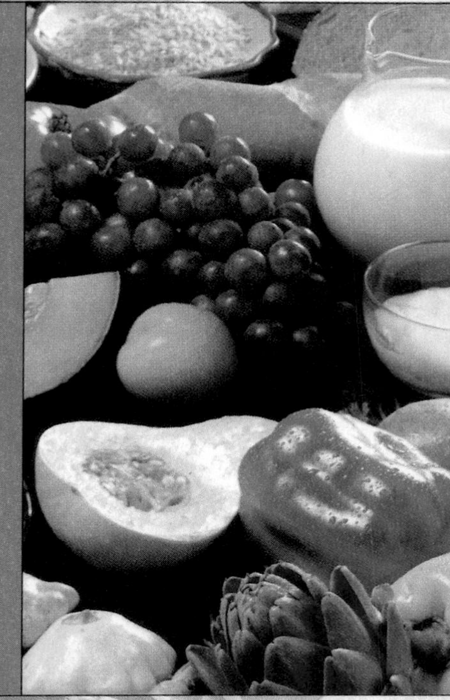

Chapter 9

Body Weight, Energy Balance, and Fitness

Do you think you're at your best weight? Do you get enough exercise? One of the following might describe your attitudes about your weight and fitness.

- You don't think much about your weight and exercise habits. You eat several times a day to satisfy your hunger, and your lifestyle naturally provides plenty of physical activity. When you have a routine physical exam, the doctor declares you to be at a good weight and at low risk of disease.
- You're among the one-fourth of the American population that is overweight and possibly inactive as well. Even though you are not obviously ill, the doctor warns you that you put yourself at risk of various diseases if you stay at this weight and don't get off the couch.
- You're at a reasonable weight and do plenty of activity, but you continually worry about your condition and work hard to maintain it. You try to eat less than you want and push yourself through very demanding workouts, because you believe that if you don't, you'll get fat in a hurry.
- You've "had it" with diets and exercise. You now eat whatever food you need to satisfy your hunger, and you've abandoned the exercise regimens you came to loathe. You've gained some weight, but you refuse to feel guilty and less worthy because of it. Having escaped the tyranny of your rigid program, you now direct your attention to other life issues.

Of course, there are other possibilities, each with its own attitudes, aspirations, and behaviors. And you may also have your own hopes about what this chapter will provide. Let's consider what you've learned so far and where we are headed.

In the last chapter, we presented the basic material you need to understand body weight issues. In this chapter, we go beyond those basics to discuss the difficulties that arise from being overweight or underweight, with a particular focus on health problems. We discuss how you can determine your best weight, and we consider various reasons why people gain weight. Of course, we discuss how to tip energy balance in a more favorable direction—and here, exercise is important.

If you think body weight is a problem for you, we hope this chapter helps you gain insight into your situation and make whatever lifestyle changes may be needed.

overweight—term usually signifying a 10–20% excess of recommended body weight

obese—term usually signifying an excess of 20% or more of recommended body weight

severely obese—term usually signifying an excess of 100% or 100 pounds of recommended body weight

underweight—term usually signifying at least 10% less than recommended body weight

Problems with Extremes in Weight

To begin, let's define some common terms as they are used in the medical literature: **overweight** is often used to mean 10–20% above ideal body weight; **obese** means more than 20% above ideal body weight. To be **severely obese** is to be either 100 pounds overweight or double the recommended weight. The term **underweight** is usually defined as body weight that is 10% less than the recommended weight.

People who are too fat or excessively thin encounter problems in almost every aspect of living (Figure 9.1).

Effects of Too Much Body Fat

According to the most recent major survey of health and nutrition in the United States, approximately 24% of adult males and 27% of adult females

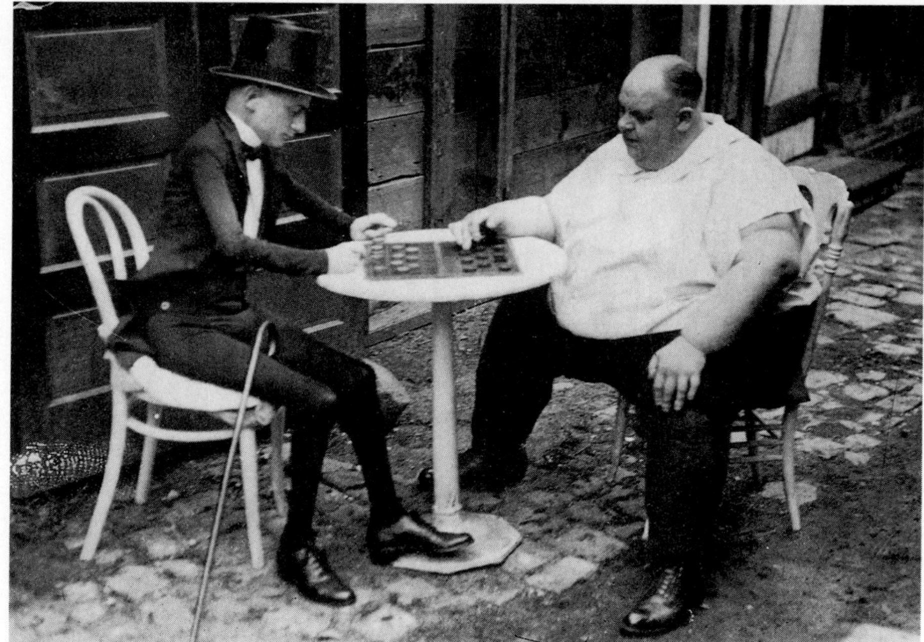

FIGURE 9.1
Body weight extremes.

It is obvious that these men, who were sideshow attractions, were severely underweight and overweight. Each of these conditions carries its own risks.

are overweight or obese (Kuczmarski, 1992). These conditions have increased markedly in American children in the last couple of decades; it is estimated that 20–23% of all school-age children are overweight or obese (Dietz, 1988). Females of all ages are somewhat more likely to be overweight or obese than are males, and people of lower socioeconomic status are more likely to be heavier.

Health Risks The likelihood of developing certain health problems is statistically greater in people who are obese than in the general population. *The Surgeon General's Report on Nutrition and Health* (1988) and the National Research Council's report *Diet and Health* (1989) link the following conditions with obesity:

- High blood pressure (hypertension)
- Stroke
- High blood LDL cholesterol
- Coronary artery heart disease
- Diabetes
- Cancer (in women, cancer of the gallbladder, breast, cervix, uterus, and ovaries; in men, cancer of the colon and prostate)
- Gallbladder disease
- Upper respiratory problems
- Arthritis and gout
- Skin disorders
- Menstrual irregularities, ovarian abnormalities, and complications of pregnancy
- Early death, if obesity is extreme

A small amount of surplus weight does not increase the risk of these problems, but obesity is associated with an increased incidence of these conditions. The severity of the risk rises with increasing obesity (Pi-Sunyer,

1991). (Remember, though, that statistical association is not proof of causation. For example, scientists debate whether obesity per se causes heart disease, or whether it is the high blood pressure that is often associated with excess body weight that causes heart disease.)

The relationship between obesity and risk of disease involves more than simply the amount of fat. The *distribution of the excess fat* also has proved to be significant. In the last couple of decades, many scientists have become convinced that excess fat at the waist and abdomen (called *upper body, central, truncal,* or *android obesity*) is more dangerous than a fat surplus in the thighs and buttocks (called *lower body, peripheral, gluteal-femoral,* or *gynoid obesity*). You may have seen these referred to as "apple" and "pear" patterns of fatness in the popular press. In general, men are more likely to develop upper body obesity, although they do not have an exclusive claim to that pattern. Women more commonly have lower body obesity; but at menopause, the amount of abdominal fat often increases (Ley et al., 1992). Some people have very evenly distributed body fat and do not fit into either category.

Some researchers have found that upper body obesity carries with it an increased risk of cardiovascular disease, stroke, hypertension, and diabetes for both men and women (Pi-Sunyer, 1991), and of breast cancer (Ballard-Barbash et al., 1990) and uterine cancer (Schapira et al., 1991) for women.

The *age at which excess weight is gained* may also affect risk, but there are fewer data on this. One report suggests that in adults, gaining surplus fat before age 50 carries more risk than adding it later (Hubert, 1988).

Psychosocial Problems Research confirms that obese people experience both psychologic and social penalties (Czajka-Narins and Parham, 1990). Obese people have experienced discrimination in all settings, including at school and in the job market. Such treatment often results in a negative self-image, feelings of loneliness, and a sense of being unable to lead a fulfilling life. Discrimination against obese women is probably greater than that against obese men.

In the opinion of many experts, the psychosocial problems can be an even greater handicap than the physical problems. A consensus panel assembled by the National Institutes of Health to consider health implications of obesity stated in its final report: "Obesity creates an enormous psychological burden. In fact, in terms of suffering, this burden may be the greatest adverse effect of obesity" (1985). Nevertheless, despite such stresses, a study of severely obese people found no more serious mental illness among the subjects than among the controls, who were people of average weight (Stunkard and Wadden, 1992).

Other Problems The health problems associated with obesity exert a financial burden. One epidemiologist assessed the annual health care costs for the diabetes, cardiovascular disease, gallbladder disease, hypertension, and breast and colon cancer that were attributable just to excess weight, and the sum was staggering: a total of $39.3 billion (Colditz, 1992). If you divide that amount by the approximate number of obese people in the United States, the amount is over $1,150 per person per year.

Obesity also brings with it many inconveniences in living, because so much of our environment is scaled for people of average size. Furniture may not be big enough or strong enough for the very fat person; he or she may find it difficult to get behind the wheel of a car or fit into a seat on an airplane; and attractive clothes that fit may be expensive and hard to find.

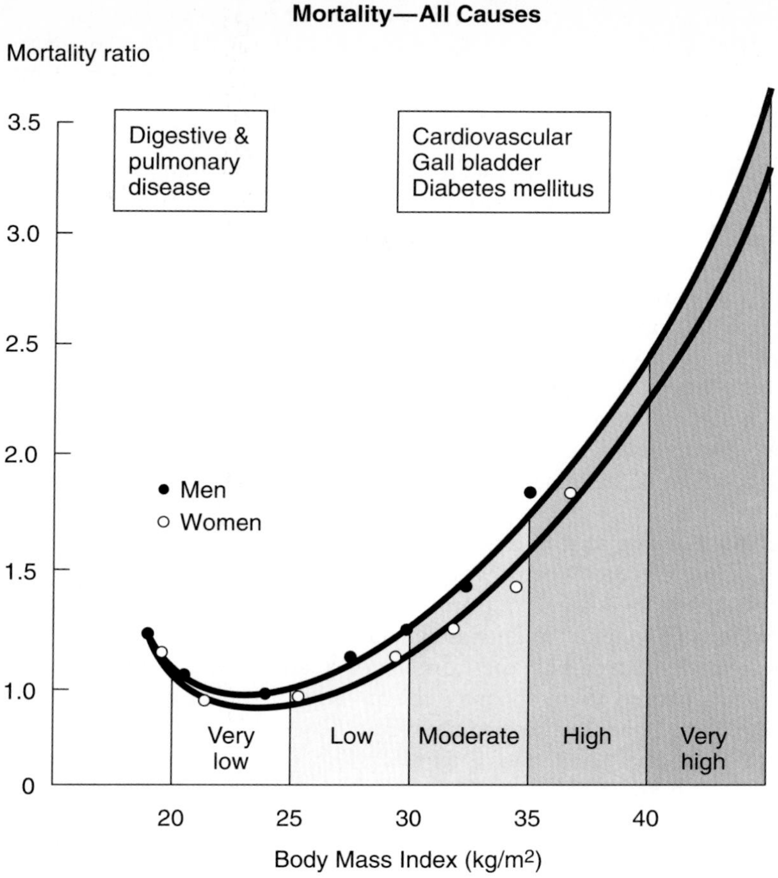

Mortality—All Causes

Mortality ratio

Digestive & pulmonary disease

Cardiovascular
Gall bladder
Diabetes mellitus

• Men
○ Women

Very low | Low | Moderate | High | Very high

Body Mass Index (kg/m²)

FIGURE 9.2
Relationship between risk of death and body mass index (BMI).

BMI is a value that indicates the relationship between a person's weight and height. Both BMIs that are very low (underweight, at the left of the figure) or very high (overweight, at the right) correlate with increased risk of death.
Source: Adapted from Bray, 1992.

Effects of Too Little Body Fat

There is less information available on the consequences of underweight in the developed countries. This, in part, reflects the fact that underweight is far less common in the industrialized nations than is obesity. As a consequence, research is less likely to be funded. Nonetheless, we know of a number of ill effects.

Health Risks Epidemiologic studies done in the more developed countries show that the relationship between mortality and body weight is U-shaped (Cornoni-Huntley et al., 1991) or J-shaped (Bray, 1992); that is, both severely underweight and overweight people are at greater risk of death. Figure 9.2 shows such a curve. (Note: the figure is based on body mass index [BMI], a measure you will learn more about on page 275. For now, be aware that BMI is a way of indicating a person's weight in proportion to height: the higher your weight in proportion to your height, the higher your BMI.)

Of course, epidemiologic data do not prove causation. Some people who are severely underweight may have lost weight due to serious illness such as AIDS; in such cases, the illness is the major cause of death, not the underweight per se. Furthermore, a study relating body weight to death rate in nonsmoking, nondrinking Seventh Day Adventist men found no increased risk associated with lower body weights (Linstead et al., 1991). This suggests that alcohol consumption and cigarette smoking might also contribute to the increased mortality of underweight people in the general public.

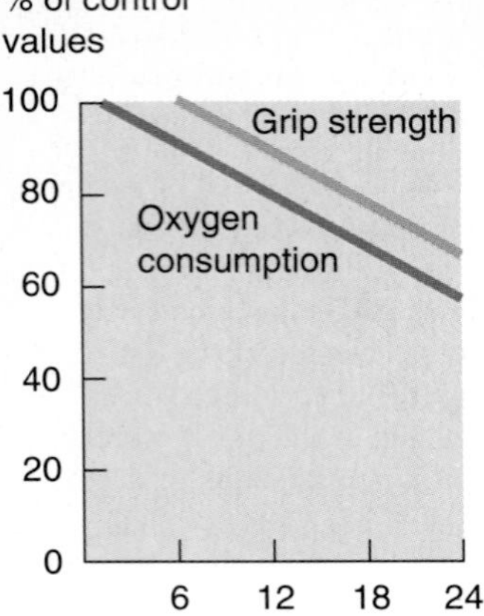

FIGURE 9.3
Effects of below-normal body weight on strength and work capacity.

When men lost more than 10% of their normal body weight, their grip strength decreased. Their capacity for aerobic work, as indicated by oxygen consumption, also fell.

Source: Adapted from Taylor et al., 1957.

Immune system function can be less effective in the underweight. Although people who are normally lean do not have a hampered immune response, a body experiencing prolonged, severe protein–energy malnutrition is less able to defend itself against infection (Myrvik, 1988).

Low body fatness in females is associated with delay or loss of menstrual function, which may lead to reproductive problems and general deterioration of health. This phenomenon occurs in an estimated 5–20% of female athletes (including dancers) who train vigorously (Mann, 1981). There may not be a direct cause-and-effect relationship, however, because menstruation does not cease at the same percentage of body fat in all cases.

Menstruation also stops in women who lose a great deal of body fat for other reasons, such as the eating disorder anorexia nervosa. Here, the *rate* of fat loss seems to have an influence: menstruation may cease even before body fat stores drop to low levels. This fact suggests that hormonal activity may be involved as well. In women who are dieting, menses may stop when 10–15% of normal weight has been lost (Frisch, 1987).

Impact on Fitness and Sense of Well-Being The Minnesota Starvation Studies, done during World War II using conscientious objectors and military volunteers as subjects, point out other effects of lower-than-normal body weight (Brozek, 1982). For six months, these men were fed diets containing approximately half the number of kcalories needed to maintain their weight; this caused them to drop about 76% of their prestarvation weights.

When they had lost approximately 10% of their weight, they had less strength than they had had formerly. The effect on endurance was even more marked: their capacity for aerobic work, indicated by oxygen consumption, also began to deteriorate rapidly after a 10% weight loss (Taylor et al., 1957). Both effects are shown in Figure 9.3.

Roughly two-thirds of these subjects reported losses in their feeling of well-being. They had a hard time concentrating, frequently felt "downhearted" and listless, and lost interest in interacting with other people. These effects eventually reversed as the men regained their original weights.

What Should You Weigh?

We receive two major types of information about what we should weigh. First, we are engulfed by cultural messages about ideal bodies. Second, researchers in the health and fitness disciplines have developed various standards for body weight.

Let's first address the cultural ideals and then discuss the health-related standards.

Current Cultural Ideals—Poor Standards for Healthy Weight

Cultures in different times and places prefer different levels of body fatness (Figure 9.4). What prompts these attitudes in a society is a complex matter, involving not only aesthetics but also economic and political considerations and other factors. For example, in some very poor societies it is considered desirable to be fat, because it demonstrates the relative wealth (and probably power) of the person who can afford enough food to become overweight. In more affluent societies, leanness may be regarded as admirable because it indicates self-control in the midst of plenty.

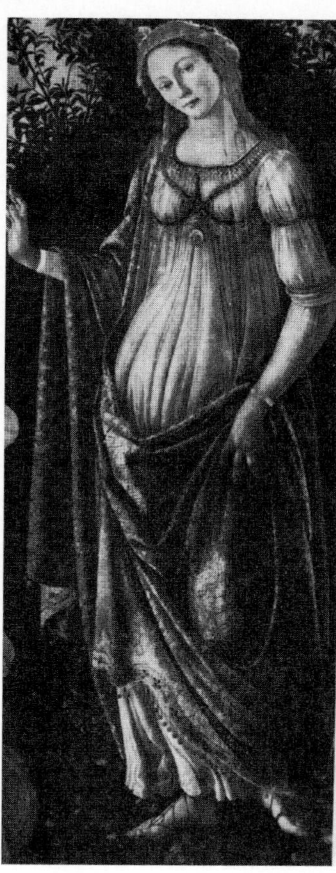
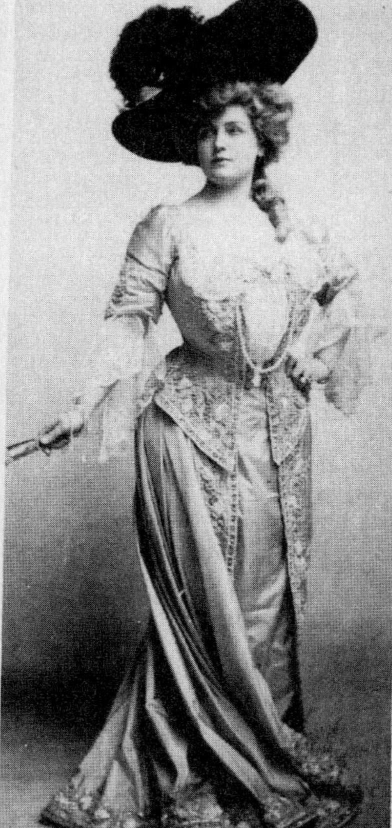
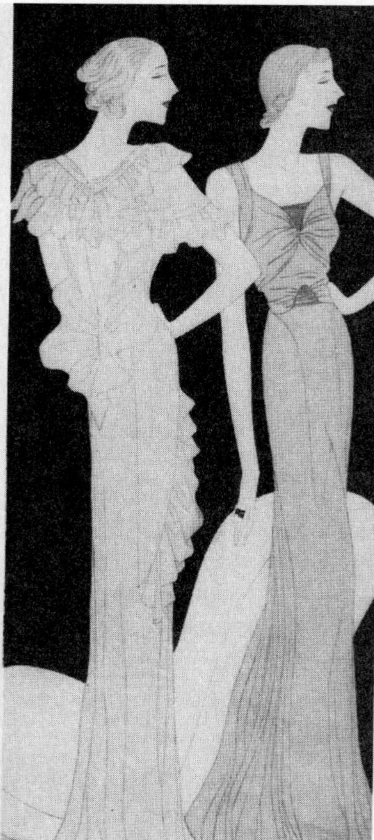
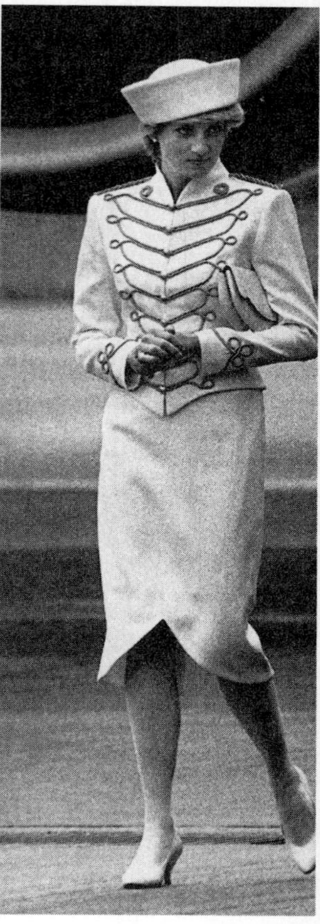

FIGURE 9.4
Various cultural ideals of body fatness for women.

Attitudes about ideal body weight vary from time to time and from culture to culture. Curves were "in" and some body fat was considered beautiful when Botticelli painted *Primavera* (ca 1478), and 186-pound soprano Lillian Russell was a popular entertainer around the turn of the century. The Art Nouveau fashion from the 1920s and the photo of Princess Diana demonstrate that extreme thinness has enjoyed popularity at other times and places. Cultural attitudes can affect people's food choices and satisfaction with their bodies but may have little to do with physical health.

Much (but not all) of the current focus on leanness in the United States seems to be directed toward females, and studies reflect this pressure on women to be slim. A survey of U.S. adults in 1989 reported that 39% of women were trying to lose weight (Williamson et al., 1992), although the actual incidence of overweight among females is about 27%. Cultural expectations for males are more in line with health standards, and men's attitudes about their weight reflect this: the study showed that 25% of men were trying to lose weight, whereas 24% of men are overweight.

This pressure affects us starting at an early age. A study of more than 450 fourth-grade children found that 60% of the girls and 38% of the boys wanted to be thinner (Gustafson-Larson and Terry, 1992). In a nationally representative sample of high school students, 44% of female and 15% of male students were trying to lose weight (National Institutes of Health, 1992). A study on a college campus regarding weight and dieting found that 37% of female and 17% of male participants stated that gaining weight was *the most powerful fear in their lives* (Collier et al., 1990).

However, the 1980s saw the beginning of a small but persistent counterculture movement. Some of the first evidence was the introduction of a new type of magazine to the newsstand—magazines maintaining that it is all right to be heavy. These publications feature articles about overweight people who are professionally successful, and they carry advertisements for fashions and other products made for large people. These magazines may help improve the self-concept and coping mechanisms of their readers.

Another expression of this movement is the organization of various groups such as Ample Opportunity, the National Association for the Advancement of Fat Acceptance, Beyond Hunger, and the Association for the Health Enhancement of Large Persons. These groups emphasize size acceptance and health maintenance for overweight people who have tried to reduce but have been unable to maintain fat losses.

To summarize, then, *current cultural ideals, especially for women, often exert pressure to weigh less than is consistent with good health.* You are better off basing your weight goals on the standards derived from health data. These standards, as described below, attempt to bring into focus the weights at which people are likely to live the longest and/or are less likely to develop disease.

Height and Weight Tables

The most familiar of the health-based standards are height and weight tables; you probably have seen these tables on the wall at your health care clinic.

Many decades ago in the United States, the insurance industry developed these tables of suggested weight for height. They were compiled from information routinely obtained from clients: age and body weight at the time a policy was purchased (usually in early adulthood) and then age at

TABLE 9.1 Good Body Weights for Adults[a]

	19–34 Years		Over 35 Years	
Height[b]	Average	Range	Average	Range
5'0"	112	97–128	123	108–138
5'1"	116	101–132	127	111–143
5'2"	120	104–137	131	115–148
5'3"	124	107–141	135	119–152
5'4"	128	111–146	140	122–157
5'5"	132	114–150	144	126–162
5'6"	136	118–155	148	130–167
5'7"	140	121–160	153	134–172
5'8"	144	125–164	158	138–178
5'9"	149	129–169	162	142–183
5'10"	153	132–174	167	146–188
5'11"	157	136–179	172	151–194
6'0"	162	140–184	177	155–199
6'1"	166	144–189	182	159–205
6'2"	171	148–195	187	164–210
6'3"	176	152–200	192	168–216
6'4"	180	156–205	197	173–222
6'5"	185	160–211	202	177–228
6'6"	190	164–216	208	182–234

[a]Body weights are given in pounds and do not include the weight of the person's clothing.
[b]Without shoes.

Source: Adapted from Bray, 1992.

However, your estimated percentage of body fat may not be very accurate because of differences in calipers, the methods of the measurers, the sites measured, your individual pattern of fat distribution, and the conversion tables used. One study pointed out how large the variation in results can be: when investigators evaluated 16 female athletes, the mean percentage of body fat for the group varied from approximately 14% to 28%, depending on the variables (Lohman et al., 1984).

Various imaging methods, such as *computed tomography (CT)* and *magnetic resonance imaging (MRI)* involve making a series of images of sites throughout the body and assessing from these images the amount of adipose tissue. These are effective methods, but they are so expensive because of the equipment, time, and expertise needed that they are rarely used except for research (Jensen, 1992).

The amount of adipose tissue can also be determined indirectly by measuring lean body mass and subtracting its weight from total body weight. One such method is *whole body counting*, which measures the total amount of K-40, a naturally occurring form of potassium present in the body. Because it occurs primarily in lean tissue in known concentration, the total K-40 value is used as a basis for calculating lean body mass.

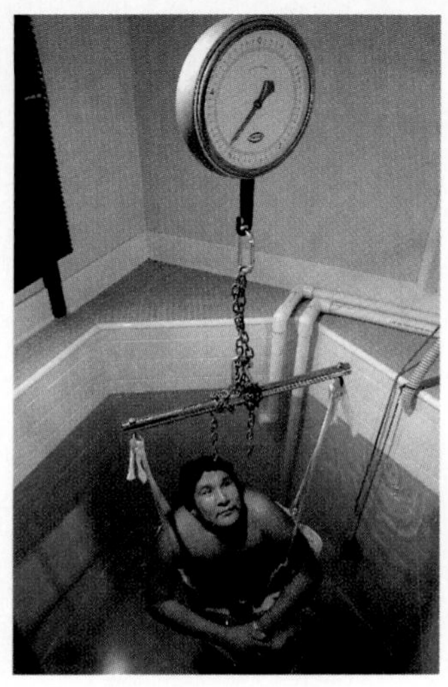

FIGURE 9.7
Underwater weighing is an accurate means of assessing body fat.

If you know what you weigh under the water and out of the water, your body fatness can be calculated. Unfortunately, the equipment for underwater weighing is not widely available.

Other methods involve introducing particular chemicals into the body, determining their concentrations in body tissues, and calculating from this the amount of adipose and lean tissue. For example, if the chemical that was used is water-soluble, then it will be distributed mainly in lean body mass, not in fat. The greater the amount of lean body mass, the more dilute the concentration of the substance in the tissues.

Ultrasonography can be used to measure the fat layer with sound waves. The probe of the ultrasound meter is placed on the skin surface. It emits pulses of high-frequency sound waves that penetrate the skin and fat layer but are reflected from the fat–muscle interface. The echoes that return to the meter are converted to a distance (skin plus fat thickness) score (Yang, 1988). Although some judgment by the operator is necessary in interpreting results, results tend to be more reliable than those obtained using skinfold calipers.

Infrared interactance involves electromagnetic radiation emitted from a probe placed on the skin. The operator analyzes energy reflected and scattered by subcutaneous fat to estimate tissue composition. The results are probably less reliable than ultrasound (Jensen, 1992).

Electromagnetic scanning (EMSCAN) measures changes in the energy of the electromagnetic field when a person is put inside a large cylindrical coil that generates an electrical current at a specific radio frequency. Because the electrical conductivity of lean tissue is far greater than that of fat tissue, the energy changes indicate the proportions of adipose and lean tissue.

Bioelectrical impedance (BEI) involves measuring the flow of a weak alternating electric current between electrodes attached to specific sites on the body (Baumgartner et al., 1989). Because lean tissue offers less resistance to the flow of the current than does adipose tissue, the rate at which the current travels can be used to determine amounts of lean and fat tissue. The process itself is simple and painless.

What About Your Weight?

You have just read about a number of methods for assessing the healthfulness of your body fat status or weight; you have probably applied some of them to yourself already. They may have yielded slightly different suggestions about what is ideal for you, but that should not be surprising—no method is perfect.

When recommendations are expressed in broad ranges, you may wonder where you belong within the range. The best way to decide is to ask yourself at what weight you function best, both physically and mentally, and what weight you tend to return to when you are not consciously trying to restrict or increase your intake.

However, you might find that your current status is above the recommended ranges. Yet you may know that this is the weight at which you function best, and it is the weight that you return to after trying to lose. If that is the case, ask yourself these questions: Does your food intake meet your nutritional needs, and with less than 30% of your kcalories from fat? Do you get at least a moderate amount of exercise? Do you have any risk factors that may have been caused by your weight, such as high blood pressure, high blood cholesterol, or Type II diabetes? If your answer to the first two questions is yes and to the last question is no, then it may be best for you to accept your current body weight and get on with other important aspects of living.

If you are above the weight ranges, have other risk factors, and seldom exercise—or if you are below the ranges and eat erratically or exercise excessively—some changes are in order. You should ask your doctor's advice about whether to attempt to gain or lose weight.

The Relationship Between Body Weight and Energy Balance

How do people come to weigh what they do? Why do people gain or lose body fat? These questions can be answered on two different levels.

On one level, the answer is very simple. *People gain fat because they consume more energy than they expend—approximately 3500 kcalories more to gain one pound of adipose tissue. Conversely, they lose a pound of adipose tissue if they expend approximately 3500 kcalories more than they consume.* Their long-term experiences with fat gains and losses (plus normal growth) bring people to their current body weights.

Keep in mind that it is the *discrepancy* between intake and output that leads to adipose tissue change. People can even gain fat when their energy intake is *lower than most people's*—that is, if their energy output is still lower than their intake. Studies have documented that many overweight people actually eat less than their peers of normal weight (National Research Council, 1989).

But we would be shortchanging you if we stopped here. There is another level at which we should discuss the matter of energy balance: it involves exploring the many factors that affect energy intake and output (Figure 9.8).

Factors Affecting Energy or Food Intake

The factors that prompt us to eat can be divided into *internal* (physiologic) and *external* (environmental) *controls or cues*. In a sense, the term *external* is a misnomer: even if an environmental cue—such as being offered an appealing food—is what initiates your interest in eating, that experience triggers some internal mechanisms as well (Weingarten, 1992). Nonetheless, we use these common terms here.

hunger—physiologic drive to consume energy in roughly the amounts expended

Internal Controls Humans, along with much of the rest of the animal kingdom, have an inborn mechanism called **hunger** that prompts energy intake sufficient to make up for recent energy output. Eating in response to

NO WEIGHT CHANGE
GAIN
LOSS
Kcalories from:
Carbohydrate
Fat
Protein
Alcohol
Kcalories for:
Basal metabolic rate
Thermic effect of food
Thermic effect of exercise
Adaptive thermogenesis
Energy In
Energy Out

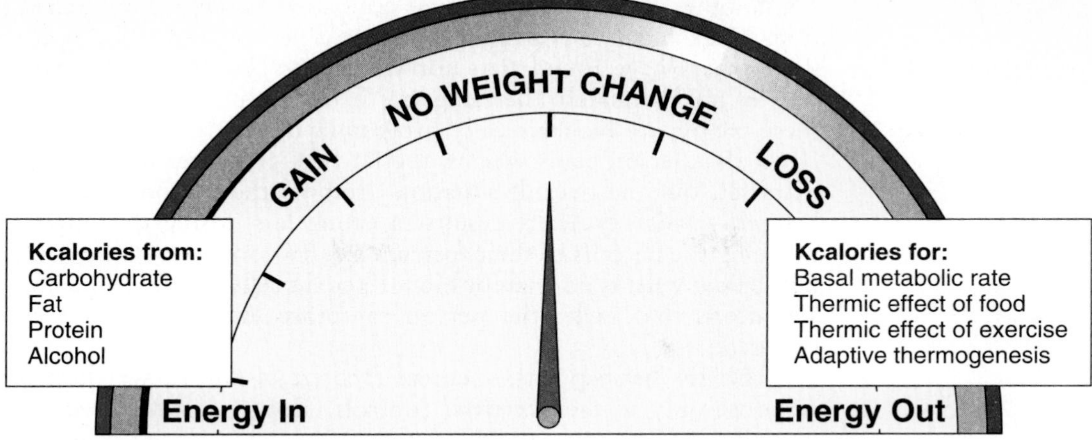

Influenced by:
Hunger and satiety
Need for sensory satiety
Emotional factors
Availability of palatable food
Social customs
Lifestyle
Determination to lose or gain body weight

Influenced by:
Genetic inheritance
Physical limitation
Attitudes about exercise
Constraints of life circumstances
Determination to lose or maintain body weight

FIGURE 9.8
Energy balance.

To maintain a stable weight, kcalories consumed and kcalories expended must be equal. A difference between intake and output of 3500 kcalories results in a pound of adipose tissue lost or gained.

hunger is referred to as *internal regulation of eating.* But what causes you to experience hunger at one time and the opposite state—**satiety** (satisfaction)—at another?

satiety—satisfaction of hunger

Scientists have studied a number of factors that may affect hunger and satiety; some are relatively short-term effects, whereas others have a longer-lasting impact. You are surely aware of the first short-term factor: when your stomach feels full, you are less likely to eat more. Nerves in the upper part of your stomach sense pressure, which makes you feel uncomfortable and disinclined to eat more. Fullness in the small intestine may produce this effect as well.

Other short-term internal controls are less obvious. Scientists theorize that levels of various chemicals circulating in the blood stimulate a hunger or satiety response. They are uncertain, however, which chemicals may be most influential and what organs they primarily affect.

Some scientists believe that two centers in the brain—one that controls hunger, the other satiety—respond to levels of circulating fat, amino acids or peptides, hormones, and/or neurotransmitters (Anderson, 1988). Other scientists believe that the liver may take a primary role in intake regulation by sensing levels of circulating macronutrients and metabolites and by initiating nervous system messages to start or stop eating.

Many women notice the effect of hormones on hunger during their menstrual cycle, and studies show variations in energy intake from one phase to another. One study documented that in the 10 days before menstruation begins, women increase their intakes by an average of 90 kcalories per day over their energy consumption in the 10 days after menstruation has begun (Lissner et al., 1988); another study showed an average daily premenstrual increase of 215 kcalories (Gong et al., 1989), and even greater increases have been documented. Such increased intakes may be offset by increases in resting metabolic rate, which have also been observed in the premenstrual phase (Solomon et al., 1982).

Another theory about hunger regulation has more long-term implications. This theory involves the size of a person's fat cells (Kolata, 1985). Researchers have found that normal-weight people usually have body fat cells of approximately the same size from one person to the next and that these people are biochemically programmed to defend this size of fat cell.

If this person gains weight, the fat cells get larger to accommodate the extra fat, but the overfill situation prompts the person to experience less hunger—which typically results in eating less, losing the surplus fat, and reducing the fat cells to their former size. By contrast, if the person's weight falls below what is normal for him or her, fat cells shrink, stimulating hunger sensations that make the person eat more until normal fat cell size is restored.

That is what happens, scientists theorize, if normal-weight people eat in response only to their *internal* controls. However, if you regularly ignore your internal controls and consistently overeat, your fat cells will increase in size until they cannot hold any more. If overeating continues, your fat cells will divide, providing you with an increased number.

Although an increase in number of fat cells is most likely to occur during growth periods, when body cells of many types are proliferating, fat cells can divide at any age (Ailhaud et al., 1992). Once a fat cell exists in the body, it is there permanently. Obesity that results from an increased number of fat cells is called **hyperplastic obesity.** It is very difficult for a person with this type of obesity to lose weight. Dr. Jules Hirsch, a physician who has devoted most of his professional life to research on this problem, talks about his findings and their implications for weight loss in the interview on page 284.

hyperplastic obesity—excess fat condition characterized by an increase in the number of fat cells

Some people who are overweight and have large fat cells (2 to 2½ times normal size) react differently from normal-weight people. When they diet to lose weight and reduce their fat cells to the normal size, they feel as though they are starving. Scientists suspect that these people may have a biochemical tendency to maintain larger fat cells.

People who have unusually large fat cells are said to have **hypertrophic obesity.** For unknown reasons, metabolic disorders such as diabetes, hypertension, and high blood cholesterol occur more often in people who have large fat cells (Bjorntorp, 1983).

hypertrophic obesity—excess fat condition characterized by an increase in the size of fat cells

Another theory about hunger and long-term body weight regulation is called the **set-point theory** (Keesey, 1988). This theory states that each person has a particular weight, or set-point, which he or she tends to maintain and at which the body handles energy intake in a metabolically normal way. Although it may be possible for a person to gain or lose weight temporarily by deliberately changing food intake, body weight will return to the set-point after the person resumes eating in response to hunger. In other words, if you force your body weight below your set-point, you will feel hungry until, eventually, you eat enough to gain back to your set-point. But if you gain weight so that you weigh more than your set-point, you will experience less hunger. Then if you eat less, you will lose weight to your set-point.

set-point theory—theory that each person tends to maintain a fairly stable, appropriate body weight by eating in response to hunger

Figure 9.9 summarizes these theories about how internal mechanisms may work together to regulate our food intake.

These theories about regulation of hunger and satiety have been partially validated, although no theory has been conclusively proved—if that is even possible. Although the theories are different, they do not necessarily conflict with each other. Actually, all of them share important points of agreement: they all acknowledge (1) that most people maintain a remarkably constant body weight over many years and (2) that there are strong biologic influences that govern your drive to eat and thereby influence your body weight.

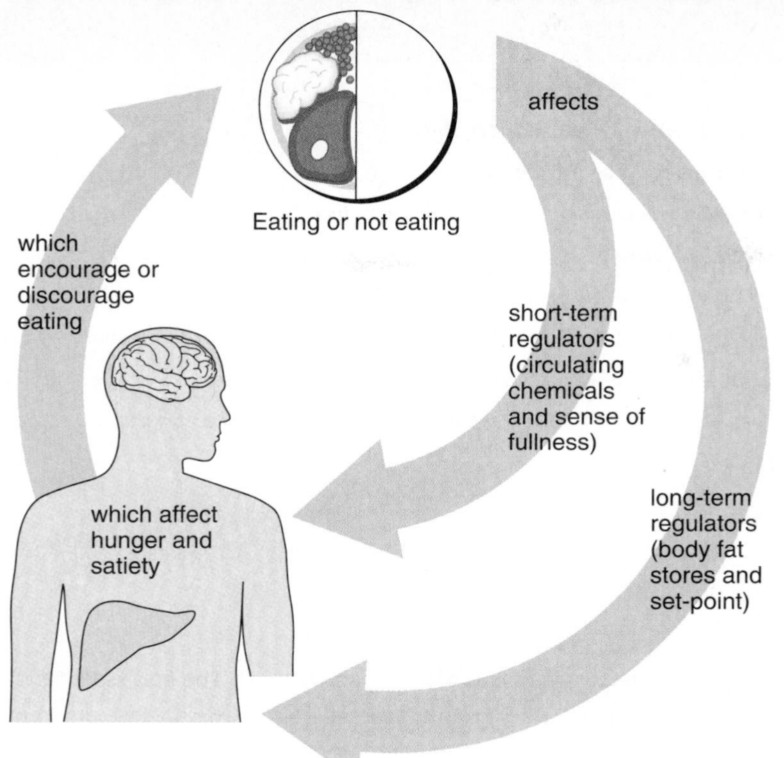

FIGURE 9.9
Internal (physiologic) effects on hunger.

Various theories suggest that hunger and satiety are influenced by short-term and long-term regulating mechanisms working together.

External Controls As you were reading about internal controls, you may have been thinking that you sometimes eat when you are not particularly hungry and that there are times when you feel hungry but do not eat. At these times, you demonstrate that external controls can influence you and even override your internal signals.

Mere *exposure to palatable food* is a powerful external control (Weingarten, 1992). Even if you have just completely satisfied your hunger with a big meal, you might also eat dessert. Just as sensory characteristics of food affect *food choices* (as was discussed in Chapter 1), palatability also influences the *amount of food* you consume.

Psychologists suggest that people may need various types of *sensory satiety* from food—such as sweetness, or fatness, or both (Drewnowski, 1991a), and that we may also seek particular smells, appearances, and textures (Rolls, 1991a). If we don't experience these with sufficient intensity, we will keep eating until we do (Herman and Polivy, 1988; Weingarten, 1992). One researcher has found that overweight people generally seek greater sensory satiety than leaner people do (Schiffman, 1986).

Other external controls are *temporal cues*, such as your usual mealtimes. *Particular locations*—such as being near a favorite restaurant—can make you want to eat. Even *food-associated sounds* can initiate eating.

Social customs influence eating as well. For example, many people have been taught to eat when a host or hostess offers something; to refuse would be to reject the person's hospitality, which is sometimes interpreted as a personal rejection. Others always "clean their plates" because they have been taught that it is wrong to waste food.

Emotional factors and psychologic states can affect eating. On the one hand, some people who suffer from clinical depression lose their appetites along with their interest in other aspects of living. On the other hand, some

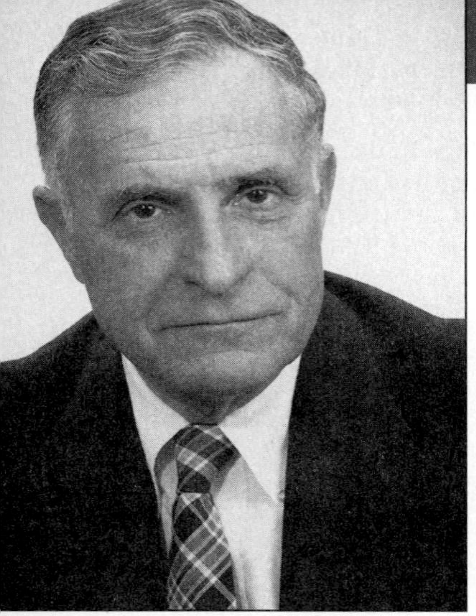

Interview with Jules Hirsch, MD

Nutrition and Weight Control

We all know people who eat whatever they like and stay slim, while others try for years to shed extra pounds. In this interview, Dr. Jules Hirsch, an expert on obesity and weight control, discusses how our genes may contribute to obesity, and whether weight loss programs are a healthy idea. Dr. Hirsch is a professor and Physician-in-Chief at the Rockefeller University in New York. His research into obesity has earned him numerous honors from scientific and medical associations in the United States and abroad.

As a physician, how did you become interested in studying weight control and adipose tissue?

I'm trained primarily in internal medicine. I came to Rockefeller University to work on the problem of serum lipids and atherosclerosis. I became interested in studying adipose tissue, which is the biggest repository of fat in the body, and in how diet affects adipose tissue. In the course of these studies, we studied obese individuals who were in the hospital losing weight, and this led me to my current interest in obesity.

What has your research in this area shown?

In obese individuals, what is obviously wrong is an extraordinary increase in the amount of stored fat. We've learned that the fat cells can only enlarge to a certain degree. After a cell enlarges by about 50%, further storage of fat requires more fat cells. What was surprising was that when individuals lost weight, the fat cell size would shrink, whereas those who began with more fat cells persisted in having these fat cells even after weight reduction.

That was a surprise, because I thought—as most people did—that if someone is obese and you get them to lose weight, they are made physically normal. That does not appear to be the case with respect to fat cells. In a reduced person you find a very different kind of adipose tissue: they have more and smaller fat cells. One thing that this strongly suggests is that there may be some biologic aspect to human obesity. There may be cellular events that make it extraordinarily difficult for the reduced obese person to maintain that "reduced obese" state.

Now, many years later, we know that there are alterations of energy metabolism in the reduced obese—they may for long periods of time, or forever, need fewer calories than a person who was never obese. There is recent evidence that there are strong genetic factors operative in at least some human obesity. One hypothesis is that the child or infant who has the genetic apparatus for obesity expresses it by super-efficient caloric storage and that the obesity comes about in that way. This has not yet been proven. But it also changes the view we have about the treatments of obesity. If it were all psychologic and an issue of nutritional information, perhaps all could be rectified by reeducating people.

What are the essentials of a good weight loss program? Is exercise an important feature?

The first essential of a good weight loss program is that it be something that someone can follow forever. There should be no such thing as a diet in the sense that you change food intake for a certain period of time, and then treatment ends and maintenance occurs. If one eats 2800 calories a day and is obese, one has to drop down by several hundred calories, slowly lose the weight, and keep it down.

Included in this very modest change in caloric intake would be an effort to increase caloric output by doing physical activity. Strangely, physical activity has an additional beneficial effect: people have reported that it is somewhat easier to comply with a diet when physical activity is increased. So it may be that the ability to adhere to a diet is greater when individuals perform physical activity.

Some health care professionals specializing in weight loss have recently questioned whether patients should be advised to lose weight, because statistics show that weight-losers are likely to regain their weight. What do you think of this attitude?

I understand this attitude, but I don't think we can afford to give up. Everyone can lose weight, but I'm not sure that everyone will lose weight and keep it off. As a matter of fact, recent studies led us to believe that after two or more years, as many as 95% of those starting a weight loss program will be back to where they were before. Does this mean that no one should be put on such a program? No, I don't think that we can give up hope.

One of the interesting points is that a very modest weight loss may create good medical events. For example, diabetes, which often accompanies obesity, may be greatly ameliorated even by small amounts of weight loss. The same is true of hypertension. On medical grounds, the compromise of a small level of weight loss may be extremely helpful.

The fact that so few people lose weight and keep it off could be attributed to the fact that we are so deluged with advertisements for good food and with the societal and psychologic aspects of eating. On the other hand, it could be related to the biologic aspect of obesity that we don't understand. I prefer the latter theory, and we need to try to understand as much as we can before we preach to the obese.

What are the risks of being obese?

The risks are great. An increase of approximately 20% above average body weight is usually accompanied by a three- to four-fold greater likelihood of developing diabetes, hypertension, and heart disease. We estimate that nearly 40 million Americans are in this category, so it is our most prevalent nutritional disorder. I don't think that diet alone as we understand it is going to be the cure; we need to do something else to prevent or treat this disorder.

What are the risks of repeatedly gaining and losing weight?

Recently there has been concern about weight cycling—where individuals repeatedly go on and off diets. Many people do that and there has been some evidence that people who cycle this way have more diseases than those who don't. Most of the animal studies that have been looking at the effect of cycling have not shown any adverse effects. In the human studies it is extremely difficult to come to any conclusion.

Probably the people who cycle and try so hard to lose weight are also those who have medical reasons for doing this. If I tell you, "You have a touch of diabetes, and it would be a good thing to take that weight off," you may try harder to do it and bounce back and forth. Cyclers may be the ones who are trying hardest, and are also the ones who show more illness. We don't have a final answer as to whether cycling has any adverse effect; my guess is that it probably does not.

Why don't more physicians become interested in nutrition? What can be done to include more nutrition in the training of physicians?

I think those are very important questions, because if more physicians and scientists had been interested in this, perhaps we would be a little further along in understanding the whole problem. First, the pressures of health care have driven physicians to see themselves as caregivers in acute situations. The structure of our health care system is to have high-tech, intensive interventions for rather definite severe illnesses over days or, at most, weeks. Obesity is exactly the opposite; there isn't anything you can do in one day. What obesity and nutrition generally speak to are lifelong habits: slowly learning, adjusting, accommodating, doing what you can with the set of genes that you have. We are not living in an age in which physicians do this. Now I think that this is being rethought, and there is a lot of talk about prevention in medicine being terribly important if we are to reduce health care costs. Increasingly physicians may see themselves as a part of this.

The other side of it is that obesity is very difficult to understand. I think that in the next century physicians are going to be increasingly concerned with diseases in which there are interwoven genetic, behavioral, developmental, and psychosocial aspects. At the moment, this is still not the medical paradigm of what doctors do but, hopefully, it will become what doctors do.

people consume extra food when they are experiencing emotional distress, such as from anger, loneliness, boredom, or depression; these people find that eating blunts their discomfort temporarily. This emotional eating is typically *episodic*; that is, it involves binging during unusually stressful times rather than overeating consistently. Stress-related binging is more likely to be a snack-time (rather than mealtime) behavior, is often done in private, and is done more often by women than by men. Although some people of normal weight may also be emotional eaters (some studies suggest one in ten normal-weight people are), the incidence in some studies of emotional eating among overweight people is as high as three out of four people (Ganley, 1989). There is currently a movement among some psychologists to define such binge-eating as an eating disorder (Spitzer et al., 1992). (See Chapter 10.)

Although less research has been done on how *positive* emotions influence eating, it is generally recognized that happy occasions usually include food as part of the celebration. In fact, this is probably the most universal connection between emotions and eating.

You Tell Me

Every day when you get home from classes, no matter what time it is and no matter when you ate your last meal, you want something to eat.

What might explain this?

FIGURE 9.10
This Pima Native American exhibits the obesity common among members of his tribe.

Lower-than-normal resting metabolic rates and low activity levels are often involved. Another factor is that the Pima abandoned their traditional diet in the 1940s, adopting a high-fat diet.

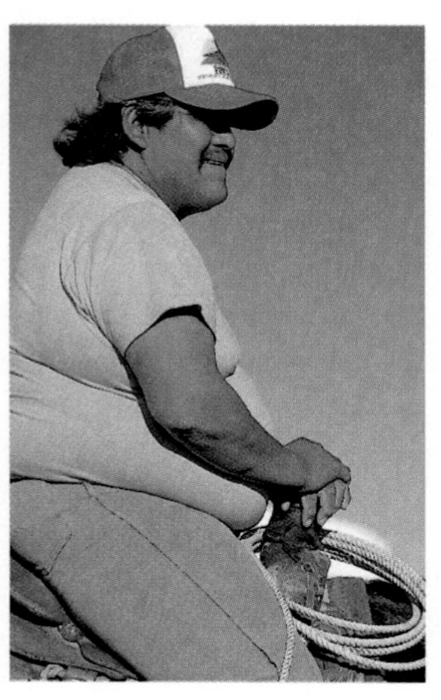

A final external factor involves people who want to change their body size. Some people deliberately eat more than they are hungry for because they want to become larger. Others, especially women, always try to eat less than they want in an attempt to control their body weight. Ironically, many such "restrained eaters" can tolerate the sense of deprivation only for limited periods, and ultimately they consume more food than they intended. In one study, the average daily kcaloric intakes of restrained eaters were actually 170 kcalories higher than the average intakes of people who were eating as much as they wanted (Kirkley et al., 1988). Some psychologists believe that restrained eaters are more responsive to external cues than are unrestrained eaters (Norvell and Kallman, 1988).

Factors Affecting Energy Output

In the case of energy output, we can also identify physiologic and nonphysiologic factors that vary among people.

Physiologic Factors In Chapter 8 (on energy), we described influences that affect your resting metabolic rate (RMR). However, we know that not all bodies function according to expectations: a few people may have RMRs that differ by as much as 30% in either direction from the metabolic rates of many of their size, sex, and age peers (Pi-Sunyer, 1988).

In a study of Pima Native Americans in the Southwest, RMRs deviated from expected levels by as much as 300 kcalories in either direction. People with the lower RMRs experienced a much higher incidence of weight gain during the four years of follow-up (Ravussin et al., 1988) (Figure 9.10). We do not know the real causes of these differences. One variable may be the amount of thyroid hormone people produce, which affects the rate at which their metabolism functions. *Hyper*thyroid individuals use more energy than those with normal thyroid activity, and *hypo*thyroid people use less energy.

Another variable may be kcalories expended for the thermic effect of food (TEF). Investigators have compared normal-weight and obese people, and obese subjects tend to use less than half the energy for TEF that normal-weight subjects use (Segal et al., 1992). When the obese people exercised after eating, their use of energy for TEF increased but did not reach the same levels expended by the normal-weight subjects who exercised after eating.

Your level of fitness may also be related to the number of kcalories you expend for TEF. People who are moderately fit seem to expend more energy for this function than do either untrained people or highly trained athletes (Poehlman and Horton, 1989). •

The extent to which our bodies may engage in adaptive thermogenesis—the "wild card" of energy use, which involves the body's thermal reaction to extreme environmental stresses—differs from one person to another. Some scientists believe that people's adaptive responses may depend on the amount of brown fat they have. (Recall from Chapter 8 that brown fat cells have more than the usual number of mitochondria.) A study done in Finland comparing the brown fat in outdoor workers and office workers found more brown fat in the outdoor workers (Sims, 1988), which might affect their ability to adapt to the cold.

Another instance of adaptive thermogenesis occurs when the expenditure of energy for RMR decreases in response to restricting kcaloric intake; that is, when you lose weight, the total number of kcalories you expend for resting metabolism decreases. Although it makes sense that RMR decreases when lean body mass is lost, some scientists believe that RMR drops to a greater extent than can be explained by losses of lean tissue (Luke and Schoeller, 1992).

Scientists disagree about whether this phenomenon actually occurs. Even those who do believe that it occurs disagree on how serious an energy deficit might cause it, or how long-lasting the effect might be. The most accurate statement we can make at this time is that the response seems to be highly individual. If you are trying to lose weight and you tend to feel chilly when others don't, and if your pulse rate has slowed down, this may be evidence that your RMR has decreased beyond the expected level.

Factors Affecting Exercise The remaining means by which we expend energy is exercise, and people are likely to vary more in this energy-use factor than in any other. Some people expend as little as a few hundred kcalories per day for physical activity, whereas others expend over a thousand kcalories for exercise per day.

What accounts for these differences? Although there are certain limiting factors, such as physical disabilities and time constraints, the amount you exercise is largely a matter of personal choice. It may be influenced by the way you feel during and after exercise. Some people feel exhilarated and increasingly powerful while exercising and pleasantly relaxed afterward. Others doing the same activity may feel breathless and inept while exercising and completely "wiped out" afterward. For the latter group, the aversive effects are likely to discourage repeat performances. Psychologists suggest that to begin to experience some benefits, these people should slow down to the point at which they can enjoy physical activity (Thayer, 1992).

Some people exercise regularly because they know it's an important factor in controlling body weight. Whatever they may think of the activity itself, they persevere with their routine because it helps them achieve or

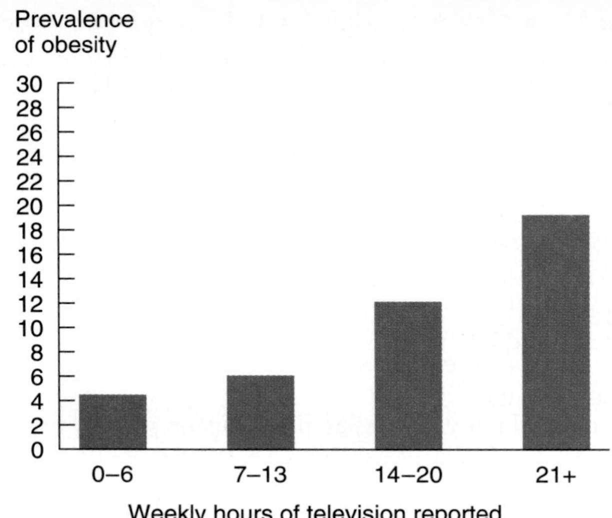

FIGURE 9.11
The more TV you watch, the more likely you are to be obese.

Among faculty, staff, and students at the Harvard School of Public Health (1986–1987), almost 20% of people who watched more than 21 hours of TV per week were obese.
Source: Reproduced from Gortmaker et al., 1990.

maintain the weight they want, or it may allow them to eat more than they could if they didn't exercise. We will say much more about the importance of exercise to weight control later in the chapter. •

People who regularly choose sedentary pursuits in preference to more physical activities are likely to have a higher body weight. A number of epidemiologic studies involving TV watching demonstrate this. Research regarding TV habits of children (Gortmaker, 1990), employed men (Tucker and Friedman, 1989), and employed women (Tucker and Bagwell, 1991) all show that the incidence of obesity is higher among people who watch more TV. Figure 9.11 shows similar data from still another study.

The authors of these studies are careful to point out that their data do not prove that the TV watching and consequent reduction in physical activity completely explain the incidence of obesity. It is possible, for example, that people who are overweight do not feel comfortable being physically active and therefore watch more TV. Another possibility is that watching TV may encourage people to increase their food intake.

Other studies have compared the energy obese people expend for physical activity to the energy normal-weight people expend. Overall, obese subjects used more kcalories for physical activity, but they used fewer kcalories per unit of body weight (Schoeller and Fjeld, 1991).

Energy expenditure patterns begin to take shape very early in life. In one study, the energy use of newborns (who were all of normal weight at birth) was assessed a few days after birth and again after three months. Although the energy intakes and resting metabolic rates of the infants were similar, their use of energy for physical activity was not: some infants used approximately 20% less energy. By one year of age, the infants who expended less energy for activity had become overweight; the others were of normal weight. It is interesting to note that the babies who were overweight at one year all had overweight mothers (Roberts et al., 1988).

The results of this study may cause you to wonder whether activity patterns could be inherited. In fact, one group of researchers does suggest there may be inherited differences in spontaneous levels of activity (Perusse et al., 1989). This leads us to our next topic—whether heredity or environment ultimately determines what you weigh.

Body Weight—A Question of Genetics or Environment?

There is no question that particular levels of body fatness tend to run in families (Figure 9.12). *This in itself does not prove that you inherit the predisposition to a certain body weight*; body weight is also affected by the environmental influences of diet and activity habits, which members of families may share.

Part of the problem in defining genetic and environmental influences on body weight is that scientists do not know enough about human genetics. They do not know how many or which **genes** ultimately affect factors that influence energy use and body mass. But scientists can classify people by a **phenotypic** characteristic, such as body weight. Then they try to design studies that separate the genetic and environmental components.

One classic approach is to study the incidence of similar phenotypes in identical twins either raised together or in separate homes that provided different environments. One such twin study showed a strong correlation in the body mass indices of twins reared apart (Stunkard et al., 1990); still another found that overfed twin pairs deposited body fat in the same places (Bouchard et al., 1990).

There has also been research involving people who were adopted as infants. When their adult weights were compared with those of their biologic parents and those of their adoptive parents, the weights of the adoptees were more similar to those of their biologic parents (Stunkard et al., 1986). Another study involved body mass index of adult adoptees and their biologic and adoptive relatives; it also found a correlation between the adoptees and their biologic relatives but not their adoptive relatives (Sorensen et al., 1992).

Various studies have attempted to determine whether genetics influences one side of the energy balance equation more than the other. One group concluded that *energy intake* is more influenced by cultural than genetic factors (Perusse et al., 1988). Other studies suggest that *energy output* may be substantially affected by genetics (Roberts et al., 1988; Ravussin et al., 1988).

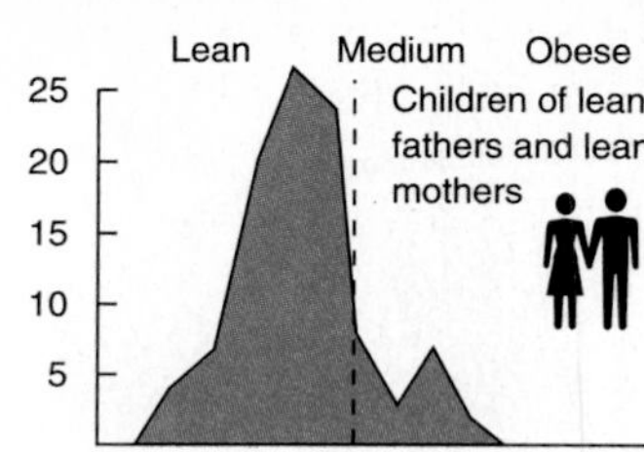

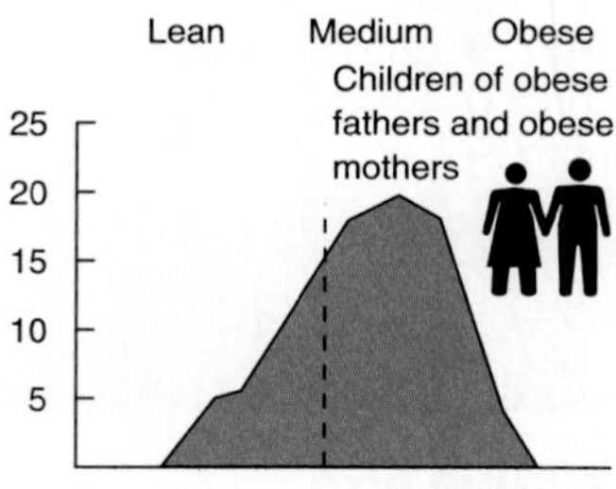

FIGURE 9.12
Body weight runs in families.

If both of your biologic parents have a similar level of fatness, the odds are that you will, too. Is this the effect of genetics or environment? Studies suggest that both factors play a role.
Source: Adapted from Garn, 1985.

gene—biologic unit of heredity within the nucleus of a cell, consisting of a segment of DNA

phenotype—an observable characteristic of a person that is determined both by genetics and environment

You Tell Me

People invest a great deal of money, time, and effort in weight-loss diets, equipment, and support services.

Assume for a moment that your weight is too high. If you knew to what extent genetics and environment were responsible for your body weight, how would that information influence your weight loss goals or the methods you would use to achieve them?

Prerequisites for Weight Loss

To begin this section, we quote from the beginning of a National Institutes of Health Statement on weight loss and control (1992): "A health paradox exists in modern America. On the one hand, many people who do not need to lose weight are trying to. On the other hand, most who do need to lose weight are not succeeding." So to start this section, it makes sense to ask, *do you really need to lose fat?* And if so, *how can you be successful?*

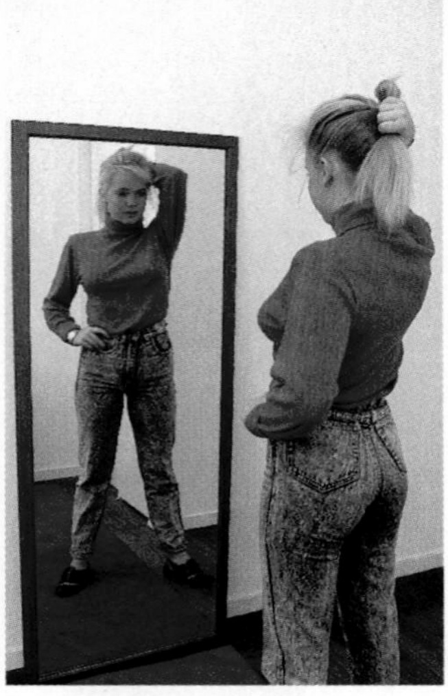

FIGURE 9.13
Be reasonable about your weight.

If your weight falls within the guidelines for good health and allows you to function well, then don't try to lose weight: you could get trapped in weight cycling, or "yo-yo dieting."

Determining Whether You Really Need to Lose Fat

If you haven't already done so, use the standards earlier in this chapter to determine whether you are overweight. If you are—and especially if you have risk factors for diseases that are related to excess fat—then you are a candidate for weight loss.

But if you are within the recommended guidelines and simply want to lose weight for cosmetic reasons, be forewarned that it is not recommended that you do so. To maintain a lower weight could mean that you would be hungry most of the time; furthermore, if you became severely underweight, you could suffer actual harm. More likely, though, you could become caught in the futile cycle of losing and regaining weight (commonly called "yo-yo dieting"), which is unhealthy both physiologically and psychologically.

Also, there are some people who should not attempt weight loss unless a physician gives the go-ahead. These include women who are pregnant or nursing, children, people over the age of 65, people with medical conditions that make weight loss dangerous, and people with psychologic problems that might be aggravated with weight loss (National Institutes of Health, 1992; Kolasa et al., 1991).

In the remainder of the material on weight loss in this chapter, we will talk directly to *you* about how to lose fat; don't think, though, that we are implying that you as an individual *need* to lose! Let's consider, then, what's involved in choosing a fat loss program.

Taking a Positive Attitude

It is amazing how many claims, theories, and treatments for losing weight have been developed: information about more than 30,000 of them has been collected at Johns Hopkins University. In the short run, all of these methods are successful for some people but unsuccessful for others. What's really important, though, is the *long-term outcome.*

When the *long-term* results of various methods have been evaluated, 80% or more of those people who lost weight regained their losses eventually (Pi-Sunyer, 1988). Even people who had so much success in commercial programs that their "before" and "after" pictures were used in newspaper advertisements have been found to backslide. In one study, 72% who had given this public testimony had regained 5 pounds or more 20 months later (Fatis et al., 1989). The data against long-term success seem so overwhelming that the American Medical Association's Council on Scientific Affairs pronounced that "it is more likely that a person will be cured of most forms of cancer than of obesity" (1988). (Although many experts may prefer to think in terms of "sustained remission" rather than a "cure" for obesity, the Council statement makes its point effectively.)

All of this seems pretty discouraging to the would-be weight loser, but you should keep several points in mind. For one thing, most available statistics are from a limited sampling of formal programs, and they may not be representative of the outcome of all weight-loss attempts. But no matter what the failure rate, the good news is that some people have succeeded in losing weight and keeping it off, and we can apply what has been learned from their experience to help others. The fact is that *weight loss is possible for most overweight people if they go about it in a way that favors success.*

Another important point is that although achieving and maintaining your best body weight is an important health goal, you do not necessarily need to drop all the way down to your recommended weight to get health benefits. Even the loss of part of the excess can improve risk factors associated with overweight. For example, a study that tested different methods of lowering blood pressure in people in the high–normal range found that a modest weight loss (averaging 8½ pounds) was more effective in lowering blood pressure than was reducing sodium intake, managing stress, or taking selected nutritional supplements (TOHP Collaborative Research Group, 1992).

Developing Combined, Gradual, Sustained Approaches

Then how can you lose weight and keep it off? First of all, realize that excess body weight is usually a multifactorial condition; like other health problems that have a number of contributing factors, you'll likely need a combination of strategies to deal with it. Studies have shown that people who succeed at weight loss are generally those who *simultaneously improve their eating habits, get a moderate amount of exercise, and use individually appropriate ways to support their gradual shift to new behaviors* (Kayman et al., 1990; Foreyt and Goodrick, 1991). In recent years, programs developed by health professionals have included these three elements, and commercial programs are being urged to follow suit (Petersmarck, 1992).

Also, realize that it took time for surplus fat to accumulate, and it will take time to lose it. *You should try to lose no more than 1 pound per week.* If you lose weight at this rate, you have a far better chance of sustaining your losses than if you try to lose faster. Remember, 1 pound of adipose tissue has the energy potential of approximately 3500 kcalories. To lose 1 pound per week, therefore, you must use 500 more kcalories per day than you take in; to lose ½ pound per week, a deficit of 250 kcalories per day is necessary. The best way to do this is to reduce your kcalorie intake moderately and increase your energy output slightly.

In addition, *for weight loss to be permanent, your lifestyle change must be permanent.* A number of the most responsible fat-loss programs screen prospective clients as to their commitment to making enduring lifestyle changes; a person who is not so determined is advised to delay attempting weight loss.

You Tell Me

An ad in the newspaper says, "Lose weight before the swimsuit season starts! Six pounds the first week and three pounds each week for a month . . . guaranteed!"

If you lose weight at this rate, is it likely to stay off?

The Three Elements of a Successful Fat Loss Program

Now let's look at the three important components of a weight-loss program: appropriate eating, moderate exercise, and support for new behaviors.

Eating to Achieve Fat Loss

The nutritional aspect of a fat-loss program should accomplish all of the following:

- Provide all the nutrients your body needs without as many kcalories as you have been eating.

- Improve your overall health.
- Keep you from being hungry or unusually tired.
- Satisfy your taste preferences and allow yourself occasional "treat" foods.
- Consist of foods that are easy to get at the grocery store and when eating away from home.
- Help you modify your eating habits for lifelong use.

You can develop your own eating plan to meet the above criteria; people who plan their own programs are more likely to lose weight and keep it off (Kayman et al., 1990). (Preplanned diets cannot take into account your individual food preferences or lifestyle, but if you prefer to use a published diet or a weight-loss service, be sure it has the characteristics described above. Many do not.)

At this point, you need to decide how to manage your energy intake—whether you will monitor kcalorie intake or fat intake (which ultimately is related to kcalorie intake). The following sections describe these different approaches.

Controlling Overall Kcalorie Intake To use this method, first you need to know what your typical energy usage is for one day. Table 8.3 and Act on Fact 8.1 give you methods of estimating your current daily kcaloric expenditure.

Then, to lose weight, plan for fewer kcalories than you now consume. Don't cut back too far; remember, an increase in exercise (discussed in the next section) should account for part of the energy deficit. Let's say that you plan to increase your energy output by 100 kcalories per day; then, to lose 1 pound per week, you need to reduce your intake by 400 kcalories per day from what it now is.

Next, use the recommendations of the Food Guide Pyramid to determine the number of servings of food from each food group you should eat daily, taking into account their kcalorie contents. Then distribute these servings among the meals and snacks you have in a typical day.

Act on Fact 9.1 on page 294 shows typical kcalorie values for servings of different kinds of foods and provides a worksheet for planning this type of program. Foods included on the chart have relatively low kcalorie values; higher-kcalorie foods are less suitable for routine use. However, you can plan for limited amounts of higher-kcalorie foods you especially enjoy by listing them in the fats, oils, and sweets section and including them as your kcalorie limit and eating pattern permit.

This is a classic approach to individualized diet planning that has been used for decades. Some people like this method because once they learn their pattern, it becomes quite easy to decide what to eat at each meal. However, others feel that it is too inflexible and restrictive, and it seems to call for limiting yourself to eating only the most simple foods and avoiding many of the combination items that provide convenience and variety.

However, the marketplace now provides an increasing number of items that combine low-kcalorie ingredients into interesting convenience foods, such as single-serving entrees and even desserts. If you want to use these products, be aware of the meaning of the terms used in labeling them. Table 9.4 defines these terms according to recent federal regulations. Many of these foods also contain low-kcalorie or no-kcalorie fat substitutes (Table 6.2) and sugar substitutes (Table 5.2) to provide levels of sweetness and perceptions of fatness that you prefer.

TABLE 9.4 Legal Label Language

By February, 1994, these terms on U.S. food product labels will have the following meanings:

Calorie-free:	Contains fewer than 5 kcalories per serving
Low-calorie:	Contains fewer than 40 kcalories per serving
Reduced-calorie:	Has 25% fewer kcalories than reference foods
Sugar-free:	Contains less than 0.5 gram of sugar per serving
Fat-free:	Contains less than 0.5 gram of fat per serving
Low-fat:	Contains 3 grams or less of fat per serving
Light or lite:	Contains at least one-third fewer kcalories or 50% less fat than the reference product

Controlling Fat Intake In the past, a number of reports from animal and human studies indicated that *the correlation between body weight and fat intake is greater than the correlation between body weight and* ***total kcalorie*** *intake* (Dattilo, 1992). In recent years, interest in this idea has been increasing, and newer studies have reinforced the earlier findings (Miller, 1991; Klesges et al., 1992).

Other studies show that when people lower their intake of fat, they lose weight without consciously restricting overall food or kcaloric intake (Sheppard et al., 1991; Kendall et al., 1991; Prewitt et al., 1991).

You can see why a low-fat diet might be a more successful method for long-term fat loss. Because fat has the highest kcalorie potential of all the energy nutrients, cutting down your intake of fat will bring about a greater reduction in kcalories than limiting any other energy nutrient. By choosing lower-fat versions of foods you already consume, you can eat the same volume of food, get fewer kcalories, and lose weight. This approach is also psychologically more comfortable, because once you have made your food choices, you do not need to be conscious of restricting your kcalorie intake.

Therefore, the idea of losing weight by focusing on dietary fat has been gaining ground. The levels of fat intake that resulted in weight loss in the studies above ranged from 20% to 25% of kcalories as fat; this can serve as a goal for people who want to lose weight. For a person who consumes 35–40% of kcalories from fat (the average American consumption), this would be a significant reduction.

Act on Fact 9.2 on page 296 guides you through planning the food part of a weight-loss program using this method. The many low-fat foods on the market provide a variety of interesting and palatable selections, and many recently published cookbooks can help you produce such foods at home.

Exercising to Achieve Fat Loss

Regular moderate exercise has many health benefits. It increases energy output and may help regulate hunger. If the exercise you do helps you retain your lean body mass, it can help maintain your resting metabolic rate as you lose weight. Exercise can also reduce stress, improve cardiovascular health, reduce the risk of Type II diabetes, and help maintain strength and flexibility. Although the extent to which exercise can achieve some of these effects is controversial, one thing that is *not* controversial is that exercise is an effective component of a weight-loss and maintenance program (Foreyt

continued on page 298

Plan for Controlling Kcalorie Intake

There are various approaches to reducing body fat; one is to reduce intake of kcalories as described in the steps below.

1. Record current daily energy use (output) from Table 8.3 or Act on Fact 8.1. (a) 2150 kcal
2. Indicate planned daily increase in exercise. + (b) 100 kcal
3. Calculate future daily energy output (a + b). (c) 2250 kcal
4. Check weight you intend to lose per week, and fill in corresponding daily decrease in kcalories required:

   Rate of Loss............................Daily decrease in kcalories

   ______ ½ pound/week.........250 kcalories/day
   __√__ 1 pound/week.........500 kcalories/day } (d) −500 kcal
5. Calculate future daily kcalorie intake (c − d) 1750 kcal
6. Choose daily number of servings to achieve both recommended number of servings and approximate kcalorie goal.

Food Group	Kcal/ Serv.	Rec. Number of Servings	Servings for You	Kcalories from Your Serv.
Bread, rice, cereal, pasta	80	6–11	8	640
Vegetables	25	3–5	3	75
Fruits	60	2–4	3	180
Milk products		2–3		
Skim milk	90		2	180
Low-fat milk	120			
Meat, poultry, fish, eggs, beans		equivalent to 5–7 oz. meat		
Lean meat (per oz.)	55		4	220
Med. fat meat (per oz.)	75			
Egg (1)	75			
Beans (½ cup)	110		1	110
Fats, oils, and sweets				
Fats (per t.)	45		2	90
Sugar (per t.)	20			
Higher-kcalorie foods:				
frozen low-fat yogurt	90		1	90
cheese, 1 oz.	110		1	110
3 t. jam	60		1	60
TOTAL KCALORIES (close to value in step 5 above)..				1755 kcal

7. Distribute the number of servings from all groups into a pattern of intended intake for the day. You do not necessarily need to plan to eat five times per day if you do not ordinarily eat that often, but it is recommended that you eat at least three times per day.
8. When you have reached your goal weight, maintain the same pattern of exercising and eating. If you continue to lose weight, gradually add a serving or two to your pattern until your weight stabilizes.

	Breakfast 1	2	Lunch 3	Dinner 4	5
Bread, rice, cereal, pasta	3	1	2	1	1
Vegetables			1	2	
Fruits	2		1		
Milk products					
Skim milk	1			1	
Low-fat milk					
Meat, poultry, fish, eggs, beans					
Lean meat, poultry, fish (oz.)				4	
Med. fat meat (oz.)					
Egg (1)					
Beans (½ cup)			1		
Fats, oils, and sweets					
Fats (per t.)			1	1	
Sugar (per t.)					
Frozen yogurt, ½ cup					1
Cheese, 1 oz.			1		
Jam, 3 t.	1				

(Items that are almost kcalorie-free can be used without restriction: for example, many beverages, sugar-free gelatin dessert, broth, and most fat-free salad dressings.)

Plan for Controlling Fat Intake

Surveys show that Americans' average intake of fat is 35–40% of total kcaloric intake. Research shows that many people can lose weight by decreasing their fat consumption to 20% of kcalories but otherwise not consciously limiting their food intake. A way to achieve this is shown below.

1. From the chart below, find the number of grams of fat that approximate 20% of your kcaloric intake. (If you have done Act on Fact 6.1 to determine 30% of calories from fat, simply calculate ⅔ of that value to get a more individualized recommendation.)

20% Fat Chart

	Men		Women	
Weight in Pounds	Ages 19–50	Ages 51+	Ages 19–50	Ages 51+
	g of fat	g of fat	g of fat	g of fat
220	86	66	81	65
210	82	63	78	62
200	78	60	74	59
190	74	57	70	56
180	70	54	66	53
170	66	52	63	50
160	62	49	59	47
150	58	46	56	44
140	54	43	52	42
130	50	40	48	38
120	47	37	44	36
110	43	34	41	32
100	39	31	37	29

This chart was derived from the 1989 Recommended Dietary Allowances for average energy allowances.
Source: Adapted from *Finding the fat in food,* 1991.

Fill in your fat budget here: 66 grams of fat/day.

2. On the form below, write down a typical day's intake for yourself, and record each item's fat content, adjusting for serving sizes. You have access to many sources of fat values: Appendix C, product labels, the chart in Act on Fact 6.1, Table 6.3, and Table 8.4. After you have recorded all values, total the grams of fat.

Food	Amount	Fat (Grams)
Granola	3/4 cup	15
2% milk	3/4 cup	5
Banana	1	0
Quarter-pound (QP) cheeseburger	1	29
Milkshake	1	9
French fries	1 regular	12
Cola	12 oz. can	0
Canned spaghetti	1-1/2 cups	15
Lettuce	1/4 head	0
Blue cheese dressing	4 T.	32
2% milk	1-1/2 cups	7
Bread and butter	1 slice, 1 t.	4
		Total Fat 128 **Grams**

Is your typical intake higher than your fat budget?

___√___ yes _______ no

If yes, by how much? ___62___ grams excess

If no, are you sure you need to lose weight?

3. In the spaces below, write down two relatively easy changes you can make immediately to decrease your fat intake, and think about other changes to implement once you have become accustomed to the first two.

	Instead of This:	Use This:	Fat (g) Less
Immediate changes	QP cheeseburger	lean QP cheeseburger	19
	granola	Wheat Chex	14
Later changes	2% milk	skim milk (2¼ c)	10
	Blue cheese dressing	(half the amount)	16

4. From now on, as you go through the day, keep track of the number of fat grams you consume. Gradually reduce your daily intake of fat until you're eating within your fat budget. (At first, you will probably need to record your intake to check your fat consumption, but as you become familiar with the values, you will probably no longer need to write down your intake.)

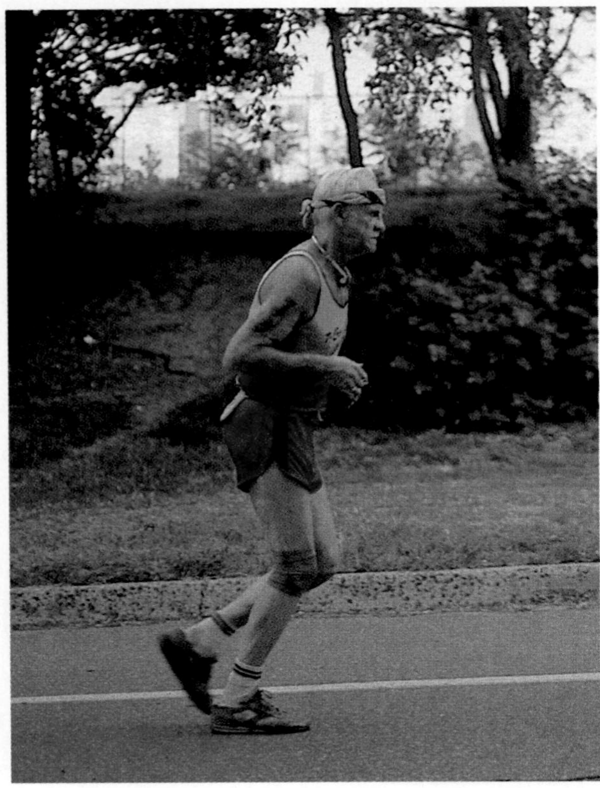

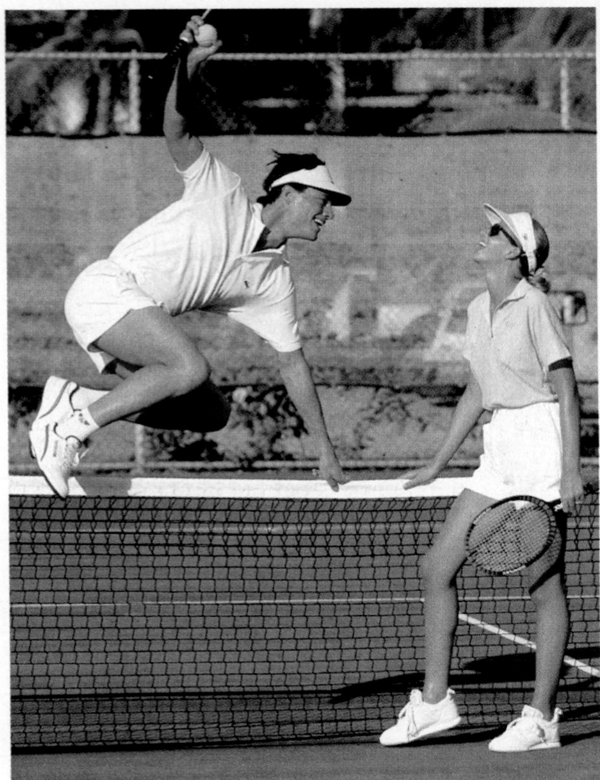

FIGURE 9.14
Easy does it.

You don't have to be on a brutal program to get the benefits of exercise; in fact, it's better if you're not. It's also important that you enjoy whatever activity you do so that you will do it regularly.

and Goodrick, 1991; National Institutes of Health, 1992). Of course, independent of weight loss, exercise is important for all people for maintaining **fitness**.

fitness—the ability to meet the physical and psychologic demands of everyday living; includes good heart and lung function, muscular strength and endurance, flexibility, and body composition

Aerobic Exercise When considering exercise to help lose body fat, you should focus primarily on aerobic exercise.

Before you begin an exercise program, it is a good idea to have a medical examination, especially if you are more than 30% overweight, smoke, have been diagnosed with health problems, or are over the age of 65. Your doctor may recommend getting professional help in planning the program and may advise you to work out in a supervised setting.

The aerobic exercise component of a fat-loss program should satisfy all of the following criteria (McArdle and Toner, 1988):

- Be a type of exercise that uses a large muscle mass in rhythmic, sustainable activity.
- Be safe and adaptable to any physical limitations you may have.
- Provide pleasure and be relatively convenient for you.
- Be done at sufficient intensity, frequency, and duration to achieve results.

Some of the types of activities that fit the first criterion are walking, jogging, running, bicycling, swimming, water walking, cross-country skiing, and aerobic dancing. Choose an activity that you enjoy, because you will be more likely to do it often enough for it to benefit you (Figure 9.14). Another important factor is that it should be relatively convenient for you; no matter how much you like swimming, it is not a practical choice if it

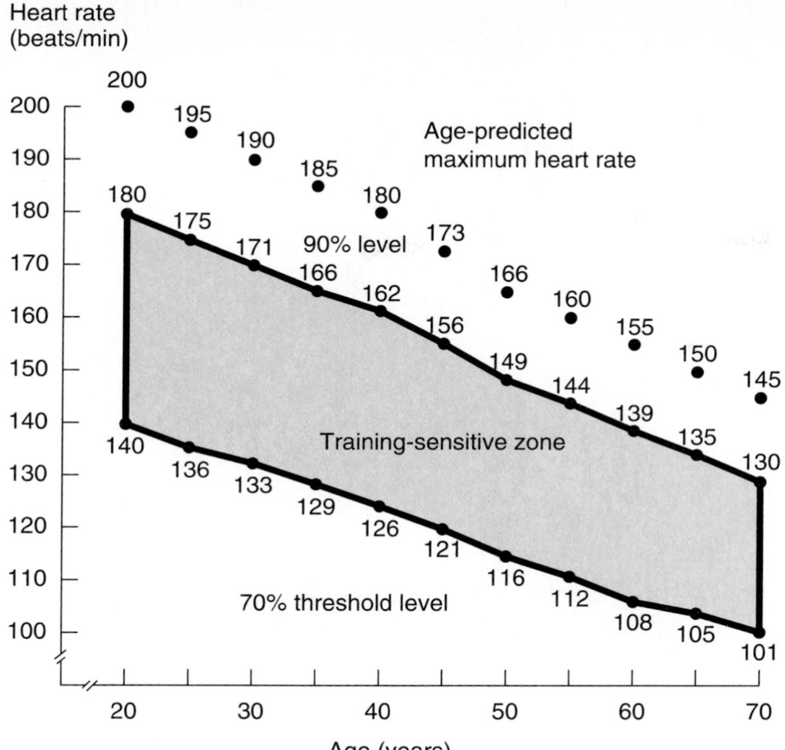

FIGURE 9.15
Recommended training heart rate ranges for age.

To get weight-loss and cardiovascular benefits from physical activity, many experts suggest that the intensity should bring your pulse within the training-sensitive zone for your age.
Source: McArdle et al., 1991.

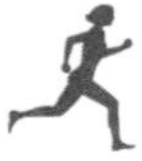

takes you 45 minutes to get to the nearest pool. Probably best of all is to have several activities that you enjoy and have easy access to, so that you can have some variety.

There are other things to consider. Do you prefer to work out alone, or would you enjoy the company of a group? There are organized programs for many of the activities mentioned above; they offer camaraderie, encourage regular participation, and provide help with monitoring your progress and modifying your program as your training state improves. However, if you like to be independent, being on your own allows you more flexibility regarding when and where you exercise.

To benefit you, your exercise program needs to meet criteria for intensity, frequency, and duration. Your workout should be at an intensity that brings your heart rate into the recommended training range for your age, as shown in Figure 9.15. If you exercise within your range, you will experience various physiologic effects over time, such as improved heart and lung function and greater metabolism of fat during exercise. Figure 9.16 illustrates how to take your pulse.

How often do you need to exercise to help lose weight? Studies have shown that you should work out at least three times per week to affect your body weight and/or skinfold thickness (McArdle and Toner, 1988). Many programs recommend three to five exercise sessions per week. People often find that if they take an occasional day off from programmed exercising, they are eager to get back to it the next day.

What about duration? The experts suggest that a workout should be long enough for you to expend about 300 kcalories. Because energy expenditure during activity is a function of the type and intensity of activity, of your body weight, and of the length of time you do it, it is best to calculate workout times for your chosen sport(s) and your own body weight. Table 8.1 (in the energy chapter) lists the energy costs of various activities

FIGURE 9.16
How to determine your heart rate.

Once you stop exercising, immediately place the middle fingers of your right hand over your carotid artery at the left side of your neck where you can easily feel the pulse, usually about 1 inch below your jaw. Do not press hard; this can slow the rate. Count your pulse for 10 seconds and multiply by 6 to get your heart rate per minute. Figure 9.15 shows training heart rates at various age ranges.

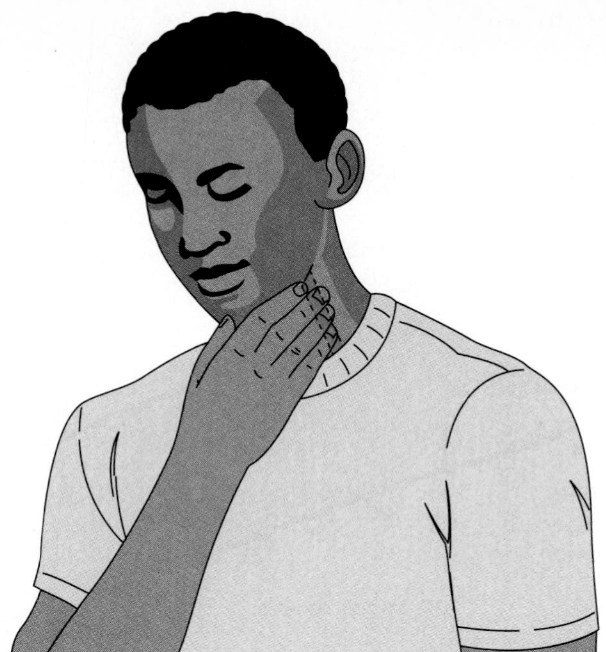

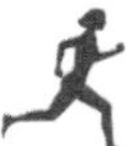

based on kcalories per kilogram per minute. In general, a person doing moderate to vigorous activity will need to exercise for 20–30 minutes to burn 300 kcalories; someone exercising at a lower intensity may need to work out for 40–60 minutes (McArdle and Toner, 1988).

If you are unaccustomed to much physical activity and you are starting an exercise program, it is best to begin at a lower intensity and duration (for example, 10–15 minutes) and eventually build up to the levels we have described here. Doing too much too soon puts you at risk of overtiredness, soreness, and injury; it is far better to work up gradually to a full program. For some people, this may take as long as 8–10 weeks.

Deliberate exercise sessions that are set apart from the performance of routine daily activities are not the only way to increase energy usage. You can, for example, walk part of the way instead of drive to school or work, take stairs during the day instead of elevators, and move around during breaks instead of sitting. Although these activities may be hard to measure and some may be of short duration, they can, if done regularly, contribute significantly to overall energy expenditure.

If you want to develop an exercise program by yourself and feel that you need more guidance about how to proceed, you can get information prepared by the American College of Sports Medicine that describes and illustrates safe and effective conditioning programs for people of various initial fitness levels: *The ACSM Fitness Book* (1992) is a paperback book available from Leisure Press in Champaign, Illinois.

Exercise for Strength and Flexibility Important as aerobic exercise is, there are other types of exercise that contribute to overall health and fitness whether you are trying to lose weight or not.

For people whose everyday activities do not involve handling heavy objects, a program of progressive weight lifting can help build strength. In its 1990 position statement on developing and maintaining fitness in healthy adults, the American College of Sports Medicine advocated strength train-

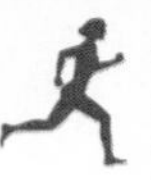

ing in addition to aerobic exercise for Americans. It is important to assess your capability first and to start your program slowly. Again, it helps to have guidelines from a responsible source such as the *ACSM Fitness Book*.

Flexibility tends to decrease with age, but doing appropriate exercises can help maintain this quality. For these types of exercises, too, see a credible fitness book. •

Providing Support for Your New Behaviors

The support part of a weight-loss program includes all the mental and psychologic aspects of developing new eating and exercise behaviors and sticking with them. These methods are called **behavior modification techniques.** They should do all of the following:

behavior modification techniques—carefully planned methods for changing living habits

- Provide training in the steps of the behavior modification process (see Chapter 2): keeping a record of your current behaviors, setting realistic goals, evaluating why you practice unwanted behaviors, planning for and implementing gradual change, rewarding yourself, thinking positively, monitoring your progress, and fine-tuning your program.
- Teach behavioral techniques for maintaining motivation, coping with temptations to deviate from your eating and exercise programs, and reducing future slip-ups.
- Help you to identify people who will support you in your new attitudes and lifestyle—as well as those who might sabotage your efforts.

One of the more recently added features of behavior modification for weight loss is **relapse prevention**. Using this technique, first you *identify which kinds of situations were likely to be high risk for you.* Situations that commonly cause people to overeat are experiencing negative emotions when alone, feeling positive emotions when with others, and being very hungry (Goodrick and Foreyt, 1991). Let's say that for you, feeling lonely is a situation that increases your temptation to overeat.

relapse prevention—method for reducing the likelihood of backsliding into unintended behaviors

Next, you *plan ahead how you might ward off overindulgence when those situations arise*. For example, you might imagine a time when you feel lonely. You want to eat to blunt your feelings; but you picture yourself deciding to react in a way that is more in keeping with your goals, and you call a friend and make plans to get together. Practice these situations repeatedly in your mind so that when they occur, the new behavior will be familiar. Even with such preparation, people sometimes lapse from their intended behaviors; a relapse prevention program teaches how to cope immediately after a lapse and get back on track.

Table 9.5 gives an example of guidelines given in a residential program. It shows that all elements of this weight-control program are interwoven—the food, the exercise, and the attitudinal and behavioral components. Together, these elements help the person cope with food cravings.

Unfortunately, relapse prevention is not successful for some people. Especially when experiencing strongly negative emotions, they may use food to blunt their feelings or to make themselves feel better (Kayman et al., 1991). At such times, they may be unable to call upon the rational techniques they have learned, much as a drug-dependent person might have difficulties in a situation of stress (Goodrick and Foreyt, 1991). When food is used excessively and frequently to deal with emotional issues, such behaviors might be classified as eating disorders, which are discussed more fully in Chapter 10.

Another important aspect of behavior modification programs is the emphasis on social support. Many people benefit considerably from having

TABLE 9.5 10 Tips for Managing Food Cravings

1 Eat at least three well-balanced meals a day. It's a normal physiological reaction to crave food if you're hungry. Even if you're trying to lose weight, don't skip meals. You'll only be hungrier for the next one, and cravings between meals can become overwhelming. Plan meals daily based on a variety of foods including plenty of whole grains, fruits and vegetables with moderate amounts of low-fat dairy products and lean meats, fish, poultry and other protein foods.

2 Give up guilt. One brownie never made anyone fat, but your attitude about eating brownies or any foods you see as forbidden can make you fat. Believing you have cheated on your diet and completely ruined your chances of succeeding produces guilt and feelings of failure. It also can cause you to give up on yourself and your attempts at managing your weight. Give yourself permission to eat favorite foods in moderation and without guilt.

3 Accept food cravings as a normal part of living in a food-oriented society. Almost everyone experiences food cravings, regardless of whether they struggle with their weight. The more you understand your cravings, the better you will be able to manage them. Food cravings occur when you are exposed to physical cues such as the sight and smell of baking bread or buffets at holiday parties. Emotional cues such as arguments with your boss can also bring on cravings. In that instance, your cravings really may be a desire to soothe unpleasant feelings with the pleasure you derive from a certain food. While you cannot control the fact that cravings occur, you can control your reaction.

4 Think "management" instead of "control." "Control" implies an adversarial relationship with food; it's generally a constant struggle to maintain control. "Management" is much easier. When we manage something, we work *with* it to achieve our desired results.

5 Look at cravings as suggestions to eat, not commands to overindulge. Overeating does not have to be an automatic response to a craving. Instead of being a helpless victim, take charge. When a craving begins, determine how you want to deal with it. Will you decide to eat now or later, or not at all? Will you choose to eat exactly what you're craving, or try something else? Will you elect to eat a little or a lot? It truly is up to you.

6 Believe that cravings will pass. Relapse prevention researchers have found that people believe a craving will continue to intensify until they give in to it. Actually, a craving is similar to a wave in the ocean. It grows in intensity, peaks and then subsides if you do not give in. Picture yourself as a surfer who is trying to "ride the wave" instead of being wiped out by it. The more you practice riding the wave, the easier it will become.

7 Disarm your cravings with the 5 D's. *Delay* at least 10 minutes before you eat so that your action is conscious, not impulsive. *Distract* yourself by engaging in an activity that requires concentration and is not compatible with eating. *Distance* yourself from the food—leave the room, ask the waiter to remove your plate, don't park at the food court entrance to the mall. *Determine* how important it really is for you to eat the craved food and how much you really want it. *Decide* what amount is reasonable and appropriate, eat it slowly and enjoy.

8 Stop labeling foods as "bad," "illegal" or "forbidden." It's not the food itself that's the problem, but the quantities you consume and how often you consume them. You can eat *some* of anything you want—even if it is high in fat, calories, sugar or salt—but if you want to reach your weight and health goals, you may not be able to eat *all* of everything you want.

9 Aim for moderation instead of abstinence. Avoiding things you fear only reinforces the fear. If you think you can never eat certain foods again, you may feel driven to eat as much as you can whenever you can. And if you think certain foods are "triggers" to overeating, you may create a self-fulfilling prophecy. Occasionally practice enjoying reasonable amounts of favorite high-fat or high-calorie foods. You may be happier and better able to stay with a well-balanced plan for healthy living. To make moderation easier to put into action, purchase single-serving sizes of favorite foods.

10 Exercise regularly. Just as it is vital to successfully managing your weight, exercise is key to managing food cravings. Rather than burning calories, the most important contribution of regular exercise may be relief from tension due to anxieties about food cravings. It's also one way to delay, distance and distract yourself from food.

(Reproduced with permission of Green Mountain at Fox Run, Ludlow, Vermont, a residentially based weight and health management facility for women.)

others around them who are aware of their efforts and provide encouragement and reinforcement; others prefer to "go it alone."

Support can come from different sources. A number of studies have shown that weight losses increase when a key family member learns how to be supportive (Buckmaster and Brownell, 1988). Others may prefer encouragement from a trained health care professional; one study showed that the people in a university-based weight loss program who were most successful were those who had made the most visits to the clinic (Fitzwater et al., 1991). Some self-help groups can also provide effective support. Those that are extensions of professionally run behavior modification programs have the best records (Buckmaster and Brownell, 1988).

One final thought on the matter of social support: some relationships can be negative. If you are trying to lose weight, consider whether anybody around you might want to sabotage your efforts, such as an overweight friend who might feel your weight loss would put pressure on him or her. You will need to consider how to get around these negative influences.

You Tell Me

Some people, in an effort to acquire weight-loss skills and get behavioral support, have hired personal nutrition coaches, or "diet cops," who take them firmly in hand and walk them through a personalized regimen. The coach might even make a house call to help a client clean the kitchen cupboards of foods not on the program, or they might go shopping together to buy foods that are acceptable.

What would be the pros and cons of having your own "diet cop"?

Preplanned Programs You may be wondering why we have not discussed the many popular books and commercial services that promise weight loss. Why not simply use one of them?

We have deliberately not identified and discussed them here, because the preplanned programs are not successful in the long run for most people. We repeat: the best way to lose weight and keep it off is to plan your own program that involves moderate changes in eating and exercise habits that you find acceptable for ongoing use, and that provides support for your new behaviors.

Fat Loss Methods Most People Should Avoid

People have tried many other methods to lose weight, but these methods either do not work in the long run, are appropriate for only a very few people, or are potentially dangerous. Several of these are discussed below. Other unusual methods are identified in the Slice of Life on page 304.

Programs Promoting More Than 1 Pound of Weight Loss per Week

Diets that cause you to lose more than 1 pound of weight per week are too drastic. They are too low in kcalories and carbohydrate, causing you to deplete your body's carbohydrate reserves and lose body water. Although

Slice of Life

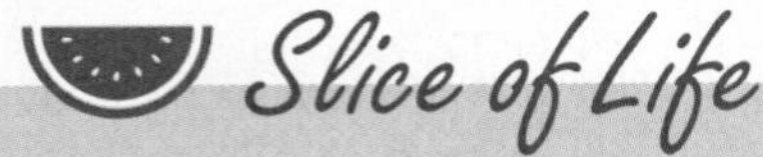

Fat Loss Fantasies

Most of us *know* that the only effective way to lose fat is to eat less and exercise more. Yet "hope springs eternal," and many people wish for ways to lose weight without having to make permanent lifestyle changes.

There is no magic bullet. Nonetheless, people have bought into many methods in hopes of losing fat, including the following:

- Weight-loss earrings that were supposed to stimulate acupuncture points to control hunger
- Flavored mouth sprays that were supposed to reduce hunger, promote vitality, and rejuvenate metabolism
- Subliminal audio tapes that were supposed to contain inaudible messages telling listeners to eat less and stick to their diets
- Wrapping of the body in plastic supposedly to mobilize fat and flush it out
- A 2-minute exercise (described in a $30 book) that was supposed to teach readers how to rub their stomachs away

WASH AWAY FAT
AND YEARS OF AGE
With La-Mar
Reducing Soap
The new discovery. Results quick and amazing—nothing internal to take. Reduce any part of body desired without affecting other parts. No dieting or exercising. Be as slim as you wish. Acts like magic in reducing double chin, abdomen, ungainly ankles, unbecoming wrists, arms and shoulders, large busts, or any superfluous fat on body.
Sold direct to you by mail, post paid, on a money-back guarantee. Price 2/- a cake or three cakes for 4/-; one to three cakes usually accomplish the purpose. Send postal or money order to-day. Surprising results. LA-MAR LABORATORIES, Ltd., 48, Rupert Street (1101.), London. W.1.
REDUCE!

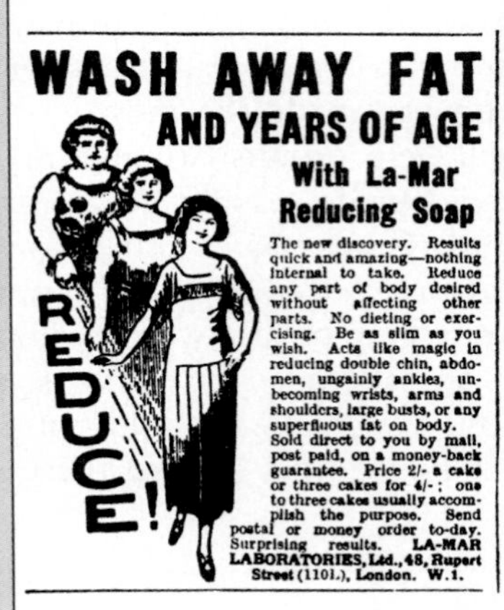

Ineffective products for reducing body fatness

People want to believe that fat can be diminished without dieting or exercising. This phenomenon is not new: over half a century ago, the ad shown here undoubtedly sparked wishful thinking in many people—with dubious results. Today's media contain hundreds of current examples.

Although you may have seen through those particular scams if they hit your area, there are hundreds of others out there waiting for you. You are vulnerable if the product is marketed in ways that appeal to you—with sophistication, or with the insinuation that only the intelligent or affluent are privy to the secret, or with a claim (unproved) of scientific authenticity.

Another ploy is the promise of fast results—but the weight you lose may not be fat. Consider the plastic wraps and various sweat suits guaranteed to make you lose weight. They make you sweat and result in temporary water loss, which registers on the scale as weight loss. Vibrating machines are marketed to wiggle the fat right off of you, but since the only energy you expend is to keep yourself upright and slightly resist the belt while it works, there is almost no benefit. Electrical muscle stimulators supposedly stimulate muscles to expend energy, but the effect is so localized and meager that benefits are negligible.

Skin creams have also been marketed for weight loss. Some of them contain irritants that cause skin to tingle and redden; you may prefer to believe the ad's claim that this is evidence that "it's working to melt away fat."

As long as there are people who want to lose weight, there will be products and services that purport to separate people from their fat. Many are only effective at separating them from their money. Let the buyer beware.

weight drops quickly in the first couple of days, only about one-fourth of the lost weight is fat, the substance you want to lose. Almost three-fourths is water, and the remainder is protein.

Furthermore, if your diet is extremely low in carbohydrate, there may not be a sufficient amount of carbohydrate to promote complete metabolism of fat, and fat fragments called *ketone bodies* or *ketoacids* are produced. Your kidneys can excrete ketoacids, but you need large amounts of water. If you don't drink enough water to compensate for urinary losses, you'll become dehydrated. Furthermore, in these circumstances you can lose electrolytes—such as potassium—in urine and accumulate ketoacids, which lower the acidity of the blood. This siutation can be life-threatening. Some people have died while on severe weight-reduction diets.

People on extreme weight-loss programs also have psychologic repercussions. These include cravings for food, which can result in mental preoccupation with food and decreased ability to concentrate on the tasks at hand. Fighting the urges to eat is stressful and can lead to mood swings and irritability.

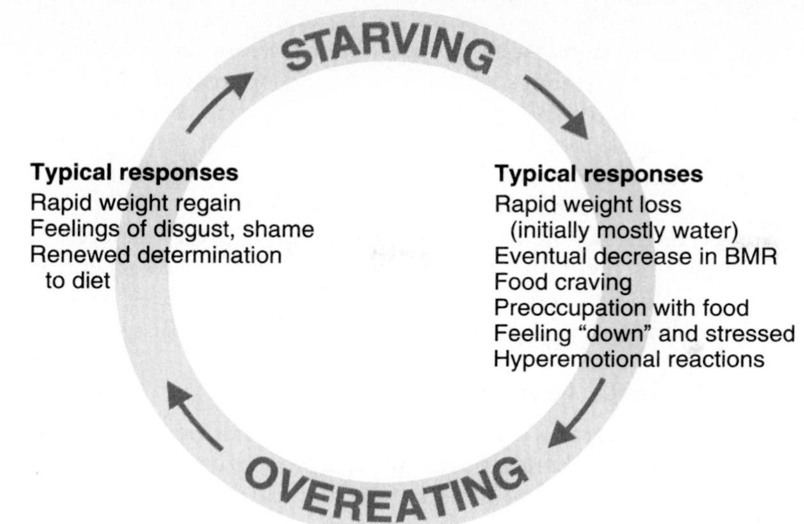

FIGURE 9.17
The vicious cycle of chronic dieting and overeating.

If a person follows a weight-loss diet that is very low in kcalories, the body and mind react against the severe deprivation, and rebound eating is likely to occur. This results in weight regain and, often, self-criticism, which may lead to another and yet another trip around the circle. A moderate approach that is more likely to succeed is described in the text.

The normal reaction to these combined physical and psychologic forces is to go off the diet and make up for the earlier food deprivation by rebound eating. If you have ever experienced this, you probably criticized yourself afterward for being weak because you could not stay on the diet. But considering how strong these physical and psychologic forces are, it's no wonder that you gave up the diet. The program failed you, not vice versa.

After regaining the weight, you may have decided to try dieting again. This can lead to a vicious cycle of dieting and overeating that makes you feel quite helpless and miserable and you may end up weighing more than you did before you started dieting. Experts call this *weight cycling* or *chronic dieting*; the popular press calls it *yo-yo dieting*. Figure 9.17 summarizes this phenomenon.

Counterproductive as it is, this chronic dieting syndrome is an eating style frequently seen in girls and women who feel pressured to be thinner than they are. It also occurs in some people with specific reasons to maintain lower-than-normal body weight, such as wrestlers, gymnasts, dancers, cheerleaders, and models.

One animal study provided a dramatic illustration of weight cycling (Brownell et al., 1986). Rats were first allowed free access to a high-fat diet that resulted in weight gain. At this point, they began the first dieting cycle, in which they were allowed only a limited amount of a low-fat diet that resulted in weight loss. Then the rats were switched back to the high-fat diet, allowing them to *regain* high weights. Here, the second cycle of weight loss and regain was initiated. In the second cycle, the animals *regained the weight three times as fast* as they had before, and it took them *twice as long to lose the weight on the subsequent kcalorie-restricted diet.*

Why does this happen? Scientists theorize that a combination of metabolic, hormonal, and enzymatic changes may be involved (McCargar and Yeung, 1991; Kern et al., 1990).

Besides the fact that weight cycling does not result in sustained, reduced body weight, there is evidence that it may be unhealthy in other ways as well. Data from 32 years of the Framingham study showed that people who had weight-cycled were more likely to die younger from all causes—and to develop coronary disease and die from it—than were people who had not weight-cycled (Lissner et al., 1991). Some other studies do not support these findings (Jeffery et al., 1992). This continues to be an active area of research.

Mental health workers also point to the damaging long-term psychologic effects of failed diets, such as loss of self-esteem, an increasing sense of ineffectiveness, and feelings of self-blame and depression. Because these consequences can seriously interfere with a person's progress in other aspects of life (school, job, interpersonal relationships), some professionals now offer programs in *undieting* to help people get out of the vicious cycle of dieting and learn to eat normally (Polivy and Herman, 1992).

Some overweight people for whom dieting has proved unsuccessful may be better off to quit trying to lose weight and work toward accepting their weight and size (Wooley and Garner, 1991). They do, however, need to learn to eat normally and get appropriate exercise (Lyons and Burgard, 1988).

Very Low Kcalorie Formula Diets

Some weight-loss programs allow only 400–800 kcalories per day, usually in the form of special formula beverages that constitute most or all of the diet. Called *very low kcalorie diets* in the medical literature, they cause a variety of problems. To begin with, unpleasant short-term effects, such as fatigue, hair loss, and dizziness often occur; an increased risk of gallstones is a more serious risk (Yang et al., 1992).

Worst of all, these programs also fail their users: they usually lead to weight regain, weight cycling, and increased difficulty in subsequently losing excess fat. If these programs are used by people who are only moderately overweight (who shouldn't be using them in the first place), they can result in large losses of body protein as well (Wadden et al., 1990).

All of this misery does not come cheap: in one study comparing various weight-loss programs, a very low kcalorie program was the most expensive, at $2,120 for a 12-week outpatient series (Spielman et al., 1992). However, some physicians recommend these programs for patients whose substantial obesity puts them at high risk for serious illness and death. To ensure safety, patients on this program need to be monitored by health care professionals who have specialized training; even then, long-term results are usually poor. In 1991, the Federal Trade Commission charged the makers of three of these products (Optifast®, Ultrafast®, and Medifast®) with making deceptive and unsubstantiated claims about the safety and long-term efficacy of their programs. The programs can no longer make such claims.

Drugs

Different pharmacologic methods have been used to promote weight loss. Many ingredients used in the past in over-the-counter preparations were not effective; therefore, starting early in 1992, over 100 such ingredients were banned by the FDA.

Drugs that *do* promote weight loss accomplish it by decreasing a person's energy intake and/or increasing energy output; however, every drug has one or more negative side effects, such as nervousness, rapid heartbeat, insomnia, or central nervous system depression (Sullivan et al., 1988). In the past, some weight-loss drugs were even found to be addictive. The best reason for looking askance at using drugs to lose weight, though, is that it doesn't work in the long run, either. Although these medications often promote initial weight loss, weight regain typically occurs after the drug is withdrawn (Figure 9.18).

Surgical Interventions

Several types of surgery can bring about weight loss. The most drastic types modify the gastrointestinal (GI) tract to restrict intake or to interfere with

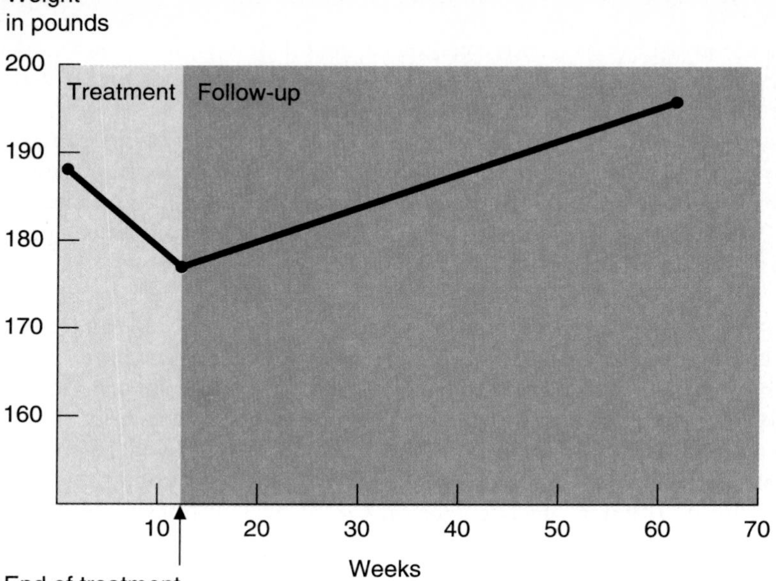

FIGURE 9.18
Lack of long-term success for weight loss using drug therapy.

This illustration shows that drugs are helpful for weight loss only as long as they are being taken. (The illustration represents data combined from five studies.) When treatment ends, weight regain begins; weight often increases to higher than pretreatment weight.

Source: Adapted from Stuart et al., 1981.

absorption. These procedures constitute major surgery; they involve risk of serious complications or even death—and substantial expense. Such methods are reserved for people whose obesity puts them at greater health risk than does surgery, and who have been repeatedly unsuccessful at weight loss by other means. Surgery may be in order if a patient has severe obesity—that is, a body mass index in excess of 40, which generally translates into being more than 100 pounds overweight or double one's recommended weight. Surgery candidates also often have hypertension or are at high risk for cardiovascular disease or Type II diabetes.

People who have had such surgery usually do not lose all of their surplus fat; weight loss averages about 50–60% of their excess weight, at which point it generally stabilizes. These individuals must also be monitored for possible nutritional deficiencies (National Institutes of Health, 1991). Ultimately, the extent of success depends on the person's motivation, because some dietary modification is still necessary (Kral, 1992).

Other, less drastic, methods to reduce intake are of dubious long-term benefit. *Jaw wiring* has been done for periods of time to limit temporarily the intake of solid foods; without behavior modification training, however, weight regain is certain. Some believe that *acupuncture* can reduce appetite, but no long-term studies support this contention.

Some methods involve direct removal of fat. With *lipectomy,* fat tissue is surgically removed. *Fat suctioning,* by contrast, involves making only a small incision where the fat is to be reduced, breaking up the excess adipose tissue, and vacuuming it out. These procedures are expensive and of uncertain benefit in the long term. They provide localized, cosmetic fat reduction; overall reduction of body fat by surgical means is not practical. Once again, if people who have had such surgery do not change their eating and exercise habits, they will regain body fat. Also, the fact that these procedures are cosmetic does not mean that they are without risk; a few patients have developed fatal blood clots after fat suctioning. Others who have had fat removed from the lower body have later accumulated a greater amount of fat on the upper body.

Techniques for Adding Body Weight

If you are considerably underweight or have lost weight without trying to you should have a thorough physical exam to be sure that there is no medical problem responsible for the low weight.

Then, to tip the energy balance in favor of gradual weight gain, develop your own three-part program, including a gradual increase in energy intake, an appropriate exercise program, and strategies to support your new behaviors. Consider these suggestions, many of which are simply the opposite of techniques suggested for fat loss:

Consume more energy Starting with a nutritionally adequate diet, eat larger meals, eat more often, and/or increase the energy density of the foods you choose. You may have noticed that there are some special supplements available for weight gain, but be wary of those that are mainly fat, because they can increase your fat intake above the recommended levels. You can be more liberal in your intake of limited extras; for you, they are really "not-so-limited" extras. However, you should still emphasize high-nutrient-density foods.

Modify your eating behaviors Set some reasonable goals for slow, gradual weight gain. Make a step-by-step plan for how to reach the goals, and implement the easiest change first.

Decrease aerobic physical activity if you do much of it Sustained aerobic activity is a substantial energy-burner, so hold such exercise to a moderate level that will achieve fitness and no more. For general maintenance of fitness, the American College of Sports Medicine (1990) recommends three to five exercise sessions per week of 20–60 minutes each, depending on the intensity of the exercise.

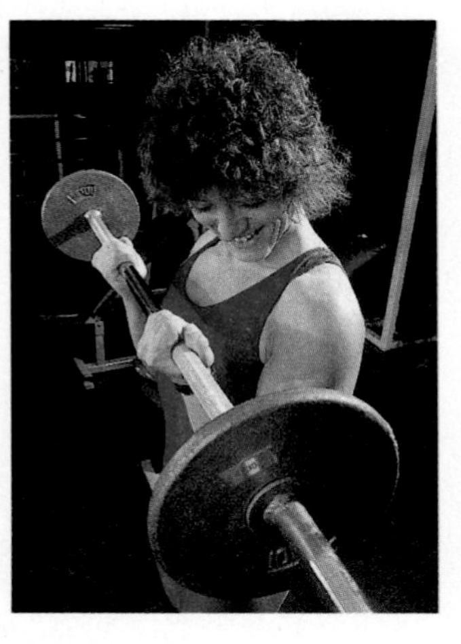

FIGURE 9.19
Weight lifting can help you gain or lose weight.

A graduated program of weight lifting can increase muscle mass. If you lift weights and increase your food intake, you should experience gains in muscle mass and weight. If you lift weights and decrease your food intake slightly, muscle mass should increase while fat decreases.

Consider body building If your muscles need further development, a moderate, progressive program of weight lifting can help you add more "muscle pounds" along with the new "fat pounds" your extra energy intake will produce (Figure 9.19). (But do be wary of the dietary recommendations of body builders; many practice poor eating habits.) •

Accept your genetically determined limits If you find that even when you implement these suggestions you do not achieve your goal weight (or you initially achieve it but then lose it quickly), you may need to accept the fact that your body is regulated at a lower level of fatness. Maintaining a larger amount of fat may require more time, effort, and expense than you consider worthwhile, and you may decide that your resources could be applied more productively to other kinds of goals.

Summary

- Certain hazards are associated with being either too fat or too thin. **Overweight, obese,** and **severely obese** people have statistically higher risks of developing many types of health problems and have to deal with numerous psychosocial and practical problems as well. People who have too little body fat have less endurance and are more susceptible to infectious diseases. Both extremely overweight and extremely **underweight** people are likely to die younger.
- You can estimate your best body weight from a combination of guidelines, all of which approximate what healthy individuals should weigh. These guidelines include height and weight tables, **body mass index,** waist-to-hip ratio, and various estimations of body fatness. A subjective assessment of the weight at which you function best can help you determine your best weight. In the United States, cultural standards for women are currently lower than generally accepted standards for good health.
- Many factors influence how people arrive at their individual body weights. Changes occur when intake and output are not equal. Energy intake is regulated both by internal controls that affect **hunger** and **satiety** and by external controls. Energy output is affected by physiologic factors and by exercise. From various traits your **genes** make possible, your environment helps express a particular **phenotype.**
- There is a theory about what happens at the cellular level during energy surplus: the body enlarges fat cells **(hypertrophy)** until they cannot expand further, and then it divides them to create more fat cells **(hyperplasia).** Energy deficits are thought to result in decreased fat cell size but not cell number. The **set-point theory** suggests that each person tends to maintain his or her unique body weight when the person eats primarily in response to internal factors.
- People have tried thousands of techniques for losing body fat, ranging from sensible to very dangerous. The programs that are most safe and effective encourage no more than 1 pound of weight loss per week through a combination of diet, exercise (which also generally promotes **fitness**), and support systems including **behavior modification** and **relapse prevention.**
- Severe weight-reduction diets and very low kcalorie formula diets lead to physical and psychologic consequences that usually result in failure of the diet and weight regain. Because such diets are often dangerous and unsuccessful in the long run and may lead to a vicious cycle of starving and overeating, they should be avoided. Drugs are also ineffective in the long run. Surgical modifications of the GI tract have a number of serious risks but may be warranted in extreme cases.
- You can also *gain* weight by applying the principles of behavior modification. Gradually increase energy intake, decrease excessive aerobic exercise while incorporating some weight training, and develop support systems for your new behaviors. Keep in mind your genetic limits so that your goals are reasonable.

References

Ailhaud, G., P. Grimaldi, and R. Negrel. 1992. Cellular and molecular aspects of adipose tissue development. *Annual Review of Nutrition* 12:207–233.

American College of Sports Medicine. 1990. The recommended quantity and quality of exercise for developing and maintaining cardiorespiratory and muscular fitness in healthy adults. *Medicine and Science in Sports and Exercise* 22:265–274.

American College of Sports Medicine. 1992. *ACSM fitness book*. Champaign, IL: Leisure Press.

American Medical Association, Council on Scientific Affairs. 1988. Treatment of obesity in adults. *Journal of the American Medical Association* 260:2547–2551.

Anderson, G.H. 1988. Metabolic regulation of food intake. In *Modern nutrition in health and disease,* ed. M.E. Shils and V.R. Young. Philadelphia: Lea & Febiger.

Ballard-Barbash, R., A. Schatzkin, C.L. Carter, W.B. Kannel, B.E. Kreger, R.B. D'Agostino, G. Splansky, K.M. Anderson, and W.E. Helsel. 1990. Body fat distribution and breast cancer in the Framingham Study. *Journal of the National Cancer Institute* 82:286–290.

Baumgartner, R.N., W.C. Chumlea, and A.F. Roche. 1989. Estimation of body composition from bioelectric impedance of body segments. *American Journal of Clinical Nutrition* 50:221–226.

Bjorntorp, P. 1983. The role of adipose tissue in human obesity. In *Obesity,* vol. 4, *Contemporary issues in clinical nutrition,* ed. M.R.C. Greenwood. New York: Churchill Livingstone.

Bouchard, C. 1991. Heredity and the path to overweight and obesity. *Medicine and Science in Sports and Exercise* 23:285–291.

Bouchard, C., A. Tremblay, J. Despres, A. Nadeau, P.J. Lupien, G. Theriault, J. Dussault, S. Moorjani, S. Pinault, and G. Fournier. 1990. The response to long-term overfeeding in identical twins. *New England Journal of Medicine* 322:1477–1482.

Bray, G.A. 1992. Pathophysiology of obesity. *American Journal of Clinical Nutrition* 55:488S–494S.

Bray, G.A. and D.S. Gray. 1988. Obesity. Part I: Pathogenesis. *Western Journal of Medicine* 149:429–441.

Brownell, K.D., M.R.C. Greenwood, E. Stellar, and E.E. Shrager. 1986. The effects of repeated cycles of weight loss and regain in rats. *Physiology and Behavior* 38:459–464.

Brozek, J.M. 1982. *The Effects of malnutrition on human behavior.* American Dietetic Association (ADA) audio cassette tape 9, 1982. Chicago, IL: ADA.

Buckmaster, L. and K.D. Brownell. 1988. Behavior modification: The state of the art. In *Obesity and weight control,* ed. R.T. Frankle and M-U Yang. Rockville, MD: Aspen Publishers, Inc.

Colditz, G.A. 1992. Economic costs of obesity. *American Journal of Clinical Nutrition* 55:503S–507S.

Collier, S.N., S.F. Stallings, P.G. Wolman, and R.W. Cullen. 1990. Assessment of attitudes about weight and dieting among college-aged individuals. *Journal of the American Dietetic Association* 90:276–278.

Cornoni-Huntley, J.C., T.B. Harris, D.F. Everett, D. Albanes, M.S. Micozzi, T.P. Miles, and J.J. Feldman. 1991. An overview of body weight of older persons, including the impact on mortality. *Journal of Clinical Epidemiology* 44:743–753.

Czajka-Narins, D.M. and E.S. Parham. 1990. Fear of fat: Attitudes toward obesity. *Nutrition Today* 23(no.1):26–32.

Dattilo, A.M. 1992. Dietary fat and its relationship to body weight. *Nutrition Today* 27(no.1):13–19.

Dietz, W.H. 1988. Childhood and adolescent obesity. In *Obesity and weight control,* ed. R.T. Frankle and M-U Yang. Rockville, MD: Aspen Publishers, Inc.

Drewnowski, A. 1991. Fats and food acceptance. In *Nutrition in the '90s,* ed. G.E. Gaull, F.N. Kotsonis, and M.A. Mackey. New York: Marcel Dekker, Inc.

Fatis, M., A. Weiner, J.A. Hawkins, and B. VanDorsten. 1989. Following up on a commercial weight loss program: Do the pounds stay off after your picture has been in the newspaper? *Journal of the American Dietetic Association* 89:547–548.

Finding the fat in food. 1991. Madison, WI: University of Wisconsin-Madison Cooperative Extension Bulletin BNEP3.

Fitzwater, S.L., R.L. Weinsier, N.H. Wooldridge, R. Birch, C. Liu, and A.A. Bartolucci. 1991. Evaluation of long-term weight changes after a multidisciplinary weight control program. *Journal of the American Dietetic Association* 91:421–426, 429.

Foreyt, J.P. and G.K. Goodrick. 1991. Factors common to successful therapy for the obese patient. *Medicine and Science in Sports and Exercise* 23:292–297.

Frisch, R.E. 1987. Nutrition, fatness, puberty, and fertility. *Nutrition and the M.D., special report: Obesity and other eating disorders.* Van Nuys, CA: PM, Inc.

Ganley, R.M. 1989. Emotion and eating in obesity: A review of the literature. *International Journal of Eating Disorders* 8:343–361.

Garn, S.M. 1985. Continuities and changes in fatness from infancy through adulthood. *Current Problems in Pediatrics* 15:1–47.

Gong, E.J., D. Garrel, and D.H. Calloway. 1989. Menstrual cycle and voluntary food intake. *American Journal of Clinical Nutrition* 49:252–258.

Goodrick, G.K. and J.P. Foreyt. 1991. Why treatments for obesity don't last. *Journal of the American Dietetic Association* 91:1243–1247.

Gortmaker, S.L., W.H. Dietz, and L.W. Cheung. 1990. Inactivity, diet, and the fattening of America. *Journal of the American Dietetic Association* 90:1247–1252, 1255.

Gustafson-Larson, A.M. and R.D. Terry. 1992. Weight-related behaviors and concerns of fourth-grade children. *Journal of the American Dietetic Assocation* 92:818–822.

Herman, C.P. and J. Polivy. 1988. Psychological factors in the control of appetite. In *Control of appetite,* ed. M. Winick. New York: John Wiley & Sons, Inc.

Hubert, H. 1988. Obesity: A predictor for coronary heart disease. In *Obesity and weight control,* ed. R.T. Frankle and M-U Yang. Rockville, ND: Aspen, Publishers, Inc.

Jeffery, R.W., R.R. Wing, and S.A. French. 1992. Weight cycling and cardiovascular risk factors in obese men and women. *American Journal of Clinical Nutrition* 55:641–644.

Jensen, M.D. 1992. Research techniques for body composition assessment. *Journal of the American Dietetic Association* 92:454–460.

Kayman, S., W. Bruvold, and J.S. Stern. 1990. Maintenance and relapse after weight loss in women: Behavioral aspects. *American Journal of Clinical Nutrition* 52:800–807.

Keesey, R.E. 1988. The body-weight set point. *Postgraduate Medicine* 83(no.6):114–127.

Kendall, A., D.A. Levitsky, B.J. Strupp, and L. Lissner. 1991. Weight loss on a low-fat diet: Consequence of the imprecision of the control of food intake in humans. *American Journal of Clinical Nutrition* 53:1124–1129.

Kern, P.A., J.M. Ong, B. Saffari, and J. Carty. 1990. The effects of weight loss on the activity and expression of adipose-tissue lipoprotein lipase in very obese humans. *New England Journal of Medicine* 322:1053–1059.

Kirkley, B.G., J.C. Burge, and A. Ammerman. 1988. Dietary restraint, binge eating, and dietary behavior patterns. *International Journal of Eating Disorders* 7:771–778.

Klesges, R.C., L.M. Klesges, C.K. Haddock, and L.H. Eck. 1992. A longitudinal analysis of the impact of dietary intake and physical activity on weight change in adults. *American Journal of Clinical Nutrition* 55:818–822.

Kolasa, K., A.C. Jobe, and C. Dunn. 1991. . . . Consult a physician before starting any weight loss . . . *Nutrition Today* 26(no.6):25–31.

Kolata, G. 1985. Why do people get fat? *Science* 227:1327–1328.

Kral, J.G. 1992. Overview of surgical techniques for treating obesity. *American Journal of Clinical Nutrition* 55:552S–555S.

Kuczmarksi, R.J. 1992. Prevalence of overweight and weight gain in the United States. *American Journal of Clinical Nutrition* 55:495S–502S.

Ley, C.J., B. Lees, and J.C. Stevenson. 1992. Sex- and menopause-associated changes in body-fat distribution. *American Journal of Clinical Nutrition* 55:950–954.

Linsted, K., S. Tonstad, and J.W. Kuzma. 1991. Body mass index and patterns of mortality among Seventh Day Adventist men. *International Journal of Obesity* 15:397–406.

Lissner, L., P.M. Odell, R.B. D'Agostino, J. Stokes III, B.E. Kreger, A.J. Belanger, and K.D. Brownell. 1991. Variability of body weight and health outcomes in the Framingham population. *New England Journal of Medicine* 324:1839–1844.

Lissner, L., J. Stevens, D.A. Levitsky, K.M. Rasmussen, and B.J. Strupp. 1988. Variation in energy intake during the menstrual cycle: Implications for food-intake research. *American Journal of Clinical Nutrition* 48:956–962.

Lohman, T.G. 1981. Skinfolds and body density and their relation to body fatness: A review. *Human Biology* 53:181–225.

Lohman, T.G., M.L. Pollack, M.H. Slaughter, L.J. Brandon, and R.A. Boileau. 1984. Methological factors and the prediction of body fat in female athletes. *Medicine and Science in Sports and Exercise* 16:92–96.

Luke, A. and D.A. Schoeller. 1992. Basal metabolic rate, fat-free mass, and body cell mass during energy restriction. *Metabolism* 41:450–456.

Lyons, P. and D. Burgard. 1988. *Great shape: The first fitness guide for large women.* Palo Alto: Bull Publishing.

Mann, G.V. 1981. Menstrual effects of athletic training. In *Medicine and sport,* ed. J. Borms, M. Hebbelinck, and A. Venerado. New York: Karger.

McArdle, W.D., F.I. Katch, and V.L. Katch. 1991. *Exercise physiology,* 3rd edition. Philadelphia: Lea & Febiger.

McArdle, W.D. and M.M. Toner. 1988. In *Obesity and weight control,* ed. R.T. Frankle and M-U Yang. Rockville, MD: Aspen Publishers, Inc.

McCargar, L.J. and H. Yeung. 1991. The effects of weight cycling on metabolism and health. *Journal of the Canadian Dietetic Association* 52:101–106.

Miller, W.C. 1991. Diet composition, energy intake, and nutritional status in relation to obesity in men and women. *Medicine and Science in Sports and Exercise* 23:280–284.

Myrvik, Q.N. 1988. Nutrition and immunology. In *Modern nutrition in health and disease,* ed. M.E. Shils and V.R. Young. Philadelphia: Lea & Febiger.

National Institutes of Health (NIH). 1985. *Health implications of obesity.* NIH consensus development conference statement, vol.5, no. 9. Bethesda, MD: NIH.

National Institutes of Health (NIH). 1991. Gastrointestinal surgery for severe obesity. *Nutrition Today* 26:(no.5):32–35.

National Institutes of Health (NIH). 1992. Methods for voluntary weight loss and control. *Nutrition Today* 27:(no.4):27–33.

National Research Council. 1989. *Diet and health.* Washington, DC: The National Academy Press.

New York City Department of Consumer Affairs, Communications Division. 1991. *Weighty issues: Dangers and deceptions of the weight loss industry.* New York: NYC Department of Consumer Affairs.

Norvell, N. and W. Kallman. 1988. Physiological and self-report responses of restrained and unrestrained eaters. *International Journal of Eating Disorders* 7:487–494.

Perusse, L., A. Tremblay, C. Leblanc, C.R. Cloninger, T. Reich, J. Rice, and C. Bouchard. 1988. Familial resemblance in energy intake: Contributions of genetic and environmental factors. *American Journal of Clinical Nutrition* 47:629–635.

Perusse, L., A. Tremblay, C. Leblanc, and C. Bouchard. 1989. Genetic and environmental influences on level of habitual physical activity and exercise participation. *American Journal of Epidemiology* 129:1012–1022.

Petersmarck, K. 1992. Building consensus for safe weight loss. *Journal of the American Dietetic Association* 92:679–680.

Pi-Sunyer, F.X. 1988. Obesity. In *Modern nutrition in health and disease,* ed. M.E. Shils and V.R. Young. Philadelphia: Lea & Febiger.

Pi-Sunyer, F.X. 1991. Health implications of obesity. *American Journal of Clinical Nutrition* 53:1595S–1603S.

Poehlman, E.T. and E.S. Horton. 1989. The impact of food intake and exercise on energy expenditure. *Nutrition Reviews* 47(no.5):129–137.

Polivy, J. and C.P. Herman. 1992. Undieting: A program to help people stop dieting. *International Journal of Eating Disorders* 11:261–268.

Prewitt, T.E., D. Schmeisser, P.E. Bowen, P. Aye, T.A. Dolecek, P. Langenberg, T. Cole, and L. Brace. 1991. Changes in body weight, body composition, and energy intake in women fed high- and low-fat diets. *American Journal of Clinical Nutrition* 54:304–310.

Ravussin, E.S. Lillioja, W.C. Knowler, L. Christin, D. Freymond, W.G. Abbott, V. Boyce, B.V. Howard, and C.

Bogardus. 1988. Reduced rate of energy expenditure as a risk factor for body weight gain. *New England Journal of Medicine* 318:467–472.

Roberts, S.B., J. Savage, W.A. Coward, B. Chew, and A. Lucas. 1988. Energy expenditure and intake in infants born to lean and overweight mothers. *New England Journal of Medicine* 318:461–466.

Rolls, B.J. 1991a. Determinants of food intake and selection. In *Nutrition in the '90s,* ed. G.E. Saull, F.N. Kotsonis, and M.A. Mackey. New York: Marcel Dekker, Inc.

Rolls, B.J. 1991b. Effects of intense sweeteners on hunger, food intake, and body weight: A review. *American Journal of Clinical Nutrition* 53:872–878.

Schapira, D.V., N.B. Kuman, G.H. Lyman, D. Cavanagh, W.S. Roberts, and J. LaPolla. 1991. Upper-body fat distribution and endometrial cancer risk. *Journal of the American Medical Assocation* 266:1808–1811.

Schiffman, S.S. 1986. Recent findings about taste: Important implications. *Cereal Foods World* 31:300–302.

Schoeller, D.A. and C.R. Fjeld. 1991. Human energy metabolism: What have we learned from the doubly labeled water method? *Annual Review of Nutrition* 11:355–373.

Segal, K.R., J. Albu, A. Chun, A. Edano, B. Legaspi, and F.X. Pi-Sunyer. 1992. Independent effects of obesity and insulin resistance on postprandial thermogenesis in men. *Journal of Clinical Investigation* 89:824–833.

Sheppard, L., A.R. Kristal, and L.H. Kushi. 1991. Weight loss in women participating in a randomized trial of low-fat diets. *American Journal of Clinical Nutrition* 54:821–828.

Sims, E.A. 1988. Exercise and energy balance in the control of obesity and hypertension. In *Exercise, nutrition, and energy metabolism,* ed. E.S. Horton and R.L. Terjung. New York: Macmillan.

Solomon, S.J., M.S. Kurzer, and D.H. Calloway. 1982. Menstrual cycle and basal metabolic rate in women. *American Journal of Clinical Nutrition* 36(no.4):611–616.

Sorensen, T.I., C. Holst, A.J. Stunkard, and L.T. Skovgaard. 1992. Correlations of body mass index of adult adoptees and their biological and adoptive relatives. *International Journal of Obesity* 16:227–236.

Spielman, A.B., B. Kanders, M. Kienholz, and G.L. Blackburn. 1992. The cost of losing: An analysis of commercial weight-loss programs in a metropolitan area. *Journal of the American College of Nutrition* 11:36–41.

Spitzer, R.L., M. Devlin, B.T. Walsh, D. Hasin, R. Wing, M. Marcus, A. Stunkard, T. Wadden, S. Yanovski, S. Agras, J. Mitchell, and C. Nonas. 1992. Binge eating disorder: A multisite field trial of the diagnostic criteria. *International Journal of Eating Disorders* 11:191–203.

Stuart, R.B., C. Mitchell, and J.A. Jensen. 1981. Therapeutic options in the management of obesity. In *Medical psychology: Contributions to behavioral medicine.* New York: Academic Press.

Stunkard, A.J. 1988. Some perspectives on human obesity: Its causes. *Bulletin of the New York Academy of Medicine* 64(no.8):902–923.

Stunkard, A.J., J.R. Harris, N.L. Pedersen, and G.E. McClearn. 1990. The body-mass index of twins who have been reared apart. *New England Journal of Medicine* 322:1483–1487.

Stunkard, A.J., T.I. Sorensen, C. Hanis, T.W. Teasdale, R. Chakraborty, W.J. Schull, and F. Schulsinger. 1986. An adoption study of human obesity. *New England Journal of Medicine* 314:193–198.

Stunkard, A.J. and T. Wadden. 1992. Psychological aspects of severe obesity. *American Journal of Clinical Nutrition* 55:524S–532S.

Sullivan, A.C., C. Nauss-Karol, S. Hogan, and J. Triscari. 1988. Pharmacological modifications of appetite. In *Control of appetite,* ed. M. Winick. New York: John Wiley & Sons, Inc.

Surgeon General. 1988. *Surgeon General's report on nutrition and health.* Washington, DC: Department of Health and Human Services.

Taylor, J.L., E.R. Buskirk, J. Brozek, J.R. Anderson, and F. Grande. 1957. Performance capacity and effects of caloric restriction with hard physical work on young men. *Journal of Applied Physiology* 10(no.3):421–429.

Thayer, R.E. 1992. Exercise and food in mood regulation. Symposium: American Psychological Association; Washington, DC; August, 16, 1992.

TOHP Collaborative Research Group. 1992. The effects of nonpharmacologic interventions on blood pressure of persons with high normal levels. *Journal of the American Medical Association* 267:1213–1220.

Tucker, L.A. and Bagwell, M. 1991. Television viewing and obesity in adult females. *American Journal of Public Health* 81:908–911.

Tucker, L.A. and Friedman, G.M. 1989. Television viewing and obesity in adult males. *American Journal of Public Health* 79:516–518.

Wadden, T.A., T.B. Van Itallie, and G.L. Blackburn. 1990. Responsible and irresponsible use of very-low-calorie diets in the treatment of obesity. *Journal of the American Medical Association* 263:83–85.

Weingarten, H.P. 1992. Determinants of food intake: Hunger and satiety. In *Eating, body weight, and performance in athletes,* ed. K.D. Brownell, J. Rodin, and J.H. Wilmore. Philadelphia: Lea & Febiger.

Williamson, D.F., M.K. Serdula, R.F. Anda, A. Levy, and T. Byers. 1992. Weight loss attempts in adults: Goals, duration, and rate of weight loss. *American Journal of Public Health* 82:1251–1257.

Wooley, S.C. and D.M. Garner. 1991. Obesity treatment: The high cost of false hope. *Journal of the American Dietetic Association* 91:1248–1251.

Yang, M-U. 1988. Composition and resting metabolic rate in obesity. In *Obesity and weight control,* ed. R.T. Frankle and M-U Yang. Rockville, MD: Aspen Publishers, Inc.

Yang, H., G.M. Petersen, M-P Roth, L.J. Schoenfield, and J.W. Marks. 1992. Risk factors for gallstone formation during rapid loss of weight. *Digestive Diseases and Sciences* 37:912–918.

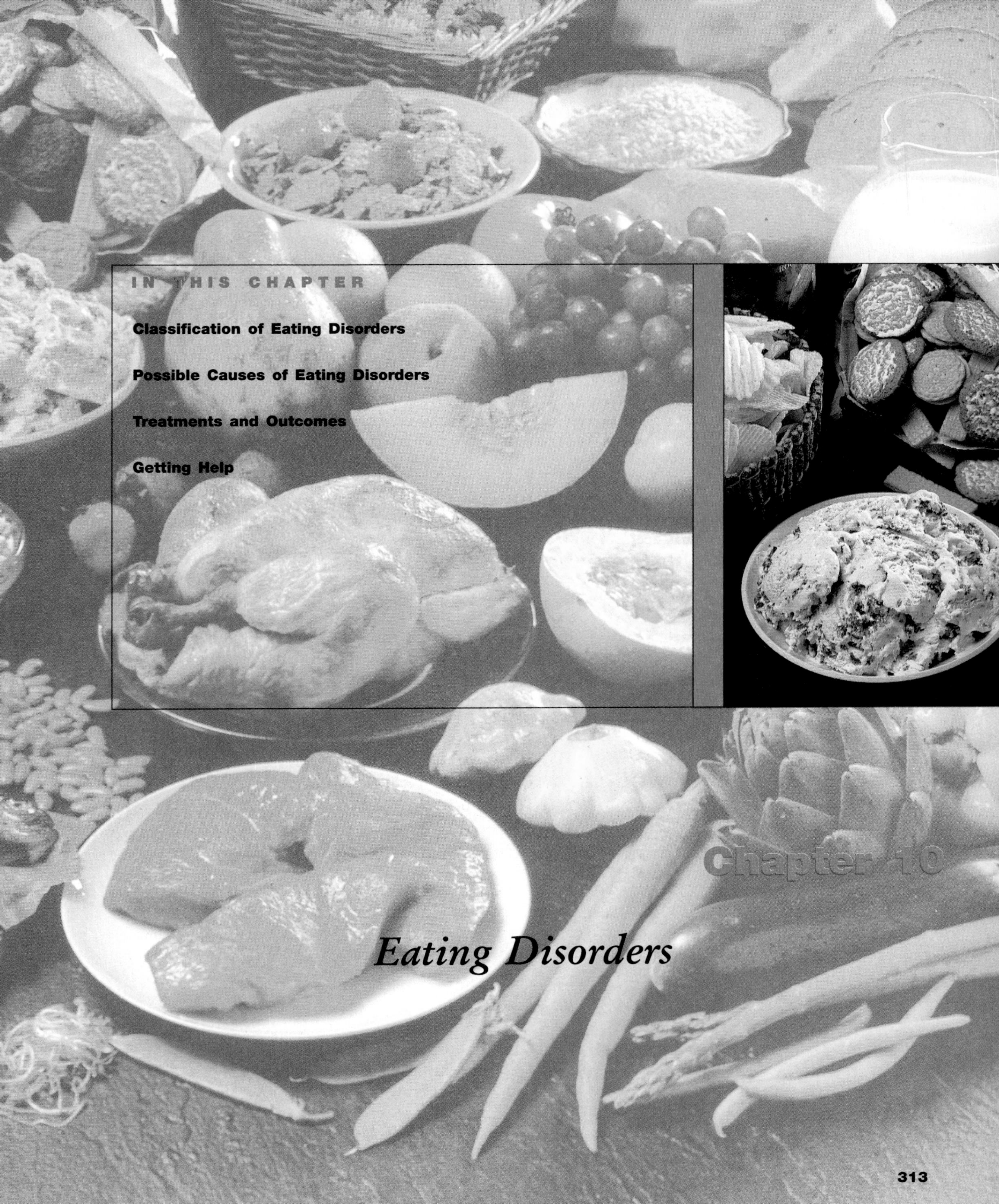

IN THIS CHAPTER

Chapter 10

Eating Disorders

eating disorder—condition in which a person's food intake deviates markedly from normal intake in a misguided effort to solve psychologic problems

anorexia nervosa—an eating disorder in which self-starvation and low body weight are prominent characteristics

bulimia nervosa—an eating disorder in which binging and purging (or other compensatory mechanisms) are prominent characteristics

Do you know somebody—or know *of* somebody—who has an **eating disorder**? Chances are very good that you do. In the last decade, publicity about these conditions and about famous people who have struggled with eating disorders has heightened public awareness of these illnesses and encouraged those affected to get help.

The two types of eating disorders that have received the most publicity are **anorexia nervosa** (which is characterized by starving and extreme weight loss) and **bulimia nervosa** (characterized by binging and purging). These problems, as you see from the term *nervosa,* are of psychologic origin; you might learn about them if you study psychology. They also warrant attention when you study nutrition, though, because they involve unhealthy eating patterns that lead to poor body functioning and even physical damage and death. Because they are most likely to occur during the adolescent years and in the 20s, eating disorders are of great concern to high school and college students and people involved with them.

Before we discuss these conditions, we need to point out that we probably all mismatch our eating to our physical needs from time to time, but this does not mean that we all have eating disorders. Eating large amounts of food on Thanksgiving Day, when your only physical activities may be helping clean up after dinner and watching football on TV, is clearly a mismatch of energy intake with energy needs; you may feel uncomfortable and even regret that you ate so much. Yet, such behavior is a typical and accepted part of feast days in all cultures and probably naturally results in eating less the next day. Another example of a mismatch of energy intake to needs would be missing a meal as you are finishing a term paper that you must turn in today; you'll make up for the energy deficit after the project has been submitted. Eating disorders, by contrast, involve *frequent, extreme departures from normal food intake behaviors; eating disorders are misguided efforts to solve psychologic problems.*

Eating disorders are serious conditions that require treatment. Some people die because of them, and many others find their lives extremely limited by their obsession with food. Reading this chapter should help you understand the difference between occasionally feasting or skipping meals and suffering from an eating disorder. You will also become aware of the physical consequences of eating disorders and learn what steps to take to get help for yourself or for others if these conditions develop.

Classification of Eating Disorders

Eating disorders are more of a challenge to classify than you might think, and they are more diverse than is commonly recognized. The American Psychiatric Association (APA) has identified four eating disorders in its *Diagnostic and Statistical Manual of Mental Disorders, Third Edition-Revised* (*DSM-III-R*) (1987), the diagnostic guide used by mental health professionals. These disorders include *anorexia nervosa*, *bulimia nervosa*, *rumination* (a rare condition characterized by involuntary vomiting after meals), and *pica* (eating of nonfood items). Because of its rarity, we will not consider rumination here. Pica is discussed in Chapter 12 (on minerals) and Chapter 15 (on pregnancy).

The *DSM-III-R* criteria for anorexia nervosa and bulimia nervosa are given in Tables 10.1 and 10.2. Because there are many similarities between these two conditions, experts debate whether they are distinct and separate disorders. Because their typical course and current treatments are different, however, it has been practical to regard them as two separate entities.

TABLE 10.1 Diagnostic Criteria for Anorexia Nervosa

A. Refusal to maintain body weight over a minimal normal weight for age and height, e.g., weight loss leading to maintenance of body weight 15% below that expected; or failure to make expected weight gain during period of growth, leading to body weight 15% below that expected.

B. Intense fear of gaining weight or becoming fat, even though underweight.

C. Disturbance in the way in which one's body weight, size, or shape is experienced, e.g., the person claims to "feel fat" even when emaciated, believes that one area of the body is "too fat" even when obviously underweight.

D. In females, absence of at least three consecutive menstrual cycles when otherwise expected to occur (primary or secondary amenorrhea). (A woman is considered to have amenorrhea if her periods occur only following hormone, e.g., estrogen, administration.)

Source: DSM-III-R, 1987.

TABLE 10.2 Diagnostic Criteria for Bulimia Nervosa

A. Recurrent episodes of binge eating (rapid consumption of a large amount of food in a discrete period of time.

B. A feeling of lack of control over eating behavior during the eating binges.

C. Regularly engaging in either self-induced vomiting, use of laxatives or diuretics, strict dieting or fasting, or vigorous exercise in order to prevent weight gain.

D. A minimum average of two binge eating episodes a week for at least three months.

E. Persistent overconcern with body shape and weight.

Source: DSM-III-R, 1987.

The two disorders overlap considerably; that is, people with anorexia nervosa might engage in periodic binging and purging, and people with bulimia nervosa might periodically starve, at least until the next binge begins (Figure 10.1). Therefore, in this section we also discuss the condition in which people exhibit characteristics of both disorders together.

Finally, we will consider an additional condition that the APA is being urged to define in its next edition of the *DSM*: *binge-eating disorder*, in which people binge frequently but do not purge.

Anorexia Nervosa

Anorexia nervosa, although it is less prevalent than bulimia nervosa, was the first eating disorder to be commonly recognized because of its very noticeable effect—extreme thinness. The anorexic person also exhibits a very obvious eating behavior—**starving.** In their pursuit of thinness, anorexics reduce their food intake drastically, often to just a few hundred kcalories per day. Laura, in the Slice of Life on page 316, serves as an example.

starving—(in the context of eating disorders) deliberately restricting total food intake to drastically low levels

Although in the past people with anorexia nervosa were generally from upper-middle- or middle-class families, the condition is now more widely distributed (Woodside and Garfinkel, 1989). Because members of other eco-

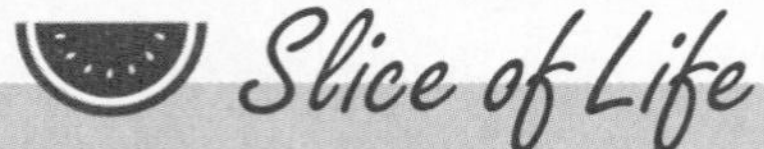

An Anorexic's Diet

Laura

I ate the same thing every day for six weeks at a time—300 kcalories a day. I'd have tea for breakfast, with artificial sweetener, and lettuce with a few green beans for lunch. I'd wash the beans so there would be no trace of salt on them; I didn't want to retain any liquid. For dinner I'd have two ounces of broiled meat, squeezed until it was like paper to get rid of the grease, and maybe a couple of bites of lettuce.

I couldn't eat in front of people and never ate with the family. I had to have my own food by myself so I could pick at it. If we went out, sometimes I could eat a lettuce salad, but that was all. If I didn't have *my* food, I wouldn't eat.

Source: Stein and Unell, 1986.

nomic groups are gaining greater access to treatment, the number of cases now reported may be more accurate.

Incidence Approximately 1% of young women in the United States and Canada develop anorexia nervosa. It usually begins in adolescence, but it has been known to occur in people 15–45 years old (Woodside and Garfinkel, 1992). People with anorexia nervosa are generally identified sooner than are those with bulimia nervosa because of their characteristic dramatic weight loss.

Males experience this condition much less often—only about 1/20 as often as females. Experts hypothesize that this may be due to the fact that males generally receive less social pressure to be thin; therefore, those who develop eating disorders may have more severe psychologic disturbances (Andersen, 1988).

Because the prevalence of eating disorders is so much higher in females, we will often use feminine pronouns in this chapter.

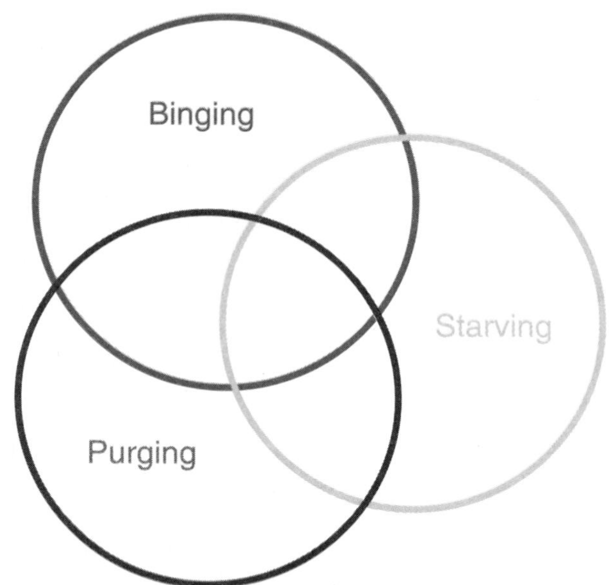

FIGURE 10.1
Overlap of disordered eating behaviors.

Frequent binging, purging, and starving are abnormal activities. A person with an eating disorder may practice just one, two, or all three of these behaviors.

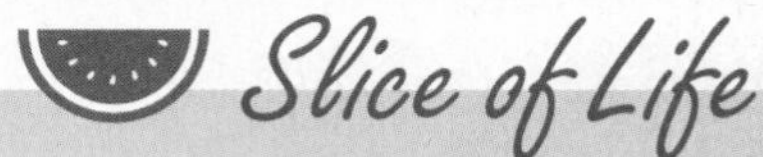

An Anorexic's Emotional Detachment

Joe

My parents were divorced when I was ten years old. . . . I was pretty crushed about the divorce, . . . but [after my mother remarried] I grew to feel that my stepbrothers and stepsisters were my actual family. There was a closeness, even though no one in our family shows much emotion. Because we didn't let our emotions show, when I would have a "big" emotion, I hadn't learned what to do with it.

I was twenty years old and a student when my relationship with a girlfriend ended. I was devastated. I became severely depressed and was suicidal during the year after this happened. The breakup happened in the spring, and I was so immobilized that I couldn't go back to school the next fall.

I started eating less and less because I was so depressed. The more weight I lost, the more obsessed I became. I was living with my mother and stepfather and brothers and sisters and would do the meal planning and preparation to help my mom. I was completely preoccupied with food. In looking back, it seems to me I was a typical, textbook anorexic.

Source: Stein and Unell, 1986.

Psychologic Characteristics As young children, most people with anorexia nervosa were cooperative, thoughtful, obedient, and eager for praise. Among their peers, they tend to be highly competitive, achievement-oriented, and perfectionist. They are often serious and not very spontaneous (Lucas and Huse, 1988); they tend to be out of touch with their emotions. Joe, an anorexic, describes his problems in dealing with his feelings in the Slice of Life above.

People with anorexia nervosa misinterpret many messages their bodies try to give them regarding hunger, temperature, pain, and fatigue. For example, when they feel the sensation that a healthy person recognizes as hunger, they do not believe it is caused by *needing* something to eat; rather, they might believe that they have a stomach ache from *having eaten* a few carrot sticks many hours before. Or, they might recognize the physiologic sensations as hunger but derive satisfaction from denying themselves food.

Although the person with anorexia nervosa avoids eating most foods, she is frantically preoccupied with food and eating. She often deliberately puts herself in proximity to food by cooking for other people.

A person with anorexia nervosa typically denies that anything is wrong; in fact, she often maintains that she is still overweight and ought to lose more weight. She is a perfectionist: if she is a student, she may study harder than ever but get less done (Sibley and Blinder, 1988). At least in the early stages of the disorder, she is likely to drive herself to perform demanding physical activities despite her low energy intake. In fact, she is likely to expend almost twice as much energy per unit of body weight in physical activity than normal controls (Casper et al., 1991). As she becomes more involved in these solitary activities, she becomes more socially isolated.

Athletes seem more prone to anorexia nervosa than the general population, although no large, well-designed studies have been conducted to establish the incidence using the APA's criteria (Brownell and Rodin, 1992). In addition to those who are technically anorexic, many athletes have lesser degrees of disordered eating. It is not known whether people who already have tendencies toward abnormal eating are attracted to certain sports, or whether the demands of certain sports to have unusually low levels of body fat might cause the anorexia.

In the case of the latter possibility, it may be that the stress of perfecting one's body for the "appearance sports" (such as gymnastics, diving, or

FIGURE 10.2
Coming soon . . . the long-term health effects of eating disorders.

In the 1960s, adolescent girls tried to get as thin as Twiggy, the most recognized model of the decade. In their quest, some developed eating disorders. Even though most were subsequently cured of the eating disorder, we do not know whether there are lingering ill effects. We will find out as the teenage girls of the 1960s become middle-aged women in the 1990s.

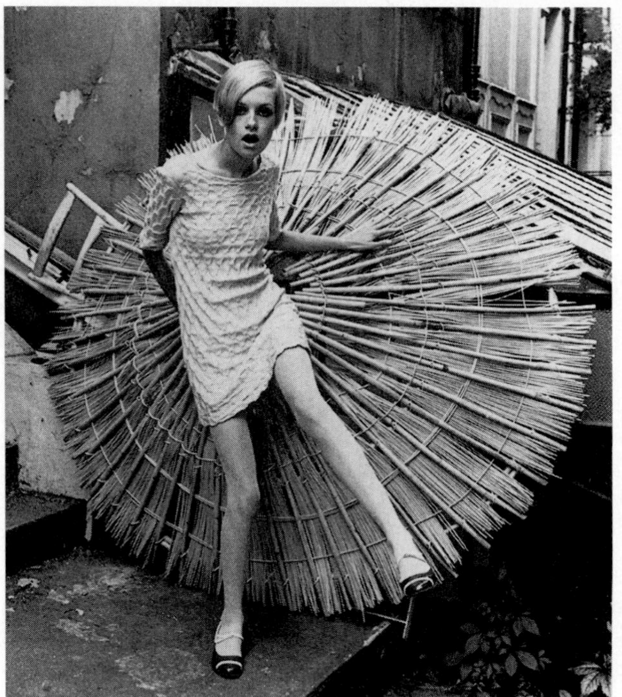

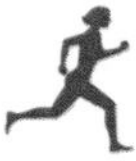

figure skating) might start behaviors which, when carried to extremes, could become eating disorders. Other athletes at risk are those who need to maintain a low weight for endurance sports (such as running or distance swimming) or for a certain weight class (such as in wrestling or rowing) (Steen, 1991). •

Physical Consequences These extreme behaviors have their consequences. Eventually, the anorexic who has been exercising excessively experiences a substantial decrease in aerobic capacity (Einerson et al., 1988), which limits physical endurance. Although anorexics commonly exercise to excess, they often have sleep disorders.

The extreme weight losses of people with anorexia nervosa are accompanied by extensive physical changes. Body functions slow down: the gastrointestinal (GI) tract works more slowly, resulting in constipation, often with abdominal pain and a sense of fullness. Resting metabolic rate goes down (Vaisman et al., 1991), as do blood pressure and pulse; cold, blue hands and feet and even dizziness commonly result. A fine body hair, called *lanugo,* may appear, and the person's complexion becomes sallow. In females, menstruation ceases.

Other, less noticeable, effects also take place. Dehydration, decreased kidney function, and abnormalities in heart function may occur. Vitamin and trace mineral deficiences may evolve. In fact, the person with anorexia nervosa has many features in common with undernourished people with marasmus (Turner and Shapiro, 1992).

Bone density also decreases as a result of reduced estrogen levels—the same factor responsible for the cessation of menstrual periods. Studies show that anorexics are more prone to fractures of the spine, hip, upper leg, and lower arm (Drinkwater, 1992). In one study, even after 2 years of treatment, anorexics experienced no restoration of bone density (Rigoti et al., 1991). We do not yet know all of the long-term consequences (Figure 10.2).

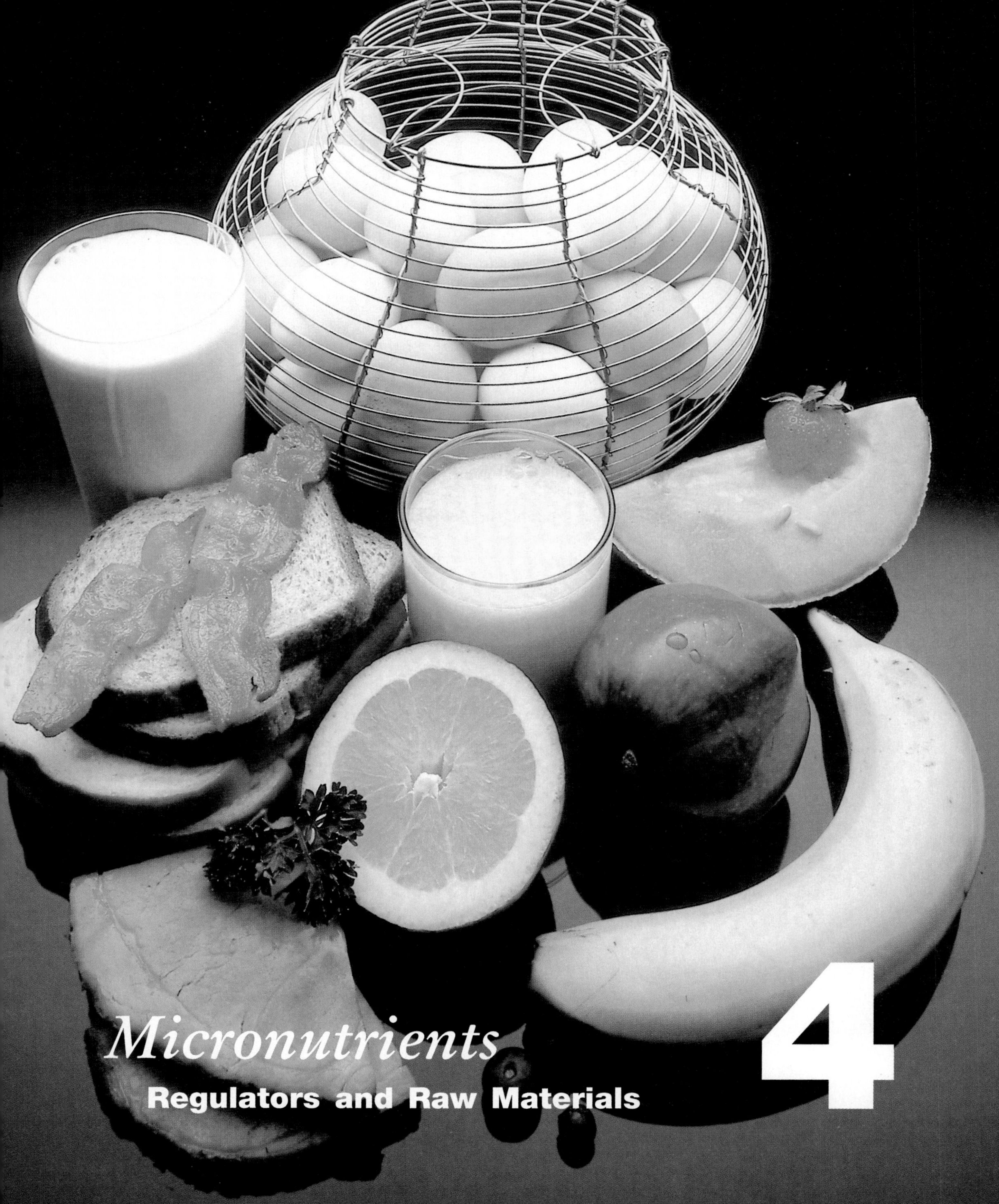

4

Micronutrients

Regulators and Raw Materials

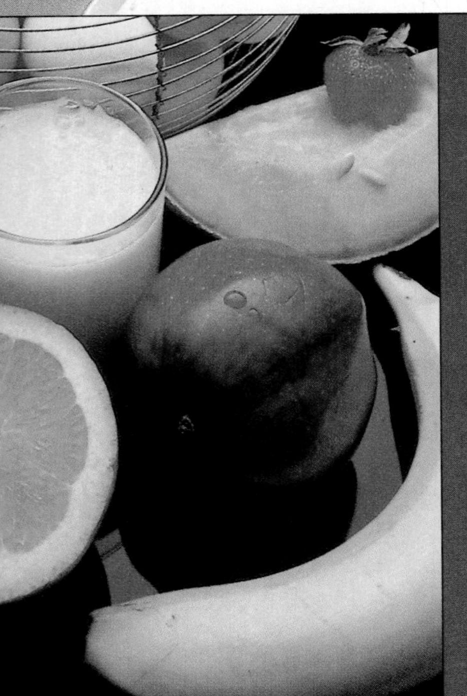

IN THIS CHAPTER

Chapter 11

Vitamins

You probably think that vitamins are important. You may even take vitamin supplements—or wonder if you should. An FDA study shows that 36% of the U.S. population takes vitamin and mineral supplements regularly (Moss et al., 1989). Ads for vitamins seem to be everywhere. It is estimated that Americans spend $2 billion each year on these products.

But do you really know what vitamins are? How do they function? The common assumption that this class of nutrients provides energy is wrong. However, it is true that vitamins are essential for your body's functioning. In this chapter, you will learn what they do.

You will also find that a *well-chosen diet can supply all the vitamins that most people need.* That may be hard to believe. Just look at the headlines on magazines at grocery checkouts. "Miracle vitamin beats tiredness" one headline claims over an article that goes on to recommend levels that are hundreds of times the RDA for certain vitamins. Another item suggests that athletes should take large multivitamin supplements. These articles give you the impression that the larger the doses you take, the better off you are.

Although supplements can be helpful in some circumstances, many nutritionists believe that they are overused. The fact is that large excesses of some vitamins can cause serious damage. You may be surprised to learn that some of your friends and family (or perhaps even you) may be at risk of consuming too many vitamin supplements.

In this chapter, you'll get the facts and have a chance to consider your intake of vitamins from food and from supplements. We want to help you find the middle ground: the point at which you take in enough vitamins to allow them to carry out the functions they perform, but not so much that they cause damage. Let's start by describing the nature of vitamins—how these substances are alike and how they differ.

Vitamins—Similar But Different

The thirteen known **vitamins** are organic substances that occur in small amounts in foods. You need them in your body in minute amounts to regulate your body's metabolic functions. Generally, you do not digest vitamins but absorb them intact through your small intestine.

vitamins—organic compounds present in small amounts in foods and needed in small amounts by the body as regulators of metabolic functions

You need relatively small amounts of these substances because vitamins are not used up in biochemical reactions; one molecule is used repeatedly. Only gradually are vitamins degraded (broken apart) and come to need replacement. Consider vitamin B-12, the vitamin needed in the smallest amount. Just 1 gram of vitamin B-12 can fulfill the RDA of one-half million people for one day. Even the vitamin we need in the largest amount, vitamin C, has a recommended intake of only 60 mg/day. A gram of it can supply 17 people for one day.

Solubilities, Absorption Efficiencies, and Storage Capacities

Traditionally, the vitamins are classified according to whether they are soluble in fat or in water. The fat-soluble vitamins are A, D, E, and K; the water-soluble vitamins are thiamin, riboflavin, niacin, vitamin B-6, folic acid, vitamin B-12, pantothenic acid, biotin, and vitamin C.

As you might expect, your body absorbs vitamins dissolved in fat differently from vitamins dissolved in water. For example, the presence of fat in the chyme in your small intestines facilitates the absorption of fat-soluble vitamins.

saturation level—the maximum amount of a substance a tissue can maintain

The maximum amount of a vitamin that your body tissues can maintain is called the **saturation level**. The saturation levels of various vitamins differ. In general, your body stores larger quantities of fat-soluble vitamins than water-soluble vitamins.

Structures, Forms, and Potencies

Aside from the fact that they are all organic, vitamins are very different structurally: there is no characteristic organization of the carbon, hydrogen, and oxygen in vitamin molecules. In addition, some vitamins also contain nitrogen, sulfur, or cobalt in their structures. You can see how dissimilar vitamin structures are by looking at Appendix E.

Some of the vitamins have several different but closely related chemical forms that can function as that vitamin. These different forms can even occur in the same food at the same time. For example, nicotinamide and nicotinic acid, two forms of niacin, can both be present in one food. (These compounds are not the same as nicotine in tobacco.)

provitamins—vitamin precursors that the body can convert into the active form of a vitamin

Sometimes your body converts a compound that is not a nutrient into a nutrient. Such early versions of nutrients are called *precursors*; vitamin precursors are called **provitamins**. For example, there are about 50 chemicals called carotenoids that are provitamins for vitamin A, one of which is beta-carotene (β-carotene). Another example is the amino acid tryptophan, which can be considered a provitamin of niacin.

Because vitamins and provitamins occur in different forms, a single vitamin can be known by a multitude of chemical names; these are alternatives to the letter names (or letter/number names) that many vitamins were given when they were first discovered. You might see any of these terms on food product or vitamin supplement labels, so we will give you the various common names and forms as each vitamin is discussed (Figure 11.1).

Different forms of the same vitamin can have different potencies (abilities to function); there are a couple of reasons for this. The various forms of vitamin A provide a good example. First, you *absorb* provitamins such as carotene much less efficiently than you absorb retinol, another form of vitamin A. Second, the ability of your body to *convert* different forms of vitamin A and carotenoids to useful forms of vitamin A in your body also varies.

You may wonder if so called "natural" and synthetic vitamins also differ in potency. Actually, "natural" and synthetic vitamins, if they are in the same form, are identical. Although they may have different origins, they are not chemically different. The Slice of Life on page 338 points out the difficulty in defining "natural" vitamins. When you reach for the package with the word *natural* on the label, you can be misled into thinking you're getting something you're not. At this time, there really is no legal definition recognized nationally and no scientific definition of *natural*.

Keep in mind that vitamins, whether in foods or in supplements, are not alone: other substances are present with them. For example, many vegetables with cartenoids also contain vitamin C, fiber, and a variety of carbohydrates. Carotenoid supplements, whether they are made from "natural" or synthetic carotene, contain fillers in addition to the carotenoids. All things considered, "natural" carotene supplements may be less pure and/or concentrated than synthetic carotene. But either type of supplement probably contains more of the carotenoids and fewer of the other substances than do good food sources of carotenoids.

These other substances can either enhance, detract from, or have no effect at all on the vitamin's activity in the body. Therefore, there's no accu-

NEW
Whole
Wheat
Flakes
NET WT. 10 OZ.
Ingredients
Whole wheat, sugar, salt, malt syrup, calcium carbonate, trisodium phosphate, sodium ascorbate (vitamin C), annato color, niacinamide, iron, vitamin A palmitate, pyridoxine hydrochloride (vitamin B-6), thiamin mononitrate (vitamin B-1), riboflavin (vitamin B-2), cyanocobalamin (vitamin B-12), vitamin D.

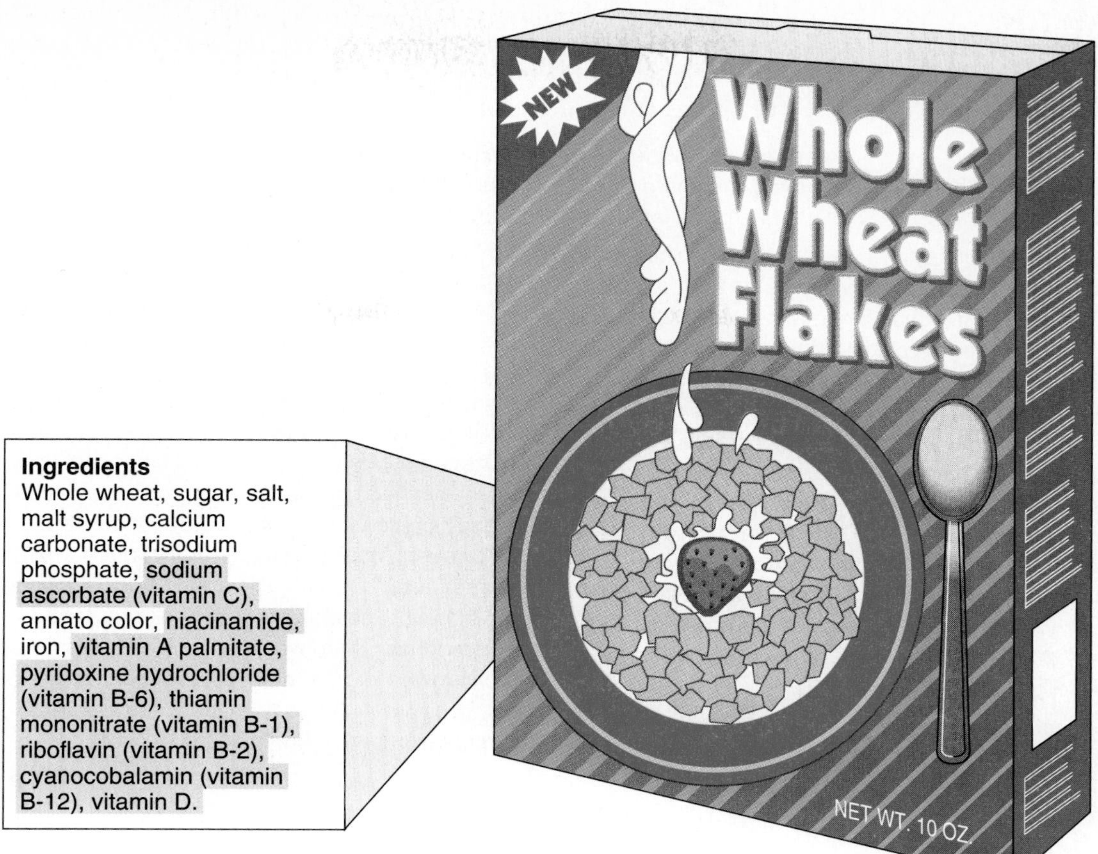

FIGURE 11.1
How added vitamins are shown on ingredient lists.

Labels of foods with added vitamins usually give both the common name and the name of the specific chemical compound used.

rate generalization about whether vitamins from "natural" supplements, from synthetic supplements, or from food will be more effective in the body.

Toxicity Levels

The level of intake at which a vitamin becomes toxic (able to harm your body) varies according to several factors. Fat-soluble vitamins have a greater potential of being toxic than do water-soluble vitamins because your body can accumulate relatively larger concentrations of fat-soluble vitamins in your tissues. In the past, it was generally assumed that you excreted in urine any excess of water-soluble vitamins, but we now know that water-soluble vitamins can also be toxic at high doses.

The potency of the form of the vitamin is another factor related to its toxicity: The more potent the chemical form, the smaller the amount required to achieve toxicity. The time frame in which the vitamin is ingested also matters. One unusually large dose of a vitamin every 6 months may not be harmful, but an intake of that same amount every day may be very toxic.

Stabilities

Generally, vitamins are less stable than other nutrients. They can be degraded, to varying degrees, by oxygen, light, various pH conditions, heat, and/or the passage of time. Practical information about how to minimize the loss of vitamins as you store and prepare your foods is included in Chapter 13 (on food processing).

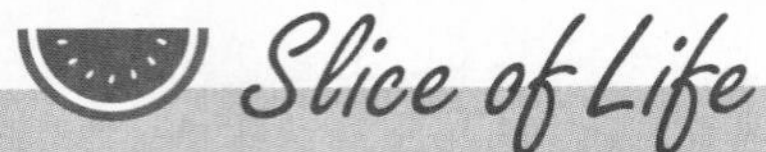

How Natural Are "Natural" Vitamins? Will the Answers Change?

The article from which this is excerpted was written two decades ago by a pharmacist with the Consumers Cooperative of Berkeley, Inc. The situation hasn't changed.

> Spurred by our growing sales . . . I visited two manufacturers of "natural" vitamins in Southern California. These companies make capsules, tablets, and other dosage forms sold under some of the most famous brand names found in "health food" stores. . . .
>
> During the visits, it became clear that many vitamin products labeled "natural" or "organic" are not really what I had imagined those terms to mean.
>
> For example, their "Rose Hips Vitamin C Tablets" are made from natural rose hips combined with chemical ascorbic acid, the same vitamin C used in standard pharmaceutical tablets. Natural rose hips contain only about 2% vitamin C, and we were told that if no vitamin C were added the tablet "would have to be as big as a golf ball" (Kamil, 1974).

Would you have guessed that the amount of vitamin C occurring naturally in rose hips was just a tiny fraction of the amount added as a synthetic chemical?

As of January 1993, the FDA was still unable to formulate acceptable definitions for the terms *natural* and *organic*. Thus, the practice described above is legal, although it is misleading.

Many individual states have worked to give meaning to these terms for use within their own borders. For a food to be labeled "organic" in these states, it must have been grown under certain conditions defined by the state. Such conditions are likely to include the avoidance of synthetic fertilizers and pesticides. It is possible to test for the presence of synthetic pesticides, so—to this extent at least—the appropriate use of the term can be verified.

However, "natural" vitamin supplements or foods to which "natural" vitamins are added pose a tougher problem. Although states could devise regulations covering these products, there would be no way to test whether the vitamins were of natural or of laboratory origin, because both types have the same chemical structure. Enforcing the regulations fairly would be impossible.

Units of Measurement

Most vitamins are quantified in milligrams (mg) and micrograms (μg). Another unit that has been used in the past for some vitamins (vitamins A and D) is the International Unit (IU).

equivalent—unit now coming into use as an indicator of the activity of certain vitamins in the body

Now that scientists are aware that different forms of some vitamins and their precursors have varying potencies, they use units called **equivalents** to reflect as accurately as possible the amount of vitamin *activity* the various forms provide. The 1989 RDA uses equivalents for recommending intakes of vitamins A, E, and niacin (see inside back cover). However, many food composition tables still express levels of these vitamins in milligrams or IUs, and until food composition tables can be completely revised to match the newer equivalent values, comparing such values is like comparing apples to oranges. We will discuss the ramifications of these temporary discrepancies at appropriate points in this chapter.

How Vitamins Function

Nutrition students typically learn about vitamins by considering each one separately—their functions, typical intakes, dietary sources, and the most significant effects of their deficiencies and excesses. Unfortunately, this approach can be somewhat misleading, because it suggests that each vitamin functions in isolation and is active only in certain tissues.

In reality, *most vitamins function in almost all body cells.* Because cells differ, the effect of a deficiency of a vitamin may be more obvious in some cells or tissues than others. But generally, a person who has any vitamin deficiency feels weak, fails to grow or reproduce, and is more susceptible to illnesses. Deficiencies of different vitamins often result in common symptoms also because most people who develop one deficiency are likely to experience several at the same time. A final, very important factor is that *vitamins do not function in isolation*. If you drastically change your intake of one nutrient, the utilization of several other nutrients is likely to be affected as well. For example, vitamin E absorption and utilization depend on the amount and type of fats you consume; if you reduce just the fat in your diet, therefore, your requirement for vitamin E will also change. You'll hear much more about the interactions of nutrients in Chapter 12.

The most common circumstances that lead to vitamin deficiencies are described below. Notice how they relate to the themes just discussed. Vitamin deficiencies occur when

1. A person just does not get enough food. This occurs most commonly for economic reasons in developing countries and generally results in multiple deficiencies.
2. A person's diet lacks variety. Children in developing countries often develop vitamin A deficiencies because economic and sociologic factors limit the types of foods available to them.
3. A person cannot absorb or utilize vitamin(s) to a normal extent because of inborn problems, disease conditions, or alcohol or other drug use.
4. A person's requirements for vitamins are unusually high because of rapid growth or disease. For this reason, children often develop symptoms of severe deficiencies more rapidly than adults.

For the sake of organization, we *will* present the vitamins one by one in this section. So as you read, keep in mind that the vitamins (and other nutrients as well) have considerable effects on each other and can influence the activities of virtually all your body cells. These themes are at least as important as the details about specific vitamins.

The Fat-Soluble Vitamins

There is much to say about the 13 vitamins. Table 11.1 gives an overview of some of the facts about them. Let's begin by discussing the fat-soluble vitamins.

Vitamin A

Vitamin A was the first vitamin to be identified. From this you might think that everything possible would have been discovered about vitamin A years ago. Far from it—there is currently an explosion of research activity about vitamin A. But before we look at that, let's get acquainted with some background on the nature of this important substance.

When we talk about vitamin A in food, we may be referring to any of several different chemical forms of vitamin A. These may be preformed (already formed) versions or provitamins of vitamin A. The most common preformed version present in food is *retinol*; others are *retinal*, *retinaldehyde*, and *retinoic acid*. The last one, retinoic acid, cannot be converted by the body into retinol, so it cannot perform all the functions retinol can.

There are hundreds of compounds called *carotenoids* that occur, for the most part, in plant materials and have some structural similarity to vitamin A. About 50 of them can be converted into retinol by the body, so only these are provitamins of vitamin A and, if converted to retinol, perform the functions of vitamin A. The most important of these provitamin A compounds is *beta-carotene* (β-carotene).

TABLE 11.1 Key Information About the Vitamins

Vitamin	RDA for Healthy Adults Ages 19–50	Major Dietary Sources	Major Functions	Signs of Severe, Prolonged Deficiency	Signs of Extreme Excess
Fat-Soluble					
A	Females: 800 RE Males: 1000 RE	Fat-containing and fortified dairy products; liver; provitamin carotene in orange and deep green fruits and vegetables	Vitamin A is a component of rhodopsin; carotenoids can serve as antioxidants; retinoic acid affects gene expression; still under intense study	Night blindness; keratinization of epithelial tissues including the cornea of the eye (xerophthalmia) causing permanent blindness; dry, scaling skin; increased susceptibility to infection	*Preformed vitamin A:* damage to liver, bone; headache, irritability, vomiting, hair loss, blurred vision *13-cis retinoic acid:* some fetal defects *Carotenoids:* yellowed skin
D	<25 years: 10 μg >25 years: 5 μg	Fortified and full-fat dairy products, egg yolk (diet often not as important as sunlight exposure)	Promotes absorption and use of calcium and phosphorus	Rickets (bone deformities) in children; osteomalacia (bone softening) in adults	Calcium deposition in tissues leading to cerebral, CV, and kidney damage
E	Females: 8 α-tocopherol equivalents Males: 10 α-tocopherol equivalents	Vegetable oils and their products; nuts, seeds	Antioxidant to prevent cell membrane damage; still under intense study	Possible anemia and neurologic effects	Generally nontoxic, but at least one type of intravenous infusion led to some fatalities in premature infants; may worsen clotting defect in vitamin K deficiency
K	Females: <25: 60 μg >25: 65 μg Males: <25: 70 μg >25: 80 μg	Green vegetables; tea	Aids in formation of certain proteins, especially those for blood clotting	Defective blood coagulation causing severe bleeding on injury	Liver damage and anemia from high doses of the synthetic form menadione
Water-Soluble					
Thiamin (B-1)	Females: 1.1 mg Males: 1.5 mg	Pork, legumes, peanuts, enriched or whole-grain products	Coenzyme used in energy metabolism	Nerve changes, sometimes edema, heart failure; beriberi	Generally nontoxic, but repeated injections may cause shock reaction

Vitamin	RDA for Healthy Adults Ages 19–50	Major Dietary Sources	Major Functions	Signs of Severe, Prolonged Deficiency	Signs of Extreme Excess
Riboflavin (B-2)	Females: 1.3 mg Males: 1.7 mg	Dairy products, meats, eggs, enriched grain products, green leafy vegetables	Coenzyme used in energy metabolism	Skin lesions	Generally nontoxic
Niacin	Females: 15 niacin equivalents Males: 19 niacin equivalents	Nuts, meats; provitamin tryptophan in most proteins	Coenzyme used in energy metabolism	Pellagra (multiple vitamin deficiencies including niacin)	Flushing of face, neck, hands; potential liver damage
B-6	Females: 1.6 mg Males: 2.0 mg	High-protein foods in general	Coenzyme used in amino acid metabolism	Nervous, skin, and muscular disorders; anemia	Unstable gait, numb feet, poor coordination
Folic acid	Females: 180 μg Males: 200 μg	Green vegetables, orange juice, nuts, legumes, grain products	Coenzyme used in DNA and RNA metabolism; single carbon utilization	Megaloblastic anemia (large, immature red blood cells); GI disturbances	Masks vitamin B-12 deficiency, interferes with drugs to control epilepsy
B-12	2 μg	Animal products	Coenzyme used in DNA and RNA metabolism; single carbon utilization	Megaloblastic anemia; pernicious anemia when due to inadequate intrinsic factor; nervous system damage	Thought to be nontoxic
Pantothenic acid	4–7 mg[a]	Animal products and whole grains; widely distributed in foods	Coenzyme used in energy metabolism	Fatigue, numbness, and tingling of hands and feet	Generally nontoxic; occasionally causes diarrhea
Biotin	30–100 μg[a]	Widely distributed in foods	Coenzyme used in energy metabolism	Scaly dermatitis	Thought to be nontoxic
C (ascorbic acid)	60 mg	Fruits and vegetables, especially broccoli, cabbage, cantaloupe, cauliflower, citrus fruits, green pepper, kiwi fruit, strawberries	Functions in synthesis of collagen; is an antioxidant; aids in detoxification; improves iron absorption; still under intense study	Scurvy; petechiae (minute hemorrhages around hair follicles); weakness; delayed wound healing; impaired immune response	GI upsets, confounds certain lab tests

[a] Estimated Safe and Adequate Daily Dietary Intake in 1989 RDAs

Sources: RDA Subcommittee, 1989; Shils and Young, 1988.

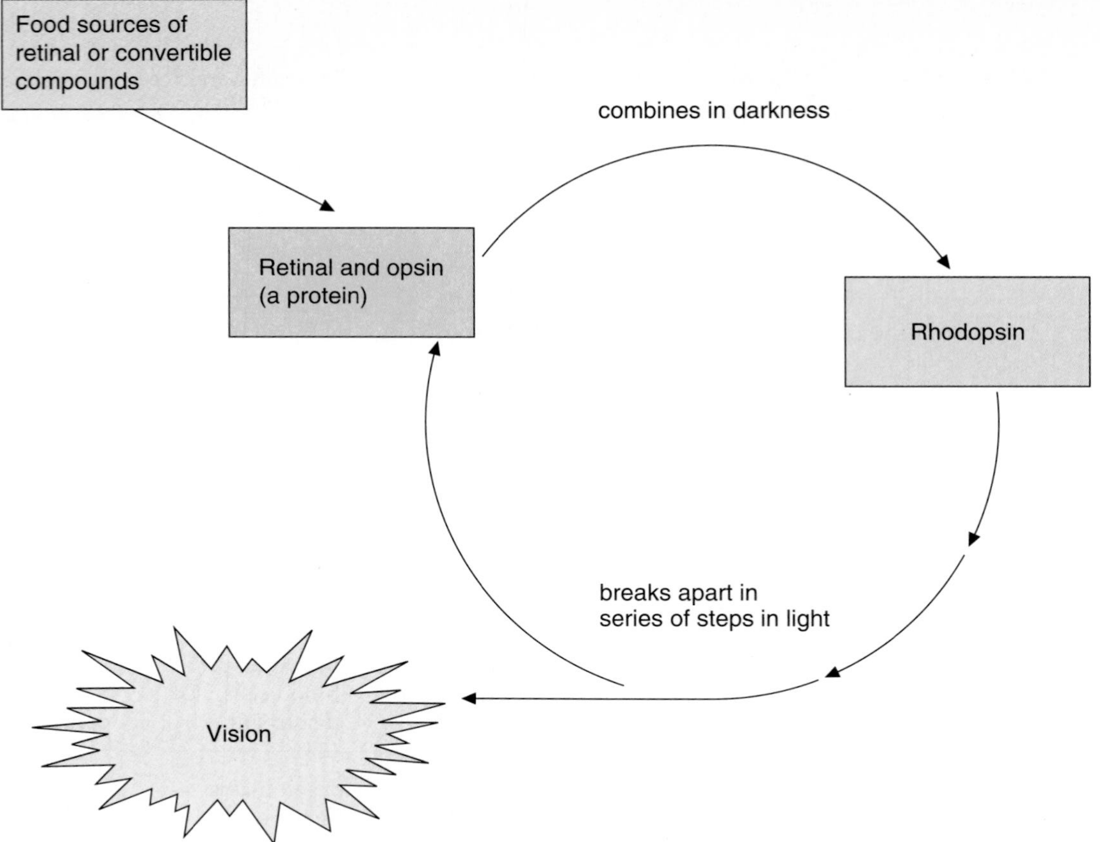

FIGURE 11.2
The visual cycle.

Retinal (a form of vitamin A) and opsin (a protein produced by your body) combine to form the visual pigment *rhodopsin*. If not enough retinal is available, your body cannot make rhodopsin fast enough, and you will have trouble seeing in dim light. This is called night blindness.

Functions and Effects of Deficiency Vitamin A plays a well-defined role in your eyes. Figure 11.2 gives a simplified explanation of the visual cycle. Vitamin A as retinal is a component of rhodopsin and iodopsin, which are colored light-sensitive substances in the retina. When light falls on these compounds, they undergo changes that are translated into messages about what was seen and are sent to the brain. Then these compounds are converted back to their original form. If vitamin A has been deficient in the diet, these conversions occur more slowly than normal, and there is a time lag before the eye can see again. Since this occurs particularly when the eye is trying to adapt from bright light to darkness, the condition is called **night blindness.** Night blindness is reversible. Only retinol or carotenoids that can be converted to retinol—not retinoic acid—can prevent night blindness.

night blindness—condition in which eyes cannot adapt quickly from bright light to darkness, leading to temporary blindness in dim light; caused by vitamin A deficiency

mRNA—(messenger RNA) form of ribonucleic acid that transmits messages from DNA to the site where proteins are synthesized

The other functions of vitamin A still puzzle scientists. Scientists think that vitamin A as retinoic acid, bound to a special protein, reacts with the DNA in the nuclei of your body's cells (Wolf, 1990). That changes the functioning of a gene in the DNA so that the production of **mRNA** is altered. The altered mRNA carries the message to ribosomes outside the nuclei where protein is synthesized. Because the mRNA is altered, the proteins synthesized are altered and often they function differently. Scientists describe this total process of altering mRNA and protein synthesis as *altering gene expression.*

If you think about it, you won't be surprised to know that retinoic acid plays a crucial role in embryo development (Smith and Eichele, 1991). Obviously, protein synthesis occurs rapidly during embryo development. This

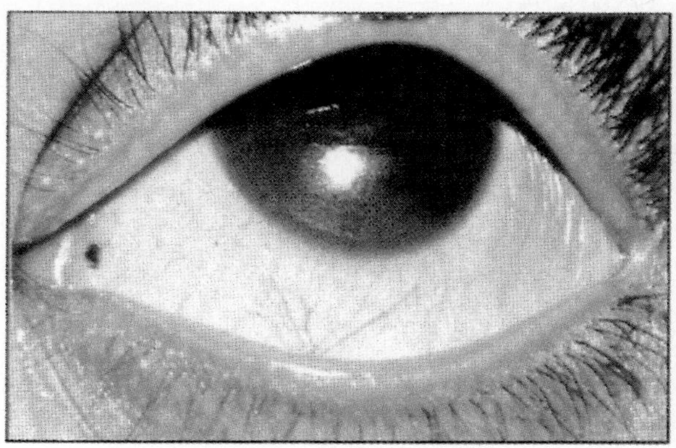

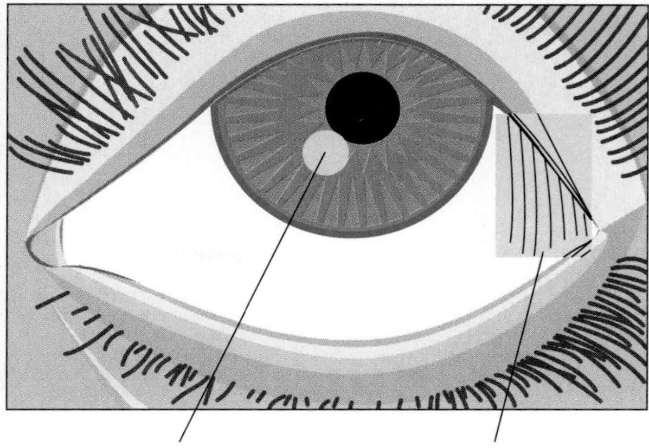

FIGURE 11.3
Changes in the cornea due to vitamin A deficiency.

Here you see one of the stages of eye damage from vitamin A deficiency. The cornea is dull and opaque, and the membrane covering the white of the eye has become wrinkled. If not treated, the membranes will tear and cause blindness.
Source: Bauerfeind, 1988.

fact also explains why both severe deficiencies and excesses of vitamin A have been associated with **teratogenesis**, the development of malformations in embryos.

Because of these effects of retinoic acid on protein synthesis, deficiencies or excesses of vitamin A affect a large number of tissues, including cartilage, bone, and body coverings and linings. These coverings and linings are called *epithelial tissues*. They include the corneas of eyes; the mucous membranes, including the linings of nasal passages, gastrointestinal (GI) tract, and genitourinary tract; and the skin. Helping keep epithelial tissue healthy is one of several ways in which vitamin A maintains immune function (Ross, 1992).

If vitamin A is deficient in your body, *keratinization* occurs—a process in which the skin becomes dry and rough and mucous membranes may crack and hemorrhage. The most devastating example of this effect occurs in the cornea of the eye (the clear covering over the front of the eyeball); in severe and prolonged cases of vitamin A deficiency, keratinization can cause blindness. The term used to refer to severe vitamin A deficiency symptoms in the eye is **xerophthalmia**. Figure 11.3 shows one stage in the development of blindness from vitamin A deficiency. Although this disease is not often seen in the developed countries, it causes blindness in an estimated one-half million children annually (Bauerfeind, 1988). Figure 11.4 shows parts of the world in which blindness due to vitamin A deficiency is common.

The immense suffering of children worldwide due to vitamin A deficiency has probably been underestimated in the past. Blindness is not the only effect of severe vitamin A deficiency. Many studies conducted in Asia and Africa during the last several years show that improving the vitamin A status of children greatly reduces death—by as much as 50%—among those exposed to infectious diseases such as measles and pneumonia (Rahmathullah et al., 1990; Hussey and Klein, 1990).

Inadequate intake of *carotenoids* may put people at greater risk of still another health problem—cancer. Several investigators have noted that the intake of more carotenoids was associated with a lower risk of cancer, particularly of the lung (Byers and Perry, 1992). The way in which carotenoids may protect us is unclear but probably involves their ability to serve as **antioxidants** without being converted to retinol (Canfield et al., 1992). Remember, though, that this statistical correlation does not *prove* that

teratogenesis—the development of malformations in embryos

xerophthalmia—condition in which cornea of the eye becomes keratinized; can result in permanent blindness if untreated; caused by severe, prolonged vitamin A deficiency

antioxidant—substance that prevents oxygen from combining with other substances to which it might cause damage

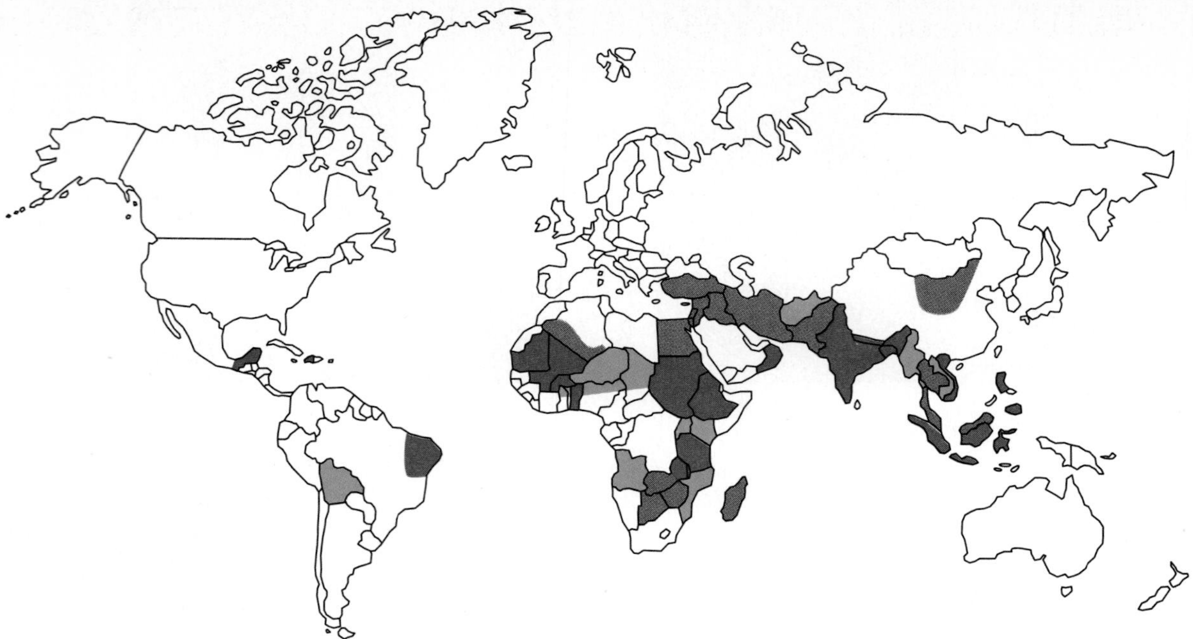

Vitamin A deficiency a significant public health problem
Vitamin A deficiency most probably a significant public health problem
Vitamin A deficiency not a significant public health problem; sporadic cases that should be monitored

FIGURE 11.4
Geographical distribution of vitamin A deficiency and xerophthalmia.
Source: Bauerfeind, 1988.

carotene reduces the risk of cancer: other components of foods that contain carotenoids (such as fiber, vitamin C, vitamin E, and other chemicals) may also affect the incidence of cancer.

Recommended and Typical Intakes Currently the RDAs for vitamin A for women and men are 800 and 1000 retinol equivalents (RE), respectively. According to survey data, the average adult male in the United States consumes more than 1400 RE of vitamin A daily (Human Nutrition Information Service, 1986). Averages are sometimes misleading: another large survey found that although the average individual from 1 to 74 years of age consumed more than the RDA for vitamin A, 42% consumed less than one-half the RDA for males on the day surveyed (National Center for Health Statistics, 1979). This is not necessarily a problem, because a large intake one day is saved for use on another day—your body stores vitamin A in the liver. This situation also demonstrates the difficulty of trying to predict the adequacy of your diet on the basis of one day's intake.

Dietary Sources As you can see in Table 11.2, the fruit and vegetable groups contain a number of foods that are outstanding sources of vitamin A. The fruits and vegetables that generally have the highest amount of vitamin A are the carotene-containing, deep orange and dark green varieties. The best among them are apricots, broccoli, cantaloupe (muskmelon), carrots, pumpkin, winter squash, sweet potatoes, and spinach and other dark, leafy greens. Another food that provides a large amount of vitamin A in one serving is liver; here, the major form of vitamin A is retinol. Dairy products and eggs provide significant amounts of both retinol and carotenoids.

TABLE 11.2 Vitamin A in Some Foods

The RDA for men is 1000 RE/day; for women, 800 RE/day.

Food	Household Measure	RE of Vitamin A (0–1000)
Bread, cereal, rice, and pasta		
Bread, white, enriched	1 slice	tr
Cornflakes	1 cup	
Total® fortified cereal	1 cup	1748
Noodles (cooked)	½ cup	
Vegetables		
Broccoli, frozen, cooked	½ cup	
Carrot, raw	7½ inches long	2025
Corn, canned	½ cup	
Green beans, frozen, cooked	½ cup	
Lettuce, iceberg	1 cup	
Spinach, frozen, cooked	½ cup	
Fruits		
Apple	1 medium	
Apricots, canned light syrup	½ cup	
Cantaloupe	½ cup	
Orange juice, frozen, reconstituted	½ cup	
Peach, fresh	1 medium	
Milk, yogurt, and cheese		
Buttermilk from skim milk, not fortified	1 cup	
Skim milk, vitamin A fortified	1 cup	
Milk, whole, not fortified	1 cup	
Cheese, cheddar	1⅓ ounces	
Meats, poultry, fish, eggs, beans, and nuts		
Beef, ground, broiled	2 ounces	
Chicken leg, roasted	2 ounces	
Eggs	2 large	
Kidney beans, canned	1 cup	
Liver, beef, fried	2 ounces	6074
Combination foods		
Bean/cheese burrito	7 ounces	
Beef chunky soup, canned	1 cup	
Cheese pizza	⅛ of 15" pie	
Nachos with cheese	6–8	
Fats, oils, and sweets		
Butter	1 teaspoon	
Carbonated beverages	12 ounces	
Dressing, salad Italian	1 tablespoon	
Sugar, honey	1 tablespoon	

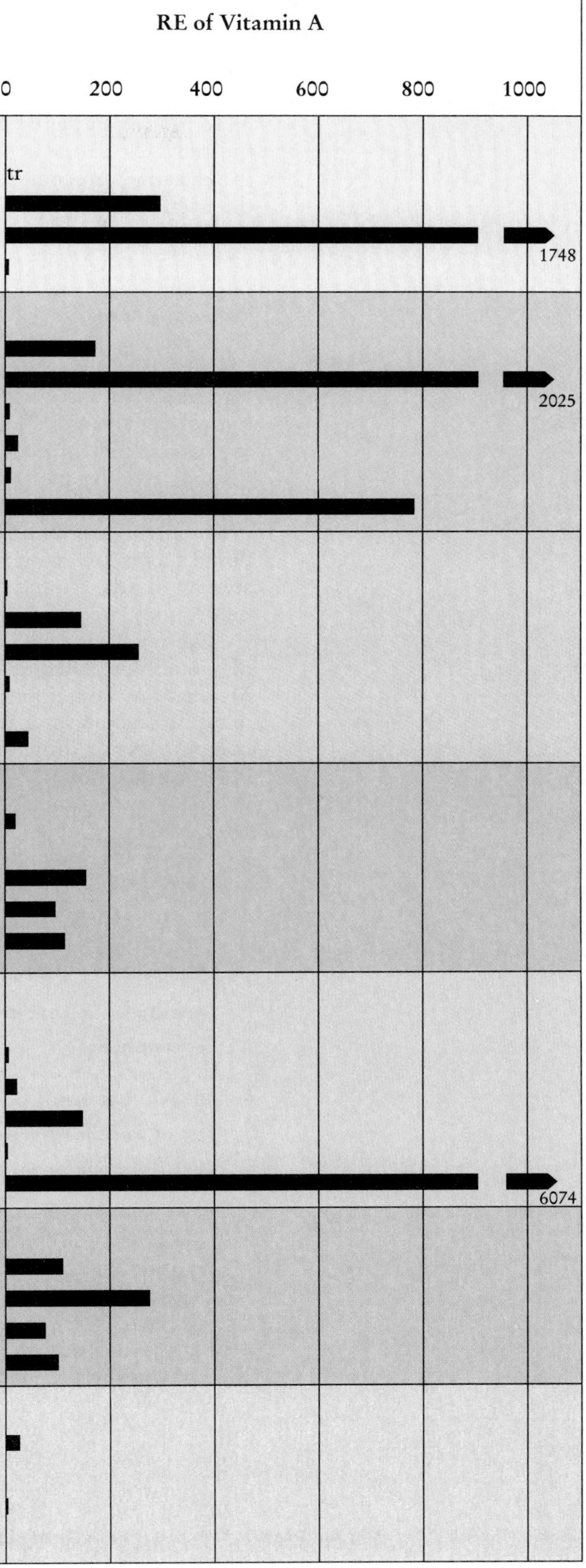

As you read in the beginning of the chapter, your body cannot use all forms of vitamin A equally well. Retinol (found mainly in animal sources) is much better utilized than carotenoids (found mainly in plant sources). Even though we generally consume more carotenoids, USDA scientists have estimated that carotenoids contribute less than one-third of the total vitamin A *activity* in the diets of Americans.

Table 11.2 and Appendix C give the vitamin A content of foods in terms of retinol equivalents (REs). Some older food composition tables still use the old IUs. Do not compare IU values for vitamin A with your RDA in REs; they are not comparable values. The REs more accurately reflect the usefulness of vitamin A compounds in food to your body than do the old IUs.

Consequences of High Intake You can consume high levels of vitamin A as carotene just by eating vegetables and fruits. The skin of people (especially children) who consume excess amounts of deep yellow and deep green vegetables with every meal may turn yellow; excess carotene has no other known detrimental consequences. The person can reverse this effect by eating less of the carotene-rich foods. However, routine overconsumption of vitamin A as retinol (more than 25,000 IUs daily) may result in toxicity (Geubel et al., 1991). Symptoms may include skin lesions, hair loss, and—eventually—liver and bone damage. A few patients who unwittingly overdosed themselves with vitamin A supplements developed such elevated pressure in fluids around the brain that physicians suspected brain tumors before they recognized the real problem (Evans and Lacey, 1986).

We must also add a caution against taking a particular synthetic form of vitamin A called *13-cis-retinoic acid,* or *isotretinoin,* during pregnancy. Medications containing this substance are sometimes prescribed for treatment of severe cystic acne. Because a number of these synthetic vitamin A compounds are known to cause malformation in animal fetuses, they should never be prescribed for a woman who is pregnant or intends to become pregnant during the course of drug use. But there have been cases in which women taking the drug have become pregnant. In studying 59 such pregnancies, researchers noted 12 spontaneous abortions, 21 malformed infants, and only 26 infants without major malformations (Lammer et al., 1985).

You Tell Me

Accutane, an oral drug containing 13-cis-retinoic acid, is used to treat severe acne.

Should you use this product if you are a woman who has the possibility of becoming pregnant? What should you consider? What are potential risks and benefits?

Synthetic vitamin A compounds are also used in certain skin creams to treat acne and/or wrinkling caused by sun damage. Their effectiveness for treating acne is better established than that for treating sun damage (Roberts, 1988). There is no evidence that such topical application for either purpose is a risk during pregnancy.

Vitamin D

Vitamin D is a unique vitamin because it can be produced by your body. This occurs when ultraviolet light from the sun changes a compound in your skin called 7-dehydrocholesterol into vitamin D. In food, vitamin D occurs as various forms of *cholecalciferol* (vitamin D of animal origin) and *ergocalciferol* (vitamin D of plant or yeast origin).

Functions and Effects of Deficiency After vitamin D is modified slightly in your liver and kidneys, it serves as a hormone. The primary roles of vitamin D are to enhance the intestinal absorption of calcium and phosphorus, to promote retention of calcium that might otherwise be lost in the urine, and to mobilize calcium from bone if necessary. All these activities work together to maintain the levels of calcium and phosphorus in your blood. This is important for normal nerve and muscle activity and to help promote calcium deposition in bone (DeLuca, 1988).

If the level of vitamin D in your body is inadequate over a period of time, your bones will fail to mineralize (incorporate bone minerals) or will progressively demineralize (lose bone minerals) in order to keep blood calcium within normal levels. This results in bone softening. The condition is called **rickets** when it occurs in children. It is characterized by abnormal bone development that may result in bowed legs and other deformities. When vitamin D deficiency occurs in adults, the condition is called **osteomalacia**.

rickets, osteomalacia—progressive demineralization of bone in children and adults, respectively; caused by vitamin D deficiency

Recommended Intakes Because vitamin D is linked closely to bone growth and maintenance, the RDA for this nutrient is highest for people who still have the potential to grow. For children and young adults through age 24, the recommended daily intake is 10 μg. At age 25 it drops to 5 μg. During pregnancy and lactation, an intake of 10 μg is again recommended.

However, it is debatable whether an RDA for vitamin D for adults is necessary. Many adults produce in their bodies as much vitamin D as they need, provided that they get enough sun. The amount of vitamin D produced in a person's skin depends on many factors: the surface area exposed to sunlight, the amount of pigment in the skin (dark skin needs more sunlight to initiate vitamin D production), the time of day, the season, the latitude, the presence of a sunscreen (sunscreens with a skin-protection factor of 8 or higher block vitamin D production), and even the person's age (production diminishes with age). Because of all these variables, it's very hard to say how much sun you need to produce sufficient vitamin D. One expert recommends that for adequate vitamin D protection, elderly white people living in Boston in the summertime should expose hands, arms, and face to doses of sun that are less than would cause reddening—usually 10–15 minutes, depending on the person's skin pigmentation, two or three times a week (Holick, 1987).

You Tell Me

Think about how you dress and how often you are outside.

Do you think that vitamin D deficiency is apt to ever be a problem for you? Under what circumstances? Do you know anyone who might be at risk?

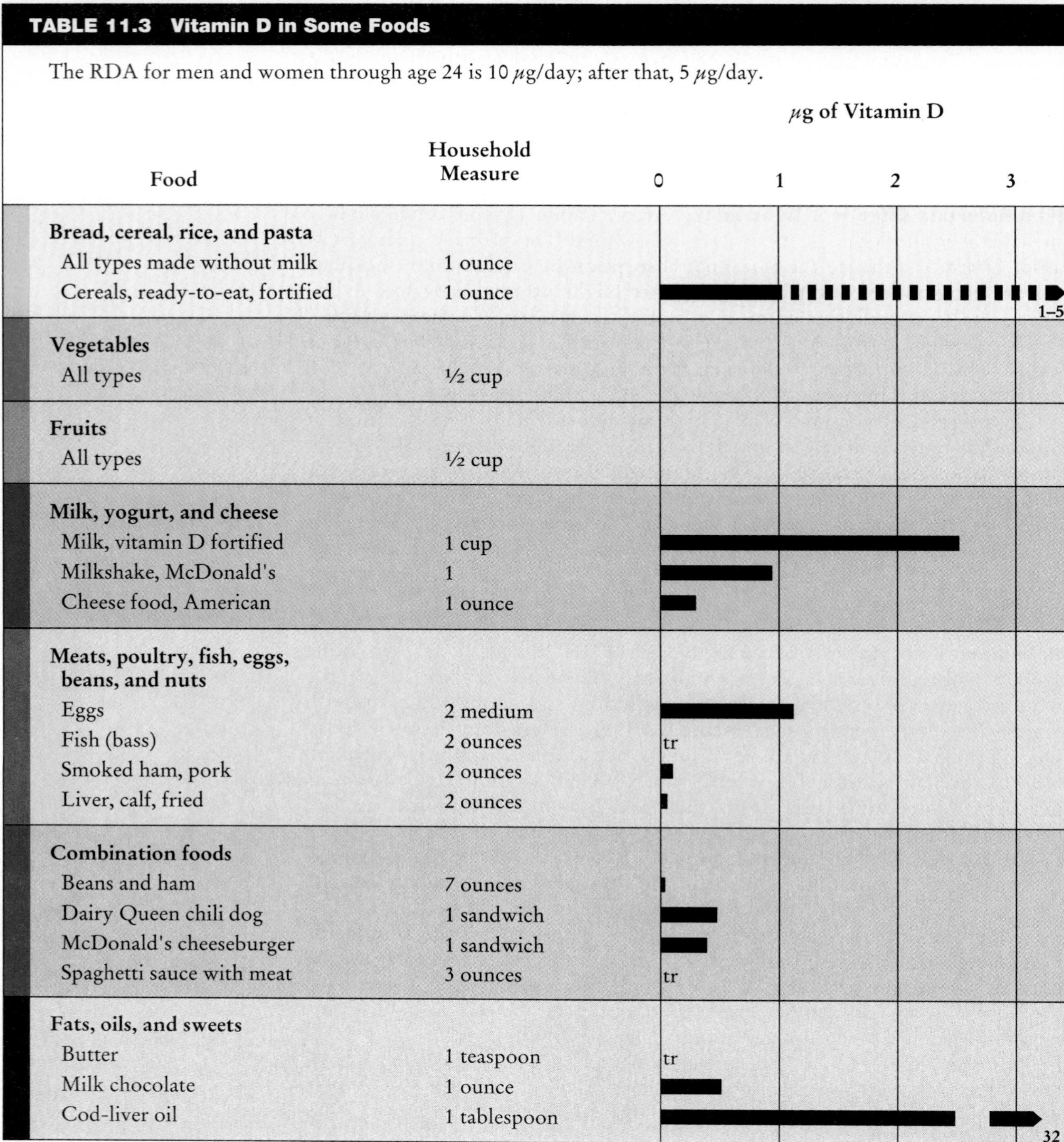

TABLE 11.3 Vitamin D in Some Foods

The RDA for men and women through age 24 is 10 μg/day; after that, 5 μg/day.

Food	Household Measure	μg of Vitamin D (0 1 2 3)
Bread, cereal, rice, and pasta		
All types made without milk	1 ounce	
Cereals, ready-to-eat, fortified	1 ounce	1–5
Vegetables		
All types	½ cup	
Fruits		
All types	½ cup	
Milk, yogurt, and cheese		
Milk, vitamin D fortified	1 cup	
Milkshake, McDonald's	1	
Cheese food, American	1 ounce	
Meats, poultry, fish, eggs, beans, and nuts		
Eggs	2 medium	
Fish (bass)	2 ounces	tr
Smoked ham, pork	2 ounces	
Liver, calf, fried	2 ounces	
Combination foods		
Beans and ham	7 ounces	
Dairy Queen chili dog	1 sandwich	
McDonald's cheeseburger	1 sandwich	
Spaghetti sauce with meat	3 ounces	tr
Fats, oils, and sweets		
Butter	1 teaspoon	tr
Milk chocolate	1 ounce	
Cod-liver oil	1 tablespoon	32

Data adapted from Pennington, 1989; Pennington and Church, 1985.

Dietary Sources There are no naturally excellent sources of vitamin D among foods that people normally eat. However, there is a good fortified source—milk fortified with vitamin D. Table 11.3 reveals that two servings will provide the adult RDA. Other significant sources are egg yolks and products made with fortified milk.

Cod-liver oil is a very potent source of vitamin D. Because of the toxicity of vitamin D, if you ingest cod-liver oil for any reason, the amount taken should be carefully controlled to avoid toxicity.

Consequences of High Intake Vitamin D is regarded as the most toxic of all the vitamins. If you consume too much vitamin D, it may lead to high blood calcium levels and deposition of calcium in your soft tissue, resulting in irreversible renal (kidney) and cardiovascular damage (RDA Subcommittee, 1989). Note this statement from the 1989 RDA: "Since the toxic level of vitamin D may in some cases be only 5 times the RDA . . . , dietary supplements may be detrimental for the normal child or adult who drinks at least two glasses of vitamin D fortified milk per day."

The importance of fortifying milk with enough, but not too much, vitamin D was emphasized in 1992. Excessively high levels of vitamin D metabolites were reported in the blood of patients who consumed milk that had been fortified with excessive amounts of vitamin D (Jacobus et al., 1992). Incidents like this make you realize how important it is that FDA and state health agencies constantly monitor our food supply.

Fortunately, there is no need to worry that excess sunlight will result in internal production of toxic levels of vitamin D. It has been found that following the initial period of sun exposure, the skin produces progressively less provitamin for vitamin D (Holick, 1987). (Of course, prolonged exposure to sun exacts a different, unrelated penalty—increased risk of skin cancer.)

Vitamin E

Vitamin E occurs in food as compounds called *tocopherols* and *tocotrienols*. The most active form of vitamin E is *alpha-tocopherol* (α-tocopherol); other forms, such as *beta-tocopherol* or *gamma-tocopherol*, are only 1–50% as active.

Functions and Effects of Deficiency Vitamin E functions in the body primarily as an antioxidant, preventing oxygen from combining with other substances and damaging them. For example, the presence of vitamin E is thought to protect vitamin A from being oxidized. Vitamin E also protects polyunsaturated fatty acids (PUFAs) from oxidation. This occurs not only in foods but also in your body, where PUFAs are part of cell membranes. Vitamin E may help protect against certain types of cancer in this way, but proving this requires much further study (Byers and Perry, 1992).

Vitamin E deficiency is so rare that for many years this vitamin was said to be in search of a disease. However, it can occur in premature infants and in people who, over a period of years, are unable to absorb fat and fat-soluble vitamins (Mino, 1992).

You Tell Me

Magazines and booklets at the checkout counter of grocery stores frequently have ads that claim that (1) vitamin E will prevent or cure heart diseases or muscular dystrophy, and (2) vitamin E will improve sexual or athletic performance.

What do you think about these claims? How can you evaluate them? Are facts from controlled studies presented? Can placebo effects occur?

Recommended and Typical Intakes Because the variation in the activity of the various forms of vitamin E is so great, recommended intakes of this nutrient are now designated in equivalents. An equivalent has the vitamin E activity equal to that of 1 mg α-tocopherol. The RDA recommends 10 α-tocopherol equivalents for adult males and 8 α-tocopherol equivalents for adult females.

Your body's actual need for vitamin E varies with the degree of unsaturation of fats in your diet. The RDA for vitamin E is based on typical intakes by Americans. Because vitamin E protects the unsaturated bonds from oxidation, if you drastically increase your intake of polyunsaturated fatty acids, you need more vitamin E.

The average daily consumption of men and women in the United States is estimated to be 9.6 and 7 α-tocopherol equivalents, respectively (Murphy et al., 1990), but people vary greatly in their intake of vitamin E. When the variable level of intake of polyunsaturated fatty acids is also taken into account, experts estimate that vitamin E intakes are less than optimal for 23% of American men and 15% of American women.

Dietary Sources Notice in Table 11.4 that the best sources of the most active form of vitamin E (α-tocopherol) are products that include plant oils. That means your major dietary sources of vitamin E (such as mayonnaise, other salad dressings, many margarines) are often foods in the fats, oils and sweets group. It just shows that variety in your diet is good for you.

A few points should be made about these outstanding vitamin E sources. First of all, because plant foods that contain high levels of polyunsaturated fats usually also contain high levels of vitamin E, the higher need for the vitamin may be automatically satisfied when the fat is eaten. However, there is some variation in the type and quantity of vitamin E compounds present in foods high in PUFAs. Second, Table 11.4 lists only the α-tocopherol content of foods. The total vitamin E activity of some foods is higher, perhaps by 20%. Finally, you may sometimes see tocopherol listed as an ingredient in bacon. It has not been put there to improve your vitamin E status; it has been approved for use as an additive in bacon to inhibit the formation of nitrosamine, a carcinogen. (Nitrosamine is discussed further in Chapter 14.) In this case, a substance we value as an antioxidant in the body can be used as an antioxidant in foods, too.

Toxicity Because of the many claims made for vitamin E, many people have consumed vitamin E supplements. There have been few side effects (Mino, 1992), but that does not mean there is *no* risk. Excess intake of vitamin E may worsen a blood-clotting defect produced by vitamin K deficiency. Also, an increased death rate was noted among low-birth-weight infants given an intravenous preparation of vitamin E. The cause was not identified, but the product was removed from the market.

Vitamin K

The vitamin K in your body comes from two sources: you eat forms called *phylloquinones*, which are synthesized by green plants, and the bacteria in your intestinal tract synthesize forms called *menaquinones*. A type of menaquinone is produced by humans when given a synthetic form of vitamin K called *menadione*, but its use is discouraged because toxic symptoms in infants have been observed from even low doses (Olson, 1989).

Functions and Effects of Deficiency Vitamin K is essential for the formation of several proteins necessary for blood clotting, as well as for the synthesis of a variety of other proteins whose functions are still undefined. When people are very deficient in vitamin K, it takes longer than normal

TABLE 11.4 Vitamin E in Some Foods

The RDA for women is 8 α-tocopherol equivalents/day; for men, 10 α-tocopherol equivalents/day.

mg of α-Tocopherol[a]: 0 | 1.0 | 2.0 | 3.0 | 4.0 | 5.0

Food	Household Measure
Bread, cereal, rice, and pasta	
Bread, white	1 slice
Pasta, cooked	½ cup
Wheat flakes	1 ounce
Vegetables	
Corn, canned	4 ounces
Greens, mustard	4 ounces
Peas, frozen	4 ounces
Potato, boiled	1 medium
Spinach, frozen	½ cup
Fruits	
Apple	1 medium
Strawberries, raw	½ cup
Milk, yogurt, and cheese	
Cheese, cheddar	1⅓ ounces
Milk, whole	1 cup
Meats, poultry, fish, eggs, beans, and nuts	
Beef steak, broiled	2 ounces
Chicken, frozen, fried	2 ounces
Eggs, cooked	2 large
Haddock, broiled	2 ounces
Peanuts, dry roasted	2 ounces
Combination foods	
Beef stew, canned	8 ounces
Cheeseburger	1 sandwich
Ravioli, chicken, canned	8 ounces
Fats, oils, and sweets	
Butter	1 teaspoon
Margarines made with soybean oil	1 teaspoon
Mayonnaise made with soybean oil	1 tablespoon
Milk-chocolate candy	1 ounce

[a]The bars on this chart represent the amount of the most active form of vitamin E (α-tocopherol) found in the specified servings of food. Since many other, less active forms of vitamin E are present at the same time, the total vitamin E activities of these foods are likely to be somewhat higher than these figures suggest.

Data adapted from Pennington, 1989; Pennington and Church, 1985.

TABLE 11.5 Vitamin K in Some Foods

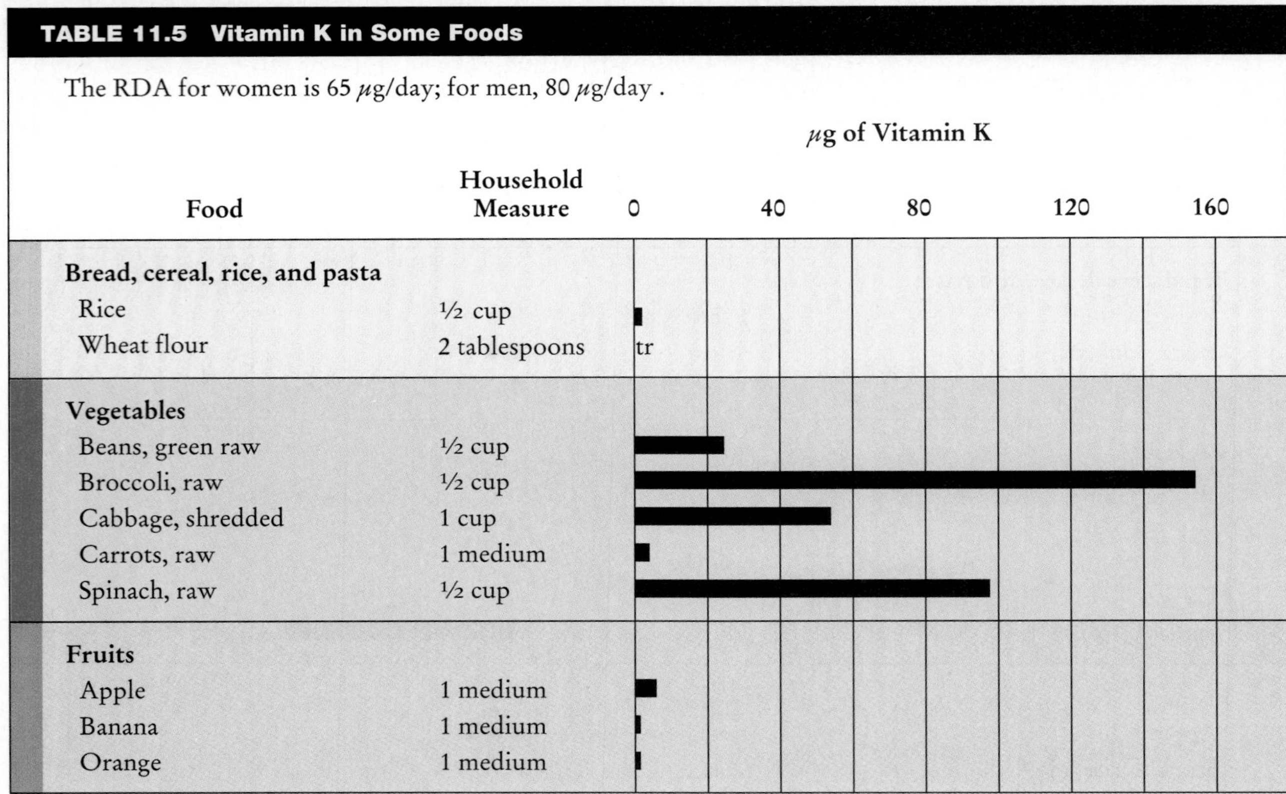

Data adapted from Suttie, 1992.

for their blood to clot when bleeding occurs. (Vitamin K is unrelated to the disease *hemophilia*; in that condition, other factors needed for blood clotting are deficient.)

Recommended Intakes In 1989, for the first time, RDAs were established for vitamin K; they are 80 μg per day for men and 65 μg per day for women. Little is known about typical intakes of vitamin K, but they have been assumed to be adequate because most people have no problem with blood clotting. In one recent survey, diets of college-age males were analyzed and found to contain an average 77 μg of vitamin K daily (Suttie et al., 1988). This suggests that some people may consume less than adequate amounts.

At birth, infants have very low levels of vitamin K in their bodies. If they become injured in some way—either internally or externally—their blood does not clot as quickly as an adult's blood, and excessive bleeding is likely. As a safeguard, it is recommended (and widely practiced) that infants be given an injection of vitamin K after birth or daily oral supplements for a short period (RDA Subcommittee, 1989).

Dietary Sources People who regularly take large doses of antibiotics (which kill useful intestinal bacteria as well as pathogenic organisms) sometimes have experienced bleeding that can be prevented by vitamin K supplements. This is one reason why scientists hypothesize that your body's need for vitamin K is met partially by absorption of menaquinones synthesized by bacteria in the gut (Suttie, 1992).

Green vegetables and tea are the leading dietary sources of vitamin K. Table 11.5 shows some of the limited information available on the vitamin K content of foods. More information on sources (both dietary sources and synthesis by the body) of vitamin K is needed.

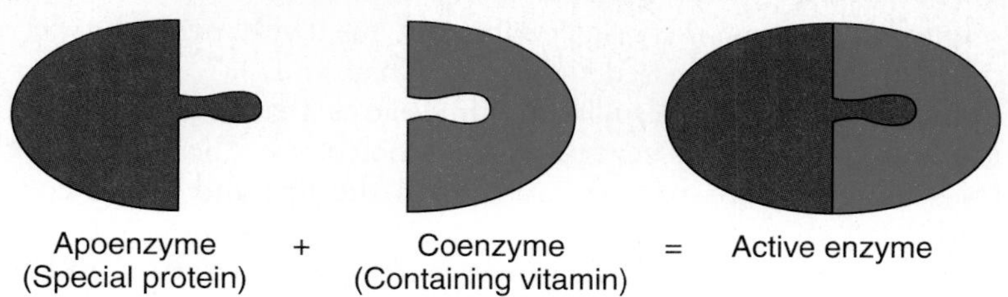

FIGURE 11.5
Vitamins, coenzymes, and enzymes.

Coenzymes containing vitamins are essential components of many enzymes. If the vitamin is deficient, the enzyme is inactive. However, an excess of the vitamin cannot create enzyme activity above a predetermined level.

coenzymes—vitamin-containing substances that unite with enzyme precursors to create active enzymes

beriberi—disease resulting from thiamin deficiency; symptoms include neuromuscular changes that can involve heart failure and edema

The Water-Soluble Vitamins

Now that you know the basics about the fat-soluble vitamins, let's discuss the water-soluble ones. Among the water-soluble vitamins, there are some natural groupings. To begin, thiamin, riboflavin, and niacin can logically be discussed together, because they are often found in the same foods and have related functions.

Thiamin, Riboflavin, and Niacin

You may have heard of some of the alternative names for thiamin, riboflavin, and niacin. Thiamin is also known as *vitamin B-1*, and riboflavin is referred to as *vitamin B-2*. The numbering scheme came about when early vitamin researchers named an important water-soluble factor in food *vitamin B*; when they later realized that this factor consisted of several different compounds, they attached the numbers to distinguish them from each other.

The term *niacin* refers to several compounds: *nicotinamide*, which is the active form of the vitamin, and *nicotinic acid*, which the body readily converts to the active form. (Neither of these compounds is the same as nicotine in tobacco.) In addition, the essential amino acid *tryptophan* can be converted into niacin by the body.

Functions and Effects of Deficiency Thiamin, riboflavin, and niacin all serve as **coenzymes**; that is, they unite with specific protein precursors called *apoenzymes* to create *active enzymes*. Figure 11.5 shows this relationship. Once an apoenzyme is fitted with coenzyme (vitamin), an additional amount of the vitamin can't increase the activity of the enzyme any further. The extra vitamin is a waste; it must be excreted, otherwise it can become toxic.

The enzymes activated by thiamin, riboflavin, and niacin have roles in energy-producing biochemical reactions involving carbohydrates, fats, proteins or amino acids, and alcohol. Figure 11.6 gives an indication of how these vitamins (and others you will read about later) enter into energy metabolism in your cells.

These vitamins often occur in the same foods, so if your intake of one of these vitamins is very poor, your intakes of the other two are also likely to be low. This is especially common in developing parts of the world.

Severe and prolonged thiamin deficiency results in the disease **beriberi** (literally, "I cannot"). It is characterized by neuromuscular changes that may result in paralysis of the legs or heart failure. Sometimes, edema occurs.

FIGURE 11.6
How vitamins are involved in metabolism.

Many of the water-soluble vitamins are involved in the biochemical pathways that produce energy from foods. Thiamin, riboflavin, niacin, biotin, and pantothenic acid are part of coenzymes for various reactions in glycolysis. Those same five vitamins—plus vitamin B-6, folic acid, and vitamin B-12—are part of coenzymes needed for conversion of protein, fat, and glycogen into compounds that ultimately can be used in the citric acid cycle and the electron transport chain.

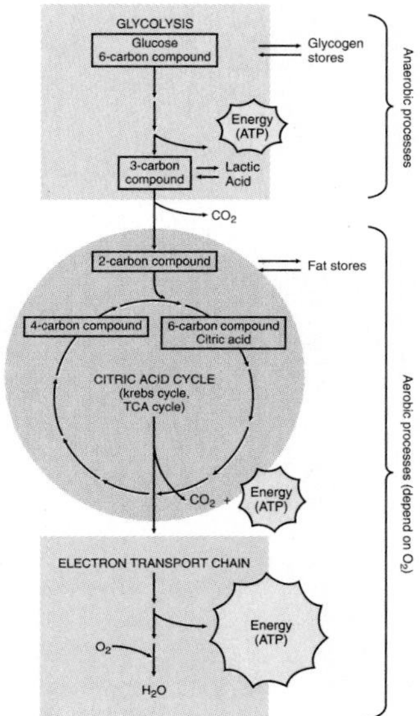

In developed countries, the only people apt to develop thiamin deficiency are alcoholics (this is discussed further in Chapter 17).

cheilosis—dry scaling at corners of mouth; sometimes attributed to riboflavin deficiency, but due to multiple causes

pellagra—disease resulting from niacin deficiency (or possibly a combination of vitamin deficiencies); symptoms include diarrhea, dermatitis, dementia, and death

Riboflavin deficiency results in skin lesions that are indistinguishable from the lesions caused by several other deficiencies. These include **cheilosis**—dry scaling with fissures that occur on the lips and at the corners of the mouth.

Another illness, **pellagra**, has been known for centuries and may be related to niacin deficiency. Its symptoms include diarrhea, dermatitis, dementia (mental illness), and death. During an outbreak in the United States between 1905 and 1910, a scientist noted that the diets of people with pellagra were lacking in meat, milk, and eggs and that when these patients increased their dietary intake of these foods, they improved. This finding suggested that pellagra was a nutritional deficiency rather than a disease caused by a microorganism. The theory was later confirmed when another researcher administered body substances including waste products from those affected with pellagra to healthy volunteers; the healthy people did not get the disease. (Such a research proposal would probably not be approved today by a committee concerned with the ethical use of human subjects.) Although pellagra is often ascribed to niacin deficiency alone, this is probably an oversimplification (Carpenter and Lewin, 1985).

Recommended and Typical Intakes In keeping with their primary roles in energy metabolism, these vitamins should be consumed in amounts directly proportional to energy intake. The more kcalories you consume, the more of these vitamins you should consume. This is accomplished fairly effortlessly, because foods that provide a lot of energy are also likely to contain these vitamins (provided they are not low-nutrient-density foods). The RDAs established for men and women reflect appropriate vitamin intakes for people in the United States with average energy usage. For thiamin and riboflavin, the adult RDAs are between 1 and 2 mg/day; for niacin, they are between 13 and 19 niacin equivalents. The average American consumes more than 100% of the RDA for these vitamins (Human Nutrition Information Service, 1985).

Niacin is one of the vitamins whose requirements are expressed in equivalents (NE). This approach makes it possible to take into account niacin that can be converted from its provitamin, the amino acid tryptophan (60 mg tryptophan = 1 NE), as well as the preformed versions.

Dietary Sources A national survey showed grain products, fruits, and vegetables to be the origin of approximately 40–60% of the thiamin, riboflavin, and niacin Americans consume. Whole grains make a significant contribution, as do enriched and fortified grain products. (We will say more about enrichment and fortification in Chapter 13.) Milk and milk products and meats and meat alternatives can also be excellent sources, as you see in Table 11.6.

Consequences of High Intake Niacin is the only one of these three vitamins for which many instances of toxic effects have been reported (McCormick, 1988). High doses of nicotinic acid, a form of niacin, can cause transient flushing (particularly of the face and neck), widespread itching, and nausea, but these symptoms often decrease with time. Occasionally, chronic use of high doses of nicotinic acid is associated with high blood sugar and uric acid and with liver damage.

TABLE 11.6 Thiamin, Riboflavin, and Niacin in Some Foods

The RDA for thiamin for women aged 19–50 is 1.1 mg/day; for men, 1.5 mg/day.

The RDA for riboflavin for women aged 19–50 is 1.3 mg/day; for men, 1.7 mg/day.

The RDA for niacin for women aged 19–50 is 15 niacin equivalents (NE/day); for men, 19 NE/day. The niacin values on this table do not account for the presence of the niacin precursor tryptophan. Foods with significant levels of protein (which contains the amino acid tryptophan) have greater niacin activity than these values show.

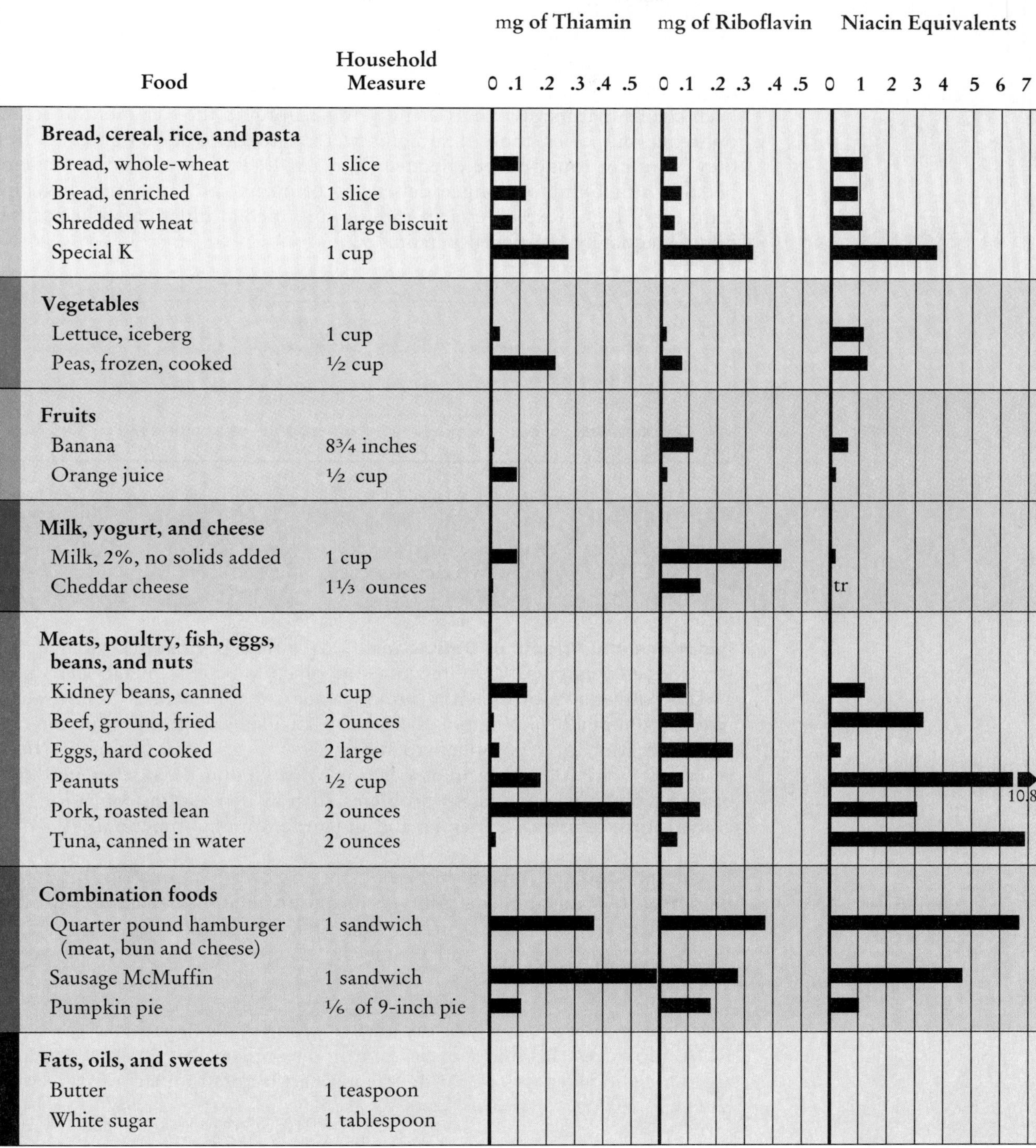

Food	Household Measure	mg of Thiamin (0 .1 .2 .3 .4 .5)	mg of Riboflavin (0 .1 .2 .3 .4 .5)	Niacin Equivalents (0 1 2 3 4 5 6 7)
Bread, cereal, rice, and pasta				
Bread, whole-wheat	1 slice			
Bread, enriched	1 slice			
Shredded wheat	1 large biscuit			
Special K	1 cup			
Vegetables				
Lettuce, iceberg	1 cup			
Peas, frozen, cooked	½ cup			
Fruits				
Banana	8¾ inches			
Orange juice	½ cup			
Milk, yogurt, and cheese				
Milk, 2%, no solids added	1 cup			
Cheddar cheese	1⅓ ounces			tr
Meats, poultry, fish, eggs, beans, and nuts				
Kidney beans, canned	1 cup			
Beef, ground, fried	2 ounces			
Eggs, hard cooked	2 large			
Peanuts	½ cup			10.8
Pork, roasted lean	2 ounces			
Tuna, canned in water	2 ounces			
Combination foods				
Quarter pound hamburger (meat, bun and cheese)	1 sandwich			
Sausage McMuffin	1 sandwich			
Pumpkin pie	⅙ of 9-inch pie			
Fats, oils, and sweets				
Butter	1 teaspoon			
White sugar	1 tablespoon			

Although excess niacin can be dangerous, physicians have found large doses of it can be useful as a drug. Patients with high blood cholesterol levels who have not responded adequately to diet modifications are sometimes given large (3–12 g/day) doses of niacin (DiPalma and Thayer, 1991). This therapy is promising, but the toxic side effects of niacin are sometimes problematic; therefore, this drug therapy use of niacin should *always be under a physician's close supervision*.

The vitamin supplement industry has promoted the idea that high intakes of B vitamins, such as thiamin and riboflavin, will help relieve psychologic stress. But one pharmaceutical company that produces a so-called stress vitamin supplement was taken to court and fined for making false and misleading claims to this effect (Nutrition Forum, 1986). There have also been claims that megavitamin therapy was helpful in the treatment of schizophrenia; but when these treatments were tested in well-designed studies, they were not found to be effective (Ban, 1981). It is important to remember that although a prolonged deficiency of niacin can cause mental symptoms, very high doses of niacin cannot cure mental illness of other causes in an adequately nourished person.

You Tell Me

The vitamin supplement industry often implies that B vitamins are sources of energy.

Can vitamins, even in megadoses, be a source of kcalories?

Vitamin B-6

Vitamin B-6 occurs in food in three forms: *pyridoxine*, *pyridoxamine*, and *pyridoxal*. They are closely related structurally and have equivalent vitamin activity.

Functions and Effects of Deficiency Like other B vitamins, vitamin B-6 serves as a coenzyme. Many reactions involved in protein metabolism, such as the conversion of essential amino acids to nonessential amino acids, require vitamin B-6. Vitamin B-6 also participates in the production and transformation of tryptophan to niacin as well as other important body reactions. Symptoms seen in association with vitamin B-6 deficiency most often involve nervous system problems such as depression, confusion, and convulsions; dermatitis; anemia; and impaired immune function.

Recommended and Typical Intakes Because of the importance of vitamin B-6 in protein metabolism, your need for this vitamin is in direct proportion to the amount of protein in your diet. The adult RDAs for vitamin B-6 of 2 mg/day for men and 1.6 mg/day for women are based on average American protein intakes.

In 1985, the average vitamin B-6 intake of adult men in the United States was slightly below the RDA, but that of women was less than 75% of the RDA. However, this does not necessarily mean that most American women are deficient in vitamin B-6; deficiency can be determined only by biochemical testing.

Dietary Sources As shown in Table 11.7, meats and some other items in that group—such as legumes—are generally good sources of vitamin B-6.

TABLE 11.7 Vitamin B-6 in Some Foods

The RDA for vitamin B-6 for women is 1.6 mg/day; for men, 2.0 mg/day.

Food	Household Measure	mg of Vitamin B-6 (0 / 0.5 / 1.0)
Bread, cereal, rice, and pasta		
Bread, whole-wheat	1 slice	
Crackers, saltines	4 squares	
Tortilla, corn	1 average	
Popcorn, popped	3 cups	
Vegetables		
Green beans, frozen, cooked	½ cup	
Potato, baked	1 large	
Spinach, chopped, raw	½ cup	
Fruits		
Apple	1 medium	
Banana	8¾ inches	
Cantaloupe	½ cup	
Prunes, cooked	½ cup	
Milk, yogurt, and cheese		
Cheese, cheddar	1⅓ ounces	
Milk, skim or whole	1 cup	
Meats, poultry, fish, eggs, beans, and nuts		
Beef, ground, fried	2 ounces	
Chicken, light meat, no skin, cooked	2 ounces	
Eggs, hard cooked	2 large	
Lima beans, canned	1 cup	
Peanut butter	¼ cup	
Tuna canned in water	2 ounces	
Combination foods		
Hot dog (frankfurter and bun)	1 sandwich	
Pie, apple	⅛ of 9" pie	
Split-pea soup, canned	1 cup	
Fats, oils, and sweets		
Butter	1 teaspoon	tr
Carbonated beverages	12 ounces	
Coffee	6 ounces	

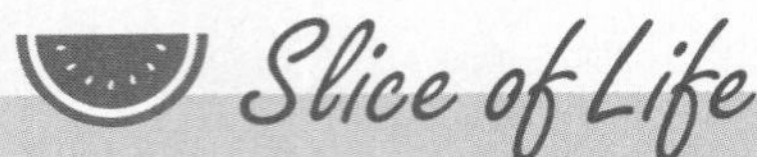

Harm from a Vitamin Rather Than Help

Two years ago, Samantha started taking vitamin B-6 supplements, hoping that they would make her problems with premenstrual syndrome (PMS) go away. She always felt bloated, tired, irritable, and depressed in the week before her period. When she read in a magazine that vitamin B-6 supplements could provide relief, she rushed to try what sounded like an easy cure.

The article said to take 1000 mg per day. She did that for the first month without results, so the second month she increased her intake to 2000 mg per day. That month, she wasn't sure it was helping; to hurry things along, she started taking 3000 mg.

Then some strange things began to happen. When she bent her head down, a tingling sensation ran down her neck and back, into her legs and to the soles of her feet. At other times, her feet felt numb, her coordination was off, and she had to steady herself. Then the numbness went to her hands as well, and she became clumsy when handling things. At this point, she knew something was seriously wrong, but she didn't suspect the supplements.

A neurologist made the connection. In addition to her muscular problems, he found that her sensations of touch, temperature, pinpricks, vibration, and joint position were severely impaired in both arms and legs. Biochemical tests confirmed his suspicion that Samantha was experiencing vitamin B-6 toxicity.

Fortunately, the damage to her nervous system was not permanent. A year after discontinuing the supplements, she felt fairly normal and could function as before.

Of course, she was still contending with premenstrual syndrome. For a new approach to her problem, she sought the help of a gynecologist, who recommended moderate measures: a balanced diet, reduction in caffeine and alcohol intake, an exercise program, and medication for the most troublesome symptoms. The physician pointed out that much remains to be learned about the cause and treatment of PMS; one of the unexpected findings along the way has been the discovery that large doses of vitamin B-6 can be dangerous (Schaumberg et al., 1983).

Some fruits and vegetables are also rich sources of vitamin B-6. If you want to increase your intake of this vitamin, consume larger or more servings of flesh proteins, nuts, and/or good fruit and vegetable sources. However, your body does not generally utilize vitamin B-6 from plant sources as well as those from animal sources (Lecklem, 1988). (We'll discuss the concept of different biologic utilization of nutrients from different foods more thoroughly in Chapter 12.)

Consequences of High Intake Excess vitamin B-6 is excreted in the urine. In the past, this led scientists to assume that it was harmless—but recently reports of toxicity started to appear in the medical literature. People who took anywhere from 200 to 6000 mg of vitamin B-6 per day, which is 100 times to 3000 times the RDA, developed sensory neuropathies (nerve disorders) (Schaumberg et al., 1983; Parry and Bredesen, 1985). Symptoms appeared 1 month to 3 years after the start of vitamin B-6 supplementation.

Why had people been taking these huge amounts of vitamin B-6? They took them for various reasons. Many thought that the supplements would give them relief from **premenstrual syndrome (PMS),** especially water retention. Others hoped for a general sense of well-being, or improvement of a psychiatric condition. However, in a well-designed clinical study, no benefits from therapy with vitamin B-6 could be shown (Mira et al., 1988).

premenstrual syndrome (PMS)—physical and/or emotional symptoms experienced by some women before menstruation that decrease or disappear during or after menstruation

The Slice of Life above describes one person's experience with vitamin B-6 supplementation.

Folic Acid and Vitamin B-12

As we continue our survey of water-soluble vitamins, we'll discuss folic acid and vitamin B-12 together because each is a part of coenzymes involved in DNA and RNA metabolism.

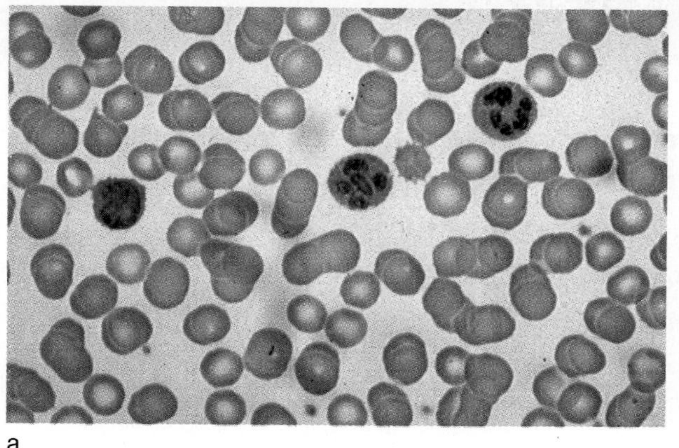

a

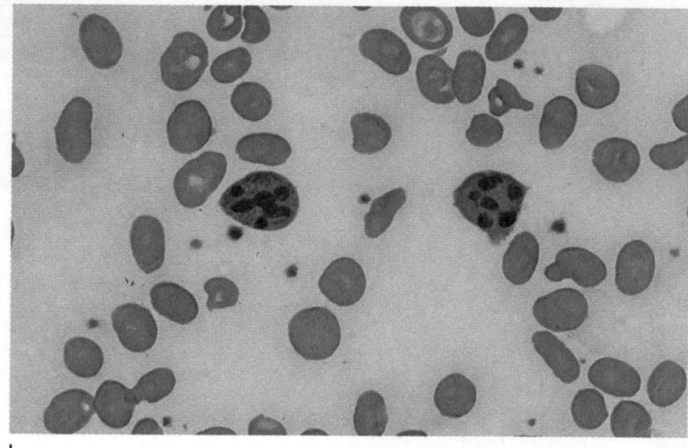

b

FIGURE 11.7
Several nutritional deficiencies can cause anemia.

A deficiency of folic acid or vitamin B-12 can produce a megaloblastic anemia. Panel (a) shows normal red blood cells; panel (b) shows the fewer, larger red blood cells characteristic of megaloblastic anemia. (In both a and b, the dark-stained cells with nuclei are white blood cells.)

Each of these vitamins includes a number of compounds. The terms *folate* and *folacin* are used to describe compounds that have nutritional properties of folic acid (also known as *pteroylglutamic acid*). Vitamin B-12 includes a group of cobalt-containing compounds known as *cobalamins*.

Functions and Effects of Deficiency Because DNA and RNA are the substances that direct cell division, you especially need these vitamins during periods of growth. In addition, folic acid and vitamin B-12 are important in the metabolism of certain amino acids and the transfer of single carbon units among various biochemical compounds in the body.

Deficiencies of either of these vitamins produce a form of **anemia** characterized by large, immature red blood cells, a condition called **megaloblastic anemia** (Figure 11.7). In cases where anemia has been produced by an inadequacy of vitamin B-12, treatment with large amounts of folic acid will normalize the red blood cells. However, B-12 deficiency can also cause nerve damage, and folic acid cannot treat this condition. In fact, taking folic acid in this case would be quite dangerous; the folic acid will mask B-12 deficiency, and the nerve damage will progress insidiously. For this reason, it is critical that the cause of the megaloblastic anemia be accurately determined so that the appropriate vitamin can be given to treat the deficiency.

anemia—general term indicating a lower-than-normal concentration of hemoglobin or of red blood cells in blood

megaloblastic anemia—form of anemia characterized by large, immature red blood cells

Large doses of folic acid appear to have therapeutic value in preventing neural tube defects (birth defects affecting the central nervous system). In a large double blind study, scientists found that ingestion of folic acid supplements (4 mg/day) during pregnancy by women at risk of having infants with these defects reduced the incidence of these birth defects (MRC Vitamin Study Research Group, 1991). The Centers for Disease Control (1991) have recommended use of folic acid supplements only for at-risk women under a physician's supervision. It's interesting to note, however, that scientists cannot induce a neural tube defect in mice by making the mother deficient in folic acid (Heid et al., 1992). Folic acid expert Lynn Bailey discusses this issue in more detail in the interview on page 360.

Recommended and Typical Intakes The RDA for folic acid for men is 200 μg; for women it is 180 μg. The 1989 RDA advises pregnant women to get 400 μg per day through careful selection of food; this recommendation contrasts with previous editions that encourage physicians to prescribe folate supplements for their pregnant patients. Except during pregnancy, Americans appear to consume amounts of folic acid that meet the RDA recommendations of 200 μg per day. But some experts question the current

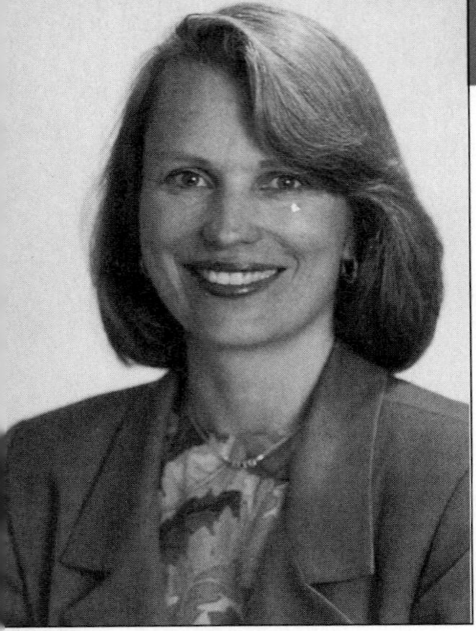

Interview with Lynn Balley, PhD

Folic Acid and Neural Tube Defects

As you've learned throughout this book, there are many correlations between health and diet. But few are as dramatic as the neural tube birth defects that sometimes can be prevented by the mother-to-be's adequate folic acid intake. Dr. Lynn Bailey is an expert on folic acid and its effects. A professor of Food Science and Human Nutrition at the University of Florida, she has been on the folic acid advisory committees of the Food and Drug Administration and the Centers for Disease Control. In this interview, Dr. Bailey describes the controversy around folic acid recommendations and explores the issue of whether to fortify flour with folic acid.

Would you describe neural tube defects?

The neural tube encapsulates the spinal cord. If the spinal cord actually protrudes through an opening in the neural tube, the defect is called spina bifida. Babies that are born with spina bifida live and are handicapped. The second major kind of neural tube defect is called anencephaly, and it relates to the opening in the area of the brain. The brain is either malformed or nonexistent, and usually those babies are born dead, or they only live a few hours. About 2,300 babies in the U.S. are born annually with either spina bifida or anencephaly; that doesn't count those that were aborted.

How strong is the connection between folic acid and these fetal defects?

While folic acid reduces one's risk, there are neural tube defects that are not responsive to folic acid. The estimation is that 50% of the neural tube defects could be prevented by folic acid in the right dose, so one must talk about reduction versus prevention.

What I'm really interested in evaluating is whether or not there is some metabolic lesion (defect) that increases the requirement of folic acid during that first 28 days. Perhaps there is a metabolic reason why these women need a higher amount of folic acid to properly close the neural tube.

The 1989 RDAs for folic acid were lower than they were in 1980. Why were they reduced?

I wrote a critique of this very question—it was published in the *Journal of the American Dietetic Association* in 1992. My concerns related to the fact that the RDA was reduced by 50%. Today the RDA for the adult woman, for example, is 180 μg per day versus the previous RDA of 400 μg per day. Among the rationales given by the National Academy of Sciences Nutrition Board was that the dietary intake of the U.S. population was close to 200 μg per day, and because not a very large percentage of the population was folic acid deficient, 200 μg should be sufficient.

The first issue here is that the dietary intake data are very flawed and there is underestimation of what is actually consumed. Their dietary intake data were based on 24-hour recalls, and the computer database is also very incomplete and inaccurate. There are now a lot of new estimates that clearly show you have more folate in the diet than was known.

Related to that is the question of whether or not there are very many people in the U.S. who are folate deficient. We really don't know the answer to that. We do know that there are sub-population groups that are folate deficient, and there are certainly high-risk groups that may need significantly more than they can get from their diets alone.

Another reason for the reduction in the RDA is that the Nutrition Board sided very strongly with a paper reporting a depletion-repletion protocol in adult women. The paper was based on a very well-controlled study to determine the minimum requirement of folic acid. The conclusion was that the minimum requirement is 200 to 250 μg. When we revisit the definition of "requirement" versus "RDA," a margin of safety is always added on the requirement to get the RDA. Here, the RDA committee took the very minimum requirement—approximately 200 μg—and established that as the RDA. I think the 180 μg is an underestimation and we should go back to the previ ous RDA of 400 or 500 μg.

Do you feel the RDA should be specificaily revised for all women or for pregnant women?

I think there should be specific revisions back to 400 μg for all women. The reason it shouldn't be limited to pregnant women is that most women do not even know that they're pregnant until after the time that the fetus' neural tube closes. In the developing embryo, the cells that are rapidly dividing to create the neural tube are forming that enclosure during the first 28 days of gestation. In a large percentage of pregnancies, it is past 28 days gestation when a woman realizes that she is pregnant. All the studies that have shown a protective effect of folate have been in what is classified as a "peri-conceptual" period, meaning just prior to pregnancy and during that first 28 days of gestation. So we want people to think about getting this into the diet of every woman—pregnant and nonpregnant—in the reproductive years.

How important is folic acid *after* the first 28 days of gestation?

During pregnancy, one certainly needs to continue to maintain an optimal level. There is new data from Ireland that indicates that during the second trimester there is a huge increase in the catabolism (breakdown) of folate, and pregnant women excrete more folate in the urine. The second issue is the huge increase in new tissue in the fetus and the mother. Folic acid is essential for cell division. Any time you have rapidly dividing cells, you're going to have an increase in the requirement for folate, so certainly during pregnancy there would by an increased requirement.

How much folic acid should a woman get once she knows she's pregnant?

I would recommend that a pregnant woman take a multi-vitamin with 400 μg folate. I think that amount, in addition to the diet during pregnancy, is sufficient. Several years ago I was pregnant, and I did take a folate supplement as a component of a multi-vitamin. As is the case for 90% of women, I was past 28 days of gestation when I realized I was pregnant. So I did not take it to protect myself from developing neural tube defect.

Can consuming high levels of folate from foods or supplements cause any problems for a pregnant woman or her fetus?

I would say it's not feasible to get "too much" folate from dietary sources. Folic acid is a very nontoxic vitamin. Even with supplements, you have to get to a high level (above 1 mg [1,000 μg] per day), and the only question is: Is it possibly interfering with the diagnosis of pernicious anemia? This is not a condition that affects very many women of reproductive age.

We don't know of any toxic effects for the fetus. One of the major studies on which these recommendations are based used 4 mg per day. They have tracked the infants that were born, and haven't seen any evidence of a problem. Also, women who develop folate deficiency in late pregnancy are routinely given 5 mg of folate, and that's never been shown to result in a problem. Dealing with the very early gestational phase, the authorities do not think that 400 μg would have a negative effect on the developing fetus.

Is it generally hard for Americans to get enough folic acid in the diet?

Folic acid is concentrated in green, leafy vegetables, citrus fruits, whole grains, and legumes. It's not difficult for most Americans to consume 200 μg per day, but it's not easy to get 400 μg in the diet unless they make a conscious effort to select very high folate foods. Most people working in this area think that food fortification is the way to go to reduce the risk of this particular birth defect. At the same time, we will work on nutrition education.

Do you think white flour should be fortified with folic acid and vitamin B-6, as it is with thiamin, riboflavin, and niacin?

The FDA brought together the Folic Acid Subcommittee of the Food Advisory Committee in 1992, and we recommended that the FDA come up with a plan for adding it to flour. Our understanding is that they are working on the mechanics of putting it in the flour. They are looking at things like how much they would have to add to a serving of flour to get 400 μg to the population at risk—women of reproductive age—while, at the other end of the spectrum, not giving them too much.

standards especially because your body cannot use folate from all foods equally well (Bailey, 1992). (We'll discuss these differences in nutrient utilization, sometimes called bioavailability, more in Chapter 12.)

For vitamin B-12, the RDA is 2 μg for both men and women. Most people's intake of this vitamin comfortably exceeds the RDA. However, if you are a vegan, you are at risk for B-12 deficiency because vitamin B-12 does not occur in plants. Vegans should consume a supplement or foods fortified with this vitamin. If a pregnant or lactating woman does not consume vitamin B-12, the baby may experience a deficiency (Specker et al., 1990).

The presence of vitamin B-12 in your diet does not guarantee that it will be absorbed. Absorption of this vitamin depends on the presence of a substance called **intrinsic factor**, which is produced by the lining of the stomach. If intrinsic factor is absent, only about 1% of dietary B-12 is absorbed; when intrinsic factor is present, amounts up to the RDA may be absorbed from one meal (Herbert and Colman, 1988). The production of intrinsic factor sometimes decreases in the elderly, so older people may become deficient in the vitamin even if their diets contain RDA levels of it. This deficiency disease is called **pernicious anemia**; people who have it are usually given periodic injections of vitamin B-12.

intrinsic factor—substance produced by the stomach lining; enhances vitamin B-12 absorption

pernicious anemia—anemia resulting from the inadequate production of intrinsic factor, which leads to the inadequate absorption of vitamin B-12 despite its presence in the diet

Dietary Sources The best sources of folic acid are fruits, vegetables, legumes, and some grain products. You can remember these sources more easily if you know that the terms related to *folic acid* come from the same root word as *foliage*. As Table 11.8 shows, the only type of basic food notably low in this vitamin is flesh protein.

The good food sources of vitamin B-12 are almost opposite from those of folic acid. Foods of animal origin are the only reliable sources of vitamin B-12.

Pantothenic Acid and Biotin

The vitamins pantothenic acid (or *pantothenate*) and biotin are both components of enzymes involved in energy metabolism. Pantothenic acid is also involved in the synthesis of other vital body substances. The Greek word from which *pantothenic* was derived means "from all sides," and the reference is appropriate because of the widespread distribution and usefulness of this nutrient. In fact, pantothenic acid is so generally available among common foods that scientists have been unable to induce a deficiency experimentally.

However, deficiency of biotin can produce diverse problems such as dermatitis and neuromuscular disorders. If you are healthy and you eat a reasonably balanced diet, you are unlikely to experience a biotin deficiency. But deficiencies of biotin do occur in patients with genetic defects (McCormick, 1988). People have induced in themselves a deficiency of biotin by consuming large quantities of raw egg whites, which contain a protein called *avidin*. This protein binds biotin in the intestine and makes it unavailable for absorption. (You would have to consume most of your diet as raw egg white to induce such a deficiency.)

Vitamin C

You've probably heard about the next vitamin already. Vitamin C (also known as *ascorbate* or *ascorbic acid*) has been promoted as the cure of the common cold and of cancer. Not surprisingly, it is the most popular single vitamin supplement (Nutrition Reviews, 1990). Even though this vitamin—

TABLE 11.8 Folic Acid and Vitamin B-12 in Some Foods

The RDA for folic acid for women is 180 μg/day; for men, 200 μg/day.
The RDA for vitamin B-12 for both women and men is 2 μg/day.

Food	Household Measure	μg of Folic Acid (0 – 100 – 200)	μg of Vitamin B-12 (0 – 1.0 – 2.0 – 3.0)
Bread, cereal, rice, and pasta			
Bread, white enriched	1 slice		
Bread, whole-wheat	1 slice		
Cake, chocolate with icing	1 wedge		
Cornflakes, fortified	1¼ cups		
Rice, brown, cooked	½ cup		
Vegetables			
Broccoli, fresh, cooked	½ cup		
Lettuce, iceberg	1 cup		
Lettuce, romaine	1 cup		
Potatoes, mashed	½ cup		
Tomato, stewed	½ cup		
Fruits			
Banana	8¾ inches		
Orange juice	½ cup		
Milk, yogurt, and cheese			
Milk, whole	1 cup		
Cheese, cheddar	1⅓ ounces		
Yogurt	1 cup		
Meats, poultry, fish, eggs, beans, and nuts			
Beans, baked, canned	1 cup		
Beef, lean, cooked	2 ounces		
Chicken, dark, fried	1 drumstick		
Salmon, canned	2 ounces		
Eggs, hard cooked	2 large		
Peanuts	½ cup		
Shrimp, fried	2 ounces		
Combination foods			
Corn dog	1 item		
Enchilada, cheese	6 ounces		
Soup, split pea	1 cup		
Pizza, cheese	1 slice		
Fats, oils, and sweets			
Butter	1 teaspoon		
Mayonnaise	1 tablespoon		

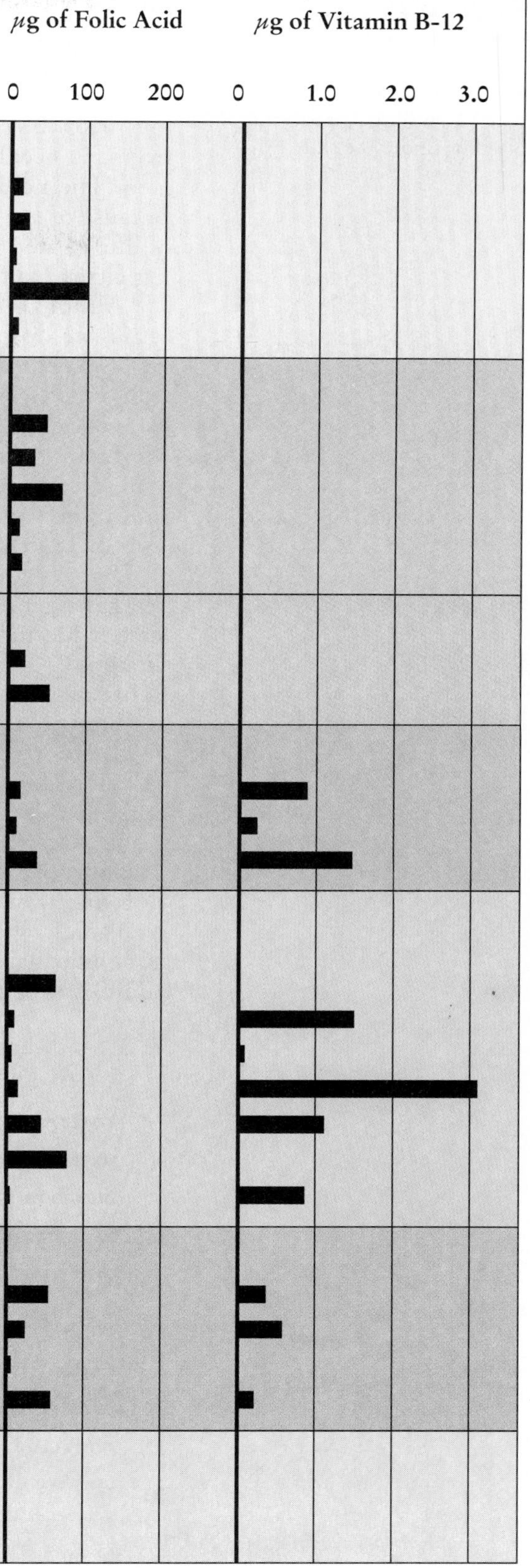

like all vitamins—is essential, whether it deserves this elevated public status is debatable.

scurvy—disease resulting from vitamin C deficiency; symptoms include edema; a spongy condition, sometimes with sores, of the gums; and bleeding under the skin

Functions and Effects of Deficiency The disease resulting from a deficiency of vitamin C is **scurvy**. It was first recognized by the Egyptians before 1500 B.C. It had been the scourge of armies and navies for centuries because typical military rations were devoid of good sources of vitamin C. Scurvy plagued the crewmen who came to America with Jacques Cartier in the 1500s. Fortunately, Native Americans knew the cure: they steeped a tea from the needles of a certain type of evergreen tree and gave it to the sick men. The needles, we now know, contained small amounts of vitamin C. Because of the lifesaving brew, the tree was named *arborvitae*, meaning "tree of life." Later, in the 1700s, British sailors cured or prevented scurvy by eating citrus fruit and so earned themselves the nickname "limeys."

Although a great deal of research has been done on vitamin C over the years, we do not yet understand exactly what vitamin C does at the cellular level (Hornig et al., 1988). We do know that it is needed for the formation of collagen, the protein that serves so many connective functions in the body. Among the body's collagen-containing materials and structures are the framework of bone; the gingivae (gums); and the binding materials in skin, muscle, and scar tissue. Vitamin C is also necessary for the production of certain hormones and neurotransmitters, as well as for the metabolism of some amino acids and vitamins.

In addition, it aids blood cells in fighting infection, the liver in detoxifying dangerous substances, and the gut in absorbing iron from foods. With such wide-ranging functions, it is not surprising that the symptoms of vitamin C deficiency are diverse: generalized feelings of weakness, bleeding gums and loosened teeth, easy bruising and small hemorrhages in the skin, and impaired immune function.

Like carotene and vitamin E, vitamin C is an antioxidant. In a number of epidemiologic studies, consumption of foods rich in vitamin C has been correlated to a reduced incidence of cancer, especially stomach cancer.

So should you consume extra vitamin C to reduce your risk of cancer? The Surgeon General's Report on Nutrition and Health sums up the situation this way: "The National Cancer Institutes suggests eating a variety of fruits and vegetables, thus ensuring an adequate supply of vitamin C. There is no adequate evidence that larger amounts of vitamin C can provide any additional benefits."

You Tell Me

Yesterday you read an article that said scientists in one study found that eating foods rich in vitamin C was associated with a lower risk of stomach cancer. Today you read another article stating that scientists at another university found no indication that high intakes of vitamin C prevented colon cancer.

What are possible reasons for inconsistencies among studies? Do foods rich in vitamin C contain other protective substances, such as fiber and carotenoids? Would you expect different body tissues to be similarly affected by intake of a nutrient? Should you continue to eat at least one serving of vitamin C rich fruits or vegetables daily?

Recommended and Typical Intakes The adult RDA for vitamin C is 60 mg/day. You probably easily consume this amount of vitamin C. The average American consumes more than 135% of the RDA for vitamin C (Human Nutrition Information Service, 1985).

This amount may not be enough for some people, though. Recent work demonstrated that to maintain serum concentration of ascorbic acid equal to that of nonsmokers, smokers had to consume at least 200 mg of vitamin C daily, because it is metabolized more rapidly in smokers (Schectman et al., 1991). If you smoke, **QUIT**. But until you do, consume *two* servings of a good source of vitamin C in your diet every day.

Vitamin C and the Common Cold As you've probably heard or read, vitamin C has been actively promoted for several years by scientist Linus Pauling for preventing and curing colds. This claim has received a lot of attention, in part because Dr. Pauling won Nobel Prizes for physical chemistry and peace. He postulated that humans, because their bodies do not produce ascorbic acid as many other animals' bodies do, need megadoses (several grams daily) of vitamin C to achieve the levels produced (and therefore assumed to be needed) by these other animals. He claimed that one of the benefits would be fewer colds. Many people, influenced by his excellent reputation and the simplicity of his recommendations, began taking megadoses of vitamin C. Subsequently, over 100 studies have been conducted to test the effect of supplemental vitamin C on the incidence and treatment of colds (Hemilä, 1992). This chapter's Thinking For Yourself on page 366 discusses this research and helps you consider options for your own use.

Dietary Sources Many common fruits and vegetables have such a high content of vitamin C that they furnish half or more of the RDA in one serving. The citrus fruits have a well-deserved reputation in this regard, but they are not alone: broccoli, cabbage, cantaloupe (muskmelon), cauliflower, green peppers, and strawberries are also excellent sources. Nature has provided very little vitamin C in other types of foods (Table 11.9).

But vitamin C is *added* to many products. Many kinds of beverages are supplemented with vitamin C: fruit juices, fruit-flavored drinks, and some carbonated beverages are fortified with it; even some cereals are.

Consequences of High Intake With all the controversy about vitamin C and the common cold, many people have taken megadoses of vitamin C, and physicians have had a chance to observe the results. Diarrhea is a typical symptom when people megadose with vitamin C. Large doses of vitamin C also interfere with several laboratory tests; for example, the standard test for colon cancer may yield a false-negative result in those who have taken large amounts of vitamin C (Hornig et al., 1988).

Large excesses of vitamin C have been accused of causing other negative effects, but such effects have not been proved in controlled studies (Hornig et al., 1988). For example, several scientists still think that some people may require more vitamin C to prevent scurvy after their bodies have become used to very large doses, but this is debatable.

Nonvitamins

Scientists and food faddists are always looking for new vitamins—although for different reasons! You may have seen claims in magazines for substances like inositol, carnitine, choline, lecithin, para-aminobenzoic acid (PABA), taurine, bioflavinoids (dubbed "vitamin P" by some), and lipoic acid. Many

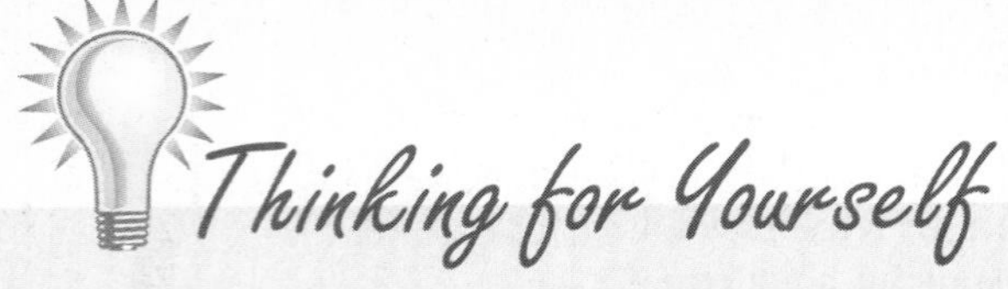

Do Vitamin C Supplements Prevent Colds?

The Situation

The person you share an apartment with has just come down with a cold and feels miserable. You are at the beginning of a very demanding couple of weeks, and catching a cold would certainly interfere with accomplishing everything you need to do. You think about what you might do to avoid the cold. One thing that crosses your mind is vitamin C; you have heard that taking vitamin C supplements can prevent a cold or cure it faster if you do get one. You wonder whether you should take some, and how much you would need.

Is Your Information Accurate and Relevant?

- Vitamin C is important to the functioning of the immune system. If a person's average intake of vitamin C remains substantially below the RDA for a long period of time, the function of the immune system becomes impaired—making the person less able to combat all types of contagions effectively, not just colds.
- Vitamin C is also an antioxidant. As such, it may react with compounds such as histamine, released by body cells during an infection, to reduce inflammatory symptoms (Hemilä, 1992).
- Other nutrients are also needed for the immune system to function effectively. If the intake of almost any of the vitamins, or of protein, remains deficient for a long period of time, immune functions become compromised.
- The effectiveness of vitamin C supplements in preventing and treating colds is debatable (see the next section).
- To maintain serum vitamin C levels similar to those of nonsmokers, smokers needed to consume 200 mg of vitamin C daily (Schectman et al., 1991).

What Else Should You Consider?

Over 100 studies have examined the effect of vitamin C on the common cold. In most epidemiologic studies, there was no *statistically significant* difference in the incidence of colds between groups that received supplemental vitamin C and those that did not.

As far as the *treatment* of colds is concerned, the evidence is somewhat more positive in a number of studies (but not all). Vitamin C supplements reduced the severity of the symptoms in some people during the first few days of the cold. Also, some people taking supplements spent less time at home with the cold—an average of half a day less. This may be due to the antihistaminic effect that vitamin C sometimes has (Hemilä, 1992).

It's interesting to note that in these studies the response to vitamin C was not proportional to the dose. One group (Baird et al., 1979) demonstrated that 80 mg of vitamin C had *a slight effect similar to the slight effect of the larger doses* of purified vitamin C used in several earlier studies. That means that drinking an extra cup of orange juice per day can provide the same benefit as consuming large supplements of vitamin C.

Another point of interest is that large epidemiologic studies of vitamin C supplements and colds often did not include an assessment of the amount of vitamin C in the diets of the subjects. It is possible that people who appeared to benefit from the supplements had been consuming inadequate levels in their diets and that the supplements made up for the dietary deficiencies.

The authors of the 1989 *RDA* provided one summary of the data noting: "Several reviewers have concluded that any benefits of large doses of ascorbic acid for these conditions are too small to justify recommending routine intake of large amounts. . . . "

Now What Do You Think?

- **Option 1** You decide to follow the Food Guide Pyramid for selecting your daily food, making sure you get one good source of vitamin C every day. You also decide to quit smoking.
- **Option 2** You decide to follow the Food Guide Pyramid for selecting your daily food and make sure you get two good sources of vitamin C every day.
- **Option 3** You decide to take a supplement of 60 mg of vitamin C every day (the adult RDA).
- **Option 4** You decide to take a daily multivitamin supplement that does not exceed 100% of the U.S. RDA for any of the nutrients.

Do you see any other safe and effective nutrition-related options? Which makes the most sense to you? What additional strategies could you use to reduce your risk of catching a cold and to reduce the severity of a cold?

TABLE 11.9 Vitamin C in Some Foods

The RDA for vitamin C for both women and men is 60 mg.

mg of Vitamin C (scale: 0 10 20 30 40 50 60 70)

Food	Household Measure
Bread, cereal, rice, and pasta	
All products, not fortified	1 ounce
Bran Buds, fortified	1 ounce
Vegetables	
Broccoli, frozen, cooked	½ cup
Green beans, frozen, cooked	½ cup
Lettuce, iceberg	1 cup
Pepper, green, raw	½ of one
Potato, white, baked	1 (5 ounces)
Spinach, frozen, cooked	½ cup
Tomatoes, canned	½ cup
Fruits	
Apple	1 medium
Cantaloupe	½ cup
Cranberry sauce	½ cup
Cranapple juice, canned	½ cup
Orange juice, frozen, reconstituted	½ cup
Strawberries, raw	½ cup
Milk, yogurt, and cheese	
Cheese, firm types	1⅓ ounces
Milk	1 cup
Meats, poultry, fish, eggs, beans, and nuts	
Eggs	2 medium
Meats, cooked	2 ounces
Walnuts	½ cup
Combination foods	
Burrito, bean (Taco Bell)	1 burrito
Club sandwich (Tomato, bacon, lettuce)	1 sandwich
Soup, tomato	1 cup
Fats, oils, and sweets	
Alcoholic beverages	1 serving
Fats, oils	1 tablespoon
Sugar, honey	1 tablespoon

of these substances are important in body reactions. But they are not essential, because most people's bodies produce as much of these substances as they need. Therefore, they cannot be called vitamins. Sometimes, though, a rare person with a metabolic abnormality cannot produce enough of one of these substances. That person needs to take a supplement.

The fact that these substances are not vitamins does not mean that they are not profitable products for dietary supplement manufacturers. They are advertised widely, and they are a significant part of the $2 billion plus in annual supplement sales.

Two nonvitamins deserve special comment. One is choline, a component of the neurotransmitter acetylcholine, which is present in lower-than-normal levels in people who have certain nervous disorders. For this reason, it is being tested as part of the treatment for those conditions. There is no evidence, however, that normally healthy people would benefit in any way from taking supplemental choline. Choline is usually found in foods as a component of the phospholipid lecithin (Chapter 6).

You Tell Me

A popular new way to sell vitamin supplements in health food stores is to call them "smart nutrients." Claims for these products include "enhances your creative thoughts," "the perfect brain food," and "like a windshield wiper for your brain." Many of these products also contain ginseng, cayenne, licorice, alcohol, and/or a variety of non-nutrient plant extracts.

Pending regulations would increase the FDA's ability to inspect and recall these products, because their health claims are unsubstantiated. Some enthusiasts for these products worry that the regulations would limit their access. They feel these products meet their "special" needs.

Do you think these products should remain available? How do you think their advertising should be regulated?

Another nonvitamin, laetrile, sometimes called "vitamin B-17," is of interest because it may actually be harmful in some instances. Laetrile contains the poison cyanide, making consumption of large amounts dangerous. Although laetrile has sometimes been used as a cancer treatment, scientific tests find it ineffective for this purpose. The primary concern is that its use may delay or substitute for treatments that *could* slow down or arrest the disease (more on laetrile in Chapter 14).

What About Vitamin Supplements?

Vitamin Toxicities

As you've probably concluded from the preceding sections, when you ingest very large amounts of vitamins, you put yourself at risk for developing health problems. In general, vitamin toxicities are more likely to occur when:

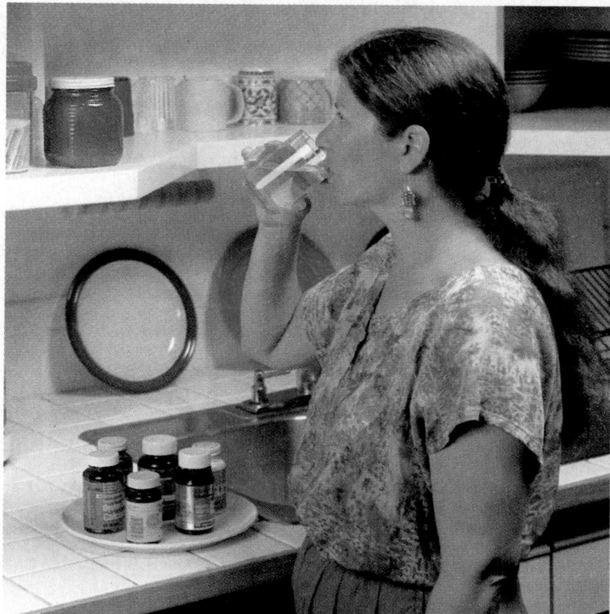

FIGURE 11.8
Vitamin supplementation.

36% of Americans take vitamin supplements routinely. In some instances, modest supplements of up to 100% of the U.S. RDA are useful; however, at high intakes there is a danger of overdose.

1. You regularly consume nutrient supplements, especially those containing large amounts of one nutrient, for several weeks or months.
2. Your body size is small. Children and women are more prone to toxicity because the dose per body mass is generally greater.
3. You are still developing. That's why fetuses and young infants are more apt to suffer permanent effects.

Although it is *possible* to incur vitamin toxicity by eating too much food with a very high vitamin density (such as liver), the most common cause of vitamin toxicity is the ingestion of vitamin supplements in excessive quantities for a long period of time. Most people who incur vitamin toxicities have been overdosing at ten or more times the RDA (often referred to as *megadosing*) for anywhere from a few months to a few years before they seek help for their vitamin-caused problems. But you can't count on it taking that long: sometimes toxicities occur more quickly and with less excessive intakes, especially in the case of vitamin D.

Every year, approximately 4000 people in the United States receive treatment for vitamin supplement poisoning. Many are unaware that substances that are essential at one level can be harmful at higher doses. This is an important concept to understand, because approximately 36% of the American public takes vitamin supplements regularly (Moss et al., 1989) (Figure 11.8).

In essence, a number of Americans are performing self-experiments with combinations and doses of single nutrients never envisioned by scientists. Vitamin supplements can be common causes of serious diseases. Researchers recently reported that in at least some western countries (excess) vitamin A consumption may represent an appreciable cause of chronic liver disease (Geubel et al., 1991). And it's not just the liver that can be affected. Toxicity can affect all your body's tissues and systems, just as deficiencies can. Just as there are classic symptoms of vitamin deficiency, typical indicators of vitamin excesses are increasingly being recognized.

When To Take Vitamin Supplements

The preceding section describes some of the risks of vitamin supplementation. But are there sometimes benefits? For whom?

You Tell Me

A few years ago researchers found that a small group of Welsh school children performed better in school after taking vitamin and mineral supplements. Other researchers could not duplicate the results in double blind trials. Then, one of the original researchers conducted another study with Belgian children. Only boys, not girls, whose diets were poor showed improvement in school when they received vitamin/mineral supplements (Benton and Buts, 1990). On the basis of limited information on dietary intake, the authors suggested that a poor diet contributed to "a poorer attitude and lack of attention" in boys. They said "the supplements are not increasing scores but rather preventing a dietary-induced decrement."

Recalling that there are about 50 required vitamins, minerals, and amino acids, do you think that the students would benefit more from supplements or an improved diet? What type of dietary and laboratory data would be needed to substantiate these authors' claims?

In 1987, the American Medical Association's Council on Scientific Affairs offered guidance in a report called Vitamin Preparations as Dietary Supplements and as Therapeutic Agents. It emphasized that most healthy adult men and women eating a typical, varied diet do not need vitamin supplements but that there are various categories of people who *do* benefit from supplements.

The types of people the report focused on were those who have pathologic conditions or diseases and those who routinely take medications that increase the need for vitamins. (We'll discuss this further in Chapter 17.) Vitamin supplements should be prescribed as a part of treatment for people in these categories according to each patient's needs.

The AMA's report also describes several groups of generally healthy people who benefit from supplemental vitamins. *Vegans* need to get vitamin B-12 from supplements because it is not generally available in their diets; *vegan children* may also need supplemental riboflavin and vitamin D. *Pregnant and lactating women* may benefit from a multivitamin supplement, because their needs are somewhat higher at these times. (However, not all experts agree with the need for vitamin supplements during pregnancy; see the footnote in Table 11.10.) A good general rule is not to take supplements that provide more than 100% of the RDA for any nutrient (National Research Council, 1989).

Newborns are generally given a single dose of vitamin K under the direction of a physician. Physicians sometimes prescribe various vitamin supplements for *infants under one year of age*, depending on what kind of milk they are fed (see Chapter 15). The *elderly*, too, may benefit from supplements, especially if their food intake diminishes. In fact, *anyone whose energy intake decreases dramatically for any reason*—and this includes

TABLE 11.10 Healthy People for Whom Vitamin Supplements Are Recommended

Advisability of Supplementation	Who Needs Supplement	Vitamin(s) to Be Supplemented
Recommended in all cases	Newborns	Vitamin K
	Vegans	Vitamin B-12; possibly riboflavin and vitamin D, especially for vegan children
Often recommended	Pregnant[a] and lactating women	Multivitamin
	Infants up to 1 year of age	Depends on what milk is used; pediatrician should advise
	Older adults	Multivitamin
	People with low energy intake, including those on weight-reduction diets	Multivitamin

[a]Moderate vitamin supplementation during pregnancy has been a long-standing medical practice. However, the Committee on Nutritional Status During Pregnancy and Lactation, of the National Academy of Sciences, stated in their 1990 report *Nutrition During Pregnancy* that the increased needs for vitamins during pregnancy could be met with a well-selected diet alone (Committee on Nutritional Status During Pregnancy and Lactation, 1990).

weight-reduction dieting—would probably benefit from a modest vitamin supplement.

These points are summarized in Table 11.10.

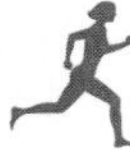

Athletes often "swear by" vitamin supplements. However, scientists are generally unable to demonstrate any effect of nutritional supplements on athletic performance of men or women in double blind trials (Telford et al., 1992). Occasionally, athletes whose diets provide less than RDA quantities of vitamins appear to benefit from vitamin supplements. The best advice for these individuals is to improve their food choices instead of taking a supplement. This chapter's Consider This on page 372 offers guidelines to help athletes (or anyone else) achieve adequate vitamin intake from food and beverages. ●

Finally, note that taking a vitamin supplement does not ensure that your nutritional needs will be met. Since there are approximately 50 essential nutrients, getting an adequate intake of only the 13 vitamins does not constitute good nutrition.

You Tell Me

A sweetened breakfast cereal is fortified with 100% of the RDA for all vitamins.

Is this product an essential part of a "good breakfast," as its makers claim? Is it better for you than a whole-grain (but unfortified) cereal that contains variable levels of vitamins and that you consume as part of a balanced diet?

To improve vitamin intake and status, instead of

This	*Consider this*
Fewer than 5 servings of fruits and vegetables daily	**At least 2 servings of fruits and 3 of vegetables daily**
Vitamin supplements for vitamin A and carotene	**At least 1 serving of a deep green, leafy vegetable or a deep yellow fruit or vegetable such as carrots, broccoli, apricots**
Nonenriched grain products	**Whole grains or enriched grain products**
Megadoses of vitamins because of "special" situations	**Evaluate situation using Table 11.10. If needed, improve diet or select supplements that provide no more than 100% RDA.**
Vitamin C supplement for smokers	**Best idea: quit smoking. If you continue to smoke, consume 2 or more servings of fruit and vegetables that are good sources of vitamin C every day.**

Remember: Gradual changes are more likely to last, and they give your body time to adjust.

Summary

- You probably don't need to be convinced that vitamins are important, but until now you may not have realized that a well-chosen diet can supply all the vitamins that you need—or that very high doses of vitamin supplements can be dangerous.
- **Vitamins** are regulators of metabolic functions. They are needed only in minute amounts. Vitamins A, D, E, and K are fat-soluble; thiamin, riboflavin, niacin, B-6, folic acid, B-12, pantothenic acid, biotin, and vitamin C are water-soluble. In general, your body can accumulate more of the fat-soluble vitamins; therefore, they have more potential to cause harm. However, toxicities due to overingestion of water-soluble vitamins can occur.
- Except in that they are all organic, the vitamins are structurally unrelated to each other. A number of vitamins exist as several slightly different chemical forms that all function in the body as that vitamin. Your body can also convert vitamin precursors, called **provitamins,** into active forms. The form in which a vitamin occurs can affect its potency, but whether the vitamin was produced naturally or synthetically makes no difference.
- Several units of measurement are used to quantify vitamins. Now that scientists are aware of the varying potencies of different forms of some vitamins and their precursors, units called **equivalents** are coming into common use to reflect as accurately as possible the amount of vitamin *activity* the various forms provide.
- Almost all vitamins are at work in almost all body cells. Every vitamin has a widespread effect

on your body, and body functions (such as energy production, growth, reproduction, and immune function) are influenced by many vitamins simultaneously. Tables 11.2 through 11.9 list common food sources of vitamins, and Table 11.1 summarizes their major functions and signs of deficiency and excess.

- Some substances that have recently been touted as vitamins are in fact produced in adequate amounts by healthy people; therefore, they technically are not vitamins and certainly need not be supplemented in the diet. Other nonvitamins are toxic and can cause harm to people who consume them.
- Extreme vitamin deficiencies are rare in the developed countries but still occur in many parts of the world. Such deficiencies usually arise in people whose food is limited in type and/or quantity, in people who cannot absorb or utilize vitamins to a normal extent, and in people whose needs for vitamins are high because of rapid growth or disease. Worldwide, most people who have vitamin deficiencies simply do not get enough to eat and are likely to have multiple deficiencies rather than a shortage of a single vitamin. There is considerable variation in both the signs and symptoms of deficiencies and the time it takes for a particular deficiency to develop.
- Large excesses of vitamins are dangerous, though it is rare for an individual to consume harmful amounts of any vitamin in ordinary foods. Vitamin toxicity is more often the result of ingesting vitamin supplements in excessive quantities over a long period of time. The level of toxicity for a given vitamin is influenced by several factors, including storage capacity in the body, level of intake, chemical form, and the length of time in which the overdose occurs. People who suffer the ill effects of toxicity have usually been taking vitamin megadoses for anywhere from a few months to a few years.
- Most healthy people do not need to take vitamin supplements at all. Vegetarians who do not eat any animal products do need supplemental vitamin B-12, and supplements can be helpful during pregnancy and lactation, periods of rapid growth, and for the elderly. Vitamin supplements may also have limited use for individuals who are taking certain kinds of drugs or whose energy intake has decreased dramatically.

References

American Medical Association, Council on Scientific Affairs. 1987. Vitamin preparations as dietary supplements and as therapeutic agents. *Journal of the American Medical Association* 257:1929–1936.

Bailey, L.B. 1992. Evaluation of a new recommended dietary allowance for folate. *Journal of American Dietetic Association* 92:463–468, 471.

Baird, I.M., R.E. Hughes, H.K. Wilson, J.E. Davies, and A.N. Howard. 1979. The effects of ascorbic acid and flavonoids on the occurrence of symptoms normally associated with the common cold. *American Journal of Clinical Nutrition* 32:1686–1690.

Ban, T.A. 1981. Megavitamin therapy in schizophrenia. In *Nutrition and behavior*, ed. S.A. Miller. Philadelphia: The Franklin Institute Press.

Bauerfeind, J.C. 1988. Vitamin A deficiency: A staggering problem of health and sight. *Nutrition Today* 23:34–36.

Benton, D., and J.P. Buts. 1990. Vitamin/mineral supplementation and intelligence. *Lancet* 335:1158–1160.

Byers T., and G. Perry. 1992. Dietary carotenes, vitamin C, and vitamin E as protective antioxidants in human cancer. *Annual Review of Nutrition* 12:139–159.

Canfield, L.M., J.W. Forage, and J.G. Valenzuela. 1992. Carotenoids as cellular antioxidants. *Proceedings of Society for Experimental Biology and Medicine* 200:260–264.

Carpenter, K.J. and W.J. Lewin. 1985. A reexamination of the composition of diets associated with pellagra. *Journal of Nutrition* 115:543–552.

Centers for Disease Control. 1991. Effectiveness in disease and injury prevention. Use of folic acid for prevention of spina bifida and other neural tube defects 1983–1991. *Morbidity and Mortality Weekly Report* 40:513–516.

Committee on Nutritional Status During Pregnancy and Lactation. 1990. *Nutrition During Pregnancy*. Washington DC: National Academy Press.

DeLuca, H.F. 1988. Vitamin D and its metabolites. In *Modern nutrition in health and disease*, ed. M.E. Shils and V.R. Young. Philadelphia: Lea & Febiger.

DiPalma, J.R., and W.S. Thayer. 1991. Use of niacin as a drug. *Annual Review of Nutrition* 11:169–187.

Evans, C.D. and J.H. Lacey. 1986. Toxicity of vitamins: Complications of a health movement. *British Medical Journal* 292:509–510.

Geubel, A.P., C. de Galocsy, N. Alves, J. Rahrer, and C. Dive. 1991. Liver damage caused by therapeutic vitamin A administration: Estimate of dose related toxicity in 41 cases. *Gastroenterology* 100:1701–1709.

Heid, M.K., N.D. Bills, S.H. Hinrichs, and A.J. Clifford. 1992. Folate deficiency alone does not produce neural tube defects in mice. *Journal of Nutrition* 122:888–894.

Hemilä, H. 1992. Vitamin C and the common cold. *British Journal of Nutrition* 67:3–16.

Herbert, V. and N. Colman. 1988. Folic acid and vitamin B-12. In *Modern nutrition in health and disease*, ed. M.E. Shils and V.R. Young. Philadelphia: Lea & Febiger.

Holick, M.F. 1987. Photosynthesis of vitamin D in the skin: Effect of environmental and life-style variables. *Federation Proceedings* 46:1876–1882.

Hornig D.H., U. Moser, and B.E. Glatthaar. 1988. Ascorbic acid. In *Modern nutrition in health and disease*, ed. M.E. Shils and V.R. Young. Philadelphia: Lea & Febiger.

Human Nutrition Information Service (HNIS). 1985. Nationwide food consumption survey: Continuing survey of food intakes by individuals. NFCS CSFII Report No. 85-1. Hyattsville, MD: U.S. Department of Agriculture.

Human Nutrition Information Service (HNIS). 1986. Nationwide food consumption survey: Continuing survey of food intakes by individuals: Men 19–50 years, 1 day, 1985. Report No. 85-3. Hyattsville, MD: United States Department of Agriculture.

Hussey, G.D., and M. Klein. 1990. A randomized, controlled trial of vitamin A in children with severe measles. *New England Journal of Medicine* 323:160–164.

Jacobus, C.H., M.F. Holick, Q. Shao, T.C. Chen, I.A. Holm, J.M. Kolodny, G.E. Fuleihan, and E.W. Seely. 1992. Hypervitaminosis D associated with drinking milk. *New England Journal of Medicine* 326:1173–1177.

Kamil, A. 1974. How natural are those "natural" vitamins? *Nutrition Reviews* (Supplement I) 32:34.

Lammer, E.J., D.T. Chen, R.M. Hoar, N.D. Agnish, P.J. Benke, J.T. Braun, C.J. Curry, P.M. Fernoff, A.W. Grix, I.T. Lott, J.M. Richard, and S.C. Sun. 1985. Retinoic acid embryopathy. *New England Journal of Medicine* 313:837–841.

Lecklem, J.E. 1988. Vitamin B-6 bioavailability and its application to human nutrition. *Food Technology* 42:194–196.

McCormick, D.B. 1988. (4 chapters) Thiamin. Riboflavin. Niacin. Biotin. In *Modern nutrition in health and disease*, ed. M.E. Shils and V.R. Young. Philadelphia: Lea & Febiger.

Mino, M. 1992. Clinical uses and abuses of vitamin E in children. *Proceedings of Society for Experimental Biology and Medicine* 200:266–270.

Mira, M., P.M. Stewart, and S.F. Abraham. 1988. Vitamin and trace element status in premenstrual syndrome. *American Journal of Clinical Nutrition* 47:636–641.

Moss, A.J., A.S. Levy, I. Kim, and Y.K. Park. 1989. Use of vitamin and mineral supplements in the United States: Current users, types of products, and nutrients. *Advance Data* 174:1–20.

MRC Vitamin Study Research Group. 1991. Prevention of neural tube defects: Results of the Medical Research Council vitamin study. *Lancet* 338:131–137.

Murphy, S.P., A.F. Subar, and G. Block. 1990. Vitamin E intakes and sources in the United States. *American Journal of Clinical Nutrition* 52:361–367.

National Center for Health Statistics. 1979. *Dietary intake source data, United States, 1971–1974.* U.S. Department of Health, Education, and Welfare (DHEW) Publication No. (PHS)791221. Hyattsville, MD: Department of Health, Education, and Welfare.

National Research Council. 1989. *Diet and health.* Washington DC: National Academy Press.

Nutrition Forum. 1986. "Stress vitamin" manufacturer agrees to stop false and misleading claims. *Nutrition Forum* 3:28.

Nutrition Reviews. 1990. Uses of vitamin and mineral supplements in the United States. *Nutrition Reviews* 48:161–162.

Olson, J.A. 1989. Upper limits of vitamin A in infant formulas, with some comments on vitamin K. *Journal of Nutrition* 119:1820–1824.

Parry, G.J. and D.E. Bredesen. 1985. Sensory neuropathy with low-dose pyridoxine. *Neurology* 35:1466–1468.

Pennington, J.A. 1989. *Food values of portions commonly used.* New York: Harper & Row.

Pennington, J.A. and H.N. Church. 1985. *Food values of portions commonly used.* Philadephia: J.B. Lippincott.

RDA Subcommittee. 1989. *Recommended dietary allowances.* Washington DC: National Academy Press.

Rahmathullah, L., B.A. Underwood, R.D. Thulasiraj, R.C. Milton, K. Ramaswamy, R. Rahmathullah, and G. Babu. 1990. Reduced mortality among children in southern India receiving a small weekly dose of vitamin A. *New England Journal of Medicine* 323:929–935.

Roberts, L. 1988. Question raised about antiwrinkle cream. *Science* 240:564.

Ross, A.C. 1992. Vitamin A status: Relationship to immunity and antibody response. *Proceedings of Society for Experimental Biology and Medicine* 200:303–320.

Schaumberg, H., J. Kaplan, A. Windebank, N. Vick, S. Rasmus, D. Pleasure, and M.J. Brown. 1983. Sensory neuropathy from pyridoxine abuse: A new megavitamin syndrome. *New England Journal of Medicine* 309:445–448.

Schectman, G., J.C. Byrd, and R. Hoffman. 1991. Ascorbic acid requirements for smokers: analysis of a population survey. *American Journal of Clinical Nutrition* 53:1466–1470.

Shils, M.E. and V.R. Young. 1988. *Modern nutrition in health and disease.* Philadelphia: Lea & Febiger.

Smith, S.M., and G. Eichele. Temporal and regional differences in the expression pattern of distinct retinoic and receptor-β transcripts in the chick embryo. *Development* 11:245–252.

Specker, B.L., A. Black, L. Allen, and F. Morrow. 1990. Vitamin B-12: Low milk concentrations are related to low serum concentrates in vegetarian women and to methylmalonic aciduria in their infants. *American Journal of Clinical Nutrition* 52:1073–1076.

Surgeon General. 1988. *Surgeon General's report on nutrition and health.* Washington, D.C.: United States Department of Health and Human Services.

Suttie, J.W., L.L. Mummah-Schendel, D.V. Shah, B.J. Lyle, and J.L. Greger. 1988. Vitamin K deficiency from dietary vitamin K restriction in humans. *American Journal of Clinical Nutrition* 47:475–480.

Suttie, J.W. 1992. Vitamin K and human nutrition. *Journal of American Dietetic Association* 92:585–590.

Telford, R.D., E.A. Catchpole, V. Deakin, A.G. Hahn, and A.W. Plank. 1992. The effect of 7 to 8 months of vitamin/mineral supplementation on athletic performance. *International Journal of Sports Medicine* 2:135–153.

Wolf, G. 1990. Recent progress in vitamin A research: Nuclear retinoic acid receptors and their interaction with gene elements. *Journal of Nutritional Biochemistry* 1:284–289.

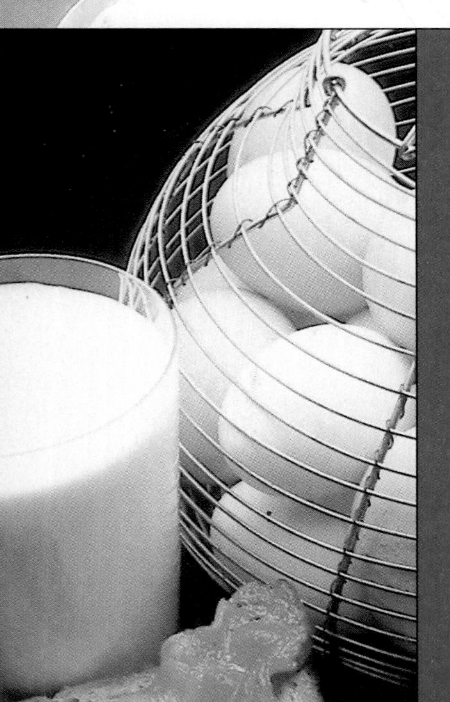

IN THIS CHAPTER

Chapter 12

Minerals

Perhaps you think minerals are almost indistinguishable from vitamins. Haven't you often heard breakfast cereal commercials refer to *vitamins and minerals* together, as though they were one large nutrient group?

It's true that there are similarities between these two groups: they are both micronutrients whose importance to humans was not appreciated before this century. Like vitamins, minerals are widespread in basic foods but are nonetheless aggressively marketed by the supplement industry. Professional nutritionists are concerned that some misleading—or even false—advertising claims about the benefits of mineral supplements encourage you to consume them at toxic levels.

There are also major differences between the two groups. Vitamins are organic (carbon-containing) compounds, whereas minerals are inorganic. In fact, minerals are single elements, not complex molecules with several constituents.

Minerals—Many Elements

Minerals are the chemical elements other than carbon, hydrogen, oxygen, and nitrogen that make up your body. Carbon, hydrogen, oxygen, and nitrogen account for 96% of body weight; minerals constitute only about 4%. Minerals in your body make up in number what they lack in gross weight: at least 20 are commonly found in humans, and as many as 60 have been identified in living organisms.

minerals—chemical elements other than carbon, hydrogen, oxygen, and nitrogen that make up the body

Categories

Minerals can be divided into two categories. Those present in the human body in amounts greater than 0.01% of body weight (or needed in the diet in amounts of 100 mg or more per day) are called **macrominerals** or **major minerals**. Calcium, phosphorus, sulfur, potassium, sodium, chloride, and magnesium are macrominerals.

macrominerals (major minerals)—those minerals present in the body in amounts greater than 0.01% of body weight

The macrominerals present in your body in the largest amounts are calcium (approximately 1 kg or 2 pounds) and phosphorus (approximately 0.7 kg or 1½ pounds). Figure 12.1 shows the amounts typically present in an adult male.

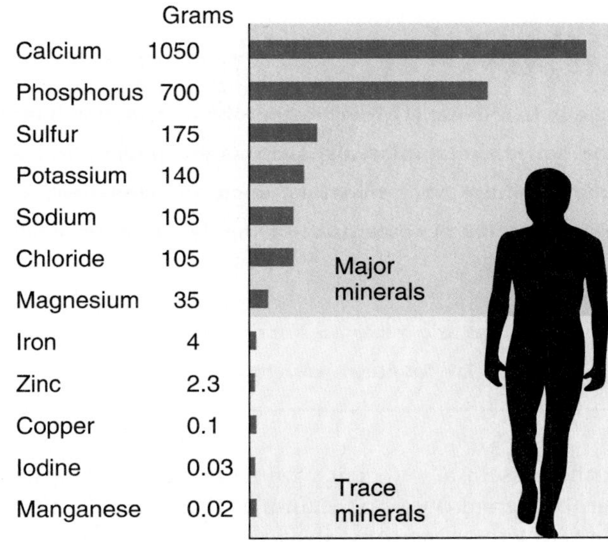

FIGURE 12.1
Some of the minerals in a 70-kg man.

Amounts of the major minerals and a few of the essential trace minerals are shown. Other trace minerals occur in the body in even smaller amounts than those listed.

trace minerals (trace elements)—those minerals present in the body in amounts less than 0.01% of body weight

The minerals that are present in your body in quantities smaller than 0.01% of body weight are called **trace minerals** or **trace elements**. They include iron, iodine, fluoride, zinc, selenium, copper, chromium, manganese, molybdenum, cobalt, silicon, arsenic, nickel, and vanadium. Iron and zinc are the most prevalent trace elements in your body; your body probably contains 2–4 grams of each of them. Most of the other trace minerals are present in much smaller quantities—perhaps just one-thousandth as much.

To help you visualize how small the amounts of trace elements in your body are, imagine that your normal body weight is one ton (2000 pounds). Assuming normal trace mineral composition, you would contain only 1.8 ounces of iron, 1.1 ounces of zinc, 0.05 ounce of copper, 0.01 ounce of iodine, 0.003 ounce of chromium, 0.001 ounce of cobalt, and 0.0004 ounce of vanadium.

Relative Importance

At this time, scientists don't think that the body requires all the chemical elements it contains: only some of the minerals found in your body have been found to be essential for growth, reproduction, and health. Although you might expect that the distinction between essential and nonessential minerals should be easy for scientists to make, it's not.

A major reason for the disagreement is that the tests to determine essentiality are difficult to conduct and interpret. A traditional test is to show that serious negative consequences result when animals' diets contain very low levels of the test nutrient. However, scientists find it difficult to study the effects of deficiencies of certain trace elements because they cannot keep all vestiges of these trace elements out of test diets and the environment of test animals.

Scientists also do not agree completely on the definition of *essential.* Some scientists regard fluoride as essential; others do not. These differing judgments arise from two facts: the presence of fluoride in the diet significantly discourages tooth decay, but poor growth and death do not result from lack of fluoride. Table 12.1 identifies the minerals some experts consider essential for animals; it's likely that humans need them as well. The fact that this table does not agree completely with the RDA listing of essential minerals underscores the differences in judgment and the limited amount of data available on several trace elements.

You Tell Me

Consider these two facts: (1) Your body probably contains a larger quantity of some nonessential minerals, such as aluminum and lead, than it has of some essential trace minerals, such as manganese and iodine. (2) Severe deficiencies of some trace elements—zinc, for example—can result in death.

Can you assume that the biologic importance of a substance is proportional to the amount found in your body?

As with other essential nutrients, mineral intakes that are in excess of your needs can be dangerous. For example, the minerals zinc and iron are essential for life, but they are toxic if ingested in very large quantities.

TABLE 12.1 Minerals—Essential and Nonessential

Minerals Believed Essential for Animals		
Calcium	Arsenic	Manganese
Phosphorus	Chromium	Molybdenum
Sulfur	Cobalt	Nickel
Potassium	Copper	Selenium
Sodium	Fluoride[a]	Silicon
Chloride	Iodine	Vanadium
Magnesium	Iron	Zinc
Minerals Not Proved to Be Required for Animals		
Aluminum	Germanium	Silver
Antimony	Gold	Strontium
Barium	Lanthanum	Thallium
Beryllium	Lead	Titanium
Bismuth	Mercury	Uranium
Bromine	Niobium	Zirconium
Cadmium	Radium	Boron[b]
Cesium	Rubidium	Lithium[b]
Gallium	Ruthenium	Tin[b]

[a]Scientists have not demonstrated that fluoride is essential for life itself, but it is well documented that its presence in the diet has a beneficial effect on dental health.
[b]Scientists have shown these elements to be essential in isolated studies. These data need to be confirmed by other investigators before these minerals are classified as essential.

Source: Nielsen, 1988.

The Bioavailability Issue

The **bioavailability** (usefulness to the body) of a given mineral you eat can vary a great deal. Many factors influence mineral bioavailability—some decrease it, whereas others increase it. As we mentioned in Chapter 11, nutritionists are beginning to learn that bioavailability is also an issue for certain vitamins, such as vitamin B-6 and folic acid. Bioavailability of minerals, by contrast, has been studied much more intensively for many years.

bioavailability—degree to which the body is able to use a substance in the form or amount present

In general, if you are healthy, you absorb more than 90% of the protein, carbohydrate, and fat in your diet, but you don't absorb minerals as efficiently. In fact, scientists have found that adults absorb an average of only 1–10% of the iron and manganese, 10–20% of the zinc, and 15–40% of the magnesium and calcium in their diets.

Differences in food composition can cause variations in the bioavailability of minerals. For example, investigators have shown that as diet composition changes, our absorption of calcium can change from less than 5% to more than 50%. Other factors can influence the bioavailability of minerals as well, such as a person's health and use of medications. These factors can alter absorption, excretion, storage, and/or transport of minerals.

Dietary Factors That Improve Mineral Bioavailability

Few dietary factors actually improve your body's use of minerals, but this section describes those that have been identified. Much of this discussion

heme iron—a form of iron that is part of hemoglobin and myoglobin; about 40% of iron in meat, fish, and poultry is heme iron

hemoglobin—the iron-containing protein in blood that carries oxygen to cells and carbon dioxide away from them

myoglobin—the iron-containing protein in muscle cells

nonheme iron—iron present in the diet other than heme iron (includes iron in milk, eggs, and plant products)

centers on iron because more is known about the bioavailability of this mineral than about that of others. The iron in your diet can be classified into two categories: heme iron and nonheme iron. **Heme iron**, as the name implies, is found in the **hemoglobin** of blood and in the **myoglobin** of animal muscle. Heme iron accounts for about 40–50% of the iron in meat, fish, and poultry. **Nonheme iron** accounts for the remaining iron in these foods. All the iron in eggs, milk, and plant foods is considered nonheme iron. These classifications are important because scientists have found that people usually absorb 15–35% of the heme iron in their diets but only 1–20% of the nonheme iron (Monsen, 1988).

What does this mean in practical terms? Let's assume that you consumed equal amounts of iron in two meals. In one meal, meat provided the iron, and in the other meal cereal provided it. You would absorb more iron from the meal containing the meat.

There are at least two ways that you can improve your absorption of nonheme iron; we discuss them in the upcoming sections. Although vegetarians are often particularly interested in this matter, it warrants general concern because nonheme iron usually accounts for more than 90% of the iron in the diets of most adults.

Ascorbic Acid One way to improve your absorption of nonheme iron is to increase the amount of vitamin C (ascorbic acid) in your diet. Scientists have found that adding 75 mg of ascorbic acid to a meal can more than double the absorption of nonheme iron from that meal. This means that if you add 6 ounces of orange juice to your breakfast of toast and eggs, you can double the bioavailability of the iron in the toast and eggs. Similarly, if you add canned tomatoes to a rice casserole you can improve the bioavailability of the iron in the rice. (Unfortunately, ascorbic acid has not been found to improve the absorption of other minerals.)

unidentified meat factor—substance present in meat that can increase the bioavailability of nonheme iron consumed at the same meal

Unidentified Meat Factor A second dietary factor that can increase the absorption of nonheme iron is known as the **unidentified meat factor**. Although scientists do not know exactly what substance in meat is responsible for this effect, they do know that adding 3 ounces of meat, fish, or poultry to a meal can more than double the absorption of the nonheme iron in the meal. In other words, if you add ham or tuna to a macaroni and cheese casserole, you will increase the bioavailability of the iron in the macaroni and cheese. At the same time, the heme iron in the meat or fish is absorbed with characteristic efficiency.

It is important to be aware of one other fact when you use these principles: ascorbic acid and/or unidentified meat factor must be consumed *at the same meal as the nonheme iron* in order to increase its bioavailability. That is, the orange juice or sausage you consume at breakfast will not influence the absorption of the nonheme iron that you eat at supper. You will improve your utilization of iron more by adding moderate amounts of foods rich in vitamin C or by including meats in each meal than by eating a large amount of these foods at just one meal during the day.

Breast Milk for Infants Nutritionists have found that infants absorb the iron and zinc in breast milk more efficiently than the iron and zinc in cow's milk or infant formulas. Reasons for this phenomenon have been suggested but not proved (Lönnerdal, 1987). In general, the balance among levels of various minerals (including calcium, iron, and zinc) and the presence of proteins, peptides, and other factors that form chemical complexes with zinc and iron appear to work together to optimize the infant's absorption of zinc and iron from human milk. (See Chapter 15 for further information on the nutrition of mothers and infants.)

ostasis), *bisphosphonates* (phosphorus-containing drugs being tested to treat osteoporosis), vitamin D derivatives, and weight-bearing exercise in conjunction with increased calcium intakes (Consensus Development Conference, 1991). Each method has been found to be beneficial for some patients, but each has limitations in effectiveness or produces side effects. Many experts think that a combination of therapies is apt to be the treatment of choice in the future. But until then, be aware that scientists do not know a sure cure nor a guaranteed preventive treatment for osteoporosis. When a woman nears menopause, she should discuss the various therapies with her physician to see which would be most appropriate.

Many experts believe that the best protection against the adverse effects of bone loss is to maximize **peak bone mass** to offset the losses of bone that occur with age. Scientists have shown that animals fed diets very deficient in calcium have smaller bones, but they are less sure of the effects of typical variations in calcium intake on bone size in humans. There are genetic limits to how much bone you can accumulate. Scientists have found that adult daughters of women with osteoporosis have lower bone densities in their spines than other premenopausal women (Seeman et al., 1989). But no matter what your genetic predisposition, you can try to maximize bone mass within your genetic potential. Experts believe that adequate intake of calcium during the teens and twenties may help you to achieve peak bone mass (Sentipal et al., 1991). So instead of thinking of osteoporosis as your grandmother's problem, take action now. We'll show you how in the Recommended and Typical Intakes, and Sources sections, below.

peak bone mass—maximum amount of bone that can be achieved; occurs during the third decade of life

Deficiency Symptoms Although calcium plays a role in blood clotting and nerve transmission, these functions are not affected when your calcium intake is low, because regulatory mechanisms maintain constant blood levels of calcium. Several hormones (one of which is a metabolite of vitamin D, another of which is called parathyroid hormone) work together when there is little dietary calcium to increase the retention of calcium by the kidneys and to withdraw calcium from bone. The vitamin D metabolite also increases calcium absorption from the gut. This means that blood calcium levels are not much affected by dietary calcium intake. For this reason, you can't use biochemical (blood or urine) tests to monitor your body's calcium status.

Several investigators have suggested that low calcium intakes may be related to a higher incidence of hypertension (Karanja and McCarron, 1986). Other investigators have suggested that high levels of calcium are protective against colon cancer (Wargovich, 1988). However, the relationships between calcium intake and hypertension and colon cancer have not been consistent; they are undergoing intensive research at this time. So although there is no doubt that calcium is essential, the consequences of taking in less than the RDA are not known for sure.

Recommended and Typical Intakes From what you have just read, you shouldn't be surprised to learn that the RDA for calcium for adults has been the source of considerable controversy in recent years. The most recent RDA committee felt that higher intakes of calcium were more apt to be beneficial in establishing maximal peak bone mass, which a person attains during the third decade of life, than in treating women with osteoporosis. Therefore, the RDAs for calcium and phosphorus are both 1200 mg (about ¼ teaspoon) daily for teens and adults through age 24. For men and women 25 and older, the RDA is 800 mg.

FIGURE 12.5
How do American adults' calcium intakes compare with recommendations?

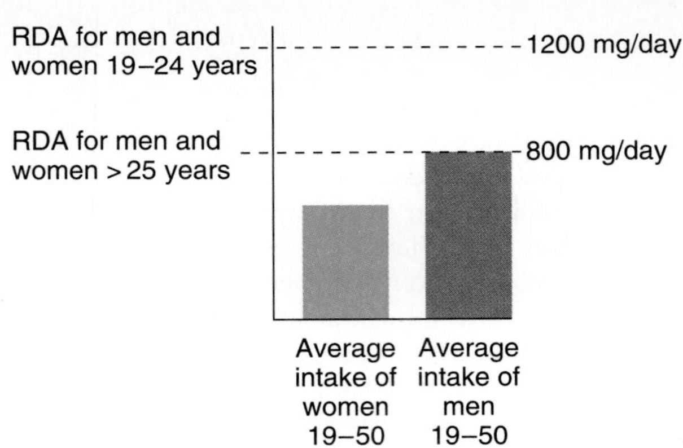

Most American women consume much less calcium than these recommended amounts (Figure 12.5). Women consumed an average of 570 mg of calcium daily in 1977 and 651 mg in 1985 (Human Nutrition Information Service, 1985). The average calcium intake of men under 50 years of age in a national survey, by contrast, was 800 mg daily; this level reflected their higher total energy intakes (Science and Education Administration, 1980).

Sources Just as certain minerals are concentrated in specific tissues of your body, so are certain minerals concentrated in particular foods. Over half the calcium (55%) consumed by Americans is supplied by milk and milk products (Block et al., 1985). Table 12.3 shows what a rich source of calcium milk is. A cup of milk provides about 300 mg of calcium; to get an equivalent amount from other dairy products, you would have to consume 1⅓ ounces of most hard cheeses (approximately ⅓ cup, shredded), 2 cups of cottage cheese, 1½ cups of ice cream, or 2 ounces of processed cheese food (approximately 3 wrapped slices). You might recognize these amounts as the serving sizes of dairy products in the Food Guide Pyramid, which were portioned that way to provide similar amounts of calcium. If you consume the three servings of milk or milk products per day recommended for teens and adults through age 24, you will ingest almost 900 mg of calcium, just 300 mg short of the RDA. The remainder is relatively easy to obtain from other foods.

It is hard to get your RDA for calcium if you don't drink milk. If you avoid milk because of lactose intolerance, you can use lactase products to help digest the lactose (See Chapter 5). To get calcium without drinking milk, (1) try different milk products, such as yogurt or cheese; (2) include milk and cheeses in sauces, casseroles, and desserts; and (3) consume vegetable products that are good sources of calcium (leafy vegetables, broccoli, legumes, and nuts). Be aware that calcium from plant sources is apt to be less bioavailable because plant sources also contain phytate, fiber, and oxalates.

You Tell Me

Sales for calcium supplements exceeded $130 million in 1985 (Uehling and Springen, 1986). Supplement users may not realize that high doses of calcium can depress the utilization of a number of other minerals (Greger, 1989a). Furthermore, some calcium supplements may have

continued on page 392

TABLE 12.3 Calcium and Phosphorus in Some Foods

The RDAs for calcium and phosphorus for adults through age 24 are 1200 mg/day; for people age 25 and older, 800 mg/day.

Food	Household Measure	Milligrams of Calcium (0 200 400 600 800)	Milligrams of Phosphorus (0 200 400 600 800)
Bread, cereal, rice, and pasta			
Bread, whole-grain	1 slice		
Bread, white enriched	1 slice		
Cereal, shredded wheat	1 biscuit		
Vegetables			
Beans, green snap, cooked	½ cup		
Peas, cooked	½ cup		
Spinach, cooked	½ cup		
Fruits			
Apple juice	1		
Apricots, canned	½ cup		
Pineapple, raw	½ cup		
Milk, yogurt, and cheese			
Milk, 2% fat	1 cup		
Yogurt, plain low fat	1 cup		
Cheese, cheddar	1⅓ ounces		
Cheese, cottage, low fat	2 cups		
Ice cream	1½ cups		
Meats, poultry, fish, eggs, beans, and nuts			
Beef, ground, broiled	2 ounces		
Eggs, fried	2		
Salmon including bones, canned	2 ounces		
Salmon, no bones, cooked	2 ounces		
Peanut butter, chunky style	¼ cup		
Combination foods			
Cheeseburger, McDonald's	4 ounces		
Pork and beans in tomato sauce	1 cup		
Cheese pizza	1 slice (4.5 ounces)		
Spinach souffle	1 cup		
Taco	1 item		
Fats, oils, and sweets			
Beer	12 ounces		
Butter, margarine	1 t.		
Candy, milk chocolate	1 ounce		
Carbonated cola beverage	12 ounces		

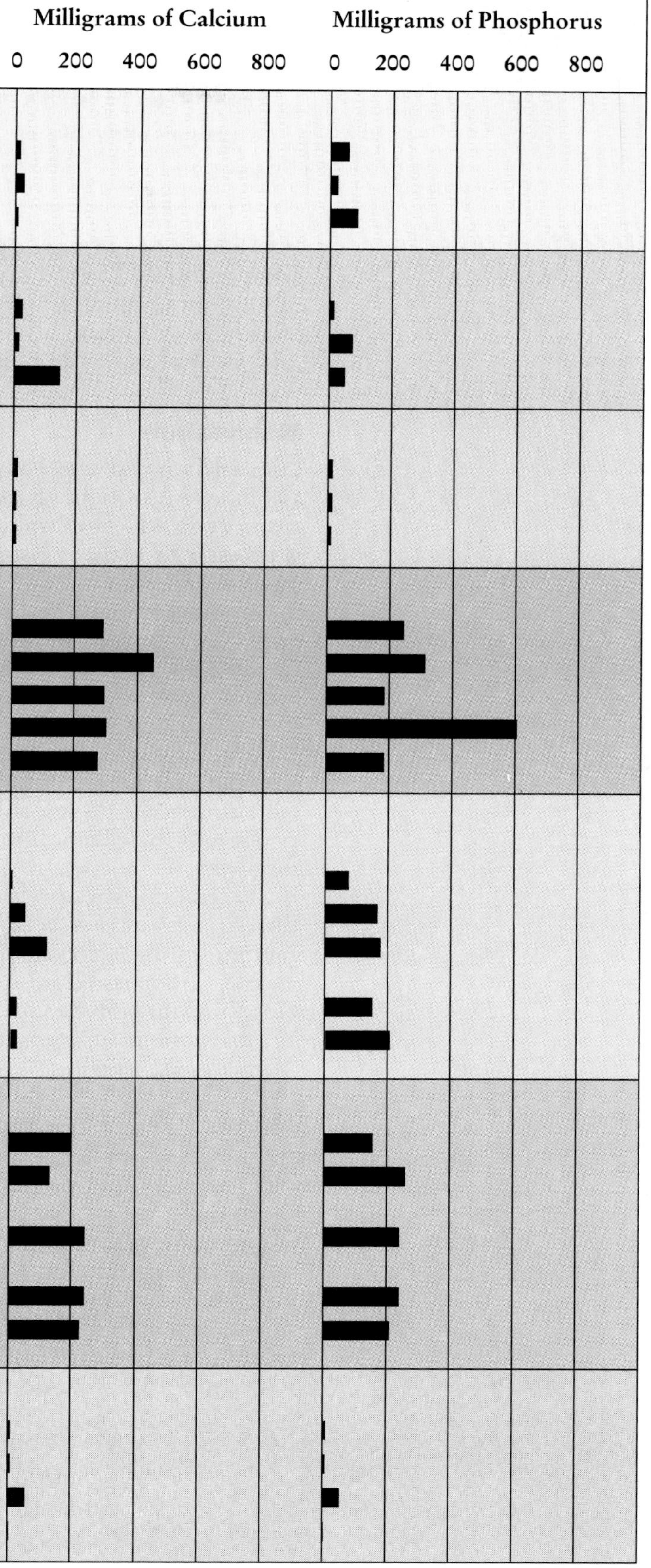

toxic components. For example, some batches of bone meal (finely ground animal bones) contain considerable amounts of lead (Miller, 1987).

Do you think the benefits of taking calcium supplements outweigh the risks? If so, for whom, or in what situations? In what other ways could a person bring his or her calcium intake up to the recommended levels?

Many foods that are good sources of calcium are also good sources of phosphorus, as Table 12.3 shows. Milk and other dairy products, fish with edible bones, legumes, and nuts are good examples. The reverse is not necessarily true: although meat, most fish, poultry, and eggs are very rich sources of phosphorus, they usually contain little calcium.

Magnesium

Like calcium and phosphorus, magnesium has diverse functions. It, too, is a component of bone. It occurs in many enzymes as well, often catalyzing reactions in which phosphorus is involved. Along with calcium, magnesium is necessary for the transmission of nerve impulses that influence the contraction and relaxation of muscles. It also helps stabilize DNA and RNA, the substances that direct protein synthesis.

Recommended and Typical Intakes The recommended intakes for magnesium are 280 mg daily for women and 350 mg daily for men. Adults in the United States usually consume less: 226 mg per day is the average for women (Human Nutrition Information Service, 1985); for men, 329 mg (Human Nutrition Information Service, 1986). Despite these dietary shortfalls, Americans do not show overt symptoms of magnesium deficiency or evidence of biochemical impairment that can be directly related to magnesium status.

Several investigators have noted that in areas with hard drinking water, there is a lower incidence of hypertension. Hard water contains high concentrations of magnesium and calcium. However, data are inconsistent, making it impossible to determine the relationship of magnesium to high blood pressure (Surgeon General, 1988). Generally in controlled clinical trials, magnesium supplements do not reduce the blood pressure of patients (Zemel et al., 1990).

Sources The richest sources of dietary magnesium are nuts, legumes, seafood, and certain leafy green vegetables (Table 12.4). Even though legumes, nuts, and products made from them are rich sources of magnesium, only 5% of the magnesium that the average American consumes comes from these sources. This fact demonstrates that a food isn't a major source of nutrients for a given individual if the person doesn't consume it in significant quantities. Grain products, which generally have less magnesium per serving, provide 21% of the average American's intake; this amount is more than any other group of foods contributes (Science and Education Administration, 1980). Of the grain products, whole grains con-

TABLE 12.4 Magnesium in Some Foods

The RDA for magnesium is 280 mg/day for women; for men, 350 mg/day.

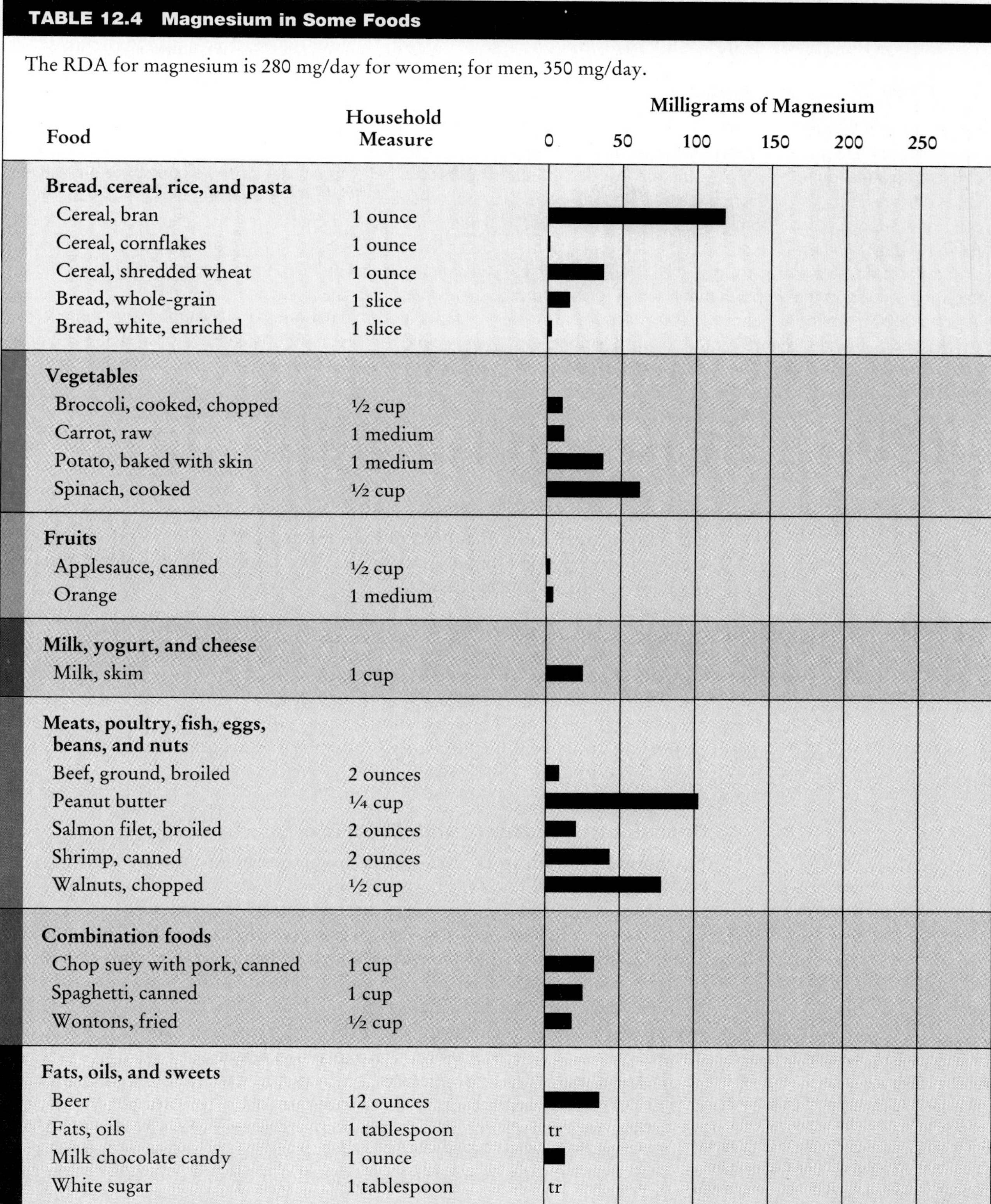

Food	Household Measure	Milligrams of Magnesium (0, 50, 100, 150, 200, 250)
Bread, cereal, rice, and pasta		
Cereal, bran	1 ounce	
Cereal, cornflakes	1 ounce	
Cereal, shredded wheat	1 ounce	
Bread, whole-grain	1 slice	
Bread, white, enriched	1 slice	
Vegetables		
Broccoli, cooked, chopped	½ cup	
Carrot, raw	1 medium	
Potato, baked with skin	1 medium	
Spinach, cooked	½ cup	
Fruits		
Applesauce, canned	½ cup	
Orange	1 medium	
Milk, yogurt, and cheese		
Milk, skim	1 cup	
Meats, poultry, fish, eggs, beans, and nuts		
Beef, ground, broiled	2 ounces	
Peanut butter	¼ cup	
Salmon filet, broiled	2 ounces	
Shrimp, canned	2 ounces	
Walnuts, chopped	½ cup	
Combination foods		
Chop suey with pork, canned	1 cup	
Spaghetti, canned	1 cup	
Wontons, fried	½ cup	
Fats, oils, and sweets		
Beer	12 ounces	
Fats, oils	1 tablespoon	tr
Milk chocolate candy	1 ounce	
White sugar	1 tablespoon	tr

Data sources: Leveille et al., 1983.

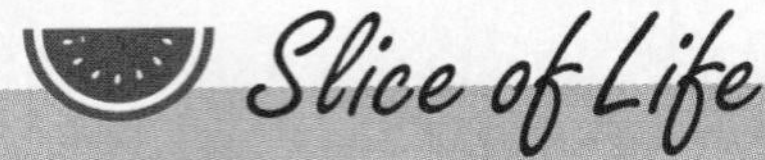

The Cure That Was a Killer

Ryan was a pleasant infant. He ate well and fell asleep soon after each feeding. One day, when he was 10 weeks old, he became quite irritable. After ruling out various other possibilities, his mother concluded he was having colic and sought advice from Adelle Davis's book *Let's Have Healthy Children.* The book suggested giving potassium supplements and reported that 653 colicky babies experienced dramatic improvement when given from 1000 to 3000 mg of potassium chloride by mouth.

Trusting this book, Ryan's mother offered him the recommended dosage of potassium from a bottle obtained at a health food store. According to the official report of the county medical examiner, Ryan received two doses of potassium chloride totaling 3000 mg along with breast milk on the first day. On the following morning, his symptoms recurred and he was given 1500 mg more. A few hours later he became listless and stopped breathing. Despite resuscitation efforts and intensive hospital treatment, he died of potassium intoxication about 36 hours later. It was calculated that Ryan had received at least four times the dose needed for treatment *if he had been deficient in potassium,* which he was not.

Many people, unfortunately, hold the belief that if a little is good, more is better. The above case report is a dramatic example that the idea is not true when it comes to nutrients.

Source: Marshall, 1983.

tain significantly more magnesium than refined grains do; therefore, an easy way to increase your magnesium intake is to consume a couple of servings of whole-grain products daily.

Sulfur

Sulfur is a component of two vitamins: thiamin and biotin. The majority of the sulfur in your body, though, is found in three amino acids: methionine, cystine, and cysteine. These amino acids are part of cellular proteins in both plants and animals. So if your diet is adequate in protein, it will also be adequate in sulfur.

Potassium, Sodium, and Chloride

electrolytes—substances that carry an electrical charge when dissolved in water

Potassium, sodium, and chloride (the ionized form of chlorine used by your body) are grouped together because they are **electrolytes** that perform similar types of functions. One important function they all serve is to aid in water balance. In Chapter 4 we discussed the role of dissolved mineral ions and soluble proteins in controlling the movement of water from one region of the body to another. Recall that water moves through a membrane from the side with the lesser concentration of dissolved particles toward the side with the greater concentration until the concentrations are equalized. The electrolytes are the minerals most involved in water balance.

Potassium (K^+) is the electrolyte found in the highest concentration within body cells; magnesium, phosphates (forms of phosphorus with oxygen), and sulfates (forms of sulfur with oxygen) are also found there. Sodium (Na^+) and chloride (Cl^-) are found in highest concentration in extracellular fluids (outside cells), such as blood plasma. On each side of the membrane, the sum of the negatively charged ions is about equal to the sum of positively charged particles. Transmission of nerve impulses and muscle contraction depend on the rapid fluxes of these ions across membranes and back.

Chloride also functions in the body in a buffering system that compensates for excess acid or alkali.

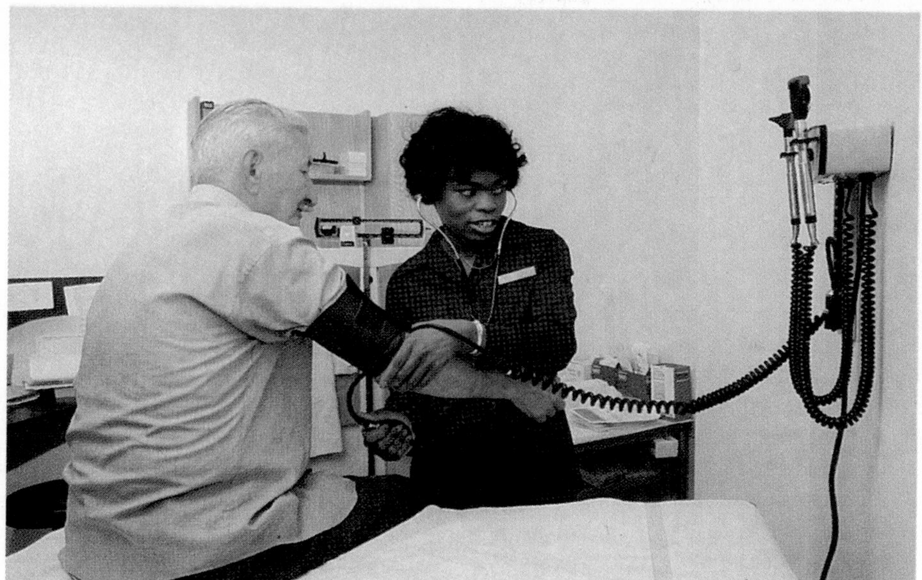

FIGURE 12.6
Blood pressure can be affected by nutrition.

If you have inherited the tendency to have high blood pressure, certain dietary factors may hasten or delay the onset of hypertension.

Problems with Excess Although your body has mechanisms for dealing with considerable variation in levels of potassium, sodium, and chloride, it is possible to overwhelm the body's systems. The Slice of Life, on page 394, about Ryan, an infant who died from potassium intoxication, is a catastrophic example of an **acute** toxicity. Excesses of sodium and chloride are more apt to be **chronic**, that is, smaller excesses are ingested over a longer period of time.

acute—having a sudden onset and a short course

chronic—persisting over a long period of time

essential hypertension—unexplained high blood pressure

Many scientists believe that chronic excess consumption of sodium may be related to the development of **essential hypertension**, or unexplained high blood pressure, which is a major risk factor for cardiovascular disease and stroke (Figure 12.6). Almost 58 million people in the United States have hypertension, including 39 million who are under the age of 65. The incidence of hypertension increases with age and is more prevalent in blacks (38%) than in whites (29%) (Surgeon General, 1988).

The Surgeon General's 1988 *Report on Nutrition and Health* notes: While some people maintain normal blood pressure levels over a wide range of sodium intake, others appear to be 'salt sensitive' and display increased blood pressure in response to high sodium intakes. Because there is no quick, practical way to identify people who are sensitive to salt, and because no one would be harmed by moderate sodium restriction, many experts recommend moderate sodium restriction for everyone.

Thinking for Yourself, on page 396, will help you consider the challenges of trying to restrict salt in your diet.

Many patients with high blood pressure use medications such as diuretics (which increase urinary sodium losses) to help control hypertension. A number of investigators have noted that the use of medication to treat individuals with mild hypertension is associated with increased risk of heart disease (Farnett et al., 1991). Physicians have found that by restricting their sodium intakes, hypertensive patients can often control their blood pressure with smaller doses of medication (Weinberger et al., 1988). However, because some types of diuretics also cause loss of potassium, patients need to be deliberate about replacing it.

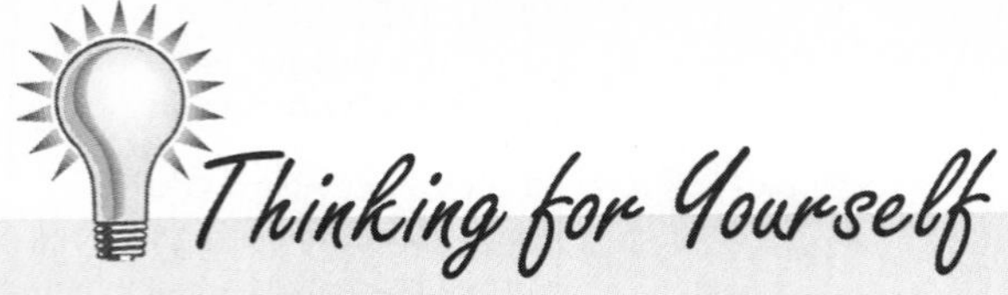

Salt: Is It a Problem?

The Situation

Alan is 23 and in excellent health and participates actively in sports. Recently, he has noticed that many dietary guidelines recommend cutting down on fat and salt. It has been fairly easy for him to make changes to lower his fat intake, but cutting down on salt has been more difficult. Although he does not usually salt his food at the table, he eats in restaurants and uses a lot of convenience foods, which he has heard are high in salt. He wonders whether he really needs to do anything about salt, because the major concern is its relationship to blood pressure, and his blood pressure was fine when it was checked about a year ago.

So Alan's question is, Should he cut down on salt?

Is Alan's Information Accurate and Relevant?

- Many dietary recommendations for the general public do suggest that people reduce their sodium intake.
- Epidemiologic and animal studies have found a connection between high sodium intake and elevated blood pressure.
- While it cannot be said that all restaurant foods are categorically high in salt, many probably are; data show that many fast-food entrees and convenience entrees have 500–1000 mg of sodium per serving, compared with a recommended limit of 2400 mg per day.

What Else Should Alan Consider?

Epidemiologic evidence that correlates salt intake with blood pressure deals with averages for large population groups. Individuals within groups vary. Some people's blood pressure is not much affected by their salt intake, no matter how much they consume; others are noticeably *salt sensitive,* although the degree to which salt affects their blood pressure varies from person to person.

Genetics plays a big role. Within some families, most of the adult members are affected by high blood pressure. Among African-Americans in the United States, the incidence of hypertension is much higher than in the general population. Furthermore, many other factors have been shown to affect blood pressure, such as levels of intake of some other minerals, body weight (Chapter 9), alcohol intake (Chapter 17), and stress.

Alan is African-American. His mother and father both have high blood pressure, and his 30-year-old brother was diagnosed with it recently. Alan's eating habits are an outgrowth of his lifestyle. He is single, has a desk job, and wants to spend most of his spare time on sports. He never learned to do more than "survival cooking"—mostly mak-

You should not assume that sodium is the only dietary factor that affects blood pressure. Increasingly, scientists are recognizing that ingesting high levels of chloride, especially with sodium as the compound sodium chloride (NaCl, or table salt), can elevate blood pressure (Kaup et al., 1991). Further, the effects of sodium chloride on the cardiovascular system may not all be due to hypertension. At least one group of researchers has shown that ingesting excess sodium chloride induced strokes in animals without elevating blood pressure (Tobian and Hanlon, 1990). Ingesting additional potassium and calcium, losing weight to alleviate obesity, and reducing alcohol intake have all been shown to reduce the incidence of hypertension in sensitive groups of people (Surgeon General, 1988).

Requirements and Recommendations The RDA Subcommittee did not establish recommended intakes for sodium, potassium, and chloride. However, it estimated that the average adult who does not sweat actively has a minimum requirement of 500 mg of sodium, 2000 mg of potassium and 750 mg of chloride per day. To discourage excess intakes of sodium and chloride, the RDA Subcommittee endorsed a previous recommendation (National Research Council, 1989) to limit intake of sodium chloride to 6 grams per day or less, which corresponds to 2400 mg of sodium and 3600 mg of chloride.

ing sandwiches or microwaving frozen dinners. He likes the taste of fast foods.

Gradually, Alan notices some ways to cut down on salt. He hears a person ahead of him at a fast-food restaurant order a hamburger without salt. Most fast-food restaurants, he learns, salt hamburgers as they cook them, and many places are willing to omit the salt on request—but they can't do anything about the salt in preseasoned items, such as breaded fish and chicken. On a quick trip to the grocery store, he sees a new product promotion for a brand of frozen dinners that has only about half the amount of sodium as those he had been eating. Then, when he is at a friend's place one night and is helping prepare dinner, he realizes that it is fairly easy to broil meat and cook frozen vegetables in the microwave.

Now What Do You Think?

How important is it for Alan to be concerned about his sodium intake? Does his reliance on restaurant and convenience food make it feasible to reduce his sodium intake, even if he wants to? If you were Alan, which of the following alternatives would you consider?

- Option 1 You make no change in salt intake, recognizing that even though you are *statistically* at risk of developing hypertension, there is no sure way of knowing whether you will get it. Further, there is no guarantee that cutting down on salt would prevent hypertension anyway.
- Option 2 You make no change in salt intake, recognizing your risk but believing that you are already doing enough of the right things—such as exercising regularly and reducing your intake of fat—both of which help keep your weight under control and thereby reduce risk of hypertension.
- Option 3 You reduce your salt intake when it is convenient, but are not slavish about it. This means buying the lower-salt frozen dinners at least some of the time, not adding salt to foods automatically before tasting them, and limiting intake of very salty foods, such as pickles and cured meats.
- Option 4 You eat only at restaurants that are willing to fix foods on request with little or no salt.
- Option 5 You learn to cook for yourself so you can limit the salt. At first, this will mean learning to broil meat, fish, and chicken; make salads; and microwave vegetables.
- Option 6 You ask your doctor or a dietitian for advice.

Do you see other options or combinations of options that are workable? What do you think would be the best choice for Alan? What is your own situation, and what makes most sense for you?

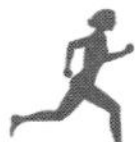

What about the electrolyte requirements of people, such as athletes, who sweat profusely? Sodium and chloride are the two primary electrolytes lost in sweat. (Potassium is lost to a much lesser degree.) But sodium and chloride are only about one-third as concentrated in sweat as in body fluids. Therefore, when you perspire, you lose relatively more water than electrolytes, and sodium and chloride become more concentrated within your body fluids. For this reason, it's important to restore water losses, but generally it's unnecessary to worry about sodium and chloride repletion. Rehydration was discussed in more detail in Chapter 4.

The use of salt tablets is not recommended, because they can make the overall situation worse. Concentrated salt in the gastrointestinal (GI) tract results in water initially moving *from* surrounding tissues into the lumen, aggravating dehydration. The key is that water must be restored first, and salt restored later if necessary. Salt tablets also occasionally resist being dissolved and stick to the lining of the stomach, where they can cause irritation. ●

Typical Intakes and Sources Foods produced by nature contain only modest amounts of sodium, with animal products having more than plant foods. Processing often adds sodium to foods. Pickles, salty snack foods, processed cheeses, and smoked meats and sausages often contain several

TABLE 12.5 Sodium and Potassium in Some Foods

Estimated minimum requirements of healthy adults are 500 mg sodium and 2000 mg potassium daily.

Food	Household Measure	Milligrams of Sodium (0 500 1000 1500)	Milligrams of Potassium (0 500 1000 1500)
Bread, cereal, rice, and pasta			
Biscuit, homemade	1 medium		
Bread, whole grain	1 slice		
Bread, enriched	1 slice		
Macaroni, cooked without salt	½ cup	tr	
Vegetables			
Beans, green, cooked without salt	½ cup		
Beans, green, canned with salt	½ cup		
Cucumber, chopped	½ cup		
Dill pickle	1 medium		
Potato, baked	1 average		
Potato chips	1 ounce (14 chips)		
Fruits			
Apple	1 medium		
Banana	1 medium		
Orange juice	½ cup		
Peach, fresh	1 medium		
Peaches, canned, heavy syrup	½ cup		

hundred milligrams of sodium per serving. Experts believe that at least one-third of the sodium that you ingest was added during processing (Surgeon General, 1988). Much of this sodium is added in the form of sodium chloride—ordinary table salt. By consulting Table 12.5, you can compare the sodium contents of processed and unprocessed foods. You can assume that the chloride contents of foods are generally proportional to their sodium contents.

Experts estimate that another one-third of the sodium you consume comes from the salt you add "to taste," but this amount varies a great deal from person to person. Nutritionists have learned that information about this added salt cannot be obtained from diet recalls or records, because people cannot accurately remember how much salt they added. However, scientists can measure sodium and chloride excretion in urine. Healthy adults excrete more than 90% of ingested sodium and chloride. Using this methodology, experts have estimated that men in Western cultures consume approximately 11 grams of salt daily. Because salt is 40% sodium and 60% chloride, that means that men might consume more than 4 grams of sodium and 6 grams of chloride daily (Sanchez-Castillo et al., 1987).

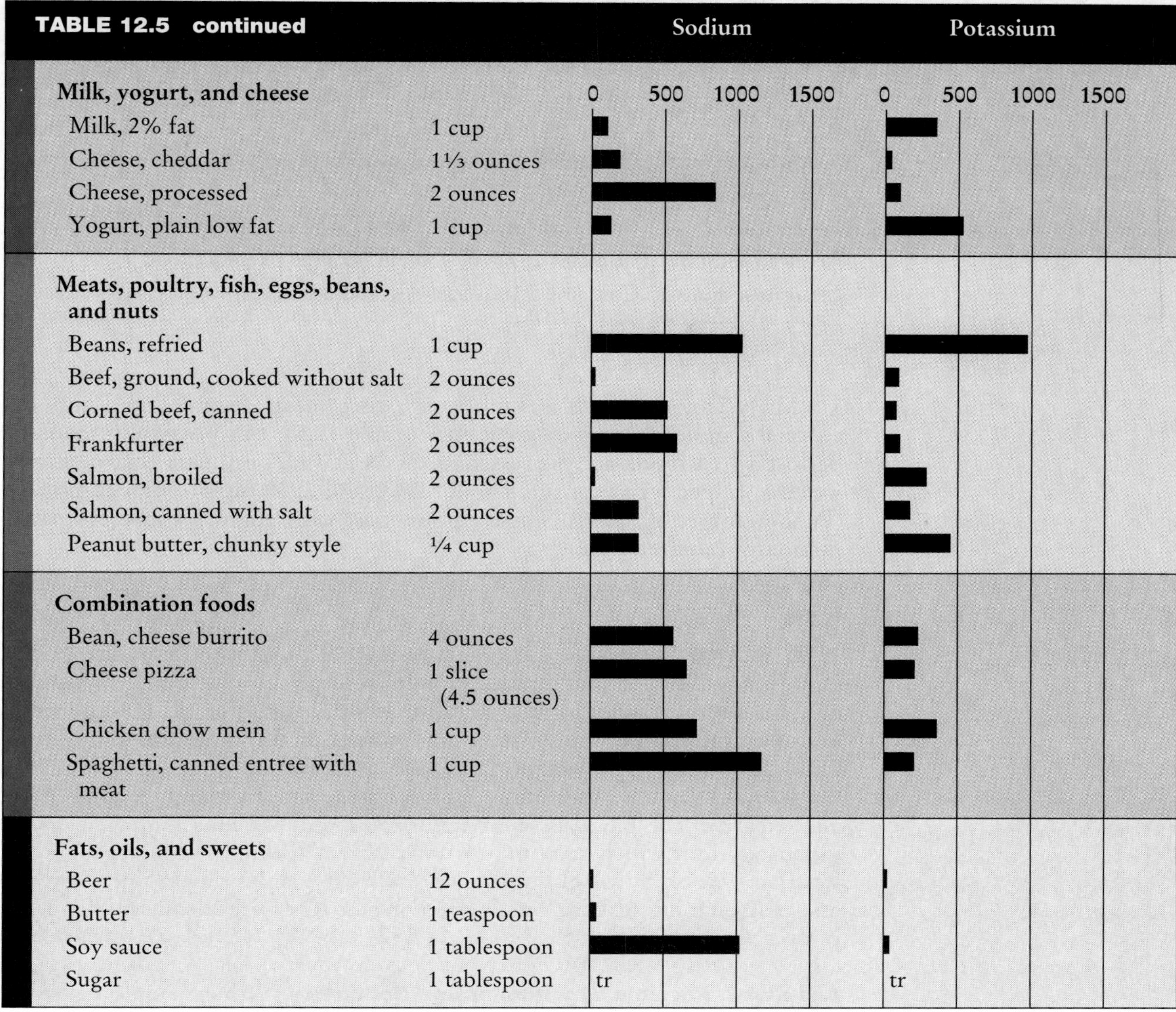

TABLE 12.5 continued		Sodium (0 500 1000 1500)	Potassium (0 500 1000 1500)
Milk, yogurt, and cheese			
Milk, 2% fat	1 cup		
Cheese, cheddar	1⅓ ounces		
Cheese, processed	2 ounces		
Yogurt, plain low fat	1 cup		
Meats, poultry, fish, eggs, beans, and nuts			
Beans, refried	1 cup		
Beef, ground, cooked without salt	2 ounces		
Corned beef, canned	2 ounces		
Frankfurter	2 ounces		
Salmon, broiled	2 ounces		
Salmon, canned with salt	2 ounces		
Peanut butter, chunky style	¼ cup		
Combination foods			
Bean, cheese burrito	4 ounces		
Cheese pizza	1 slice (4.5 ounces)		
Chicken chow mein	1 cup		
Spaghetti, canned entree with meat	1 cup		
Fats, oils, and sweets			
Beer	12 ounces		
Butter	1 teaspoon		
Soy sauce	1 tablespoon		
Sugar	1 tablespoon	tr	tr

You can reduce your sodium intake considerably by restricting the amount of salt you add to food and reducing your intake of certain processed salts. Food labels can help you select foods with reduced sodium levels (Table 12.6). To avoid confusing claims, the Food and Drug Administration (FDA) has approved the use of five terms that the food industry can use to identify foods with reduced amounts of sodium.

Water naturally contains some sodium. Home water softeners add more sodium to water; the softening process substitutes sodium for the calcium and magnesium that made the water hard. Nonetheless, water is usually only a minor source of sodium, and you probably will ingest less than 100 mg of sodium daily from water (assuming whatever water you use for drinking and food preparation contains approximately 20 mg of sodium per quart) (Safe Drinking Water Committee, 1980).

Foods and water are not the only sources of sodium. Many medications, including some over-the-counter drugs, contain more than 200 mg of sodium per dose.

TABLE 12.6 Label Language about Sodium

By February 1994, these terms will have the following meanings on U.S. food product labels:

Sodium-free	Contains less than 5 mg of sodium per serving
Very low-sodium	Contains less than 35 mg of sodium per serving
Low sodium	Contains less than 140 mg of sodium per serving
Reduced sodium	Contains 25% less sodium than the reference food
Light in sodium	Contains at least 50% less sodium than the reference product

Many fruits, vegetables, milk and yogurt, meats, legumes, and nuts are especially good sources of potassium (Table 12.5). But potassium tends to be lost when foods are processed. Experts at FDA estimate that men and women, respectively, consume about 2000 and 2900 mg of potassium daily (Pennington et al., 1989). These amounts are only slightly above estimated minimum requirements.

Iron

Now that you've gained an understanding of why your body needs the major minerals and what amounts you should get in your diet, let's turn to a discussion of trace minerals. Recall that although some of these minerals are essential to your body, they are present in tiny amounts—less than 0.01% of your body's weight. Let's look at iron first.

Iron, like many other minerals, is a component of many enzymes. It is also a part of the blood protein hemoglobin and the muscle protein myoglobin, both of which can bind (carry) oxygen. Although iron accounts for less than 1% of the weight of these proteins, it enables them to perform the essential ongoing tasks of moving oxygen to and carbon dioxide from all body cells.

Anemia: A Possible Symptom of Iron Deficiency When people consume too little iron to meet their needs, they become anemic. Iron deficiency is not the only cause of anemia, however.

hematocrit—concentration of red blood cells in blood

Anemia is a condition in which a person's blood hemoglobin level, or **hematocrit,** is lower than normal. When this condition occurs, body cells receive less oxygen, and carbon dioxide wastes are removed less efficiently. These compromised functions cause the person to feel tired or run down.

Anemia can result from a number of causes, such as loss of blood due to surgery, accidents, or disease, including duodenal or stomach ulcers or cancers, genetic conditions, and various vitamin or mineral deficiencies. The most common cause of anemia is iron deficiency. This type of anemia, a microcytic anemia, results in smaller red blood cells that contain less hemoglobin than usual (Figure 12.7).

About 10% of the nonpregnant women (11–44 years of age) in the United States are anemic (Life Science Research Office, 1991). (As we'll discuss in Chapter 15, the incidence of low hematocrits is much higher in pregnant than nonpregnant women.) Although the incidence of anemia among children in the United States used to be higher, it has declined steadily during the last 20 years, and only 2.9% of children ages 6 months to 5 years were anemic in 1985 (Dallman and Yip, 1989). In the United States, people whose family incomes are below the poverty level are more apt to have low

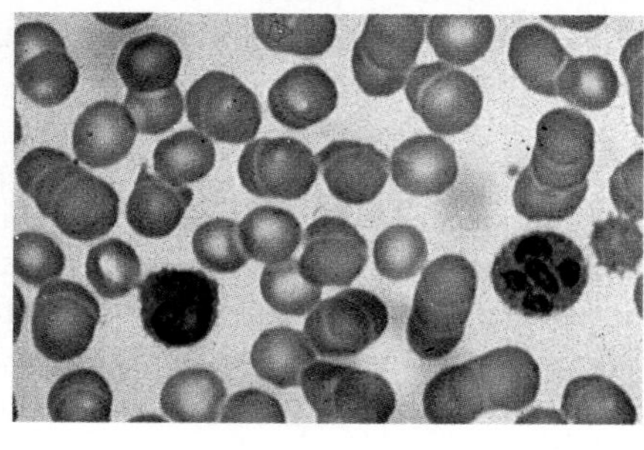

a

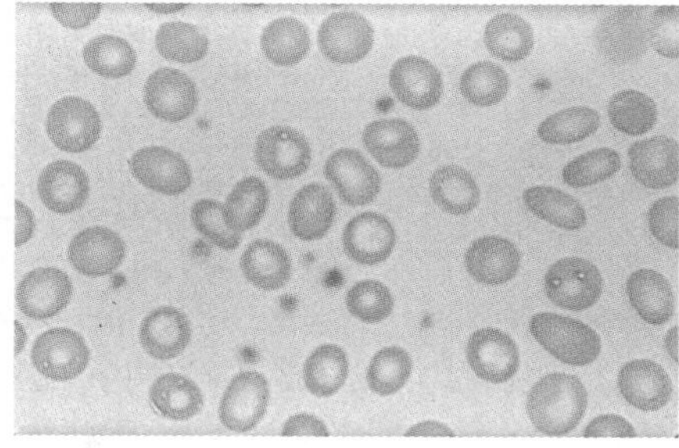

b

FIGURE 12.7
Iron deficiency produces a microcytic anemia.

Panel (a) shows normal red blood cells; panel (b) shows the small red blood cells with less hemoglobin than normal that characterize iron deficiency anemia. (In a, the dark-stained cells with nuclei are white blood cells.)

hemoglobin levels than members of more affluent families. For example, in one study of more than 300 Alaskan native children whose families lived below the poverty level, 23% were anemic (Thiele et al., 1988).

The decreased incidence of anemia in the United States during the last 40 years reflects a number of factors, including iron supplementation of formulas and cereals. Major public health efforts, such as the Supplemental Food Program for Women, Infants, and Children have also been important (Chapter 15).

Within the last decade, a number of physicians have noted anemia among women athletes (Duester et al., 1986). Although the anemia may be related to decreased iron absorption or increased iron losses in some women, many of the athletes reported low intakes of iron.

Other Symptoms of Iron Deficiency People with iron deficiency also have depressed levels of iron-containing enzymes. This results in decreased work efficiency and decreased ability to maintain body temperature (Beard and Smith, 1992).

Iron deficiency is also associated with depression of immune function (Dallman, 1987). Iron repletion must be carried out carefully in severely malnourished children, because bacteria also need iron for growth. If too much iron is given too soon, it may cause bacteria in the children's bodies to proliferate faster than their immune functions recover, causing uncontrolled infections if antibiotics are not available. This is a concern particularly in the developing countries.

Iron Toxicity Although nutritionists are more concerned about iron *deficiency*, iron *toxicity* can also occur. Every year, about a dozen young children die from acute iron toxicity caused from having taken a large number of their mothers' iron supplements.

Chronic iron toxicity can occur in people with a genetic predisposition—especially men, because they do not experience losses of iron in blood during menstruation and childbirth. Even when they consume fairly typical levels of iron, these men can experience iron overload, which can cause liver damage and, sometimes, heart failure. Excess use of alcohol exacerbates the problem in susceptible individuals. Recently, researchers reported that men with large amounts of stored iron were more prone to heart attacks (Salonen et al., 1992).

Recommended and Typical Intakes Iron is an exception to the general rule that RDA values are higher for adult males than for adult females.

Males, on the average, have larger bodies and more lean body mass, so they require more nutrients. However, the adult male RDA for iron is 10 mg, and that for females is 15 mg, because women in their reproductive years lose iron during menstruation.

The RDA for iron is 12 mg for adolescent males and 15 mg for adolescent females. These high iron recommendations reflect physiologic changes that occur during the teen years. For males, the extra iron is used primarily to form additional lean body mass; for females, it is used both for additional lean body mass and to replace iron lost in menstruation.

The recommended intake of iron during pregnancy is 30 mg daily because of the large amount of iron needed by growing fetal, placental, and maternal tissues. It is impossible to obtain this level through diet alone, and the 1989 RDA Subcommittee recommended daily supplemental iron for pregnant women.

In the general population, iron intakes do not parallel recommendations. The average adult male under 65 years in United States Department of Agriculture (USDA) surveys consumed more than 15 mg daily (Science and Education Administration, 1980), but the average female consumed 11 mg daily (Human Nutrition Information Service, 1985). That means most men had adequate intakes of iron, but the average woman consumed only 74% of the RDA.

Sources Foods contain very uneven quantities of iron (Table 12.7). Meat, fish, and poultry are superior sources because the heme iron and unidentified meat factor they contain make the iron in those foods very bioavailable. Eggs, legumes, nuts, whole grains, enriched cereal products, and leafy vegetables can also contribute significant amounts of iron to the diet.

Several foods are questionable sources of iron. For example, certain dried fruits, such as raisins and apricots, contain significant amounts of iron only if eaten in large amounts. (The drying process doesn't add iron to these foods; it just concentrates the iron and all other substances that were in the fresh product by removing most of the water.)

Before you become too concerned about the *quantity* of your iron intake, consider the *quality* (that is, the bioavailability) of your intake. A recent study of college-age women emphasizes the importance of bioavailability (Davis et al., 1992). Small increases (<1 mg/day) in heme iron intake were consistently associated with higher hematocrits. In contrast, consuming more (10–20 mg) nonheme iron did not consistently elevate hematocrits.

You Tell Me

Several laboratories have demonstrated that iron-deficient women tend to have slightly lower body temperatures than nonanemic women. Their plasma levels of thyroid hormones are often lower, too.

Are you ever cold for no apparent reason when everyone else is comfortable? Perhaps in a few years scientists will be able to offer better advice to women who are always "chilly." Until then, by what means can you determine whether your iron intake is adequate?

Iodine

Iodine makes its principal contribution to human functions as a component of thyroid hormones, primarily T3 and thyroxin (T4). (T3 has three iodines

TABLE 12.7 Iron in Some Foods

The RDA for iron for women is 15 mg/day; for men, 10 mg/day.

Food	Household Measure	Milligrams of Iron (0, 2, 4, 6, 8, 10)
Bread, cereal, rice, and pasta		
Bread, whole-grain	1 slice	
Bread, white enriched	1 slice	
Cereal, bran flakes	1 ounce	
Cereal, wheat flakes, iron-fortified	1 ounce	
Cereal, shredded wheat	1 ounce	
Spaghetti, enriched	½ cup	
Vegetables		
Beans, green snap, cooked	½ cup	
Broccoli, chopped, cooked	½ cup	
Lettuce, iceberg	1 cup	
Peas, green, cooked	½ cup	
Potatoes, mashed with milk	½ cup	
Spinach, chopped, cooked	½ cup	
Fruits		
Apricots, raw	3 medium	
Apricots, dried	6 large halves	
Orange juice, frozen, rehydrated	½ cup	
Milk, yogurt, and cheese		
Milk, 2% fat	1 cup	
Cheese, cheddar	1⅓ ounces	
Meats, poultry, fish, eggs, beans, and nuts		
Almonds, chopped	½ cup	
Beans, refried	1 cup	
Beef, ground, fried	2 ounces	
Chicken breast roll, cooked	2 ounces	
Eggs, hard-boiled	2	
Liver, beef, cooked	2 ounces	
Peanut butter, chunky style	¼ cup	
Shrimp, canned	2 ounces	
Combination foods		
Cheeze pizza	1 slice (4.5 ounces)	
Pork & beans with tomato sauce	1 cup	
Taco	1 item	
Fats, oils, and sweets		
Beer	12 ounces	
Butter, margarine	1 teaspoon	tr
Carbonated beverage, cola type	12 ounces	
Molasses, light	1 tablespoon	
Sugar, white	1 tablespoon	tr

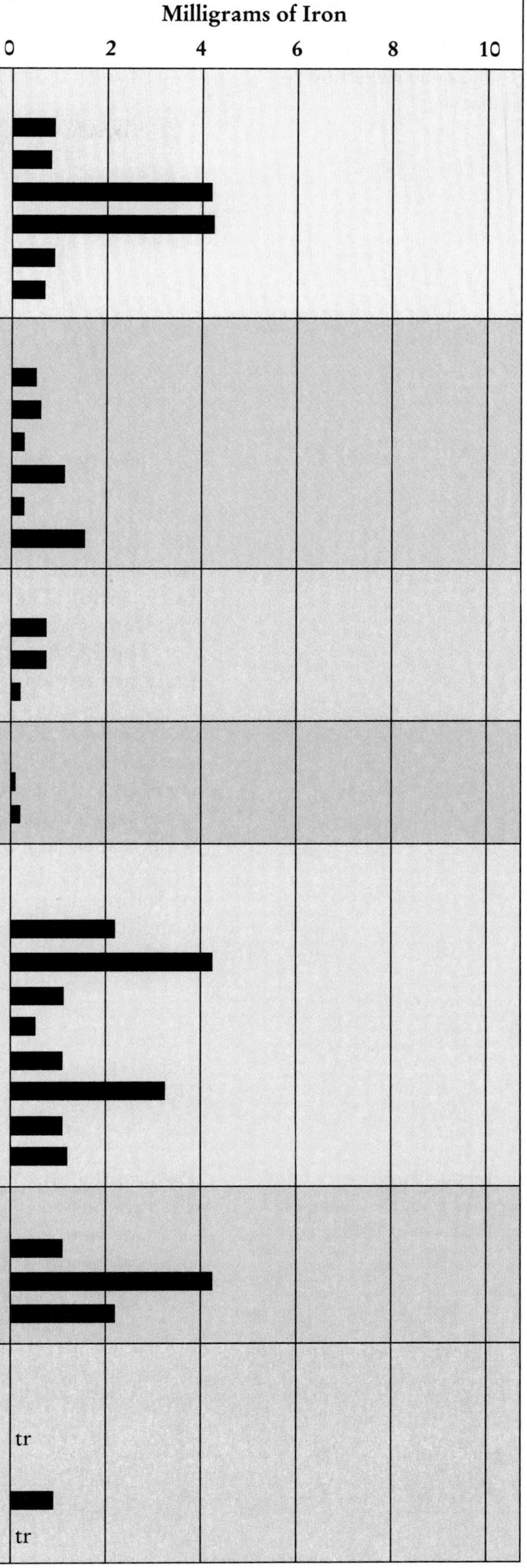

FIGURE 12.8
Goiter.

Severe, long-term iodine deficiency results in enlargement of the thyroid gland, as you see in this woman.

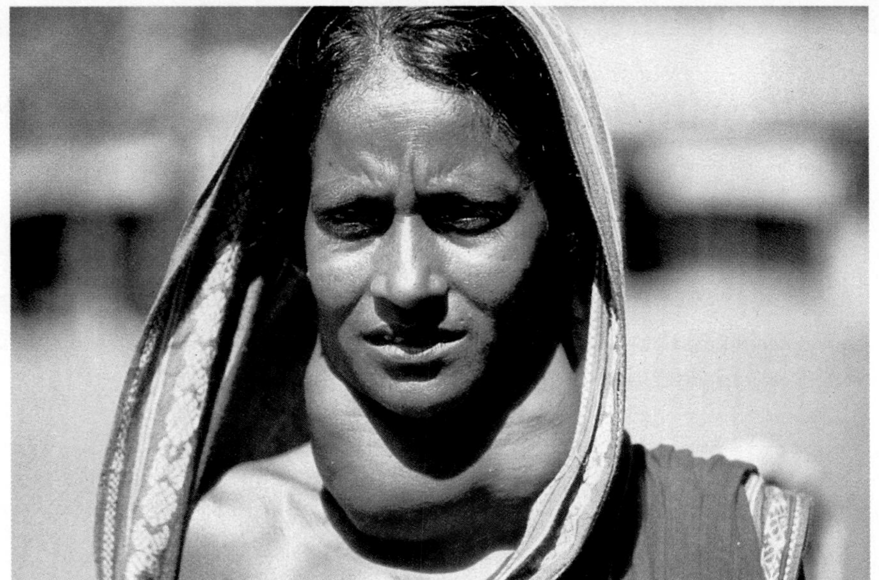

attached; thyroxin has four.) These hormones stimulate oxygen consumption and basal metabolic rates in tissues by a variety of mechanisms (Stanbury, 1988). They also affect cell development and growth in fetuses and children.

The RDA for adults for iodine is only 150 μg (0.15 mg) daily. This is truly a trace amount.

Sources Traditionally, the best dietary sources of iodine were ocean fish, other seafoods, and crops grown on land near the ocean. To supplement the diets of Americans who did not live near salt water, iodine was added to table salt. This made iodized salt the major source of iodine for many Americans, especially those living in the Midwest.

In the 1970s, milk and grain products became the major dietary sources of iodine. Dairy cows were being fed more iodine, and iodine-containing dough conditioners and other additives were used in commercially baked products.

Because of these new sources of iodine, during the 1970s adult Americans may have consumed levels of iodine more than five times the 150 μg suggested in the RDAs. The FDA has successfully encouraged the food industry to reduce the use of iodine-containing compounds in recent years; FDA officials recently estimated a young man's typical intake to be 470 μg (313% of the RDA) for iodine (Pennington et al., 1989).

goiter—enlargement of the thyroid gland, resulting primarily from iodine deficiency

Deficiency and Toxicity Enlargement of the thyroid gland, or **goiter**, is the most obvious symptom of iodine deficiency (Figure 12.8). When iodine is inadequate in the diet, the thyroid gland does not have enough of this mineral to produce a normal amount of thyroid hormones. In an attempt to produce more of them, the thyroid gland enlarges. However, even with a larger mass of thyroid tissue, the gland may be unable to produce enough additional thyroid hormones.

In the early part of the twentieth century, goiters were very common in inland areas in the United States, especially in the Midwest. After iodized salt was accepted as a public health measure designed to increase iodine to

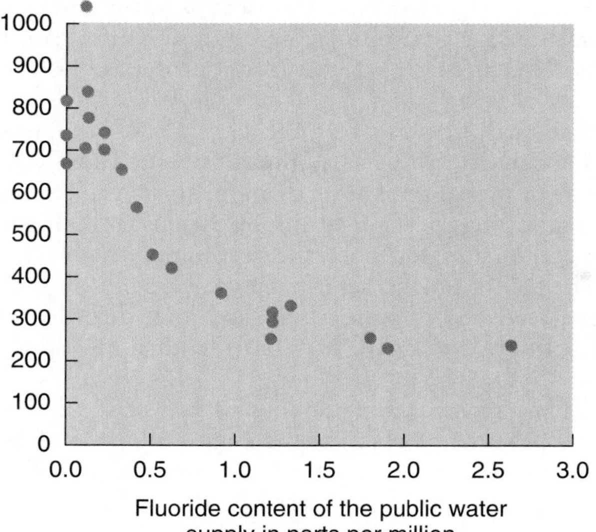

FIGURE 12.9
The effect of fluoride on dental health.

Here, you see the beneficial effect of adequate levels of fluoride intake. Children who did not ingest fluoride had two to three times more decayed, missing, and filled teeth than those who received at least 1 part per million of fluoride in their water supply.

Source: Sweeney and Shaw, 1988.

recommended levels, the incidence of goiters dropped markedly. However, goiters are still **endemic** in inland areas of South America, Africa, and Asia.

endemic—very common in a population

Dietary factors and drugs that prevent the normal incorporation of iodine into thyroxin can also promote the development of goiters. This effect is accentuated in people who consume low or marginal levels of iodine.

If a pregnant woman takes in too little iodine, her child may be born with **cretinism**, an irreversible condition characterized by both mental and physical growth retardation.

cretinism—irreversible condition involving both mental and physical growth retardation; can occur in children of mothers who were severely iodine-deficient during pregnancy

People who chronically ingest very high amounts of iodine may also develop goiter. This condition occurs among residents of certain areas of Japan who consume large amounts of iodine-rich seaweed (Stanbury, 1988).

Fluoride

Fluoride (the ionized form of fluorine used by your body) functions in your teeth and bones by becoming part of the hydroxyapatite crystals and making them larger and less soluble. A certain minimal level of fluoride in the diet, therefore, increases resistance to dental caries.

For adults, the estimated safe and adequate intake range for fluoride is 1.5–4 mg daily. The major source of fluoride in most people's diets is water and (to a lesser extent) tea and the soft edible bones of fish. Topical application of fluoride by dentists and fluoride-containing toothpastes and powders are other sources of fluoride.

Fluoride is naturally present in the water supplies of some areas, but in regions where less than 0.7 parts per million of fluoride occurs naturally in water, public health agencies encourage that it be added to the level of 1 part per million. This level is equivalent to 1 ounce of fluoride in over 7750 gallons of water.

This small concentration of fluoride is associated with a reduced rate of dental caries (Sweeney and Shaw, 1988). Figure 12.9 shows the dramatic effect of adequate fluoride on the rates of decayed, missing, and filled teeth in children. Although fluoridation of water has had a very positive public health effect, the addition of fluoride to water remains controversial in some areas (Jones et al., 1989). However, concerns about municipal water fluoridation programs causing environmental pollution (Osterman, 1990) or being related to a higher incidence of cancer (Mahoney et al., 1991) have not been substantiated.

The fact that small amounts of fluoride can lower the incidence of dental caries does not mean that *excess* fluoride is beneficial. People who habitually drink water that contains four or more times the recommended level may develop slight *mottling* (spotty discoloration) of their teeth. When the water supply contains eight times the recommended level, *fluorosis* may develop; this is a condition characterized by severe mottling of the teeth and eventual degenerative and crippling bone and joint disorders. Evidently, the safety range for fluoride is small, and fluoride must be added to water supplies carefully.

During the last few years, a number of physicians have tried to treat osteoporosis in postmenopausal women with fluoride (Kleerekoper and Balena, 1991). Fluoride was associated with increased mineral density of some bones but, paradoxically, increased bone fragility; furthermore, many patients experienced side effects, such as GI distress and rheumatic (bone and joint) complications. Therefore, the use of fluoride to treat osteoporosis is not currently recommended.

Zinc

Zinc is a component of over 70 of your body's enzyme systems that have a wide variety of functions. It is also a structural component of proteins in your body that allow steroids, including hormones, to interact with DNA in genes (Luisi et al., 1991). Zinc is also necessary for adequate immune functions.

Zinc Deficiency and Excess Zinc deficiency was first discovered in adults in villages in Iran and Egypt about 30 years ago. Investigators found adults who were unusually short and sexually immature—the abnormalities that were corrected by zinc supplementation. It is not surprising, in retrospect, that the deficiency occurred: the local staple diet was low in zinc; the bioavailability of the small amount of zinc present was poor; and a high incidence of infections and gut infestations resulted in high excretion of zinc.

Zinc deficiency is not limited to the Middle East. The symptoms of poor growth in children, poor wound healing in adults, scaly dermatitis, and impaired resistance to infections have also been seen in other parts of the world, including patients in North America. Some experts are particularly concerned about the zinc status of elderly people (Greger, 1989b), low-birth-weight infants, and infants with genetic defects (Hambidge et al., 1986). Figure 12.10 shows an infant with severe skin symptoms from zinc deficiency.

You Tell Me

Severe zinc deficiency prevents sexual maturation in adolescents and impairs the reproductive capacity of adults. Serious zinc deficiency is occasionally seen in the United States, but it's more common in the developing countries.

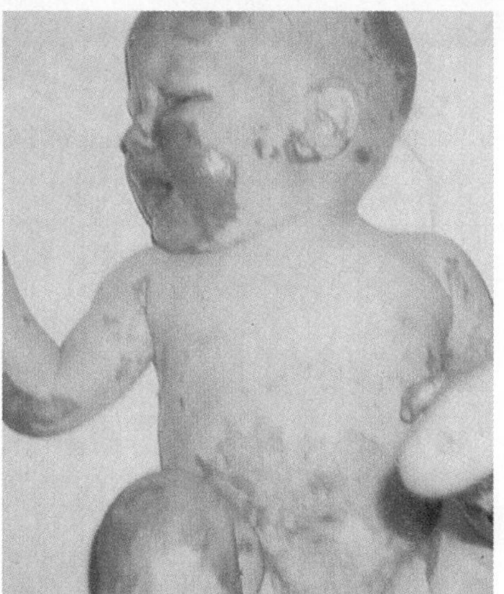

FIGURE 12.10
Zinc deficiency.

The skin of this infant shows the scaly dermatitis characteristic of severe zinc deficiency.
Source: Hambidge et al., 1978.

Zinc supplements have sometimes been marketed in the United States as a way to improve sexual performance. Do you think they would help well-nourished people?

At the other end of the spectrum, zinc toxicity can occur either as an acute or a chronic problem. Acute zinc toxicity with nausea and vomiting has been reported in some people who drank acidic beverages (such as lemonade) stored in galvanized (zinc-coated) containers. More frequently, chronic zinc toxicity has been reported among people who consumed high levels of zinc in supplements. The chronic ingestion of excess zinc depresses copper absorption and eventually *impairs* immune function and induces anemia (Fosmire, 1989).

Recommended Intakes and Sources The adult RDA for zinc is 15 mg for men and 12 mg for women. The average North American consumes fewer than 12 mg of zinc daily (Hambidge et al., 1986). Vegetarians, especially those who do not eat legumes frequently, and dieters with low energy intakes are likely to have low intakes of zinc.

As Table 12.8 shows, the best dietary sources of zinc are seafood, red meats, nuts, and legumes. Other meat products, milk, and whole-grain products also contribute significant amounts to the diet. Of course, the bioavailability of zinc from some of these products—especially whole grains, legumes, and nuts—is lessened by the fiber and phytate they contain.

Selenium

Selenium functions as a cofactor of an important enzyme called *glutathione peroxidase* that helps prevent **oxidative stress or damage** to cell structures. It is probably also a cofactor for an enzyme necessary for thyroid function (Nutrition Reviews, 1991b). A number of animal and epidemiologic studies have shown that adequate selenium has a protective effect against certain

oxidative stress or damage—process by which oxygen reacting with membranes and cell structures results in reduced function or structural damage

TABLE 12.8 Zinc in Some Foods

The RDA for zinc for men is 15 mg/day; for women, 12 mg/day.

Food	Household Measure	Milligrams of Zinc (0, 5, 10, 15)
Bread, cereal, rice, and pasta		
Bread, white	1 slice	
Bread, whole-grain	1 slice	
Macaroni	½ cup	
Vegetables		
Corn, frozen, cooked	½ cup	
Peas, frozen, cooked	½ cup	
Spinach, frozen, cooked	½ cup	
Fruits		
Apple	1 medium	tr
Banana	1 medium	
Milk, yogurt, and cheese		
Milk, 2% fat	1 cup	
Meats, poultry, fish, eggs, beans, and nuts		
Beef, ground, cooked	2 ounces	
Chicken, dark meat—thigh	2 ounces	
Chicken, light meat, cooked	2 ounces	
Eggs, hard boiled	2	
Beans, refried	1 cup	
Oysters, canned	2 ounces	51
Peanut butter, chunky style	¼ cup	
Shrimp, canned	2 ounces	
Fish, perch	2 ounces	
Combination foods		
Cheeseburger, McDonald's	4 ounces	
Cheese pizza	1 slice (4.5 ounces)	
Pork and beans in tomato sauce	1 cup	
Taco	1 item	
Fats, oils, and sweets		
Butter, margarine	1 teaspoon	tr
Gum drops, jelly beans	1 ounce	

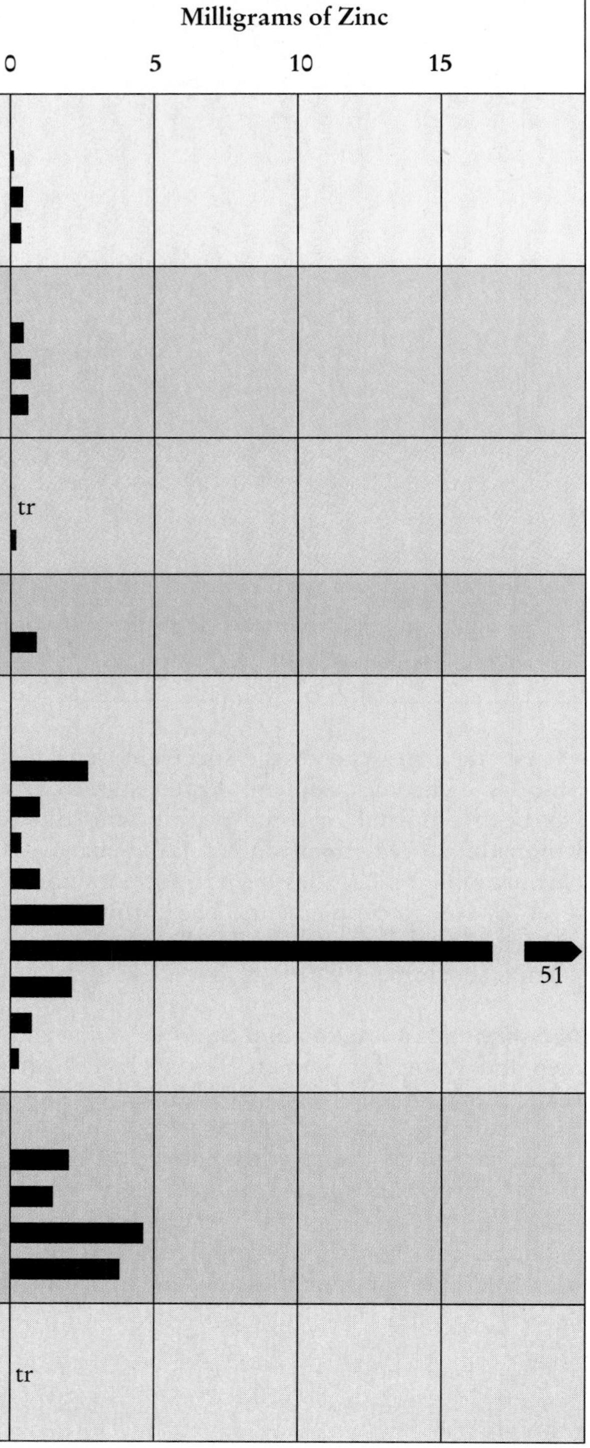

cancers (Surgeon General, 1988), but the mechanism of this protective effect is not known. In some cases, symptoms of selenium deficiency can be prevented by adequate vitamin E intakes.

Selenium Deficiency and Excess The selenium content of grains varies with the selenium content of the soil on which they are grown. Livestock that graze in regions with very low or high soil selenium levels suffer selenium deficiency and excess, respectively. But human diets, especially in the United States, are generally based on foodstuffs grown in a variety of areas; therefore, the overall selenium content of the diet is not much affected by the selenium content of the soils on which individual foods were grown.

There is one important exception. In a large area of western China, selenium intake is very low. There, a potentially fatal condition called *Keshan disease*, which is characterized by heart damage, is endemic in children and young women. In large studies in the 1970s, selenium supplements were given to thousands of children. The incidence of Keshan disease dropped to about 5% of the rate in controls. Despite this impressive response to raising selenium levels, the cause of Keshan disease is probably more complex than simple selenium deficiency. This belief is based on a number of observations; for one, Keshan disease is not found in other locations with low selenium levels in foods (Levander, 1991).

Although selenium is an essential element, it can also be very toxic. Selenium toxicity has also been found in some areas in China in which very high levels of selenium were found in local crops. In California, wildlife at the reservoir of a nature preserve suffered malformations due to very high levels of selenium in irrigation waters that drained into the reservoir. Toxicity has also occurred among people in the United States and Europe who consumed excess amounts of selenium supplements (Levander, 1991). Hair and nail loss were the most common symptoms that occurred with chronic ingestion of more than 1 mg of selenium daily.

Recommended Intakes and Sources An RDA was set for selenium for the first time in 1989. For men, the recommended daily selenium intake is 70 μg (.07 mg); for women, it is 55 μg (.055 mg). These recommendations are based on extensive studies worldwide. Experts at the FDA estimate that men and women in the United States typically consume 100 μg and 70 μg of selenium, respectively; therefore, American diets appear to be adequate in selenium (Pennington et al., 1989).

Selenium is obtained primarily from grains, seafood, and meats. As mentioned above, the selenium content of grains is quite variable, depending on the selenium content of the soil on which they are grown. The bioavailability of different forms of selenium that occur in foods also varies.

Other Trace Elements: Copper, Manganese, Cobalt, Chromium, Molybdenum, and Boron

Both copper and manganese function primarily as components of enzymes. Copper-containing enzymes are important in the synthesis of collagen, normal cardiovascular function, and normal immune function. Because copper influences iron metabolism, copper deficiency can result in anemia. Copper and manganese are cofactors of two forms of an enzyme, *superoxide dismutase,* that prevents oxidative damage in body tissues.

You Tell Me

Health-food stores now sell products labeled "stress vitamins." These are advertised as a means of reducing risk of heart disease and cancer by preventing oxidative stress in tissues. Some of the products sold contain carotenoids, vitamin E, selenium, and the enzyme superoxide dismutase.

Do you think that any of these products are needed by individuals consuming a well-balanced diet? And what will probably occur to an enzyme during the digestion process?

Cobalt also is needed in the diet, but only insofar as it is a component of vitamin B-12. Other cobalt that may be present in the diet does not have any biologic function. Chromium aids in normal glucose metabolism, apparently by working with insulin. Molybdenum is best known as a component of three key enzymes.

Boron is essential for plants, but it has not been established as essential for animals. Some researchers have observed that ingestion of additional boron increased circulating estrogen levels and reduced urinary calcium losses in postmenopausal women (Nielsen, 1992). It is too early to draw conclusions from these limited data.

Estimated Safe and Adequate Intakes and Typical Intakes The most recent *RDA* gives safe and adequate daily dietary ranges for these trace elements. The recommended range of intake for copper is 1.5–3 mg daily. The typical daily copper intake of most adult North Americans is believed to be 0.8–1.2 mg (Pennington et al., 1989). Experts are concerned, but recognized symptoms of copper deficiency are rarely seen.

The recommended range of intake for manganese is 2–5 mg per day. Typical intakes of adults in the United States are believed to be within the lower part of this range, approximately 2–3 mg/day (Pennington et al., 1989).

Recommended intakes for adults for chromium are 50–200 μg daily. Those for molybdenum are 75–250 μg daily. Reliable data on typical intakes are not available. As yet, no recommendation for boron intake has been made.

Sources For several reasons, it's not possible to give reliable data for the copper, manganese, chromium, and molybdenum content of foods. First, the analyses for chromium, molybdenum, and boron are difficult to perform, and those that have been done have resulted in only a limited amount of usable information. Second, the amounts of trace minerals in many foods are extremely variable, depending on the minerals' concentration in the soil, in the water, and in the fertilizer involved in food production. The amounts of certain trace minerals in root vegetables can vary by severalfold (Allaway, 1986); the trace mineral content of seafood is also affected by environmental conditions. For these reasons, no single value can be regarded as representative of any of these minerals in a particular food.

Despite analytical problems and natural variation, these trace minerals are thought to be widely distributed in foods as they come from nature;

people who eat a wide variety of foods are likely to get what they need. Furthermore, because the foods available in any given part of North America have come from many different regions, the likelihood is great that at least some good sources of these minerals will be present.

Because refinement processes generally remove much of the trace mineral content of foods, you'll get more trace minerals from minimally processed items such as whole grains, and you'll get very little from such foods as white flour, sugars, and fats.

Nonetheless, it's a mistake to think that food processing always decreases the trace mineral content of foods. Trace elements are sometimes added intentionally and unintentionally during processing. You'll learn more about the effects of processing on minerals in Chapter 13.

Your Intake: Staying Near Recommended Levels

We've mentioned that different mineral deficiencies produce different results; for example, low iron intake can lead to a type of anemia; low iodine can result in goiter; and prolonged low calcium intake by children and young adults may result in a lower peak bone mass that increases the risk of osteoporosis. But is *your* mineral intake likely to be a problem?

Deficiencies

Generally speaking, deficiencies are more likely to occur if several precipitating factors are present at the same time. The following factors, usually in combination, are likely to cause mineral deficiencies:

1. The diet is limited in overall quantity, resulting in low intake of minerals and all other nutrients.
2. The diet is poorly selected for mineral content because of lack of knowledge, unavailability of certain foods, or poverty.
3. Bioavailability of minerals is low, for any of the many reasons discussed earlier in this chapter.
4. The individual cannot absorb, utilize, or maintain minerals normally because of inborn metabolic problems, disease conditions, or alcohol or other drug use.
5. Requirements for minerals are unusually high because of rapid growth or disease.

Given these factors, you can probably predict which groups of people will be most at risk of mineral deficiency. As one example, the total food intake of some elderly people is limited because of medical, social, or psychologic problems, resulting in low intakes of zinc. Elderly people are more apt to be at risk of marginal zinc deficiency if they selectively avoid meat, a good source of zinc, because they have trouble chewing it; if they suffer from a variety of conditions that cause zinc to be used inefficiently; and/or if they use a variety of medications that interfere with zinc utilization (Greger, 1989b). Keep in mind that being at risk does not *guarantee* that a deficiency will occur; it means only that it is statistically *more likely* to occur.

As with vitamin deficiencies, mild mineral deficiencies are not apt to produce distinct symptoms; rather, they may have certain common consequences, such as a decline in reproductive performance and compromised ability to deal with injury or infection.

You Tell Me

Vegans consume diets that often contain low levels of minerals such as zinc, and large amounts of such factors as phytate and fiber that reduce mineral absorption.

Which vegans would be most apt to have problems with consuming enough zinc to meet their requirements: adult men, pregnant women, or young children? Why?

Excesses

The old saying "If a little is good, more is better" is not true for any nutrient, including minerals. As you've learned in this chapter, it's definitely possible for you to ingest quantities that are too large. Finding the range between too little and too much is the key to good mineral nutrition.

Interference with Other Minerals We've already mentioned one way in which mineral excess may be damaging: a large dietary intake of one mineral, such as zinc, can depress the absorption of another mineral, such as copper. And if the intake of copper is already low, the excess of zinc, although not toxic itself, will interfere with copper status.

Such imbalances rarely occur when you get your minerals in food, but they can occur fairly easily if you supplement your diet with individual minerals. You should be very cautious about taking a mineral supplement to ensure your health; you may do more harm than good.

Toxicities As we mentioned earlier, there are two general types of toxicities: acute and chronic. Acute toxicities occur when very large doses of a mineral are consumed; the effects are rapid and severe. We've already mentioned examples, such as the toxicities that occur when picnickers store lemonade in galvanized (zinc-coated) containers or when a child consumes a bottle of her mother's iron supplements. Acute poisonings of this sort usually cause nausea, vomiting, and diarrhea; they are occasionally fatal.

Most cases of mineral toxicity occur more gradually and are due to chronic exposure to lower-level excesses of the mineral. You've already read about three examples—iodine, fluoride, and iron. Other minerals are also known for their toxicity; these include lead, cadmium, and mercury. Although many of the reported cases of such toxicities were due to industrial exposure, occasionally these minerals enter the food supply in sufficient quantities to be toxic. We'll discuss this topic in Chapter 14.

A number of factors can affect the development of toxicity. In general, children are more sensitive than adults to toxic doses of minerals, partially because of their smaller size. Also, there is considerable individual variation in sensitivity. Genetics also plays a role; as we mentioned earlier, some people have a genetic predisposition to accumulate iron to abnormally high levels over time.

The Consider This for this chapter gives you quick, practical advice on how to avoid deficiencies and toxicities of minerals.

Ways to Evaluate Your Mineral Intake

Because we've discussed the difficulties in setting nutritional requirements and determining contents of foods in regard to several minerals, you might

To improve mineral intake and status, instead of

This	. Consider this
Consuming large amounts of fats, oils, and sweets	**Consume additional foods from the basic Pyramid food groups and fewer from the "fats, oils, and sweets" group**
Eating refined, highly processed foods	**Consume whole grains and choose vegetables and meats that are not highly processed**
Taking supplements to get trace elements	**Eat a wide variety of foods**
Taking megadoses of minerals	**Consider nutrient interactions and your needs. If needed, improve diet or select a supplement that provides no more than 100% of the RDA**
If you're a vegan, having a limited intake of legumes and grains	**If you're a vegan, eat a variety of legumes and whole grains**
If you're a woman, putting off thinking about calcium and osteoporosis until you reach menopause	**No matter your gender, select calcium-rich foods and exercise regularly in teens and early 20's to maximize peak bone mass**

Remember: Gradual changes are more likely to last, and they give your body time to adjust.

wonder whether there is any reliable way to evaluate your mineral intake. The answer is yes: we do have enough information to estimate with some accuracy the adequacy of diets in regard to several minerals.

Methods You Have Already Used

You've been encouraged to use the Food Guide Pyramid (Act on Fact 2.1) to evaluate the quality of your diet quickly. Although the Pyramid is somewhat less useful for promoting adequate intakes of minerals than for most other nutrient groups, a diet that follows the recommendations of the Food Guide Pyramid is likely to contain at least two-thirds of the recommended levels of the essential minerals.

You've also had experience using food composition tables to assess more specifically the level of nutrients in your diet. When you did Act on Fact 2.2, one of the things you determined was the status of your diet in regard to those minerals for which reliable food composition data exist (information about these minerals is listed in Appendix C).

There is another way of looking at mineral intake that can be useful, especially for those minerals that some people find difficult to consume in adequate amounts. This method involves determining nutrient density.

Calculation of Nutrient Density

Nutrient density, as you learned in Chapter 2, is a term used to describe whether a food is a good source of a nutrient relative to the kcalories it contains. Usually, nutrient density is expressed as the quantity of a particular nutrient in 100 kcalories of the food. For example, a ground beef patty has a nutrient density for zinc of 1.7 mg per 100 kcalories; this was calculated from the food composition information that 244 kcalories of ground beef contain 4.2 mg of zinc.

Act on Fact 12.1 will help you learn more about the concept of nutrient density and help you decide whether it's a useful concept for you.

Summary

- Both vitamins and minerals are important micronutrients that are widespread in basic foods; the main difference between them is that vitamins are organic (carbon-containing) and **minerals** are inorganic, being simply individual chemical elements. Depending on the amounts present in your body, essential minerals are categorized as either **macrominerals** or **trace minerals**. Some minerals present in the body are needed for growth, reproduction, and maintenance of health, and they are considered essential. Minerals are not present in proportion to their importance; both trace mineral and macromineral deficiencies can be damaging to health.
- Many factors can influence the **bioavailability** of minerals, making specific intake recommendations difficult to establish. For example, **heme iron** is better absorbed than **nonheme iron**. Both vitamin C and **unidentified meat factor** can increase the absorption of nonheme iron in the diet, and vitamin D is needed for optimal absorption of calcium and phosphorus. Dietary fiber, **phytate, tannins**, and **oxalates,** by contrast, can depress the absorption of minerals. Minerals can also compete with each other for absorption, so supplementing a diet with individual minerals may adversely alter the bioavailability of other minerals. Medications, **pica**, and physiologic factors can affect mineral absorption and excretion, too.
- Minerals function in four structural and regulatory ways: (1) they form part of tissue structure, (2) they help maintain water and acid–base balance, (3) they form components of enzymes and hormones, and (4) they facilitate the function of nerve and muscle cells. Tables 12.3, 12.4, 12.5, 12.7, and 12.8 list food sources for essential minerals, and Table 12.2 summarizes key information about their RDAs, major functions, and signs of deficiency or excess.
- Mineral deficiences are most likely to arise when the following combination of circumstances exists: (1) the overall diet is limited in quantity, (2) the diet is poorly selected for mineral content, (3) mineral bioavailability is low, and (4) mineral requirements are unusually high because of rapid growth or disease. All of these factors are less likely to occur simultaneously in the developed countries than in less developed parts of the world. The most common mineral deficiencies worldwide are for iron, iodine, and zinc.

continued on page 417

Calculating Nutrient Density for a Selected Mineral

Because calcium, zinc, and iron are three minerals many people have trouble getting in the quantities suggested by the RDA, it makes sense to consider their density in various foods. The procedure and a partial example are provided below.

1. Decide whether to evaluate your diet for its nutrient density of calcium, zinc, or iron. Check Act on Fact 2.2 to see whether your intake of one of these was low; if so, use that nutrient.
2. Circle the name of the mineral you have chosen to assess in the third column heading of a form for Act on Fact 12.1
3. Copy your menu from Act on Fact 2.2 onto the assessment form for Act on Fact 12.1, and transfer to the appropriate columns the contents of the mineral in the foods you ate, the total, and your RDA for that mineral. In addition, copy the energy content of the foods.
4. Divide the mineral content of each food by the kcalorie value of the food; this will give you the nutrient density of the mineral per kcalorie of food. Since nutrient density is usually expressed in nutrient content per 100 kcalories of food, multiply your answer by 100, and enter the product in the nutrient density column.

(continued)

Sample Act on Fact 12.1

Calculating nutrient density for a selected mineral.

Food or Beverage	Approximate Measure	Absolute (Calcium), Zinc, or Iron Content	Energy (Kcal)	Nutrient Density (mg/100 kcalories)
Egg bagel	1	23	163	14
Jelly	2 T.	8	110	7
Fruit punch	12 oz.	30	175	17
McDonald's cheeseburger	1	199 (A)	310	64
French fries	regular	10	220	5
Brownie	1 square	25	243	10
Cola drink	12 oz.	5	151	3
Pork chop—lean only	2½ oz.	5	169	3
Barbecue sauce	2 T.	6	24	25
Biscuit	2 avg.	68 (C)	240	32
Frozen peas, cooked	½ c.	19	63	30
Butter	2 t.	2	72	3
Salad: Iceberg lettuce	½ c.	5	4	125 (3)
Spinach	½ c.	28	6	467 (1)
French dressing	2 T.	3	134	2
2% milk	½ c.	148 (B)	60	246 (2)
Graham crackers	2 squares	6	55	11
Total		590	2169	
RDA		1200		

5. Scan the nutrient densities of all foods in the column. Rank your top three sources next to their nutrient density values as (1), (2), and (3).
6. Now scan the column of absolute content for the mineral. Rank the top three next to their absolute values as (A), (B), and (C). These rankings will not automatically correspond with the nutrient density rankings, but they might.
7. Now that you've gathered the facts, answer these questions.
   a) One way to improve your intake of this mineral is to increase your consumption of the foods that have the highest density of the mineral; you labeled them (1), (2), and (3). If you doubled your intake of these foods, how much would your intake of the mineral and of energy increase in an absolute sense?
   b) Another way to improve your intake of this mineral is to increase your consumption of the foods that have highest absolute amounts of the mineral; you labeled them (A), (B), and (C). If you doubled your intake of these foods, how much would that increase your intake of the mineral and of energy? Would the extra kcalories be a problem for you?
   c) Do either or both of these methods of evaluating mineral intake consider the bioavailability of the mineral you are studying?
   d) What factors, then, do you need to take into account when you increase your intake of a problem mineral?

• It is definitely possible to consume mineral overdoses; overdoses can both interfere with the absorption of other minerals and cause either acute or chronic toxicity symptoms, depending on the type and duration of exposure. The minerals necessary to health can be obtained in almost all cases by simply eating a balanced and varied diet; most people don't need mineral supplements.

References

Allaway, W.H. 1986. Soil-plant-animal and human interrelationships in trace element nutrition. In *Trace elements in human and animal nutrition,* volume 2, ed. W. Mertz. Orlando, FL: Academic Press.

Beard, J.L., and S.H. Smith. 1992. Re-evaluation of apparent hypometabolism in iron-deficient rats. *Journal of Nutritional Biochemistry* 3:298–303.

Bergkvist, L., H.O. Adami, I. Persson, R. Hoover, and C. Schairer. 1989. The risk of breast cancer after estrogen and estrogen-progestin replacement. *New England Journal of Medicine* 321:293–297.

Block, G., C.M. Dresser, A.M. Hartman, and M.D. Carroll. 1985. Nutrient sources in the American diet: Quantitative data from the NHANES II Survey. I. Vitamins and minerals. *American Journal of Epidemiology* 2:13–26.

Consensus Development Conference. 1991. Consensus development conference: Prophylaxis and treatment of osteoporosis. *American Journal of Medicine* 90:107–110.

Dallman, P.R. 1987. Iron deficiency and the immune response. *American Journal of Clinical Nutrition* 46:329–334.

Dallman, P.R. and R. Yip. 1989. Changing characteristics of childhood anemia. *Journal of Pediatrics* 114:161–164.

Davis, C.D., and J.L. Greger. 1992. Longitudinal changes of manganese-dependent superoxide dismutase and other indices of manganese and iron status in women. *American Journal of Clinical Nutrition* 55:747–752.

Davis, C.D., E.A. Malecki, and J.L. Greger. (1993). Interactions among dietary manganese, heme iron and nonheme iron in women. *American Journal of Clinical Nutrition* 56:926–932.

Dawson-Hughes, B. 1991. Calcium supplementation and bone loss: a review of controlled clinical trials. *American Journal of Clinical Nutrition* 54:274s–280s.

Deuster, P.S., S.B. Kyle, P.B. Moser, R.A. Vigersky, A. Singh, and E.B. Shoomaker. 1986. Nutritional survey of highly trained women runners. *American Journal of Clinical Nutrition* 45:954–962.

Ettinger, B., H.K. Genant, and C.E. Cann. 1987. Postmenopausal bone loss is prevented by treatment with low-dosage estrogen with calcium. *Annals of Internal Medicine* 106:40–45.

Fairbanks, V.F. and E. Beutler. 1988. Iron. In *Modern nutrition in health and disease,* ed. M.E. Shils and V.R. Young. Philadelphia: Lea & Febiger.

Farnett, L., C.D. Mulrow, W.D. Linn, C.R. Lucey, and M.R. Tuley. 1991. The J-curve phenomenon and the treatment of hypertension. *Journal of the American Medical Association* 265:489–495.

Fosmire, G.J. 1989. Possible hazards associated with zinc supplementation. *Nutrition Today* 24(no. 3):15–18.

Greger, J.L. 1989a. Effect of dietary protein and minerals on calcium and zinc utilization. *Critical Reviews of Food Science and Nutrition* 28:249–271.

Greger, J.L. 1989b. Potential for trace mineral deficiencies and toxicities in the elderly. In *Mineral homeostasis in the elderly*, ed. C.W. Bales. New York: Alan R. Liss, Inc.

Greger, J.L., C.E. Kryzkowski, R.R. Khazen, and C.L. Krashoc. 1987. Mineral utilization by rats fed various commercially available calcium supplements or milk. *Journal of Nutrition* 117:717–724.

Hambidge, K.M., C.E. Casey, and N.F. Krebs. 1986. Zinc. In *Trace elements in human and animal nutrition,* volume 2, ed. W. Mertz. Orlando, FL: Academic Press.

Hambidge, K.M., P.A. Walravens, K.H. Neldner. 1978. Zinc and acrodermatitis enteropathica. In *Zinc and copper in clinical medicine.* ed. K.M. Hambidge and B.L. Nichols. New York: Spectrum.

Heaney, R.P., J.C. Gallagher, C.C. Johnson, R. Neer, A.M. Parfitt, B. Chir, and G.D. Whedon. 1982. Calcium nutrition and bone health in the elderly. *American Journal of Clinical Nutrition* 36:986–1013.

Hernandez-Avila, M., G.A. Colditz, M.J. Stampfer, B. Rosner, F.E. Speizer, and W.C. Willett. 1991. Caffeine, moderate alcohol intake, and risk of fractures of the hip and forearm in middle-aged women. *American Journal of Clinical Nutrition* 54:157–163.

Horner R.D., C.J. Lackey, K. Kolasa, and K. Warren. 1991. Pica practices of pregnant women. *Journal of the American Dietetic Association* 91:34–38.

Human Nutrition Information Service (HNIS). 1985. *Nationwide Food Consumption Survey, Continuing Survey of Food Intake by Individuals.* Report 85-1. Hyattsville, MD: U.S. Department of Agriculture.

Human Nutrition Information Service (HNIS). 1986. *Nationwide Food Consumption Survey, Continuing Survey of Food Intake by Individuals.* 1 Day. Report 85-3. Hyattsville, MD: United States Department of Agriculture.

Johnson, M.A. and C.L. Murphy. 1988. Adverse effects of high dietary iron and ascorbic acid on copper status in copper-deficient and copper-adequate rats. *American Journal of Clinical Nutrition* 47:96–101.

Jones, R.B., D.N. Mormann, and T.B. Durtsche. 1989. Fluoridation referendum in LaCrosse, Wisconsin: Contributing factors to success. *American Journal of Public Health* 79:1405–1408.

Karanja, N. and D.A. McCarron. 1986. Calcium and hypertension. *Annual Review of Nutrition* 6:475–484.

Kaup, S.M., J.L. Greger, M.S.K. Marcus, and N.M. Lewis. 1991. Effect of chronic ingestion of various chloride salts on blood pressure, fluid compartments and utilization of chloride. *Journal of Nutrition* 121:330–337.

Kleerekoper, M., and R. Balena. 1991. Fluorides and osteoporosis. *Annual Review of Nutrition* 11:309–324.

Lane, H.W., and L.O. Schultz. 1992. Nutritional questions relevant to space flight. *Annual Review of Nutrition* 12:257–278.

Levander, O.A. 1991. Scientific rationale for the 1989 Recommended Dietary Allowance for selenium. *Journal of the American Dietetic Association* 91:1572–1576.

Leveille, G.A., M.E. Zabik, and K.J. Morgan. 1983. *Nutrients in foods.* Cambridge, MA: The Nutrition Guild.

Life Science Research Office. 1991. Guidelines for the assessment and management of iron deficiency in women of childbearing age. Bethesda, MD: Federation of American Societies of Experimental Biology.

Lönnerdal, B. 1987. Protein-mineral interactions. In *Nutrition 1987*. Washington DC: Federation of American Societies of Experimental Biology.

Luisi, B.F., W.X. Xu, Z. Otwinowski, L.P. Freedman, K.R. Yamamoto, and P.B. Sigler. 1991. Crystallographic analysis of the interaction of the glucocorticoid receptor with DNA. *Nature* 352:497–505.

Marshall, C.W. 1983. *Vitamins and minerals: Help or harm?* Philadelphia: George F. Stickley Company.

Mahoney, M.C., P.C. Nasca, W.S. Burnett, and J.M. Melius. 1991. Bone cancer incidence rates in New York state: Time trends and fluoridated drinking water. *American Journal of Public Health* 81:475–479.

Merhav, H., Y. Amitai, H. Patti, and S. Godfrey. 1985. Tea drinking and microcytic anemia in infants. *American Journal of Clinical Nutrition* 41:10–13.

Miller, S.A. 1987. Lead in calcium supplements. *Journal of the American Medical Association.* 257:1810.

Monsen, E.R. 1988. Iron nutrition and absorption: Dietary factors which impact iron bioavailability. *Journal of the American Dietetic Association* 88:786–790.

Muñoz, L.M., B. Lönnerdal, C.L. Keen, and K.G. Dewey. 1988. Coffee consumption as a factor in iron deficiency anemia among pregnant women and their infants in Costa Rica. *American Journal of Clinical Nutrition* 48:645–651.

National Research Council. 1989. *Diet and Health.* Washington DC: National Academy Press.

Nielsen, F.H. 1988. Ultra trace minerals. In *Modern nutrition in health and disease,* ed. M.E. Shils and V.R. Young. Philadelphia: Lea & Febiger.

Nielsen, F.H. 1992. Facts and fallacies about boron. *Nutrition Today* 27:6–12.

Nutrition Reviews. 1991a. More people are fracturing more bones more often. *Nutrition Reviews* 49:24–25.

Nutrition Reviews. 1991b. Type 1 iodothyronine deiodinase is a selenium containing enzyme. *Nutrition Reviews* 49:247–249.

Osterman, J.W. 1990. Evaluating the impact of municipal water fluoridation on the aquatic environment. *American Journal of Public Health* 80:30–35.

Pennington, J.A., B.E. Young, and D.B. Wilson. 1989. Nutritional elements in U.S. diets: Results from the Total Diet Study, 1982–1986. *Journal of the American Dietetic Association* 89:659–664.

Prince, R.L., M. Smith, I.M. Dick, R.I. Price, P.G. Webb, N.K. Henderson, and M.M. Harris. 1991. Prevention of postmenopausal osteoporosis: A comparative study of exercise, calcium supplementation, and hormone-replacement therapy. *New England Journal of Medicine* 325:1189–1195.

RDA Subcommittee. 1989. *Recommended dietary allowances.* Washington, DC: National Academy Press.

Riis, B., K. Thomsen, and C. Christiansen. 1987. Does calcium supplementation prevent postmenopausal bone loss? *New England Journal of Medicine* 316:173–177.

Safe Drinking Water Committee. 1980. *Drinking water and health,* volume 3. Washington, DC: National Academy of Sciences.

Salonen, J.T., K. Nvyssöne, H. Korpela, J. Tuomilehto, R. Seppänen, and R. Salonen. 1992. High stored iron levels are associated with excess risk of myocardial infarction in Eastern Finnish men. *Circulation* 86:803–811.

Sanchez-Castillo, C.P., S. Warrender, T.P. Whitehead, and W.P. James. 1987. An assessment of the sources of dietary salt in a British population. *Clinical Science* 72:95–102.

Science and Education Administration. 1980. *Food and nutrient intakes of individuals in 1 day in the United States, Spring, 1977.* Nationwide food consumption survey 1977–78; preliminary report No. 2. Washington, DC: United States Department of Agriculture.

Seeman, E., J.L. Hopper, L.A. Bach, M.E. Cooper, E. Parkinson, J. McKay, and G. Jerums. 1989. Reduced bone mass in daughters of women with osteoporosis. *New England Journal of Medicine* 320:554–558.

Sentipal, J.M., G.M. Wardlaw, J. Mahan, and V. Matkovic. 1991. Influence of calcium intake and growth indexes on vertebral bone mineral density in young females. *American Journal of Clinical Nutrition* 54:425–428.

Shils, M.E. 1988. Magnesium. In *Modern nutrition in health and disease,* ed. M.E. Shils and V.R. Young. Philadelphia: Lea & Febiger.

Snead, D.B., C.C. Stubbs, J.Y. Weltman, W.S. Evans, J.D. Veldhuis, A.D. Rogol, C.D. Teates, and A. Weltman. 1992. Dietary patterns, eating behaviors, and bone mineral density in women runners. *American Journal of Clinical Nutrition* 56:705–711.

Solomons, N.W. 1988a. Physiological interaction of minerals. In *Nutrient interactions,* ed. C.E. Bodwell and J.W. Erdman. New York: Marcel Dekker.

Solomons, N.W. 1988b. Zinc and copper. In *Modern nutrition in health and disease,* ed. M.E. Shils and V.R. Young. Philadelphia: Lea & Febiger.

Stanbury, J.B. 1988. Iodine. In *Modern nutrition in health and disease,* ed. M.E. Shils and V.R. Young. Philadelphia: Lea & Febiger.

Surgeon General. 1988. *Surgeon General's report on nutrition and health.* Washington, DC: United States Department of Health and Human Services.

Sweeney, E.A. and J.A. Shaw. 1988. Nutrition in relation to dental medicine. In *Modern nutrition in health and disease,* ed. M.E. Shils and V.R. Young. Philadelphia: Lea & Febiger.

Thiele, M., M.E. Geddes, E. Nobmann, and K. Petersen. 1988. High prevalence of iron deficiency anemia among Alaskan native children. *Journal of the American Medical Association* 259:2532.

Tobian, L. and S. Hanlon. 1990. High sodium chloride diets injure arteries and raise mortality without changing blood pressure. *Hypertension* 15:900–903.

Uehling, M.D. and K. Springen. 1986. Cashing in on a booming new market. *Newsweek* Jan. 27, p. 52.

Wargovich, M.J. 1988. Calcium and colon cancer. *Journal of American College of Nutrition* 7:295–300.

Weaver, C.M., B.R. Martin, J.S. Ebner, and C.A. Krueger. 1987. Oxalic acid decreases calcium absorption in rats. *Journal of Nutrition* 117:1903–1906.

Weinberger, M.H., S.J. Cohen, J.Z. Miller, F.C. Luft, C.E. Grim, and N.S. Fineberg. 1988. Dietary sodium restriction as an adjunctive treatment of hypertension. *Journal of the American Medical Association* 259:2561–2565.

Underwood, E.J. 1977. *Trace elements in human and animal nutrition.* New York: Academic Press.

Zemel, P.C., M.B. Zemel, M. Urberg, F.L. Douglas, R. Geiser, and J.R. Sowers. 1990. Metabolic and hemodynamic effects of magnesium supplementation in patients with essential hypertension. *American Journal of Clinical Nutrition* 51:665–669.

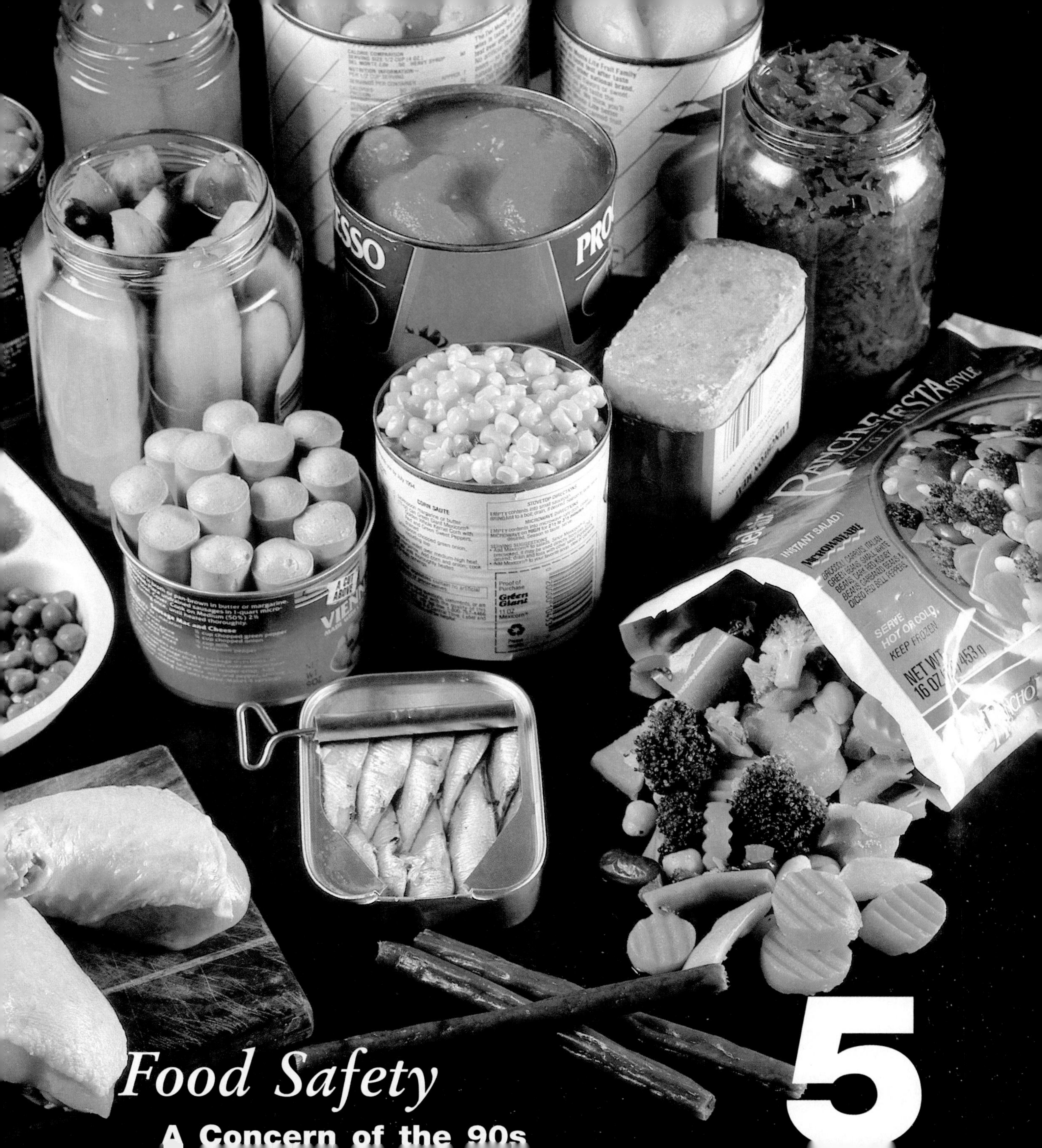

5

Food Safety

A Concern of the 90s

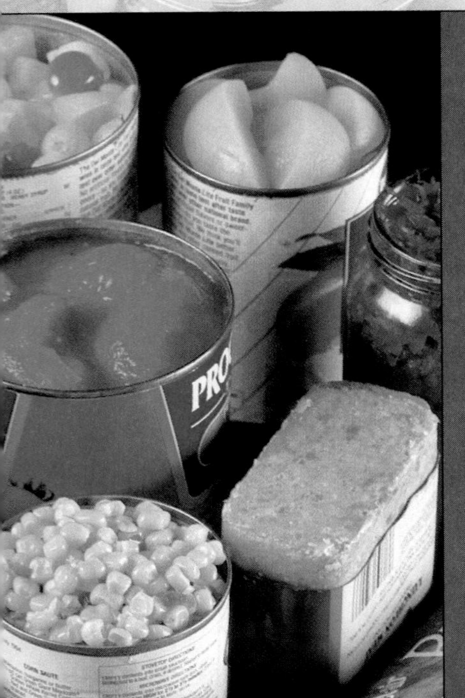

IN THIS CHAPTER

Chapter 13

Effects of Food Production and Processing on Nutrients

We Americans have high expectations of food. First and foremost, we want it to taste good. Recently, in a large U.S. food marketing survey, 96% of shoppers said that taste is an important factor in food selection—but almost as many also rated nutrition, price, and product safety as important. In addition, storability and convenience were influential in the food choices of more than three-fourths of those surveyed (Food Marketing Institute, 1992).

The food industry takes such survey results seriously (Figure 13.1). Some consumer expectations are relatively easy for food producers to define and satisfy, but, as you can imagine, others—such as what makes a food "taste good" or what makes it "nutritious"—are open to a variety of interpretations. For example, you might regard products with added vitamins and minerals or fiber as nutritious. Somebody else, whose main concern is to lose weight, may think "nutritious" means low-kcalorie products that taste sweet and feel rich without containing the sugar or fat that the traditional versions of such foods contain. Another person might assess a food's nutritional value according to whether it appears fresh or contains little salt.

From this you can see why food processors who want to stay in business have had to develop an extensive array of foods just to satisfy the public's concept of good nutrition, to say nothing of the additional characteristics consumers want. All of these expectations have driven the average supermarket to stock 25,000 different items. Each year, thousands of new products—more than 12,000 in 1991—are introduced into the American food supply (Gallo, 1992). Many do not survive, making way for next year's new batch of hopefuls.

In this chapter, first we identify consumers' major concerns about nutrition. Then, to see how American food systems have responded to these concerns and to the concerns of experts, we look at how nutrients in food are affected by farm production and harvesting methods, by processing and storage, and by home preparation.

Consumers' Major Nutrition Concerns

Two large national consumer surveys give insight into consumers' nutrition concerns.

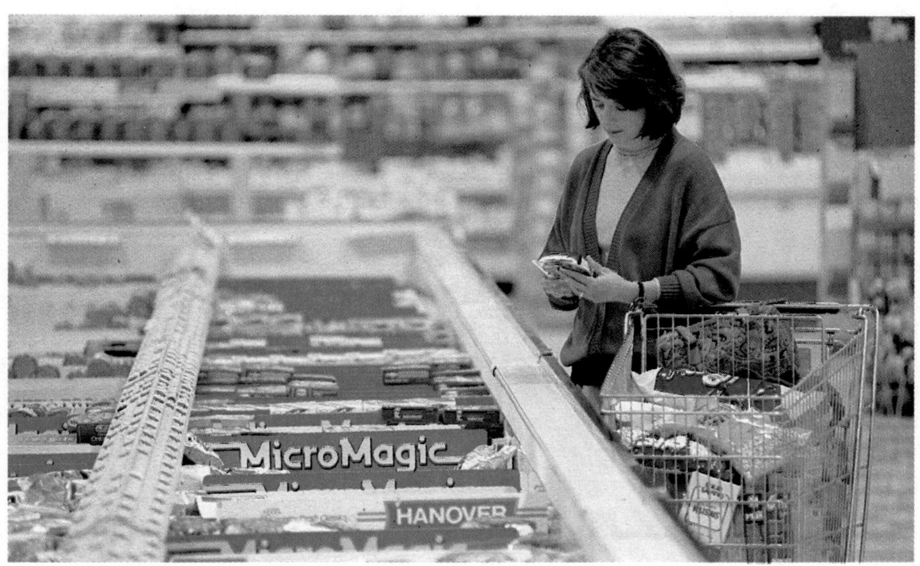

FIGURE 13.1
When consumers talk, food processors listen.

Urban consumers have the most clout in effecting changes in today's food marketplace. For example, the fast-paced urban lifestyle has encouraged a huge expansion of frozen microwavable foods in single-serving packages.

TABLE 13.1 Most Important Nutrition Concerns: Two American Consumer Surveys

Consumer Nutrition Concerns	Percent of respondents	
	American Dietetic Association Survey (1991)[a]	Food Marketing Institute Survey (1992)[b]
Fat content	21	50
Cholesterol levels	23	30
Salt or sodium content	9	21
Sugar content	—[c]	13
Kcalories	12	9
Vitamins/minerals	21	8
Fiber	9	2
Other/don't know	5	—[d]

[a]Instructed to choose only one item from list
[b]Allowed multiple responses to open-ended question
[c]Not on list of choices
[d]18 other matters were listed here; some were not nutrient concerns, and others were nutrient issues that concerned fewer than 4% of the respondents

Data sources: American Deitetic Association, 1991; Food Marketing Institute Survey, 1992.

In the American Dietetic Association's *Survey of American Dietary Habits* (1991), 1000 adults aged 25 and older were interviewed by telephone in June 1991. The sample was representative for gender, age, race, and geography. None of the participants was on a medically prescribed diet.

When asked to choose which single nutrition issue from a list of six possibilities was of greatest personal concern, two-thirds of the respondents cited cholesterol, fat, or vitamin and mineral content of food. These three topics were almost tied as the issues of top concern (Table 13.1). Salt, kcalorie, or fiber content of food were top concerns for the remaining one-third of the group questioned.

The second survey is *Trends 92: Consumer Attitudes & the Supermarket*, one of an annual series conducted by the Food Marketing Institute (1992). Two thousand shoppers from a representative, nationwide sample were surveyed by telephone in January 1992. One in five respondents was on a medically prescribed diet. Ninety-six percent of all respondents said that nutrition was somewhat or very important to them in buying food.

These 96% were asked an open-ended question regarding what concerned them most about the nutritional content of food. Many respondents gave more than one answer. Fully half answered fat, followed at some distance by cholesterol, salt, kcalories, and vitamins and minerals (Table 13.1).

Clearly, both surveys show that fat and cholesterol contents of food are primary nutrition concerns of people in the United States. There's no way to know for sure why the other results of these two broadly based surveys were not more uniform, but the nature of the questions may have influenced the responses.

You Tell Me

What would be your "spontaneous" responses to these survey questions? Here's the Food Marketing Institute's question: "What is it about the nutrient content of what you eat that concerns you and your family most?" And the American Dietetic Association's question: "Which ONE of these, or any other that you can think of, is most important to you personally: cholesterol, fat, vitamins and minerals, kcalories, fiber, or sodium or salt?"

Did you give different answers to the two questions? What factors might have affected your responses? Do you think that current advertising campaigns and public health messages might affect people's answers?

You might wonder why salt—composed of the mineral ions sodium and chloride—is listed separately from vitamins and minerals in the survey question above. The reason probably is that people's attitudes about salt are very different from their attitudes about the other micronutrients. With salt, as you learned in Chapter 12, people worry that they take in too much rather than not enough. People associate salt with *health problems,* such as high blood pressure and heart disease, whereas they associate the other micronutrients with *good health.*

Because these studies show that most of us have a few key concerns about our nutrition, you can better plan your diet if you know how food processing affects those aspects of food. We devote this chapter to discussing how the fat, cholesterol, salt, and vitamin and mineral contents of food are affected by production and processing, both commercial processing and processing done at home. Sugar, kcalories, and fiber, which were also of some concern in these surveys, have been discussed in Chapters 5 and 9.

The Effects of Farm Production and Harvesting

Of the food components we're considering here—fat, cholesterol, salt, vitamins, and minerals—which do you suppose can be most affected on the farm?

The answer is different for animal products from that for plants. For some animal products, lipids can be modified; for plants, though, the major variables are vitamin and mineral content. Farm practices do not significantly affect the salt content of any food, so it is not considered in this section.

Effects of Farm Production on Fat and Cholesterol

A considerable amount of agricultural research has focused on ways to reduce the fat and cholesterol in animal products. Some experiments have been very successful, as we'll discuss below, and now you can find those products in your supermarket. Other efforts to modify fat and cholesterol in animal products have not proved practical.

FIGURE 13.2
Fatness of meat animals "then" and "now."

In recent decades, cattle and hogs have been genetically selected and raised to be less fat.

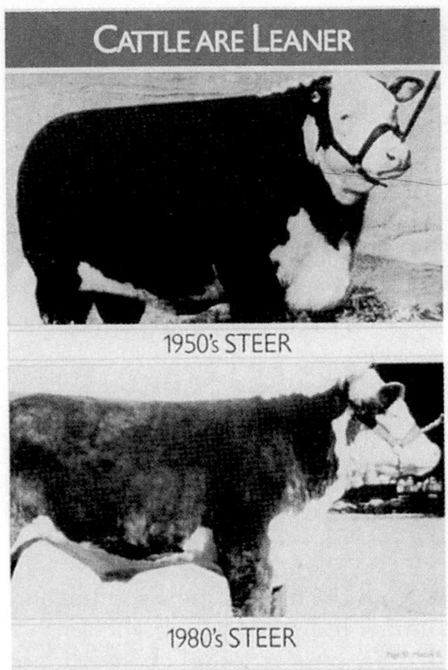

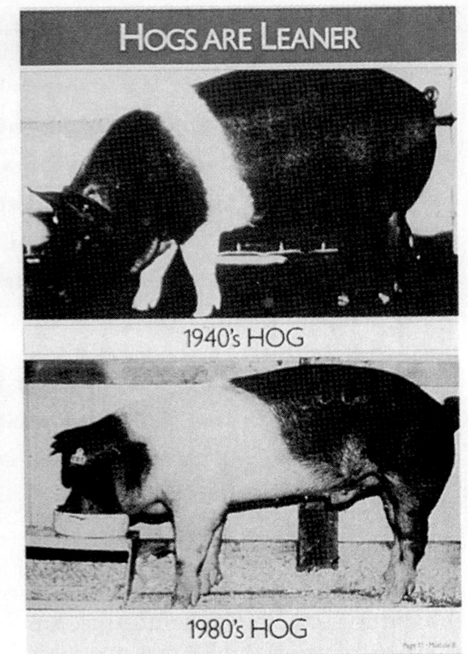

Meats and Poultry The amount of fat and lean tissue on animals—whether beef cattle, hogs, lambs, or poultry—depends first of all on genetics: inherited traits establish patterns, limits, and types of growth (Byers et al., 1988). Nonetheless, the types and amounts of food the animals are fed can affect gains in fat and lean tissue. By altering the character of the feed, it is possible even to change the proportion of saturated and unsaturated fats produced in some animals.

Another way of promoting the development of more lean and less fat is to stimulate the animal's own hormone system or to administer additional hormones. These techniques are not equally effective with all types of animals, and some have not yet been accepted for commercial use.

On the whole, though, the efforts to lower fat content of animal products have paid off. Today, beef cattle and lambs average about 6% less body fat than their counterparts of three decades ago, and pork has about 30% more lean meat per animal (National Livestock and Meat Board, 1987). Figure 13.2 shows some dramatic "before" and "after" pictures of this development.

These technologies could be used to lower fat content even further, but there are factors that stand in the way of their widespread adoption. A key problem is that many people don't like very lean meats as well: they are often perceived as less tender, juicy, and flavorful than fatter meats (Savell and Cross, 1988). Another stumbling block is the grading system established by the United States Department of Agriculture (USDA). Because meat grades were developed many decades ago—before we understood the connection between high fat intake and various chronic health problems—grading standards have placed a premium on higher fat content of meat. Meats earning the higher quality designations (e.g., *prime* and *choice*) bring higher prices to the farmer; therefore, the grading system has been an incentive to overfeed and excessively fatten animals before slaughter (Committee on Technological Options, 1988).

A positive step was taken in 1987 when a lower-fat grade of meat, formerly labeled *good*, was renamed *select*, which has a more positive connotation. Experts suggest, however, that more changes are needed to remove the grading biases that currently favor production and marketing of fatter meats.

Milk The milk pricing system also is out of step with current health concerns: it favors production of milk that contains the maximum content of fat and protein. The percentage of fat in milk naturally ranges from 3.4 to 5.6% of the milk's total weight, depending primarily on the cow's breed.

Experiments show that modifying their diet can make cows produce milk containing as little as 1% fat (Gorewit, 1988). This method also increases the proportion of unsaturated fatty acids in the milk. However, the experimental diet causes health risks to the cow and so is unacceptable. It's much more practical to lower the fat content of milk after it has left the farm. (This is discussed in the section on food processing.)

Eggs Because egg yolks are high in cholesterol, some poultry scientists have altered the hens' diets to lower the cholesterol content of eggs. The methods these scientists use have negative effects on other nutritional values of the egg or on the hen's egg production. Drugs added to hens' diets can reduce cholesterol in eggs, but those tested thus far also have harmful side effects for the hens and are therefore not a good solution (Gyles, 1988).

As with milk, post-farm processing methods for eggs are more practical at this time. In a later section we'll discuss various lower-cholesterol egg products.

Effects of Farm Production on Vitamins and Minerals

In large part, the micronutrient content of both animals and plants depends on genetics (you should be getting used to this concept); that is, the vitamin and mineral contents of animals and plants of a given species or variety generally tend to be similar to others in their group. Scientists are beginning to develop new varieties of plants with higher values of some nutrients—for example, a carrot with twice the usual amount of carotene. Someday farmers will be able to improve the nutritional value of their crops simply by planting varieties with this characteristic.

However, the conditions under which animals and plants are grown can also affect to some degree their vitamin and mineral makeup. Animals fed unusual diets sometimes depart from the norm in the micronutrient makeup of their tissues, but plants grown in varying environments are likely to show greater differences. In this section, we focus on plants.

Plants and Vitamin Content Vitamin C is sensitive to a variety of changing conditions; therefore, vitamin C is often measured as a marker to show whether various production factors affect the overall vitamin content of fruits and vegetables. Also, because vitamin C is a nutrient we count on getting from these foods, it's important to find out to what extent various production factors might diminish it.

Environmental conditions, such as climate, soil, and fertilizer, can influence vitamin levels of plants. For example, tomatoes that are vine-ripened outdoors in summer sunlight have twice as much vitamin C as tomatoes grown in greenhouses in winter (Agricultural Research Service, 1977), and grapefruit grown in the cooler coastal areas of California contain more vitamin C than those picked on the same date in the hotter desert areas of Arizona (Nagy and Wardowski, 1988).

FIGURE 13.3
Soil composition affects crop growth and nutrient content.

This farmer is taking a sample of soil to have it analyzed for mineral content. No matter what kind of agricultural methods are used—conventional or alternative—it is important to monitor soil composition, because it can have a dramatic effect on total yield and on the nutritional quality of crops.

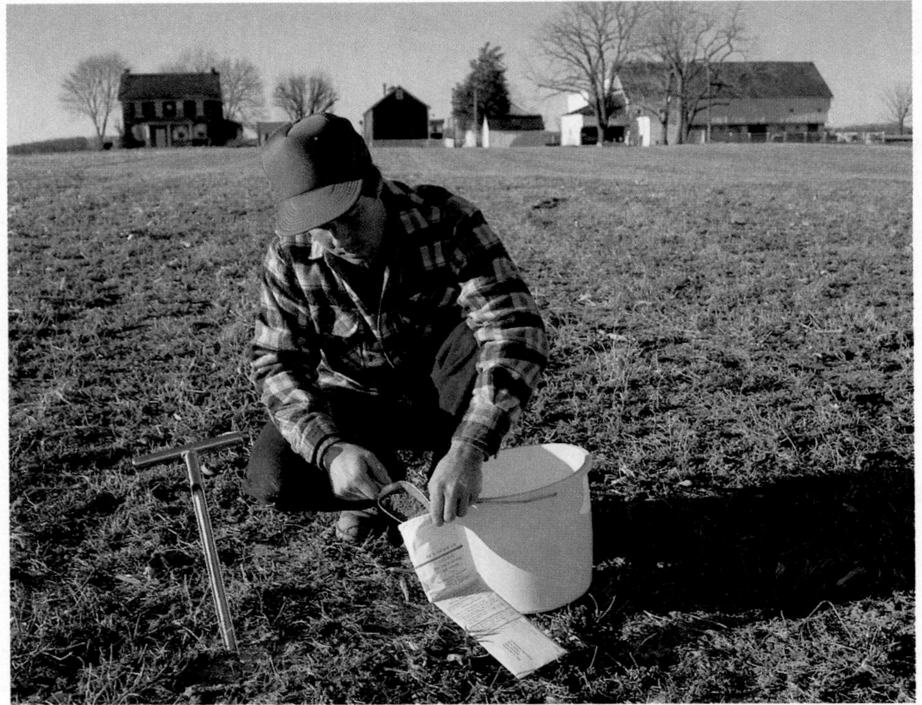

The *mineral content of the soil* can influence the vitamin content of plants as well. The vitamin C levels in citrus fruits grown on sandy Florida soils (which are naturally deficient in zinc, magnesium, manganese, and copper) are lower than citrus fruits grown in soil containing adequate amounts of minerals (Nagy and Wardowski, 1988). Even moderate adjustments are sometimes enough to optimize vitamin C levels, but, of course, using excessive fertilizer cannot make them higher than genetic limits allow.

Adequate nitrogen is necessary for achieving healthy crops with a good yield and nutritive quality. Nitrogen deficiency is unquestionably the most common chemical deficiency of soils. However, in vegetable farming, applying *too much* nitrogen can *decrease* the vitamin C content in some vegetables by as much as 30% (Salunkhe and Desai, 1988).

Carrots that were not fertilized with nitrogen, phosphorus, potassium, or magnesium have been found to have lower carotene levels than those that were fertilized (Salunkhe and Desai, 1988). Just as in earlier discussions about nutrient supplementation for humans, scientists have learned that plants need adequate amounts of minerals, but excesses are actually damaging. It is important for farmers to have their soil tested periodically so that they can add the right amounts of minerals needed for healthy crops (Figure 13.3).

Does it matter whether the minerals come from natural fertilizer (such as decomposed plant material or animal manure) or synthetic fertilizer (specific pure chemicals)? The Thinking for Yourself on page 429 gives you the opportunity to answer this question and to use other bases for comparing "organic foods" with foods produced by conventional practices.

The maturity of fruits and vegetables at harvest can also affect vitamin levels. Some fruits and vegetables reach their highest nutritive value while they are still immature, others when mature, and still others when overripe (Nagy and Wardowski, 1988; Salunkhe and Desai, 1988). Most often,

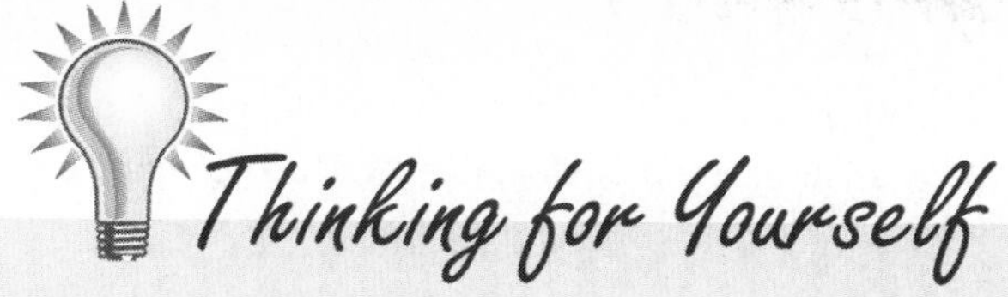

Is Organic Food Better?

The Situation

While on your way to the food store, you run into an acquaintance headed in the same direction. Walking along together, he asks you whether you shop in the new "organic foods" section that the store has recently opened. You say that you do not. He says that he has decided to buy "organic foods" because they are more nutritious and do not contain any synthetic chemicals. Although "organic foods" are more expensive, he says he has decided that they are worth the money.

The conversation moves on to other topics. As you head in different directions a few blocks later, you begin to think about what he said. You wonder: "Should I buy 'organic foods'?"

Is Your Information Accurate and Relevant?

- As is the case with "natural vitamins" (Chapter 11), it's difficult to say anything definitive about "organic foods," because the term is still waiting for a nationally recognized definition. The 1990 Farm Bill created the National Organic Standards Board and charged it to work with the USDA to determine the criteria for organic foods and how to market and label them. Until then, the nature of foods labeled "organic" is uncertain.
- When people buy "organic food," they may think they are getting foods produced without synthetic fertilizers and pesticides, but grown with organic fertilizer (such as decomposed plant material or animal manure). This may indeed be what they are getting, especially if the food was grown in one of the 26 states that have their own organic laws or regulations; unfortunately, however, these laws are not uniform, and it's difficult to determine whether prescribed practices are being followed.
- There is no evidence that foods produced with organic fertilizers are more nutritious than those that are conventionally grown; in fact, studies comparing cabbage and carrots fertilized with organic materials to those fertilized with synthetic materials found no difference in their in vitamin C or carotene contents (Salunkhe and Desai, 1988).
- There isn't now, and cannot be in the future, any guarantee that "organic" produce will be completely free of residues from synthetic fertilizers or pesticides, because once used, these substances persist in the environment and may contaminate other crops. However, the amounts of these chemicals allowed in organic produce will be lower than amounts allowed in their conventionally grown equivalents. It's expected that when tolerance limits are set for "organic foods," only 10% of the levels allowed in conventionally grown produce will be allowed in organic produce (Lynch, 1991).
- It's true that "organic foods" are usually more expensive. It's not unusual for these foods to cost more than double the price of conventionally produced foods (Larkin, 1991). Once the federal program is in operation, industry-shared costs of the program may push prices of organic foods still higher.

What Else Should You Consider?

Some people have promoted "organic foods" by saying that they are safer than conventionally grown foods. These people fear that the synthetic materials used in conventional agriculture may be carcinogenic. Experts in cancer research say that the chance of your developing cancer from eating foods that have the amounts of chemicals allowed by the Environmental Protection Agency (EPA) is very remote (Ames and Gold, 1989) (see Chapter 14, Table 14.2). Most conventionally grown foods contain even less than the amounts of pesticides allowed by the EPA.

In fact, many conventionally grown foods contain no detectable pesticide residues at all. Surveys conducted by the National Food Processors Association, the California Department of Food and Agriculture, and the Food and Drug Administration showed that 93%, 79% and 60% of these foods, respectively, were *free* of pesticide residues (Institute of Food Technologists, 1990).

Experts at estimating the cancer-causing potential of various pesticides judge the risk to be much greater to the farmer who applies these chemicals than to the consumer (see Table 14.2). Farmers handle these materials in much higher concentrations than the concentrations that may be present on the food that was treated. To minimize their risk, farmers need to follow recommended procedures for the use of pesticides. Some farmers simply prefer to use agricultural methods that avoid the use of concentrated chemicals.

Some people prefer "organic food" because they believe that the methods of producing such foods are kinder to the environment. They believe that conventional agricultural practices are not sustainable—that is, they don't foster the continued productivity of the ecosystem—but that organic methods are. The challenge is to find agricultural methods that simultaneously are sustainable and provide adequate yields of good quality. Some experts believe that today's purely "organic farms" can exist because many are surrounded by farms where more aggressive pest control is practiced, providing some protection to neighboring farms.

There's no doubt that all of us need to be concerned about agricultural sustainability, but organic farming is not the only effective option. There is a spectrum of alternative methods that farmers can use to work toward sustainability. They might use techniques that reduce the use of chemicals without entirely eliminating them, or they might till their fields (plow the weeds under) rather than use a synthetic herbicide. They might rotate crops (vary the crops planted in a field from one growing season to another), a practice that can better maintain the nutrient contents of the soil and reduce the need for fertilizer. There's no one set of methods for sustainable farming; each farm ecosystem, and even each field within a farm, has different requirements (World Resources Institute, 1992). (Chapter 18 discusses sustainable agriculture more extensively.)

Now What Do You Think?

- Option 1 You decide to seek out and buy "organic food."
- Option 2 You decide not to use "organic food," considering it to be just another high-priced specialty market.
- Option 3 You decide to use either conventionally grown or "organic food," whichever is available, affordable, and of good quality, now and in the future.
- Option 4 You decide to buy, when feasible, from area farmers who use sustainable practices, but otherwise to buy whatever is sold at your favorite market.
- Option 5 You decide to pressure your market to stock more food from area farmers who use sustainable agricultural practices.

What other options do you see? Which do you choose?

though, you will get higher nutritional value from a just-mature fruit or vegetable than from one that was harvested either long before ripe or well past its prime.

Be aware that often fruits and vegetables marketed as "fresh" have been harvested and transported from a distance several weeks before they are purchased and consumed. Their nutritional values are very likely to be lower than a ripe, recently picked product. You may have assumed that the term *fresh* means recently picked, but on a food label, it doesn't. According to new labeling regulations, *fresh* simply means that the fruit or vegetable is raw: it has never been frozen or heated through (Congressional Federal Register, 1993).

Plants and Mineral Content Plants need certain minerals, such as potassium and magnesium, for survival; the level of these minerals found within a given variety of plant is usually quite constant. If the levels of these minerals in the soil are not high enough for the plants to achieve their genetically determined levels, the plants will not thrive, and the crop yield will be smaller.

The genetic makeup of some plants allows them to take up and store certain minerals for later use; for example, legumes store phosphorus in a form called *phytate* (as we discussed in Chapter 12), but grasses do not. Some plants can accumulate minerals, such as selenium and aluminum, in amounts that would be highly toxic to other plants. Tea plants grown in aluminum-laden soil, for instance, may contain levels of aluminum high enough to impair or kill other kinds of plants.

As we pointed out in Chapter 12, when certain minerals are in low concentration in soil, plants grown in that soil will be low in those minerals. Some elements that occur in plants in levels relative to amounts present in the soil are iodine, copper, manganese, cobalt, chromium, and molybdenum. Although the lack of these minerals apparently is not a problem to the plants themselves, mineral deficiency can become a problem to animals (including humans) that eat the plants. Ruminant animals that feed on forage grown in soil deficient in cobalt are thin and "poorly fleshed" (Ockerman, 1988), and people who consistently eat food grown in soil low in iodine develop goiters (see Figure 12.10).

Because most of us now eat foods that were produced in many different regions, it is quite unlikely that you would experience mineral deficiencies due to low levels in soil. Eating foods of different geographical origins is another dimension of eating a varied diet.

The Effects of Processing and Storage on Nutrients

Chances are that many of the foods you eat are not straight from the farm. Many have been processed first, either commercially or by you at home.

You Tell Me

Scientists define food processing as anything done to food after harvest to delay spoiling or to make food safer, more nutritious, more palatable, or more convenient. Technically, processed foods include not only highly processed convenience foods, such as single-serving entrees, but also minimally processed foods, such as a fresh fruit or vegetable that has been waxed.

According to this definition, which foods that you ate yesterday were minimally processed? Which were highly processed convenience foods? Which do you think were not processed in any way?

food processing—any method of food handling that discourages spoilage of food or enhances its safety, nutrition, palatability, and/or convenience

Although the number of processed foods—especially convenience foods—has skyrocketed in the last few decades, the practice of food processing is ancient (Koskinen, 1989). Grinding grain into flour and making cheese from various animal milks are processes of prehistoric origin, as are salting and drying meat, brewing, and wine-making. Evidence of bread-making dating back to about 5000 B.C. has been found in Europe and Asia.

We assume that many of these practices were discovered accidentally, but more recent developments have been intentional. For example, **canning** was developed in the early 1800s by confectioner Nicholas Appert, who was lured by the French government's offer of a prize to whoever developed a method of preserving food for Napoleon's army (Parmley, 1991). **Freezing** became feasible for retail foods in the 1920s when Clarence Birdseye invented a commercial process for freezing packaged foods quickly, and **pasteurization** was commercially implemented during the 1930s for improving the safety of milk.

Today's food processing methods are the result of many scientific advances. In 1989 the Institute of Food Technologists, the professional organization for food scientists, identified the following to be among the most important developments in food processing during their organization's half-century of existence:

- *High-temperature–short-term (HTST) processing and packaging* **High-temperature–short-term (HTST) processing** is used for practical ster-

canning—heating a food and its rigid container sufficiently to sterilize the contents

freezing—lowering a temperature of a food so far that enzymes and microorganisms are almost inactivated but not destroyed

pasteurization—heating a product at a temperature below its boiling point for less than a minute to kill most pathogens

high-temperature–short-term (HTST) processing—heating a product at higher temperatures and shorter times than are used in conventional pasteurization; practically sterilizes the product

FIGURE 13.4
Food processing is not new.

Although technology has advanced, this ancient limestone sculpture from a tomb at Giza, Egypt, of a woman grinding grain shows that food processing has been a common practice for thousands of years.

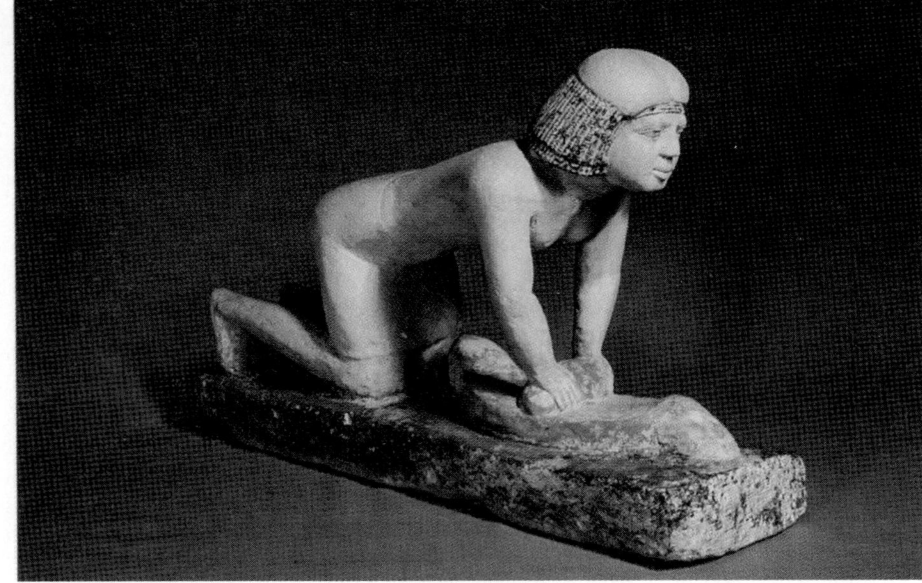

ilization of boxed fruit juices and allows for greater retention of aesthetic and nutritional quality; progress in plastics technology helped make it possible.

- *Refinement of commercial canning methods for vegetables* To ensure safety, specific procedures have been developed for different types of vegetables.
- *The microwave oven* By the year 2000, 90% of U.S. households are expected to have this convenient appliance.
- *Frozen concentrated citrus juices* This technology makes possible year-round access to food with a high vitamin C content.
- *Controlled-atmosphere packaging for fresh fruits and vegetables* In **controlled-atmosphere packaging,** fruits and vegetables are packaged, not in air, but in a harmless blend of gases that delays ripening and spoilage.
- *Freeze-drying* **Freeze-drying,** a moisture removal process, helps preserve product quality and retention of nutrients to a greater extent than other methods of drying. It can be used for a wide variety of foods and beverages.
- *Frozen meals* Specific conditions have been developed for different foods to maintain their aesthetic and nutritional quality.
- *Food fortification* **Fortification** makes it possible to guarantee that foods contain significant amounts of selected nutrients.
- *Ultra-high temperature (UHT), short-term sterilization of milk* **Ultra-high temperature (UHT)** is a variation of pasteurization that allows milk or cream to be stored unopened at room temperature for more than 90 days.

A process the food scientists did not put on their list is **irradiation,** which can be used to rid food of pests or to preserve food for longer-term storage. When food is irradiated, it is exposed to gamma rays, x-rays, or electron beams; this controls various food spoilage factors, conserves nutrients better than some other processes, but does *not* make the food radioactive.

controlled-atmosphere packaging—process in which proportions of oxygen and carbon dioxide within a storage facility or package are modified from proportions in air; delays ripening and rotting

freeze-drying—removal of moisture from food at very low temperatures

fortification—any addition of nutrients to foods during processing

ultra-high temperature (UHT) processing—sterilizing a food by using higher temperatures than are used for HTST processing

irradiation—using gamma rays, x-rays, or electron beams to kill microorganisms and control certain factors that cause food spoilage

Irradiation has been approved in the United States for only limited uses: disinfecting herbs and spices, controlling insects in wheat and wheat flour, inhibiting the sprouting of potatoes, controlling maturation and insects in fresh fruits and vegetables, reducing the risk of trichinosis from pork, and reducing the microorganisms on poultry. These processes require lower dosages of radiation than do longer-term preservation uses.

Although studies of irradiation of food began in the late 1940s, applications to the U.S. food supply have been few for a number of reasons: government regulations have not been fully developed; other effective and less expensive technologies for food preservation can be used; some scientists have reservations about certain chemicals formed in irradiated foods; and the general public has not been very receptive to the process (Schutz et al., 1989). Further, effective regulation would be very difficult, because irradiation leaves no easily measurable unique markers. Inspectors would therefore not be able to identify irradiated foods. Irradiation is used more extensively in some other countries, especially in the processing of seafood.

You Tell Me

In January 1992, a company called Vindicator opened its doors in Florida for the purpose of large-scale irradiation of food. After 9 months, the business had lost close to a million dollars (Community Nutrition Institute, 1992). Industry watchers speculated that business was poor because food processors and distributors feared that consumers would not buy irradiated products.

Would you buy food that you knew had been irradiated? If not, why not? Are there questions you would like answered before using irradiated foods? Do you think that irradiated foods should be labeled as irradiated if they are not nutritionally different from their nonirradiated counterparts?

Food technologists have data to show that, overall, all of these processes result in foods that are high in nutritional quality as well as convenient, safe, and appealing. However, some people dispute this conclusion. They claim that commercially processed food is not of good nutritional quality, pointing to the fact that most processes cause some degree of nutrient destruction. Others question the safety of some processes, a topic we cover in Chapter 14. Still others criticize processed food because of its higher cost or the environmental problems created by its packaging.

It is difficult to say whether processed or unprocessed foods are "better," because your values come into play along with the facts. For example, are you willing to trade off more convenience for the somewhat reduced levels of nutrients that often come with it? In this section, we discuss how food processing impacts the nutritional matters consumers are most concerned about—fat and cholesterol, sodium, and other vitamins and minerals.

The Effects of Food Processing on Fat and Cholesterol

The level of lipids, including cholesterol, in food can be increased or decreased, depending on the processing methods used. Because many of us are particularly concerned about having less fat in food, we'll focus on ways processors can reduce fat in various types of food.

Meats and Poultry An easy way to eat less fat is to trim off obvious layers of fat from meat. Whereas meat cutters used to leave a border of approximately half an inch of fat around a cut of fresh meat, they have reduced it to about one-eighth of an inch. Producers of processed meat have also responded to this consumer demand. Products such as hams and sliced sandwich meats that are 95% fat-free (by weight) are very popular; the small amount of fat that remains is within or between the muscle cells (Rust, 1988).

But not all products have easily lent themselves to fat reduction; the fat content of sausages has been more difficult to modify. In traditional cooked sausage, such as a frankfurter, fat usually is 25–30% of the weight of the product. Early attempts to lower the fat content significantly resulted in a rubbery product. Another approach was to use a lower-fat meat. Frankfurters made from poultry contain 18–22% fat (by weight), which is lower than the amount in their beef counterparts, but still relatively high (Mast and Clouser, 1988). New regulations allow versions in which water, starch, and milk proteins that have been subjected to hydrolysis are combined with lean ground meats, bringing the fat content to as little as 3%. Because of their additional ingredients, these products are moist, tender, and flavorful.

Another meat of concern is fried chicken—the mainstay of many restaurants, carry-out food shops, and retail frozen foods—because fat can account for as much as 60% of its kcalories. In response to consumer interest, the food industry has developed new cooking systems, such as removing the skin of the chicken and cooking the meat in hot air, which can reduce the proportion of kcalories derived from fat to less than 30% (Mast and Clouser, 1988).

Prepared Meals and Entrees You can find prepared meals and entrees that range from high to low in fat, depending on the ingredients used. A portion of frozen lasagna could have 20 grams of fat, whereas a serving of chicken teriyaki with rice might have only 3 grams. If you're looking for less fat, check the nutrition facts panel on the product.

You Tell Me

You can get a false sense of security from seeing terms such as *reduced-calorie* or *light* on product labels. If you're looking for a low-fat food, will products that make these claims fill the bill?

Do you remember what these two terms mean? (If not, check Table 9.4.) Are products that carry a "reduced-calorie" or "light" claim necessarily low in fat?

Eggs Various methods are used to lower the cholesterol content of processed (out of the shell) eggs; these products represent about 15% of all eggs consumed. Because the yolk of the egg contains the cholesterol, some low-cholesterol egg products are made by removing the yolk and then mixing the egg white with vegetable oil, food coloring, and other ingredients to yield a product that resembles blended whole eggs.

CONTAINS: Sugar, enriched bleached flour [bleached flour, niacin, iron, thiamin mononitrate (vitamin B-1), riboflavin (vitamin B-2)], partially hydrogenated soybean oil with BHA, BHT and citric acid added to protect flavor, corn starch, dextrose, modified tapioca starch, baking powder (baking soda, sodium aluminum phosphate, monocalcium phosphate), propylene glycol monoesters, salt, mono- and diglycerides, artificial flavor, sodium phosphate, calcium acetate, cellulose gum, xanthan gum, polysorbate 60, lecithin, artificial color and FD&C Yellow No. 5.

INGREDIENTS

Enriched flour (bleached flour, niacin, reduced iron, thiamin mononitrate, riboflavin), sugar, animal and/or vegetable shortening (contains one more of the following partially hydrogenated fats: cottonseed oil, beef fat, lard, palm oil) freshness preserved with BHA and citric acid, dextrose, leavening (baking soda, sodium aluminum phosphate, dicalcium phosphate), modified corn starch, salt, propylene glycol mono esters, mono- and diglycerides, guar gum, artificial flavor, soy lecithin, FD&C Yellow No. 5&6.

FIGURE 13.5
Want to stay in control of what you're eating?

Then read labels: with lots of choices on the market, you can often find a convenience food that contains what you want. The ingredient lists above (from cake mixes) are for products made with different kinds of shortening.

A newer version does not include the vegetable oil, making the product virtually fat-free as well as cholesterol-free. Other approaches are to extract some of the cholesterol from a whole-egg mixture by using a solvent or cornstarch, or to add extra egg white to a whole-egg mixture.

Because some products are only partially reduced in cholesterol, you need to read food labels to determine the content of a given product.

Milk and Dairy Products You can now find most dairy products in a range of fat contents: milk, yogurt, cheese, frozen desserts, and even sour cream are available with varying fat levels. For example, the fat content of frozen dairy desserts ranges from 24 grams per cup for "premium" ice creams to almost no fat in some frozen yogurts and ice milks. Although natural cheeses generally have 7–9 grams of fat per ounce, you can buy cheese products that contain only a few grams of fat or almost none. These products may have a different *mouth-feel* (sensations of texture and consistency) and may behave differently from traditional cheeses when used as ingredients in recipes, especially if you need to cook or bake the product.

Dairy products are also a source of cholesterol: a cup of whole milk contains 33 mg. Because 85% of the cholesterol in milk is associated with the milk fat, removing all or part of the fat also reduces the cholesterol. A cup of skim milk has an insignificant 5 milligrams of cholesterol.

Baked Grain Products Baked grain products vary considerably in fat content, from 1 gram in a slice of most yeast-raised breads to more than 20 grams in a piece of rich cake. Besides the quantity of fat in these products, you may want to consider the *type* of fat they contain. Some products use butter or hydrogenated fats, which are more saturated; liquid vegetable oils are less saturated.

You can influence the market with your choices: when producers become aware of consumer concern about certain food constituents, food companies usually respond with new products that provide a wider range of options within their product lines. As usual, label reading is key to getting what you want (Figure 13.5).

Effect of Food Processing on Sodium Content

As you learned in Chapter 12 and Table 12.5, nature puts relatively little sodium in food. Most of the sodium you consume comes from salt that is added to food, and 75% of Americans' salt intake comes from processed food (National Academy of Sciences, 1989). Other sodium compounds—such as monosodium glutamate, sodium nitrite, sodium bicarbonate (baking soda) and sodium citrate—probably account for less than 10% of the sodium in your diet. Therefore, as you would expect, our discussion of how to lower the sodium content of food focuses on processed foods.

If you want to keep track of your sodium intake, the new food labeling regulations work in your favor. As of May 1994, nutrition facts, including sodium content, are to be listed on all processed food product packages, and descriptors such as *sodium-free* and *reduced sodium* may be displayed when appropriate (Table 12.6).

Processed Meats The level of sodium in processed meats today is approximately 15 times the level in fresh meats, largely because of the addition of salt and sodium nitrite. Salt has three major functions in these products: preservation, promotion of stability, and flavor enhancement. Nitrites aid in preservation and coloring. Because these compounds serve multiple purposes, and because consumers seem to prefer the taste of foods that contain them, the industry has not wanted to reduce their levels to a very great extent.

Two concerns in recent decades have led to the reduction of sodium nitrite in most processed meat products. In the late 1970s, the food industry voluntarily reduced levels when the safety of nitrites was questioned. (We discuss this further in Chapter 14.) In the 1980s, interest in reducing sodium in the food supply led the industry to reduce the levels in cooked sausage by an estimated 20% (Rust, 1988).

Another approach to reducing sodium is to use compounds such as potassium chloride as a partial substitute for sodium chloride. Substituting more than about one-third of the salt, however, results in unacceptable flavors (Mast and Clouser, 1988).

Canned Soups and Vegetables USDA data published in 1980 indicate that the amounts of sodium in 8 ounces of ready-to-eat canned soup range between 900 and 1100 mg, and reconstituted dehydrated soups usually contain 1000–1300 mg per serving. This is a huge amount of sodium for one food item, considering that the recommended upper limit for sodium intake is 2400 mg per day from salt (Committee on Diet and Health, 1989).

Some commercial soup companies have lowered the sodium content of their products since 1980 when the USDA data were published; according to information from labels, one popular brand of canned soup now ranges between 700 and 900 mg per serving. The same soup maker markets an additional line of soups with one-third less salt, but even these products are significant sources of sodium (450–600 mg/serving).

Canned vegetables generally have about 300 mg of sodium per 1/2-cup serving, most of it from added salt. (Fresh vegetables usually contain less than 10 mg/serving.)

Vegetables pickled in brine are very high in sodium. One dill pickle contains about 930 mg of sodium, and the 1/2 cup of sauerkraut you have on your Reuben sandwich has a similar amount.

You Tell Me

A local diner offers a daily lunch special of a ham and cheese sandwich with a dill pickle and potato chips. Check Appendix C for the sodium content of these lunch items.

Which two items have the most sodium? Suggest two ways of altering the menu, to substantially reduce the sodium content. (Make changes you would accept.)

Effects of Food Processing on Vitamin and Mineral Contents

The body of scientific literature regarding the effects of processing on nutrients is huge. A respected reference on these matters, *Nutritional Evaluation of Food Processing* by E. Karmas and R.S. Harris (1988), is a volume of almost 800 pages—and it claims only to summarize the work in this field. Our approach here is even more general: to discuss *principles* that affect micronutrients rather than to deal with the details of particular products processed under specific conditions.

Generally speaking, a product loses a portion of vitamins and minerals during processing, and the losses are cumulative when multiple processes are used. Vitamins are more vulnerable to destruction than minerals are; of the vitamins, vitamin C and thiamin break down and lose their function most readily. Losses can occur from exposure to oxygen, light, or heat; a particular pH; the passage of time; or physical separation, such as the removal of bran layers from grain. Table 13.2 indicates which micronutrients are unstable in the presence of some of these conditions.

Notice that heat negatively affects the greatest number of nutrients. This is an important point, because most methods of food processing involve heat in some way. (An exception is irradiation, which involves little increase in

TABLE 13.2 Stability of Vitamins

	Effect of pH					
Vitamin	Neutral pH	Acid pH	Alkaline pH	Air or Oxygen	Light	Heat
Vitamin A	S	U	S	U	U	U
Carotene (pro-A)	S	U	S	U	U	U
Vitamin D	S		U	U	U	U
Vitamin E	S	S	S	U	U	U
Vitamin K	S	U	U	S	U	S
Thiamin	U	S	U	U	S	U
Riboflavin	S	S	U	S	U	U
Niacin	S	S	S	S	S	S
Vitamin B-6	S	S	S	S	U	U
Folic acid	U	U	S	U	U	U
Vitamin B-12	S	S	S	U	U	S
Biotin	S	S	S	S	S	U
Pantothenic acid	S	U	U	S	S	U
Vitamin C	U	S	U	U	U	U

S = stable (no important destruction)
U = unstable (significant destruction)
Source: Adapted from Karmas and Harris, 1988.

temperature.) But heat is widely used because it serves many very beneficial purposes. It is the most common way of killing pathogenic organisms and controlling spoilage; it makes many foods more digestible; and it may protect against "off" flavors, loss of color, and poor texture (Dietz and Erdman, 1989). Commercial processors are careful to use only enough heat to achieve the benefits, because energy is expensive. This financial thrift results in nutritional savings as well.

To retain the food's sensory and nutritional quality, commercial processors also carefully choose the most suitable packaging materials and storage conditions.

Because of the advanced technology and precise controls used in most commercial processing operations, such products are likely to contain a higher proportion of the original nutrients than the same food processed at home. For example, you are not likely to be able to pick, clean, process, package, and freeze the peas in your garden as quickly or under as carefully controlled conditions as the workers in a commercial plant can—and this is likely to be reflected to some degree in lower nutrient values in your home-frozen peas.

Passage of time is another factor that affects nutrients. The micronutrient content of processed foods tends to decrease gradually during storage, but these losses occur much more slowly than would have occurred in the fresh food. You can minimize losses in processed foods by storing them at lower temperatures. Canned foods retain over 90% of their vitamin C during one year of storage, provided that the storage temperature doesn't exceed 20°C (68°F) (Gilbert, 1988). Frozen foods should be stored at −18°C (0°F) or below; if they are stored at −7°C (20°F), losses of vitamin C are substantially higher (Fennema, 1988).

Although nutrient loss is characteristic of processing, there are also situations in which processing actually *increases* the food's nutrient contents. Nutrients are sometimes deliberately added—for example, in the fortification process. A broad array of products, from baked products to soft drink mixes, now contain added nutrients. The process of **fermentation** also increases the levels of some nutrients in certain products. For example, in the production and aging of cheese, niacin and folic acid levels increase (McFeeters, 1988).

fermentation—process in which microorganisms metabolize components of a food, changing the composition and taste of the product

Probably the greatest positive impact of food processing on nutritional value is that processing has made many foods year-round commodities rather than just seasonal ones available only after harvest. This means that your diet can be more varied during all 12 months of the year—and a varied diet is likely to be more nutritious than one that relies only on the limited number of foods in season. For this reason, the development of the canning process may have been the most significant advance toward decreasing nutritional deficiency diseases (Dietz and Erdman, 1989).

Now that you understand these general principles, let's look at some types of foods whose micronutrients are particularly affected by processing.

Fruits Processed fruits can retain high levels of vitamins because of their acidic nature. Freezing does a better job of retaining vitamin activity in these foods than does canning or **dehydration**. Frozen orange juice, one of the most commonly consumed processed fruit products, loses only 5% of its vitamin C; most other frozen fruit products retain over 70% of their original amounts (Fennema, 1988). Losses of vitamins in canned fruit are generally somewhat higher.

dehydration—removal of moisture from food; can be accomplished by various methods

It is more difficult to generalize about vitamin losses in dried fruits, because there are many different processes causing different amounts of loss.

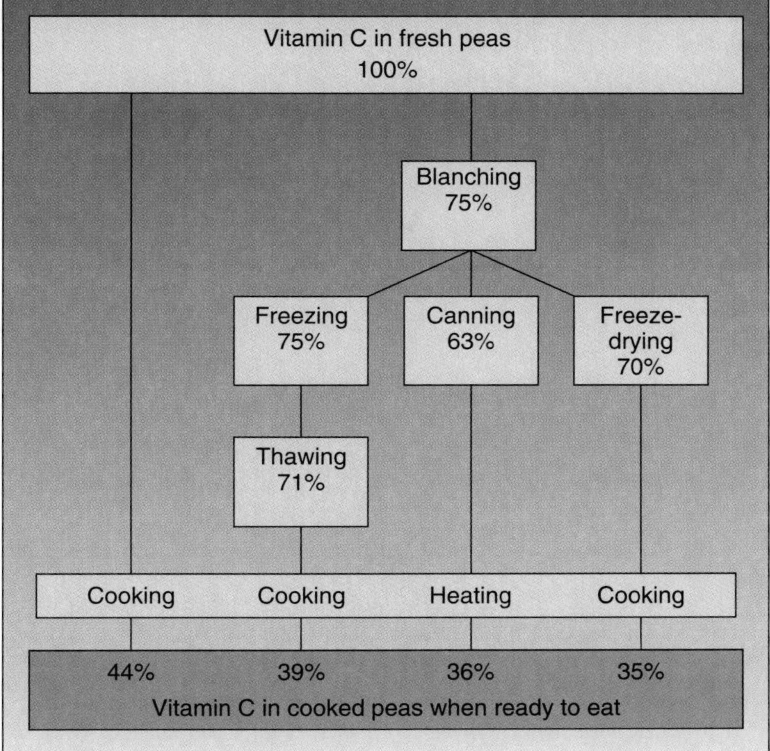

FIGURE 13.6
The bottom line: the nutrient value of a food as you eat it.

Different food preservation techniques decrease nutrient content by varying amounts. However, by the time you have cooked the food and are ready to eat it, there may not be much difference in nutritional value. This illustration indicates the percentage of vitamin C retained in peas processed by currently common methods and then prepared for eating. Remember that fresh peas that are not used immediately after harvest start losing vitamin value quickly; after 2 days of refrigeration, fresh vegetables are likely to have *lower* values than their commercially preserved counterparts.
Source: Tannenbaum et al., 1985.

A major factor is the amount of water removed; the *drier* the final product, the *better* the vitamin C retention. Freeze-drying, which is quick and thorough, causes very little vitamin C loss (Bluestein and LaBuza, 1988). Sun-drying, a more lengthy process that does not dry a product very thoroughly, by contrast, leaves little vitamin C intact (Adams and Erdman, 1988). When an elaborate series of processes is involved, vitamin losses can be high. For example, apple flakes made by slicing, **blanching**, pureeing, and finally drying the product between hot drums have only about 30% of the apple's original vitamin C (Bluestein and LaBuza, 1988).

blanching—heating a food with boiling water, steam, and/or microwaves for just long enough to destroy many of the enzymes that reduce palatability and nutritive value; often followed by further processing

Vegetables You usually get the best nutrient quality from vegetables if you harvest them at their prime and consume them soon after. The micronutrients in vegetables are more vulnerable than those in fruits because vegetables are less acidic. Their less-stable vitamins start losing activity quickly, even when vegetables are kept cool after harvest: after 2 days of refrigeration, nutritional values of fresh vegetables generally have fallen below what the same vegetable, preserved right after harvest, would contain (Fennema, 1988).

Does it matter what method of food preservation was used—whether canning, dehydration, or freezing? Not much, if you compare the nutritional contents of different processed forms of the same vegetable *when they are ready to eat.* As Figure 13.6 shows, although common commercial processing methods differ somewhat in destruction of nutrients, vegetables, once they've been cooked or heated prior to being served, are quite similar in nutritional content. Because the data in this figure are for highly destructible vitamin C, they show more substantial losses than would occur with most other nutrients. Of course, if you cook your fresh or frozen vegetables so they're still crisp, you'll lose less vitamin C than if you cook them until they're as tender as canned vegetables.

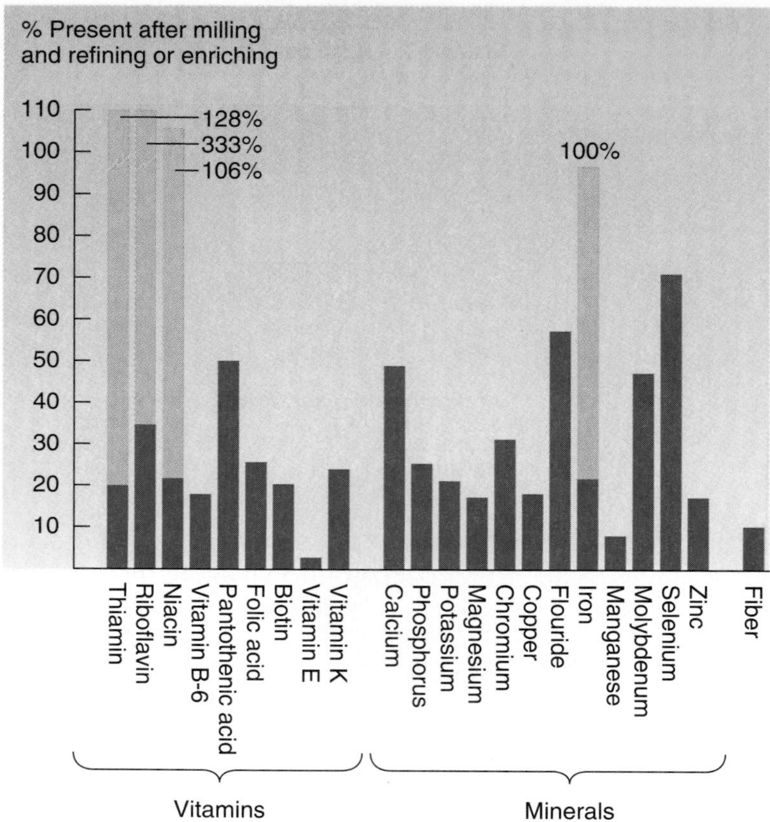

FIGURE 13.7
Proportions of some nutrients present in wheat flour after refining and enrichment.

On this graph, 100% represents the nutrients found in whole wheat. The most commonly used refined flour (darker bars) contains less than half the amount of many nutrients present in whole wheat. Enriched flour (lighter extension of bars) has had only four nutrients added: thiamin, riboflavin, niacin, and iron. *Source:* Data from Davis, 1981.

Grain Products The way grain is processed has a major impact on its nutritional value. Whole grains have three major portions. The tough, darker, outer layers are the *bran* layers; the region toward the end of the kernel from which sprouting occurs is the *germ*; and the lighter, larger, inner starchy portion is the *endosperm.* (Figure 5.10, in the chapter on carbohydrate, shows these areas in a kernel of wheat.)

milling—the grinding of grain into flour

refining—separation of the coarser bran and germ particles from the endosperm early in the milling process

Milling is the grinding of grain into flour. The bran layers and the germ do not break down as readily as the endosperm does. This characteristic makes them relatively easy to separate from the powdered endosperm early in the milling process. Such separation is called **refining.**

Different types of flour are produced by controlling the relative proportions of powdered endosperm, ground bran layers, and germ. Whole-grain flour contains all parts; refined flours have had some or all of the bran and germ sifted out. This is significant because the germ and bran layers contain most of the vitamins, minerals, and fiber that are in the grain, whereas the endosperm is largely starch.

The method of milling wheat into refined flour in the United States results in losses of 50–90% of approximately 20 nutrients (Sebrell, 1992). Figure 13.7 shows the percentages of micronutrients found in refined flour compared with whole-wheat flour. Other whole-grain products readily available in the United States are brown rice, dark rye flour, and rolled oats.

enrichment—the addition of nutrients already present in a food to levels that meet a specific FDA standard

Some of the nutrients lost during milling and refining of flour are replaced by **enrichment,** a process in use since 1941. In this process, thiamin, riboflavin, niacin, and iron are added to specific levels established by FDA standards. In the United States, refined grain products such as wheat flours, bread, rolls and buns, farina, cornmeal, corn grits, pastas, and rice are commonly enriched.

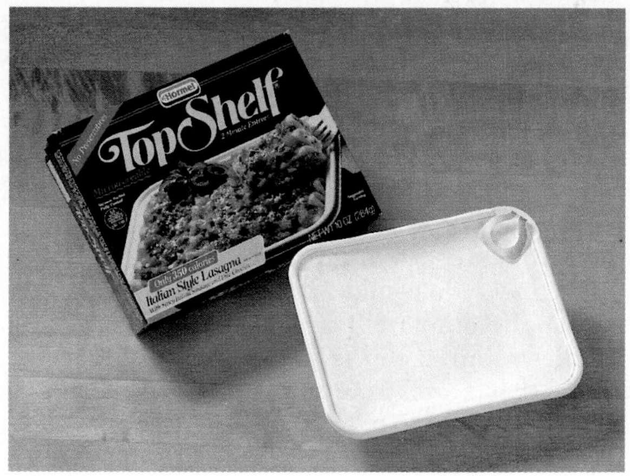

FIGURE 13.8
A new form of packaging that helps preserve nutrients.

Food that is processed in a flexible, laminated retort container and sterilized as a unit can be stored at room temperature. Because these packages are quite flat, less time is required to heat the contents, and less loss of heat-vulnerable nutrients occurs.

Figure 13.7 also shows how enriched wheat flour compares nutritionally with refined and whole-wheat flours. Enriched products are clearly second best to whole grain products, because only four nutrients are added back. Although it is feasible to restore other nutrients to grain products—and this was proposed by the National Academy of Sciences almost 20 years ago—the proposal has never been acted on by the FDA (Sebrell, 1992).

Milk Fresh milk is typically pasteurized, a heating process that kills most pathogenic organisms but does not destroy all microorganisms or their spores. Because the treatment is not very severe or very long, nutrient damage does not exceed 10% of vitamins present in significant quantities. Even lower losses occur with high-temperature–short-time (HTST) processing, which ensures the same degree of safety. Because these two processes produce safer but not sterile products, the milk must be refrigerated to discourage growth of remaining microorganisms.

Yet another variation of pasteurization, ultra-high temperature (UHT) processing, produces a sterile product because of the still higher temperature used. UHT-processed milk can be stored at room temperature for many months as long as it is unopened. Because of the very short time during which heat is applied, nutrient losses are as low as those of traditional pasteurization (Lund, 1988). UHT milk is more heavily marketed in Canada and Europe than in the United States, although it has also been used by the U.S. military (Baird, 1991).

Prepared Meals and Entrees The use of prepared meals and entrees has increased tremendously in recent years. Canned convenience foods have long been available, but the most dramatic new increase has been in frozen meals and entrees. A more recent innovation is foods processed in a **flexible retort pouch** or similar flat, laminated container that can be stored at room temperature (Figure 13.8). These were highly visible as the MREs (Meals, Ready-to-Eat) eaten by U.S. troops in Operation Desert Shield in Saudi Arabia in 1990 (Baird, 1991).

flexible retort pouch—a multilayered food package that can be sealed by heat; can withstand high temperatures needed to sterilize contents

Generally, when you eat prepared meals and entrees—whether they've been frozen, canned, or sealed in a retort container—you should expect to get somewhat lower levels of nutrients than you would get from a comparable product that was freshly made and immediately served. Processing the product and reheating the food before you eat it both take their toll on nutrient content.

Some people think of flexible retort containers as similar to cans; in both processes, the product is sealed into the container and sterilized afterward. However, because the retort container is quite flat compared with a can, heat can completely penetrate the product in only one-half to two-thirds the time needed for the same item in a can; this shorter processing time leads to less nutrient destruction (Dietz and Erdman, 1989).

Imitation Foods Advances in food technology have enabled the food industry to produce food look-alikes that are very different substances from the foods they attempt to imitate. For example, you can buy a product that looks and tastes like crabmeat but is actually a less expensive fish; you may also see something that seems like mayonnaise but isn't. Such foods are sometimes produced as a cheaper alternative to the real thing, or they may be designed to avoid an undesirable constituent, such as the fat and cholesterol in mayonnaise. In either case, the nutritional value of the new product may be considerably different from that of the food it resembles.

If a food producer markets a product that has significantly less protein and micronutrients than the food it looks like, and if the producer wants to use on the label the name of the food it mimics, then the product must be labeled as an **imitation** food.

imitation food—product that has measurably less protein or other nutrients than the reference food

It is not possible to make a blanket statement about whether imitation foods are better or worse for you than the foods they resemble. It depends on what the product is made of, how much of it you eat, and what your needs are.

You Tell Me

Because egg yolks are removed from imitation egg mixtures, they lose much of the vitamin A, folic acid, vitamin B-12, iron, and zinc as well as all of the cholesterol found in the original eggs. Although some of these losses are restored with additives, the imitation eggs still are nutritionally inferior. However, this product can be very useful to some people.

For whom are imitation egg mixtures most valuable? For whom do they seem unnecessary? Would they be useful to you?

Sugars Some people believe that "less refined" or "more natural" sources of sugar are substantially more nutritious than white sugar. Although it is true that there are differences in the nutritional values of various sweeteners, these differences are minor. As Table 13.3 shows, white sugar, brown sugar, honey, maple syrup, and molasses are all very low in nutrients and contribute only a tiny amount of the nutrients we need every day.

Foods of the Future Considering the variety of processed foods that are currently available, what new developments could possibly be ahead? Some food futurists believe that the sky's the limit. They suggest that the foods of the future will be whatever you want: consumers will have only to define what "bundles of characteristics" they want in their foods, and food scientists will be able to design products to satisfy consumer interests.

Is that scenario likely to be realized soon? Would such products be nutritious and safe? Find out what food scientist Susan Harlander forsees in the expert interview on page 444.

TABLE 13.3 Nutritional Content of One Tablespoon of Various Concentrated Sweets

Food (1 tablespoon)	Nutrients	% of the U.S. RDA: 0 — 25 — 50 — 75 — 100
White sugar	Calcium	
	Iron	
	Thiamin	
	Riboflavin	
	Niacin	
Brown sugar	Calcium	
	Iron	
	Thiamin	
	Riboflavin	
	Niacin	
Light molasses	Calcium	
	Iron	
	Thiamin	
	Riboflavin	
	Niacin	
Honey	Calcium	
	Iron	
	Thiamin	
	Riboflavin	
	Niacin	
Maple syrup	Calcium	
	Iron	
	Thiamin	
	Riboflavin	
	Niacin	

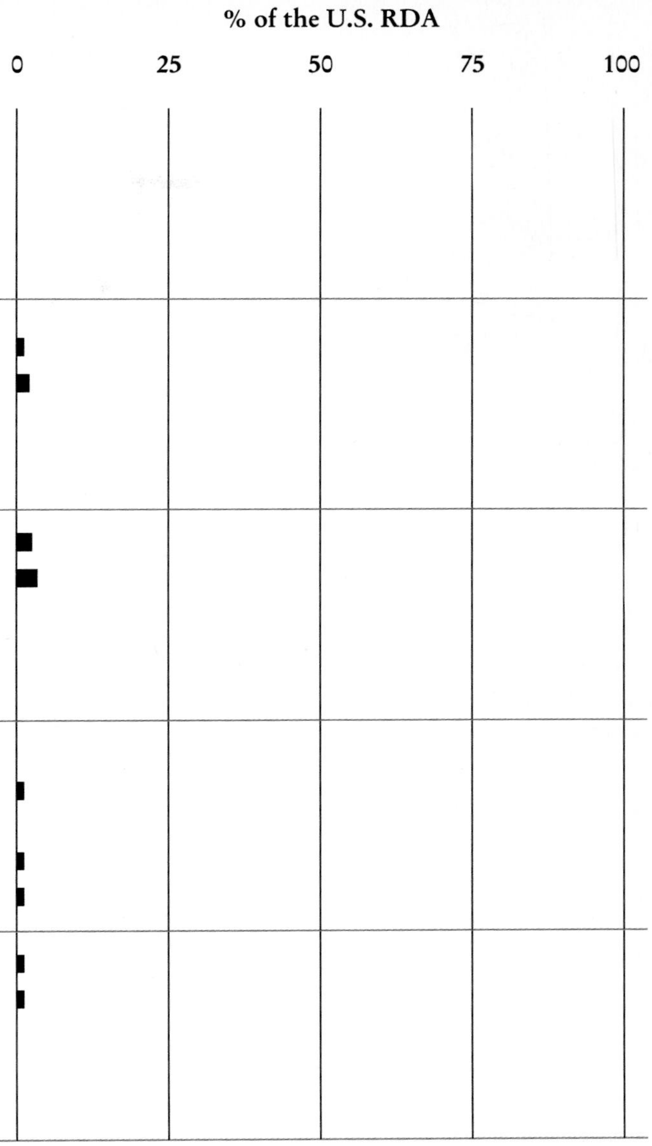

Of the foods commonly used as sweeteners, none is a significant source of protein, vitamin A, or vitamin C— but they all contain from 42 to 56 kcalories per tablespoon.

Data sources: Pennington, J. 1989; Science and Education Administration, 1985.

Retaining Nutrients at Home

Once you bring food home, what happens to its nutritional value is up to you. In the remainder of this chapter you'll learn how your handling of food at home affects its content of minerals and vitamins.

As you read, keep in mind the techniques for reducing fat and cholesterol and controlling sodium during home preparation of food, which we discussed in Chapters 6 and 12, respectively. One reminder as you try to find alternative ways to flavor your foods: remember that many flavoring agents contain significant amounts of sodium.

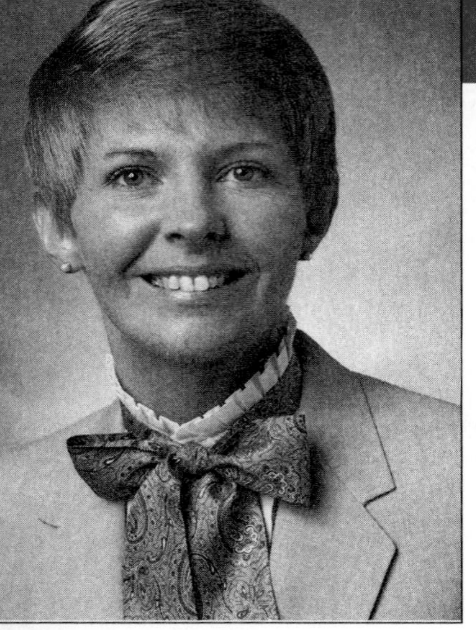

Interview with Susan Harlander, PhD

Foods of the Future

What foods will we eat in the twenty-first century? And how will we know that they are safe and nutritious? For several years Dr. Susan Harlander has been committed to explaining to the public how biotechnology is being used to create the foods of the future. As she describes in this interview, more nutritious, less wasteful, and less expensive foods may be the result. Formerly a faculty member in the department of Food Science and Nutrition at the University of Minnesota, Dr. Harlander is currently Director of Dairy Foods Research and Development at Land O'Lakes, Inc.

How did you get involved in the demanding schedule of public lectures on food biotechnology that you've had for several years?

From 1985 to 1992 I was an assistant professor and then an associate professor of food biotechnology. I decided at that point to move into an administrative position, because I felt that the scientists in the university were not responding to what society needed. As scientists, we need to spend a lot more time educating the public about what we are doing. And as we move toward applying science and technology to agriculture, it is going to be even more important. It was very important to me to talk to people about food, about agriculture, about the genetic modification that has been going on in nature for hundreds of years with our traditional techniques. With that understanding, I felt people could make better decisions about the new technology that is going to be used to improve the food supply in the future.

What are the most exciting trends in the food industry right now?

I think the food industry is going to be driven by what the consumer wants, and the consumer is going to be driven by a number of factors, including health consciousness. I think more and more kids have recognized the connection between food and health. So you're going to see a lot of foods that are rich in the nutrients that nutritionists tell us are important.

I think the ultimate trend will be for each of us to have a diet based on our own genetic make-up. Even if we're the same size, sex, and age, we probably metabolize foods very differently. Right now our recommended dietary allowances for foods are based on what the general population needs. As we understand more about human metabolism, we are going to find the genetic markers that will tell us how you and I metabolize food differently. Therefore, I think that in the future—probably 20 years from now—we'll be designing individual diets based on my body's needs, not the population's needs.

Another driving force in the food industry is going to be convenience. I'm not willing to spend more than ten minutes cooking dinner anymore; I don't think most people are. So demographics, such as the number of women in the work force who have children, are also going to drive the food industry.

What are some examples of how biotechnology can be used by the food industry in response to these trends?

Corn, like all cereal grains, is deficient in certain amino acids. In countries that rely on corn as their main source of protein, that protein is not sufficient to sustain growth. Biotechnology can be used to modify the biochemical pathways for the production of those amino acids so that we can get an increased amount of the amino acids that are normally deficient in those grains.

Many of the oils that we consume are too high in saturated fats. By making very small genetic changes, we can modify the fatty acids that are present in those oils. If nutritionists tell us that the best oil we can consume has a particular fatty acid composition, then we should be able to modify the plant so that it produces that fatty acid profile.

The first genetically modified food to be approved will probably be a tomato that has a single gene that's been deactivated. That single gene codes for an enzyme that breaks down the tomato fruit when it is ripening. Although it isn't a direct nutritional improvement, extension of shelf life and maintaining flavor and texture are also important.

What other aspects of biotechnology do you think will be important in the food industry?

We add literally hundreds of ingredients to different food products: acids, flavors, sweeteners, thickeners, antioxidants, vitamins, amino acids, and enzymes. All of those things are derived from microorganisms. Many people don't realize that. Biotechnology can be used to make those processes more efficient and less expensive, so ultimately I think it will decrease the cost of food.

Biotechnology is also being used in waste management.

For example, in the dairy processing industry, for every ten pounds of milk, we get nine pounds of whey and one pound of cheese. So when we make cheese, nine-tenths of the material is waste. Up until several years ago, the whey used to be pumped out onto fields with the assumption that microorganisms in the soil would digest all the protein and it wouldn't be an environmental problem. Now we know that we need to convert that whey into something of value. The Japanese have taken the genetically engineered bacterium that produces the hepatitis B vaccine and they grow it on whey.

How do we detect microorganisms that can cause disease in foods, or agricultural residues, or pesticides or herbicides that are present in fruits? Using two different techniques of biotechnology—DNA probes and monoclonal antibodies—we can develop rapid detection systems that will tell us if there is a pathogenic microorganism present and the food isn't safe to eat. Although now there are quality control tests done in the lab, the ultimate goal is to have something like a dipstick—you take a little strip of paper, stick it in the food, and it changes color. The farmer can test his or her own milk right on the farm using dipstick tests. If there are any agricultural chemicals or any pathogenic organisms there, the strip turns a different color, and that milk never gets into the food supply.

Are guidelines suggested by the FDA adequate to control biotechnology in the food industry? Does it take too long to gain approval from the FDA for new processes and products?

RIght now I think the guidelines are appropriate. I think the public needs to be assured that someone is taking a look at these foods and that they are okay. For the first companies going through that FDA process it is going to be arduous, but at this stage I think we still need to continue to regulate on a case-by-case basis. As we gain experience, those guidelines can be relaxed.

Few people realize that you and I could breed a vegetable in our backyard and we could market that vegetable without getting FDA approval—in fact, without getting any regulatory approval—because food is food, and food is considered safe. As long as we are not creating some very unusual thing that's never been in the diet before, there has never been any approval process. We regulate food by the product. The controversy has existed because we are now producing food by a new process. What the FDA is being asked is: Shouldn't you be regulating the process of genetic engineering, not the final product?

To me, genetic engineering is safer than the breeding that we've been doing for hundreds of years. When we breed crops, we take the fifty or sixty thousand genes from one corn plant and we mix it with the fifty or sixty thousand genes from another plant, and we have no idea what all those genes encode. With genetic engineering, we take a single gene and put it into a crop that we've already had a lot of experience with.

When can we expect the first genetically engineered foods to be in our supermarkets?

The FDA is looking at the tomato with extended shelf life, and I anticipate that that's probably going to be approved this year. That will be one of the first products, but there are lots of them in field trials. They are already testing potatoes with a higher starch content that prevents them from absorbing a lot of oil when you make French fries or potato chips. I would guess the potatoes will be one of the next foods for which approval will be sought. But I think that within the next five years, we're going to have a whole variety.

Vitamins and Minerals

As you learned in the section on commercial processing, exposing food to oxygen, light, heat, and various levels of pH results in micronutrient losses, and these losses increase with time. Other factors, such as loss of moisture, can also be damaging. These factors continue to affect food during home storage and preparation. Careless handling of food at home can bring about more micronutrient losses than are caused by commercial processing.

This section gives you suggestions for how to keep these losses to a minimum.

Storage of Fresh Foods When you refrigerate fresh foods such as milk, meat, fruits, and vegetables, you probably do it to keep them safe to eat. At the same time, you get another benefit: refrigeration helps retain nutrients. For example, refrigerated vegetables lose only one-fourth to one-third of the amount of vitamin C they would have lost at room temperature.

You also need to protect food against moisture loss. The faster a product loses moisture, the greater its micronutrient losses will be. Vegetables are most vulnerable, because, unlike most fruits, many are not equipped with the heavy peels that reduce moisture loss. If the vegetables you buy are not wrapped, wrap them as air-tight as possible before refrigerating them. Storing vegetables and fruits in your refrigerator's produce drawers also helps them retain moisture.

As you learned in the discussion of commercial processing, the micronutrients in fresh vegetables deteriorate more readily than those in meats and fresh fruits. If you don't eat fresh vegetables soon after harvesting, progressive vitamin deterioration occurs; vitamin C and the fat-soluble vitamins are most vulnerable to loss in typical oxygen-containing environments. This is another reason to wrap food well. But even with proper storage, don't let food sit too long: you'll get better nutrition from refrigerated foods if you eat them as soon as possible.

Preparing Food Down to the last minute—even while you are doing final preparation of your food—you need to take measures to preserve micronutrients. If you're not careful, the greatest micronutrient losses of all can occur during this stage.

Cutting away edible parts of fruits and vegetables causes nutrient losses, both because you are throwing away some of the food and because you are exposing the rest to oxygen. The vitamin values of the discarded parts may be higher (per unit weight) than those of the parts kept to eat. For example, the vitamin C in potatoes is present in highest concentrations in the layer just beneath the skin, and the vitamin A content of leafy green vegetables is highest in the outer, darkest leaves.

Cutting or chopping food partially destroys any vitamins that are vulnerable to oxygen. Dividing food into smaller pieces produces a larger total surface area that comes in contact with oxygen and leads to vitamin destruction. It makes sense to wait as long as possible before cutting food up for a meal.

Cooking or heating food just before serving is the final assault on its micronutrients. Heat, as you've learned, has a damaging effect on most nutrients; the higher the temperature and the longer the heat is applied, the greater the losses. The best approach for protecting nutrients is to use as low a temperature for as short a time as possible, but you have to cook food hot enough and long enough to ensure that what you have prepared is safe to eat. (More on this in Chapter 14.)

To retain micronutrients in foods at home, during storage of

This	*Consider this*
Fruits and vegetables that have a rind or peel	**Refrigerate in the produce drawer (except bananas); eat peels if edible; remove inedible peels just before eating or cooking**
Fruits and vegetables that do not have a rind or peel	**Wrap with moisture barrier and refrigerate in produce drawer; do not cut up until just before using**
Frozen foods	**Keep in freezer at -18°C (0°F) or below**
Canned foods	**Keep at 20°C (68°F) or below, but do not freeze**
Grain products	**Keep package tightly closed; store in dark place**
Fresh meats, fish, and poultry	**Refrigerate, or freeze at -18°C (0°F) or below**

Because a food's water-soluble nutrients can leach (dissolve) into the water it's cooked in, it is better to cook food without immersing it in water, especially if you plan to throw away the water. That's why **steaming** and **pressure-cooking** allow for greater nutrient retention than boiling. For the same reason, cooking with dry heat (by roasting, grilling, stir-frying, or baking), is nutritionally better than cooking in water. Of course, you have to consider which cooking method will yield a high-quality product. If you are cooking a less tender cut of meat, for example, you may decide you need to stew it; but you can recover nutrients that leach into the cooking water by eating the juices as well.

steaming—using vapor from boiling water to cook foods while keeping the food out of the water

pressure-cooking—using superheated steam under pressure in an airtight utensil to cook foods quickly

microwave cooking—using short electromagnetic waves to cook foods quickly

How does **microwave cooking** rate? Studies show that the effects of microwaving vary with the product type; cooking time; internal temperature; and oven size, type, and power (Institute of Food Technologists, 1989). Experiments show that vegetables retain more vitamin C after they're microwaved than after they're cooked by conventional methods, provided that cooking time was shorter and little water was used (Klein, 1989). But because various conditions affect nutrient retention, you can't count on superior performance from microwaving in all situations. Therefore, the best general statement about microwaving is that it is no more destructive than conventional cooking methods—and in some cases is much less so.

The Consider This features above and on page 448, summarize advice about how to retain the best vitamin and mineral contents during home storage and during final preparation.

To retain micronutrients in foods at home, during preparation of

This	*Consider this*
All foods that require cooking	**Cook at as low a temperature and for as short a time as possible to achieve safety and palatability; eat immediately**
Frozen foods	**For whatever cooking method you use, follow package directions exactly**
Fresh or frozen vegetables	**Learn to like crisp cooked vegetables; steam them or cook in minimum amount of water**
Canned foods	**Heat just enough to bring to temperature you like for eating**
Meats, fish, poultry	**Use dry heat methods, such as roasting or broiling, when possible; otherwise, eat cooking juices too**

Summary

- Advances in agricultural and **food processing** technologies have led to a rapid expansion of the number of products available. The food industry is responsive to consumer interest in good taste, nutrition, affordable price, safety, storability, and convenience. More and more, it is becoming possible to create foods that have the characteristics we want.
- We can affect the nutritional properties of raw agricultural products to some degree. Animals are now fed in ways that yield leaner meats. Plants vary somewhat in certain vitamin and mineral values according to environmental conditions and soil mineral content.
- Beyond the farm, food is subjected to various food processing methods designed to delay spoilage and to make food more safe, nutritious, palatable, and convenient. Among the processes used to preserve foods are **canning, blanching, freezing, pasteurization, high-temperature–short-term (HTST) processing, ultra-high temperature (UHT) processing, irradiation, controlled-atmosphere packaging,** and **freeze-drying,** as well as other methods of **dehydration.** Food preservation provides year-round access to a wide variety of foods, thereby making better nutrition possible.
- However, every processing technique, whether done commercially or at home, inevitably causes some loss of micronutrients. Losses occur as a result of physical separation, heat, oxygen, light, certain conditions of pH, and the passage of time. Food preservation techniques control these factors and substantially slow down nutrient losses. Without preservation, a harvested "fresh" product might be nutritionally inferior to its commercially harvested and preserved counterpart within a couple of days. The vitamins most vulnerable to destruction are vitamin C and thiamin.

• Some foods *gain* nutrients during processing. In **fortification,** nutrients are deliberately added; **fermentation,** originally designed to preserve food, incidentally increases certain nutrients. Grains that have undergone **milling** and **refining** may later be **enriched** to restore the levels of thiamin, riboflavin, niacin, and iron that the whole grain had originally. Salt is often added to meet taste expectations; processed foods account for most of the salt in our diets, and eating large amounts of them may result in excessive intakes. Because there is increasing interest in less salty foods, some processors of lunchmeats, soups, canned vegetables, and frozen entree items have created new product lines with less salt.

• There are differences between nutritional values of a fresh food and those of its various processed forms, and final preparation methods also cause different amounts of nutrient destruction. It is difficult to generalize about the effects of **microwave cooking,** but **steaming** and **pressure-cooking** cause the least nutrient losses. Nonetheless, by the time different process forms of a food have been prepared for the table, nutritional values are quite similar. Attention to home storage and preparation are important, since the largest nutritional losses can occur here.

• Food technologists have developed various **imitation foods,** which resemble traditional products but are made from different ingredients. They do not have the same nutrient values as the items they mimic. Nonetheless, imitation foods are not necessarily inferior products; each should be evaluated on its individual merits.

• New packaging techniques that help conserve nutrients may represent the next wave of changes in food processing. An example is the **flexible retort pouch,** which allows for greater nutrient retention and convenience over the metal can.

References

Adams, C.E. and J.W. Erdman, Jr. 1988. Effects of home food preparation practices on nutrient content of foods. In *Nutritional evaluation of food processing,* ed. E. Karmas and R.S. Harris. New York: Van Nostrand Reinhold Company.

Agricultural Research Service. 1977. *Conserving nutritive values in foods.* Home and Garden Bulletin No. 90. Washington, DC: United States Department of Agriculture.

American Dietetic Association. 1991. *Survey of American dietary habits.* Chicago: The American Dietetic Association.

American Dietetic Association. 1993. Position of The American Dietetic Association: Biotechnology and the future of food. *Journal of the American Dietetic Association* 93:189–192.

Ames, B.N. and L.S. Gold. 1989. Pesticides, risk and applesauce. *Science* 236:755–757.

Baird, B. 1991. Hot meals in a hot spot: How we feed our troops in Saudi Arabia. *Food Technology* 45:52–56.

Bluestein, P.M. and T.P. LaBuza. 1988. Effects of moisture removal on nutrients. In *Nutritional evaluation of food processing,* ed. E. Karmas and R.S. Harris. New York: Van Nostrand Reinhold Company.

Byers, F.M., H.R. Cross, and G.T. Schelling. 1988. Integrated nutrition, genetics, and growth management programs for lean beef production. In *Designing foods.* Washington, DC: National Academy Press.

Committee on Diet and Health. 1989. *Diet and health: Implications for reducing chronic disease risk.* Washington, DC: National Academy Press.

Committee on Technological Options. 1988. *Designing foods.* Washington, DC: National Academy Press.

Community Nutrition Institute. 1992. Vindicator looks to Iraq after poor poultry sales. *Nutrition Week* November 20, 1992.

Congressional Federal Register. 1993. Food labeling. *Congressional Federal Register*, January 6, 1993. Washington, DC: U.S. Government Printing Office.

Davis, D.R. 1981. Wheat and nutrition. *Nutrition Today* 16:16–21.

Dietz, J.M. and J.W. Erdman. 1989. Effects of thermal processing upon vitamins and proteins in foods. *Nutrition Today* 24:6–15.

Fennema, O. 1988. Effects of freeze preservation on nutrients. In *Nutritional evaluation of food processing,* ed. E. Karmas and R.S. Harris. New York: Van Nostrand Reinhold Company.

Food Marketing Institute. 1992. *Trends: Consumer attitudes & the supermarket 1992.* Washington, DC: Food Marketing Institute.

Gallo, A.E. 1992. Record number of new products in 1991. *Food Review* 15(no.2):19–21.

Gilbert, S.G. 1988. Stability of nutrients during storage of processed foods. In *Nutritional evaluation of food processing,* ed. E. Karmas and R.S. Harris. New York: Van Nostrand Reinhold Company.

Gorewit, R.C. 1988. Lactation biology and methods of increasing efficiency. In *Designing foods.* Washington, DC: National Academy Press.

Gyles, R. 1988. Technological options for improving the nutritional value of poultry products. In *Designing foods.* Washington, DC: National Academy Press.

Institute of Food Technologists. 1989. Microwave food processing. *Food Technology* 43:117–124.

Institute of Food Technologists. 1990. Organically grown foods. *Food Technology* 44(no.6):26–29.

Karmas, E. and R.S. Harris. 1988. *Nutritional evaluation of food processing.* New York: Van Nostrand Reinhold Company.

Klein, B.P. 1989. Retention of nutrients in microwave-cooked foods. *Contemporary Nutrition* 14(no.2.)

Koskinen, E.H. 1989. Future developments and research priorities in food technology. In *Food technology in the year 2000,* ed. S. Lindroth and S.S. Ryynanen. Basel: Karger.

Larkin, M. 1991. Organic foods get government "blessing" despite claims that aren't kosher. *Nutrition Forum* 8:25–29.

Lund, D. 1988. Effects of heat processing on nutrients. In *Nutritional evaluation of food processing,* ed. E. Karmas and R.S. Harris. New York: Van Nostrand Reinhold Company.

Lynch, L. 1991. Congress mandates national organic food standards. *Food Review* 14(no.1):12–15.

Mast, M.G. and C.S. Clouser. 1988. Processing options for improving the nutritional value of poultry meat and egg products. In *Designing foods.* Washington, DC: National Academy Press.

McFeeters, R.F. 1988. Effects of fermentation on the nutritional properties of food. In *Nutritional evaluation of food processing,* ed. E. Karmas and R.S. Harris. New York: Van Nostrand Reinhold Company.

Nagy, S. and W.F. Wardowski. 1988. Effects of agricultural practices, handling, processing, and storage on fruits. In *Nutritional evaluation of food processing,* ed. E. Karmas and R.S. Harris. New York: Van Nostrand Reinhold Company.

National Academy of Sciences. 1989. *Recommended dietary allowances,* 10th edition. Washington, DC: National Academy Press.

National Livestock and Meat Board. 1987. *Exploring meat and health.* Chicago: National Livestock and Meat Board.

Ockerman, H.W. 1988. Effects of agricultural practices, handling, processing, and storage on meat. In *Nutritional evaluation of food processing,* ed. E. Karmas and R.S. Harris. New York: Van Nostrand Reinhold Company.

Parmley, M.A. 1991. A brief history of food preservation. *Food News for Consumers* 8(no.1):8–9.

Pennington, J.A.T. 1989. *Food values of portions commonly used.* New York: Harper & Row.

Rust, R.E. 1988. Processing options for improving the nutritional value of animal products. In *Designing foods.* Washington, DC: National Academy of Sciences.

Salunkhe, D.K. and B.B. Desai. 1988. Effects of agricultural practices, handling, processing, and storage on vegetables. In *Nutritional evaluation of food processing,* ed. E. Karmas and R.S. Harris. New York: Van Nostrand Reinhold Company.

Savell, J.W. and H.R. Cross. 1988. The role of fat in the palatability of beef, pork, and lamb. In *Designing foods.* Washington, DC: National Academy Press.

Schutz, H.G., C.M. Bruhn, and K.V. Diaz-Knauf. 1989. Consumer attitude toward irradiated foods: Effects of labeling and benefits information. *Food Technology* 43:80–84.

Science and Education Administration. 1985. *Nutritive value of foods.* Home and Garden Bulletin no. 72. Washington, DC: United States Department of Agriculture.

Sebrell, W.H. 1992. A fiftieth anniversary—Cereal enrichment. *Nutrition Today* 27(no.1):20–22.

Tannenbaum, S.R., V.R. Young, and M.C. Archer. 1985. Vitamins and minerals. In *Food chemistry*, ed. O.R. Fennema. New York: Marcel Dekker.

World Resources Institute. 1992. *World resources 1992–93.* Oxford: Oxford University Press.

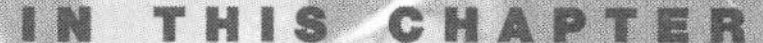

IN THIS CHAPTER

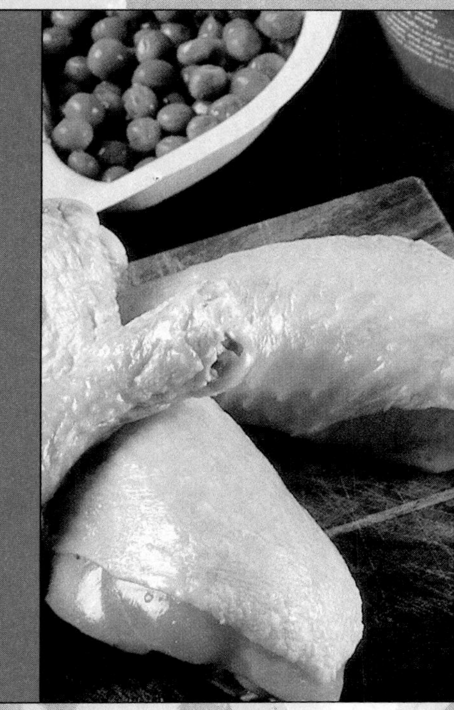

Chapter 14

Beyond Nutrients: What Else Is in Your Food?

You've probably seen many headlines questioning the safety of our food supply. Arsenic in Chilean grapes, Alar in apples, benzene in Perrier water, lead in drinking water and wine, and bovine somatotropin in milk are some of the concerns that have surfaced in recent years. As one food industry executive stated, "Food safety and food labeling are *the* issues of the 90's" (Boynton, 1990).

Many people feel a generalized anxiety about "the chemicals in our food." But as you know from preceding chapters, the essential nutrients themselves are chemicals, as are thousands of other naturally occurring substances that do not harm us.

However, foods do contain substances that are potentially harmful. Why doesn't our government protect us against all harmful chemicals? Unfortunately, this is not always possible. For one thing, scientists haven't yet identified all the substances in common foods. For another, many laboratory techniques have become so sensitive that scientists now find trace amounts of many chemicals in almost everything they test. In other words, ensuring an absolute zero amount of a given chemical in food is probably unrealistic. Scientists can detect some chemicals when they're present in food in just 1 part per million, which is equivalent to 1 ounce in 32 tons of food; for a few chemicals, scientists can even detect 1 part per trillion, which is 1 drop in 5,000,000 gallons. Depending on the substance, such concentrations may be harm*less,* even if higher concentrations are harm*ful.* Therefore, the relevant question often is not "*Could* this given substance harm us?" but "*At what level* is the substance harmful?"

Potentially dangerous substances can enter your food by various routes. Sometimes such chemicals occur naturally in plants and animals as they grow. Sometimes such chemicals accidentally enter the food supply through manufacturing or packaging. Sometimes they are added to foods deliberately (in small amounts) to accomplish an important and useful purpose, such as preservation. In some instances it may be difficult to determine by what means—singly or in combination—a harmful amount of a substance gained entry; therefore, it may be difficult to find out how to prevent it from happening again.

Food safety is important. You'll be hearing much more about it in the future, and as a consumer, you need to have enough scientific background to put food safety concerns into perspective. This chapter will help you learn how to evaluate critically the food safety issues you hear about in your daily life.

Let us emphasize from the start that many experts believe the food supply in the United States and Canada to be generally the safest in the world. However, this does not mean that the food supply is risk-free or that it is even possible for the food supply to be totally risk-free. Sometimes, in recent years, consumer groups, the media, food processors, and regulatory agencies have appeared to view each other as enemies. This is unfortunate, because the dialogue among these groups is important to you. Only discussions based on scientific studies—not those based on fear and misinformation—can prompt the food production, processing, and service industries to make changes that will ultimately improve our food supply.

Another major purpose of this chapter is to help you do your share in keeping your own food safe. As a consumer, you are responsible for carefully selecting, storing, and preparing food to ensure that it is safe to eat. A food that met standards for safety when you purchased it can become unsafe if you handle it improperly.

Toxicology: A Scientific Perspective on Harmful Substances

Food toxicology is the science that establishes the basis for judgments about the safety of foodborne elements (Hall and Taylor, 1989). Toxicology includes detecting **toxicants,** identifying their actions, and treating the conditions they produce. The following terms are commonly used in toxicologic discussions:

food toxicology—the scientific study of harmful substances in food, including detecting them and defining their modes of action

toxicant—a substance with the ability to cause harm

safety—a practical certainty that a substance will not cause injury

hazard—the probability, based on the dose and conditions of exposure, that a substance will cause injury

toxicity—the capability of a substance to produce injury at some level of intake

toxicant, toxin, poison (used almost synonymously)—a substance with the ability to cause harm

detoxification—the process of converting a dangerous substance into a harmless one

mutagen—a type of toxicant that causes a change in cells' genetic material (These changes are called *mutations.*)

carcinogen—a type of toxicant that stimulates a cell to multiply out of control, eventually resulting in cancer (Even if the risk of cancer is small—such as one case resulting per million exposures—a substance that has this effect is still called a carcinogen.)

You should realize that all substances are toxic at extreme intakes, but most are not hazardous under normal conditions. The types of problems induced by hazardous chemicals range from minor symptoms, such as a slight, short-term skin rash, to permanent damage of the nervous system, kidneys, or liver, or even death.

Possible Relationships Between Dosage and Effect

Toxicologists view substances as having one of the following four effects:

1. *no effect:* there is no negative effect at any *practical* level of intake.
2. *threshold effect:* the substance can be ingested without effect up to a certain amount; after that, negative effects increase as levels of intake increase.
3. *no threshold:* all levels of intake produce harm; the greater the intake, the greater the harm.
4. *low-dose beneficial threshold:* low levels of intake produce desirable effects; increasing levels eventually cause negative effects.

Figure 14.1 illustrates these four possibilities, which are called **dose-response curves.** Nutrients generally have a low-dose beneficial threshold. Vitamins and minerals that are essential for life at low levels of intake can be very toxic at higher levels. Many other food toxicants show a threshold effect. Unfortunately, scientists do not know which curve best describes the responses to many chemicals in our food supply.

dose-response curve—graph that shows the relationship between the dosage of a substance and its effect

Testing for toxic effects is a complex issue, and results can be difficult to interpret. Scientists can expose animals to high doses of the substance by feeding or injecting it and then monitoring acute effects, or they can feed

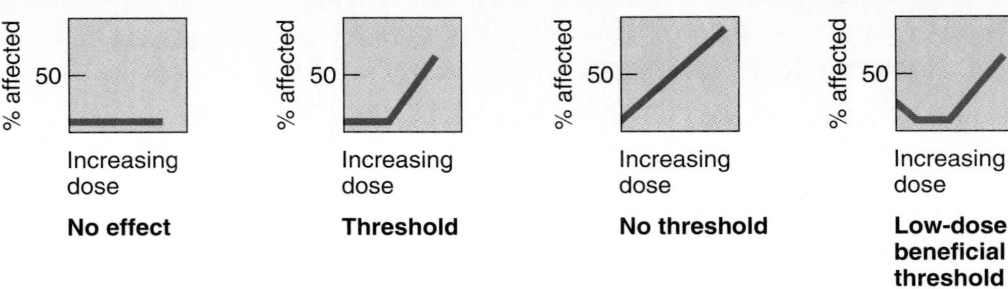

FIGURE 14.1
Possible forms of the dose-response curve.

(Adapted from Murphy, 1979. Copyright © by the Institute of Food Technologists.)

the animals low doses of the substance for years and monitor the gradual development of chronic effects. The advantage of the high-dosage trials is that results become apparent more quickly; however, these responses may be different from those induced in chronic feeding trials, in which the bodies of the test animals have time to adjust to the substance. Besides, as we've mentioned, substances can be essential or harmless at one level of intake and toxic at another. The advantage of the low-dosage trials is that they resemble more closely the way people are usually exposed to the substances in food; however, chronic toxic effects are occasionally missed in these studies. Generally, in trying to define the toxicity of substances, scientists use a combination of both types of trials in several species of animals.

Additional Factors That Influence Toxicity

In addition to the level of intake, a number of other factors influences the activity and effects of food toxicants.

Detoxification One reason that low levels of some toxicants cause no harm is that your body has a means of detoxifying small amounts of them. Your liver is most directly involved in changing toxicants into harmless metabolites.

Time Your liver is able to detoxify substances at only a limited rate. As an extreme example, you can safely ingest 10,000 mg of the toxicant solanine, which is present in the 120 pounds of potatoes the average American consumes annually, provided that your consumption of the potatoes is spread out over a year. The same amount of solanine in one dose, however, would be enough to kill you—or even a horse.

Storage Toxicants that cannot be degraded easily by your body often slowly accumulate in your liver, bone, adipose, or other tissues. After many years they may be present in amounts large enough to cause serious problems. Cadmium and certain organic compounds, such as polychlorinated biphenyls (PCBs), are examples of toxicants that accumulate in your body with time.

Nutritional Status If your diet is deficient in either energy intake or specific nutrients (for instance, protein) your body will probably be less able to deal with toxicants.

Growth and Body Size During periods of rapid growth, such as childhood and pregnancy, absorption of some toxicants is increased. Furthermore, a given amount of toxin usually has a greater effect on a smaller person, because there is more toxin present per unit of body weight.

Interactions Among Substances The toxicities of individual substances are generally not additive; that is, if you ate 1/100 of the lethal dose of each of 100 different toxic food components, the mixture would probably be harmless.

Some toxicants have **antagonists** that render the toxicants ineffective. In fish, for example, selenium tends to decrease the potential toxicity of any mercury present. Also, the addition of calcium, iron, and other trace elements to the diet has been found to depress the absorption and therefore the toxicity of cadmium and lead.

antagonist—a substance that can render another substance inactive

anticarcinogen—a compound in food that can counteract the effect of cancer-causing substances

There are also components in food that counteract the effect of cancer-causing substances. These are called **anticarcinogens.** One of the goals of current cancer research is to identify these chemicals and learn how they work. For example, foods of the cabbage family are believed to contain anticarcinogens. Vitamin A (at least carotene), vitamin C, and vitamin E also have anticarcinogenic functions.

Ranking of Food-Related Problems

Experts generally agree that the major public health problems associated with our food supply are due to microbiologic, not chemical, contamination of food (Miller, 1991). Of the chemical contamination problems, environmental contaminants and naturally occurring food toxicants affect more people than problems due to food additives (Wodicka, 1977). Let's begin with the most important problem: microbes.

Microorganisms and Parasites: The Most Common Foodborne Problems

An expert panel of the Institute of Food Technologists (IFT) estimated that between 24 and 81 million cases of foodborne diarrheal disease caused by microorganisms occur each year in the United States, costing between 5 and 17 billion dollars in medical treatment and lost productivity (IFT Expert Panel on Food Safety and Nutrition, 1988). As high as these estimates seem, the true numbers are even higher; it is probable that only 10–15% of cases are reported. But when compared with the number of times people eat, even this incidence of illness is very low.

Foodborne bacteria can cause the problems known as "food poisoning" through either *infection* or *intoxication*.

Common Foodborne Infections

If environmental conditions are favorable for their growth, bacteria and viruses can reproduce in food in large numbers, surpassing the threshold tolerated by most people. The resulting illnesses are called **foodborne infections.**

foodborne infection—illness produced by food containing large numbers of bacteria or viruses

In the past, *Salmonella* was believed to be the most common culprit in foodborne infections. However, *Campylobacter jejuni* causes even more **gastroenteritis** in the United States than *Salmonella* (Doyle, 1988). Other organisms implicated in foodborne infections are *Yersinia, Vibrio,* and even certain strains of *Escherichia coli (E. coli),* a bacterium that normally plays a healthy role in human gastrointestinal (GI) tracts (Ryser and Marth, 1989).

gastroenteritis—inflammation of the stomach and intestines

These bacteria are fairly ubiquitous (widespread), occurring in human and animal intestines, skin, soil, and water. They thrive in any setting that provides essential nutrients (high-protein foods, in particular), moisture, oxygen (or absence of oxygen, depending on their particular needs), and suitable temperature (especially 4–60°C, or 40–140°F).

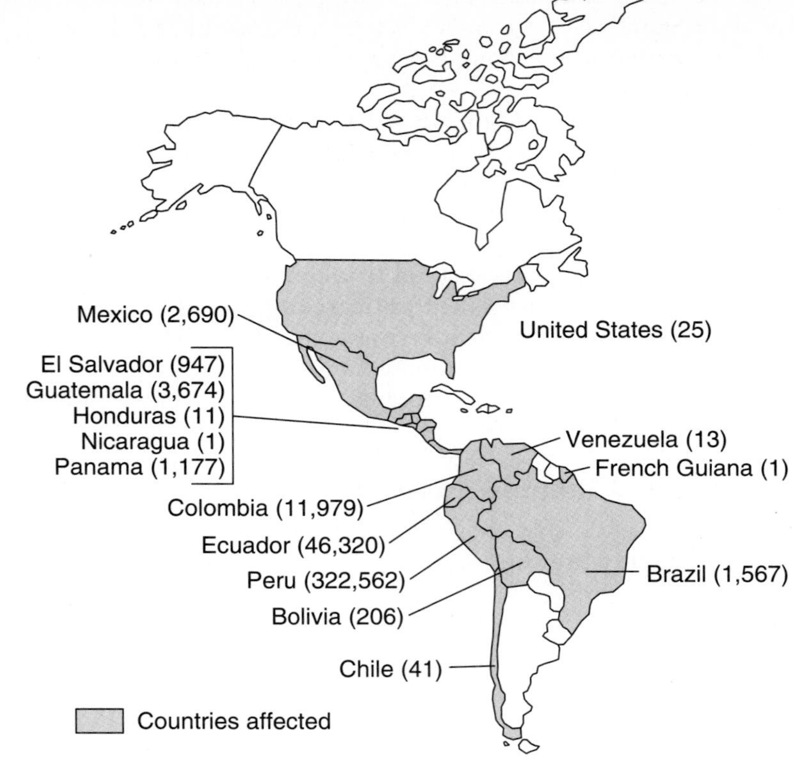

FIGURE 14.2
Cholera cases in the Americas.

Map indicates the number of cholera cases in 1991 reported to the Pan American Health Organization.
(Reprinted from Glass et al., 1992.)

All of these organisms produce GI distress in the form of nausea, vomiting, and diarrhea, anywhere from 12 hours to 5 days after ingestion (Ryser and Marth, 1989). How quickly and seriously you become ill depends on which organism you're harboring and how healthy you are to begin with. Although these illnesses tend to be short-term and are not usually severe, they occasionally cause death to a person already in weakened health.

One of these bacteria, a form of *Vibrio,* causes **cholera,** a form of GI distress that leads to such severe dehydration that death can result. In 1991, a cholera **epidemic** occurred in South and Central America; almost 400,000 cases were reported (Glass et al., 1992) (Figure 14.2). Sewage contamination of drinking water, vegetables, and shellfish appeared to be the sources of the infection, but experts felt that the decision of officials in Peru not to chlorinate water supplies accounted for the spread of the epidemic (Anderson, 1991).

cholera—an acute infectious disease caused by *Vibrio cholerae* that results in a profuse, watery diarrhea

epidemic—a disease attacking many people in a community in a short time

You Tell Me

Chlorine is an effective disinfectant. Unfortunately, it can sometimes also react with by-products of organic decay in water to create suspected, very weak, carcinogens (Anderson, 1991). Because of concerns about slight cancer risks, Peruvian officials did not chlorinate water in their country—and over 322,000 cases of cholera occurred there in 1991. Even with modern therapies, it is estimated that at least 1% of people with cholera die (Glass et al., 1992); history suggests that the typical death rate, before such aggressive treatment became available, was around 20%.

If you had to make the decision, would you have chlorinated the water?

If you opted for chlorination, you would be in agreement with experts in the United States and in the Pan American Health Organization. They do suggest careful monitoring of chlorine by-products to avoid exceeding suggested limits, however.

The primary symptom of at least one foodborne infection, *Listeria monocytogenes,* is not GI distress but a systemic (whole-body) infection that leads to death in 23% of patients whose immune systems are not functioning normally and in fetuses (Schuchat et al., 1992). This infection is therefore of serious concern to people who are very ill (such as AIDS patients) and to pregnant women (for the sake of the fetus). It is not generally dangerous to healthy adults. One food to which a number of cases of this disease was traced was non-aged cheese made from unpasteurized milk.

foodborne bacterial intoxication—illness produced by food containing bacterial toxins

botulism—an uncommon but sometimes fatal food intoxication

Foodborne Intoxications

Some bacteria cause illnesses by producing toxins in the foods they contaminate. These illnesses are called **foodborne bacterial intoxications.** *Staphylococcus aureus* is the most common cause of food intoxication. *Clostridium perfringens* frequently causes foodborne illness by both infection and intoxication. These organisms are most often found in cooked foods that were cross-contaminated with the bacteria from raw foods and then stored improperly. Both organisms cause abdominal pain and diarrhea, but *Staphylococcus* also causes nausea and can cause symptoms more rapidly than other foodborne bacteria—anywhere from 30 minutes to 8 hours after ingestion (Newsome, 1988).

You Tell Me

Tom held an unforgettable picnic last year. He cut up raw chicken on a cutting board and then—without washing the board—cut up celery, hard-boiled eggs, and cooked potatoes for the potato salad. He let the potato salad ingredients sit on the picnic table for a couple of hours while he started the fire and barbecued the chicken.

What symptoms do you think the guests developed? How could their symptoms have been prevented?

One form of bacterial intoxication is particularly important because of its severity. The *Clostridium botulinum* organism, when it produces its toxin in food, may cause the sometimes fatal disease **botulism.** *C. botulinum* is found in soil and in the sediments of many freshwater lakes and rivers. The organism by itself is not hazardous; probably everybody has consumed it at one time or another without noticeable effects. But dire consequences can occur when it is present in an environment where circumstances allow it to thrive: anaerobic conditions (the absence of oxygen), the presence of low-acid foods, and room temperature. In time, the bacteria—or their protected resting forms, called *spores*—become active and produce the potentially deadly toxin. The affected food will not necessarily look or smell unusual, making the toxin impossible to detect.

Low-acid canned foods that have been improperly processed are most often the cause of botulism. Foods with a pH higher than 4.6 are regarded as low-acid. (Figure 14.3 shows the acidity of various foods.) Products improperly canned at home are more often the source of this toxin than commercially canned foods.

FIGURE 14.3
The pH values of various canned foods.

Low-acid foods must be processed under pressure at temperatures greater than 212°F to ensure the destruction of *Clostridium botulinum*.

(Adapted from Leveille and M.A. Uebersax, 1979.)

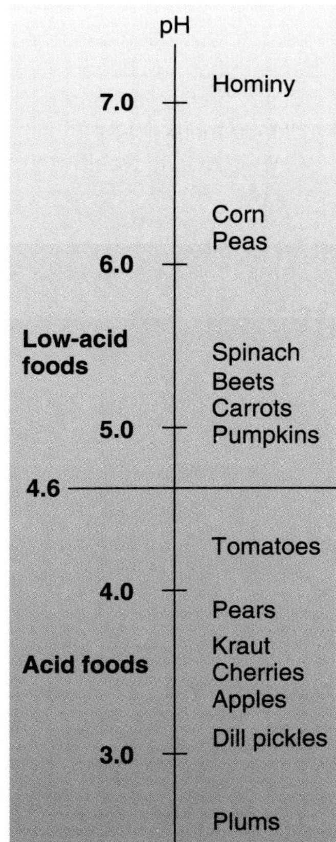

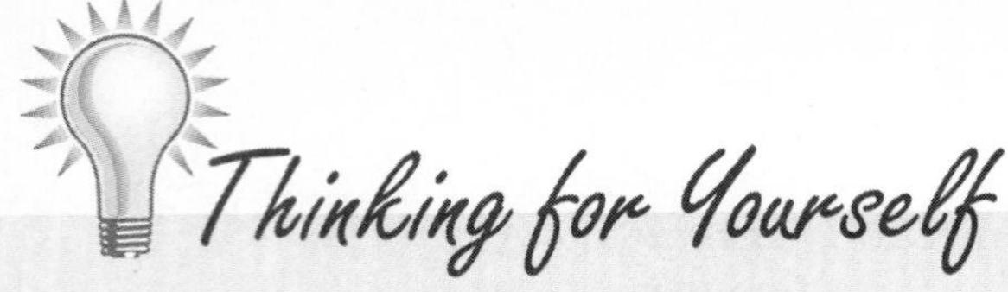

Food Safety of Poultry: Whose Job?

The Situation

The *Washington Post* of May 2, 1990, carried an article titled "FDA Approves Irradiation of Poultry." Here are excerpts from the article:

> The Food and Drug Administration yesterday approved the use of irradiation to control salmonella and other bacteria in fresh and frozen poultry products. This is the first time the process has been approved in this country to control bacteria that cause illness to humans.
>
> According to the Centers for Disease Control (CDC), there are approximately 40,000 reported cases of salmonella poisoning a year. But since most foodborne disease outbreaks are not reported, the CDC estimates the actual number of annual cases could be anywhere from 400,000 to 4 million.
>
> . . . The poultry industry is not anxious to use the technology. "It amounts to consumer acceptance. At least at this time we do not have a sense that there's wide consumer demand for irradiated foods of any kind," said Stephen Pretanik, director of science and technology for the National Broiler Council.

In short, irradiation can now be used to lower the risk of a disease that has become an increasing problem; yet, the industry hesitates, because it fears loss of business in reaction to the process.

What action would you, the consumer, like to see taken?

Is Your Information Accurate and Relevant?

- It is true that the FDA approval of irradiation for poultry was the first attempt at reducing risk from bacteria; however, in 1985 irradiation was approved for control of another pathogen, the *Trichina* worm, in pork. It has also been approved for selected other purposes of food safety and pest control.
- It is true that reported *Salmonella* infections have reached 40,000 cases per year and have been increasing at a rapid rate; unreported cases are probably many times higher.
- It is likely that the increase in the use of poultry is part of the reason for the increase in *Salmonella* infections; however, there may be other reasons, such as an increase in the use of delicatessen foods, or inadequate cooking or handling of food in restaurants or at home.
- There is evidence that some consumers reject the idea of eating food that has been irradiated; New York, New Jersey, and Maine have banned the sale of irradiated foods.

What Else Should You Consider?

Salmonella organisms are present on much raw poultry. Estimates range from one-fourth of poultry purchased to virtually all raw poultry. Current mass-production and processing methods are thought to contribute to the spread of contamination in poultry processing plants. Changing these processing methods would cost a great deal of

A type of botulism can also occur in babies less than a year old. Unlike an adult's mature GI tract, a baby's stomach or colon seems to provide the conditions that allow *C. botulinum* to produce toxins. Botulism in infants produces neurologic distress, a condition sometimes called "limp baby disease." Although more than 500 cases have been reported, there have been very few deaths (Liska et al., 1986). The means by which babies get this disease is not known, but honey and corn syrup were believed to be the sources of *C. botulinum* spores in a couple of cases. Therefore, these sweeteners should not be given to infants.

Prevention Strategies

How can you protect yourself against food poisoning? When should you be able to depend on the food industry and regulatory agencies? The Thinking for Yourself above serves as a basis for discussion of this issue. It is

money, and this cost would ultimately be borne by consumers.

Irradiation of foods is a process that has been approved by 33 countries around the world and is used more extensively in many countries than it is in the United States. Irradiation of food does not make food radioactive; the major scientific question that is raised about the process is whether other potentially dangerous chemical compounds might be formed in the food as a result of irradiation. (See Chapter 13 for more information on irradiation as a food preservation technique.)

Proponents of irradiation point out that traditional processes, such as canning, also produce some of these same chemical substances and that irradiation produces similar amounts. Furthermore, some of these chemicals also *occur naturally* in foods. Since the doses of irradiation approved for poultry are lower than those approved for some other applications, they are less likely to lead to the production of these chemical substances.

Because of the low levels of irradiation that have been approved, the number of *Salmonella* organisms on poultry would be reduced but not eliminated. With *Salmonella* organisms still present, proper refrigeration and cooking of poultry would still be critical in order to ensure a safe product. *Salmonella* organisms are destroyed when poultry is cooked to an internal temperature of 185°F.

Now What Do You Think?

There are a number of ways to address the concern about *Salmonella* infection from poultry. Taking all of the above points into consideration, what do you think is the best action to take?

- Option 1 You think that low dose irradiation of poultry at the processing plant as approved by the FDA is the best action to take; it offers a good cost/benefit ratio.
- Option 2 You think that the poultry industry should change to smaller operations with slower production lines and more inspection to reduce contamination, despite higher costs to the consumer.
- Option 3 You think that poultry should be treated with FDA-approved chemicals, such as trisodium phosphate, to kill *Salmonella*.
- Option 4 You think that since *Salmonella* are killed by adequate cooking, uncooked poultry in the retail market should be labeled with instructions for safe cooking.
- Option 5 You decide to urge the expansion of relevant educational programs of the Cooperative Extension service and other agencies that teach consumers about safe food handling and preparation.
- Option 6 You decide that the status quo is satisfactory.
- Option 7 You decide that no matter what others do, you will thoroughly cook all poultry that you eat.

Do you see other options or combinations of options? Which makes the most sense to you?

imperative that the food industry, you, and other consumers share the responsibility for food safety. The way to make food safe is to practice the following:

Start with Clean Food Choose food that looks clean. Wash produce thoroughly. Avoid food cans with leaky seams or bulging ends, which indicate gas formation by bacteria living in the food.

Drinking raw (unpasteurized) milk—even if certified (monitored for contamination by some bacteria)—increases your risk of getting microbial infections. Some people who drink raw milk regularly appear to develop immunities to its pathogens (Blaser et al., 1987). However, experts don't advise you to drink raw milk, because it offers no proven advantages.

Cook Animal Products Adequately Cook raw meats, poultry, fish, and eggs thoroughly before you eat them, because the raw forms can harbor dis-

FIGURE 14.4
Trichina.

The curled worms shown in this micrograph are the parasite *Trichinella spiralis* encysted in pig muscle. Cooking pork to 170°F destroys these parasites, should they be present. If they are alive when a person ingests the pork, they can result in the disease trichinosis.

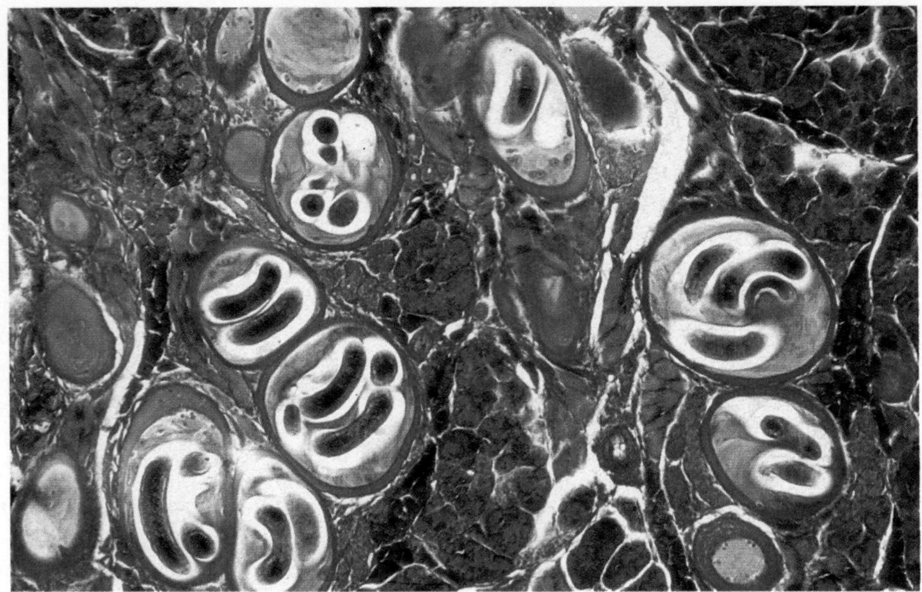

ease-causing microorganisms. Cook pork to an internal temperature of 72°C (170°F): the heat kills parasites called *Trichina* that occasionally are found in muscles of swine (Figure 14.4) and that cause the painful disease *trichinosis*. Although trichinosis is rare today, you should still follow this good advice.

Nowadays, there is a much greater risk of getting sick from eating inadequately cooked chicken than from inadequately cooked pork. In one study, 23% of 862 raw chicken samples purchased from grocery stores tested positive for *Campylobacter jejuni* (Harris et al., 1986). Some officials estimate the percentage of chicken contaminated with this and other bacteria to be *much* higher. Handle chicken properly before cooking, and cook it thoroughly; refer to cookbooks for cooking times and temperatures.

Recent cases of food poisoning due to *E. coli* contamination of beef has led the FDA to suggest that even ground beef should be cooked to an internal temperature of 71°C (160°F). That means it's wise to order your hamburger "medium" to "well done."

In the past, the contents of uncracked eggs were assumed to be sterile; therefore, it was considered safe to use them in uncooked foods and beverages, such as eggnog. Now it is known that eggs can be contaminated with *Salmonella* through the hen (St. Louis et al., 1988) and that it is therefore risky to eat any uncooked (or less than thoroughly cooked) egg product. The risk is particularly high for people whose immune function is already compromised by illness or age.

The risks of eating raw or incompletely cooked seafood also have been highlighted in recent years. Between 1978 and 1987, almost 6000 cases of illness due to seafood contamination were reported to the Centers for Disease Control (Nutrition Reviews, 1991). This constitutes about 4% of the reported cases of foodborne illness.

The most typical problems are due to consumption of raw or improperly cooked mollusks (such as oysters, clams, and mussels) that were contaminated with viruses or bacteria from sewage. The symptoms include mild to severe gastroenteritis and, in a few cases, **hepatitis** and liver disease (Desenclos et al., 1991). To prevent these problems, many states have

hepatitis—inflammation of the liver

adopted rules to prevent the harvesting and distribution of shellfish from water contaminated with human fecal pathogens. Federal agencies have also increased their monitoring of these products. But ultimately, you as a consumer need to take responsibility.

The best way for you to enjoy such seafood safely is to be sure to cook it thoroughly. The usual procedure—to steam mollusks until the shells open—may be inadequate to inactivate viruses they contain (DuPont, 1986). Many cookbooks don't take this new information into account.

Parasitic roundworms can infect fin fish and cause chronic gastroenteritis in humans who eat raw fish (such as that in sushi and ceviche) or inadequately cooked fish. Freezing and holding fish at −23°C (−10°F) for 7 days can make it safe from these parasites (Jackson et al., 1990), but freezing does not prevent all the problems, such as viruses and bacteria, that can be associated with ingesting raw fish.

Avoid Recontamination of Food After Cooking Once you have properly cooked a food, *it is critically important to keep from recontaminating it.* Cooked food, with its low population of microorganisms, provides a medium in which newly introduced organisms can thrive without significant competition. To prevent this, thoroughly wash between uses any cutting boards, knives, blenders, or other equipment that contacts food. Plastic or glass cutting boards are easier to keep clean than are wooden cutting boards.

Careless personal sanitation practices can also cause recontamination of food. Wash your hands before handling food and after touching your clothes, face, hair, the baby, the dog, or anything else likely to carry organisms. Avoid sneezing and coughing onto food, and do not handle food if you have cuts or sores on your hands.

Keep Food Out of the Temperature Danger Zone The temperature range most conducive to the reproduction of microorganisms that cause foodborne illnesses is called the *danger zone.* Moist foods and foods high in protein are most likely to promote growth of microorganisms. For storage and holding purposes, 4–60°C (40–140°F) is the range to avoid. Figure 14.5 shows the effects of different temperatures on microorganisms.

Between preparation and consumption, food should be kept either hotter than 60°C (140°F) or colder than 4°C (40°F). When cooling large amounts of cooked foods for cold storage, spread the food out in thin layers to allow faster cooling. When allowing foods to sit at room temperature, such as on the table during meals or for a buffet, try to maintain safety by using ice-lined bowls for cold food and warmers for hot food. If you don't take these precautions, foods can be exposed to danger zone temperatures. It is impossible for experts to tell you exactly how long the foods remain safe to eat. You'd probably be wise to discard moist, high-protein foods that were in the danger zone for two hours or more (United States Department of Agriculture, Food Safety and Inspection Service, 1984). In hot weather, one hour is a safer guideline. Keep in mind the old adage: "When in doubt, throw it out."

The Slice of Life on page 463 describes a case of food poisoning caused by food left at room temperature.

Follow Canning Instructions to the Letter If you can foods at home, be sure to use methods recommended in the most recent brochures published by the United States Department of Agriculture (USDA). This is particularly important for protection against botulism. Such brochures are avail-

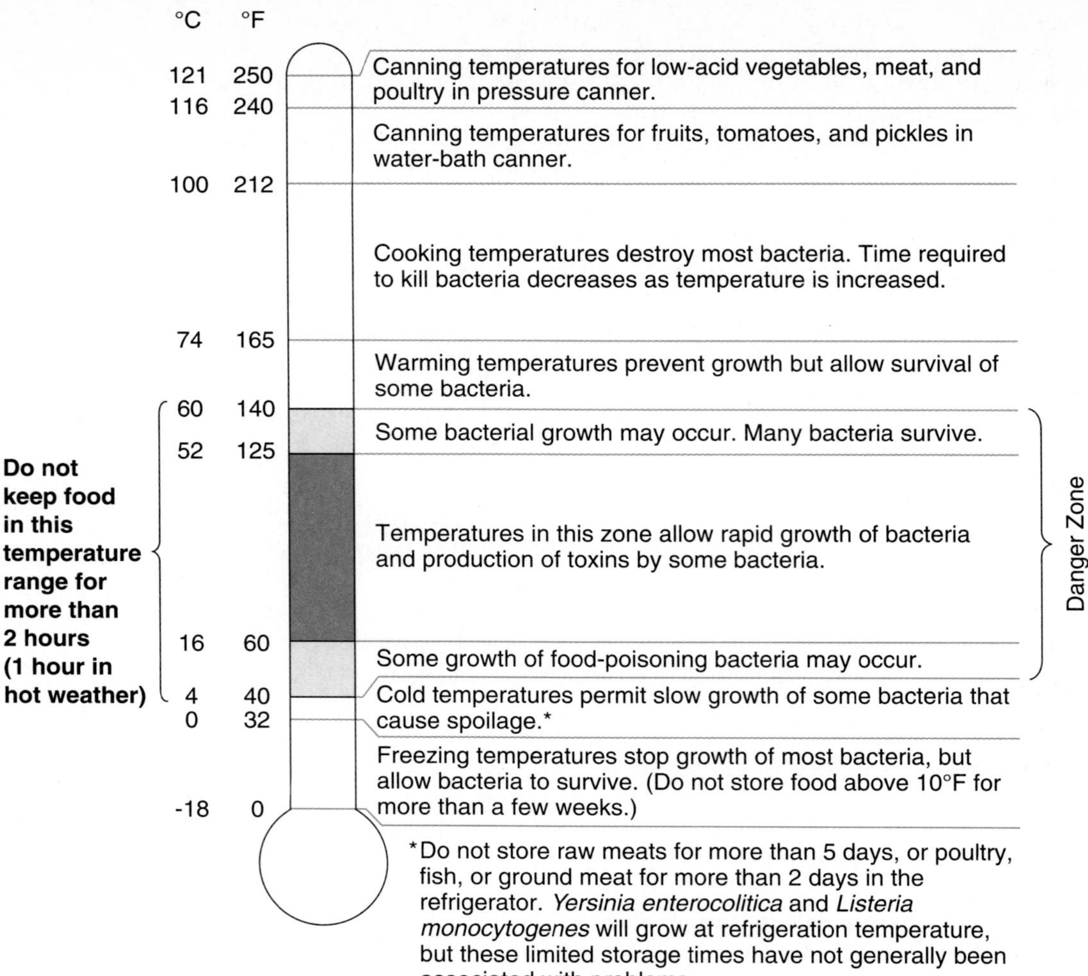

FIGURE 14.5
Effects of temperature on microorganisms.

(Adapted from United States Department of Agriculture, Food Safety and Inspection Service, 1984.)

able through the Cooperative Extension system in your state. It is critical to use the right method for each product you are preserving. Recommended substances to add to the product, processing times, and whether to heat in boiling water or in a pressure cooker may seem like picky details, but they may literally make the difference between life and death.

This section has emphasized the harm that some bacteria and other organisms present in food can cause, but it's only fair to point out that certain microorganisms can also play a positive role and are deliberately and safely added during processing. Bacteria are used to make yogurt, some cheeses, vinegar, and wine; yeast is used to make beer; and specific molds are cultured on certain varieties of cheese. Keep in mind, though, this important difference: the time-tested, deliberate use of microorganisms in food processing is likely to be safe, but random or accidental introduction of microorganisms into food is more likely to create hazards.

Environmental Contaminants: Common but Seldom Harmful

Toxic minerals, toxic organic compounds, and even radioactive substances can get into food. Some popular media have sensationalized situations in

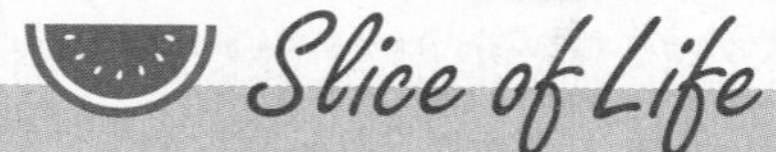

An Easter Egg Hunt That Led to the Hospital

A neighborhood church invited area children to an Easter egg hunt. Three to five days before the hunt, a cook boiled and dyed numerous batches of eggs and rinsed them in cold water. While most were still warm, he removed them from the water and left them unrefrigerated in the church kitchen.

The day of the hunt, the eggs were hidden on the church grounds, and approximately 850 children turned out to retrieve them. Many eggs were eaten at the hunt or on the way home.

Several hours later, children began showing up at local hospital emergency rooms with severe GI symptoms. Some required intravenous fluids and electrolyte replacement. Although most children did not need to go to the hospital, almost 300 of them experienced some GI symptoms from eating the eggs.

County health department officials, on learning of the outbreak from an emergency room physician, began their sleuthing. Their investigation revealed that *Staphylococcus aureus* organisms were present in the eggs; the same type of bacteria were cultured from various sites on the cook's body.

Apparently, *Staphylococcus* organisms from the cook got into the rinse water and through the shells of the cooked eggs. By the time the children ate the eggs, the bacteria had multiplied and produced toxin.

If you're ever acting as the Easter bunny, don't make the same mistake. It might be smart to substitute plastic Easter eggs or wooden eggs for the real thing during the hunts.

which environmental contaminants caused serious problems, suggesting that such hazards are widespread. The truth is that environmental contaminants rarely enter your food and water supply in sufficient quantities to be of practical significance; nevertheless, it's important to be aware of their sources and possible, although unlikely, consequences.

Mineral Contaminants

Although a number of minerals enter your food and water during storage and processing, few ever cause problems. The most potentially toxic are lead, aluminum, tin, mercury, and cadmium.

Lead Lead can cause anemia, kidney disease, and damage to the nervous system. It is particularly dangerous to children for two reasons. First, children absorb a higher percentage of the lead that they ingest than adults do. Second, the effects of exposure to low levels of lead in childhood persist into young adulthood. Children exposed to low (but nonetheless excessive) levels of lead have a greater incidence of reading disabilities, lower class standings in high school, and poorer eye–hand coordination as young adults (Needleman et al., 1990).

Table 14.1 illustrates the severity of the problem. A significant number of children in a national survey were found to have high levels of lead (30 μg per 100 ml) in their blood—levels high enough to require medical treatment. In this 1976–1980 survey, the prevalence of high lead levels was much greater among black children, especially those living in low-income homes.

Since this survey, experts have demonstrated that even blood levels lower than those considered toxic had negative effects. Infants with little more than 10 μg of lead per 100 ml of cord blood (from the umbilical cord at birth) were found to have permanent mental impairment. Mental development index scores for these children at 12 months and 24 months of age were below average, even though their lead levels were then below 10 μg per 100 ml of blood (Bellinger et al., 1987). Where did this lead come from?

TABLE 14.1 Percentage of American Children with Elevated Lead Levels in Blood[a]

	% of Children	
	White	Black
Annual Family Income		
Under $6,000	5.9	18.5
$6,000–14,999	2.2	12.1
$15,000 or more	0.7	2.8
Degree of Urbanization of Place of Residence		
Urban, 1 million persons or more		
Central city	4.5	18.6
Non-central city	3.8	3.3
Urban, fewer than 1 million persons	1.6	10.2
Rural	1.2	10.3

[a]This table gives the percentage of children ages 6 months to 5 years who have blood lead levels of 30 μg or more per 100 ml (1976–1980). Many experts now consider blood lead levels greater than 10 μg per 100 ml to be an indication of excess exposure to lead.
Source: Adapated from Annest, et al., 1982.

Lead can get into soil and water from such sources as paint chips from buildings being demolished, solid waste sludges used as fertilizers, and the airborne products of fuel combustion. The exhaust from vehicles requiring leaded gasoline also contributes lead to the air. Contaminants in soil, water, and air can, in turn, accumulate in food.

Many children, especially those living in old, low-income areas, are believed to ingest lead by chewing paint chipped from walls. (Indoor paint sold in the U.S. no longer contains lead.) Preventing pica would be the best strategy, but adequate nutrition helps: sufficient calcium and iron intakes reduce the amount of lead absorbed (Mahaffey et al., 1986).

Commercially canned foods contain very little lead. The food industry has eliminated lead by rolling the seams of cans instead of soldering them with lead, by developing cans with no side seam, and by packaging more foods in glass. All baby foods, except for infant formulas, are now sold in glass containers. Despite these advances, other containers could contaminate food with lead, as the following You Tell Me points out.

You Tell Me

Lead can leach from leaded crystal and glazed pottery into food and beverages, especially if acidic liquids are stored in the containers. Food and Drug Administration (FDA) regulations prevent the sale in the U.S. of ceramicware that can leach significant amounts of lead into food.

If you bought glazed pottery in another country or at a craft fair, do you think the vendors could tell you whether the glaze contained lead? If the answer were yes or unclear, would you use the pottery as a food or beverage container, or strictly as a decoration? Do you think storing alcoholic beverages in leaded containers for a month or more is smart?

Drinking water can be a significant source of lead intake if the pipes or solder with which they were joined contain lead (Bois et al., 1989). Building codes in many jurisdictions are being modified to prevent this problem. The Thinking for Yourself in Chapter 4 discusses lead and other contaminants in drinking water. If you live in an old house and are concerned about lead levels in your water, call your local health department for advice.

Aluminum Perhaps you've seen headlines on the potential neurotoxicity of aluminum. At this time, researchers believe that levels of aluminum commonly present in the diet do not adversely affect people with normally functioning kidneys.

However, there are several ways aluminum may enter food. Aluminum is one of the most common elements in the earth's crust and is therefore naturally present in plant foods. Although some aluminum enters the diet as a component of additives in certain processed cheeses and some baked goods, people who routinely take aluminum-containing medications consume 100 times more aluminum than can be obtained through food. Aluminum-containing drugs (for example, antacids) have been found to affect bones and nervous tissue in some people with kidney failure (Greger, 1992).

Last on the list of contributors to aluminum intake are cooking implements and foil. Only a very small amount of the aluminum that you consume can be attributed to aluminum cookware or aluminum foil (Greger, 1992).

Tin The main source of dietary tin is the coating on "tin" cans (which are mainly steel). The tin content of a canned food increases dramatically if the can is opened and the food is stored in it in the refrigerator (Greger, 1987). Excess tin ingestion may depress absorption of essential minerals, such as zinc and copper. For this reason, don't store unused foods in the cans; use glass or plastic containers. If cans are lacquered or polymer-coated inside, however, only barely detectable levels of tin leach into food.

Mercury The burning of fossil fuel and industrial wastes can add considerable amounts of mercury to the environment. But there are government standards that limit the exposure of industrial workers and the general population to mercury. This has not always been the case; the phrase "mad as a hatter" is derived from the bizarre symptoms exhibited by hat makers who treated furs with mercury during the 1700s and 1800s.

Fortunately, very little industrial mercury waste enters the food supply; however, problems can occur if microorganisms in soil and water add organic compounds to inorganic mercury. This produces a variety of organic substances, including **methyl mercury,** which is more readily absorbed by and more toxic to biologic systems than is inorganic mercury (Clarkson, 1987). Ingesting methyl mercury in toxic quantities can cause progressive loss of coordination, vision, and hearing; mental deterioration; and death. Infants born to mothers who ingested large amounts of methyl mercury during pregnancy suffer from a variety of neurologic disorders.

methyl mercury—an organic form of mercury, highly toxic to biologic systems

Recently, experts recognized that tiny amounts of mercury are released from "silver" dental amalgams used to fill cavities (Aposhian et al., 1992). Most dentists believe that the amount of mercury absorbed, even by people with many fillings, is insignificant. But this is apt to remain a controversial topic until scientists collect more convincing data.

Cadmium Most foodstuffs contain little cadmium naturally (Kostial, 1986). However, oysters and other seafood, especially those grown in industrially contaminated water, can contain very high levels of cadmium. Some vegetable crops can also accumulate cadmium when grown in soil to which sewage sludge has been heavily applied. Cigarette smoke can be another major source of cadmium for some people.

Ingested cadmium damages the kidneys and reproductive organs and interferes with absorption of essential elements, such as zinc and iron (Kostial, 1986). In laboratory animals, cadmium causes hypertension, but it is not known whether it could do the same to you.

Other Contaminants

Agricultural and other industrial technologies add many different organic contaminants to the food supply. You've probably seen newspaper and magazine headlines proclaiming the toxicity of some of these contaminants. These situations are generally more complex than most people realize.

Antibiotics In addition to their use in treating human infections, antibiotics are used to treat animal infections and to increase the weight gain of food-producing animals. This makes it possible to produce greater quantities of meats and eggs at lower cost.

There is some concern that antibiotic residues may remain in animal tissues and cause allergic or other adverse reactions in the people who eat the meat. The USDA, particularly the Food Safety and Inspection Service (FSIS), conducts more than 1½ million analyses annually to check for residues of antibiotics and pesticides in meats, poultry, and eggs. Fewer than 1% of tests show excessive levels; the limits generally provide a 100- to 1000-fold safety margin, according to USDA officials (Russell, 1990).

A more far-reaching concern is the buildup of antibiotic-resistant bacteria—*Salmonella,* for example—in the intestinal tracts of humans. Physicians fear that infections caused by these antibiotic-resistant bacteria would be very difficult to treat medically. However, it is likely that the fairly indiscriminate use of antibiotics in treating patients and livestock is a more important contributor to resistant strains of bacteria than is the inclusion of low levels of antibiotics in animal feedstuffs (DuPont and Steele, 1987).

Hormones A variety of hormones is naturally present in animal and plant tissues. Bovine somatotropin (BST), or bovine growth hormone (BGH), is a naturally occurring hormone that increases milk production. Scientists using biotechnology have developed ways to manufacture large quantities of this hormone by splicing the gene for BST into bacteria and growing huge vats of these "engineered" microbes; cows injected with the synthetic BST produce more milk. Experts believe that the composition and nutritional value of milk from cows treated with BST is "essentially the same" as milk from untreated cows (NIH Technology Assessment Conference, 1991).

However, some consumers and activists have not been reassured by the available data. In addition, farmers in the United States and Europe, where there is already a surplus of milk, doubt its economic value, and question its long-term effects on cows. Therefore, several state legislatures and the European Economic Community have restricted the use or sale of milk produced in this way (Collins et al., 1989). For all of these reasons, the future use of BST to increase milk production appears questionable, even though all government panels have reported the milk to be safe.

Pesticides The need to produce sufficient food for a growing world population has led to increased use of pesticides, particularly herbicides (Figure 14.6). Experts estimate that every dollar farmers spend on pesticides earns three to six dollars as a result of increased yields and improved quality of food products (Bruhn, 1991).

Pesticides (including insecticides, herbicides, fungicides, and rodenticides) vary greatly in their chemical structures, their modes of action, the manner in which they are applied, and their potential toxicities; therefore, evaluating the effects of these products on your health is complex. The amounts of pesticide residues that remain in food when consumed is important; these residues can be due to direct application of pesticides to growing plants and animals or due to environmental contamination resulting from previous applications. The effect of pesticides also depends on your body's ability to absorb, excrete, and/or detoxify them and on the breakdown products and metabolites that remain in your body (Coats, 1987). For example, if you cannot excrete a pesticide, it may accumulate over time in your tissues. If threshold doses of toxins are reached, toxic effects will occur.

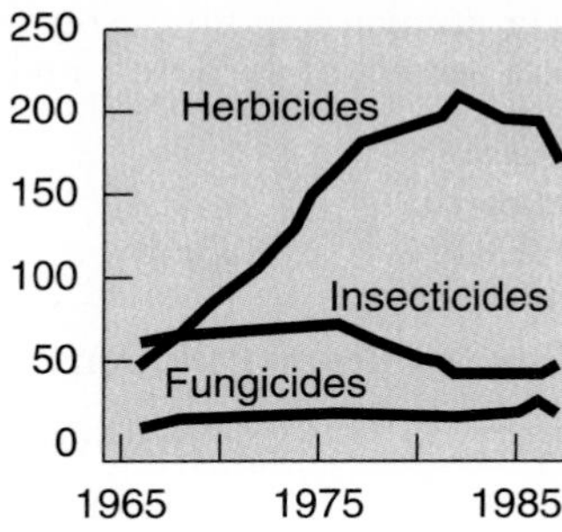

FIGURE 14.6
Pesticide use in the United States.

(Reprinted from United States Department of Agriculture, 1990.)

Pesticides affect various tissues differently. Some are neurotoxins and can affect behavior; other pesticides or impurities within them have been demonstrated to be carcinogens or **teratogens.** Some affect the immune system.

teratogen—an agent or factor (such as industrial chemicals, drugs, radiation, excessive level of a nutrient, or disease) that causes a physical defect to an embryo

To compare the risks of various substances, scientists have proposed a variety of toxicity scales. Bruce Ames, a well-known cancer researcher, and his associates have developed HERP scores; HERP is the acronym for *h*uman *e*xposure dose/*r*odent *p*otency dose (Gold et al., 1992; Ames and Gold, 1989). These scores take three factors into consideration: Americans' typical exposure to the tested substance during a lifetime, body size, and the amount of the tested substance that was fed to rodents to produce tumors in 50% of the animals tested. This complex ratio makes it possible to compare the relative risk associated with exposure to a wide variety of substances. Table 14.2 gives HERP scores for a number of substances. As you can see, drinking 12 ounces of beer is potentially more hazardous than exposure to pesticides, such as DDT or EDB, in food at typical dose levels. However, it is interesting to note that the use of DDT or EDB in the United States is now banned.

Compounds naturally present in foods are often much more carcinogenic at the levels consumed than intentional food additives or environmental contaminants are. You may think of pesticides as substances added by farmers and food processors, but actually more than 99% of those we consume are natural constituents of plants and animals (Ames and Gold, 1989). Plants and animals produce these compounds to survive pests' attacks. In addition, some added pesticides or spoilage inhibitors reduce production of more toxic compounds. For example, Alar is a synthetic growth regulator that delays ripening of apples so that they do not drop prematurely and overripen in storage. This prevents the growth of molds that produce compounds that are much more carcinogenic than Alar.

All evaluations of pesticide safety are subject to review as new data become available. For example, ethylene dibromide (EDB) is a compound that was used in the United States for more than 40 years to control insect infestation in stored grain and citrus fruit (Sun, 1984). Originally, this compound was assumed to dissipate quickly after application, but later evidence showed that residues lasted for many months in agricultural products. And although the amount of EDB in food posed only a weak carcinogenic risk

TABLE 14.2 Ranking of Possible Carcinogenic Hazards: The HERP Index

The *H*uman *E*xposure/*R*odent *P*otency index is calculated as human exposure (daily lifetime dose per kg body weight) as a percent of the dose found to induce tumors in half of the rodents tested.

Possible Hazard: HERP%	Daily Human Exposure	Potential Carcinogen
Environmental Pollution		
0.001	Tap water, 1 liter	Chloroform
0.008	Swimming pool, 1 hour (for child)	Chloroform
1.4	Mobile home air (14 hr/day)	Formaldehyde
Pesticides and Other Residues in Food		
0.00008	DDT and related compounds: daily dietary intake in 1990	DDT/DDE
0.0002	Apple, 1 whole (based on 1988 use of Alar)	Breakdown product of Alar
0.0004	EDB: daily dietary intake (from grain products before 1984 ban)	Ethylene dibromide
Natural Dietary Toxicants		
0.003	Bacon, cooked (100 g)	Dimethylnitrosamine
0.03	Peanut butter (one sandwich)	Aflatoxin
0.1	Mushroom (one raw)	Hydrazines
2.8	Beer (12 ounces)	Ethyl alcohol
Food Additives		
0.06	Diet cola (12 ounces)	Saccharin
Drugs		
16	Phenobarbital, one sleeping pill	Phenobarbital
Occupational Exposure		
4.0	Formaldehyde workers' average daily exposure	Formaldehyde
140	EDB workers' daily exposure	Ethylene dibromide

Source: Adapted from Gold et al., 1987.

polychlorinated biphenyls (PCBs)—types of industrial compounds, some of which have entered the food supply by accident, that are of concern because they may accumulate in biologic tissues over time

halogenated compounds—organic chemicals with chloride, fluoride, or bromide attached. PCBs and the pesticide DDT are examples of halogenated compounds

to consumers, occupational exposure risks of workers who produced EDB were very large (see Table 14.2).

Halogenated Compounds **Polychlorinated biphenyls (PCBs)** and related **halogenated compounds** are used for a variety of industrial purposes. Through improper disposal and accidents, many of these compounds have entered the food chain. Fish, especially sport fish, pick up high levels of PCBs if they live in polluted water. Although PCBs are no longer manufactured in United States, they continue to be a problem because they do not degrade easily.

DDT, a highly effective pesticide, is another example of a halogenated compound that was banned in the United States (in 1972) but still occurs in the environment. Its persistence is due to its slow rate of degradation (i.e., its long *half-life*) and its continued use overseas; some DDT enters the United States in imported products.

The effects of halogenated compounds vary (Stone, 1992). Some are toxic to the liver and can thereby adversely affect the metabolism of some nutrients, drugs, and other toxicants; others appear to affect the immune system, potentially making animals more susceptible to carcinogens.

You Tell Me

PCBs accumulate in body fat and are not easily excreted, except in breast milk (Jacobson et al., 1989). Many federal and state agencies monitor fish and the lakes from which they come, particularly the Great Lakes, for PCB contamination (Foran et al., 1989). Experts generally advise mothers who routinely consume fish caught in PCB-polluted waters to feed commercial formula to their infants rather than breast milk.

Do you think that a pregnant woman should be concerned if she had several fish meals while on a fishing vacation? Should this information affect *your* consumption of fish? (Remember the benefits of consuming fish.)

Radioactivity

More than 40 naturally occurring kinds of radioactive atoms have been identified in rocks and soils; many occur in the cells of plants and animals as well. You are also exposed to cosmic radiation. In fact, experts estimate that 82% of the radioactivity that you are exposed to is from natural sources (Marshall, 1990).

But there are sources of radioactivity other than nature. Fallout from tests of nuclear weapons, mining of certain ores, nuclear fuel processing, reactor installations, and applications of radioisotopes in medicine, industry, and agriculture can also add radioactivity to the environment. For example, medical x-rays are the source of 11% of Americans' radiation exposure (Marshall, 1990).

The nuclear accident at Chernobyl in the former USSR in 1986 demonstrated that an accident at a nuclear power plant can greatly increase the radioactivity in foods over a wide region (Anspaugh et al., 1988). Experts estimate that radiation-induced cancer mortality rates will increase 0.02% over natural occurrence in Europe because of this accident. Table 14.3 puts the relative risk due to various radiation sources in perspective.

Naturally Occurring Substances That Can Be Toxic

Among the myriad of natural chemicals that you eat daily, some are potentially toxic substances, as Table 14.2 suggests. Because you usually consume only low levels of these substances, however, they are not generally regarded as a problem.

TABLE 14.3 Comparison of Several Common Radiation Risks

Action	Dose (mrem/[a] year)	Estimated Cancers If All U.S. Population Exposed
Medical x-rays	40	1100
Radon gas (1.5 pCi/liter, equivalent dose)[a]	500	13,500
Cosmic radiation at sea level	40	1100
Cosmic radiation at Denver[b]	65	1800
Dose to average resident near Chernobyl first year	5000	Not relevant
One transcontinental round trip by air[b]	5	135
Average within 20 miles of nuclear plant	0.02	>1

[a]mrem and pCi are measures of exposure to radioactivity.
[b]The atmosphere protects you from cosmic radiation. Therefore, when you are at high altitudes as occurs in mountainous areas or during a flight, you are less protected from this radiation.
Source: Adapted from Wilson and Crouch, 1987.

Even so, there are certain situations in which you could be injured by eating compounds that occur naturally in plant and animal materials. This could occur if you consume abnormally large quantities of these toxicant-containing foods, if you consume foods highly contaminated with highly toxic substances from fungi or algae, if you consume food look-alikes containing highly toxic substances, or if you are unusually sensitive to the toxicants' effects.

Consumption of Abnormally Large Quantities of Natural Toxicants

If you eat large amounts of a single food (especially if you eat less of other foods at the same time), you may experience effects from naturally occurring toxicants. This can happen to people who deliberately emphasize just a few foods in their diets or to people experiencing famine, when minor foodstuffs may of necessity become major dietary components. Certain naturally occurring toxicants have caused problems at times, but often there are ways to avoid such problems, as the rest of this section explains.

methylxanthines—group of compounds that occur naturally in many plant species; coffee, tea, and cola beverages are common sources

Caffeine and Related Compounds Caffeine, theophylline, and theobromine are members of a group of compounds known as **methylxanthines.** They occur naturally in about 63 species of plants. Products containing these compounds are used daily in almost all cultures worldwide. The most common sources of these compounds are coffee, tea, chocolate, cola beverages, and a variety of over-the-counter and prescription drugs. Table 14.4 indicates the amounts of caffeine in products that you may consume.

Caffeine is a drug. It is well documented that low doses of it enhance alertness and increase the amount of time it takes for a person to fall asleep. Some studies in the 1970s indicated that caffeine can also aid performance in prolonged, exhaustive exercise, but research in the 1980s found that caffeine did not improve performance by well-trained marathoners during treadmill running (Casal and Leon, 1985).

TABLE 14.4 Caffeine Content of Selected Food Products

Product	Amount	Range (mg)	Average (mg)
Roasted and ground coffee (percolated)	5 ounces	39–168	74
Roasted and ground coffee (drip)	5 ounces	56–176	112
Instant coffee	5 ounces	29–117	66
Roasted and ground coffee, decaffeinated	5 ounces	1–8	2
Instant coffee, decaffeinated	5 ounces	2–8	3
Tea	5 ounces	8–91	27
Instant tea	5 ounces	24–31	28
Cocoa	5 ounces	2–7	4
Milk chocolate	1 ounce	1–15	6
Chocolate milk	8 ounces	2–7	5
Baking chocolate	1 ounce	18–118	60
Soft drinks	12 ounces		
Regular colas		30–46	—
Decaffeinated colas		trace	
Diet colas		2–58	—
Other soft drinks		0–trace	

Source: Adapted from Roberts and Barone, 1983. Copyright © by Institute of Food Technologists.

The average adult American consumes 3 mg of caffeine per kilogram of body weight daily (Roberts and Barone, 1983). (If you weigh 150 pounds and consume two to three cups of coffee per day, you get approximately this dose.) Doses at this level (3–5 mg/kg/day) can produce mild anxiety, respiratory stimulation, cardiovascular effects, diuresis (increased urine production), and increased gastric secretions. But you can develop a tolerance to methylxanthines if you consume them consistently over a period of time. Long-term intake of more than 600 mg per day may lead to chronic insomnia, persistent anxiety, paranoia, depression, and stomach upset.

Weak correlations between coffee drinking and coronary heart disease have been observed in some, but not all, studies. The correlation probably reflects coffee drinkers' different habits regarding alcohol consumption, diet, smoking, and exercise—not the effects of caffeine (Puccio et al., 1990). Moreover, although caffeine does cause blood pressure to rise slightly, most people develop a tolerance to its continued ingestion, and blood pressure then returns to baseline (Myers, 1988).

Similarly, studies attempting to link coffee consumption and cancer have also yielded mixed results (Nomura et al., 1986). Some physicians have suggested that caffeine and related compounds may promote symptoms of cyclical fibrocystic breast disease in women who are susceptible to it. (This condition involves the development of hard, nonmalignant breast lumps.) However, most physicians doubt that methylxanthine consumption is related to breast cancer (Phelps and Phelps, 1988).

In general, you shouldn't consider drinking two to three cups of coffee or tea per day a threat to health. But if you find that your consumption of coffee, tea, and/or colas is making you irritable and keeping you from sleeping, it's time to change your habit.

TABLE 14.5 Nitrate and Nitrite Content of Selected Vegetables and Cured Meats

	Concentration, mg/kg fresh weight			Concentration, mg/kg fresh weight	
	Nitrate	Nitrite		Nitrate	Nitrite
Asparagus	44	0.6	Melon	360	nd
Bacon, fried	32	7.0	Mushroom	160	0.5
Beans: green	340	0.6	Peas	28	0.6
lima	54	1.1	Pepper: sweet	120	0.4
Beet	2400	4.0	Potato: white	110	0.6
Broccoli	740	1.0	Pumpkin and squash	400	0.5
Cabbage	520	0.5	Rhubarb	2,100	nd
Carrot	200	0.8	Salami	78	13.0
Celery	2300	0.5	Spinach	1,800	2.5
Corn	45	2.0	Tomato	58	nd
Ham, nitrite cured	150	10.0	Turnip greens	6,600	2.3
Lettuce	1700	0.4	Wieners	96	10.0

nd = no data reported
Source: Adapted from the Committee on Nitrite and Alternative Curing Agents in Food, 1981, with the permission of the National Academy Press, Washington, D.C.

nitrate, nitrite—compounds of nitrogen and oxygen that occur naturally in many foods and can also be added during processing

nitrosamines—chemical products of certain reactions involving nitrates and nitrites

Nitrates, Nitrites, and Nitrosamines Elemental nitrogen and oxygen combine in various proportions to form **nitrate** and **nitrite.** Both occur *naturally* in foods and in your body, where some interconversions occur between them. (The major difference between these compounds is that nitrate has more oxygen in its structure.) Nitrite is also used as a food additive to cure meats and to prevent the growth of *Clostridium botulinum.* Nitrites can react with other substances in food or in your body to form other compounds called **nitrosamines.**

Levels of nitrate and nitrite vary widely among foods (Table 14.5). A number of factors, including agricultural practices and storage conditions, can affect the nitrate levels in food. In the average diet, vegetables contribute 87% of the *nitrate* ingested. And although you may have assumed that all the nitrite in foods is added during food processing, only about 39% of the nitrite in the U.S. food supply is added intentionally, mainly to cured meats (Committee on Nitrite and Alternative Curing Agents in Food, 1981). The rest occurs naturally. Actually though, all these figures on dietary sources of nitrite and nitrate are somewhat misleading, because your body produces nitrate in a quantity that may *exceed* the amount of nitrite and nitrate in your diet (Lee et al., 1986).

So what's the concern about these compounds? Epidemiologic studies have implicated foods containing high levels of nitrate, nitrite, and nitrosamines in the development of cancer, particularly of the stomach and esophagus. Later, animal studies showed that only the nitrosamines were carcinogenic (Committee on Nitrite and Alternative Curing Agents in Food, 1981). Fortunately, some foods contain substances that inhibit the formation of nitrosamines and therefore reduce this risk of cancer. For example, the presence of vitamin C, α-tocopherol, and other antioxidants (substances that prevent reactions between oxygen and certain food constituents) can block the formation of nitrosamines from nitrites.

You Tell Me

In response to concerns about nitrites and nitrosamines, the food industry in the United States now uses smaller amounts of nitrite to cure foods than it did in the past. Processors also use more antioxidants to prevent the formation of nitrosamines (IFT, 1987).

Do you think that commercially cured meats constitute a carcinogenic risk in the diets of Americans today?

The ingestion of large amounts of nitrate is sometimes a health concern for another reason. It can cause a condition called *methemoglobinemia,* which involves the production of abnormal hemoglobin unable to carry the usual amount of oxygen. This condition is most likely to occur in infants, who may become cyanotic (turn blue from lack of oxygen) if they consume well water contaminated with high levels of nitrate (Committee on Nitrite and Alternative Curing Agents in Food, 1981). In most states, there are county and/or state facilities that can test well water for its nitrate content.

Polycyclic Aromatic Compounds One difficulty in assessing the cancer risk from exposure to one substance—such as the nitrosamines discussed above—is that these compounds may not occur in isolation in food. Other potential mutagens and antimutagens which can affect the outcome of experiments may also be present.

For example, some carcinogens may be introduced into foods by normal cooking procedures. Two common classes of mutagens produced in foods by cooking are **polycyclic aromatic hydrocarbons** and **polycyclic aromatic amines.** These complex organic compounds are also found in some uncooked foods.

polycyclic aromatic hydrocarbons, polycyclic aromatic amines—common classes of mutagens produced in foods by certain types of dry heat cooking, especially if charring occurs

Polycyclic aromatic hydrocarbons are most likely to be produced in high-protein foods, such as meats, particularly when they are pan-fried or broiled, and especially if charring occurs. Some experts believe you should avoid ordering well-done charbroiled meats on a very frequent basis (Bjeldanes, 1983).

However, other experts note that these mutagenic compounds cause fewer cancers in test animals than might be expected, based on the amounts present. One explanation may be that anticarcinogens are also present in cooked food that lessen the risk from the polycyclic aromatic compounds (Hargraves, 1987). One such substance appears to be a derivative of linoleic acid, called *conjugated linoleic acid* or *CLA,* which occurs naturally in grilled ground beef and in milk products (Ha et al., 1990).

Consumption of Toxins from Molds and Other Fungi

Certain fungi that can grow on food may produce toxins. For example, **ergot** is a toxin produced by a fungus that can grow on grains, especially rye. The toxin can cause hallucinations—ergot is a natural source of LSD—and constrict capillaries, causing gangrene (death of tissue).

ergot—a fungal toxin that can cause hallucinations and blood vessel constriction

Before the development of modern milling processes that remove the part of the plant harboring the fungus, there were periodic outbreaks of the disease *ergotism*. Some historians believe that ergotism may have been the cause of the peculiar behavior of colonial Americans in the Salem witch trials. It probably was not the "devil" that made them act erratically; moldy rye may have been the cause.

Mold toxins of current importance are the **aflatoxins,** which are produced by some molds of the genus *Aspergillus;* many experts believe them to be the most potent liver toxins and carcinogenic agents known. Although aflatoxins have been found in many different foods, they most commonly contaminate peanuts, grains, and vegetables.

Note in Table 14.2 the slight risk of cancer from eating a peanut butter sandwich every day of your life. This does *not* mean that you should quit eating peanut butter. But it emphasizes the importance of carefully monitoring the food supply for aflatoxin, as is done routinely in North America for peanuts and grains. As a result of these tests, your exposure from commercially processed foods is low. However, aflatoxin contamination is thought to be more prevalent in developing countries.

Are other mold toxins hazardous? Very likely, but because they have not been as thoroughly studied as aflatoxin, scientists aren't sure. Your best bet is simply to discard food that has become moldy, because it is difficult to estimate how far into the food's interior the mold's toxin may have penetrated. If you want to salvage a large solid block of refrigerated cheese that has a slightly moldy surface, cut away at least ½ inch of cheese from every moldy surface to avoid toxins (IFT, 1986).

Consumption of Toxic Substances in Nonfood Materials

Young children are the most common victims of poisoning by nonfood materials. If you've ever watched a baby or toddler explore his or her environment by seeing, touching, and tasting everything, this will not surprise you.

In recent years, state health departments and the Centers for Disease Control (CDC) have also received data on a number of adults who have been poisoned by natural products that resemble food products but are not foods themselves. Consuming poisonous mushrooms or herbs for tea that are "look-alikes" of edible varieties can be a fatal mistake.

If you are interested in collecting and consuming natural products, you should obtain authoritative information from the experts in state hygiene laboratories and state horticulture Cooperative Extension offices. If there is any doubt about a plant you are considering for use as food, do not consume it.

Treating people who ingest toxic plant material is often difficult because the poisonous substances in plants and the symptoms they produce vary so greatly. Some substances may irritate the GI tract and rapidly induce nausea and vomiting; others damage the liver or central nervous system. This variety of consequences makes diagnosis difficult. If somebody starts to become ill after consuming an unusual natural product, call your local poison control center immediately (Figure 14.7). If you are advised to go the hospital emergency room, take along a sample of the plant material (if you have it); this will aid in diagnosis and treatment.

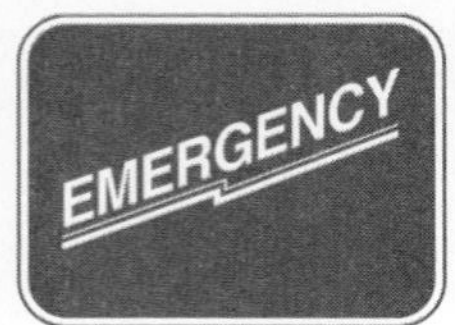

9-1-1

Or dial "0" (operator). Tell the operator the exact location including the community name, street number and the type of help needed. Stay on the telephone.

Police

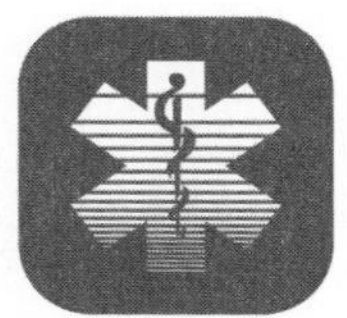

Ambulance

Fire

Sheriff

Poison Center

FIGURE 14.7
The phone number of your local poison center.

This valuable number can be found in the front of your telephone book with other emergency numbers.

Additives: A Risk to Few People

The FDA defines *additives* as "substances added directly to food, or substances which may reasonably be expected to become components of food through surface contact with equipment or packaging materials, or even substances that may otherwise affect the food without becoming a part of it" (Jukes, 1981). Despite that rather overwhelming formal definition, in the discussion that follows we'll consider only substances that are directly and deliberately added to food.

aflatoxin—a group of mold toxins believed by some to be the most potent liver carcinogens known

Government Monitoring

The federal government first concerned itself with food additives in 1906, when the Pure Food Law was enacted. This law (and the ensuing regulations that were used to enforce it) called for truth in labeling and gave the government the authority to seize and destroy hazardous foods. A primary concern at that time was to rid the food supply of foreign or misrepresented substances that some food processors were using in lieu of the pure, more expensive product that they claimed to be marketing. For example, pepper sometimes was polluted with ground wood, raspberry jam with alfalfa seeds, ground mustard with flour, and candy with plaster of paris. In 1938, the Federal Food, Drug, and Cosmetic Act improved on the earlier law, with stronger and more specific prohibitions against adulteration and misbranding.

In 1958 and 1960, with hundreds of additives already in use, the Food, Drug, and Cosmetic Act was amended in several important ways:

- Any company wanting to use a new food additive is now required to present to the FDA proof of its safety. The additive cannot be used until the FDA gives its approval.
- A listing, called the **GRAS list,** was made of hundreds of additives already in use that were *G*enerally *R*ecognized *A*s *S*afe (GRAS), based on their innocuous presence in the food supply for many years. (The GRAS list has now grown to thousands and includes items such as salt and sugar.) A list of *prior sanctioned substances* was also prepared, consisting of additives that the FDA or USDA had approved before 1958. (The status of additives on these lists can be challenged by new evidence; some substances have lost their places on the original lists in that way.)
- A *margin of safety* was established. For most additives, there is an *acceptable daily intake* of 1/100 of the amount thought to be hazardous. This applies only to substances that are not carcinogenic; carcinogenic substances may not be added at all.
- The **Delaney Clause** specified that no substance could be added to the food supply if it had been shown to cause cancer in people or animals. Now that sensitive testing can identify minute, probably inconsequential levels of carcinogens in common foods, this legislation is not logical (Curran, 1988). Even so, although modifications of the Delaney Clause are often discussed, no changes in legislation have occurred. If consumers and legislators really understood the problem and cost of guaranteeing zero amounts of substances in foods—as the sensitivity of the tests has increased by more than a thousand-fold—they would demand changes in the legislation.

GRAS list—list of thousands of additives in current use that are *G*enerally *R*ecognized *A*s *S*afe, based on their long-standing innocuous presence in the food supply

Delaney Clause—law specifying that no substance can be added to the food supply if it has been shown to cause cancer in people or animals

Purposes and Prevalence of Additives

Additives must have purposes that will benefit the consumer. There are four broad categories of legitimate use recognized by FDA: to maintain product quality, to help in processing or preparation, to make food more appealing, and to maintain or improve nutritional value. The addition of nutrients to

Ingredients
Specially processed degerminated white corn grits, salt, niacin, reduced iron, BHA (a preservative), thiamin mononitrate, riboflavin.
SHAKER'S
Instant
GRITS
Grandma's
Gourmet
Soups
Split
Pea
Ingredients
Cooked split peas, carrots, potatoes, potato starch, celery, bacon, salt, sugar, monosodium glutamate, yeast extract, natural flavoring, and smoke flavoring.

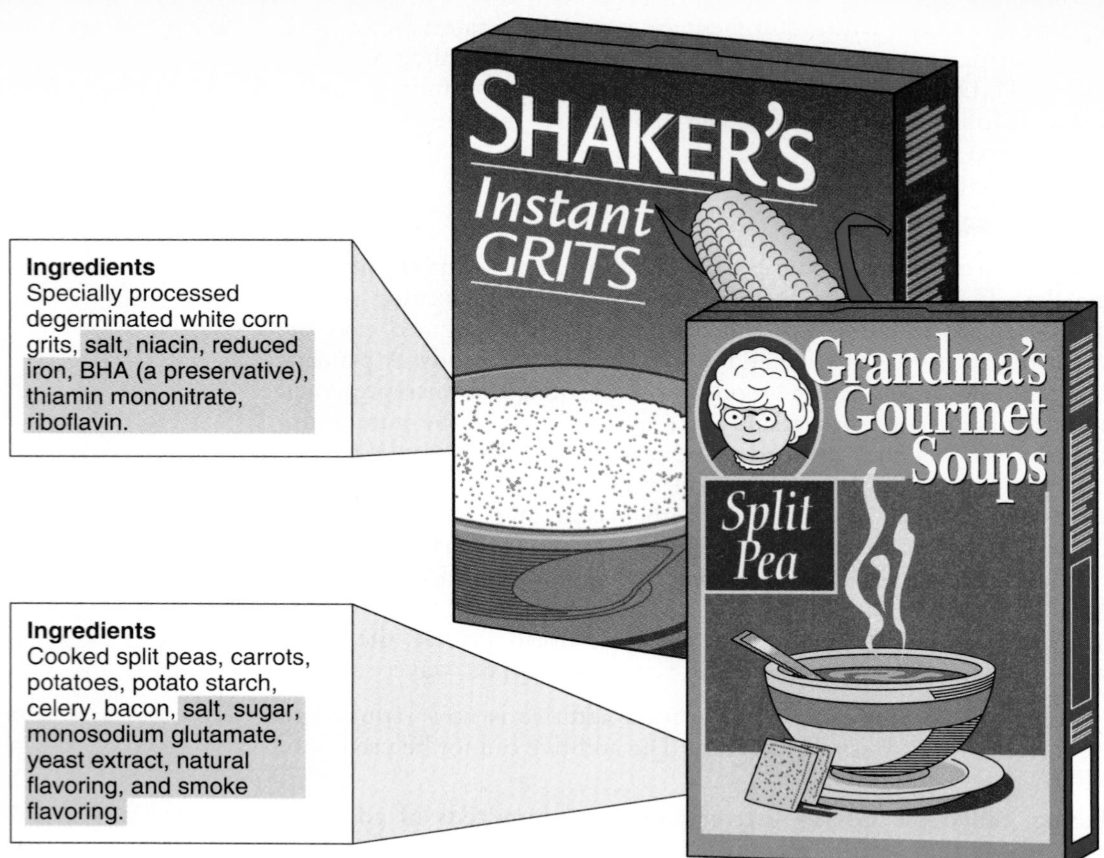

FIGURE 14.8
Examples of additives in two processed foods.

improve nutritional value has been discussed in earlier chapters; this section focuses on the first three purposes.

There are currently over 2900 additives approved for use in the United States. You, as an average American, consume approximately 73 kg (160 pounds) of additives per year: over 64 kg (140 pounds) of sweeteners, including sucrose; 7 kg (15 pounds) of sodium chloride (table salt); and 2–5 kg (5–10 pounds) of all the others. This means that flavorings, colorings, and preservatives constitute up to 0.6% of the estimated 759 kg (1670 pounds) of food you consume in a year (Welsh and Marston, 1982).

Figure 14.8 shows examples of additives as they might appear on labels of processed foods.

Additives That Maintain Product Quality You benefit from the addition to foods of substances that eliminate or control microorganisms and other living contaminants. For example, sodium and calcium propionate, sodium benzoate, potassium sorbate, and sulfur dioxide are used in baked goods and other products to prevent growth of bacteria, yeast, and mold.

Another important group of additives that preserve product quality are the antioxidants: the additives BHA (butylated hydroxyanisole), BHT (butylated hydroxytoluene), propyl gallate, and vitamin E protect against oxidation of fats (rancidity). Antioxidants often function by being easily oxidized themselves, thereby sparing other compounds in the food.

Other additives are used to inhibit the enzymes that cause browning reactions in fruits and vegetables. Vitamin C is sometimes used for this purpose, especially to prevent the browning of fruits.

One group of compounds used to prevent browning—*sulfites*—has gained notoriety in the last decade. Since 1982, the FDA has received more than 20 reports of deaths alleged to be due to ingestion of food processed with sulfur dioxide, sodium sulfite, sodium or potassium bisulfites, or metabisulfites (Taylor, 1987). The people who died were known to have *asthma,* a condition in which the airways constrict under certain conditions. Experts believe that only a small percentage (5–10%) of severe asthmatics are sensitive to sulfites, and most of those who are sensitive develop hives and shortness of breath that is not life-threatening. Certainly, people who are severely affected need to become experts at avoiding sulfites.

Packaged foods that have typically been treated with sulfites are light-colored dried fruits (such as apricots and pears), dried potatoes, and wine. FDA regulations require all packaged foods containing significant sulfite residues (10 or more micrograms per gram of food) to be labeled accordingly. Over-the-counter medications may also contain sulfites.

You Tell Me

The FDA has banned the use of sulfites on fresh fruits and most vegetables. But regulations regarding the use of sulfites, especially to treat cut potatoes, continue to change.

If you were sulfite-sensitive, what would be a good strategy when buying a packaged potato product—or any other consumable, for that matter? What defensive dining behaviors would be needed in restaurants?

Additives That Aid in Processing or Preparation Many additives are useful in the processing and preparation of food. For example, sodium bicarbonate (baking soda), calcium phosphate, and sodium aluminum phosphate are leavening agents used in baked products raised without yeast, such as biscuits, muffins, cornbread, and cakes. Calcium and aluminum silicate and iron-ammonium citrate are anticaking agents used in salts and many powdered products. Emulsifiers, such as mono- and diglycerides, lecithin, carrageenan, and polysorbates, are used in salad dressings, processed cheese, and ice cream. Various gums, pectin, and alginates are used to thicken jellies, candies, and ice cream. Acetic acid, citric acid, lactic acid, phosphates and phosphoric acid, and sodium acetate are used to adjust the acidity in such foods as pickles and carbonated beverages.

Other additives serve as humectants (moisturizers), maturing agents (factors that speed ripening), bleaching agents, and dough conditioners. Some of the tongue-twisting terms you see toward the end of ingredient lists refer to these various processing aids.

Additives That Make Food More Appealing Any additive that makes food more pleasing to taste or look at is a member of this group. Three principal categories are flavorings and flavor enhancers, sweeteners, and colorings.

Flavorings and Flavor Enhancers *Flavorings* include condiments, spices, concentrated fruits and juices, process flavors (such as "roasted"), or flavor elements concentrated from the above. Compounds extracted from food sources (natural flavorings) are often chemically identical to those produced in the laboratory (artificial flavorings). In such cases, these flavorings are also indistinguishable in terms of their safety (Smith, 1981). *Flavor en-*

hancers, such as monosodium glutamate (MSG) and hydrolyzed vegetable proteins, heighten existing flavors in foods (see Chapter 7).

Sweeteners Other groups of additives that make food more appealing are caloric sweeteners (including beet and cane sugars, syrups, honey, molasses, and purified sweet carbohydrates such as sucrose, glucose, fructose, sorbitol, and mannitol) and noncaloric sweeteners (including saccharin, aspartame, and acesulfame-K).

One of these additives—saccharin—has had a controversial history. It was included on the GRAS list in 1958 because of its long-standing use without apparent problems. But its status was challenged in 1977 because saccharin was found to cause bladder cancer in rats (although not in humans). According to the Delaney Clause, this evidence was sufficient for FDA to ban saccharin. However, saccharin is still on the market today because Congress has repeatedly declared a moratorium on the ban in response to public pressure to keep saccharin available (Miller and Frattali, 1989). Many observers believe the controversy about artificial sweeteners helps make the case that the Delaney Clause is outdated.

There are also scientific reasons to defend the continued availability of saccharin. For one, differences in the metabolism of rats and humans make it unlikely that saccharin is a carcinogen in humans. For another, experts believe that the best policy is to have several low-calorie sweeteners (including saccharin, aspartame, and others) available for public use to lessen the chance of overuse of any one product (Gelardi, 1987). For information on the safety of aspartame, see Chapter 7.

Colorings *Colorings* are the final group of additives that improve sensory appeal. Approximately 30 food colorings are used in the United States. Others can be used in specified circumstances.

More questions have been raised about the safety of colorings than about most other categories of additives. Many synthetic dyes formerly used in foods are no longer allowed, in some cases because they were found to be carcinogenic. Future use of other synthetic dyes will hinge on individual tests. Natural colorings present problems, because they do not hold up in foods as well as the synthetic colorings do (Meggos, 1984).

Just as with some other scientific issues, experts disagree about the interpretation of studies on food colorings. For example, at about the same time that the FDA banned Red No. 2 and suggested using Red No. 40 as a substitute, Canada banned Red No. 40 and in its place used Red No. 2 (IFT Expert Panel on Food Safety and Nutrition and the Committee on Public Information, 1980). As part of the new nutrition labeling regulations (published on January 6, 1993), all colors used as food additives must be individually listed on food labels. If you read the label, therefore, you can avoid these food additives if you wish.

The Consider This box on page 479 summarizes how best to avoid taking in a hazardous amount of any substance.

To avoid excess amounts of toxicants in food, instead of

This	*. Consider this*
Avoiding all foods that might contain toxicants at any level	**Eating a variety of foods as suggested in the Food Guide Pyramid.**
Unsafe handling and disposal of yard and household chemicals	**Following instructions on labels of pesticides, fertilizers, and all yard and household chemicals. Contact local sanitation department for more information on disposal of hazardous chemicals.**
Relying on others to ensure the safety of your food	**Taking an active role in your own food safety. Be alert to both print and electronic media for information on food recalls and improved food-handling procedures.**

Summary

- Thousands of substances besides nutrients occur naturally in foods, and most are harmless in the amounts typically consumed. Among those substances that do have the potential to cause harm, some occur naturally, others find their way into the food supply by accident, and still others may be added intentionally to achieve some other effect. Unfortunately, it is not possible to simply make lists of harmful and harmless chemicals and avoid the former, nor is it necessary to avoid all potentially harmful substances entirely, because at low levels of intake and under typical conditions many are harmless.
- **Food toxicology** is the science that establishes the basis for judgments about the safety of foodborne chemicals. Common toxicologic terms are *safety, hazard, toxicity,* **toxicant** (also *toxin* or *poison*), *detoxification, mutagen, teratogen,* and *carcinogen*. It is important to remember that all substances that make up foods are toxic at extreme levels of intake, but most are not hazardous under normal conditions of use. Furthermore, some foods contain **antagonists** to toxic substances such as **anticarcinogens.**
- **Dose-response curves** illustrate the relationship between the dosage of a substance and its effect. Some substances have no effect; others have a threshold effect or no threshold (are harmful at all levels of intake). Most nutrients have a low-dose beneficial threshold. Many factors influence toxicity, including detoxification processes, time, storage in the body, nutritional status, growth and body size, and interactions among substances.
- Microorganisms are responsible for the majority of food-related health problems, such as **gastroenteritis, hepatitis,** and even **cholera.** If such a condition affects a large number of people, the result is an **epidemic. Foodborne infections** (caused by large numbers of bacteria in food) and **foodborne bacterial intoxications** (caused by bacterial toxins) can be very unpleasant but are not usually severe. **Botulism,** a less common intoxication, can be fatal, as can infection with *Listeria monocytogenes.*
- Environmental food contaminants are common but not always harmful. Lead, aluminum, and tin can migrate into food from metal food preparation equipment and storage containers and from other

environmental sources. Mercury (in the form of **methyl mercury**) and cadmium can also enter the food supply in various ways. The harm they produce depends on many factors, including chemical form, dosage, length of exposure, and age and health status of the person(s) involved.

- Organic contaminants, such as antibiotics, hormones, pesticides, and other industrial **halogenated compounds,** such as **polychlorinated biphenyls (PCBs),** can be toxic in certain situations, particularly if they accumulate in animal tissues over time. The effects of these compounds vary greatly. Some are toxic to nervous tissue, some to liver, some to the immune system, and some are carcinogens.
- Radioactivity is another possible food contaminant. Natural radiation comes from the soil and cosmic sources. Other sources are radioactive substances from medical and industrial uses and from nuclear power generation.
- Many naturally occurring substances can also be toxic. Problems can arise if an individual consumes abnormally large quantities of such substances as **methylxanthines** (including caffeine), **nitrosamines** and related compounds, and **polycyclic aromatic hydrocarbons** and **amines.** Consuming the mold toxins **ergot** and **aflatoxins** can have dire consequences. Poisonings resulting from the ingestion of nonfood items, such as misidentified mushrooms and certain herbal teas, also occur periodically.
- Governmental monitoring of the U.S. and Canadian food supplies is routine and ongoing. Federal laws regulate the introduction of new additives and their margin of safety. The **GRAS list** includes thousands of additives that are generally recognized as safe, and the **Delaney Clause** specifies that substances shown to cause cancer in animals or humans cannot be added to the food supply. Regulations are continually being reviewed and revised.
- Additives must benefit food consumers in at least one of the following ways: (1) by maintaining product quality (controlling microorganisms, preventing oxidation); (2) by aiding in processing or preparation (leavening, emulsifying, thickening); (3) by making food more appealing (flavoring, sweetening, coloring); or (4) by maintaining or improving nutritional value.

References

Ames, B.N. and L.S. Gold. 1989. Pesticides, risk and applesauce. *Science* 236:755–757.

Anderson, C. 1991. Cholera epidemic traced to risk miscalculation. *Nature* 354:255.

Annest, J.K., K.R. Mahaffey, D.H. Cox, and J. Roberts. 1982. Blood lead levels for persons 6 months–74 years of age: United States 1976–80. *NCHS Advance Data* 79:1–24.

Anspaugh, L.R., R.J. Catlin, M. Goldman. 1988. The global impact of the Chernobyl reactor accident. *Science* 242:1513–1519.

Aposhian, H.V., D.C. Bruce, W. Alter, R.C. Dart, K.M. Hurlbut, and M.M. Aposhian. 1992. Urinary mercury after administration of 2,3-dimercaptopropane-1-sulfuric acid: Correlation with dental amalgam score. *FASEB Journal* 6:2472–2476.

Bellinger, D., A. Leviton, C. Waternaux, H. Needleman, M. Rabinowitz. 1987. Longitudinal analyses of prenatal and postnatal lead exposure and early cognitive development. *New England Journal of Medicine* 316:1037–1043.

Bjeldanes, L.F. 1983. Hazards in the food supply: Lead, aflatoxins and mutagens produced by cooking. *Nutrition Update* 1:105–119.

Blaser, M.J., E. Sazie, and L.P. Williams. 1987. The influence of immunity on raw milk-associated *Campylobacter* infection. *Journal of the American Medical Association* 257:43–46.

Bois, F.Y., T.N. Tozer, L. Zeise, and L.Z. Benet. 1989. Application of clearance concepts to the assessment of exposure to lead in drinking water. *American Journal of Public Health* 79:827–831.

Boynton, R. 1990. *California Farmer,* June 2, 1990.

Bruhn, C.M. 1991. Pesticide use in California. *Food Safety Notebook* 2:13–15.

Casal, D.C. and A.S. Leon. 1985. Failure of caffeine to affect substrate utilization during prolonged running. *Medicine and Science in Sports and Exercise* 17:174–179.

Clarkson, T.W. 1987. Mercury. In *Trace elements in human and animal nutrition,* 5th edition, ed. W. Mertz. San Diego, CA: Academic Press.

Coats, J.R. 1987. Toxicology of pesticide residues in foods. In *Nutritional toxicology,* volume II, ed. J. Hathcock. Orlando, FL: Academic Press.

Collins, S.S., K.E. Belk, H.R. Cross, and G.C. Smith. 1989. The EEC ban against growth-promoting hormones. *Nutrition Reviews* 47:238–246.

Committee on Nitrite and Alternative Curing Agents in Food. 1981. *The health effects of nitrate, nitrite, and N-nitroso compounds.* Washington, DC: National Academy Press.

Curran, W.J. 1988. Cancer causing substances in food, drugs and cosmetics: The de Minimis Rule versus Delaney Clause. *New England Journal of Medicine* 319: 1262–1264.

Desenclos, J.C.A., K.C. Klontz, M.H. Wilder, O.V. Nainan, H.S. Margolis, and R.A. Gunn. 1991. A multistate outbreak of hepatitis A caused by consumption of raw oysters. *American Journal of Public Health* 81: 1268–1272.

Doyle, M.P. 1988. *Campylobacter jejuni. Food Technology* 42(no. 4):187–188.

DuPont, H.L. 1986. Consumption of raw shellfish—is the risk unacceptable? *New England Journal of Medicine* 314:707–708.

DuPont, H.L. and J.H. Steele. 1987. Use of antimicrobial agents in animal feeds: Implications for human health. *Review of Infectious Diseases* 9:447–460.

Foran, J.A., M. Cox, and D. Croxton. 1989. Sport fish consumption advisories and projected cancer risks in the Great Lakes basin. *American Journal of Public Health* 79:322–325.

Gelardi, R.C. 1987. The multiple sweetener approach and new sweeteners on the horizon. *Food Technology* 41:123–124.

Glass, R.I., M. Libel, and A.D. Brandling-Bennett. 1992. Epidemic cholera in the Americas. *Science* 256: 1254–1255.

Gold, L.S., T.H. Slone, B.R. Stern, N.B. Manley, and B.N. Ames. 1992. Rodent carcinogens: Setting priorities. *Science* 258:261–265.

Greger, J.L. 1987. Aluminum and tin. *World Review of Nutrition and Diet* 54:255–285.

Greger, J.L. 1992. Dietary and other sources of aluminum intake. In *Aluminum in Biology and Medicine*. Ciba Foundation Symposium 169. Chichester: John Wiley & Sons.

Ha, Y.L., J. Storkson, and M.W. Pariza. 1990. Inhibition of benzo(a)pyrene-induced mouse forestomach neoplasia by conjugated dienoic derivatives of linoleic acid. *Cancer Research* 50:1097–1101.

Hall, R.L. and S.L. Taylor. 1989. Food toxicology and safety evaluation: Changing perspectives and challenge for the future. *Food Technology* 43(no. 9):270–279.

Hargraves, W.A. 1987. Mutagens in cooked foods. In *Nutritional technology,* volume II, ed. J.N. Hathcock. Orlando, FL: Academic Press.

Harris, N.V., D. Thompson, D.C. Martin, and C.M. Nolan. 1986. A survey of *Campylobacter* and other bacterial contaminants of pre-market chicken and retail poultry and meats, King County, Washington. *American Journal of Public Health* 76:401–406.

Institute of Food Technologists (IFT). 1980 *Food colors. Food Technology* 34(no. 7):77–84.

Institute of Food Technologists (IFT). 1986. Mycotoxins and food safety. *Food Technology* 40(no. 5):59–66.

Institute of Food Technologists (IFT). 1987. Nitrate, nitrite and nitrosocompounds in food. *Food Technology* 41(no. 4):127–135.

Institute of Food Technologists (IFT) Expert Panel on Food Safety and Nutrition. 1988. Bacteria associated with foodborne diseases. *Food Technology* 42(no. 4):181–200.

Jackson, G.J., J.W. Bier, and T.L. Schwartz. 1990. More on making sushi safe. *New England Journal of Medicine* 322:1011.

Jacobson, J.L., H.E.B. Humphrey, S.W. Jacobsen, S.L. Schantz, M.D. Mullin, and R. Welsh. 1989. Determinants of polychlorinated biphenyls (PCBs), polybrominated biphenyls (PBBs) and dichlorodiphenyl tricholorethane (DDT) levels in the sera of young children. *American Journal of Public Health* 79:1401–1404.

Jukes, T.H. 1981. Organic foods and food additives. In *Controversies in Nutrition,* ed. L. Ellenbogen. New York: Churchill Livingstone.

Kostial, K. 1986. Cadmium. In *Trace elements in human and animal nutrition,* 5th edition, ed. W.J. Mertz. Orlando, FL: Academic Press.

Lee, K., J.L. Greger, J.R. Cansaul, K.L. Graham, and B.L. Chinn. 1986. Nitrate, nitrite balance, and de novo synthesis of nitrate in humans consuming cured meats. *American Journal of Clinical Nutrition* 44:188–194.

Leveille, G.A. and M.A. Uebersax. 1979. Fundamentals of food science for the dietitian: Thermal processing. *Dietetic Currents* 6(no. 3). Columbus, OH: Ross Laboratories.

Liska, B.J., E.M. Foster, J.H. Silliker, and D.L. Archer. 1986. New bacteria in the news: A special symposium. *Food Technology* 40(no. 8):16–26.

Mahaffey, K.R., P.S. Gartside, C.J. Glueck. 1986. Blood lead levels and dietary calcium intake in 1- to 5-year old children: The second National Health and Nutrition Examination Survey, 1976 to 1980. *Pediatrics* 78:257.

Marshall, E. 1990. Academy panel raises radiation risk estimate. *Science* 247:22–23.

Meggos, H.N. 1984. Colors—key food ingredients. *Food Technology* 38(no. 1):70–74.

Miller, S.A. 1991. Technology, food safety and federal regulations. In *Nutrition in the '90s,* ed. G.E. Gaull, F.N. Kotsonis, and M.A. Mackey. New York: Marcel Dekker, Inc.

Miller, S.A. and V.P. Frattali. 1989. Saccharin. *Diabetes Care* 12:75–80.

Murphy, S.D. 1979. Toxicological assessment of food residues. *Food Technology* 33(no. 6):35–42.

Myers, M.G. 1988. Effects of caffeine on blood pressure. *Archives of Internal Medicine* 148:1189–1193.

Needleman, H.L., A. Schell, D. Bellinger, A. Leviton, and E.N. Allred. 1990. The long-term effects of exposure to low doses of lead in childhood: An 11-year follow-up report. *New England Journal of Medicine* 322:83–88.

Newsome, R.L. 1988. *Staphylococcus aureus. Food Technology* 42(no. 4):194–195.

NIH Technology Assessment Conference. 1991. NIH technology assessment conference statement on bovine somatotropin. *Journal of the American Medical Association* 265:1423–1425.

Nomura, A., L.K. Heilbrun, and G.N. Stimmermann. 1986. Prospective study of coffee consumption and risk of cancer. *Journal of the National Cancer Institute* 76:587–590.

Nutrition Reviews. 1991. Highlights of the executive summary of the report by the Committee on Evaluation of the Safety of Fishery Products of the Food and Nutrition Board, Institute of Medicine, National Academy of Sciences. *Nutrition Reviews* 49:357–363.

Phelps, H.M. and C.E. Phelps. 1988. Caffeine ingestion and breast cancer. *Cancer* 61:1051–1054.

Puccio, E.M., J.B. McPhillips, E. Barrett-Conner, and T.G. Ganiats. 1990. Clustering of atherogenic behaviors in coffee drinkers. *American Journal of Public Health* 80:1310–1313.

Roberts, H.R. and J.J. Barone. 1983. Biological effects of caffeine: History and use. *Food Technology* 37(no. 9):32–39.

Russell, L. 1990. Consumers face little danger from residues in meat and poultry. *Food News* 6(no. 4):10–11.

Ryser, E.T. and E.H. Marth. 1989. "New" foodborne pathogens of public health significance. *Journal of the American Dietetic Association* 89:948–954.

Schuchat, A., K.A. Deaver, J.D. Wenger, B.D. Plikaytis, L. Mascola, R.W. Pinner, A.L. Reingold, C.V. Broome, and Listeria Study Group. 1992. Role of foods in sporadic listeriosis. *Journal of the American Medical Association* 267:2041–2045.

Smith, M.V. 1981. Regulation of artificial and natural flavors. *Cereal Foods World* 26:278–280.

St. Louis, M.E., D.L. Morse, M.E. Potter, T.M. Demelfi, J.J. Guzewich, R.V. Tauxe, and P.A. Blake. 1988. The emergence of grade A eggs as a major source of *Salmonella enteritidis* infections. *Journal of the American Medical Association* 259:2103–2107.

Stone, R. 1992. Swimming against the PCB tide. *Science* 255:798–799.

Sun, M. 1984. EDB contamination kindles federal action. *Science* 223:464–466.

Taylor, S.L. 1987. Allergic and sensitivity reactions to food components. In *Nutritional toxicology,* volume II, ed. J.N. Hathcock, Orlando, FL: Academic Press.

United States Department of Agriculture. 1990. *Chartbook.* Agriculture Handbook No. 689. Washington, DC: United States Department of Agriculture.

United States Department of Agriculture, Food Safety and Inspection Service. 1984. *The safe food book.* Home and Garden Bulletin No. 241. Washington, DC: United States Department of Agriculture.

Welsh, S.P. and R.M. Marston. 1982. Review of trends in food use in the United States, 1909–80. *Journal of the American Dietetic Association* 81:120–125.

Wilson, R. and E.A.C. Crouch. 1987. Risk assessment and comparisons: An introduction. *Science* 236:267–270.

Wodicka, V.O. 1977. Food safety—rationalizing the ground rules for safety evaluation. *Food Technology* 31(no. 9):75–79.

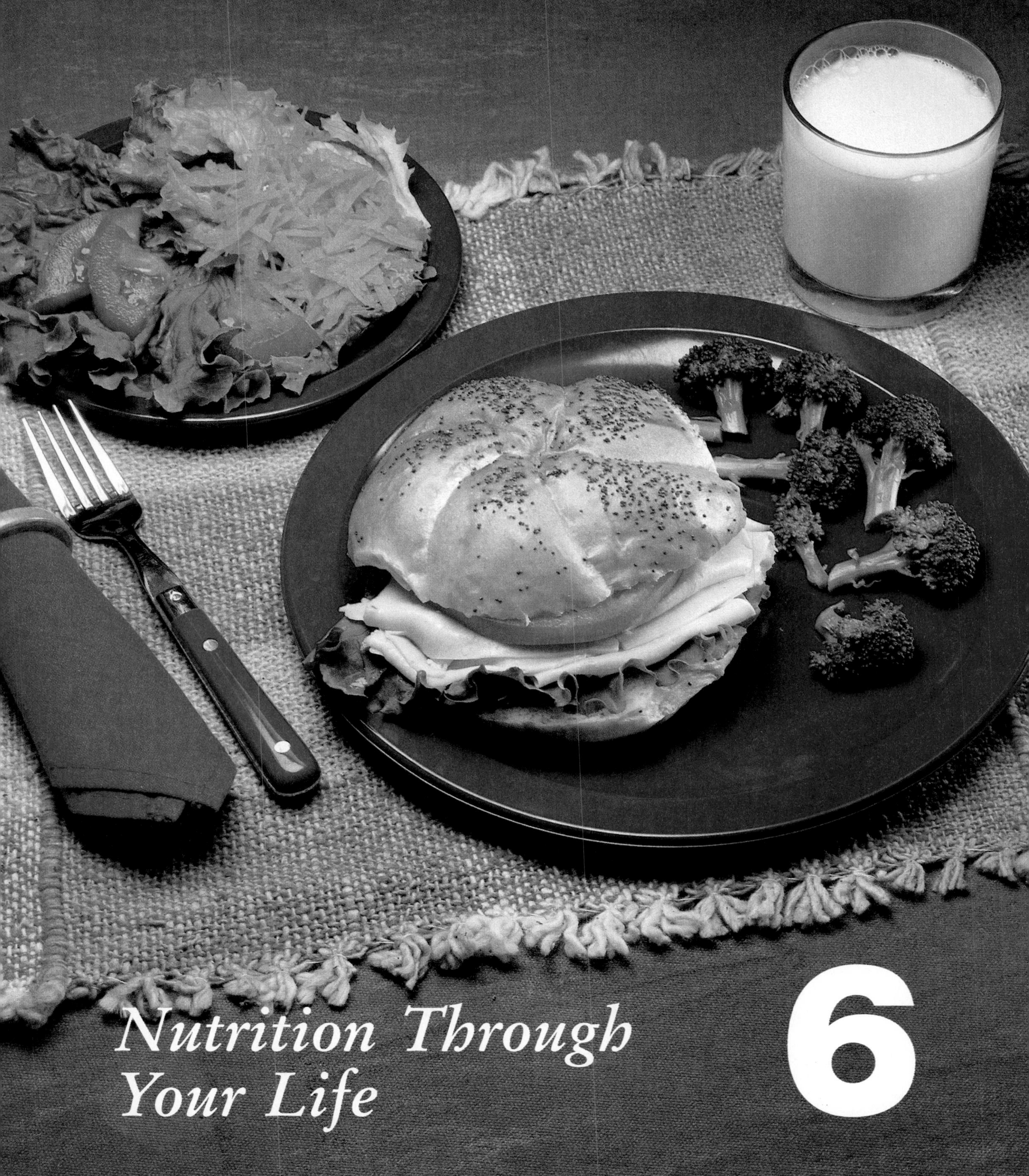

6 Nutrition Through Your Life

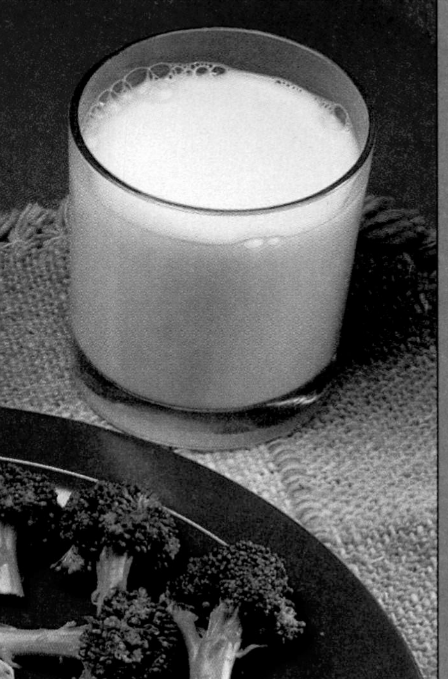

IN THIS CHAPTER

Chapter 15

Nutrition for Pregnancy, Lactation, and Infancy

You're *what*? You're *pregnant*?

What's happening here? A happy young husband could be responding to the news from his elated wife, both delighted that their plans for starting a family are on target. Or a couple could be facing the news with mixed reactions—expecting that parenthood will enrich their lives, but wondering how much they will need to change their career-oriented lifestyle. A teenage boy could be recoiling in fright and anger at the news from his panicky girlfriend. Or an older father who has enjoyed his parenting role but is now looking forward to having the children go out on their own could be reacting in shock to the announcement of his equally stunned middle-aged wife.

Whatever the circumstances, pregnancy has a major emotional impact on the lives of the prospective mother and father and the people close to them. It also has a considerable physiologic impact that affects nutritional needs.

During pregnancy, all the raw materials for the development of what becomes the baby must be taken from the supply of nutrients circulating in the mother's bloodstream; the mother is truly eating for two. Her increased hunger may give her the message to eat more, but she may need information about what foods will best satisfy her nutrient needs: many people have misinformation about nutrition for pregnancy (Carruth and Skinner, 1991).

Before delivery, the mother and father must decide whether they will nourish their baby by breast-feeding or bottle-feeding. Breast-fed infants continue to rely on their mothers' bodies as their main source of nourishment. Bottle-fed babies consume substitutes for breast milk, in the form of various specially designed formulas created by modern technology.

The questions of when to start adding other foods and what these other foods should be are other important parental considerations. In the past, most parents simply adopted the usual practices of their culture, but now scientific data are available to help parents decide about these issues. But feeding is not just about nutrition: parents also need to be aware that feeding times are of prime importance in their child's social development as well.

In this chapter you'll learn about all of these topics.

The Importance of Gaining Enough Weight

Nutrition has a great effect on the health of the baby and mother; however, it is not the only thing that matters. Table 15.1 lists major factors that pose risks to the developing fetus.

One factor that is very important in every pregnancy—and one over which the mother has considerable control—is weight gain. Gaining enough weight is essential: if the mother doesn't gain sufficient weight during **gestation,** her baby may be too small. This puts her infant at risk of death or, if it survives, increases the risk of various health problems. *Infant birth weight is more closely related to infant mortality than is any other variable* (Brown, 1989).

gestation—development of the future baby from fertilization to birth; pregnancy

How Much Weight Should a Pregnant Woman Gain?

Mothers who have gained either too little or too much weight are more likely to face poor birth outcomes. Generally, for a mother who was at her recommended weight at conception, a weight gain of 11–16 kg (25–35 pounds) for a single pregnancy will produce the healthiest baby (Committee on Nutritional Status During Pregnancy and Lactation, 1990).

TABLE 15.1 Risk Factors in Pregnancy

Risk Factors Present at the Beginning of Pregnancy
Age
15 years or younger
35 years or older
Frequent Pregnancies: three or more during a 2-year period
Medical problems during previous pregnancies
Poverty
Bizarre or faddist food habits
Use of nicotine, alcohol, or certain other drugs
Therapeutic diet required for a chronic disorder
Abnormal weight
Less than 85% of standard weight
More than 135% of standard weight
Risk Factors Occurring During Pregnancy
Low levels of iron in blood (according to special standards for pregnancy)
Any weight loss during pregnancy
Inadequate weight gain: less than 2 pounds/month after the first 3 months
Excessive weight gain: more than 2.2 pounds/week after the first three months

Source: Adapted from Williams, 1988.

There are many exceptions to this standard, though. Because a woman who is 10% below recommended weight for height at conception is more likely to have problems during pregnancy and to have a poor birth outcome, a larger weight gain might be better for her. Conversely, for a pregnant woman who is either very overweight or quite petite, a somewhat lower weight gain may be in order.

Figure 15.1 shows what amounts and patterns of weight gain are recommended for pregnant women, based on their prepregnancy body mass index (BMI). Note that even an obese woman needs to gain some weight during pregnancy; *this is not the time to try to shed excess pounds,* because

FIGURE 15.1 Recommended weight gain ranges for single pregnancies, based on body mass index (BMI).

A mother's weight status at conception determines how much weight she should gain during pregnancy. The graph at the left represents gains recommended for normal-weight women with a prepregnancy BMI of 19.8–26.0. Recommended weight gain ranges for overweight and underweight women are shown in graphs at middle and right.

(Adapted from Committee on Nutritional Status During Pregnancy and Lactation, 1990.)

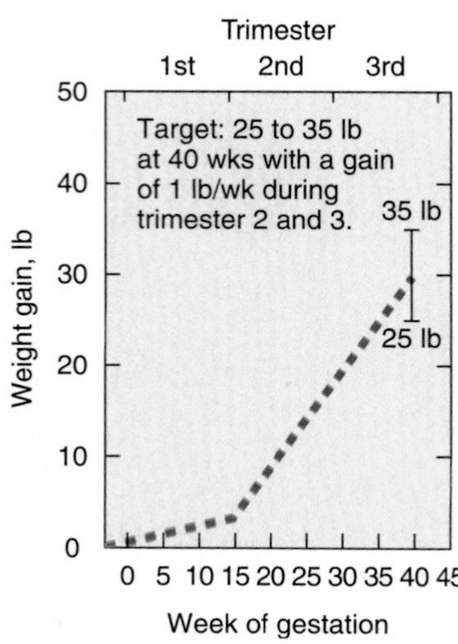

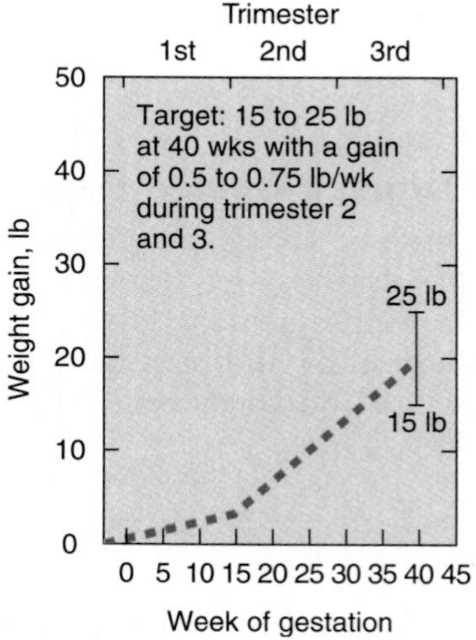

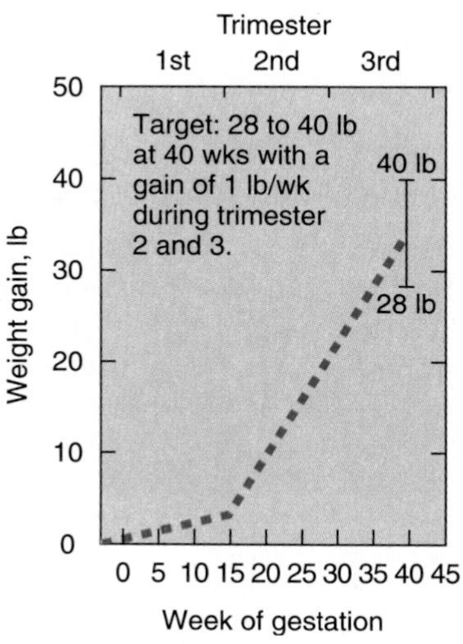

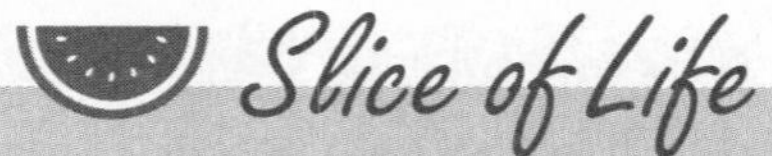

Weight Gain During Pregnancy

In her book *Child of Mine,* Ellyn Satter, who is both a registered dietitian and a mental health worker, describes the pattern of her own weight gain during pregnancy:

> I found in my pregnancies that I lost two or three pounds immediately when I became pregnant, probably because of a shift in water balance, then gained seven pounds in each of the fourth and fifth months. I blamed that on a shift in body fluid as well, because I know I wasn't overeating, at least to that extent. I kept my fingers crossed and tried not to do any mathematics in my head (you know, the type where you say "seven pounds times four more months is—") and just kept on eating. Sure enough, by the sixth month the monthly gain had leveled off to a nicely respectable three pounds, and it actually dropped during the last trimester to only about two pounds per month. (Satter, 1986a.)

Although her weight wavered slightly above and below the standard gain during her three pregnancies, she gained about 25 pounds each time, and all three babies were in excellent health.

doing so may have a negative effect on the development and health of the fetus. Notice in the figure that the pattern of weight gain during pregnancy is not a straight line from conception to delivery. There is likely to be little (perhaps 2–4 pounds), if any, gain in the first **trimester,** but the weight gain in the second and third trimesters should make up for it. During those phases, the mother should gain an average of almost 1 pound per week. It is not unusual for the weekly gain to be slightly higher in the second trimester than in the third.

trimester—the first, second, and third 3-month periods of pregnancy

Individual cases may deviate somewhat from this pattern and still be safe, but it is important that a health care professional monitor the mother's progress and recommend action if there is any indication of a problem. The Slice of Life above gives an example of the pattern of weight gain in one woman's pregnancies.

For multiple pregnancies, the mother needs to gain more weight than she would if she were carrying a single fetus. The recommended weight gain for a woman carrying twins is 16–20 kg (35–45 pounds) (Committee on Nutritional Status During Pregnancy and Lactation, 1990).

What Makes Up the Weight?

The growth that takes place between conception and birth is truly phenomenal. A single fertilized egg cell is so small and multiplies so rapidly that after only 4 weeks it is 7000 times larger than its original size, yet it is still only one-fifth of an inch long and weighs less than 1 ounce.

During the first 2 weeks after conception, the fertilized egg is called a **zygote.** Approximately 2 weeks after fertilization, the zygote attaches itself tightly to the wall of the **uterus,** the chamber in which it will grow until delivery. At this stage, it is called an **embryo.** In the area of attachment, an organ called the **placenta** develops; this organ contains the network of blood vessels that allows for the exchange of oxygen, nutrients, and waste products between the blood supplies of the mother and developing baby. Eight weeks after fertilization, when organs are beginning to develop and tissues are assuming distinct functions, the organism is called a **fetus,** the term used until birth (Figure 15.2).

zygote—the name given to a fertilized egg during the first 2 weeks after conception

uterus—the organ in which the baby develops during gestation

embryo—a zygote that has attached to the wall of the uterus

placenta—organ that forms at the site of embryo attachment and contains the blood vessel network that supplies the developing baby

fetus—a developing baby from 8 weeks after egg fertilization until birth

The average infant at birth weighs 3.2–3.5 kg (7–7½ pounds). Then why does the mother need to gain 11–16 kg (25–35 pounds)?

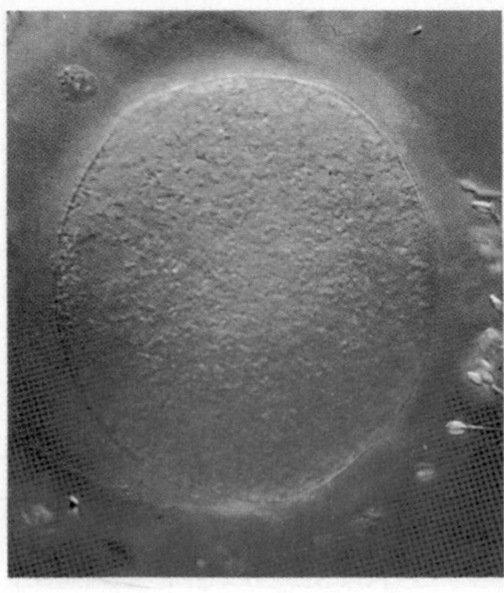
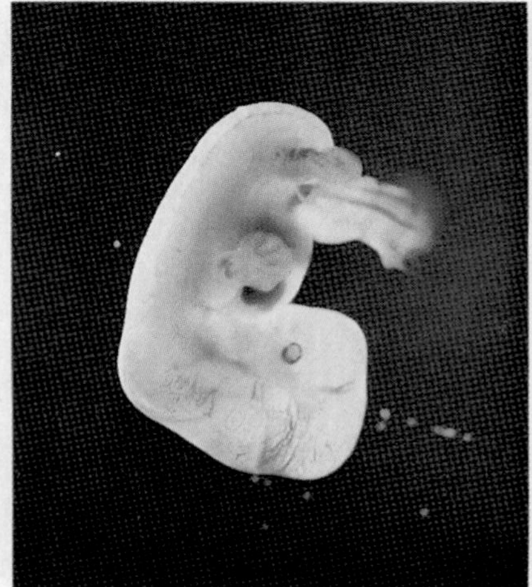
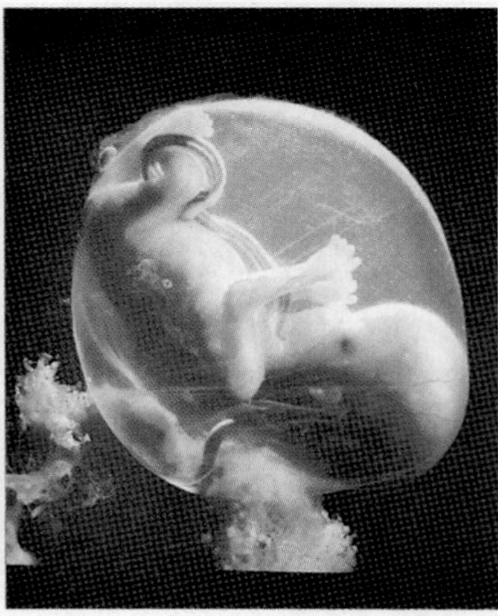

FIGURE 15.2
Stages of development between conception and birth.

Human sperm surrounds a human egg (left). The organism pictured in the center is 5 weeks old, representing the embryonic phase. The photo on the right was taken during the fetal stage at 14 weeks.

lactation—milk production

The answer is that many additional materials are needed to support healthy development. The weight of the uterus increases by almost 2 pounds by the time of delivery; amniotic fluid surrounding the developing baby takes up another 2 pounds; and by the end of pregnancy, the placenta accounts for an additional 1–2 pounds.

That's not all: the mother's blood supply increases by about 3 pounds, and her breast tissue increases in preparation for **lactation.** In addition, she needs to store extra body fat so that late in pregnancy, when the fetus's need for kcalories is very high but the mother is not likely to be able to eat enough to meet these needs entirely, the fetus can draw from her body fat reserves; the fat also provides energy that may be needed later for breast-feeding the baby. Finally, the mother is likely to accumulate more extracellular fluid (which, if excessive, results in edema). Table 15.2 shows the typical weights of these tissues and other materials.

Some women attempt to restrict their weight gain during pregnancy in order to avoid accumulating extra fat. This is not a good idea, because such restriction can affect the normal development of the fetus (Worthington-Roberts, 1988).

When the baby is born, the typical mother loses only part of the weight she gained during a normal, healthy pregnancy.

You Tell Me

When a baby is born, the amniotic fluid and placenta leave the mother's body along with the fetus.

What is the typical weight that is lost at the time of delivery? What tissues that were developed during pregnancy remain with the mother? What is their weight?

A new mother needs to realize that immediately after delivery, the right weight for her is about halfway between her prepregnant weight and her weight just before delivery. In the weeks following delivery, she will lose the fluid her tissues retained during pregnancy (Committee on Nutritional Status During Pregnancy and Lactation, 1990). Accumulated fat is generally lost more gradually.

TABLE 15.2 Composition of Weight Gain at the End of a Single Pregnancy

Type of Tissue	Weight Gain (Pounds)	Weight Gain (Kilograms)
Fetus	7–7½	3.2–3.4
Amniotic fluid	2	0.9
Placenta	1–2	0.5–0.9
Increase of		
Uterus	2	0.9
Maternal blood supply	3	1.4
Breast tissue	1	0.5
Other materials (fat, extracellular fluid, and possibly some lean mass)	9–17	4.1–7.7
Total	**25–35 pounds**	**11–16 kg**

Possible Problems from Inadequate Weight Gain

You learned earlier that if the mother does not gain enough weight, her baby could be too small, and very small babies may not live. This section describes more specifically the problems that result from inadequate weight gain.

Effect on Birth Outcome Babies weighing less than 2.5 kg (about 5½ pounds) at birth are referred to as **low-birth-weight babies.** These infants are 20 times more likely to die in their first year than are babies of higher birth weight.

low-birth-weight babies—infants who weigh less than 2.5 kg (5½ pounds) at birth

There are two types of low-birth-weight babies. One type consists of infants who were born prematurely and didn't have the chance to develop fully in the womb. These infants are more likely to die at birth or in their first few weeks of life than the second type of low-birth-weight infants.

The second type consists of babies who were carried to term (the full 9 months) but are small for their age. They exhibit two types of growth retardation. Some of these babies have poorly developed muscles and almost no body fat but are of typical length, with normal head circumference and skeletal development. Others are growth-retarded in both length and weight. Studies of low-birth-weight laboratory animals show that body organs, such as the liver and brain, often are growth-retarded as well, resulting in structural and functional abnormalities (Worthington-Roberts, 1988). The same can happen with human babies.

Weight gain during pregnancy is not the only critical influence on the weight of the baby; the mother's prepregnant weight is also important. A woman who is underweight when she becomes pregnant is more likely to have a small-for-age baby. One study showed that 18% of the babies of underweight mothers were small-for-age at birth. The risk was somewhat less for mothers who gained at least 1 pound per week during the last two trimesters, but even then their risk of having a small baby was three times higher than that of normal-weight women (Van der Spuy et al., 1988).

The effect of low birth weight can extend to the next generation. Mothers who themselves were low-birth-weight babies are at greater risk of having low-birth-weight babies. Their babies are more likely to require intensive care, experience respiratory difficulties, and die (Hackman et al., 1983).

FIGURE 15.3
Vulnerable periods for various parts of the developing body.

Different tissues, organs, and systems develop at different times during pregnancy. The critical period theory of development states that injury from nutrient extremes or teratogenic agents is more likely to occur during these periods of rapid development. The red parts of the bars indicate periods when damage is likely to be more severe; in periods indicated by blue bars, damage is less likely to be severe.
(Adapted from Moore, 1988. Reprinted by permission.)

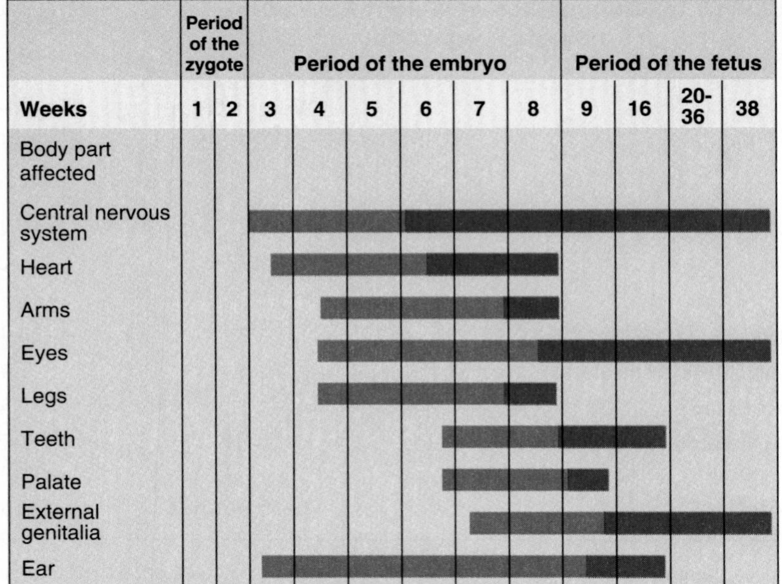

Effect of Timing The problems that occur as a result of malnutrition depend to some degree on the phase(s) of pregnancy during which nutrition was inadequate. The normal sequence of tissue formation in the fetus follows a pattern. Typically, the basic structure is established first by cells dividing rapidly (a process called *hyperplasia*). In the next phase, cell division continues, and existing cells simultaneously increase in size. Finally, increase in cell size *(hypertrophy)* predominates.

Some experts believe that the consequences of malnutrition are more likely to be serious during the stages of rapid cell division. Because the basic structures of body organs are being developed by **cell differentiation** and proliferation during the embryonic phase, this stage is often referred to as a **critical period.**

cell differentiation—progressive development of the features of specific types of cells

critical period—developmental stages involving rapid cell division, during which maternal nutrient intake can have the greatest consequences for the fetus

Figure 15.3 shows during which weeks of pregnancy some body structures are most vulnerable to injury. Although the embryonic period is of primary importance, it is certainly not the only time during which damage can occur. Although the *structure* of an organ may not be noticeably affected at later stages, malnutrition may result in less than optimal *function*.

In general, if severe undernutrition occurs only in the early months of pregnancy, when cell division should be rapid, the embryo does not develop normally and is less likely to survive. If severe deprivation is limited to the end of pregnancy, when cell enlargement takes place, the survival rate is better, although low birth weight can occur.

Many effects of maternal malnutrition on pregnancy have been studied in women who experienced food shortages during war and famine (Abrams, 1991; Susser, 1991). However, it is very difficult to separate the effect of undernutrition from other conditions (Walker et al., 1991).

You Tell Me

The military forces occupying Holland during World War II imposed a severe 6-month famine on the Dutch people, who had previously been well-nourished. During this time and for a short time thereafter, the birth rate dropped dramatically.

What other factors do you imagine might have affected the birth rate in this situation? Do you think it is appropriate to generalize from this situation to that of a developing country in which food intake is less than optimal most of the time?

Nutritional Needs During Pregnancy

To gain enough weight, a pregnant woman needs to consume a diet higher in kcalories than she did before pregnancy; however, simply to take in more energy without regard for the nutrient composition of the food that provides it is not the best approach. To be optimally nourished, the mother-to-be should eat a diet of high nutrient density.

The Need for Extra Kcalories

The energy cost of supporting a full-term pregnancy is approximately 80,000 kcalories (RDA Subcommittee, 1989). This is the approximate number of extra kcalories required over the course of 9 months for gaining the recommended 25–35 pounds.

Because a mother-to-be is expected to gain little if any weight during the first trimester, she does not need additional kcalories at this time. During the remainder of the pregnancy, though, she should increase her intake by approximately 300 kcalories per day. If she ordinarily consumed about 2200 kcalories per day before pregnancy, for example, she needs about 2500 kcalories (about 14% more) during most of pregnancy.

Scientists have based these estimates on certain assumptions about the amount and type of tissue gained during a typical pregnancy, about the average pregnant woman's basal metabolic rate (it's likely to increase), and about her usual activity level. If a woman's pregnancy doesn't follow the norm, her need for extra kcalories may be either higher or lower than 300 per day. For example, although pregnant women are encouraged to be appropriately physically active during pregnancy, a woman might be considerably less active, especially during the last trimester; at that time, the number of extra kcalories she needs may not be as high.

The Increased Recommendations for Specific Nutrients

The Recommended Dietary Allowances generally increase during pregnancy, but there are exceptions (Figure 15.4). For vitamin A, vitamin D, calcium, and phosphorus, the recommendations for the pregnant woman don't increase at all over those of the nonpregnant 19- to 24-year-old woman. Scientists advise pregnant women not to increase their intakes of vitamins A and D because excess levels can cause toxicity and damage to the developing baby.

During pregnancy, the recommended intakes for most other nutrients (that is, protein and many vitamins and minerals) increase by between 10% and 38% above the needs of nonpregnant 19- to 24-year-old women. The extra nutrients are required to supply the raw materials for building all of the fetal and maternal tissues and for increased energy needs. Because the recommended kcaloric increase is only 14%, a pregnant woman needs to choose her extra kcalories carefully to achieve these higher nutrient intakes.

The recommendations for intakes of iron and folic acid increase by 100% or more. The extra iron is needed for several tissues: the expanded maternal blood supply, the fetal blood supply, and the fetal liver. The large

FIGURE 15.4
Nutrient increases recommended for adult pregnancy.

During pregnancy, intakes of most nutrients should increase above prepregnancy recommendations. Because the needs for some micronutrients and protein increase substantially more than the recommended energy intake, the mother should choose more high-nutrient-density foods.

(Data from RDA Subcommittee, 1989.)

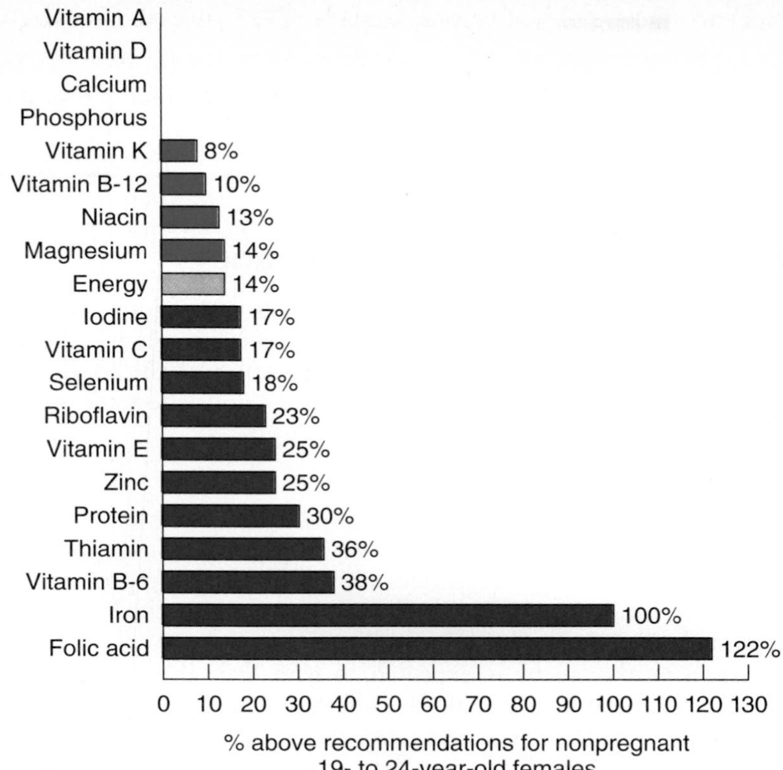

increase in folic acid is needed for production of red blood cells and for cell division in general.

Eating to Meet the Increased Needs

If you have known many pregnant women, you may have noticed that they vary considerably in their enthusiasm for eating. Some experience nausea and vomiting, usually early in their pregnancies. (We discuss this in more detail later in this chapter.) A pregnant woman's appetite often increases naturally in the second and third trimesters, when the expected weight gain and nutritional needs are highest.

Women not only find themselves eating more, but also often acquire new food preferences and aversions. A study of pregnant middle-income Americans found that they substantially increased their intake of milk and frequently craved ice cream, sweets and candy, fruits, and fish. The foods to which they most often developed aversions were coffee, red meat, poultry, and certain sauces (Rosso, 1988).

Many pregnant women believe that when they crave a certain food, their bodies need it and therefore they should eat it (Carruth and Skinner, 1991); however, there is no evidence for this. Some women believe that aversions to certain foods help them steer clear of harmful substances, but there is no proof of this, either. It is better for pregnant women to follow eating guidelines for meeting their recommended nutrient intakes.

The Food Guide Pyramid can be adapted for selecting an adequate diet for pregnancy and lactation (Table 15.3). Because the needs for many micronutrients increase more than does the need for extra energy, the extra food should be of high nutrient density—that is, from the basic groups rather than from fats, oils, and sweets. The recommended increase of 300

TABLE 15.3 Food Guide Pyramid Adapted for Pregnancy and Lactation

Food Group	Servings Daily		
	Nonpregnant 19- to 24-year-olds	Pregnant and Lactating Females	Pregnant Vegans[c]
Bread, rice, cereal, and pasta	6–11	add 1 or 2[a]	7–12
Vegetables	3–5	add 1[a]	5–6
Fruits	2–4	add 1[a]	3–5
Milk, yogurt, and cheese	2–3	3[b]	4 (as soy milk)
Meat, poultry, fish, beans, eggs, and nuts	5–7 ounces	add 1[a] ounce	3 (as legumes, nuts, and seeds)

[a]Add to prepregnant intake.
[b]For pregnant teenagers, increase to at least four servings daily.
[c]Adapted from Mutch, 1988; and RDA Subcommittee, 1989.

kcalories per day can be met with two additional servings of grain products, another vegetable, an additional serving of fruit, and one more ounce of meat. Another nutritious approach is to add one serving of each group, including dairy products.

Vegans, who avoid all foods of animal origin, need to be especially careful to eat a good diet during pregnancy and to supplement their diets with vitamin B-12. Bioavailability of minerals is also a concern, because the insoluble fiber content of vegan diets is high. Because vegans often avoid fortified and enriched foods and vitamin and mineral supplements, they particularly are at risk of nutrient deficiency. Recommendations for food intake for pregnant vegans are given in Table 15.3. Nonetheless, a pregnant vegan should seek the advice of a qualified nutritionist or dietitian to be sure that her diet is adequate.

Are Supplements Needed During Pregnancy?

Most pregnant women (especially omnivores) can meet their needs for almost all nutrients by eating a balanced and varied diet. However, one nutrient unlikely to be obtained from foods in the amount suggested by the RDA is iron: the recommended intake increases from 15 mg before pregnancy to 30 mg during pregnancy. Because it is a challenge for many women to consume even 15 mg of iron from their diets, the RDA recommends a daily iron supplement during pregnancy.

The RDA for folic acid during pregnancy can generally be met from ordinary foods; nonetheless, scientists are currently debating whether folic acid supplements should be taken during pregnancy. As you learned in Chapter 11, doses of folic acid much larger than those recommended in the RDA have been used to prevent neural tube defects (birth defects involving the central nervous system) in fetuses of women who previously had borne babies with such defects (MRC Vitamin Study Research Group, 1991). The question is whether similarly high doses should be recommended for *all* women in their reproductive years. (Folic acid expert Lynn Bailey discussed this issue in the interview in Chapter 11.)

Although a well-chosen diet can fulfill the other nutritional needs of most pregnant women (Committee on Nutritional Status During Pregnancy and Lactation, 1990), many physicians recommend that their pregnant patients take a moderate multivitamin and mineral supplement. Doing so may be useful and is not hazardous unless the amounts of nutrients are excessive or unbalanced; vitamin supplements that are too potent are toxic to the fetus.

A pregnant woman must not regard the moderate supplement recommended by her doctor as a replacement for a balanced diet. Because some essential nutrients are not likely to be included in supplements, a nutritious diet is still critically important.

A Special Program for High-Risk Pregnant Women

Supplemental Food Program for Women, Infants, and Children (WIC)—national federally funded program that provides nutrition and medical support for low-income women who have high-risk pregnancies

The **Supplemental Food Program for Women, Infants, and Children (WIC)** is a nationwide, federally funded program that provides access to specific foods, nutrition education, and medical referral services for low-income women who have high-risk pregnancies. Several studies have demonstrated its effectiveness in decreasing the incidence of premature births, stillbirths, and maternal anemia and in increasing birth weight (American Dietetic Association, 1989). Providing for healthier babies also holds down other health care expenses. Studies show that every dollar spent for WIC saves $2 to $4 in Medicare costs (United States Department of Agriculture, 1991).

The most positive effects of the WIC program are seen among women who had the poorest nutritional status at the time they joined the program. Adequate length of time in the program is also important; a study of the program in Missouri showed that mothers needed to receive benefits for at least 7 months before increased birth weights were seen (Stockbauer, 1987).

One group of people the WIC program serves is pregnant teenagers. We'll focus on this group in Chapter 16.

Coping with the Physiologic Changes of Pregnancy

Physiologic changes occur in virtually every system of a woman's body to accommodate and support a pregnancy. Some of these changes are related to nutrition. This section discusses how pregnant women can cope with the lesser problems and discomforts that have a nutritional component, but we emphasize the importance of seeking medical intervention for more serious conditions.

Nausea and Vomiting Over half of pregnant women experience some degree of nausea and vomiting during pregnancy, whether it occurs as "morning sickness" or at other times of day. This condition is not an indication that anything is wrong; oddly, it seems to be a good sign, if it is not severe. Studies show that there are fewer spontaneous abortions among women who have experienced nausea (Stein and Susser, 1991).

Many women experiencing nausea say it helps to keep some food in their stomachs much of the time. They do this by eating small, frequent meals; by drinking fluids between meals rather than with them; and by eating something bland, such as a few crackers or toast, before getting out of bed in the morning.

For a very few women, these suggestions do not help. If a pregnant woman vomits more than twice a day, she should seek help from the health care professional who is monitoring her pregnancy. Without intervention, the severely affected woman's risk of having a low-birth-weight baby is many times higher than that of a woman with less severe vomiting. If nothing else can be found to ease her problem, nutrients in solution can be given intravenously to provide what she and her fetus need (Levine and Esser, 1988).

Heartburn Heartburn (reflux of acidic stomach contents into the lower part of the esophagus) bothers some women during pregnancy. It is especially common in the later stages, when the fetus is large enough to exert pressure on the stomach. Avoiding fatty or greasy foods, heavily spiced dishes, and coffee can help reduce heartburn. Eating smaller meals and not lying down soon after eating can also help (see Chapter 3).

Constipation During pregnancy, hormonal changes relax the muscles of the colon, slowing down the movement of solid waste. Constipation may be aggravated in the later stages of pregnancy, when the rapidly growing fetus crowds the colon. Some women believe that iron supplements contribute to constipation.

Usually, increasing the amount of fiber in the diet by eating more fruits, vegetables, and whole grains and by drinking more fluids solves the problem (see Chapter 5). Moderate exercise, such as walking, also helps.

Pregnancy-Induced Hypertension (PIH) Some pregnant women develop a unique form of hypertension known as pregnancy-induced hypertension (PIH). Along with the increase in blood pressure, they are likely to excrete abnormally high levels of protein in their urine and experience fluid retention. Intervention is important for preventing more serious consequences, such as damage or even death to the fetus or, in rare cases, to the mother. PIH may also put the mother at increased risk of cardiovascular or renal disease later in life (Zeman and Ney, 1988).

Although experts do not know for certain why this condition occurs, they know that certain groups of pregnant women are at higher risk of PIH. It is most common in women who are pregnant for the first time and who are under 20 or over 35 years of age. Because it occurs more often among low-income and among underweight women, experts believe that poor general nutritional status and quality of prenatal care may contribute to its development (Zeman and Ney, 1988).

In the past, physicians commonly advised women to restrict their sodium intake during pregnancy, believing that this would help women avoid PIH. But we now know that *severe* sodium restriction can interfere with the development of the fetus and that it is not effective in preventing PIH. *Moderate* sodium restriction (avoiding added salt and obviously salty foods) and bed rest can usually help control PIH if it develops (Zeman and Ney, 1988). Fortunately, the condition resolves after delivery.

Toxic Substances to Avoid During Pregnancy

Getting enough of the essential nutrients is only one concern during pregnancy; it is also important to avoid taking in substances that could cause fetal damage. As you learned in Chapter 14, such substances are known as *teratogens.*

Tobacco, alcohol, and many other drugs are known teratogens; other substances are suspected of being dangerous. We will discuss them in this section.

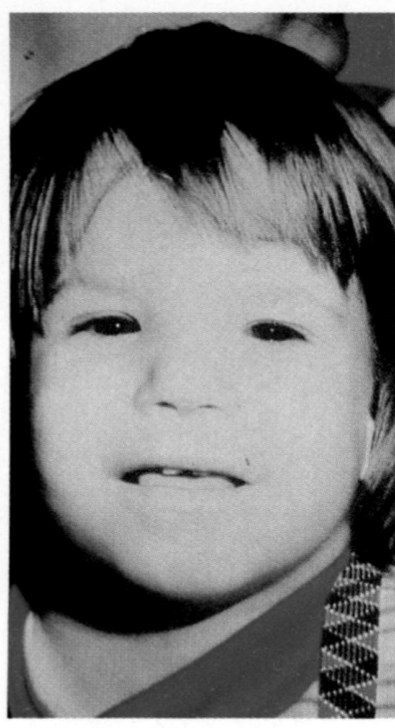

FIGURE 15.5
A child with fetal alcohol syndrome (FAS).

This child shows several facial characteristics of FAS: wide space between the eyes, small nose, and thin upper lip.

fetal alcohol syndrome— condition occurring in some children of alcoholic mothers, involving certain characteristic mental and physical abnormalities

Alcohol

Like many other substances, some of the alcohol in a mother's bloodstream crosses the placenta and circulates in her developing baby's bloodstream. At some level, alcohol interferes with the growth processes in the embryo or fetus, possibly by reducing the supply of oxygen flowing through the placenta and/or by blocking the activity of essential nutrients. It is estimated that as many as 2% of all babies born alive in the Western world may be suffering from the effects of alcohol exposure in utero (Miller, 1986).

Animal studies and observations of humans show that one or more episodes of binge-drinking during the early stages are most likely to produce low-birth-weight babies and children with impaired mental functions (Wright et al., 1983). Experts believe that the effects of alcohol are dose-related and vary according to the stage of pregnancy: excess alcohol during the first trimester is most often associated with the development of physical abnormalities in the fetus; alcohol in the second trimester can increase the risk of miscarriage; and during the third trimester, it reduces the rate of fetal growth (American Medical Association, 1983). Even heavy alcohol use by the mother *before* conception has been associated with low birth weight (Little et al., 1980).

In the 1960s, the name **fetal alcohol syndrome (FAS)** was given to the set of abnormalities seen among some children of women who consumed large amounts of alcohol during pregnancy. FAS is now considered a prime cause of developmental disability in the Western world. The typical abnormalities of FAS include characteristic facial features (Figure 15.5); poor growth before and after birth; and central nervous system disorders, including mental retardation and deficiencies in fine motor skills.

Although experts agree that frequent heavy drinking during pregnancy is dangerous to a developing baby, studies regarding the effect of light-to-moderate use of alcohol have produced conflicting results. This is due in part to difficulty in separating the effects of alcohol from those related to other factors, such as smoking and poor diet.

One study found that the children of mothers who consumed 1.5 ounces of alcohol per day (about three drinks) before they knew they were pregnant had lower IQ scores than the children of nondrinkers. Measured at the age of 4 years, IQ scores were 5 points lower in the children of the mothers who drank early in their pregnancies (Streissguth et al., 1989).

It is important to note that no threshold level has been defined; that is, *there is no level of alcohol consumption known to be completely risk-free during pregnancy.* The American Medical Association advises: "Physicians should be explicit in reinforcing the concept that, with several aspects of the issue still in doubt, the safest course is abstinence" (American Medical Association, 1983). Other reports concur: the *Dietary Guidelines for Americans* (United States Department of Agriculture and United States Department of Health and Human Services, 1990), *The Surgeon General's Report on Nutrition and Health* (1988), and *Diet and Health* (National Research Council, 1989) recommend avoiding alcohol during pregnancy.

Data suggest that the father's drinking habits before conception also may be related to his child's birth weight. Infants whose fathers drank two drinks or more per day in the month prior to conception weighed almost 6 ounces less than the babies of men who drank only occasionally (Little and Sing, 1986). This topic deserves more study.

Other Drugs

Various pharmaceuticals can damage the developing baby. Some of these are prescription medications, and others are over-the-counter drugs. The pregnant woman should check with her health care professional before using *any* medications.

Street drugs can also have serious negative effects. For example, more and more data are indicating that pregnant women who use cocaine are more likely to have spontaneous abortions, premature labor, or small-for-age babies; its teratogenic effects are less clear (Committee on Nutritional Status During Pregnancy and Lactation, 1990). As with alcohol, it is difficult to separate the effects of illicit drugs from the effects of other lifestyle factors that may be practiced simultaneously, such as smoking tobacco, use of other drugs, poor nutrition, and inadequate health care.

Caffeine

Caffeine is a drug naturally present in coffee, tea, and chocolate. It is also added to colas and other soft drinks and to certain medications (see Chapter 14).

Because caffeine is a stimulant that crosses the placenta and circulates in the fetal bloodstream, there has been concern that its use during pregnancy may harm the fetus or even cause spontaneous abortion. Animal studies using *very* high doses of caffeine have shown that it can cause fetal abnormalities.

Several studies have been conducted to determine whether these effects occur in humans as well; the results have generally been negative. A recent study showed that moderate caffeine consumption (less than 300 mg/day) was not associated with increased risk of spontaneous abortion or problems with fetal growth. Although women who consumed more than 300 mg of caffeine per day during pregnancy had smaller babies, this effect disappeared when other risk factors—especially smoking—were taken into account (Mills et al., 1993).

Smoking

Smoking during pregnancy has many negative effects. Babies of mothers who smoked are shorter and lighter and have a higher prevalence of signs suggesting growth retardation in utero. One study showed that infants of mothers who smoked weighed 5% less than those whose mothers did not smoke (Brooke et al., 1989). Complications of pregnancy—bleeding, premature rupture of membranes, spontaneous abortion, and infant death—are also more likely (Hoff et al., 1986). In addition, children of mothers who smoked during pregnancy are at greater risk of developing cancer as young children (Stjernfeldt et al., 1986). These effects are dose-related; that is, the more a woman smokes, the higher the risk of these negative consequences.

Pica

Another dietary practice thought to be dangerous during pregnancy is pica, a pathologic craving for and consumption of substances that are not food (see Chapter 12). Clay is the historical favorite, but some people substitute materials such as laundry starch, baking soda, or chalk. Members of certain socioeconomic and racial groups—especially black women from the rural South—are more likely to eat these substances, and culture influences the practice as well. Some people believe that pica is a *response* to deficiency of iron or other nutrients; many others believe pica is the *cause* of the poor status of iron that is often associated with the condition (Blinder et al., 1988).

The significance of pica in nutrition depends on the type and amount of nonfood items consumed. Clay can bind dietary minerals into a nonabsorbable form. Ingested clay can result in intestinal obstructions or can be the source of parasites that cause disease (Blinder et al., 1988). In addition, clay, chalk and paint chips can contain dangerously high levels of such toxicants as lead.

You Tell Me

Some pregnant women eat laundry starch—as much as a pound each day. Others consume baking soda (sodium bicarbonate).

How many kcalories are in a pound of starch? How might eating it affect your intake of food? What health problems could be caused (or aggravated) by the substances in laundry starch and baking soda?

It's hard to guess what nonfood items pregnant women might choose to eat; who would have thought that some would crave and consume burned matches, hair, mothballs, tire inner tubes, or air-freshener blocks, as has been documented (Worthington-Roberts, 1988)? Pregnant women should not eat any nonfood items. Pica can pose health risks to both a mother and her fetus, even causing death.

The Consider This box on page 499 summarizes recommendations for diet during pregnancy.

Rapid Infant Growth and High Nutrient Needs

During the first year of life, growth in both length and weight is more rapid than at any other period of life outside the womb. (Look at the changes in a chronologic series of baby pictures up to the first birthday!) A normal infant birth weight doubles by 4–6 months and triples by the end of the first year. Height at 1 year is usually 150% of birth length. This rapid growth gives infants the highest nutrient needs per unit of body weight of any age group.

Continuing Growth

The growth taking place in an infant involves all types of tissue; insufficient nutrient intake during the first few months of life can cause growth to be slower than normal. If adequate nourishment is provided later in the first year, partial or even complete catch-up growth can occur (Pipes, 1989).

Body growth is important for its own sake, but it's also critical because of its relationship to brain growth. One expert notes that the best way to ensure good *brain* growth is to encourage optimal overall *body* growth from conception until the second birthday (Dobbing, 1984).

Physical Status

Although a healthy baby is sufficiently developed to survive as an independent biologic entity at birth, its tissues, organs, and systems are still developing. Therefore, what a baby consumes must not only provide adequate nutrition, but also be consistent with its physiologic and metabolic capabilities.

A baby's gastrointestinal (GI) tract is immature and of small capacity at birth, and the production of gastric secretions, stomach acid, and certain

During pregnancy, instead of

This	*Consider this*
Eating the same amount as before pregnancy	**Increasing intake by about 300 kcal/day during second and third trimesters.**
Ignoring nutritional quality of the food eaten	**Eating more servings from the five basic groups of the Food Guide Pyramid, without increasing consumption of fats, oils, and sweets.**
Scheduling meals as before	**Eating meals and snacks in amounts and at times that are most comfortable.**
Emphasizing foods that are craved	**Including some craved foods, provided that they make a reasonable contribution to the total diet.**
Forcing down food that doesn't appeal	**Substituting foods of similar value that you can enjoy.**
Drinking alcoholic beverages, smoking, and pica	**Totally avoiding these practices during pregnancy.**

enzymes is low (Hendricks and Badruddin, 1992). A newborn's stomach, which can hold less than 1 ounce at birth, will be able to hold about 7 ounces of food at 1 year of age. The kidneys are also immature at delivery: they do not have the ability to concentrate urine as the older child's and adult's kidneys do. Because of these conditions, an infant's food must be dilute and easy to digest. Breast milk and formulas that simulate it meet these requirements.

Nutritional Status

A healthy full-term infant (one who was born to a well-nourished mother after 9 months of normal gestation) has a reserve supply of some nutrients. For example, iron stored in a newborn's liver can meet its needs for several months if the baby's intake of iron is low.

Even so, a steady supply of energy and nutrients is essential for proper growth and development. Experts have estimated infants' needs for individual nutrients by monitoring the average amount consumed by thriving infants who were breast-fed by healthy, well-nourished mothers (RDA Subcommittee, 1989). Energy requirements of the normal infant, per unit of body weight, are three to four times that of the normal adult (Heird and Cooper, 1988). Adequate intake of nutrients is especially critical for babies who are born without adequate reserves; low-birth-weight babies are usually more vulnerable to poor diet and disease.

Psychosocial Status

A baby's social development begins at birth, with its first human contact. Because so much of the time spent with a baby involves feeding, the feeding relationship is the primary route by which babies find out about themselves and the world.

At birth, infants are thought to be able to distinguish positive from negative sensations, but not what caused them. It takes a sensitive caregiver to identify what is causing an infant's discomfort (such as hunger), to get rid of the cause (feed the baby), and to read the cues from the baby that the problem has been solved (satiety). Such two-way communication between the infant and caregiver helps babies gain self-awareness, assures them that they can make their wants known, and teaches trust (Satter, 1986b).

If, however, babies are consistently frustrated or thwarted in their demands for food or have food forced upon them when they do not want it, they learn a very different lesson about their world: they may perceive it as a hostile place. For them, hunger is associated with anxiety rather than with pleasurable anticipation.

The best way for a caregiver to promote healthy psychosocial development through feeding is to feed the infant "on demand"; that is, when the baby gives cues that it's hungry. One cue is persistent crying; of course, an infant may also cry because of some other discomfort, but if the crying continues after other needs have been met, the baby probably needs to eat. Another cue is the baby sucking on anything available—its fist, the blanket, your shirt, and so on. Caregivers should respond to these signals, rather than adhering to the rigid feeding schedules used in the past.

Considering Whether to Breast-Feed or Bottle-Feed

The two common options most parents consider for feeding their infants are breast-feeding or bottle-feeding a commercially prepared infant formula. Is one clearly better than the other?

Breast milk sets the nutritional standard for what an infant needs in the first several months of life, and it is less allergenic and more protective against infection than formulas. Today's commercially produced infant formulas are made to mimic the nutrient composition of human milk as much as possible, but they cannot duplicate human milk's other advantages.

From this information, you might think that breast-feeding is always preferable to formula-feeding—but it would be an oversimplification to give such a categorical answer. Consider the following You Tell Me to sense some of the dimensions of this issue.

You Tell Me

In the early 1970s, only about 25% of new mothers in the United States nursed their babies; by the early 1980s, the proportion rose dramatically to 62% (Ryan et al., 1991). Then, in the late 1980s, breast-feed

ing started to decline, and by 1989, only 52% of new mothers nursed their babies. As these major shifts took place, there were no large corresponding changes in infant health indicators or survival rates.

Does this suggest that one approach to feeding may be markedly better than the other? Do trends necessarily indicate what is best or what should be done in specific cases? Does the experience in one country provide a good model for all other countries?

You could expect that if breast-feeding were always the better option, health and mortality statistics would change as infant feeding practices shifted; however, this has not been the case. In the United States and other developed countries, although breast-feeding—the method provided by nature—is recommended in most cases, a properly chosen infant formula is considered a reasonable alternative. Even the American Academy of Pediatrics (AAP), traditionally a proponent of breast-feeding, says so (American Academy of Pediatrics, Committee on Nutrition, 1992).

That brings us back to square one. If you were expecting a child, what would you consider when making such a decision? The next sections provide more information about what breast milk and formulas offer an infant from nutritional and health perspectives. Then, the Thinking for Yourself later in this chapter discusses a wider variety of factors to consider, including social and lifestyle issues.

Considerations Regarding Breast-Feeding

From the time of delivery, a mother's mammary glands produce fluids for the infant. For the first few days, a fluid called **colostrum** is produced; this is a watery substance that is higher in protein and some minerals than the milk that will come later. It also contains antibodies and special cells that increase the baby's immunity to several diseases.

colostrum—watery liquid produced by the breasts (mammary glands) of mothers during the first few days after delivery

Beneficial Factors in Mature Milk Mature breast milk replaces colostrum about 4 or 5 days after delivery. It, too, provides unique benefits for the infant beyond supplying nutrients needed for growth.

- The proteins in breast milk are less likely to provoke allergic reactions than the milks of other animals. This is an especially important consideration for the infant with a family history of allergies. However, even some breast-fed babies develop allergies; researchers have tried to find ways to reduce this effect (Arshad et al., 1992), but more research is needed.
- Mature milk contains antibodies from the mother, certain proteins, and other substances that help protect the baby against GI and respiratory infections (Subcommittee on Nutrition During Lactation, 1991). In the developing countries, where sanitation is poor, this immune protection is an important safeguard, but it is not as important in the industrialized countries (Wray, 1991).
- Breast milk contains substances that may promote the maturation of a baby's GI tract (Hendricks and Badruddin, 1992).
- The proteins in breast milk are mostly lactalbumins, which are easier for an infant to digest than the casein proteins of non-heat-treated cow's milk.

- Lactose is the main carbohydrate in human and animal milks. There is more lactose in human milk than in cow's milk, and it promotes the absorption of calcium and some other minerals.
- Fats supply about half of the kcalories in breast milk, and the structure of the triglycerides makes them easy for the baby to absorb.
- The mineral content of breast milk is well suited to the infant's needs. The ratio of calcium to phosphorus facilitates the minerals' absorption. Although the iron content is low, the infant very readily absorbs almost half of it.
- If the mother is well nourished, the vitamin content of her milk is usually adequate for her baby's needs, but inadequacies in her diet are reflected in lower quantities of some vitamins in her milk. A number of water-soluble vitamins are affected in this way (Whitehead, 1988).
- In the first few weeks of life, when stomach capacity is tiny, infants should nurse between 8 and 15 times per day. After the first month, infants are likely to want to nurse 5–12 times per day (Subcommittee on Nutrition during Lactation, 1991).

A Breast-Fed Infant's Need for Supplements Although breast milk from a well-nourished mother generally meets the nutritional needs of her infant (Figure 15.6), there are a few exceptions.

At birth, an infant's body does not have enough vitamin K for normal blood clotting should the baby be injured. For this reason, experts advise giving infants an injection or oral supplements of vitamin K after delivery. In the weeks after birth, infants get some vitamin K from breast milk and some that is produced by their colonic bacteria. Current practice is not to give further supplements, but some experts call for more research on this matter (Jensen et al., 1992).

Supplemental vitamin D is usually recommended for the breast-fed infant, because breast milk does not supply the amount the RDA recommends (Jensen et al., 1992). Although sun exposure leads to some internal production of vitamin D, dark-skinned babies in northern climates are unlikely to produce enough and therefore should be given the supplement. Whether light-skinned babies who get some sun exposure need a supplement is debatable, but vitamin D is often recommended as a safeguard (Pipes, 1989).

Fluoride supplements also should be given to breast-fed infants (Subcommittee on Nutrition During Lactation, 1991). This is necessary because very little fluoride transfers from the mother's plasma into breast milk. Fluoride is important for developing healthy teeth and probably bones as well.

A case can be made either for or against iron supplementation. Because almost half of the iron in breast milk is bioavailable, few breast-fed babies become anemic. When babies begin eating solid foods, however, they consume less breast milk, and their risk of anemia increases. Therefore, at this time an iron supplement should be considered (Subcommittee on Nutrition During Lactation, 1991). If the mother stops breast-feeding when she starts giving her baby solids, she should give iron-fortified formula in place of the breast milk.

If a lactating mother is a vegan (total vegetarian), she should give her baby supplements of vitamin B-12, as well as taking such supplements herself.

Change in Composition of Breast Milk During a Feeding The composition of a mother's milk changes somewhat within a feeding period. The water content of breast milk is initially high, giving her infant relatively

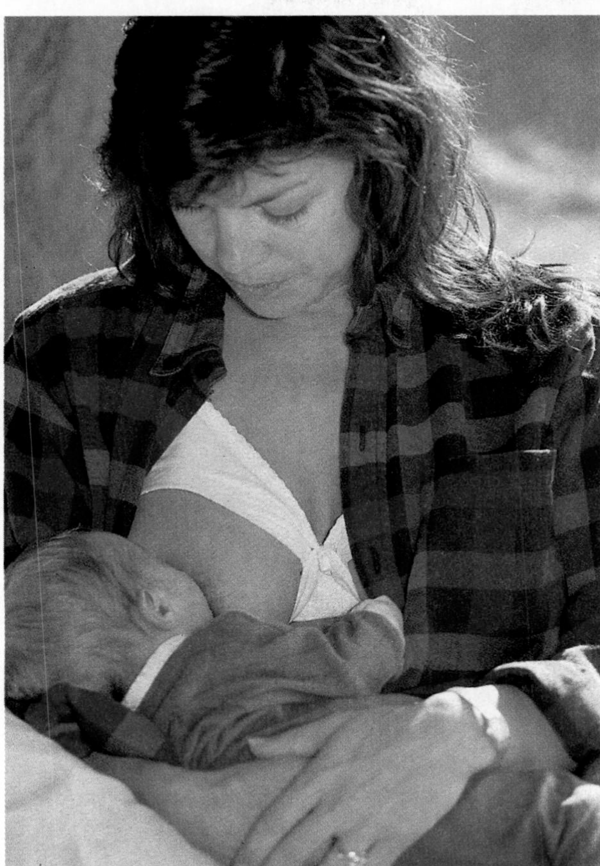

FIGURE 15.6
Is breast-feeding best?

In many cases, breast-feeding—the natural method—is the best choice. Breast milk provides most of the nutrients an infant needs; it also provides immune factors and is less likely to provoke allergies than formula-feeding.

dilute milk at the beginning of a feeding session, when the baby is very thirsty. This provides the amount of water the infant's kidneys need. As the feeding continues, the milk's fat content increases, water content decreases, and the baby's hunger is satisfied more quickly (Jensen et al., 1992).

Volume Influenced by a Baby's Intake During the first 6 months, nursing infants consume an average of 750 ml (approximately 3 cups) of breast milk per day; newborns consume much less, and they progressively take more. A well-nourished mother is able to meet this increasing demand because the amount of milk she produces for upcoming feedings is largely determined by the extent to which her baby emptied her breasts at previous feedings.

After solids have been added to their diets, infants do not need as much milk. From 6 months to 1 year of age, babies take an average of 600 ml (about 2½ cups) per day (RDA Subcommittee, 1989). The feedback mechanism works at this time as well; decreased emptying of a mother's breasts causes them to make less milk. That also explains why a mother who frequently supplements her infant's nursing with formula finds that her own supply of milk decreases. Some mothers and infants find it very satisfactory to combine the use of breast milk and formula.

Because milk production increases with frequent and thorough emptying of her breasts, even a mother of twins may be able exclusively to breast-feed her babies. However, supplementing with formula can work well for these mothers and infants, too.

Volume Influenced by a Mother's Energy Balance In some instances, a mother may not produce enough milk to satisfy her baby's needs. If she is

During lactation, instead of

This . . . . . . Consider this

This	Consider this
Eating whatever you want after baby is born	**Continuing to eat the nutritious diet recommended for pregnancy.**
Ignoring fluid needs	**Drinking enough fluids—especially water, juices, and milk—to satisfy thirst.**
Using unlimited amounts of caffeine and alcohol	**Consuming these in moderate amounts only (see text).**

severely underweight and her energy intake is inadequate, as are many women in developing countries, her milk output may be low despite her infant's deliberate message about wanting more (Rasmussen, 1992).

In the developed countries, lactating women who try to lose weight too rapidly or find themselves "too busy to eat" may compromise the volume of milk they could produce. Following the first month after delivery, they should not lose more than 2 kg per month (4.5 pounds); another rough guideline is that mothers should consume *at least* 1800 kcalories per day for adequate milk production (Subcommittee on Nutrition During Lactation, 1991).

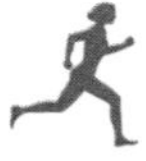

In the United States, women who like to exercise regularly have wondered whether their activity levels would interfere with milk production. A study showed that activity is not a problem; in fact, very active lactating women produced somewhat *more* milk than did less active women (Lovelady et al., 1990). ●

A Mother's Increased Needs for Lactation Milk production calls for a mother to consume more protein, vitamins, and minerals; recommended intakes increase by as much as 65% above the amounts needed before pregnancy. Compared with recommendations during pregnancy, most of the nutrient recommendations for lactation are slightly higher; others stay the same, and those for iron and folic acid are lower. The RDAs for a nursing mother during the first 6 months are slightly higher than from 6 months to 1 year, reflecting the decrease in a baby's intake of breast milk as it increases its consumption of solids.

A nursing mother needs more water, proportional to the volume of milk the baby drinks—anywhere from ½ quart to over 1 quart per day. When a mother satisfies her own thirst, she generally meets her fluid needs.

The Consider This box above summarizes intake recommendations for food and fluids during lactation. Normally, women do not need nutritional supplements at this time (Subcommittee on Nutrition During Lactation, 1991).

Effects of Maternal Substance Use A mother who breast-feeds her baby should limit her use of substances that are known to be transmitted via the breast milk and to have negative effects on babies. She should also limit her intake of substances known to reduce milk production.

Caffeine is one of the substances to limit, whether from coffee, other beverages, or medications (see Table 14.4). The caffeine-equivalent of 1–2 cups of regular coffee per day is acceptable, but more may make her baby irritable and wakeful.

Some of the alcohol the mother consumes also enters her milk; a nursing mother should not consume more alcohol than 0.5 g/kg of her body weight per day. This guideline would allow a 60-kg (132-pound) woman to drink up to 2½ ounces of liquor, 8 ounces of table wine, or 2 cans of beer in a day. However, one study showed that when mothers consumed even 0.3 g/kg of their body weight before nursing their babies, their babies drank approximately 20% less milk at that feeding (Mennella and Beauchamp, 1991). The alcohol in the milk peaked 30 minutes to 1 hour after the mother consumed the alcohol.

Smoking decreases milk production and also has many other negative health effects on mothers and babies; therefore, mothers should not smoke. Similarly, mothers using illicit drugs should get help to stop their habit.

Effects of Lactation on a Mother's Body Lactation affects a woman's whole body. When a baby nurses, the suckling stimulates muscle contractions in the mother's uterus, which helps her uterus return to its prepregnant size.

Lactation uses some energy from a mother's fat stores; on average, during the first 4–6 months, nursing mothers lose a total of 2.8–4.2 kg (6 to 9 pounds), with losses slowing down after that. (Interestingly, the amount of weight lost by mothers who do not breast-feed is very similar [Potter et al., 1991].) However, there is much individual variation in weight changes in lactating women; one in five actually *gain* weight instead of losing.

Lactation also has a long-term effect on health: nursing mothers have a lower risk of breast cancer than do other women.

What Formulas Offer an Infant

In a few situations, *bottle-feeding is clearly preferable to breast-feeding.* Obstetricians and pediatricians advise mothers who have certain illnesses, who are receiving certain treatments, or who are taking particular medications to bottle-feed instead of breast-feed.

More commonly, parents who prefer bottle-feeding have other reasons: they find it more convenient and more equitable. For example, mothers may decide that their time and schedule constraints make breast-feeding too difficult, and fathers may feel they want more involvement with their baby than breast-feeding would allow (Figure 15.7). An example of how one couple weighed such factors is described in Thinking for Yourself on page 508.

A variety of infant formulas is available. Let's take a look at some of the options.

Cow's Milk Formulas Most infant formulas are made from cow's milk that has been modified to resemble breast milk as closely as possible. However, the major protein in cow's milk—casein—is difficult for a baby to digest: it makes a tough curd in the stomach. For that reason, most milk-based formulas have been heat-treated in a way that improves the digestibility of the

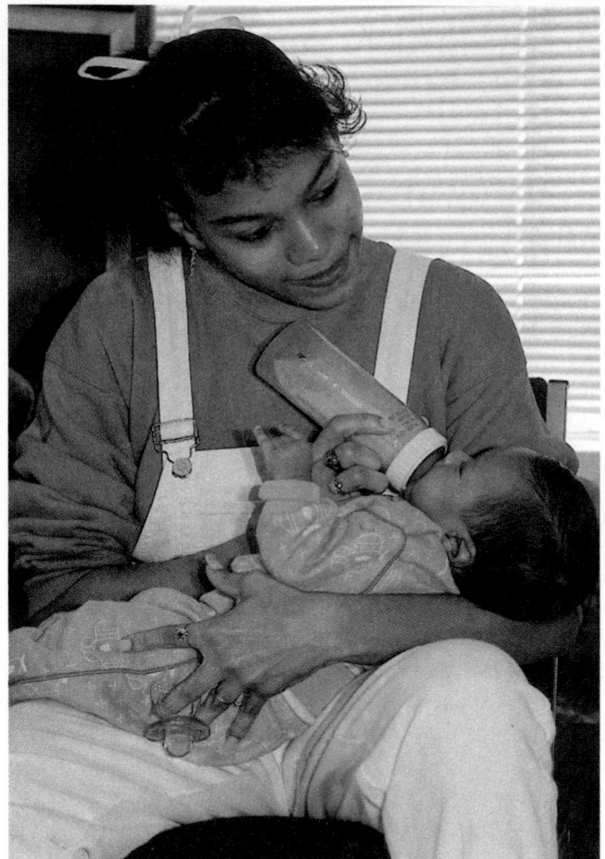

FIGURE 15.7
Bottle-feeding is a reasonable option for many parents and their babies.

Nutritionally, formulas are similar to breast milk, although they are more likely to provoke allergies in susceptible infants. Bottle-feeding has various social advantages, such as allowing greater participation by the father and allowing the mother more flexibility in her activities and schedule.

casein. Whey proteins, which babies digest easily, are also added to many formulas. The butterfat is replaced by blends of plant oils that babies readily digest and absorb. Additional lactose or other carbohydrate is added. Table 15.4 shows how formulas compare with human milk and cow's milk.

Vitamins and minerals are added to formulas to mimic the levels in human milk, but one ingredient whose addition has been seriously debated is iron. Should it be added? The fact that you can still buy some formulas that have been iron-fortified, and some that have not, reflects this lingering difference of opinion.

Taking the *pro* position, the American Academy of Pediatrics (AAP) states that "the only acceptable alternative to breast milk is iron-fortified infant formula" (American Academy of Pediatrics, Committee on Nutrition, 1992). The AAP bases its recommendation on the fact that iron-fortified formulas have helped reduce considerably the rates of anemia among formula-fed infants in the United States.

Taking the opposite position, some parents prefer to give their infants formula that has not been iron-fortified, believing that the fortified formula causes GI distress in their babies. Nevertheless, research does not show this relationship (Nelson et al., 1988). Some physicians are concerned that high iron intakes may encourage the growth of pathogenic organisms in some infants. However, this is a greater problem in developing countries, where babies who are iron-deficient often also have low-grade infections; when iron is supplemented, their infections can actually *worsen,* because the pathogens make use of the iron more rapidly than the infant's body does.

TABLE 15.4 Composition of Human Breast Milk, Cow's Milk, and Some Infant Formulas

Component	Human Milk	Cow's Milk	Formulas[a]				
			1	2	3	4	5
Protein (g/dl)	1.0	3.4	1.5	1.5	1.5	1.6	1.5
Casein (% of total protein)[b]	40	82	40	82	40	0	40
Fat (g/dl)	3.9	3.3	3.8	3.6	3.6	3.3	3.4
Lactose (g/dl)	6.8	4.8	7.0	7.2	7.2	7.2	7.6
Kilocalories/dl	72	75	68	68	68	65	67

[a]1 = Enfamil, Mead Johnson; 2 = Similac, Ross; 3 = SMA, Wyeth; 4 = Good Start, Carnation; 5 = NAN, Nestle. All are for healthy term infants.
[b]Proteins in all except (4) are cow's milk whey and casein; (4) contains only hydrolyzed whey.
Source: Adapted from Jensen et al., 1992.

Soy Formulas Some commercially produced infant formulas are made from soybeans; both iron-fortified and non-iron-fortified forms are available. Soy formulas tend to have somewhat higher protein and lower carbohydrate levels than cow's milk formulas. Also, the bioavailability of some minerals may be lower, because these products are of plant origin. For these reasons, such products should be used only on a pediatrician's advice.

Soy formulas may be useful for infants who are potentially allergic to cow's milk proteins and for infants who are sensitive to lactose. However, soy formulas are not usually recommended for infants who have already shown signs of allergy, because soy protein, like cow's milk protein, is a common allergen. Infants who have reacted strongly to cow's milk protein may react strongly to soy protein as well.

Other Formulas Unmodified cow's milk or homemade cow's milk formulas are *not recommended for the first year of life* (Subcommittee on Nutrition During Lactation, 1991). You have already learned many ways in which unmodified cow's milk differs nutritionally from human breast milk. In addition, it has larger concentrations of electrolytes and proteins than immature kidneys can easily handle. Some young infants become anemic on cow's milk because it is a poor source of iron and may cause low-level intestinal bleeding. The milk of other animals, such as goats, should be avoided as well, unless the baby's pediatrician advises their use.

A Bottle-Fed Infant's Need for Supplements As you learned earlier, all newborns should initially receive supplemental vitamin K. In addition, babies fed commercially produced infant formula may benefit from supplemental fluoride if they do not get adequate amounts from the water they drink. Because an infant's fluoride intake from water can vary widely, and because excess fluoride is toxic, fluoride is not added to infant formulas. Parents should follow the advice of their baby's pediatrician on whether to supplement, and if so, with how much.

Safety Considerations with Bottle Feeding Most formulas are available as a powder, a liquid concentrate, or a ready-to-use beverage. The first two

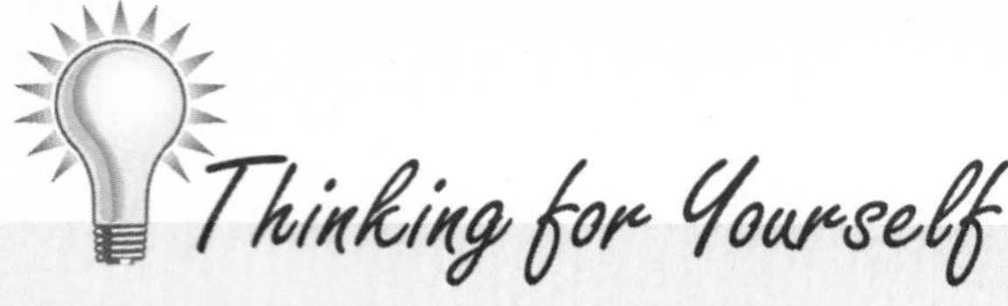

To Breast-Feed or to Bottle-Feed?

The Situation

Angie and John are expecting a baby in 3 months. John is a policeman, and Angie is an elementary school teacher. They both intend to continue to work after the baby is born, although Angie will take a maternity leave of 2 months.

When they first started talking about having a family, they had planned that Angie would breast-feed their baby for about a year. They believed the adage that "Breast is best"; they believed that besides providing good nutrition, breast-feeding would promote **bonding** between Angie and the baby, and that the baby would be less likely to be "colicky," get sick, or have allergies if he were breast-fed.

Now, as the time is getting closer and Angie is coping with the rigors of teaching plus the stresses of late pregnancy, she privately wonders whether she will have the time or energy to nurse the baby. She knows that she herself was bottle-fed as an infant, and she was healthy; couldn't bottle-feeding work for their baby too? But she assumes that John is counting on her, and she thinks that her best friends, who breast-fed their infants, will think less of her if she doesn't nurse her baby. She feels guilty even thinking about bottle-feeding.

John also remembers their commitment and still basically believes in their decision. However, he's been thinking about the fact that breast-feeding will make it more difficult for him to be as involved with the baby as he would like. He's reluctant to bring this up; it seems pretty self-centered. Furthermore, he doesn't want Angie to misconstrue his motivation; he doesn't want her to think that he has lost confidence in her ability to breast-feed the baby and to be a "good mother."

Is Their Information Accurate and Relevant?

- It's true that the milk of a well-nourished mother sets the standard for nutrition for the baby. However, commercial infant formulas closely mimic the nutrients in human milk.
- It's true that breast-feeding does encourage bonding, which can promote an infant's healthy development; but if a caregiver holds and interacts with the baby during feeding, bonding can be fostered during bottle-feeding as well.
- It is not true that breast-feeding prevents **colic;** up to 30% of all babies, both breast-fed and bottle-fed, experience these periods of crying caused by spasms of abdominal pain. In some cases, breakdown products of cow's milk in formula or in mother's milk have been thought to be the cause of colic (Nutrition Reviews, 1988); however, changing the feeding techniques (Davidson, 1983) or trying various responses to the baby's crying (Taubman, 1988) may be more effective than changing the nature of the milk feeding.
- The immune factors in breast milk are very important for infant health in the *developing* countries; but in the *developed* countries, where sanitation is generally good and infections not as common, breast-feeding does not provide the same clear advantage (Wray, 1991).
- It is true that allergies are less likely to occur in breast-fed babies; this is an important factor in families with a history of allergies. There is no such history in either Angie's or John's family.

What Else Should They Consider?

When Angie and John made their decision about breast-feeding some time ago, they planned that Angie would quit working when they had a baby. As things are turning out, as happy as she is about having the baby, she now realizes how committed she is to teaching . . . and how much they like the double income. They decided together

bonding—special feelings of love and attachment between caregiver and baby

colic—periods of crying, apparently from spasms of abdominal pain in an otherwise healthy infant

need to be reconstituted with appropriate amounts of water before use, making them less convenient but usually less expensive. It is critical that the formula be of the correct concentration when given to the baby. If it is not dilute enough, the baby's body can become stressed; if it is too dilute, the baby will not be adequately nourished.

If you have mixed formula in advance, store it in the refrigerator until you use it. Then, if the baby prefers it warmer, take the chill off by putting the bottle into a container of warm water for a few minutes. It is probably

that Angie should continue teaching. Since their circumstances will be different from what they had originally thought, and since their thinking and feelings about breast-feeding are in flux, they should reopen the topic for discussion.

There are things that they didn't consider earlier, when they thought Angie would be at home with the baby. Angie knows that some mothers who work away from home also breast-feed their babies. Although she would not find it possible to come home for feedings as one of her friends did, she knows that some mothers pump their breasts and leave the milk for the baby. She does not know how to do this, so she decides to ask her obstetrician about it. Another source of information would be a local chapter of the La Leche League, an international organization that provides education about and promotion of breast-feeding. They have clearly written print materials, well-informed leaders, and members who share their experiences and encourage each other.

Angie and John are also somewhat concerned about the issue of toxins in breast milk. Angie has totally avoided alcohol during her pregnancy, but one of the things she has been looking forward to when she is no longer pregnant is being able to relax with friends and have a beer. She makes a mental note to ask the baby's doctor whether her drinking one or two beers would pose a problem for the baby. Pediatricians give different advice on this question.

She and John are also beginning to wonder whether there is any problem with the fact that about once every 2 weeks she has been eating fish that John caught in the local lake. The lake is fed by a river that flows through agricultural areas, and they wonder whether runoff chemicals could have been in the fish they've been eating. If so, were they absorbed into her body, and would they be secreted into her milk? In some states, departments of natural resources periodically publish recommendations regarding the safety of consuming fish taken from state waterways. John plans to check on this; such information could help in estimating whether Angie has been accumulating levels of toxins in her body that could get into her breast milk. Angie will talk with her doctor about this, too.

As they discuss again the issue of how to feed their baby, they realize that their early decision to breast-feed was based on some correct information, some misinformation, and some emotion. They are learning that there are other responsible feeding options from which "good parents" can choose. They know that breast-feeding has certain physical and emotional benefits, but now they understand that bottle-feeding is also a healthy option. It is important to take practical matters into account as well when making their decision.

Now What Do You Think?

If you were advising Angie and John, what would you recommend? Some options are listed below; do you see others?

- Option 1 You advise Angie and John exclusively to breast-feed their baby for the first year, as they had planned. You suggest ways to ensure that Angie gets enough relaxed time to nurse the baby and that John gets regular quality time with the baby as well.
- Option 2 You advise that their baby should be exclusively breast-fed while Angie is on leave for 2 months; then, as she prepares to go back to work, she should make a transition to formula-feeding.
- Option 3 You advise that their baby should be breast-fed during the first year whenever Angie is home and be given a bottle of either breast milk or formula when she is away.
- Option 4 You advise that their baby should be formula-fed exclusively from the beginning.

better not to heat the formula in a microwave oven, because it is easy to overheat it or produce "hot spots" in the formula. Some infants have suffered burns in the mouth and/or esophagus from drinking formula heated with microwaves that was not well-mixed and tested before serving.

When bottle-feeding their babies, caregivers need to take measures to avoid **baby bottle tooth decay** (sometimes called *nursing bottle caries*). This condition involves rampant dental decay in children around the age of 2 years (Figure 15.8). It is most likely to occur in children who are put to bed

baby bottle tooth decay—tooth decay resulting from prolonged exposure to sweet beverages (even infant formula) consumed from baby bottles

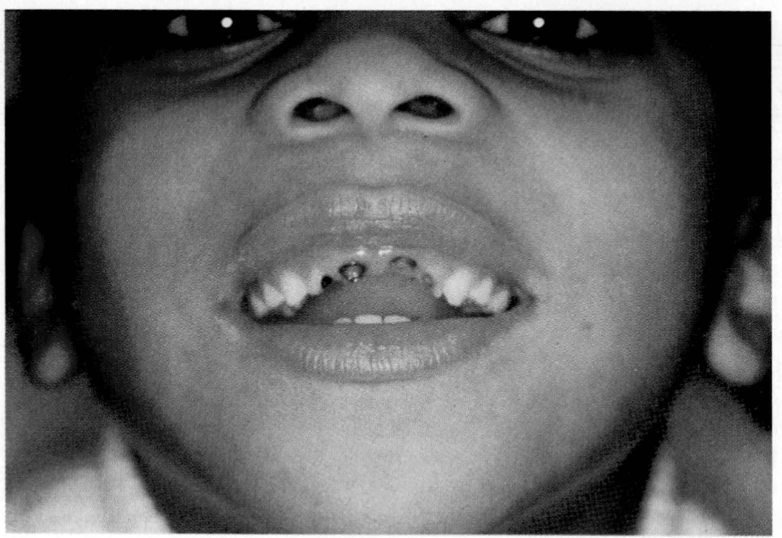

FIGURE 15.8
Baby bottle tooth decay.

Infants who are put to bed with bottles of sugar-containing fluids may develop rampant dental decay.

with a bottle containing sweet liquids, such as milk, juice, or any sugar-sweetened drink. As the child falls asleep, saliva flow (which ordinarily helps cleanse the teeth of sugar) diminishes; with sweet liquids pooled in the mouth, mouth bacteria have the opportunity to metabolize the sugars, producing acids that cause decay. To prevent the condition, don't put babies to bed with bottles. Also, experts recommend weaning children from the bottle at about 1 year of age (Johnsen and Nowjack-Raymer, 1989).

Solid Foods for Older Infants

"Only 3 weeks old, and he's eating cereal already? Your little guy is way ahead for his age! He must be awfully smart!"

Several decades ago, proud parents loved to hear such praise. They looked on a baby's early eating of solid foods as a sign of accelerated physical and intellectual development. However, not all infants who were given solid foods were ready for them. Some parents actually resorted to using "feeders" that squirted food into the back of their baby's mouth because the baby was unable to swallow it otherwise.

Now we know that solids should be introduced in infants' diets only when they are physically ready to handle those foods and when they need the nutrients that such foods can provide. In this section, you'll learn when these stages occur and what foods are appropriate at each.

Introducing Solid Foods

An infant's physical readiness and nutritional need for solid foods occur at approximately the same time: 4–6 months of age. Until this time, mother's milk and/or formula constitute the baby's total diet.

Physical Readiness Physical development is the most reliable indicator of a child's readiness for solid foods. Somewhere between 4 and 6 months of age, babies undergo many changes that enable them easily to eat solid foods from a spoon (Figure 15.9): they learn to use their tongues to move solids to the back of their mouths for swallowing; their kidneys concentrate urine more efficiently; they become able to sit in a high chair; they show their

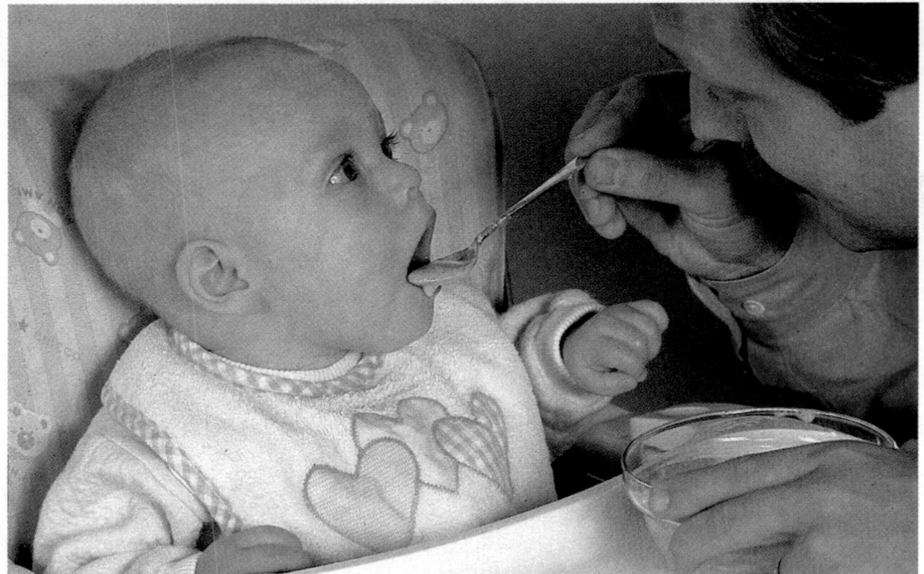

FIGURE 15.9
Adding solids to an infant's diet.

The appropriate time to begin giving solid food to infants is between 4 and 6 months of age, when they are physically ready and need the nutrients.

eagerness for more food when they're hungry, keeping an eye on the food and opening their mouths as the spoon approaches; they can turn their heads away or otherwise refuse food when their hunger is satisfied. Encouraging these physical activities when babies become able to do them improves their skills and prepares them for their next stage of physical development.

Nutrient Needs At 4–6 months of age, a rapidly growing infant can benefit nutritionally as well from eating some solid foods. Solids tend to be more concentrated in energy and protein than breast milk or formula.

A separate set of RDAs applies to babies in the latter 6 months of the first year. In most cases, these RDAs are higher—sometimes as much as double the recommendations for newborns—reflecting the larger size and continuing growth of the older baby.

Social Implications When a baby starts on solids, the feeding routine changes somewhat. Now babies' tasks are to experience the food, move it back in their mouths, swallow it, sense how it feels to have it in their stomachs, and then communicate whether they want more or not. The caregiver still needs to give the same time and attention as before to the baby's signals of hunger and satiety and to respond appropriately to them.

If a caregiver short-circuits the process by simply spooning food into a baby until the dish is empty (irrespective of cues from the infant), the baby gets the message that its hunger and satiety signals are not being taken seriously. Depending on the baby's personality, different responses may be exhibited. Placid babies who are overfed may accept the situation and open their mouths each time the spoon advances; more determined infants might resist the spoon frantically in a fight for their right to determine their intake.

The problem with overfeeding or restricting food during infancy is that children are likely to learn not to trust their internal messages. Some experts believe that if children learn to override their internal hunger and satiety signals, they may initiate lifelong problems with eating behaviors.

Sequence and Timing Because a baby needs more iron at this time than breast milk or formula provide, iron-fortified infant cereals should be the first solid food. Some pediatricians recommend that parents give rice or barley cereals until 7–9 months of age, because they are less likely to provoke an allergic response than wheat, corn, or mixed cereals. Families with a history of allergies may benefit from waiting to start their infants on *any* solids until around 6 months of age (McBean, 1992).

Once cereals have been successfully incorporated into a child's diet and the infant has mastered the skill of taking cereal from a spoon and swallowing it, the infant is ready for other textures. Cooked and pureed, fork-mashed, or diced fruit and vegetables fed by spoon or self-fed by fingers offer a developmentally and nutritionally logical next step. Add pureed or ground meat after fruits and vegetables, or wait to offer meat until the child begins eating from the table, somewhere near the first birthday.

When you add a new food to an infant's diet, give only small amounts for several days before you try another new food. In this way, you can easily identify the offending food if the baby has an allergic reaction.

When solid foods represent a large part of a baby's intake, give extra liquids as well, because solids contain less water than the breast milk or formula that they are partially replacing.

Table 15.5 summarizes the guidelines for introducing solid foods into an infant's diet. Don't follow the table slavishly, because normal babies can develop at different rates. The important principle is to modify an infant's diet gradually as you see changes in developmental readiness.

Commercial Versus Homemade Baby Foods Many parents rely on commercial baby foods until their child can eat with the rest of the family. The commercial products come in ready-to-eat form, and some are also available as dehydrated flakes to which liquid must be added. Others prefer to prepare their own baby foods "from scratch."

The commercially prepared infant foods are convenient and safe but are often more expensive than home-prepared foods. Furthermore, because of their smooth texture, they don't offer much developmental challenge to the child who is ready to progress to a more mature eating style.

Many people believe that commercially prepared baby foods are high in sugar, salt, and preservatives, but most manufacturers now use little or none of these ingredients in their basic pureed foods. If you make your own baby food out of foods being prepared for the rest of the family, you can take out the baby's portion before adding seasoning or sauces. In this way, you will minimize the level of sugar, salt, and spices that the baby receives. For future convenience, freeze some in ice cube trays and then store the cubes in plastic bags.

Do not make baby food from canned food: most canned vegetables and meats contain added salt, and most canned fruit has added sugar. Furthermore, canned foods may contain lead if lead solder was used in making the can (see Chapter 14). It is better to buy baby food or ingredients for baby food that are packaged in glass or plastic containers.

A good rule of thumb for those who buy prepared baby food is to stick to simple, single-ingredient items. If the food does not agree with the baby, it is easier to identify the problem. Furthermore, foods such as strained chicken are cheaper and more concentrated in nutrients than fancier combination foods, such as chicken dinners.

Safety Baby foods prepared from the family's meals can be just as nutritious as commercial types, but you need to take special care to make them as safe. One potential problem is microorganisms. The safest approach is to make and serve the baby's food, on the spot, from what is being served to

TABLE 15.5 Recommendations for Feeding Infants

Age	Foods to Introduce	Physical Development	Comments
Birth	Breast milk or commercially produced formula; no other foods.	Baby can suck liquids from birth but thrusts tongue forward to push solids from mouth (extrusion reflex). Kidneys cannot concentrate urine. Digestive secretions produced at low levels. Little control of head and neck.	Breast-feeders should get supplemental fluoride and vitamin D; if the mother is a vegan, the infant needs supplemental vitamin B-12 as well. Formulas are usually adequate in vitamins and most minerals, although fluoride may need to be supplemented.
4–6 months	Iron-fortified cereal[a] mixed with formula or breast milk.	Baby learns to swallow solids. Control of head and neck allows child to sit up for eating and to indicate hunger and satiety. Kidneys are able to concentrate urine.	If there is a family history of allergies, delay solids until 6 months. Delay wheat cereals until 7–9 months.
6–9 months (starting 6 weeks after cereal was added)	Strained, mashed, or diced fruits and vegetables. Either bottled baby foods or table foods prepared without sugar, honey, or seasonings.	Baby can grasp and route food from hand to mouth. Teeth begin to come in.	Babies at this age accept many tastes and can learn to accept a variety of textures. Allow 3–4 days between introduction of new items.
9–12 months	Juices from a cup. Finger foods, whole pieces of soft fruits and vegetables. Pureed, milled, or finely chopped meats. Eggs. Casseroles from family table. Bread and crackers.	Chewing pattern has begun. Child can drink from cup.	This is a transitional period from soft, mushy foods to table foods. Older babies usually prefer to feed themselves and to examine their food by handling it.
12 months	Table foods. Finely cut meats. Most finger foods, except items that are hard to chew (such as popcorn, nuts, and raisins), or small, slippery, rounded foods (such as hot dogs, grapes, and candy), because of the risk of choking.	Biting, chewing, and swallowing are well developed. Pincer grasp (thumb and fingers) enables child to pick up small objects. Good spoon control begins.	Delay use of honey and corn syrup until after 12 months: they may cause infant botulism. Infant should be weaned from the bottle and may be weaned from the breast.

[a]Continue iron-fortified infant cereal until at least one year of age, to help restore dwindling iron reserves.

the rest of the family. Family fare can be changed to baby food by grinding, fork-mashing, or dicing. Baby food that is pureed or ground in quantity ahead of time and not properly stored is a perfect medium for bacterial growth because of its large surface area. Make sure that all equipment used in preparation is scrupulously clean; keep hot foods hot and cold foods cold until you serve them. Do not reheat leftover baby foods more than once, and if a baby food has been at room temperature for more than half an hour, throw it away.

Do not give honey and corn syrup to infants under 1 year of age. These products sometimes contain spores of *Clostridium botulinum* (see Chapter 14). Because an infant's immature GI tract might allow the spores to become active and produce their lethal toxin (Liska et al., 1986), it is better not to risk giving these products to a baby.

A final safety issue has to do with the form of food served to young children. Although we have suggested offering more challenging foods as soon as children are ready for them, don't overshoot in this regard. Children can choke to death on food: in a study of over 100 choking cases involving babies through 9-year-olds, the most common offending foods were hot dogs, candy, nuts, grapes, cookies, meats, and carrots, in that order (Harris et al., 1984). This shows that round, slippery, and small foods pose greater risk for young children. If you allow them to eat such foods, be especially attentive. You can make some of these foods safer by cutting them into pieces that will not block the child's airway. For example, carrots or hot dogs cut into thin strips are safer than big cylindrical chunks, which could plug a child's airway.

Self-Feeding Usually between 7 and 9 months, babies reach another milestone in their development: they start to feed themselves. Self-feeding begins with easy-to-hold foods, such as teething biscuits, and progresses to soft foods, such as pieces of cooked vegetables. Anything that sticks together long enough for the baby to get it from the high-chair tray to the mouth is fair game.

At about this time, a baby can also begin to drink liquids from a cup. Many experts recommend waiting until this stage to give a baby fruit juices, because fruit juices from a bottle are a possible cause of baby bottle tooth decay.

How Much Is Enough?

Parents chronically worry about whether their baby is getting the right amount to eat. On the one hand, even if a baby is eating normally, grandparents might cast some doubt by commenting that "a fat baby is a healthy baby." On the other hand, some of today's parents want to keep children too slender; even when the child's intake is normal, these parents worry that their baby is overeating.

The soundest approach is to abandon preconceived ideas about how thin or fat a particular child should be and to provide, from the beginning, appropriate food in response to the child's hunger and satiety messages. Babies fed in this way have the chance to attain their individually appropriate body weights. Some babies will be naturally fatter or leaner than others, but this does not predestine their size for life: a fat baby usually does not become an obese child. We'll discuss this topic more thoroughly in Chapter 16.

Babies differ in the quantity of food they require for their normal growth and in how often they want to be fed. Newborns need to be fed at least 8 times per day—and some may prefer 15 or more times per day—until their stomach capacities increase enough to have fewer and larger feedings. A month-old infant will take about 20 ounces of breast milk or

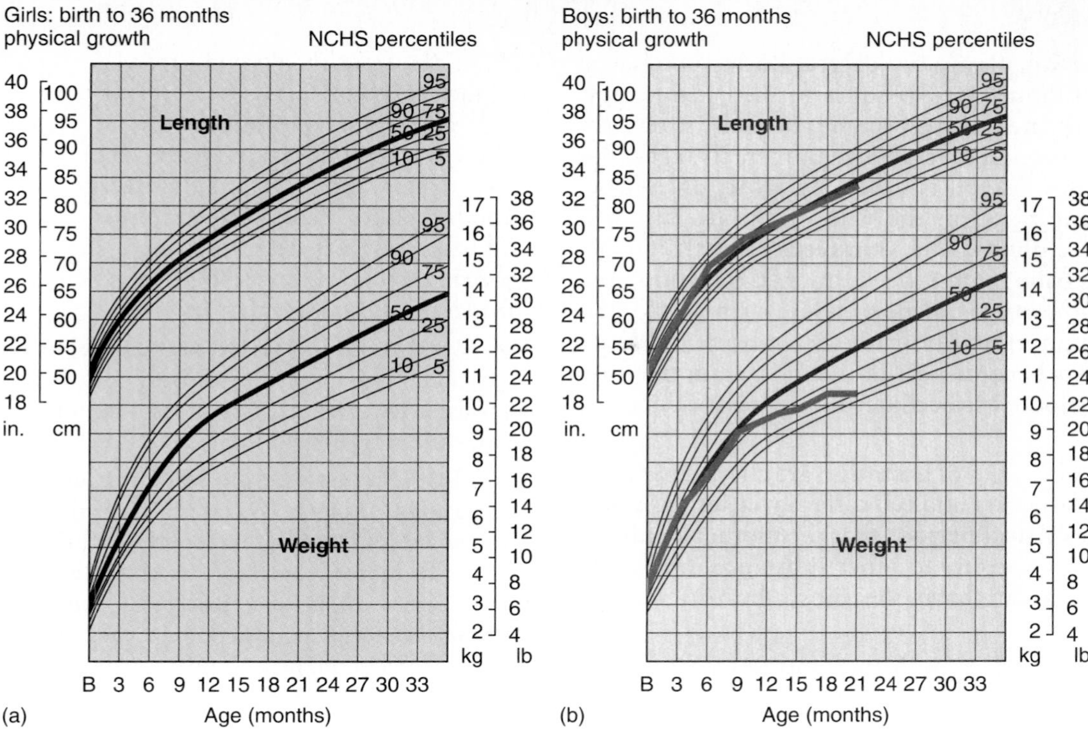

FIGURE 15.10
(a) Normal growth curves for girls. (b) Normal growth curves for boys.

The red lines in part (b) show one child's poor growth.

(Adapted from National Center for Health Statistics, 1976. Data from The Fels Research Institute, Yellow Springs, Ohio. © 1976 Ross Laboratories, Columbus, Ohio 43216.)

formula each day in 5–12 feedings, although the amount may vary considerably from day to day. This often increases to well over a quart per day by around 4–6 months, at which time a few teaspoons of solid food are added to the diet. By the time a child is 1 year old, a variety of table foods accounts for a large part of the diet, and milk intake should have decreased to 20–32 ounces (2½–4 cups) per day.

The best way to check whether a baby's intake of food is on target is to measure the child's growth in length and weight. Parents should take their babies to health care providers for regular health checkups, which include growth monitoring. Charts from the National Center for Health Statistics (Figure 15.10) show the typical length and weight distributions for American children. The 50th percentile for weight is the point at which 50% of the infants weigh more and 50% weigh less. The 90th percentile is the point at which 10% weigh more. Once a child has settled into particular length and weight bands on the growth charts, he or she is likely to stay and progress in those "canals" or close to them.

Babies are very individual in the rates at which they grow and in the eventual body sizes they attain. Don't be alarmed if your child does not keep up with the growth of another youngster of the same age; what is important is to keep up with the child's own previously established pattern. Most children do this naturally, but there are occasional exceptions.

Figure 15.10(b) shows an example of a child who "fell off his growth curve." Such **failure to thrive** is serious and can be the result of an underlying illness, a structural problem, or misunderstanding on the part of the caregivers about how to feed the baby. In any case of failure to thrive, it is extremely important that parents seek the help of health care professionals to determine the cause and to aid in the treatment of poor growth.

failure to thrive—inability to maintain a previously established growth curve

Summary

- Nutrition plays a critical role during pregnancy because so much new tissue is formed at this time. Some of the new tissue becomes the baby, after progressing through several developmental stages. For the first 2 weeks, it is called a **zygote;** once it becomes implanted in the wall of the **uterus,** it is called an **embryo.** The term **fetus** refers to the developing baby from 8 weeks after fertilization until birth. Other types of new tissue, such as the **placenta,** support and nourish the embryo and fetus. Still others become part of the mother, in the form of extra blood, extracellular fluid, breast tissue, and body fat.

- Certain stages of **gestation** are characterized by rapid cell division and **cell differentiation;** it is during these **critical periods** that the mother's nutrient intake and exposure to other substances (including teratogens) can have the most dramatic consequences.

- The weight of both the mother-to-be and the new baby are important; total desirable gain for the normal-weight mother is 25–35 pounds, although a fairly wide range can be normal, depending on the woman's prepregnant weight and height. The birth weight of the baby should be at least 5½ pounds; an infant weighing less is a **low-birth-weight baby.** To achieve these weight gains, the woman should choose foods for nutritional adequacy, balance, and variety, because the need for many nutrients is high at this time, especially in the last 2 **trimesters.** A carefully planned diet can meet these needs, except for iron, which should be supplemented. Although physicians recommend multivitamin and mineral supplements in some cases, pregnant women should practice the principle of adequate but not excessive intake. Good nutrition also provides reserves for **lactation.** The **WIC** program helps low-income women who have high-risk pregnancies to meet their nutrient needs.

- Pregnant women should be careful to avoid ingesting dangerous levels of dietary toxicants. A set of abnormalities called **fetal alcohol syndrome** has been observed in some children of women who consumed alcohol heavily during pregnancy. (Less is known about the risks of drinking alcohol in smaller amounts.) Practices such as pica and smoking may also affect the fetus, so pregnancy calls for an evaluation of many lifestyle factors besides nutrition.

- Because of their rapid growth, infants have the highest nutrient needs per unit of body weight of any age group. Deciding what to feed a baby is therefore an important matter. The immature GI and urinary tracts of infants do not handle adult foods well for the first few months of life. Healthy full-term infants do have reserve supplies of some nutrients that can meet their needs during the time when milk is their only food.

- Infants should be fed on demand until they are satisfied. This practice not only allows them to establish their own natural growth pattern but also allows them to develop trust.

- Both breast-feeding and bottle-feeding offer certain advantages. Breast milk is uniquely adapted to the infant's nutritional needs, and the **colostrum** contains factors that increase the infant's immunity to various infections. Both the composition and volume of milk produced can vary in response to the baby's demands. Iron-fortified formulas can provide nutritionally satisfactory substitutes for breast milk and are available in several different varieties. Factors other than nutrition—such as psychologic factors (e.g., **bonding**), convenience, economy, safety, the risk of **baby bottle tooth decay,** and lifestyle of the parents—can also influence the decision of how to feed a baby. Some babies receiving each type of feeding are likely to experience **colic.**

- Older infants need the nutrients that solid foods provide; such foods should be introduced when the baby is physically ready for them, usually between 4 and 6 months of age. Iron-fortified cereals are usually the first solid food and should be followed by others introduced gradually. Commercially prepared baby foods are convenient and safe, though often more expensive than those prepared at home. Between 7 and 9 months of age, babies are usually able to begin feeding themselves and to drink from a cup. At this stage of life (as at others), it is probably best to provide appropriate food in response to the child's hunger and satiety messages. A reliable way to check whether the baby is getting enough nutrients is to keep track of the baby's height and weight, which can then be compared with population norms and the child's own past growth pattern. A few children exhibit **failure to thrive,** but most grow normally.

References

Abrams, B. 1991. Maternal undernutrition and reproductive performance. In *Infant and child nutrition worldwide,* ed. F. Falkner. Boca Raton, FL: CRC Press.

American Academy of Pediatrics, Committee on Nutrition, 1992. The use of whole cow's milk in infancy. *Pediatrics* 89:1105–1109.

American Dietetic Association. 1989. Ambulatory nutrition care: Pregnant women. *Journal of the American Dietetic Association* 89 (Supplement):S10–S14.

American Medical Association. 1983. Fetal effects of maternal alcohol use. *Journal of the American Medical Association* 249:2517–2521.

Arshad, S.H., S. Matthews, C. Gant, and D.W. Hide. 1992. Effect of allergen avoidance on development of allergic disorders in infancy. *Lancet* 339(no.8808):1493–1497.

Blinder, B.J., S.L. Goodman, and P. Henderson. 1988. Pica: A critical review of diagnosis and treatment. In *The eating disorders,* ed. B.J. Blinder, B.F. Chaitin, and R. Goldstein. New York: PMA Publishing Corp.

Brooke, O.G., H.R. Anderson, J.M. Bland, J.L. Peacock, and C.M. Stewart. 1989. Effects on birth weight of smoking, alcohol, caffeine, socioeconomic factors, and psychosocial stress. *British Medical Journal* 198:795–801.

Brown, J.E. 1989. Improving pregnancy outcomes in the United States: The importance of preventive nutrition services. *Journal of the American Dietetic Association* 89:631–638, 641.

Carruth, B.R. and J.D. Skinner. 1991. Practitioners beware: Regional differences in beliefs about nutrition during pregnancy. *Journal of the American Dietetic Association* 91:435–440.

Committee on Nutritional Status During Pregnancy and Lactation. 1990. *Nutrition during pregnancy.* Washington, DC: National Academy Press.

Davidson, M. 1983. Causes and management of colic in infancy. *Nutrition and the M.D.* 9(no.11):1–3.

Dobbing, J. 1984. Infant nutrition and later achievement. *Nutrition Reviews* 42:1–7.

Hackman, E., I. Emanuel, G. vanBelle, and J. Daling. 1983. Maternal birth weight and subsequent pregnancy outcome. *Journal of the American Medical Association* 250:2016–2019.

Harris, C.S., S.P. Baker, G.A. Smith, and R.M. Harris. 1984. Childhood asphyxiation by food: A national analysis and overview. *Journal of the American Medical Association* 251:2231–2235.

Heird, W.C. and A. Cooper. 1988. Nutrition in infants and children. In *Modern nutrition in health and disease,* ed. M.E. Shils and V.R. Young. Philadelphia: Lea & Febiger.

Hendricks, K.M. and S.H. Badruddin. 1992. Weaning recommendations: The scientific basis. *Nutrition Reviews* 50(no.5):125–133.

Hoff, C., W. Wertelecki, W.R. Blackburn, H. Mendenhall, H. Wiseman, and A. Stumpe. 1986. Trend associations of smoking with maternal, fetal, and neonatal morbidity. *Obstetrics and Gynecology* 68:317–321.

Jensen, R.G., A.M. Ferris, and C.J. Lammi-Keefe. 1992. Lipids in human milk and infant formulas. *Annual Review of Nutrition* 12:417–441.

Johnsen, D. and R. Nowjack-Raymer. 1989. Baby bottle tooth decay (BBTD): Issues, assessment, and an opportunity for the nutritionist. *Journal of the American Dietetic Association* 89:1112–1116.

Levine, M.G. and D. Esser. 1988. Total parenteral nutrition for the treatment of severe hyperemesis gravidarum: Maternal nutritional effects and fetal outcome. *Obstetrics and Gynecology* 72:102–107.

Liska, B.J., E.M. Foster, J.H. Silliker, and D.L. Archer. 1986. A new bacteria in the news: A special symposium. *Food Technology* 40(no.8):16–26.

Little, R.E. and C.F. Sing. 1986. Association of father's drinking and infant's birth weight. *New England Journal of Medicine* 314:1644–1645.

Little, R.E., A.P. Streissguth, H.M. Barr, and C.S. Herman. 1980. Decreased birth weight in infants of alcoholic women who abstained during pregnancy. *Journal of Pediatrics* 96:974–977.

Lovelady, C.A., B. Lonnerdal, and K.G. Dewey. 1990. Lactation performance of exercising women. *American Journal of Clinical Nutrition* 52:103–109.

McBean, L.D. 1992. Infant nutrition in the 1990s. *Dairy Council Digest* 63:31–36.

Mennella, J.A. and G.K. Beauchamp. 1991. The transfer of alcohol to human milk. *New England Journal of Medicine* 325:981–985.

Miller, M.W. 1986. Effects of alcohol on the generation and migration of cerebral cortical neurons. *Science* 233:1308–1311.

Mills, J.L., L.B. Holmes, J.H. Aarons, J.L. Simpson, Z.A. Brown, L.G. Jovanovic-Peterson, M.R. Conley, B.I Graubard, R.H. Knopp, and B.E. Metzger. 1993. Moderate caffeine use and the risk of spontaneous abortion and intrauterine growth retardation. *Journal of the American Medical Association* 269:593–597.

Moore, K.L. 1988. *The developing human,* 4th edition. Philadelphia: W.B. Saunders Co.

MRC Vitamin Research Group. 1991. Prevention of neural tube defects: Results of the medical research council vitamin study. *Lancet* 338(no.8760):131–137.

Mutch, P.B. 1988. Food guides for the vegetarian. *American Journal of Clinical Nutrition* 48:913–919.

National Center for Health Statistics. 1976. *NCHS Growth Charts, 1976.* Monthly Vital Statistics Report vol. 25, no. 3, Supp. (HRA) 76–1120. Rockville, MD: Health Resources Administration.

National Research Council. 1989. *Diet and health.* Washington, DC: National Academy Press.

Nelson, S.E., E.E. Ziegler, A.M. Copeland, B.B. Edwards, and S.J. Fomon. 1988. Lack of adverse reactions to iron-fortified formula. *Pediatrics* 81:360–364.

Nutrition Reviews. 1988. Is colic in infants associated with diet? *Nutrition Reviews* 46:374–376.

Pipes, P.L. 1989. Nutrition in infancy and childhood. St. Louis: Times Mirror/Mosby College Publishing.

Potter, S., S. Hannum, B. McFarlin, D. Essex-Sorlie, E. Campbell, S. Trupin. 1991. Does infant feeding method influence maternal postpartum weight loss? *Journal of the American Dietetic Association* 91:441–446.

Rasmussen, K.M. 1992. The influence of maternal nutrition on lactation. *Annual Review of Nutrition* 12:103–117.

RDA Subcommittee. 1989. *Recommended dietary allowances.* Washington, DC: National Academy Press.

Rosso, P. 1988. Regulation of food intake during pregnancy and lactation. In *Control of appetite,* ed. M. Winick. New York: John Wiley & Sons, Inc.

Ryan, A.S., D. Rush, F.W. Krieger, and G.E. Lewandowski. 1991. Recent declines in breast-feeding in the United States, 1984 through 1989. *Pediatrics* 88:719–727.

Satter, E. 1986a. *Child of mine.* Palo Alto, CA: Bull Publishing Company.

Satter, E. 1986b. The feeding relationship. *Journal of the American Dietetic Association* 86:352–356.

Stein, A. and M. Susser. 1991. Miscarriage, caffeine and the epiphenomena of pregnancy: The causal model. *Epidemiology* 1991(no.2):163–167.

Stjernfeldt, M., K. Berglund, J. Lindsten, and J. Ludvigsson. 1986. Maternal smoking during pregnancy and risk of childhood cancer. *Lancet* I(no.8494):1350–1352.

Stockbauer, J.W. 1987. WIC prenatal participation and its relation to pregnancy outcomes in Missouri: A second look. *American Journal of Public Health* 77:813–816.

Streissguth, A.P., P.D. Sampson, H.M. Barr, B.L. Darby, and D.C. Martin. 1989. IQ at age 4 in relation to maternal alcohol use and smoking during pregnancy. *Developmental Psychology* 25:3–11.

Subcommittee on Nutrition During Lactation. 1991. *Nutrition during lactation.* Washington, DC: National Academy Press.

Surgeon General. 1988. *The Surgeon General's report on nutrition and health.* Washington, DC: United States Department of Health and Human Services.

Susser, M. 1991. Maternal weight gain, infant birth weight, and diet: Causal sequences. *American Journal of Clinical Nutrition* 53:1384–1396.

Taubman, B. 1988. Parental counseling compared with elimination of cow's milk or soy milk protein for the treatment of infant colic syndrome: A randomized trial. *Pediatrics* 81:756–761.

United States Department of Agriculture. 1991. (Addendum to) The savings in Medicaid costs for newborns and their mothers from prenatal participation in the WIC Program. Washington, DC: United States Department of Agriculture.

United States Department of Agriculture and United States Department of Health and Human Services. 1990. *Nutrition and your health: Dietary guidelines for Americans.* Washington, DC: U.S. Government Printing Office.

Van der Spuy, Z.M., P.J. Steer, M. McCusker, S.J. Steele, H.S. Jacobs. 1988. Outcome of pregnancy in underweight women after spontaneous and induced ovulation. *British Medical Journal* 296:962–965.

Walker, A.R., B.F. Walker, and D. Labadarios. 1991. Nutritional needs in pregnancy: Why is the state of knowledge still speculative? *Nutrition Today* 26(no.6):18–24.

Whitehead, R.G. 1988. Pregnancy and lactation. In *Modern nutrition in health and disease,* ed. M.E. Shils and V.R. Young. Philadelphia: Lea & Febiger.

Williams, S.R. 1988. Nutrition for high-risk populations. In *Nutrition throughout the life cycle,* ed. S.R. Williams and B.S. Worthington-Roberts. St. Louis: Times Mirror/Mosby Publishing Company.

Worthington-Roberts, B.S. 1988. Maternal nutrition and the course and outcome of pregnancy. In *Nutrition throughout the life cycle,* ed. S.R. Williams and B.S. Worthington-Roberts. St. Louis: Times Mirror/Mosby Publishing Company.

Wray, J.D. 1991. Breast-feeding: An international and historical review. In *Infant and child nutrition worldwide,* ed. F. Falkner. Boca Raton, FL: CRC Press.

Wright, J.T., I.G. Barrison, I.G. Lewis, K.D. MacRae, E.J. Waterson, P.J. Toplis, M.G. Gordon, N.F. Morris, and I.M. Murray-Lyon. 1983. Alcohol consumption, pregnancy and low birth weight. *Lancet* I(no.8326):663–664.

Zeman, F.J. and D.M. Ney. 1988. *Applications of clinical nutrition.* Englewood Cliffs, NJ: Prentice-Hall.

Chapter 16

Nutrition for Children and Adolescents

IN THIS CHAPTER

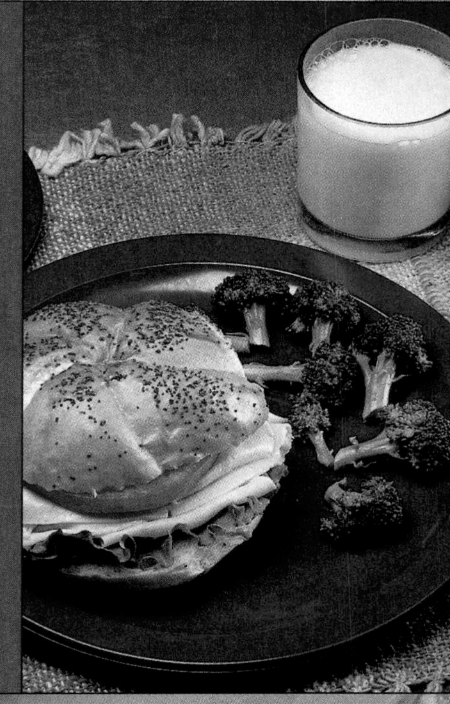

The growing years are about change. Physical changes are the most obvious, especially in the early years, but impressive mental development is taking place at the same time. Children's behavior—including their eating behavior—reflects both of these realms of growth.

Think of the young children you know, and recall how their eating behavior changed in the first year of life. If you watched them learn to eat solid foods, you may have seen them progress from simply opening their mouths as food came their way, to holding their mothers' hands as the mothers held the spoon, to feeding themselves (hit-or-miss), and eventually to delivering the goods in a fairly reliable way. The advance from one to the next of these seemingly simple tasks actually represented substantial increases in the capacity of the children's musculoskeletal and nervous systems and, at the same time, may have been triggered by the first stirrings of their drive for independence.

Food preferences can reflect both physical and mental changes. A toddler may like a particular food because she has just learned to handle it or because she is increasingly aware of its taste or texture. A preschooler or elementary school child might be influenced to some degree by his peers' preferences or by repeated TV advertising. Surely, adolescents are also affected by various social influences.

The changes in all kinds of behavior that take place throughout the first two decades of life make these years very dynamic, exciting, and challenging. How can you, an adult in a child's life—whether as a brother or sister, day-care worker, neighbor, teacher, coach, parent, or health care provider—help a child to cope with these changes? It's important that you learn first what is normal during each stage in a child's development and what opportunities can help a child make transitions from one stage to the next more easily. With some basic guidelines in mind, you can help children develop sound eating habits. This is the most important influence any adult can have on a child's nutrition.

Helping you appreciate this is an important goal for this chapter.

Development Through the Elementary Years

The examples above show that food and eating are closely interwoven with a child's development. Let's take a more detailed look at those interrelationships during the preschool and elementary school years.

Physical Development and Activity

Rates of growth are not constant in children. In Chapter 15, you learned that a baby is likely to triple its birth weight by the first birthday, so it is not uncommon for a child to gain 12–15 pounds or more during its first year. By contrast, a child 3–5 years old probably will not gain more than 4 pounds per year. Figure 16.1 shows average gains in weight and height for girls and boys. You can see that rates of growth decrease dramatically after the first year and then increase markedly in the preteen and teen years.

Body tissues and organs continue to develop throughout the years of childhood (Figure 16.2). The gastrointestinal (GI) tract develops more rapidly than many other systems. As a baby's GI tract gradually matures, it can handle more complex foods. Because gastric secretions and most enzymes are produced at nearly adult levels by the end of the first year, it is reasonable to offer a wide variety of foods by this time. More teeth (eight molars by about 2 years of age and four permanent molars around age 6)

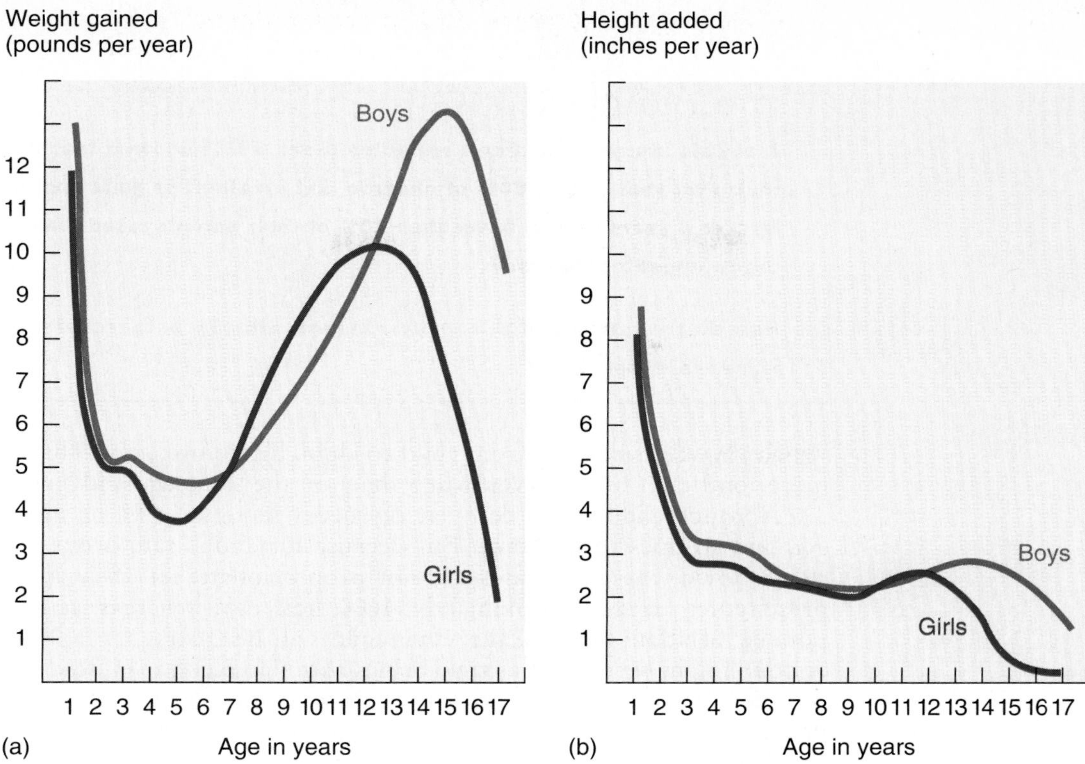

FIGURE 16.1
(a) Average gains in weight for girls and boys. (b) Average additions to height for girls and boys.
(Data source: RDA Subcommittee, 1989.)

provide the equipment to break apart meats and other chewy foods. Nutrition is very important during these years: in addition to meeting immediate needs, nutrients must be stored in preparation for the next surge of growth.

Young children's food intakes vary considerably, reflecting peaks and valleys in appetite. Appetites, in turn, often reflect the rate at which children are growing.

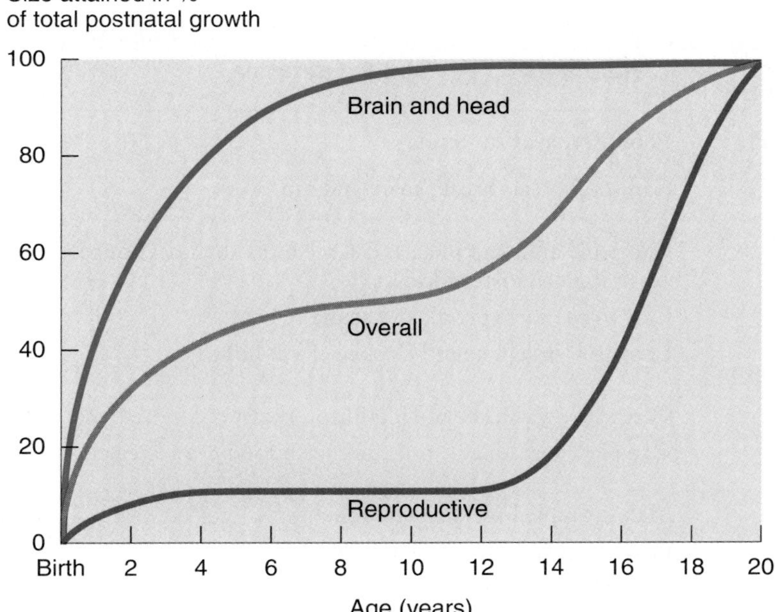

FIGURE 16.2
Growth of body components.
(Adapted from Scammon, 1927.)

Children's energy needs are also partly determined by activity levels,

> ### *You Tell Me*
>
> **A classic study of children's appetites (Beal, 1957) showed that during their first year of life, 80% of children had excellent or good appetites. By 3 or 4 years of age, fewer than 20% of their parents rated their children's appetites that way.**
>
> **How do the findings of this study compare with the patterns of growth shown in Figure 16.1?**

which vary considerably from child to child. Therefore, some children need more food than others, even when they are the same age and size.

A young child's total daily energy needs increase as he or she gets bigger, and so does food intake. But because metabolic rate drops as growth slows down, these increases are not proportionate: an 18-kg (40-pound) preschooler needs approximately 1600 kcal/day, whereas at 36 kg (80 pounds, at about age 11), the same child will need roughly 2000 kcal/day. A doubling in weight at this time brings about an increase in need for energy of only 400 kcal/day. Or look at it this way: during the first several years of life, children need 40–45 kcal per pound per day, whereas at age 11, they need only 20–25 kcal per pound per day.

Coordination

Just as a child's rate of physical *growth* is not constant, development of physical *skill* is not uniform, either. A child's physical development generally takes this pattern: from trunk to extremities (arms and legs) and from head to toe. Large muscles develop before smaller muscles, so coordination and control over fine movements tend to follow increases in size and strength.

TABLE 16.1 Physical Abilities of Preschool-Aged Children in Relationship to Food Preparation

Age (yr)	Food Preparation Skills
2	Can scrub, tear, break, snap, and dip
3	Can pour milk and juice and serve individual portions from a serving dish if given instructions Can wrap, mix, spread, and shake Feeds self independently, especially if hungry
4	Can wipe, wash, set table, pour premeasured ingredients Can peel, spread, cut, roll, and mash foods; crack eggs
5	Makes simple breakfast and lunch Can measure, cut, grind, and grate

Source: Adapted from Hertzler, 1989; Sigman-Grant , 1992.

TABLE 16.2 Observed Emotional, Eating, and Feeding Behaviors of Preschoolers

Age (yr)	Emotional Behaviors	Eating Behaviors	Feeding Behaviors
1–2	Neophobia Sharing is difficult Requires constant supervision Enjoys helping but can't be left alone Curious Often defiant Eager for attention	"Finicky" eater Food jags Holds food in mouth without swallowing	*One-year-old* Uses spoon with some skill (especially if hungry) Has good control of cup—lifts, drinks, sets it down, holds with one hand Helps self-feed *Two-year-old* Masters big arm muscle movements
3	The "me too" age—wants to be included in everything Responds well to options rather than demands Sharing is still difficult Somewhat rigid about the "right" way to do things	Eats most foods except for certain vegetables Dawdles over food when not hungry Comments on how foods are served	Uses spoon in semiadult fashion; may spear with fork Medium hand muscle development Feeds self independently especially if hungry
4	Shares well Needs adult approval and attention—shows off Understands; needs limits Follows rules most of the time Still rigid about the "right" way to do things	Eating and talking get in the way—prefers to talk Strong food likes and dislikes Refuses to eat to the point of tears	Uses all eating utensils Small finger muscle development
5	Helpful and cooperative with family chores and routines Still somewhat rigid about the "right" way to do things Very attached to mother, home, and family	Likes familiar foods, prefers most vegetables raw Latches on to food dislikes of family members and declares these as own	Fine coordination in fingers and hands

Source: Sigman-Grant, 1992.

Intermittently throughout childhood, therefore, a child's fine motor skills and physical coordination improve. At age 3, a child may be able to use a fork and spoon quite well but may not learn to use a knife for spreading and cutting until somewhat later (Table 16.1). You can help children develop better coordination by encouraging them to practice at mealtimes the skills for which they seem physically ready.

You can also help children develop coordination by involving them in simple food preparation tasks. As early as age 2, they may be able and willing to help you wash and prepare some vegetables, but don't expect too much at this age (Table 16.2). A somewhat older helper can stir the batter for a batch of muffins or peel an orange. Children are likely to be much more interested in eating a food they helped prepare; this can sometimes

FIGURE 16.3
Fixing food = trying food.

Children are more likely to try a new menu item if they have helped prepare it. The activities must be matched to the child's developmental level. Here nursery school children demonstrate some kitchen skills.

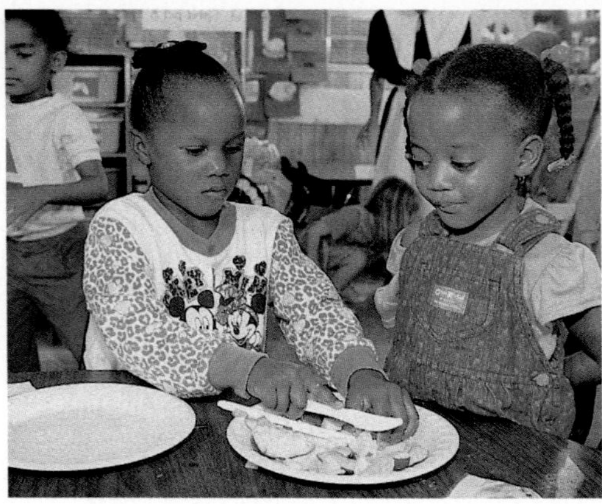

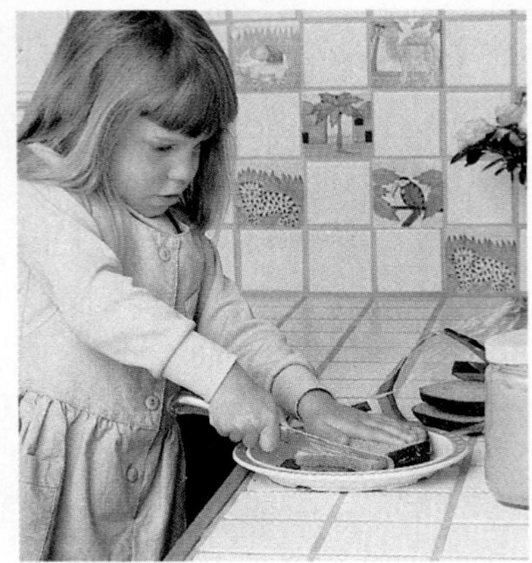

mean the difference between acceptance and rejection of a particular food (Figure 16.3). Of course, adequate supervision and teaching safe use of age-appropriate kitchen equipment is essential (Tang et al., 1992).

Psychosocial Development

Psychosocial changes are part of the mix of interactions that affect eating. Between 18 months and 3 years, children begin to recognize that they are separate from others (Sigman-Grant, 1992). They may demonstrate their emerging sense of individuality by engaging in power struggles with their caregivers at mealtimes, such as by refusing to eat a certain food or even refusing to eat at all.

Even though parents may understand exactly what is going on in this situation, they still feel responsible for nourishing their child well and feel frustrated if their child won't eat. It's important to have a sense of humor at such times and to realize that no child has had a serious setback from missing an occasional meal. The child is very likely to make up for it at the next couple of opportunities to eat.

After children pass through this challenging phase into the preschool years, they develop more maturity and are ready to explore their world. "No" changes to "me too." Children are able to learn simple routines and may become quite compulsive about them. If a child hasn't yet become involved in helping in the kitchen, this is a good time to start. However, the process of gaining independence continues to include an element of struggle, because it conflicts with the need to be, at least in part, cared for by adults. A 4-year-old may resist any parental efforts to help ("Let *me* do it") and then suddenly demand that the parents do everything ("Daddy, *you* put butter on my bread. I can't.")

Although children's appetites may lag and cause them to dawdle at the table, consistent with their slower rate of growth at this phase, they generally accept most foods. It's fun to see children become more aware of details at this stage. However, they may try to use their eating behavior to control others. They may throw tantrums to get foods they want or to avoid what they don't want. In some cases, children who sense their parents' concern over whether they eat their vegetables may learn that agreeing to eat them is a way of negotiating for things they want. Children may even go so far as to insist on a reward *before* eating such foods. This is another of those power struggles that are in one sense unpleasant, but in another sense, encouraging: it shows that the child is becoming more sophisticated about social relationships. Maintaining a sense of humor and anticipating children's table behavior may help during these confrontations.

It's good to know that emotions usually stabilize during the elementary school years.

The Child's Food Environment

Think back to the influences (discussed in Chapter 1) that affect *your* food choices: food availability and inborn, cultural, and individual factors. Children experience these same influences, although they have not yet been exposed to as extensive an array of them as you have. This section deals with cultural factors that affect children in particular.

The Effect of Working Mothers on Nutrition In recent decades in the United States, more mothers than ever before have taken jobs outside the home. From 1960 to 1988, the proportion of all children under age 6 whose mothers worked outside the home exploded from 19% to 57% (United States Bureau of the Census, 1990), with the percentage expected to climb to 66% by 1995 (Johnston and Packer, 1987). Experts have wondered whether mothers' employment status affects the nutrition of children.

When a mother works outside the home, she devotes less time to food-related activities for her family than she would if she were at home; families with working mothers eat out more often and use more prepared food. Studying this situation in the mid-1980s, experts found that these circumstances did not negatively affect the nutrition of young children unless they ate out very frequently—such as seven meals in 3 days (Morgan and Goungetas, 1986).

A more recent study also evaluated the effect of mothers' employment status on children's nutrition. The food intakes of 216 children (ages 2–5) were analyzed from questionnaires completed by their parents. Children with mothers employed full-time outside the home ate an average of five to six meals away from home in 4 days, compared with one to two meals eaten away from home by those whose mothers did not work. The diet quality of the children in the two groups did not differ significantly (Johnson et al., 1992).

Even when children eat some meals away from their parents, parents still have the responsibility of being sure that someone will provide regular, nutritious meals and snacks for their children. Parents need to know

FIGURE 16.4
Typical meals . . . then and now.

Decades ago, most meals were major family social events: several generations gathered for home-prepared meals. Now the average household size is much smaller, and most families eat together less often. More food is eaten away from home or purchased as convenience items.

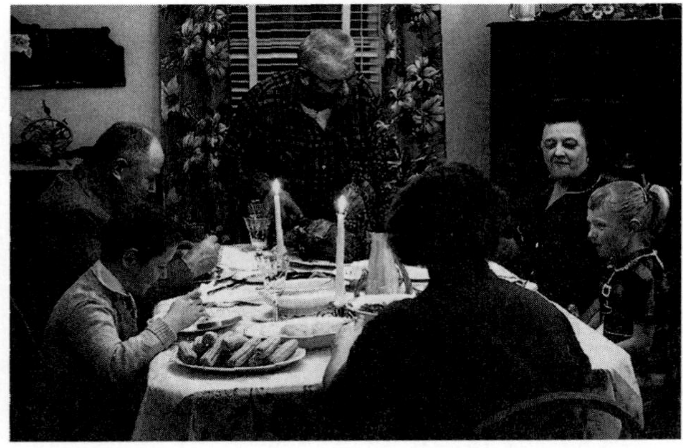

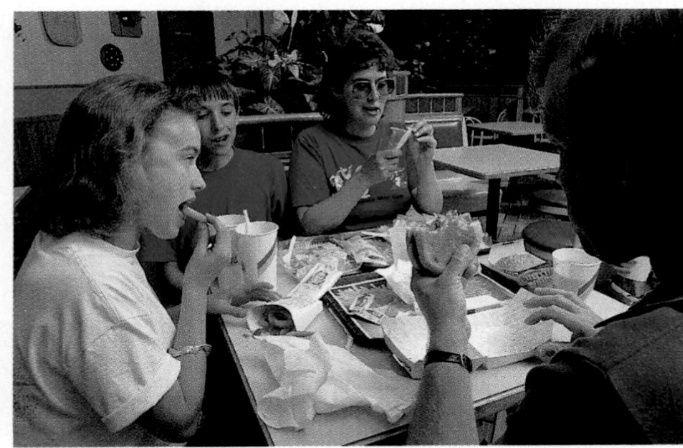

what food is provided at day care, school, and after school. When picking up a child at the end of the day, the parent should ask what and how much the child actually did eat in order to plan for what to offer later at home. (Thinking for Yourself, later in this chapter, suggests some options for parents who are not happy with food provided for their children.)

Most families with children eat their dinner meal together. Over 90% of children 6–9 years old, when asked how often they eat dinner with their families, said three to four times a week; and 69% reported doing so every day (International Food Information Council, 1992).

Who fixes the child's dinner when a child does not eat with the family? In many cases, the child does. Among U.S. children ages 6–14, 65% prepare food for themselves at least once per week (American Dietetic Association, 1992). If a meal needs heating, the child is more likely to use the microwave oven than the conventional oven: 38% of parents surveyed allowed their children between the ages of 5 and 8 years to use a microwave oven unsupervised, whereas only 6% of parents allowed their children to operate a conventional oven (Wilkes, 1991).

You Tell Me

Many food companies are marketing microwaveable foods for children between the ages of 3 and 12 years.

If you were a parent, what conditions would your child have to meet before you would allow the child to use the microwave oven unsupervised? Consider factors such as the child's reading ability, understanding of microwaving safety, and the location of the oven. What else should you consider? At what age do you think a child could meet your criteria?

The Effect of Other People on Children's Preferences Children may adopt the food preferences of other people in their world. A child in school or day care is affected by what his peers eat. Brian may think that broccoli is a perfectly delicious food, until he realizes that his friends say it's "yucky" or that one of his adult role models (Uncle Bill or a hero from a comic book) doesn't like it.

Many parents believe that they have a very strong influence on what their children will and will not eat. But there's little need to blame your own lack of enthusiasm for a certain food if your child rejects it, too: experts say that parents' food preferences have only a weak influence on their child's food preferences (Borah-Giddens and Falciglia, 1993).

The Effects of Television TV can be a strong influence on what a child wants to eat. This is due partly to the extensive exposure time: the average child in elementary school spends more time in front of a television set each year than in the classroom. A child watches about 20,000 television commercials each year, many of which promote foods that are high in sugar, salt, and/or fat.

One study found that during prime time, food was mentioned almost five times per half hour, and 60% of those references were for sweets or beverages of low nutrient density (Story and Faulkner, 1990). Another researcher analyzed 225 commercials during 12 hours of Saturday morning children's TV programming; 80% of those ads were for foods of low nutritional value (Cotugna, 1988).

Some groups of nutrition professionals, aware of the number of negative nutrition messages children receive between cartoons, have tried to counterbalance it. Recently, both the American Dietetic Association and the Society for Nutrition Education helped prepare cartoon-style public service messages that promote good nutrition. With funding by the McDonald's Corporation, they were aired on Saturday mornings on network TV. Encouraging as such initiatives are, it is difficult to combat effectively the barrage of frequently repeated commercials children see.

The amount of time children watch TV is also related to their body weight. As is the case with adults, investigators found that children who spent more time watching TV had a higher incidence of being overweight (Dietz and Gortmaker, 1985). Another study provided an interesting insight into why this might be: researchers found that when children watch TV, their metabolic rate can actually drop *below* their usual resting metabolic rates (Klesges et al., 1993). Of course, additional factors could contribute to energy imbalance and weight gain of TV watchers.

There is yet another health risk to children who watch a great deal of TV: elevated blood cholesterol. In a study involving over 1000 children, those who watched more than 4 hours of TV per day were almost five times as likely to have elevated blood cholesterol (200 mg/dl or higher) compared with those who watched less than 2 hours of TV per day (Wong et al., 1992).

Establishing a Division of Responsibility

Throughout childhood, there are occasions when eating becomes a battleground for parents and children. When this occurs, the issue is usually one of control: who will make the decisions regarding what, when, where, and how much to eat? Deciding who should attend to which aspects of eating can help lessen food-related hassles substantially (Satter, 1987).

Essentially, when children are young, *parents and other caregivers* should be responsible for the following:

- Serve food that is nourishing, that the child will eat, and that is manageable and safe for the child
- Serve food at regular times and at appropriate intervals to meet the child's needs
- Serve food in an environment that encourages attention to eating (generally in a chair at a table)

At all ages, *children* are responsible for eating enough to satisfy hunger.

If this division of responsibility is carried out, a healthy child will usually eat adequately and with minimal fuss. (A chronically sick child may need special help, which a pediatric dietitian can design and explain.)

Remember: caregivers should not try to influence how much the child eats. Pressuring a child on this matter simply is *not* in the best interest of the child. Pressure tells children that they cannot trust their own sense of how much food they need, that they should regularly override their sense of hunger and satiety, and that they need to check with an outside authority (the caregiver) about how much they need. This can undermine the child's self-confidence and emerging sense of self-control.

Training a child to ignore inner signals about how much to eat can also set the stage for a lifetime of weight regulation problems. A child who complies with the pressure to eat more may become too fat; a very assertive child under the same circumstances may resist and eat less than ever. Conversely, a compliant child whose intake is restricted may mutely accept the limitation and fail to grow normally; a more assertive sibling might demand more food and become overweight as a result.

All of this means that if a child is not particularly hungry at a meal and eats less than usual, the caregiver should accept that situation without fuss. However, if the child claims to be hungry an hour later and asks for ice cream, then the answer must be no; the child has to wait until the next usual meal or snack time for something to eat and cannot expect a bottomless bowl of ice cream. Even young children can learn to function within these limits.

As children get older, they need to take on gradually more responsibility for their own eating. Each family has to judge when an individual child is ready to start assuming more of his or her own food-related responsibilities. A child's needs and capabilities and the family's situation will help guide these decisions.

The Nutritional Status and Needs of Today's Children

The recommended intakes of nutrients for children according to age and sex are shown in the 1989 RDA table. Figure 16.5 shows how the RDAs for various ages compare to the adult male RDA. In general, the older the child, the higher the nutrient intake recommendations. These increases reflect the demands of maintaining a larger body and furnishing raw materials for further growth.

Notice that even young children sometimes need as much or more of some nutrients as adult males need; that is true for vitamin D and calcium. These nutrients are important for promoting the greatest possible bone mass that the child's genetic limits will allow.

Nutritional Status of North American Children

Compared with children in other parts of the world, children in North America do quite well in meeting minimum nutritional requirements. A 1986 national survey evaluated the nutritional intakes of young children in the United States. Information was collected from mothers on as many as six separate occasions. The study found that the average intakes of children ages 1–5 met the RDA for all nutrients except iron and zinc, which were 82% and 79% of the RDAs, respectively. The average intakes of calcium for nonwhite groups of children were 80–88% of their RDAs (Human Nutrition Information Service, 1988). Even for children of impoverished families, average intakes were at least 100% of their RDAs except for iron (84%), zinc (78%), and calcium (97%) (Human Nutrition Information Service, 1988). Of course, these are averages; these data do not show that all the children in the survey were well-nourished. Furthermore, homeless children were not included in this survey because of the difficulty in collecting data (see Chapter 18); it is unlikely that their needs are consistently met. Let's look at the consequences of undernutrition—whether for hungry children in the United States or for the 14 million beyond our borders who die each year due, in part, to shortage of food.

Children who have been severely malnourished in infancy experience growth deficits. Usually children who have been nutritionally deprived have also lacked social stimulation, so experts are not sure to what extent each influences poor growth. Some growth deficits may be partly made up for

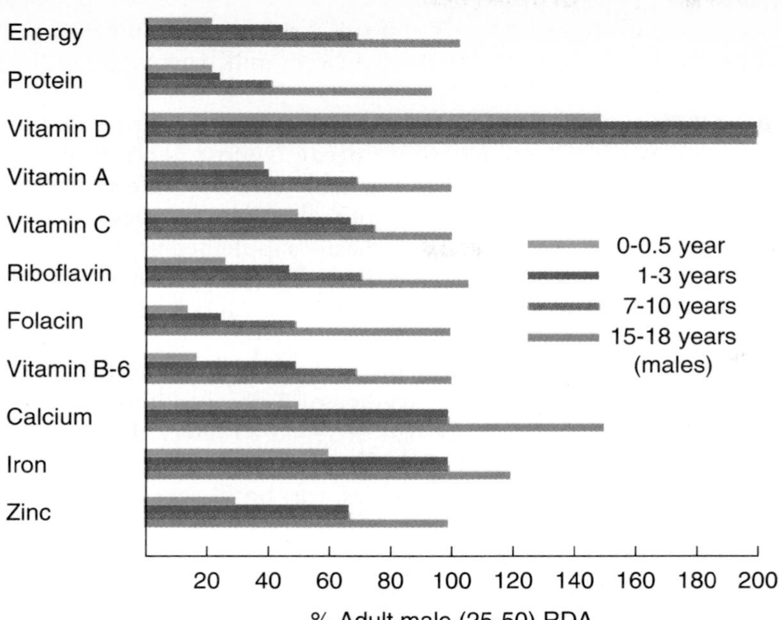

FIGURE 16.5
RDAs in childhood and adolescence.
(Data source: RDA Subcommittee, 1989.)

later; how much can be corrected depends on the developmental age at which adequate nutrition is provided, the length and severity of the previous inadequacy, and the composition of the rehabilitation diet. Similarly, the intellectual impairment that results from malnutrition in early childhood may be partly or mostly restored when nutrition improves, if it takes place soon enough and if it is accompanied by adequate social stimulation.

Poor and homeless children are not the only ones who may be undernourished; undernutrition also has been seen in mid- to high-level income families in the United States. For example, some parents who have adopted a strict low-fat diet for their own use have imposed the same diet on their young children. A low-fat diet for children under the age of 2 years old clearly does not provide enough energy for proper growth and development. After age 2, restriction of fat to 30% of kcalories is recommended, but intake should not drop below that level (Committee on Nutrition, 1992).

Physicians have also noted that some preteen children, especially girls, are so afraid of gaining weight that they restrict their food intake to very low levels. Over a period of time, this can interfere with growth in height and sexual maturation, even if the problem does not progress to the extreme disorder of anorexia nervosa (see Chapter 10). The problem emphasizes the need for children to develop good eating habits and establish realistic expectations of themselves and their bodies.

Less Anemia In the past, iron deficiency anemia has been a serious problem in young children; it affected almost 15% of 1-year-olds. Fortunately, this situation has been changing.

A study of low-income U.S. children ages 1–5 found that the overall prevalence of anemia decreased from almost 8% in 1975 to approximately 3% in 1985 (Yip et al., 1987). This decrease has been attributed to the use of iron-fortified formulas for bottle-fed infants (Committee on Nutrition, 1989).

Children who are given unmodified milk in place of iron-fortified formula may develop anemia due to the lower level of iron in milk. Further, if children drink so much milk that they do not eat enough solid foods, which are better sources of iron, they may develop "milk anemia."

Decreasing Dental Decay Dental caries are another significant problem in children. As you learned in Chapter 5, tooth decay is most likely to occur in susceptible teeth with the presence of fermentable carbohydrate and acid-producing bacteria. Important factors in the control of dental caries are adequate fluoride intake (from water or appropriate supplements) or topical application; restricted intake of fermentable carbohydrates, such as sticky, sweet snacks; and adequate dental hygiene to remove carbohydrates, acid, and bacteria.

The prevalence of caries has declined in the last 20 years. In the early 1970s, children 5–17 years of age had an average of 7 decayed, missing, and filled teeth. A decade later, this number had dropped to fewer than 5. Statistics show the prevalence of caries to be highest in the Northeast, in females, and in lower socioeconomic groups for both sexes (National Research Council, 1989).

Increasing Obesity The body weight status of American children is alarming. In a 15-year period, the percentage of obese 6- to 11-year-olds has increased by more than 50%; the number of severely obese children has increased by almost 100% (Gortmaker et al., 1987). In the first 11 years of another long-term investigation, the Bogalusa Heart Study, the prevalence of overweight among 5- to 14-year-olds increased from 15% to 24% (Shear et al., 1988). Overweight children are also at increased risk of obesity in adulthood. Obese children usually experience a great deal of psychologic distress because they are often teased or even socially isolated by their peers; this can be very detrimental to a child's self-concept.

Helping Overweight Children

A physician should evaluate the overweight child to make sure there is no underlying physical problem. Next, a plan for dealing with the weight issue should be developed.

If a child is only moderately overweight, most experts think it is better to *stabilize* the weight rather than to try to get the child to lose the excess. They believe that as the child gets taller, the height/weight relationship becomes more normal and relative body fatness decreases. But if the child is severely overweight, a weight reduction program is in order. Moderate programs are more successful than very aggressive programs at any age, but for children, moderation is even more crucial; severe programs can interfere with normal growth in height (Dietz and Hartung, 1985).

The cause(s) of the obesity, if it can be determined, will suggest what the treatment program should emphasize. When *inactivity* is a problem, the most logical and satisfactory intervention is to encourage physical activity that the child will find pleasurable and not regard as punishment for being overweight. In some instances, it may be feasible to bring together a number of overweight children for exercise, but such groupings need to be done with considerable tact to avoid negative labeling. One of the best approaches is for the child's family to find activities they enjoy doing together and can do often. Walks after supper, frequent bike rides, and regular backyard volleyball games would be excellent, but the nature of the activity is not as important as simply getting away from sedentary pastimes (Dietz, 1988). •

Some obese children overeat for comfort, for self-reward, or to relieve boredom. Eating is a reliable and convenient source of pleasure, and some

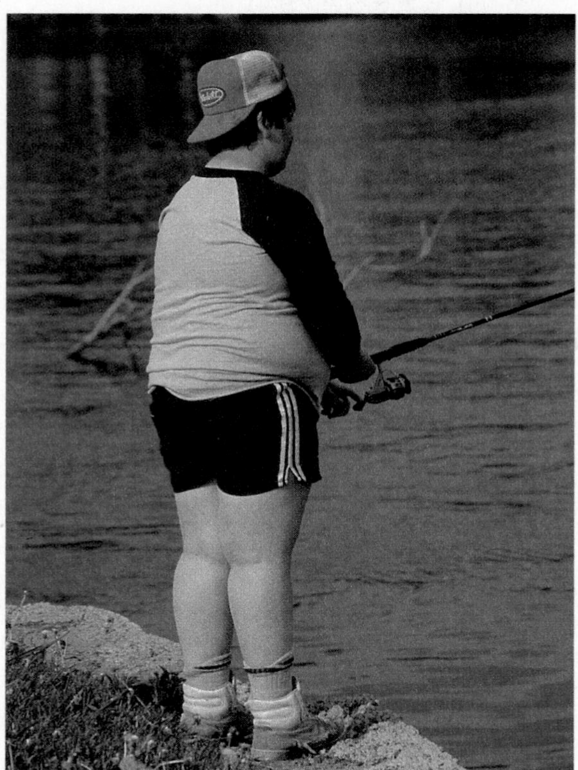

FIGURE 16.6
The incidence of obesity among children is increasing.

In a recent 15-year period, the incidence of obesity increased by over 50%.

children are not very resourceful about finding positive alternatives for themselves. In such cases, it is useful to help a child find other gratifications to substitute for the excessive eating. Although it is important to help a child not to *overeat,* the child should be allowed to eat enough to satisfy hunger at regular meal and snack times. The obese child, like all children, needs to determine how much to eat at each eating occasion. Pressure on the child to restrict eating is likely to backfire, as the Slice of Life on page 532 demonstrates.

The issue of *what* the child eats requires more parental involvement, particularly for the younger child. The child should be encouraged to eat fewer foods that are high in fat and sugar. Foods that should not be a regular part of a child's diet are fried potato chips and other snacks, candy, most cookies and cakes, sugar-sweetened beverages, butter or margarine, and oil-based salad dressings. The best way to accomplish this is to avoid having these items in the house, or to provide lower-fat substitutes.

There are ways to increase the chances of successful weight control for children without professional intervention. If a parent is concerned about a child's weight and the issue has not become a highly emotional one, it is possible that the parent(s) and child can together work out some changes that will address the problem. It may be helpful for the parent first to get an outside resource, such as the booklet produced by the University of California's Cooperative Extension Program (Ikeda, 1989). Publications such as this help parents to talk about the issue with their children without hurting their self-concepts, to provide the best kinds of foods, and to plan activities their children might enjoy.

In some homes, the problem can escalate to the point where emotions are highly charged and family members cannot deal with them effectively on their own. It is possible that the child's problems stem from deep-seated

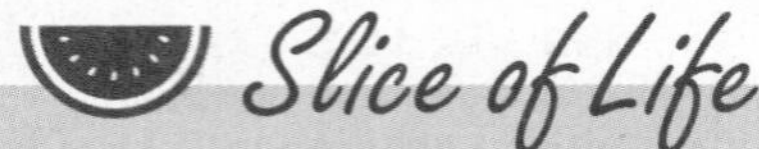

Withholding Food from the Overweight Child Can Backfire

Ellyn Satter (1987) recounts the following:

> When Melissa was three and a half, they visited their pediatrician, who told them she was too fat and they should do something about it. They started cutting back on her food, and over the next eighteen months her rate of weight gain again increased. It appeared their attempts to withhold food, which I'll call restrained feeding, was currently at the heart of the problem. Her preoccupation with food that was resulting from the restrained feeding was making her eat more and actually making her gain more weight than when they had just been feeding her normally.
>
> We set out to reestablish normal feeding and get rid of the restrained feeding. The first step was to reassure Melissa that she would get enough to eat. We let her know she could have snacks and what times those snacks would be. We told her she could have as much as she wanted at meals and at snacks. And we told her she would not be allowed to eat between times.
>
> Melissa's parents were ahead of the game, because they were doing a good job of having good meals. However, they were giving food handouts instead of having planned snacks, so they started to work on that. They set up regular snack times, and started choosing some food for snacks that she liked and was likely to [find] filling and satisfying.
>
> The structure and reassurance worked. At first she ate quite a bit, and she pestered them for food in between. But they held firm and kept their bargain about allowing her to eat as much as she wanted, and after a couple of weeks her pressure on food began to drop off. She still wanted a lot on her plate (it seemed she needed that to reassure herself she would get enough), but she often didn't finish it. She would go off and play, and occasionally she would even play through snack time.
>
> Now Melissa's eating is more positive and relaxed, and her weight has leveled off.

difficulties within the family. A practitioner who treats children with eating disorders notes, "Eating is a sensitive barometer of emotional state and parent-child interaction" (Satter, 1986). For example, a parent who is very concerned about his or her own body weight may be determined to prevent a similar problem in a child. The overweight parent may prohibit the child from eating enough to satisfy hunger in a misguided attempt to make the child thin. The hungry child, then, looks for every opportunity to get more to eat to satisfy hunger and even to hedge against anticipated deprivation later on.

In such cases, the family may well profit from family counseling or from a program designed to help overweight children and their families. SHAPEDOWN is one such comprehensive program that is available around the country; the program addresses issues of nutrition, exercise, self-concept, the child's food environment, and family interactions (Mellin, 1988). Many programs for overweight children will not accept a child for treatment unless the parents participate as well; this greatly increases the child's chances of success.

Basic Nutritional Goals and Guidelines

The Food Guide Pyramid is suitable for planning diets for children as well as for adults. Table 16.3 lists the food groups and their recommended numbers of servings.

Portion sizes should be varied according to the age of the child. For example, a 1- or 2-year-old boy may barely manage 4 ounces of milk with a meal or snack; at age 7 or 8, he may easily drink an 8-ounce glass; and at age 15, that same boy may drink a 12-ounce tumblerful and reach for more.

TABLE 16.3 Daily Food Intake Recommendations for Young Children Through Preteens

Adjust serving sizes according to the age and appetite of the child. For young children, offer 1 tablespoon per year of age for most foods.

Food Group	Recommended Servings	Comments
Bread, rice, cereal, and pasta	At least 6	Offer whole-grain and enriched breads, pastas, crackers, and cereals. Ready-to-eat breakfast cereal, milk, and juice or fruit constitute a nutritious breakfast.
Vegetables	At least 3	For young children, be sure to provide the right form for the child's level of development, for example, cooked carrot sticks rather than raw.
Fruits	At least 2	Again, be careful about the form for the age of child; for example, cut grapes in fourths instead of offering them whole.
Milk, yogurt, and cheese	*Under age 2:* whole milk *Preschoolers:* at least 16 oz. (2 cups); low-fat OK after age 2 *Older children:* 24 oz. (3 cups)	Children who do not like to drink much milk may accept other dairy products, such as cheese, low-fat yogurt, puddings, or frozen dairy desserts.
Meat, poultry, fish, beans, eggs, and nuts	2–3	Prepare these in ways that are easy for children to eat: tender, ground up, or cut small and thin enough to make them easy to chew. Avoid nuts for children under 4 years old.
Fats, oils, and sweets	Go easy!	Underplay these, but don't prohibit them, or they will become even more appealing. Moderation is the key.

For serving solid foods to young children, an easy standard to keep in mind is to put 1 tablespoon (standard measuring-spoon size) per year of age on the child's plate. Children may not be able to eat that much or may want more, but until they're old enough to serve themselves or tell you how much they want, this ratio can serve as a guideline.

Remember that the Pyramid suggests totals for the day and does not specify how many times to eat per day; this can be varied with the child's needs and the family's schedule. Because young children have a small stomach capacity, they need to eat more often; besides meals, they may need one, two, or even three snacks per day. Caregivers should plan snacks that will make a nutritional contribution, because snacks usually provide 15–20% of a child's energy intake (Human Nutrition Information Service, 1988).

Table 16.3 suggests kinds of food in each group that can help children avoid nutritional shortfalls some children experience. It also considers safety issues for young children. Most of the time, these simple guidelines provide sufficient information for feeding a healthy child well.

Common Questions and Answers

Even if you "do everything right" regarding a child's eating, questions might arise. The next section discusses some of the questions most often asked by parents and other people who are involved with children.

Won't Kids Get What They Need If You Just Let Them Eat What They Want? This idea probably originated from the studies of pediatrician Clara Davis, who in the 1920s and 1930s published at least a dozen papers on the self-selection of diets by infants and children up to the age of about 5 (Story and Brown, 1987). The young children she studied were orphans housed in a hospital unit in Chicago; they did amazingly well at meeting their nutritional needs by choosing each meal from a tray of ten foods and two types of milk. An essential point—which most people are not aware of—is that the children chose from simply prepared, uncombined, basic foods such as oatmeal, beef, eggs, haddock, bananas, spinach, peaches, and carrots. No sweeteners were added to any of the foods.

The foods from which these children chose were very different from what is available to most children today. Many of our foods are combinations of ingredients that have substantial amounts of added sugar, fat, and salt. Recent studies show that when children are allowed to choose freely from an assortment of foods including both basic items and more processed items including low-nutrient-density foods, they choose a disproportionate number of low-nutrient-density foods (Klesges et al., 1991; Birch, 1992). Because such foods are low in micronutrients and tend to be high in fat, sugar, and salt, you can't count on a hunger-satisfied child being a well-nourished child.

How Can I Convince My Child to Try New Things? First of all, we have to acknowledge that children prefer familiar foods. Therefore, it helps to expose children gradually to an expanding assortment of nutritious foods so that more and more foods *become* familiar.

What does it take for a food to become familiar enough for a child to accept it? Experts estimate that a minimum of at least eight to ten opportunities to taste it are needed (Birch, 1992). It isn't effective for a child just to see or smell the food; the child must actually ingest it. (Beware: if tasting the food has *negative postingestion consequences*—for example, if it makes the child feel sick—you can save yourself the effort of offering the food again within the child's memory of the experience.)

You may be wondering whether there is some way to shorten this process. You can try some subtle techniques to overcome children's neophobia (fear of something new). Sometimes, special treatment of a new food might encourage a child to try it. Cutting sandwiches into interesting shapes, decorating the food, or telling a story about it may help the child to overcome initial resistance. Another strategy is to involve children in helping prepare the food; this, along with their pride in seeing others eat and enjoy the food, may heighten their interest enough that they try it themselves. Of course, the job has to be appropriate to the child's developmental level (Figure 16.3).

One strategy clearly doesn't work in the long run: bribing a child to eat a new food by offering a reward ("Eat that spinach, and you can have some candy"). If you bribe the child, you may win the battle but lose the war: although the child may try the spinach once, bribing makes the child less willing to eat it again later and makes the candy even more appealing than before. Bribing suggests to the child that you yourself think the new food is undesirable. This is true even if the reward is not another food ("Finish your sandwich, and you can watch TV"). When food is used as a bribe other than at mealtime ("Be good while I'm on the phone and I'll give you a cookie"), it may suggest that food is a suitable reward, distraction, or time-filler.

Is a "Food Jag" a Serious Problem? Sometimes children like a food so much that they want it to be the mainstay of every meal. Such temporary food fixations are common during the toddler years as a child begins to discriminate between different sensory characteristics of food and to develop preferences. But nutritious though it may be, peanut butter for breakfast, lunch, and dinner cannot be accepted as a balanced diet. Thankfully, children themselves usually limit a food jag so parents do not have to make an issue of it unless it persists for more than a couple of weeks.

What Foods Are Good Snacks? Snacks should make a good nutritional contribution to a child's diet. Because foods from the basic food groups are the most nutritionally dense, they offer good snack possibilities. Every food group has some items that lend themselves to being convenient as well as nourishing. Fresh fruits and vegetables (what could be more convenient than half of a banana?), milk and crackers, cereal in big enough pieces to pick up by hand, cheese curds, yogurt with fruit, and peanut butter on half of a bagel are easy to prepare. You're not looking for whole meals, just something to tide the child over until the next meal.

Kids may not want the same foods that they eat at mealtimes, so it may help to have certain items that are specifically used for snacks at your house. Offer juices frozen onto a stick or particular kinds of crackers or cereal that you don't otherwise bring to the table.

Table 16.4 shows how some commonly used snacks compare nutritionally. Notice that sugared foods are generally at the bottom of the list because of their lower nutrient density. Although it's fine to have a cookie *with a meal* when there are a lot of other things to help satisfy hunger, at snack time kids may be more inclined to overeat when given sweets. It may be better to offer the less-sweet foods for snacks.

Should All Children Take Supplements? Statistics suggest that parents believe their children need supplements to be well-nourished. In 1985, 60% of children between the ages of 1 and 5 took supplements regularly or occasionally (Wotecki, 1992). Although children beyond infancy can get the nutrients they need from a good diet, a multivitamin and mineral supplement at RDA levels can provide a nutritional safeguard, especially during phases when a child's appetite is finicky.

However, parents should not count on supplements to correct major dietary flaws. As a source of nutrients, supplements are an inferior second choice to a well-balanced diet; they do not contain all the dietary essentials. Of course, if a qualified health care provider diagnoses a medical condition (such as a malabsorptive disease) and recommends appropriate supplements, follow that person's advice.

Does Sugar Affect Children's Behavior? Some popular articles have claimed that refined sugars cause behavioral and emotional problems in children. The authors of such articles often suggest that parents put their children on "natural" or "sugar-free" diets.

Let's examine this recommendation by looking at some facts and some evidence. When high-carbohydrate foods are eaten alone—whether the food is sucrose or any other readily digestible carbohydrate—digestion and

TABLE 16.4 Snack Food Rankings

Food Class	
Raw vegetables	High nutrient density
Fruit or vegetable juice	
Cereal	
Milk	
Fresh fruit	
Pumpkin or sunflower seeds	
Yogurt, flavored	
Cheese	
Milkshake	
Peanuts	
Rolls, bread, bagels	
Pudding	
Peanut butter	
Graham crackers	
Ice cream	
Dried fruit	
Crackers, pretzels	
Cookies or cake	
Canned fruit	
Granola bars	
Potato chips	
Pies, pastry, doughnuts	
Jello	
Candy	
Soft drinks	Low nutrient density

Source: Adapted from Gillespie, 1983.

absorption are relatively rapid, and blood sugar rises. This stimulates the pancreas to secrete extra insulin, the action of which causes glucose to move from the bloodstream into the body's cells, and brings about a decrease in blood sugar that is generally still within the normal range. These physiologic changes may be accompanied by some perceived energy differences but do not normally involve major mood changes. By contrast, people who have reactive hypoglycemia (a rare condition, described in Chapter 5, in which blood glucose drops to abnormally low levels after eating carbohydrates) may experience anxiety along with the physical symptoms of this condition.

Some uninformed individuals have tried to make a connection between the possible emotional effect of carbohydrate ingestion in people with hypoglycemia and the effects of carbohydrates on children's emotions and behavior. To support their claims, they use theories and anecdotal reports rather than evidence from well-designed scientific double blind studies. There is now considerable evidence to disprove these theories (Kanarek and Marks-Kaufman, 1991).

When well-controlled studies have been conducted to determine the relationship between sugar consumption and behavior, the association has usually been found to be very weak, if present at all. Over a dozen studies have failed to find that sugar increased children's level of activity; in some studies, sucrose ingestion actually had a calming effect (Greenwood, 1989). Of five studies that included cognitive measures, three found no differences in mental performance, one found improvement, and only one found poorer performance (Kruesi and Rapoport, 1986). Similarly, despite theories and some poorly designed studies to "prove" that consuming sucrose causes violent or delinquent behavior, well-designed studies do not show such a connection (Gans, 1991).

Do Other Food Substances Affect Attention Deficit Disorder? Another popular theory linking food to behavior was published in 1975 by the late Dr. Benjamin Feingold, an allergist with the Kaiser-Permanente medical system in California. Among his patients were children with **attention deficit disorders** (also called *ADD, hyperkinetic syndrome,* or simply *hyperactivity*). Children with this condition are more physically active, fidgety, excitable, impulsive, and distractible, and they have shorter attention spans, lower tolerance for frustration, and more difficulty in learning than most children of their age. (These children nonetheless tend to be of normal or above normal intelligence according to standardized tests.)

attention deficit disorder—condition occurring in some children who tend to be more physically active, excitable, and distractible than their peers

According to Dr. Feingold's theory, certain food additives and *salicylates* (which are naturally occurring chemicals in many fruits, vegetables, herbs, and spices and also constitute the drug aspirin) are responsible for these behaviors. He reported that 50–70% of hyperactive children improved when they were placed on a diet free of foods containing salicylates and artificial flavors and colors (some of which are chemically related to salicylates). This type of diet received so much publicity that many controlled scientific experiments were conducted to determine whether such a relationship does exist. An analysis of 23 studies, however, provided negligible support for the effectiveness of the Feingold diet; at most, only a very small percentage of children may be affected by additives (Kanarek and Marks-Kaufman, 1991).

Megavitamin therapy has also been suggested to be useful for reducing hyperactive behavior in children, but most well-designed experiments fail to support this hypothesis. Although some children in a few studies seemed to experience benefit, it is possible that the supplements corrected nutritional deficiencies that had affected their behavior. In other studies, behavior of some subjects actually worsened during megavitamin therapy; others experienced evidence of vitamin toxicity in the form of GI complaints (Kanarek and Marks-Kaufman, 1991). Megavitamin therapy is a questionable and potentially dangerous treatment for hyperactive behavior.

Do Children Really Need Breakfast? Some children would rather sleep late than get up in time to have breakfast before school. Does it matter whether kids have breakfast, as long as their overall intake for the day is adequate? Some studies suggest that skipping breakfast has a negative effect on the quality of children's schoolwork. On a test that involved matching familiar figures (Pollitt et al., 1981), investigators found that skipping breakfast impaired children's late morning problem-solving performance. Another study showed poorer performance in arithmetic and in continuous performance tasks on days when breakfast was not eaten (Kruesi and Rapoport, 1986). Although the studies varied in their methods and the ages of children tested, they showed that, even for well-nourished children, hunger can have significant, measurable, negative impacts on their attention span and school performance (Meyers, 1989).

Are Vegetarian Diets Healthy for Children? The diets of lacto-vegetarians and lacto-ovo-vegetarians can provide adequate amounts of nutrients for most children, provided that these are well planned. Milk, cheese, eggs, and legumes usually can provide the protein, vitamins, and minerals that meat provides in an omnivore's diet.

A study comparing the heights of lacto-ovo-vegetarians 7–18 years old with meat-eating children of the same ages found that the vegetarians generally grew as well as their meat-eating peers. However, lacto-ovo-vegetarian girls were 1 inch shorter at ages 11–12 years, but their growth caught up later (Sabate et al., 1992). The researchers attribute the lower preadolescent height to delayed onset of the growth spurt; the vegetarian girls also experienced later **menarche.** This may be a health advantage: the investigators point out that a later age of menarche is associated with decreased risk for breast cancer.

menarche—the beginning of menstruation

However, strict vegetarian (vegan) diets are not recommended for preschool children, because following these diets makes it difficult to provide adequate protein, vitamins, minerals, and energy for normal growth. One problem is that the child must eat a large volume of food to get the recommended amounts of nutrients. An additional problem is that the bioavailability of minerals from plant sources is relatively low. However, older children can usually thrive on properly planned vegan diets. Vegan children need to eat three meals and three snacks every day to get enough nutrients. Their growth should be carefully monitored to ensure that their diet is adequate (Jacobs and Dwyer, 1988).

What Can Parents Do if They Are Not Happy with the Food Others Are Serving to Their Child? Some parents are concerned about the quality of the food served to their children in day care, nursery school, or after-school care. They may not agree with the kind or amount of food being served, or they may find it difficult to coordinate the care provider's schedule with their family schedule.

These are legitimate concerns. The quality of care programs is inconsistent, as is the food they provide (Spedding, 1989). It is not uncommon for these programs to serve food that provides less energy and other nutrients than parents would expect (Briley et al., 1989). Some programs do consistently provide enough food, but parents may have other concerns, such as you'll note in the Thinking for Yourself on page 539.

The Challenges of the Teen Years

As you have no doubt experienced, the adolescent years are unique in many ways. During this time, teenagers make a concerted effort to separate themselves from younger children and from their parents by identifying with a teen culture that looks, acts, and functions differently. Perhaps you, like many teens, adopted some new eating practices as one of these lifestyle changes. These changes may compromise nutrient intake, and because they occur at the time when physical growth and nutritional needs are greater than at any time since infancy, the adolescent years are a period of considerable nutritional vulnerability.

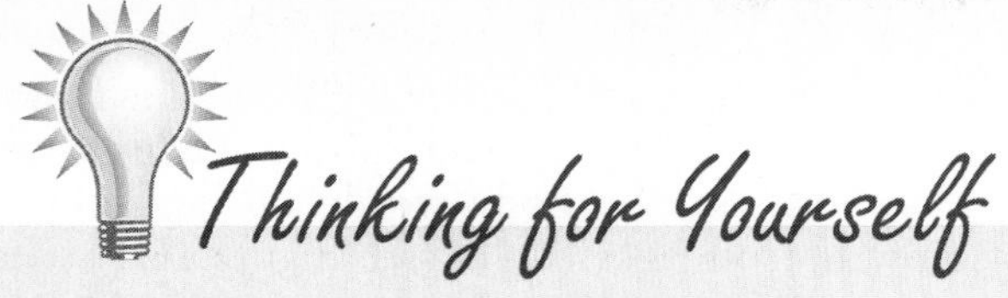

When Day-Care Snacks Ruin Dinner

The Situation

Elise and Sam, both of whom work full-time, take their 4-year-old daughter Mollie to a day-care center. Overall, Elise and Sam are very happy with the arrangement: Mollie likes it there; the staff relates very well to the children: and the environment is safe and comfortable, and it provides indoor and outdoor space and equipment for creative play.

There's just one sticking point. Sam picks Mollie up at the end of the day, and when they get home, Elise is generally already there fixing dinner. They eat about 15 minutes later, but Mollie usually just picks at her dinner without eating much. Recently they have been asking Mollie what kind of snack she had in the afternoon, and invariably she says it was cookies or candy.

It appears to Elise and Sam that Mollie may be eating a lot of sugary things in the afternoon that spoil her dinner. They are not sure what to do about the situation.

Is Their Information Accurate and Relevant?

- It's hard to know whether Mollie's report of the snacks is totally accurate; preschoolers can have an active imagination, or they might report their favorite things rather than what was actually served that day. It would be a good idea to check with the day-care providers regarding what was actually served for snacks.
- Elise and Sam have noticed that on weekends, when they provide all of Mollie's meals and snacks, she eats well at the evening meal. This adds to their belief that her day-care snacks may be the problem during the week.

What Else Should They Consider?

The problem might have more to do with the *timing* of the snack than the *nature* of it. If the snack is served late in the afternoon, Mollie may be so hungry that she eats enough to interfere with her appetite for dinner. If the snack were eaten earlier, she might eat less and therefore be hungrier for her evening meal.

Another condition that can negatively affect a child's appetite is being overtired. It is possible that Mollie is more tired after playing all day with other children than she is while at home with her parents on the weekend. Maybe what she needs is a chance to rest quietly before dinner.

To begin, Sam decides to find out what snacks are actually being offered. When he picks up Mollie, he asks one of the day-care workers or the college student helper what the snack was that day. After a week, he has found that they had cookies twice, peanut butter and crackers once, birthday cupcakes one day, and candy that was provided by a parent for an upcoming holiday on the other day. He asks about the timing of the snack, and finds that it is usually between 3:30 and 4:00. One of the day-care workers mentions that Mollie enjoys the snacks a lot, especially when they have something sweet.

With this information, Elise and Sam consider some options.

Now What Do You Think?

If you were in their situation, which of the following alternatives would seem best to you?

- Option 1 Explain your concern to whoever plans the snacks, and ask the person to consider serving fewer sugary things; have some examples in mind of items you would find more acceptable, or volunteer to be part of a parent committee that plans the snack menu.
- Option 2 Give a good guidebook to the center, such as *Meals Without Squeals: Child Care Feeding Guide and Cookbook* (Berman and Fromer, 1991). Mark the information regarding snacks, and offer to provide an appropriate snack for one day.
- Option 3 Suggest that the center use candy, birthday treats, or cookies as a dessert item with lunch rather than as a snack, when children might want to eat more of it.
- Option 4 Suggest that a memo be sent to parents recommending items that make good treats (for birthdays, holidays, and so on) but are not excessively sugary.
- Option 5 Ask whether the snack could be served earlier.
- Option 6 Postpone dinner for an hour, allowing everybody some time to relax after the day and allowing Mollie time to get hungry for dinner.
- Option 7 Leave things as they are if Mollie seems to be growing normally; even without much dinner, she may be getting enough to eat during the rest of the day.

Do you see other options or combinations of options? Which do you think makes the most sense?

Growth

Approximately 20% of adult height and 50% of adult weight are added during the teen years (Lucas et al., 1989). The average American girl adds more than 10 inches in height and 40–50 pounds in body weight during the five adolescent years of greatest growth, from ages 10–14 (see Figure 16.1). The average adolescent boy experiences his greatest growth from ages 12–16, during which time he is likely to add approximately 12 inches in height and 50–60 pounds in weight.

As many middle-school and junior-high school students have observed with dismay, the growth spurt in girls generally occurs 2 years earlier than it does in boys, although there is tremendous individual variation. In fact, the age at which puberty begins and growth spurts occur in teens is so variable that growth charts based on age are of limited value for teenagers; teenagers' weights should be interpreted in relationship to their heights rather than to their age (Underwood, 1991). Some health care providers find it useful to evaluate teenagers' growth in relation to sexual maturation rather than to chronologic age.

Another generalization is that the gains in weight are much more marked than the increases in height. At the end of the growth spurt, teens weigh 65% more than they did at the beginning and have gained 15% in height. Weight gain in girls is attributable to increases in blood volume, muscle mass, skeletal mass, and adipose tissue. Boys have greater increases in blood volume, skeletal mass, and muscle mass than girls and actually become leaner during adolescence (Figure 16.7). Girls achieve their maximal lean body mass by age 18, about 2–3 years earlier than do boys (Forbes, 1991).

The increased blood volume and muscle mass raise the requirement for iron (for hemoglobin and myoglobin). Although girls add less of these materials than boys, they have a high need for iron to replace what is lost in menstrual flow.

There is evidence that nutritional status affects the age of puberty. More data are available for females than males; it is more difficult to measure sexual maturity in males, because there is no easily identifiable event comparable to menarche. Within any culture, there is a range of ages during which it is normal for a woman to begin to menstruate. But young women from Western cultures, who are generally better nourished, usually begin to menstruate at an earlier age than women in less developed countries.

Also, girls who have minimal levels of body fatness—such as runners, gymnasts, ballet dancers, swimmers, and cyclists—are likely to begin menstruating later or to menstruate less often than other young women who have a greater percentage of body fat (Loucks and Horvath, 1985). This is often associated with abnormally low levels of certain hormones and can be a result of kcaloric restriction, excessive activity, or both.

Some preliminary studies suggest that the low hormone levels may allow larger losses of calcium from the body, increasing the risk of osteoporosis later in life. Evidence is accumulating that female athletes whose menstrual periods are irregular or entirely absent have lower bone densities than peers who have regular periods (Henderson, 1991). Further studies are needed to determine the interrelated effects of body weight, *amenorrhea* (absence of menstrual periods), undernutrition, athletic training, and eating disorders (which some athletes develop), all of which affect the health of bone.

Just as body weight seems to affect reproductive capability, the reverse may also be true. One group of researchers has documented that women who start to menstruate at a younger age are almost twice as likely to be

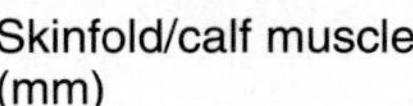

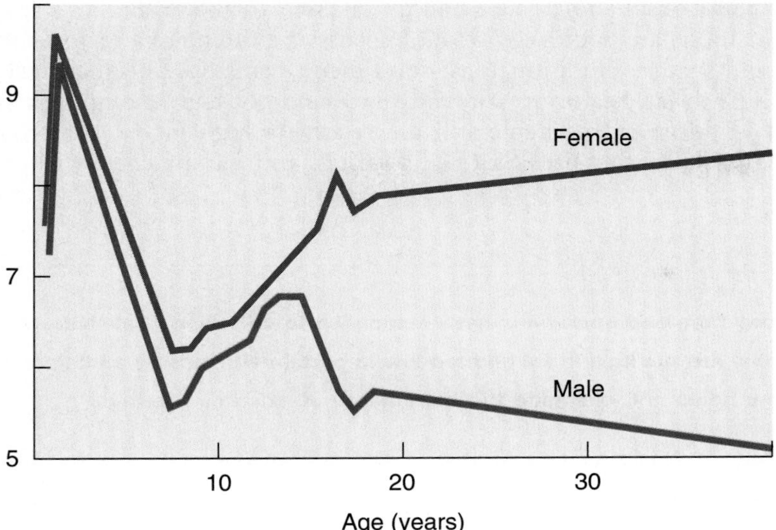

FIGURE 16.7
Fat accumulation between childhood and adolescence.

Measurements of skinfold thickness in the calf indicate that the deposition of fat during adolescence varies greatly according to sex.
(Adapted from Valadian and Porter, 1977.)

obese later in life. Data revealed that women who had started menstruating before age 11 had nearly 30% more fat by age 30 than those who began menstruating after age 14 (Garn, 1986).

Psychosocial Development

During the teen years, children not only grow bigger, stronger, and more mature physically but also develop traits that are not common in younger children. They push for greater independence but still seek reasonable and supportive limits. Emotional volatility often replaces the more easygoing disposition of the elementary school years. The tendency to reject traditions as they search for their own identity can lead to some bizarre eating habits. In some teens, decreased growth or even eating disorders may be caused by fear of becoming fat, by fear of the physical and social consequences of maturing, or by a sense of ineffectiveness (see Chapter 10).

Teens tend to think in terms of the present; they are not much influenced in their behavior by what might happen in the future. For anyone trying to educate teens about nutrition, it is more effective to promote good nutrition on the basis of how it can improve current appearance and performance than on how it can reduce risk of heart disease, cancer, and osteoporosis at age 50 or 60.

The Teen's Food Environment

During the teen years, factors outside the home have an increasing impact on food habits and nutrition beliefs. Although peer pressure is probably at its peak during these years, coaches and other adult role models can also significantly influence adolescents' nutrition beliefs and food practices.

Outside activities, such as jobs and school functions, may keep teens away from home, leading these teens to take part in family meals less frequently. Even dinner, which is the meal families most often eat together, may be disrupted during the teen years.

Adolescents commonly skip meals, usually breakfast or lunch. Girls are most likely to skip breakfast. Partly because of their irregular meals, most teenagers snack; in one study, 91% of teens had snacked at least once on the preceding day (Farthing, 1991). Typically, snacks account for approximately 20% of an adolescent's energy intake (Story, 1989).

Fast foods are popular with adolescents and often are a major source of meals and snacks. Traditional fast-food menu items have been criticized for being high in fat, kcalories, salt, and sugar, and not high enough in vitamins A and C. Most entree items still are relatively high in fat, kcalories, and salt—especially the breakfast sandwiches and sandwiches with special sauces.

You Tell Me

Many fast-food operations have responded to criticisms that their menu items are too high in fat and too low in certain vitamins by adding some new items and changing the ingredients of existing offerings.

What changes have you noticed on fast-food menus that show a greater concern about good nutrition? Have you tried these items? What additional changes could help further?

Despite all the factors that tend to separate teens from their families, there is still some degree of interdependence in the nutrition realm. Most teens value eating dinner with their families. In some families, teenage children participate in routine food-related tasks, such as grocery shopping and food preparation. In 70% of households where both parents work, teenagers do much of the grocery shopping (American Dietetic Association, 1992). One-third of teens surveyed by *Food and Beverage Marketing* and *Forecast* magazines reported cooking for their family more than once a week (Mennes, 1992).

The best ways for parents to influence the nutrition of their teenagers are to provide family meals that are nutritious, relaxed, and enjoyable as often as possible; to be good models of healthy eating behaviors; and to be sure there are plenty of healthy, convenient, appealing snacks in the house. This is as far as a parent can go at this stage in overcoming the barriers that teens say interfere with their eating well—lack of time, inconvenience, lack of self-discipline, and lack of a sense of urgency about reducing the risks of developing chronic diseases (Story, 1989).

Appearance

At no time in most people's lives is physical appearance of greater concern than during adolescence. The majority of teenagers are unhappy with their bodies. In one study, 70% of the girls surveyed wanted to lose weight, although the proportion that was obese was only 15% (Lucas et al., 1989); even the thinnest girls want to be thinner (Moses et al., 1989). Many of the methods adolescents use to lose weight—including fasting, vomiting, and using diet pills, laxatives, and diuretics—are harmful (Berg, 1992). The wide variety of methods of weight control adolescent girls and boys use is shown in Table 16.5. The methods at the top of the list, used in moderation, are reasonable, but the others are not recommended and can be dangerous. We provide suggestions for healthy weight reduction in a later section and in Chapter 9.

TABLE 16.5 Methods Teenagers Use to Lose Weight

The first four behaviors at the top of the list, practiced in moderation, are reasonable. The methods lower on the list are dangerous.

	Females (% of total)	Males
Eat less food	57	23
Exercise more (than usual)	57	26
Avoid sweets	53	22
Eat low calorie foods/sodas	50	18
Skip a meal	45	19
Consume salads only	41	16
Consume fruits only	39	18
Hardly eat or fast	33	12
Eat only high protein foods	30	16
Consume liquids only	27	13
Use diet pills or diet candies	11	3
Vomit after eating	8	3
Take laxatives	4	3

Source: American School Health Association et al., 1989.

Although some boys want to lose weight, 59% want to *gain* weight to achieve a strong, muscular look. For them, bogus products are being marketed that promise to speed their development and ease their growing pains. We'll say more about products marketed for athletes in a later section.

The strength of these concerns is such that fad diets and special body-shaping products have great appeal to many teens. The psychologic discomforts associated with maturing and the impatience of many teenagers make them vulnerable to trying products that promise an easy way to make their bodies what these teens want them to be. Furthermore, the fact that many teens have discretionary money makes them prime targets for quacks (Food and Drug Administration and Better Business Bureau, 1988).

Acne

The hormonal changes that trigger the onset of puberty are also largely responsible for acne, a common teenage problem that affects about 85% of teens and young adults to some degree.

Acne begins with the excessive secretion of *sebum,* an oily substance that lubricates the skin. This fosters the proliferation of bacteria that cause inflammation and clogging of ducts and glands beneath the skin. Anxiety, lack of sleep, and hormonal fluctuations during the menstrual cycle can aggravate the condition (Willis, 1992).

acne—skin condition especially common during adolescence; caused by proliferation of bacteria that produce inflammation in ducts and glands beneath the skin

Scientific studies have not found that over-the-counter products cure acne; similarly, most dietary changes do not bring about significant improvement. However, because certain products and food restrictions have helped some people, physicians may suggest this approach, making sure that the diet is nutritionally adequate at the same time. Fortunately, whether acne is treated or not, spontaneous improvement occurs in almost all cases before the end of the teen years.

For people with cystic acne, a severe form of the disease in which large abscesses cause pits and scars, help is now available. A synthetic form of vitamin A called *13-cis-retinoic acid* has proved helpful in many of the most serious cases. This drug is not as toxic as other forms of vitamin A, but it can produce side effects, including elevated levels of blood lipids, reduction of normal body secretions, and birth defects. For these reasons, it is available by prescription only, and patients using it should be carefully monitored by a physician. No female at risk for becoming pregnant should use this drug.

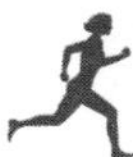

Physical Performance

Physical performance is another common motivator of adolescent eating behavior. Many teens try to boost their athletic capabilities by using food supplements or eating foods claimed to improve performance or to bring good luck.

There is no doubt that good nutrition is critical to top-level performance; however, of the staggering number of available special sports nutrition products and supplements, most have no demonstrable benefit beyond what a person can obtain from a well-balanced diet (Williams, 1992). In addition to various nutrients, many of these products also contain substances with no known benefit whatsoever (Philen et al., 1992). Furthermore, these products can be very expensive; taken as directed, they can cost over $100 per week (Kris-Etherton, 1989).

Participants in some sports are more likely than others to use supplements; one study found that weight lifters most often used them (Schultz, 1990). For some athletes, supplements and special foods may contribute to their "psych up" and result in a placebo effect.

When you physically exert yourself, especially in endurance activities, your needs for water and carbohydrate increase the most (see Chapters 4 and 5), and you need somewhat higher levels of micronutrients. Generally, because many athletes consume more food than their less active peers, they easily meet these micronutrient needs; however, when athletes restrict their intake to maintain low body weight (for such sports as gymnastics, volleyball, dancing, running, cheerleading, and waterskiing) they cannot assume that their nutrient intakes are adequate. If an athlete's food intake is low, a diet evaluation is in order.

Some of the regimens athletes use can be very dangerous; the fasting or fluid restriction that some wrestlers practice to "make weight" is an example. In its "Position Stand on Weight Loss in Wrestlers" (1976), the American College of Sports Medicine points out the many risks of such practices (Table 16.6). Such effects not only jeopardize athletic performance but also could interfere with normal growth and development. Some experts suggest that a wrestler who repeatedly fasts and later overeats (and therefore weight-cycles) may be a candidate for weight problems later in life. A study that compared the resting metabolic rates (RMRs) of wrestlers who weight-cycled with those who did not found that the weight cyclers averaged 12% lower RMRs (Steen et al., 1988).

How can athletes be convinced of what really is in their best interest? Nutrition counselors acknowledge that simply advising athletes to eat from the basic food groups doesn't have much appeal when compared to the glitzy testimonials of famous athletes paid to promote special products. Alvin R. Loosli, a physician who researches the nutritional practices of athletes, also counsels Olympic athletes. He has found that reformatting basic nutrition information into eight discussion points better addresses the inter-

TABLE 16.6 Risks of Drastic Weight Loss by Severe Dieting and Dehydration in Wrestlers

Reduction in muscular strength
Decrease in endurance
Lower blood volume
Reduction in cardiac functioning during submaximal effort
Lower oxygen consumption, especially with food restriction
Impairment of body heat regulation
Decrease in kidney function
Depletion of liver glycogen stores
Increase in electrolyte losses

Source: American College of Sports Medicine, 1976.

ests of athletes (Loosli, 1990). These eight concerns are complex carbohydrates, simple sugars, protein, fats, vitamins, minerals (especially calcium and iron), fiber, and water. •

Alcohol and Other Drug Intake

It's not unusual for teens to use alcohol and street drugs. By 18 years of age, over 90% of teenagers have had some experience with alcohol (Lucas et al., 1989). Over 33% of Americans over age 12 have experimented with some sort of illegal drug (Mohs et al., 1990).

Alcohol can interfere with nutrient absorption and utilization, in addition to providing empty kcalories that displace nutritious foods. Because nutrient needs are high during the teen years, alcohol-induced nutrient shortages cause the classic ill effects of alcohol to be accentuated among teenagers. (We discuss these effects in Chapter 17.) Another serious concern regarding alcohol consumption is that approximately 50% of fatal automobile accidents involve a driver who is intoxicated.

The effects of street drugs on nutrition have not been studied as intensively. However, animal and human studies of marijuana, morphine, heroin, cocaine, and nicotine all show nutritional effects (Mohs et al., 1990). Drugs can affect not only appetite and intake but also the way in which the body handles nutrients. Most of the effects are negative.

Teenage Pregnancy

One of every five infants born in the United States has a teenage mother. Almost 1 in 5 of these babies is a low-birth-weight (LBW) infant (Stevens-Simon and McAnarney, 1988). LBW babies are more likely to be a product of pregnancies that occur within 2 years of menarche (Olson, 1987). (Chapter 15 discusses the problems of low-birth-weight infants in greater detail.) Other possible medical consequences of teenage pregnancy include infant respiratory distress, pregnancy induced hypertension (see Chapter 15), difficult deliveries due to small pelvic size, and higher maternal and fetal death rates.

Many factors make teenage pregnancy more likely to have a poor outcome. One is the mother's physical immaturity; pregnancy puts great demands on the teenager's own body, which should be undergoing its own rapid growth. In addition, the teen mother may have other kinds of problems, such as inadequate medical care; tobacco, alcohol, or other drug abuse; or various sociologic problems.

Sociologic difficulties common in teenage pregnancy include interrupted and incomplete education, poverty and welfare dependence, social disapproval, unstable families, and child abuse and neglect. Because most teenage mothers are unmarried, another disruptive factor may be a lack of emotional and financial support from the baby's father. Alienation from family and friends may be another problem for the pregnant teenager.

Nutrition is often a significant problem; teenage girls are the most poorly nourished age/sex group in the United States. Like other teens, a pregnant teenager may choose food based more on what she likes and what her peers eat than on what is best for her and her developing fetus. Furthermore, in the teen mother, the transfer of nutrients to the fetus seems to be reduced, so the developing infant may derive less benefit from a given nutrient intake than would the fetus of an adult mother (Stevens-Simon and McAnarney, 1988). And teen mothers, who often live in impoverished circumstances, may not have access to adequate food.

Teenage mothers can increase their likelihood of delivering a healthy baby by gaining enough weight during pregnancy. Fetal mortality from teenage mothers who gain 26–35 pounds during pregnancy is only half the rate as for those who gained less than 16 pounds (American Dietetic Association, 1989). A committee of the National Academy of Sciences advises that young adolescents strive for weight gains at the higher end of the ranges recommended for adult mothers (Committee on Nutritional Status During Pregnancy and Lactation, 1990). However, a recent study suggests that pregnant adolescents who gain the same amount of weight as adult mothers will have babies of similar size (Johnston et al., 1991). Suggestions that pregnant teens should gain more than pregnant adults relate in part to the teens' own higher needs for continued growth and development.

People who work with teenagers should be alert to the possibility of teenage pregnancy and help the pregnant teen seek prenatal health care at the earliest possible opportunity. In addition to medical and social services, care should include two important nutrition goals: to ensure adequate access to food and to encourage the consumption of nutrient-dense foods that the mother enjoys (American Dietetic Association, 1989). Nutrition counseling is more likely to be successful when the teenager's present diet is used as the basis for the diet during pregnancy and when she is urged to add gradually foods dense in nutrients whose intake had previously been inadequate. Bringing a partner, relative, or friend with her for the counseling will help build mutual nutritional support. Chapter 15 contains additional information on nutrition during pregnancy.

Few studies have been done regarding the number of teenage mothers who nurse their babies. However, among teen mothers who do lactate, milk production appears to be adequate, because most of the babies grow well (Subcommittee on Nutrition During Lactation, 1991).

Various public and private agencies offer programs to help pregnant teenagers. Many school districts operate special classes in parenting, nutrition, infant care, and similar topics of concern to young mothers. Many services include day-care assistance to help the young mother complete her high school courses and earn a diploma. The March of Dimes provides information and counseling in health and nutrition for prospective parents and often provides referral to other agencies when they need special assistance. Nutrition services are also available through the WIC program, which is discussed in the upcoming section.

The Nutritional Status and Needs of Today's Teens

Compared with teenagers in the developing countries, American teenagers are relatively well-nourished. But compared with what *optimal* nutrition would be, the diets of many teens are short on certain nutrients and long on kcalories, sugar, fat, cholesterol, and sodium (Story, 1989).

Although this assessment comes from data collected in the late 1970s and the RDAs have changed since that time, today's findings probably would be similar: the nutrients most likely to be deficient are iron, calcium, magnesium, zinc, and vitamin B-6. Teens of low socioeconomic status and females are prone to having the lowest nutrient intakes (Story, 1989).

Girls 11–16 tend to have the poorest diets of any age/sex group in the United States, a problem accentuated in those on weight-reduction diets. The diets of teenage boys usually are better, although when their intakes fall short of the RDA, they are generally low in the same nutrients as those of girls.

The 1989 RDA table (inside the back cover of this book) gives the recommended intakes of nutrients for teens in the 11- to 14-, 15- to 18-, and 19- to 24-year-old age groups. Figure 16.5 shows how the nutrient recommendations for 15- to 18-year-old males compare with those of younger and older males; from this comparison, you can see that recommended intakes of some nutrients are higher during the adolescent years than at any other age. For teenage girls, the same generalization holds. Of course, a pregnant teenage girl has greater nutrient needs than she would have otherwise.

Table 16.7 suggests ranges of intakes from the food groups for the teenager and the pregnant teenager. A teenager who is tall or physically active needs intakes at the upper end of the ranges.

The more common nutritional problems of teenagers are discussed below.

Anemia

Between 5% and 10% of some subgroups of teenagers are anemic. Low hemoglobin levels have been found more often in 12- to 14-year-old boys than in girls of the same age, but in the later teen years, more girls than boys are anemic (National Center for Health Statistics, 1982). Blacks, especially males, are anemic more frequently than whites. Interestingly, there is little correlation between low hemoglobin levels and dietary intake of iron; other factors, such as iron absorption and utilization, growth rates, and menstrual losses, are important in determining iron status.

Hypertension

High blood pressure may affect up to about 10% of teenagers (Gong and Heald, 1988). Because hypertension is a major risk factor for cardiovascular disease, prompt intervention in the teen years can help forestall or reduce later, more serious problems. As is true for adults, nonpharmacologic methods are recommended for initial treatment of high blood pressure. Those related to nutrition include weight reduction (if the teen is overweight), moderate dietary restriction of salt, and reduction of dietary saturated fat.

Obesity

Obesity in younger children and its incidence and treatment were discussed earlier in this chapter. Obesity is a serious problem with teenagers as well;

TABLE 16.7 Daily Food Intake Recommendations for Teenagers and Pregnant Teens

Number of servings needed depends on the teenager's size, growth rate, and activity level.

Food Group	Recommended Servings	Comments
Bread, rice, cereal, and pasta	6–11	Encourage consumption of whole-grain and enriched products. Consume good source of vitamin C with enriched products to increase iron absorption. Avoid frequent use of high-fat snack chips and crackers.
Vegetables	3–5	Teens' diets are likely to be inadequate in these. Try to include a couple of servings at dinner, and include mixed dishes. Having vegetable juices and raw vegetables (ready to eat) available in the refrigerator may increase their use.
Fruits	2–4	Keep fresh fruit and juices available for snacks and bag lunches.
Milk, yogurt, and cheese	*Most teens:* 24 oz. (3 cups) *Pregnant teens:* 32–40 oz. (4–5 cups)	Many teens don't get enough dairy products. Keep refrigerator stocked with low-fat dairy products: milk, yogurt, cheese, and ice milk.
Meat, poultry, fish, beans, eggs, and nuts	*Most teens:* equiv. of 5–7 oz. of meat *Pregnant teens:* equiv. of 6–8 oz. of meat	These are important for adequate iron and zinc intakes. When eating starchy beans and peas, eat some meat or a good vitamin C source to increase iron bioavailability.
Fats, oils, and sweets	Go easy!	Limited amounts are fine, but these should not be staples of the diet. For example, don't consistently drink carbonated beverages in place of milk.

in a 15-year period, the prevalence of obesity among 12- to 17-year-olds increased by 39%, and severe obesity increased by 64% (Gortmaker et al., 1987).

It is a challenge to get teenagers to use weight-loss methods that are safe and provide the best likelihood of long-term success. The principles of treatment that apply to younger children also apply to teenage obesity. It is necessary to encourage greater energy output (more exercise) and less input (especially by decreasing the amount of energy-dense foods consumed and increasing food of lower kcaloric density).

A critically important factor to keep in mind when dealing with overweight teenagers is their extreme sensitivity regarding their bodies. Teens who are obviously fatter than the norm suffer acutely. One of the most important aspects of programs for overweight teenagers is to help them develop a more positive self-image; this increases confidence that they can gain control over their problem. Even normal-weight teens need help with their self-image; many of them see themselves as overweight.

Group programs can be very helpful. SHAPEDOWN, which also has a program for younger children, is an example of an effective program for overweight teens and their parents. Offered by trained leaders in many parts of the country, it involves a thorough individual assessment. The program guides teens toward gradually improving their eating and exercise habits by helping them change the way they think about themselves, the way they communicate their feelings, and the way they make decisions about their lives (Mellin et al., 1987). In contrast, many commercial programs focus primarily on overly restrictive dieting and ignore the other components; recidivism and dropout from such programs are common (Mellin, 1989).

Some overweight teenagers can tackle their problem without a group, although not alone. Books such as *Winning Weight Loss for Teens* by Joanne Ikeda (1987) recommend a comprehensive individual program and suggest how parents and friends can be important allies instead of adversaries as teens try to normalize their weight.

Eating Disorders

Chapter 10 is devoted exclusively to eating disorders, but because these conditions are more prevalent during the teen years than at any other time of life, we remind you of them here. In an eating disorder, a person—usually female—dramatically departs from recommended levels of food intake. She preoccupies herself so completely with her disorder that she avoids dealing with other life issues.

Whether the disorder involves severe food restriction or excessive intake; vomiting, laxative or diuretic abuse; or excessive exercise, the person needs help. An eating disorder is an especially urgent concern if it involves cessation of the menstrual cycle or includes other troubling behaviors such as abuse of alcohol or other drugs, or sexual abuse.

Any type of eating disorder threatens health and possibly life itself. The most useful thing you can do for a person with an eating disorder is to help her seek treatment as promptly as possible; the earlier the intervention, the more likely the treatment will be successful.

Help for Undernourished Children and Teens

In 1986, data were collected in the United States on a large number of children ages 1–5 and women ages 19–50. Women and their children were categorized into three groups: the top group had incomes in excess of 300% of the poverty standard; the incomes of the middle group ranged from 131% to 300% of the poverty standard; and the poorest had incomes below 131% of the standard. A comparison of the nutritional intakes of these groups of women revealed significant differences between the middle- and lowest-income groups: the nutrient intakes of the lowest-income group averaged approximately 10% lower than that of the middle group. (Some people criticize the 1986 statistics, noting that possibly the neediest of people—the homeless—were not adequately represented in the survey. Chapter 18 deals more thoroughly with this issue.)

The children in the 1986 study did not fare as badly as their mothers. The nutrient consumption of children in the lowest-income group was on average only 2% less than that of the middle group; and for a few nutrients, the lowest-income group's average intakes were actually higher. The more moderate effect of poverty on the nutrition of children can be attributed, in part, to various government programs that help people provide food for low-income children. This section discusses domestic food programs that benefit children. Some also help low-income adults.

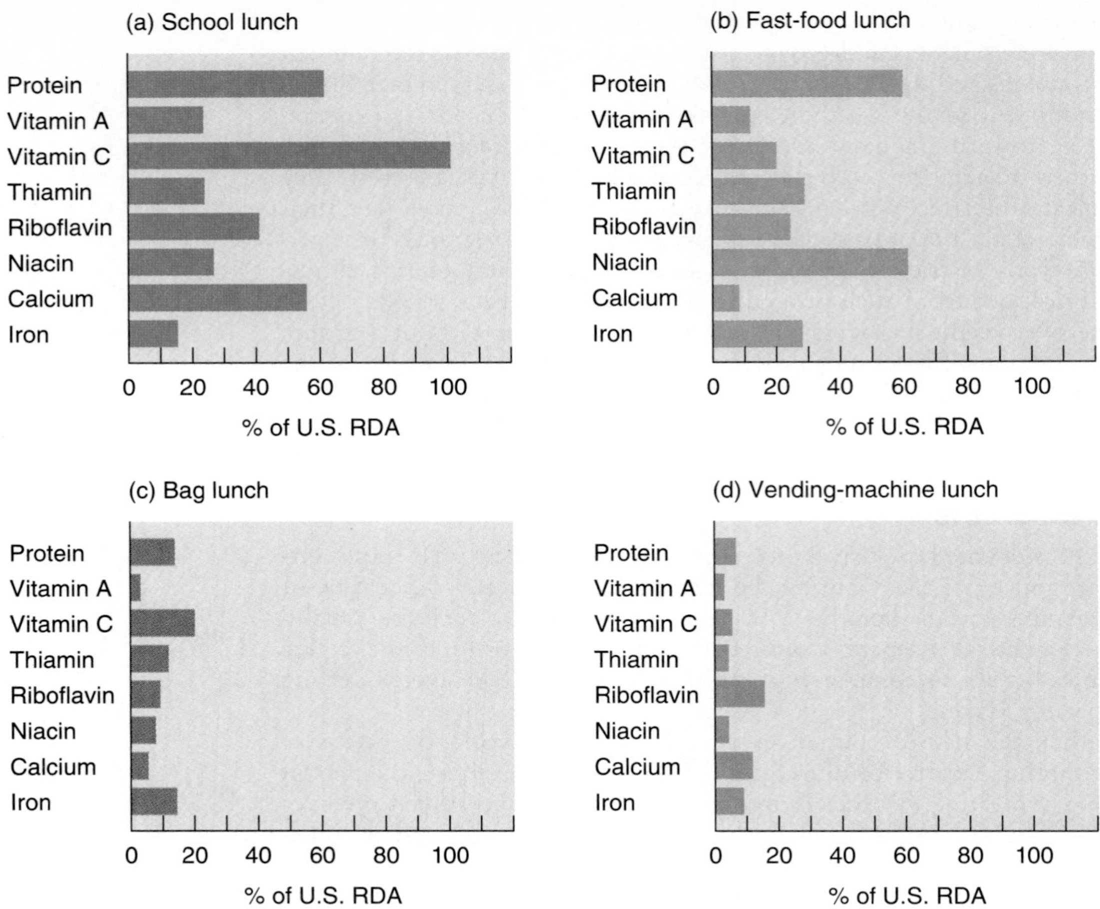

FIGURE 16.8
Nutrient and kcalorie profiles of various lunches.

(a) Profile of a typical school lunch: turkey-and-cheese sandwich, celery sticks, cranberry sauce, fried potatoes, mixed fruit, whole milk, million-dollar cookie. (b) Profile of a typical fast-food lunch: quarter-pound hamburger, fries, cola beverage. (c) Profile of a typical bag lunch: bologna sandwich, cookies, sweetened fruit drink. (d) Profile of a typical vending-machine lunch: potato chips, chocolate candy bar, soda.

(Courtesy of the National Dairy Council.)

The National School Lunch Program

Since the 1940s, the National School Lunch Program (NSLP) has provided full-price, reduced-cost, or free lunches to millions of U.S. schoolchildren according to nationwide eligibility criteria. At present on each school day, approximately 27 million children eat a school lunch (Lytle and Snyder, 1993).

One of the original goals of the program was to improve the nutritional intakes of American children, and data consistently show that it has done that. According to a study by the United States Department of Agriculture's Consumer Nutrition Center and the University of North Carolina, the lunches from the NSLP were superior in nutrient content to other options (Figure 16.8). Children 6–11 in school lunch programs were found to consume 70% more vitamin A, 6% more energy, and 19–21% more calcium, iron, and vitamins B-6 and C than those who ate other kinds of lunches. The positive impact of the school lunch program was even greater for low-income children (Akin et al., 1983).

The high nutritional quality of meals served in the NSLP is no accident: the meals are required to provide about one-third of the RDAs for protein, vitamins, minerals, and energy. This is not to say that the NSLP is the only possible nutritious choice. The typical fast-food lunch (quarter-pound hamburger, fries, cola beverage) has many nutritional strengths but would be improved by replacing the cola beverage with milk. A typical sack lunch (bologna sandwich, cookies, sweetened fruit drink) could be improved by substituting fruit for the drink and purchasing milk at school. It is more difficult to suggest how to improve the vending machine lunch, because the items stocked are so variable.

In recent years, the NSLP has had to meet a variety of new challenges. Many school systems now require their food services to modify their menus according to the Dietary Guidelines; at the same time, they must conform to the federal NSLP nutrition requirements and stay within their budgets. Some school lunch districts have collaborated, as did those in Minnesota, in planning and implementing lunches lower in fat and sodium and in developing educational materials for students and parents about the new program (Snyder et al., 1992).

Another challenge for the NSLP to face is the competition that vending machines in schools and nearby commercial establishments pose. With the availability of other attractive food options and money to spend, participation in NSLP in some schools has dropped off to the extent that the program may be threatened in those schools (American Dietetic Association, 1991). Various solutions are being tried. Some strategies are to incorporate salad bars, family-style lunches, fast foods, ethnic foods, or school-prepared bag lunches to increase the attractiveness of the meals to students and regain their participation.

Other Child Nutrition Programs

The *School Breakfast Program,* which began in the late 1960s, provides breakfast at full price, reduced cost, or no cost according to specific eligibility criteria. The number of meals it serves per year is approximately 11% of that of the NSLP (Lytle and Snyder, 1993). A study indicated that participants in the School Breakfast Program improved their scores on basic skills tests and had fewer absences and tardiness (Meyers et al., 1989).

The *Special Milk Program* provides milk to schoolchildren. It expanded in 1987, when federal legislation included kindergartners who attend school for just a half-day and do not have access to other meal-service programs. The *Child Care Food Program* provides cash and commodity assistance to nonprofit child-care centers and day-care homes. This program demonstrated the greatest growth of any of the child nutrition programs during the 1980s, with almost 125,000 sites participating in 1988 (Matsumoto and Smith, 1989).

The Supplemental Food Program for Women, Infants, and Children (WIC)

The WIC program provides nutrition education and vouchers for certain foods to high-risk pregnant women, nursing mothers, and children up to the age of 5 who meet the program's criteria. Most pregnant teenagers qualify for this program. Studies have shown the program was effective in decreasing premature births, stillbirths, and maternal anemia, and in increasing birth weight.

Participation in WIC has increased steadily since it was established in 1974 (Matsumoto, 1992). Although the cost of the program has also risen, the increases have not always been proportional. For example, participation in 1989 was 13% higher than in 1988, but costs increased by only 5% (Matsumoto, 1989). This efficiency was made possible by infant formula manufacturers, who had entered into agreements with various states to provide rebates in exchange for being the sole providers of the formula in their region.

The situation changed in 1990, when states with expiring contracts sought new bids from formula manufacturers; the producers all offered *lower* rebates than they had formerly. This threatened to increase the program cost per client and to force the program to reduce services. Congress acted quickly to maintain the service level by passing legislation allowing state WIC programs to spend a portion of the funds allotted for the next fiscal year, but this was only a stop-gap measure. (This situation is a good example of how economic and political factors can affect nutrition.) Since that time, public and congressional support has been sufficient to continue the growth of the WIC program.

The Food Stamp Program Another important program affecting the food intake of low-income families is the Food Stamp Program. The federal government sponsors this program, which issues food stamps that can be used to buy food at any approved grocery store. The monetary value of the food stamps issued depends on the income and size of the family. The amount of money granted is designed to supplement a family's other resources so they can meet their basic nutritional needs when carefully choosing from economical foods. Average monthly benefits in early 1991 were approximately $64 per person (Matsumoto, 1991).

Programs that provide access to food can make a critical difference to a child. Good nutrition is important throughout life, of course, but its impact during childhood can have lifelong consequences. Just as physiologic, psychologic, sociologic, political, and economic factors all affect a child's nutritional intake and status, getting enough good food to eat can optimize the functioning of each child's mind and body.

Summary

- The most important influence that caregivers can exert on a child's nutrition during the growing years is to help the child develop sound eating habits. This challenge demands patience, a sense of humor, and some knowledge about what is normal during these transitional times.
- The changes that take place in children's bodies and minds affect the amounts of nutrients they need and what foods they can eat. The nutrients from the food they eat, in turn, affect their further physical and mental development.
- The food intake of young children is variable and not strictly proportional to their weight. As children's motor skills and coordination improve, they should be encouraged to participate in food preparation. Children often assert themselves by rejecting certain foods or using their eating behavior as a negotiating tool. Advertising, family circumstances, and peer influence all contribute to a child's nutritional socialization. Anticipating a child's behavior and the many influences on it can help put this issue in perspective.
- Children in the U.S. and Canada do not have the same nutritional problems that children in some other parts of the world have; in general, children in the U.S. and Canada are more likely to be *over*nourished than *under*nourished. Obesity, a common and increasing problem for children, can predispose a person to various health problems both during childhood and in the future. Iron deficiency anemia and dental caries, although decreasing in prevalence, continue to be significant problems.
- A healthy diet for children is similar in many ways to that for adults and should include a wide variety of nutritionally dense foods. Because children tend to like familiar foods more than unfamiliar ones, it is important to expose them to an increasing assortment of foods that can *become* familiar. A child's sense of hunger and satiety should determine the amount of food consumed. Caregivers are responsible for deciding what, when, and where children should eat.
- Many popular articles have attempted to link children's diet with their behavior, although no meaningful scientific evidence supports such claims. There appears to be no association between sugar consumption and negative behavior in normal children; nor have food colorings and salicylates been proved to cause **attention deficit disorder,** except in a very few cases.

• The dramatic growth of the adolescent years produces high nutrient demands at the very time when many other factors seem to adversely affect nutrition. Intense preoccupation with physical appearance can inspire strange eating habits, compromised growth, or—in extreme cases—eating disorders. **Acne** afflicts most teens, who sometimes try to deal with it by restricting certain foods. The desire to improve athletic performance also motivates adolescent eating behavior and may lead teenagers to use unnecessary supplements and special dietary products. Peer pressure, the time demands of outside activities, and the use of alcohol and other drugs can affect eating habits as well.

• Teenage pregnancies present many medical and nutritional problems for both the mother and the baby and are often considered high-risk situations. The mother's nutritional status both before and after conception is very important to the baby's health. Various agencies sponsor programs to counsel teenage mothers about health, nutrition, and child care and to help them finish school.

• The diets of teenage boys appear to be better than those of girls; teenage girls on weight-reduction diets tend to be less well-nourished than almost any other North American population group. Nutrition and health problems seen during the teen years include iron deficiency anemia, hypertension, obesity, and eating disorders. In girls, anemia is more likely to occur after the age of **menarche.**

• Because nutrition during the childhood and teen years has such an impact on the person's current and future health and well-being, it is fortunate that there are programs that provide food assistance to children at risk for malnutrition. Some of these programs are the National School Lunch Program, the School Breakfast Program, the Special Milk Program, the Child Care Food Program, the Supplemental Food Program for Women, Infants, and Children (WIC), and the Food Stamp Program.

References

Akin, J.S., J.S. Bass, D.K. Guilkey, P.S. Haines, and B.M. Popkin. 1983. Evaluating school meals. *The Community Nutritionist* 2:4–7.

American College of Sports Medicine. 1976. Position stand on weight loss in wrestlers. *Medicine and Science in Sports and Exercise* 8(no.2):xi–xiii.

American Dietetic Association. 1989. Position of the American Dietetic Association: Nutrition management of adolescent pregnancy. *Journal of the American Dietetic Association* 89:104–109.

American Dietetic Association. 1991. Position of The American Dietetic Association: Competitive foods in schools. *Journal of the American Dietetic Association* 91:1123–1125.

American Dietetic Association. 1992. Family ties: Who's doing the cooking? In *Eat right America, a supplement to the Journal of the American Dietetic Association.* Chicago: American Dietetic Association.

American School Health Association, Association for the Advancement of Health Education, Society for Public Health Education, Inc. 1989. *The national adolescent student health survey: A report on the health of America's youth.* A cooperative project of U.S.D.H.H.S., P.H.S., Office of Disease Prevention and Health Promotion, Centers for Disease Control, National Institute on Drug Abuse.

Beal, V.A. 1957. On the acceptance of solid foods and other food patterns of infants and children. *Pediatrics* 20:448–456.

Berg, F.M. 1992. Harmful weight loss practices are widespread among adolescents. *Obesity and Health*, July/August, 1992.

Berman, C. and J. Fromer. 1991. *Meals without squeals: Child care feeding guide and cookbook.* Palo Alto, CA: Bull Publishing Company.

Birch, L.L. 1992. Children's preferences for high-fat foods. *Nutrition Reviews* 50:249–255.

Birch, L.L., S.L. Johnson, F. Andresen, J.C. Peters, and M.C. Schulte. 1991. The variability of young children's energy intake. *The New England Journal of Medicine* 324:232–235.

Borah-Giddens, J. and G.A. Falciglia. 1993. A meta-analysis of the relationship in food preferences between parents and children. *Journal of Nutrition Education* 25:102–107.

Briley, M.E., A.C. Buller, C.R. Roberts-Gray, and A. Sparkman. 1989. What is on the menu at the child care center? *Journal of the American Dietetic Association* 89:771–774.

Committee on Nutrition. 1989. Iron-fortified infant formulas. *Pediatrics* 84:1114.

Committee on Nutrition. 1992. Statement on cholesterol. *Pediatrics* 90:469–473.

Cotugna, N. 1988. TV ads on Saturday morning children's programming—what's new? *Journal of Nutrition Education* 20:125–127.

Dietz, W.H. 1988. Childhood and adolescent obesity. In *Obesity and weight control,* ed. R.T. Frankle. Rockville, MD: Aspen Publishers, Inc.

Dietz, W.H. and S.L. Gortmaker. 1985. Do we fatten our children at the TV set? Television viewing and obesity in children and adolescents. *Pediatrics* 75:807–812.

Dietz, W.H. and R. Hartung. 1985. Changes in height velocity of obese preadolescents during weight reduction. *American Journal of Diseases of Children* 139:705–707.

Farthing, M.C. 1991. Current eating patterns of adolescents in the United States. *Nutrition Today* 26(no.2):35–39.

Food and Drug Administration and Better Business Bureau. 1988. Quackery targets teens. *FDA Consumer,* February, 1988.

Forbes, G.B. 1991. Body composition of adolescent girls. *Nutrition Today* 26(no.2):17–20.

Gans, D.A. 1991. Sucrose and delinquent behavior: Coincidence or consequence? *Critical Reviews in Food Science and Nutrition* 30:23–48.

Garn, S.M. 1986. Maturational timing as a factor in female fatness and obesity. *American Journal of Clinical Nutrition* 43:879–883.

Gillespie, A. 1983. Assessing snacking behavior in children. *Ecology of Food and Nutrition* 13:167–172.

Gong, E.J. and F.P. Heald. 1988. Diet, nutrition, and adolescence. In *Modern nutrition in health and disease,* ed. M.E. Shils and V.R. Young. Philadelphia: Lea & Febiger.

Gortmaker, S.L., W.H. Dietz, A.M. Sobol, and C.A. Wehler. 1987. Increasing pediatric obesity in the United States. *American Journal of Diseases of Children* 141:535–540.

Greenwood, C. 1989. The role of diet in modulating brain metabolism and behavior. *Contemporary Nutrition* 14(no.7). Minneapolis: General Mills.

Henderson, R.C. 1991. Bone health in adolescence: Anorexia and athletic amenorrhea. *Nutrition Today* 26(no.2):25–29.

Hertzler, A.A. 1989. Preschooler's food handling skills—motor development. *Journal of Nutrition Education* 21:100B–C.

Human Nutrition Information Service (HNIS). 1988. *CSFII: Continuing survey of food intakes by individuals.* Washington, DC: United States Department of Agriculture.

Ikeda, J. 1987. *Winning weight loss for teens.* Palo Alto, CA: Bull Publishing Company.

Ikeda, J.P. 1989. *If my child is too fat, what should I do about it?* Oakland, CA: ANR Publications.

International Food Information Council (IFIC). 1992. *Parents set the menu, kids set the table.* Washington, DC: International Food Information Council.

Jacobs, C. and J.T. Dwyer. 1988. Vegetarian children: Appropriate and inappropriate diets. *American Journal of Clinical Nutrition* 48:811–818.

Johnson, R.K., H. Smickilas-Wright, and A.C. Crouter. 1992. Effect of maternal employment on the quality of young children's diets: The CSFII experience. *Journal of the American Dietetic Association* 92:213–214.

Johnston, C.S., F.S. Christopher, and L.A. Kandell. 1991. Pregnancy weight gain in adolescents and young adults. *Journal of the American College of Nutrition* 10:185–189.

Johnston, W.B. and A.H. Packer. 1987. *Workforce 2000.* Indianapolis: Hudson Institute.

Kanarek, R.B. and R. Marks-Kaufman. 1991. *Nutrition and behavior.* New York: Van Nostrand Reinhold.

Klesges, R.C., M.L. Sheldon, and L.M. Klesges. 1993. Effects of television on metabolic rate: Potential implications for childhood obesity. *Pediatrics* 91:281–286.

Klesges, R.C., R.J. Stein, L.H. Eck, T.R. Isbell, and L.M. Klesges. 1991. Parental influence on food selection in young children and its relationships to childhood obesity. *American Journal of Clinical Nutrition* 53:859–864.

Kris-Etherton, P.M. 1989. Nutrition and athletic performance. *Contemporary Nutrition* 14(no.8). Minneapolis: General Mills.

Kruesi, M.J. and J.L. Rapoport. 1986. Diet and human behavior: How much do they affect each other? *Annual Reviews of Nutrition* 6:113–130.

Loosli, A.R. 1990. Athletes, food and nutrition. *Food & Nutrition News* 62(no.3):15–18. Chicago: National Livestock and Meat Board.

Loucks, A.B. and S.M. Horvath. 1985. Athletic amenorrhea: A review. *Medicine and Science in Sports and Exercise* 17:56–72.

Lucas, B., J.M. Rees, and L.K. Mahan. 1989. Nutrition and the adolescent. In *Nutrition in infancy and childhood,* ed. P.L. Pipes. St. Louis: Times Mirror/Mosby.

Lytle, L. and M.P. Snyder. 1993. Feeding school children. *Food & Nutrition News* 65(no.2):7–9. Chicago: National Livestock and Meat Board.

Matsumoto, M. 1989. Recent trends in domestic food programs. *National Food Review* 12(no.2):33–39.

Matsumoto, M. 1991. Domestic food assistance costs are rising. *Food Review* 14(no.4):40–42.

Matsumoto, M. 1992. The WIC program meets a special need. *Food Review* 15(no.1):40–42.

Matsumoto, M. and M. Smith. 1989. Food assistance. *National Food Review* 12(no.2):33–39.

Mellin, L.M. 1988. *SHAPEDOWN: Just for kids: Level 1 (6–8 years); Level 2 (8–12 years); Parent's guide: A guide for supporting your child.* Anselmo, CA: Balboa Publishing.

Mellin, L.M. 1989. Adolescent obesity: Implications for action. *Food & Nutrition News* 62(no.5):32–33. Chicago: National Livestock and Meat Board.

Mellin, L.M., L.A. Slinkard, and C.E. Irwin. 1987. Adolescent obesity intervention: Validation of the SHAPEDOWN program. *Journal of the American Dietetic Association* 87:333–338.

Mennes, M.E. 1992. New generation foods and new generation cooks: Interface for concern. *Food & Nutrition News* 64(no.2):7–9. Chicago: National Livestock and Meat Board.

Meyers, A.F. 1989. Undernutrition, hunger, and learning in children. *Nutrition News* 52(no.2):5–7. Rosemont, IL: National Dairy Council.

Meyers, A.F., A.E. Sampson, M. Weitzman, B.L. Rogers, and H. Kayne. 1989. School breakfast program and school performance. *American Journal of Diseases of Children* 143:1234–1239.

Mohs, M.E., R.R. Watson, and R. Leonard-Green. 1990. Nutritional effects of marijuana, heroin, cocaine, and nicotine. *Journal of the American Dietetic Association* 90:1261–1267.

Morgan, K. and B. Goungetas. 1986. Snacking and eating away from home. In *What is America eating? Proceedings of a symposium.* Washington, DC: National Academy Press.

Moses, N., M. Banilivy, and F. Lifshitz. 1989. Fear of obesity among adolescent girls. *Pediatrics* 83:393–398.

National Center for Health Statistics. 1982. *Diet and iron status, a study of relationships.* DHHS Publication No. (DHS)83-1679. Hyattsville, MD: U.S. Department of Health and Human Services.

National Research Council. 1989. *Diet and health.* Washington, DC: National Academy of Sciences.

Olson, C.M. 1987. Pregnancy in adolescents: A cause for nutritional concern? *Professional Perspectives* no.1: 1–5. Ithaca, NY: Cornell University Division of Nutritional Sciences.

Philen, R.M., D.I. Ortiz, S.B. Auerbach, and H. Falk. 1992. Survey of advertising for nutritional supplements in health and bodybuilding magazines. *Journal of the American Medical Association* 268:1008–1011.

Pollitt, E., R.L. Leibel, and D. Greenfield. 1981. Brief fasting, stress, and cognition in children. *American Journal of Clinical Nutrition* 34:1526–1533.

RDA Subcommittee. 1989. *Recommended dietary allowances.* Washington, DC: National Academy Press.

Sabate, J., M.C. Llorca, and A. Sanchez. 1992. Lower height of lacto-ovo vegetarian girls at preadolescence: An indicator of physical maturation delay? *Journal of the American Dietetic Association* 92:1263–1264.

Satter, E. 1986. Childhood eating disorders. *Journal of the American Dietetic Association* 86:357–361.

Satter, E. 1987. *How to get your kid to eat . . . but not too much.* Palo Alto, CA: Bull Publishing Company.

Scammon, R.E. 1927. The measurement of the body in childhood. In *The Measurement of Man,* by J.A. Harris, C.M. Jackson, and R.E. Scammon. Minneapolis: University of Minnesota Press.

Schultz, L.O. 1990. Nutrient supplement use by athletes. *Food & Nutrition News* 62(no.3):19–20. Chicago: National Livestock and Meat Board.

Shear, C.L., D.S. Freedman, G.L. Burke, D.W. Harsha, L.S. Webber, and G.S. Berenson. 1988. Secular trends of obesity in early life: The Bogalusa heart study. *American Journal of Public Health* 78:75–77.

Sigman-Grant, M. 1992. Feeding preschoolers: Balancing nutritional and developmental needs. *Nutrition Today* 27(no.4):13–17.

Snyder, M.P., M. Story, L.L. Trenkner. 1992. Reducing fat and sodium in school lunch programs: The LUNCHPOWER! intervention study. *Journal of the American Dietetic Association* 92:1087–1091.

Spedding, O. 1989. Day care: Safe or sorry? *Human Ecology Forum* 17(no.3):16–18.

Steen, S.N., R.A. Opplinger, and K.D. Brownell. 1988. Metabolic effects of repeated weight loss and regain in adolescent wrestlers. *Journal of the American Medical Association* 260:47–50.

Stevens-Simon, C. and E.R. McAnarney. 1988. Adolescent maternal weight gain and low birth weight: A multifactorial model. *American Journal of Clinical Nutrition* 47:948–953.

Story, M. 1989. A perspective on adolescent life-style and eating behavior. *Nutrition News* 52(no.1):1–3. Rosemont, IL: National Dairy Council.

Story, M. and J.E. Brown. 1987. Do young children instinctively know what to eat? The studies of Clara Davis revisited. *The New England Journal of Medicine* 316(no.2):103–105.

Story, M. and P. Faulkner. 1990. The prime time diet: A content analysis of eating behavior and food messages in television program content and commercials. *American Journal of Public Health* 80:738–740.

Subcommittee on Nutrition During Lactation. 1991. *Nutrition during lactation.* Washington, DC: National Academy Press.

Tang, W., A.A. Hertzler, and D. Stewart. 1992. Survey of kitchen equipment usage, kitchen accidents, and kitchen safety awareness of four-year-olds. *Journal of Nutrition Education* 24:316–319.

Underwood, L.E. 1991. Normal adolescent growth and development. *Nutrition Today* 26(no.2):11–16.

United States Bureau of the Census. 1990. *Statistical abstract of the United States: 1990.* Washington, DC: United States Bureau of the Census.

Valadian, I. and D. Porter. 1977. *Physical growth and development from conception to maturity: A programmed text.* Boston: Little, Brown & Co.

Wilkes, A.P. 1991. Frozen and shelf stable meals. *Food Engineering* 63:69.

Williams, M.H. 1992. *Nutrition for fitness and sport.* Dubuque, IA: William C. Brown, Publishers.

Willis, J.L. 1992. Acne agony. *FDA Consumer* 26(no.6): 23–25.

Wong, N.D., T.K. Hei, P.Y. Qaqundah, D.M. Davidson, S.L. Bassin, and K.V. Gold. 1992. Television viewing and pediatric hypercholesterolemia. Pediatrics 90:75–79.

Woteki, C.E. 1992. Nutrition in childhood and adolescence: Part I. *Contemporary Nutrition* 17(no.1). Minneapolis: General Mills.

Yip, R., N.J. Binkin, L. Fleshood, and F.L. Trowbridge. 1987. Declining prevalence of anemia among low-income children in the United States. *Journal of the American Medical Association* 258:1619–1623.

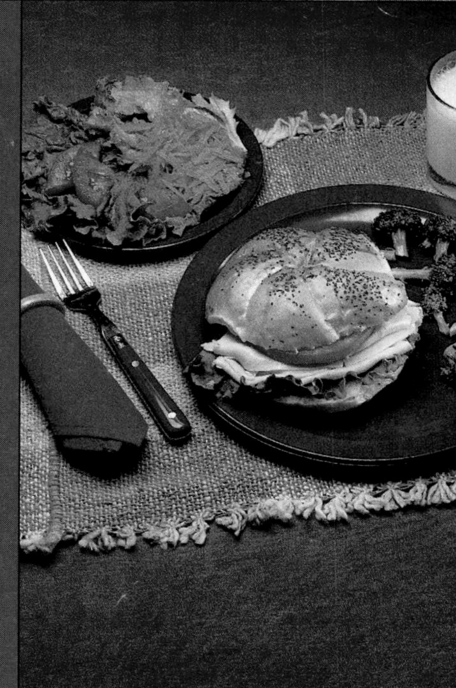

IN THIS CHAPTER

The Gradual Changes of Aging

How Nutrition and Fitness Affect Health and Longevity

How Drugs Interact with Nutrients

Influences of Alcohol on Nutrition and Health

Live Well in the 1990s!

Chapter 17

Nutrition for Adults of All Ages

What are the mental images you have of yourself in the future? Are you training for a profession? Headed for a career in business? Hoping to raise a family? Looking forward to involvement in the performing arts? Expecting to participate in sports? No matter what you choose to do in life, good nutrition is among the factors that can help equip you physically and mentally to accomplish your goals.

The issue of how to stay as healthy as possible during adulthood is exceptionally important, because we now have more adult years to live than at any time in history. Around 1900 in the United States, life expectancy was 48 years (Kinsella, 1992); now it is over 75 years. Demographic forecasters predict that the proportion of our population that will live into old age will increase progressively during the next century (Figure 17.1). Currently, one of *eight* Americans is at least 65 years old; in 100 years, one in *four* is expected to be that age.

As we noted in the beginning of this book, nutrition has three basic functions throughout life. First, nutrients equip our body cells to produce energy; second, nutrients enable cells to regulate metabolic processes. These ongoing processes result in wear and tear on cells, causing them to deteriorate gradually, whereupon new cells are produced to replace them. This emphasizes the third basic function nutrients perform for us: they become the constituents of those new cells.

At some time during the adult years, cell replacement no longer keeps pace with the rate of cell breakdown; our mass of most types of tissue decreases, as does the level of tissue function. Scientists have found that there is no rigid timetable for the rate at which these changes of aging take place. In fact, the variable rates at which we age make us more different from our peers during the elder years than we are at any other phase of life. Clearly, there are some 75-year-old people who are healthier than some 50-year-olds.

Experts in the field of aging research (called *gerontology*) are working to discover how various environmental factors—including nutrition—can influence aging. Physical fitness, the function of the immune system, the presence or absence of disease, psychologic state, and even the ability to think and learn are all involved. Scientists have a great deal yet to learn on

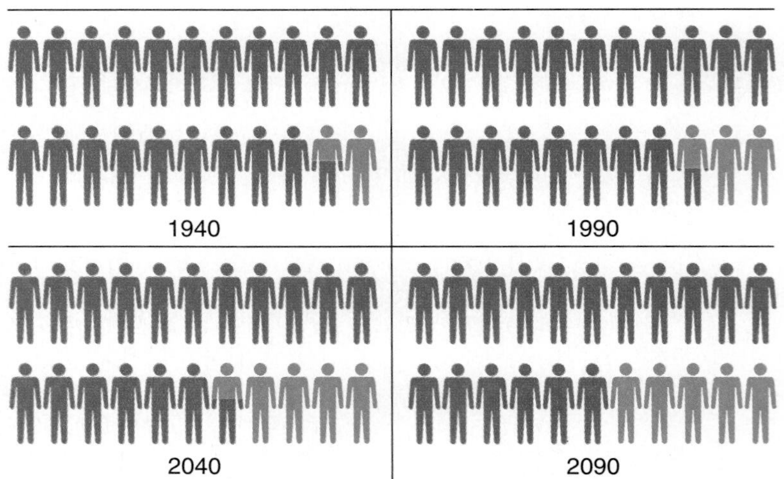

FIGURE 17.1
The aging of America.

In 1940, 6.8% of the population was 65 or older. By 1990, 12.7% of us reached age 65; by 2040, 21.7%; and a century from now, nearly one out of four Americans will be 65 or older. An estimated 25,000 Americans now living are 100 years old or older.
Source: Flieger, 1988.

these topics; they suggest that optimizing these factors may make the difference between "successful aging" and "usual aging" (Rowe and Kahn, 1987).

The Gradual Changes of Aging

The status of body cells, tissues, organs, systems, and their functions changes with time. Although many people consider 21 years of age as the *chronologic* beginning of "adulthood," 40 as the start of "middle age," and 65 as the year in which a person becomes "elderly," the *physiologic* changes during adulthood are neither so abrupt nor even very uniform.

Physical Changes During Adulthood

Figure 17.2 shows some of the changes in body composition that occur with aging. Levels of body calcium, potassium, and protein are likely to remain fairly stable, or decrease slowly, for decades and then rather quickly decrease in mass (Heymsfield et al., 1989). Similarly, losses in organ function do not usually follow a straight line (Figure 17.3). From age 30 to age 75, body systems decrease in function by from less than 10% to more than 50% of young adult values.

Overall, the most influential physiologic change that affects nutrition is the decrease in lean body mass and the concurrent reduction in energy need (Rosenberg, 1991; Vaughan et al., 1991). Although various changes in the gastrointestinal (GI) tract can occur with age (thereby affecting nutrition),

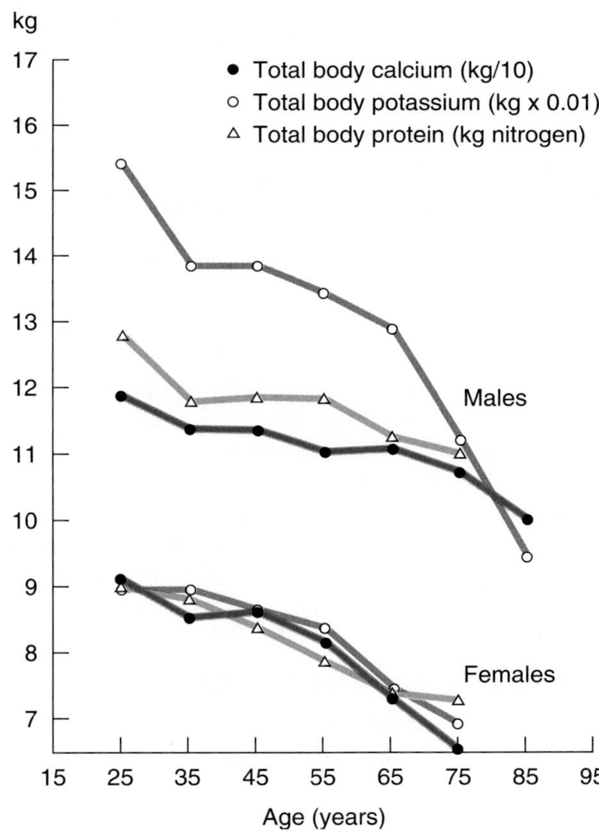

FIGURE 17.2
Body composition changes during adulthood.

This figure shows how average levels of certain substances differ among groups of people of different ages. Calcium is an indicator of bone mass; potassium and protein are indicators of lean tissue (Heymsfield et al., 1989).

FIGURE 17.3
Average loss of function with age.
(Leaf, 1973.)

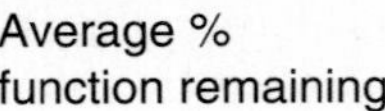

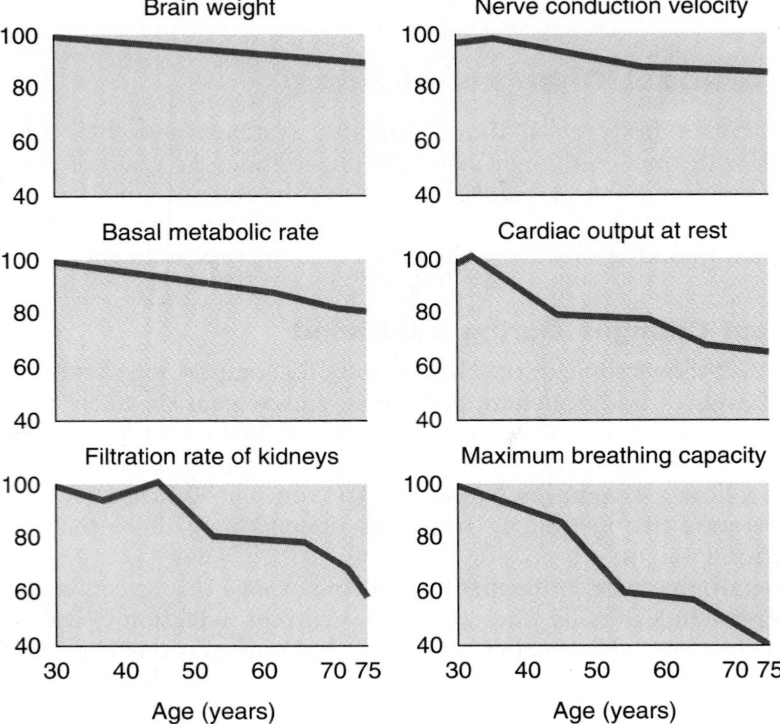

the tract's functions remain largely intact. Any impairment that does occur is not usually evident until the elder years; it is more likely to be evident if the person is ill (Chernoff, 1991; Russell, 1992).

Some of the changes that can occur are reduced production of saliva and decreased senses of taste and smell (Schiffman, 1991), which may change food preferences. People with missing teeth or ill-fitting dentures are likely to avoid chewy, crunchy, or hard foods. Gastric secretions of acid and enzymes decrease to some degree with age; if stomach acid decreases substantially, less calcium, iron, and some other nutrients can be absorbed. If large decreases in production of intrinsic factor occur, vitamin B-12 will not be well absorbed.

The size of a person's liver decreases with age, and its blood flow diminishes (Russell, 1992); nonetheless, most elderly people's GI tracts handle fat very well, unless they are stressed by illness (Russell, 1992). In some aging people, muscular changes may occur in the lower GI tract, making the person vulnerable to constipation. Because kidneys function less efficiently with age, electrolyte and water balance are more difficult to maintain. As with other changes of aging, this effect is more pronounced during periods of illness. Most elderly people have a diminished sense of thirst, which may result in dehydration (Chernoff, 1991).

Theories Concerning Age-Related Changes

Although we can observe many physical changes as people age, scientists are not sure to what extent these changes are *inevitable.* To explain what we mean by this, let us consider the two general classes of theories about why and how we age.

One class of theories says that the changes of aging are genetically predetermined. Cells may be programmed to divide a certain number of times and then die, or they may be programmed to increase the number of physiologic "mistakes" in cell production.

The other class of theories suggests that repeated assaults from environmental factors such as viruses, malnutrition, pollutants, or solar radiation cause our bodies to initiate such changes in cell production and function. Some of these factors may increase your body's production of **free radicals,** highly reactive molecules that can unite with body cells, causing oxidative stress or damage (Blumberg, 1992). Although your body has a network of defenses against free radicals, these defenses may become less efficient with age, allowing damage to accelerate (Monti et al., 1992).

free radicals—oxygen molecules and other highly reactive compounds that can damage body cells

The first class of theories suggests that your fate is sealed by your genetic makeup and that you can't alter your course of aging, no matter what you do. The second group more optimistically suggests that you can do things to reduce the rate at which the changes of aging occur, such as getting enough exercise and sleep, not smoking, avoiding excessive environmental and psychologic stresses, maintaining a good attitude about life, getting medical help when you need it, and—of course—nourishing yourself well. Some scientists suggest that certain nutrients, such as the antioxidant vitamins (beta-carotene, vitamin C, and vitamin E) may help maintain the network of defenses against free radicals and thereby reduce aging (Blumberg, 1992; Monti et al., 1992).

Which theory is correct? Actually, scientists find evidence that both of these scenarios together describe the aging process (Flieger, 1988).

Nutritional Needs During Adulthood

Scientists have learned a considerable amount about the nutrient needs of young adults, but they have done less of such research on middle-aged and elderly adults. Therefore, nutrition recommendations for young adults are probably more reliable than those for older adults. Besides, the fact that older people vary so extensively in their physical status complicates the assessment of their nutritional needs.

Energy Studies show that lean body mass generally declines after early adulthood at a rate of 2–3% per decade; *resting metabolic rate* declines proportionately (Vaughan et al., 1992). A study of healthy men showed that, beginning in their 20s, their *total energy usage* declined each year by about 12 or 13 kcalories per day. Of this amount, falling basal metabolic rate accounted for approximately 5 kcalories, and the remainder were attributable to declining physical activity levels (McGandy et al., 1966). In keeping with this decrease in usage, men and women tend naturally to reduce their total *intake* of kcalories as they age (Figure 17.4).

The energy RDA for men ages 19–50 is 2900 kcalories; for women, it is 2200 kcalories. For adults over age 50, the RDA for energy is only 80–85% of that for younger adults (RDA Subcommittee, 1989). Keep in mind that energy RDAs are average figures; some people need more kcalories, others fewer.

It is also possible that the same person will experience dramatically different energy needs and intakes within the broad age range of ages 19–50.

FIGURE 17.4
Average daily kcalorie intakes of adults.
Data source: National Center for Health Statistics, 1977.

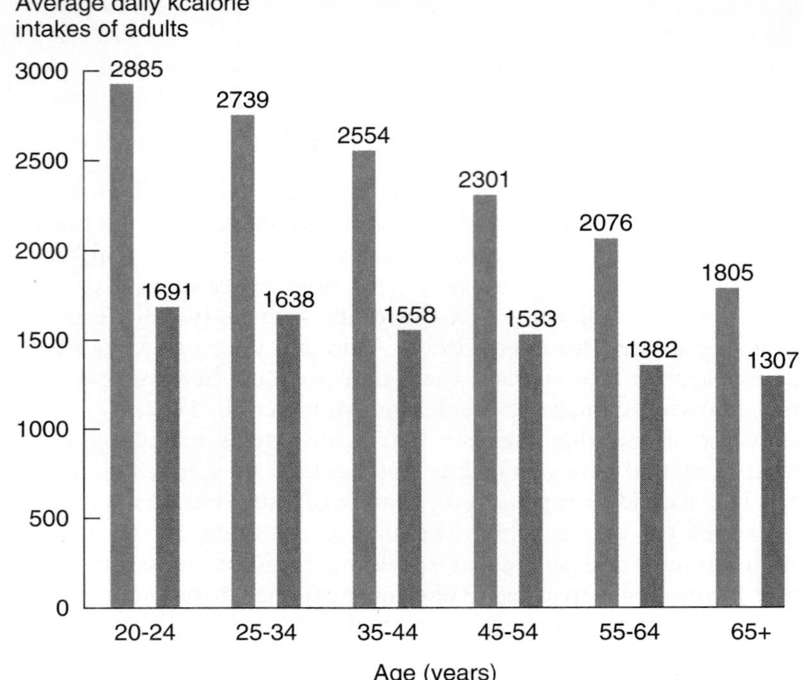

You Tell Me

Suppose that you are a college student in your early 20s who walks everywhere—to classes, to a part-time job, to your apartment—and that you take part in recreational sports a couple of times a week. Suppose that after graduation you get a job that demands long hours at a desk, that you commute to and from work by car, and that you spend your evenings reading or watching TV.

What will this do to your energy expenditure? What will it do to your energy needs? What will happen if you don't bring your energy intake in line with your needs?

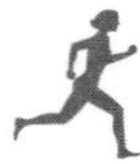

Although population studies generally show that energy usage decreases with advancing age, in recent years a small but increasing number of people have been enjoying vigorous activity late into adulthood. Consider that many community sports events—such as competitive running, swimming, and tennis—now include a "masters" category for older adults . . . and that it is not uncommon for some of these participants to cross the finish line ahead of some of their younger competitors. ●

Other Nutrients for Young and Middle-Aged Men and Women Most nutrient needs remain constant or decline somewhat from the late teen years into the early and middle adult years, because the major periods of growth are over. However, because bone mass can accumulate through the 20s and possibly into the 30s, the experts who developed the 1989 RDAs decided that the highest calcium, phosphorus, and vitamin D recommendations for the teen years should also apply through age 24. These intakes may help people reach their genetic potential for bone mass and thereby reduce their risk of osteoporosis in later years.

Because women are typically smaller than men, and because women have proportionately less lean tissue, RDAs for many nutrients are lower for women than for men. Generally, the difference is 20–25%, similar to the difference in energy needs. Of course, nutrient needs increase substantially if a woman becomes pregnant or is lactating; in fact, the RDAs for pregnant and lactating women are higher than the RDAs for men. (We discuss the specific needs during those unique times in Chapter 15.)

Other Nutrients for Older Adults Why do the needs of older adults change? Many factors can affect nutrient requirements with advancing age (Greger, 1989). Consider all of these: some people's bodies become less efficient at absorbing nutrients; these people may need to consume more to get enough. Some people may choose more foods that lower bioavailability of minerals and vitamins, such as high-fiber foods. Because of decreases in tissue mass, the body may need less of certain nutrients. The rates at which nutrients are excreted in urine and feces can change with age. Chronic illness and/or routine use of medications also may affect nutrient needs.

With such a complex set of interactions, any of three scenarios is possible: the need for a particular nutrient may go up; it may stay the same; or it may go down. And because of usual physiologic and dietary changes, the needs of 50-, 70-, and 90-year-olds are likely to be different.

What nutrient intakes, then, do experts recommend to older adults? Because the amount of research on this issue (especially that regarding the micronutrients) has been inadequate, scientists have had to make estimates. The table inside the back cover of this textbook shows what judgments the 1989 RDA Subcommittee made. In general, for most nutrients, the recommended intakes for older adults are the same as for 25- to 50-year-old adults. There are exceptions to this, however: recommended intakes of thiamin, riboflavin, and niacin are somewhat smaller because of decreased energy metabolism. Also, the RDA for iron is lower for women over age 50, when menopause halts the monthly iron losses previously occurring during menstruation.

Research under way today may change recommendations in the future regarding levels of intake of some micronutrients. For example, epidemiologic studies show that populations with higher dietary intakes of the antioxidant vitamins (C, E, and beta-carotene) have lower incidences of certain forms of cancer, cataracts, and cardiovascular disease (Blumberg, 1992). However, until these effects have been demonstrated under well-controlled conditions and are well understood, scientists cannot give responsible advice about increasing these RDAs.

Are U.S. Adults Well-Nourished?

How do the diets of American adults compare with their RDAs? Just as energy intake declines with age, so do the intakes of most vitamins and minerals. Average intakes of calcium, magnesium, zinc, and vitamin B-6 were reported to be less than 100% of the 1980 RDAs for men and women included in the Nationwide Food Consumption Survey in the late 1970s. For women in their reproductive years, iron was also low; however, because women need less iron after menopause, inadequate intakes of this nutrient are not as frequent in elderly women.

Determine Your Nutritional Health

The warning signs of poor nutritional health are often overlooked. Use this checklist to find out if you or someone you know is at nutritional risk. Read the statements below. Circle the number in the yes column for those that apply to you or someone you know. For each yes answer, score the number in the box. Total your nutritional score.

	Yes
I have an illness or condition that made me change the kind and/or amount of food I eat.	2
I eat fewer than 2 meals per day.	3
I eat few fruits or vegetables, or milk products.	2
I have 3 or more drinks of beer, liquor or wine almost every day.	2
I have tooth or mouth problems that make it hard for me to eat.	2
I don't always have enough money to buy the food I need.	4
I eat alone most of the time.	1
I take 3 or more different prescribed or over-the-counter drugs a day.	1
Without wanting to, I have lost or gained 10 pounds in the last 6 months.	2
I am not always physically able to shop, cook and/or feed myself.	2
Total	

Total your nutritional score. If it's—

0–2 **Good!** Recheck your nutritional score in 6 months.

3–5 **You are at moderate nutritional risk.** See what can be done to improve your eating habits and lifestyle. Your office on aging, senior nutrition program, senior citizens center or health department can help. Recheck your nutritional score in 3 months.

6 or more **You are at high nutritional risk.** Bring this checklist the next time you see your doctor, dietitian or other qualified health or social service professional. Talk with them about any problems you may have. Ask for help to improve your nutritional health.

Remember that warning signs suggest risk, but do not represent diagnosis of any condition.

FIGURE 17.5
Determining your nutritional health.

Use this checklist to find out if someone you know is at nutritional risk.
Source: White et al., 1992.

The results of a 1986 survey, which focused on the intakes of women 19–50 years of age, were more alarming. For this group of almost 1200 women, average intakes of the following were below the 1980 RDAs: energy, vitamin E, vitamin B-6, folic acid, calcium, magnesium, iron, and zinc. This study indicates that the poor dietary habits of many teenage girls continue into adulthood. Nutrient intakes generally are also lower than the average for women who are poor and nonwhite (Human Nutrition Information Service, 1988).

Assessing the nutritional adequacy of older Americans is more difficult, as you might expect. The number of health problems differ dramatically from one person to another. One may take several medications that affect nutrients; another may take no drugs at all. Their activity levels may be very different. They may or may not eat well or take nutritional supplements.

A striking demonstration of the difference between groups of elderly adults involves protein status. Whereas clinical protein deficiency is unusual among the community-dwelling elderly in the United States, it is much more frequently seen in the hospitalized elderly and those living in nursing

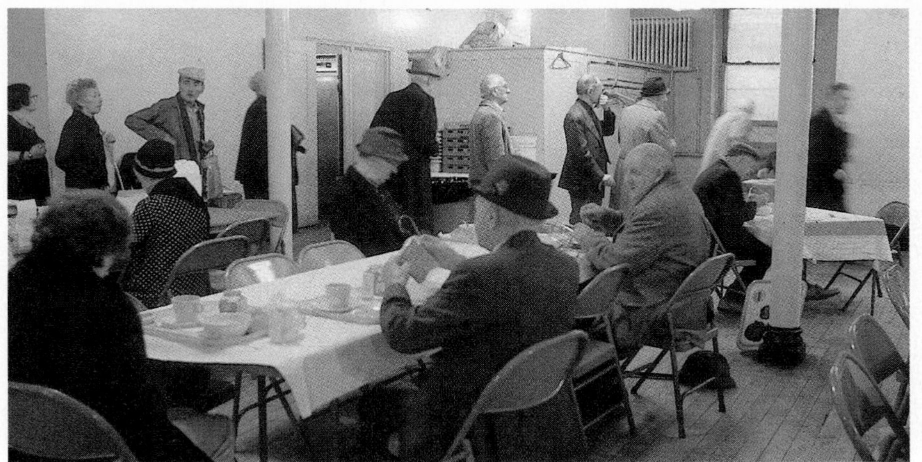

FIGURE 17.6
Congregate meals for the elderly.

The Nutrition Program for Older Americans provides a nutritious meal and a social opportunity for many mobile people.

homes (Zheng and Rosenberg, 1989). Further, shut-ins are much more likely to have low vitamin D status than people who freely go outdoors.

The National Health and Nutrition Examination Survey II (NHANES II) collected data from noninstitutionalized elderly people between 1976 and 1980. Analysis of this survey shows that living arrangements and economic conditions can have a substantial impact on nutrient intakes. Men who lived with spouses had much better nutrient intakes than those who did not, and low-income men without a spouse were at highest risk of dietary inadequacy (Ryan et al., 1989). For women, the factor most closely associated with lower nutrient intakes was poverty.

Because some elderly adults living in the community are sure to be at nutritional risk, nutrition professionals have developed a simple screening tool to identify people who may need help. This tool is a public awareness checklist called *Determine Your Nutritional Health;* it can be used by elderly people themselves as well as by those who are involved with them (Figure 17.5). A person who gets a high score is encouraged to contact an agency that can provide help (White et al., 1992).

Programs to Improve the Status of Adults at Nutritional Risk

Various programs are in place to help adults of different ages and situations meet their nutritional needs. As you learned in Chapters 15 and 16, the Supplemental Food Program for Women, Infants, and Children (WIC) provides nutrition education and vouchers for certain nutritious foods to low-income pregnant and lactating women and their children. The Food Stamp Program serves low-income individuals and families.

The Nutrition Program for Older Americans (Title III-C), established in 1973 by the federal government, is specifically targeted to the elderly population. It provides for people over age 60 community-based noon meals at a nominal fee that is often optional. The largest component of this program is the congregate meal service at senior-citizen centers, churches, schools, and other locations (Figure 17.6). These meals are designed to provide one-third of the RDAs; health and welfare counseling and nutrition education are also provided regularly. Participants' evaluations show that the program provides other important benefits as well, namely, increased socialization and improved life-satisfaction (Roe, 1992).

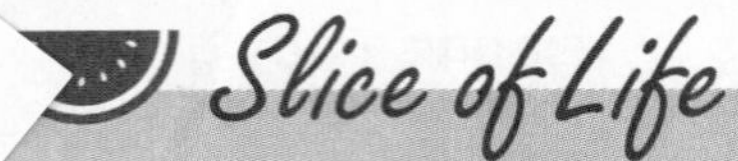

A Delivery Service with Mutual Benefits

Nearly every weekday morning Ed Meyer can be found loading warm lunches and cold dinners into the back of his Mercury Marquis. Ed, who is 78, drives a regular route for the Milwaukee, Wisconsin, Visiting Nurse Association's Mobile Meals program, which provides meal service to people for whom this program makes the big difference. Without it, they might not be able to live independently.

At his age, he is older than almost everybody on his route. He explains why he does it: "My wife and I were married 50 years, and after she died two years ago I couldn't stay home alone. Doing this every day is what keeps me alive."

With meals, Ed delivers his own brand of humor and concern. After Rosalie did not answer her door for two days in a row, Meyer greeted her with, "I'm gonna scold you! Where were you Thursday? Where were you yesterday? With your boyfriend?" She holds up her arm in quiet protest, revealing a cast. "I broke my wrist," she explains.

At another stop along his 25-mile route, Ed lets himself in. The thin man in the chair brightens immediately. "How are you, Ed? Any snow on the highway?" he asks. "No," Meyer tells him, "but if you want me to bring you snow, I'll bring it." After a minute or two of visiting, Ed is on his way to the next stop. "Take care now," the man in the chair says. "Don't slip. Thanks. I'll see you later."

Traveling with Ed for a day makes it clear—essential as his services are to the clients on his route, the help he provides adds an important element to his own life at the same time.

Adapted from *The Milwaukee Journal,* Monday, December 8, 1986.

Elderly people who cannot leave their homes may be able to get help in meeting their nutrition needs from various local organizations. Some organizations deliver ready-to-eat meals, often using a combination of federal and local funds; others supply frozen dinners; and others provide grocery service to people in their homes. Although most federally funded meal programs originally provided service only 5 days per week, now almost half offer 7-day service (Balsam et al., 1992). Some local programs also serve the needs of younger home-bound adults who do not qualify for programs for the elderly (Roe, 1989).

A study of the elderly's use of community services showed that approximately 10% of noninstitutionalized older adults made use of meals programs, either at senior centers or by receiving home-delivered meals (Stone, 1986). The greatest value of such programs is that they help older people continue to live in their own homes. The Slice of Life above describes how one meal delivery program benefits both its clients and their volunteer driver.

How Nutrition and Fitness Affect Health and Longevity

Good health is more than the absence of obvious physical and mental illness; it also involves minimizing the modifiable risk factors for chronic diseases and, in addition, achieving and maintaining physical fitness. In a book called *Biomarkers: The 10 Determinants of Aging You Can Control,* the authors discuss how to enhance the factors that correlate with good health (Evans and Rosenberg, 1991). Table 17.1 lists the ten biomarkers.

Research shows how important and how interrelated some of these factors are. For example, exercise increases energy expenditure; when a person increases kcalorie intake to achieve energy balance, nutrient intakes improve. Adequate exercise helps achieve and maintain physical fitness and

TABLE 17.1 Determinants of Aging You Can Influence

These health indicators often change with age (some up, some down). Adequate exercise and healthy nutrition can minimize these changes.

1. Your muscle mass
2. Your strength
3. Your basal metabolic rate
4. Your body fat percentage
5. Your aerobic capacity
6. Your blood-sugar tolerance
7. Your total cholesterol/HDL ratio
8. Your blood pressure
9. Your bone density
10. Your body temperature regulation

Source: Evans and Rosenberg, 1991.

also helps reduce many risk factors (Astrand, 1992). Even late in life, weight lifting and low-impact aerobic exercise enhance strength, flexibility, and cardiorespiratory fitness (Work, 1989). Furthermore, large epidemiologic studies in recent years suggest that getting enough exercise helps us to live longer.

In one such study, approximately 17,000 Harvard alumni were categorized according to the amount of exercise they had done in ordinary daily activities, such as walking and stair climbing, as well as in sports; then, death rates of the group were compared. Death rates declined steadily as energy expended on activity increased; death rates were one-fourth to one-third lower among alumni expending 2000 or more kcalories during exercise per week than among less active men (Paffenbarger et al., 1986).

In a more recent study, over 13,000 men and women were evaluated for fitness using a maximal treadmill exercise test at the Institute for Aerobics Research in Dallas, Texas. Anybody with obvious present or past illness (such as hypertension, diabetes, or a heart attack) was excluded from the study. In the 8 years of follow-up, approximately 280 deaths occurred. When the deaths were evaluated based on five fitness categories, the death rate among the least fit was several times higher than that of the most fit: the least fit men were 3.4 times more likely to die than the most fit; the least fit women, 4.6 times more likely (Blair et al., 1989). •

Nutrition, Health, and Disease

Some nutrition experts believe that the most important things that good nutrition can do are to help delay the onset of chronic diseases (those persisting over a long period of time) and to reduce the amount of medication needed in early stages of chronic illnesses. With fewer years of severe disease, people could enjoy a better *quality* of life and perhaps even a somewhat *longer* life (Browner et al., 1991).

Many of the effects of nutrition on chronic diseases have already been discussed in this text:

- atherosclerosis (see Chapter 5, section on fiber, and Chapter 6)
- cancer (see Chapters 6, 11, 12, 14)

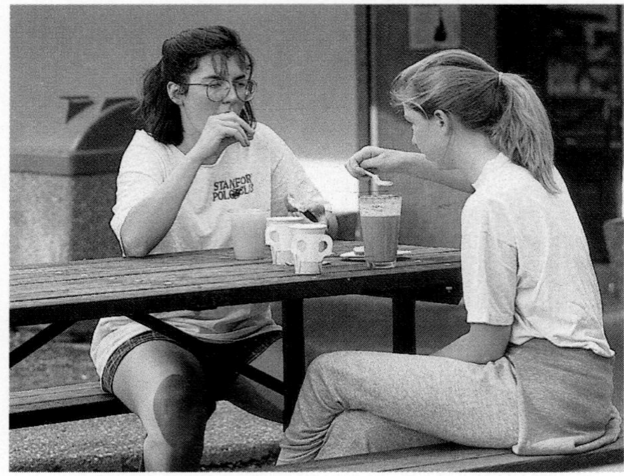

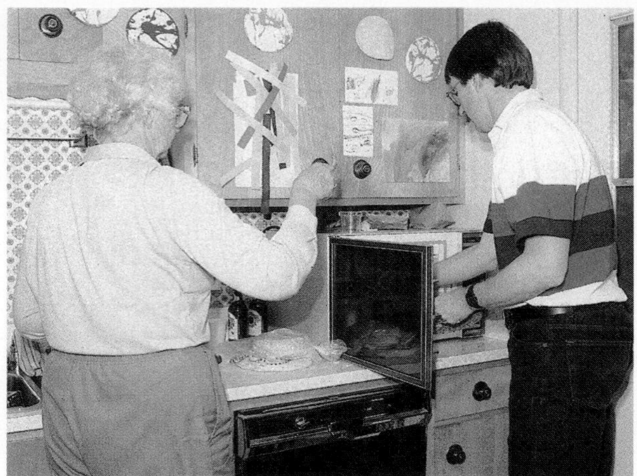

FIGURE 17.7
Good nutrition . . . health enhancing at every age.

What you eat now affects your health not only today but also in the future.

- constipation (see Chapter 5, section on fiber)
- diverticular disease (see Chapter 5, section on fiber)
- diabetes (see Chapter 5)
- overweight (see Chapter 9)
- hypertension (see Chapter 12, section on sodium, potassium, and chloride)
- osteoporosis (see Chapter 12, section on calcium)

In addition to the conditions listed above, those discussed below are evident in adults. The following sections summarize what we know about how nutrition affects them.

Infectious Diseases In the early part of this century, infectious diseases caused the greatest number of deaths. By the middle of the century, immunization and improved sanitation had dropped such diseases to a very low place on the list of direct causes of death. Now, the trend has shifted: with no effective treatment available for infection with the human immunodeficiency virus (HIV), deaths due to acquired immune deficiency syndrome (AIDS) are causing the number of deaths from infections to rise.

Another infectious disease that has been getting attention recently is tuberculosis (TB); it has been increasing since 1988, after three previous decades of decline. Public health experts believe that its resurgence is related in large part to AIDS, because people infected with HIV are more vulnerable to TB as well (Landesman, 1993). Other possible reasons for its spread are the influx of immigrants suffering from the disease and the crowded living conditions of other vulnerable groups, such as the homeless, the elderly, and the imprisoned, among whom contagions are more likely to spread.

Researchers continue to study the degree to which nutrition influences the ability of the immune system to combat viral and bacterial diseases. Scientists have already learned that inadequate intake of many of the micronutrients weakens the function of the immune system, making infections of all kinds more likely; however, there is no evidence that taking doses larger than the RDA offers greater protection.

You Tell Me

Although getting *adequate* levels of nutrients is critical to optimal immune function, consuming a large overload of nutrients is not. For certain nutrients there is evidence that overzealous supplementation actually has a *counterproductive* effect. Zinc, which is required for immune system function, *interferes* with immune function when taken in very large doses (Chandra, 1989), as do excesses of selenium, vitamin E, vitamin A, and others.

For adults who want to take micronutrient supplements to *help* their immune system function, what would be the best advice? Does this apply to adults of all ages—young, middle-aged, and elderly?

Currently, some unscrupulous promoters are marketing megavitamin and mineral supplements to people infected with HIV. With no scientific proof, they claim that such supplements will restore and bolster immune function, inhibit or delay progression of Kaposi's sarcoma (a cancer sometimes found in people with HIV), or act as anti-infective agents (Dwyer et al., 1988). Rather, appropriate nutritional support consists of eating a nutritious diet that will prevent malnutrition, maintain weight, and promote normal GI function. Health care providers have developed guidelines for nutritional support for patients in various stages of HIV infection (Task Force on Nutrition Support in AIDS, 1989). In an expert interview on page 570, Donald P. Kotler discusses nutritional considerations regarding AIDS.

A recent review states that although immune system function generally decreases in older people, making them more vulnerable to all types of infection, this change may not be totally inevitable (Rosenberg and Miller, 1992). When scientists have simultaneously assessed nutritional status and immune responses, they have found that some cases of impaired immunity in the elderly may be associated with nutritional deficiencies. Furthermore, a few studies of undernourished adults whose intakes were subsequently improved showed an increase in immune function (Chandra, 1989; Meydani et al., 1989). Interestingly, some studies showed that adequate exercise correlates with higher immune function, and loss of a spouse correlates with decreased immune response (Chandra, 1989).

Nervous System Function There is a great deal of public interest in how nutrition affects nervous system function. Some of the questions involve short-term effects of nutrition on cognitive functioning (perception, thinking, and memory); others have to do with whether nutrition can prevent or relieve psychologic stress; and still others relate to long-term disability in the elderly.

Some of the information on nutrition and *mental acuity* centers on amino acid and carbohydrate metabolism. Although this research is very interesting, it is equivocal; therefore, it is too early to come to conclusions or to apply much of this research. It is not possible, then, to guarantee that eating certain foods before an exam will sharpen your mental abilities or that eating a high-protein "power lunch" will guarantee a business executive success in closing the deal. There may be gender-related, age-related,

Interview with Donald P. Kotler, MD

Nutrition and AIDS

As the AIDS epidemic continues to grow with no cure in sight, many people have wondered how special nutritional therapy might help patients cope with symptoms, including the extreme weight loss frequently associated with AIDS. In this interview, Dr. Donald Kotler describes the relationship between AIDS and nutrition as it is currently understood, and as it relates to other chronic diseases. An expert in this field, Dr. Kotler is an Associate Professor of Clinical Medicine at the Columbia University College of Physicians and Surgeons, and Associate Chief of the Gastrointestinal Division of St. Luke's-Roosevelt Hospital Center in New York.

As a physician, how did you become interested in nutrition?

I've been interested in nutrition for a long time. Starvation by itself is enough to bring people to the point of death; and starvation may be avoided or treated so easily compared to the complexities of other diseases in the world. The fact that it progresses on to death seems to me such an incredible human waste.

My training was in medicine, in gastroenterology (the study of the GI tract) related to malabsorption syndrome and progressive wasting. In my training, I naturally veered toward diseases of absorption. That was all before AIDS came along. In 1981, when I began to see patients with AIDS, what I saw were the wasting illnesses, the diseases that cause diarrhea and weight loss.

Readers have learned that nutrient deficiencies can compromise immunity. In terms of AIDS, does this mean that a poor diet could shorten the period between the time a person is infected with HIV and the time that person develops an active case of AIDS?

Before I answer that, let me make a couple of important points. Number one, people can develop AIDS without having pre-existing malnutrition; malnutrition is not a cause of AIDS. Number two, people can have AIDS for a while and not be malnourished, so AIDS does not automatically lead to malnutrition. Therefore, when malnutrition occurs, it's not simply because of AIDS, but rather because of a complication of AIDS.

AIDS is a state of being, if you will; it is a state of immune dysfunction. By itself, it doesn't mean anything, but it does lead to consequences. For example, the immune deficiency leaves one vulnerable to an intestinal infection. If the infection involves those cells of the intestine that are involved with absorption, then that complication of AIDS will be malabsorption, and with it, malnutrition.

In fact, it is not known whether poor nutrition may hasten the development of an active case of AIDS, but it is certainly suspected. In fact, in the Third World it appears (although it is not well studied) that patients will die from complications of the disease when laboratory testing would suggest that their immune function is not nearly so bad as, for example, some people in America who are still working. It is well known that people walk around with severely depleted lymphocytes (disease-fighting white blood cells) and are still doing quite well, so the absolute level of lymphocytes doesn't automatically predict one's function.

Are there realistic ways in which you think good nutrition may help patients with AIDS? For example, would it help them to withstand chemotherapy more easily?

Again, that's suspected, but not proven. Good nutrition certainly can help people with AIDS. Malnutrition brings weakness and a decrease in quality of life, in whatever disease it appears. Uncomplicated starvation affects quality of life; there is no reason to believe that with AIDS it would do so any less.

It depends on specifically what is wrong. Let me give you a very specific example of how a malnutrition process can affect responsive therapy. Let's say the malnutrition is caused by intestinal disease with malabsorption. The medication you use to treat the disease is oral medicine and the oral medicine is malabsorbed. Blood levels of the medicine will then be much less than actually given because of the malabsorption. Under the circumstances, the medicine might not be effective at all.

Nutrition support in AIDS, just like in any other disease, has to be individualized for each patient. If the problem is poor food intake, what could be done to try to stimulate food intake? If the problem is poor absorption, what could be done to alter the diet or treat the underlying cause, to try to improve absorption? If the problem is a metabolic alteration related to the disease, the first thing to do is find the disease that is causing the problem and try to treat it effectively. If that's done, that may be all that is needed.

What is the most exciting prospect for nutrition in patient care that you see on the horizon?

The most exciting prospect is people becoming interested in nutrition. Nutrition is usually tacked on the basic therapy, because nutrition is usually considered a secondary phenomenon and all attention is placed on the primary problem. But in most chronic diseases malnutrition plays a role. For example, if you go to a dialysis unit, people who are getting hemodialysis for kidney failure are usually very skinny. If you look at a ward of people with chronic lung disease, they are often scarecrows. Or look at patients who have chronic neurologic disorders—they very often die as a result of a wasting illness. If you take people who have bad arthritis, the same phenomenon occurs. If you look at people who are elderly and have difficulty getting out of the house to get food, poor food intake and malabsorption is not so uncommon.

So in fact, many chronic problems might have malnutrition superimposed on them, and these receive very little attention from physicians who specialize in pulmonary, cardiac, and GI diseases. It takes a disease as complicated as AIDS for people to see that nutrition really may have a rehabilitative benefit.

Are new nutritional therapies for AIDS being investigated? Or are there therapies that are being tried to help wasting in AIDS patients?

Clearly we are way off in coming up with the most appropriate ways of treating HIV. We may have all the nutritional products we need on the shelf right now if we could learn to use them correctly. And learning to use them correctly in somebody with AIDS is not so different, I believe, than learning to use them correctly in patients with kidney failure, lung failure, neurologic disease, or progressive arthritic disease. I think it's all the same: finding out what's wrong and then bypassing the abnormality. Someone who can't eat for any reason is going to lose weight and feel bad. Somebody who malabsorbs for any reason is going to have a wasting illness.

One of the therapies on the horizon is the use of anabolic steroids to affect metabolism so as to build muscle and protein in patients with AIDS. The drugs have been available for many years, but they are mostly drugs of abuse by weightlifters and others. In fact, the early results seem to show that one can accelerate the repletion of protoplasm by using anabolic agents. There's one multicenter clinical trial going on here and several other places looking at the drug "growth hormone," and there are other studies looking at an anabolic agent called IGF. In Australia, yet another anabolic agent is being used.

Now throughout the community, more and more physicians treating AIDS patients are realizing that AIDS patients have testicular failure, with low testosterone levels. Testosterone is the original anabolic steroid, and more and more physicians are detecting the low testosterone levels and are replacing testosterone. In doing so, they are probably preventing, in some patients, progressive loss of protein.

Nonetheless, one should always look for a cause for malnutrition. For example, malnutrition related to tuberculosis in a patient with low testosterone level should be treated by finding and treating the tuberculosis—not just by giving testosterone. There are really no simplistic answers, just like there's not one nutritional regimen that is good for every AIDS patient. It all has to be tailored to what is wrong.

and individual differences in people's responses to particular nutrient intakes. The following study is an example of an effect found within one well-defined group.

You Tell Me

A study of college-age women (18–30 years old) compared the effects of drinking 12 ounces of a sugar-sweetened beverage, an aspartame-sweetened drink, or plain water. The students were more sleepy and less alert 1 hour after drinking the sugared beverage than after the unsugared drinks (Pivonka and Grunewald, 1990). The test drink contained 50 grams of sugar and no caffeine.

What characteristics of the *subjects* could have made their response to the drinks different from what it might be in other groups? (Consider such factors as age, body size, and foods that were recently consumed.) What characteristics of the drinks could have affected their response? Describe the circumstances under which someone might make use of the findings of this study.

Psychologic stress can affect people throughout their adult years as they make life-shaping decisions and experience social, occupational, and health changes. Little scientific information suggests that nutrition can be used to allay *mental and emotional stress,* even though we know that nutrient needs can increase in response to certain *physical stresses,* such as illness or injury (see Chapter 11 on vitamin supplements). Therefore, there is no basis for recommending unusual diets or nutrient supplements for people dealing with the psychologic ups and downs of everyday life. Some nutritional supplements on the market claim to do just that; not only are such products of unknown benefit, but many also may cause risk if they contain megadoses of vitamins. If you want to take a supplement, a multiple-nutrient supplement containing levels that do not exceed 100% of the U.S. RDA would be the best choice.

Before we discuss the role of nutrition on the long-term mental condition of the elderly, some background is in order. As Figure 17.3 suggests, small changes in brain mass and function typically occur in the healthy adult between ages 30 and 75. Despite these decreases, reasonably good nervous system function normally continues into the elder years. Among some individuals, however, pathologic changes that result in **dementia** may occur. Up to 6% of the elderly over age 65 have severe dementia, and up to 15% may have a mild form (Gray, 1989). Dementia has various causes.

dementia—impairment of memory, thinking, and/or judgment to a degree that affects daily activities and relationships with others; may be accompanied by personality changes

Over half of the cases represent people with *Alzheimer's disease,* a progressive, incurable loss of mental function. The cause of Alzheimer's disease is unknown, although a genetic component exists. Certain proteins accumulate and the neurotransmitter acetylcholine decreases in brains of people with Alzheimer's disease (Hooper, 1992); but increasing the dietary intake of choline and lecithin (precursors of acetylcholine) does not relieve the condition. Aluminum also accumulates in the brains of patients with the disease, but scientists do not think this is part of its cause (Greger, 1992). Several scientists speculate that a *nerve growth factor* might be a useful therapy (Marx, 1990).

The second most common type of dementia in the elderly is *multi-infarct dementia,* the result of multiple strokes. Nutrition therapy can reduce the risk of this condition in ways similar to those used to reduce hypertension: that is, treatment of obesity and moderate restriction of sodium intake (Gray, 1989). Third in prevalence is *dementia associated with alcoholism;* abstinence from alcohol use is a sure preventive technique. Severe, prolonged nutritional deficiencies are an additional, but very rare, cause of dementia in the United States.

Scientists have known for many decades that severe deficiencies of many of the water-soluble vitamins result in neurologic and behavioral problems. Although severe deficiencies are rare among older people in the United States, some scientists believe that even mild deficits may cause brain function to decline as people age (Rosenberg and Miller, 1992). The challenge for the future is to determine the biochemical markers for these subtle deficiencies so that people with these problems can be identified and treated.

Arthritis The major symptom of **arthritis** is pain in the joints, which fluctuates in severity from time to time without obvious reason (Bollet, 1988). Although arthritis is an ancient and common disease, its causes have not been clearly defined. The disease cannot be cured, but patients can usually be helped.

arthritis—painful condition resulting from the distortion or inflammation of joint surfaces due to degeneration or mineral deposits

Over 100 different forms of arthritis exist. *Osteoarthritis,* the type very common among the elderly, is characterized by the distortion of joint surfaces apparently due to lifelong wear and tear. *Rheumatoid arthritis,* which is less common and more prevalent in young adults, is characterized by joint inflammation and other systemic changes of unknown origin. The only widely accepted dietary treatment is weight loss (for overweight arthritics) to relieve stress on joints.

Other dietary modifications have often been promoted in the popular press, but they have not usually proved to be effective treatments in controlled studies. (One expert suggests that most popular books on arthritis should be listed in the "fiction category" [Bollet, 1988].) Furthermore, many such programs do not take overall nutritional needs into account: they may be either nutritionally inadequate or excessive in some regard (Jarvis, 1990). Any arthritic person contemplating the use of a special diet or dietary product should check first with a dietitian, who can analyze the proposed program for nutritional adequacy and possible nutrient toxicity (Wolman, 1987).

Gout is a type of arthritis that has been thought to have a closer relationship to diet. In this condition, crystals of uric acid (a breakdown product of certain protein components) form in the joints, causing pain. In the past, foods containing certain chemicals from which large amounts of uric acid are produced were limited in the diet. However, we now know that the body can produce uric acid precursors from fragments of any of the macronutrients. Even for gout, then, diet is not the primary cause or treatment method: genetic factors are probably the major cause, and drug therapies are the most effective treatment.

Periodontal Disease Degeneration of the tissues supporting the teeth is referred to as **periodontal disease.** It generally affects both gum tissue and the bony arches in which the teeth are situated.

periodontal disease—degeneration of the gum and bone tissues supporting the teeth

Periodontal disease is the major cause of tooth loss in Americans. Although experts don't know with certainty what causes it, periodontal disease is important to a discussion of adult nutrition for two reasons; first, poor nutrition may contribute to the bone loss that occurs. Second, deterioration of the bony arches makes it difficult to fit dentures properly, which may lead to chewing problems and reduced nutrient intake. A diet deficient in vitamin C for several months can produce symptoms of periodontal problems; but because vitamin C intake is adequate for most people in North America, good dental hygiene is the primary recommendation for dealing with this problem.

The Impact of Nutrition on Length of Life

The search for a way to live longer is as ancient as the quest for the Fountain of Youth. Periodically we hear stories of people in remote places, such as the mountains of Russia, the former Soviet Georgia, Pakistan, or Ecuador, who reach a vigorous old age. To try to understand what might be responsible for their longevity, scientists have studied the cultures of these people; you will read about them in the next section.

Another type of research on aging has been the study of the effects of nutrition and various other lifestyle factors on laboratory animals. Each species of animal—including humans—has a **maximum life span,** which is the *oldest age* to which some members of the species have been known to survive (approximately 115 years for humans). Life span appears to be limited genetically and is therefore unlikely to be influenced by nutrition.

maximum life span—oldest age to which a member of a species has been known to survive

Life expectancy, or **average life span,** is not the same thing; it represents the *average length of life* statistically shown for a specific group. For people born in the United States in 1990, life expectancy was over 75 years; it is 7 years higher for women than for men (Kinsella, 1992). **Longevity,** by contrast, is the length of time *actually lived* by an individual member of a species. Nutrition may have a role in life expectancy and longevity.

life expectancy (average life span)—average length of life for a given group of animals

longevity—length of time an individual animal actually lives

Human Epidemiologic Studies on Longevity Regions of the world in which many of the inhabitants are claimed to live to a very old age have been studied to determine what factors might account for their longevity. In such regions of Russia, Pakistan, and Ecuador, several cultural characteristics stand out. First, all are agrarian societies in which people labor in the fields all their lives to sustain themselves; second, they all consume largely vegetarian diets, out of necessity rather than choice; and third, all of these communities provide strong psychologic support for their elderly (Leaf, 1988).

As early reports of these people's diets were published, many people in the United States hoped that they could live longer by consuming foods indigenous to these areas; this led some people to add yogurt, exotic fruits and juices, and other products to their diets. But later comparisons among the nutritional composition of the diets of these cultures showed no uniformity, so the nutritional content of their diets did not explain their longevity.

Other surprises were found to interfere with the theory that particular diets led to long life: many people had represented themselves as older than they were. In some regions of Russia, citizens admitted that during World War II, many men had taken their father's names and ages to avoid conscription into the military; these men had acquired an impressive number of years by the time the research on aging was conducted (Figure 17.8). Another research team in Vilcabamba, Ecuador, discovered that many people older than 65 routinely exaggerated their ages, sometimes by as much as 20 to 40 years (Mazess and Forman, 1979). This practice was socially acceptable in a culture where village elders were esteemed in proportion to their ages.

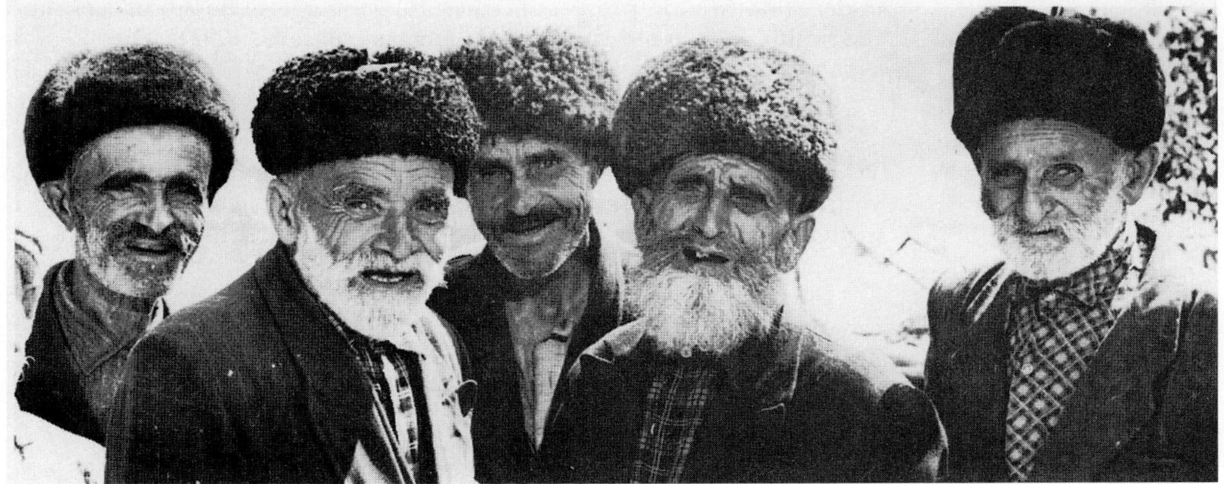

FIGURE 17.8
Diet and longevity.

Claims have been made that in certain isolated regions of the world, many people live to extraordinary ages. Investigation casts doubt on whether these people are as old as first thought and on the theory that their diets may have been responsible. The Russian men pictured are from a district legendary for its inhabitants' longevity; these five men claim that their ages total over 600.

Careful evaluation showed that the life expectancy of Vilcabambans was actually the same as that of other Ecuadorans—and it was approximately 15% lower than that of Americans. In addition, the researchers learned that many elderly people had gravitated to this village for sociability's sake, as has happened in some communities in the United States, and that younger people had left.

Therefore, the initial excitement regarding a provable association between diet and human longevity collapsed. Neither these investigations nor any other scientifically valid studies have been able to show that supplements or special foods can prolong human life more than a balanced diet of ordinary foods.

All of that notwithstanding, researchers in Vilcabamba noted that the older adults there enjoyed apparent good health: they were not overweight and had hypertension only rarely, and they had lower than usual blood cholesterol values, lower heart rates, and fewer fractures from osteoporosis. Although their longevity was not impressive, these aspects of health were. For this reason, research on these populations continues.

Animal Studies About Longevity A number of animal studies, conducted over more than half a century, have looked at the effects of food restriction on longevity. These studies have shown that diets providing only about half the energy needed for the animals to achieve maximal growth increased the average age to which they lived and slowed down many of the physiologic changes seen with aging (Weindruch and Westford, 1988; Masoro, 1992). As part of their low-kcalorie diets, the animals received optimal levels of micronutrients.

The studies also showed that underfeeding had drawbacks, however. Severely restricted animals had increased infant mortality and growth retardation. In several studies, certain aspects of immune function improved; in others, certain aspects declined (Good and Lorenz, 1988).

Do these studies suggest that humans would benefit from severe kcaloric restriction? Experts don't think that such restrictions are wise in children or the elderly (Widdowson, 1992), but the consequences of kcaloric restriction in middle-aged adults is debatable. Several large trials with animals, including nonhuman primates, are now being conducted. These and other animal studies and cell culture research provide information that may help scientists uncover the mechanisms of the aging process. Once these are understood, we can progress further in learning how nutrition can improve the health and extend the lives of humans (Masoro, 1992).

How Drugs Interact with Nutrients

When you take medication, you are looking for a health benefit. But along with the help you get, you may experience some side effects, which may include changes in the way your body handles nutrients. Drugs can potentially affect any process relating to nutrition, from ingestion to excretion.

Interactions between drugs and nutrients cut both ways: just as drugs can affect nutrition, food and its constituents can affect your body's utilization of medications. Let's start by looking at the effect of drugs on nutrition.

How Medications Interfere with Nutrients

Medications can affect nutrition by influencing appetite, decreasing the absorption of nutrients, interfering with nutrient metabolism, and/or affecting excretion. People whose nutrition is most at risk for experiencing negative effects of drugs are those who (1) use medicines for long periods of time, (2) take several kinds of drugs at the same time (whether prescription or over-the-counter types), and (3) have marginal nutritional status to begin with.

People of any age may need medications from time to time, but older adults are more likely to develop chronic conditions that require ongoing treatment with drugs. For this reason, the elderly are generally more likely to experience negative effects from nutrient–drug interactions than are people in other age groups.

Nutrient intake and general nutritional status can affect your body's use of drugs in many ways, such as how well the drug dissolves and is absorbed, transported, and distributed; how rapidly it is metabolized; and how readily it is excreted. Common drugs with consequences for nutrition are discussed below.

Aspirin Aspirin is one of the medicines used most frequently in the United States by people of all ages. Many people are chronic users of high doses of aspirin because its anti-inflammatory and pain-relieving properties are helpful in treating arthritis. Some people take aspirin routinely to slow down blood clot formation, especially if they have had a heart attack, because aspirin reduces the risk of further blockage of coronary vessels.

Aspirin causes a small amount of blood (and therefore iron) loss via the GI tract. People who routinely use aspirin should include good sources of iron in their diets.

Oral Contraceptives Most women who take low-dose oral contraceptives have approximately the same requirement for vitamins and minerals as those who are not taking them; therefore, routine supplementation is not called for. However, a small proportion of the women taking oral contraceptives, especially if the doses are high, develop biochemical evidence of vitamin B-6 deficiency. They may experience mental depression, high blood glucose levels, and/or general malaise. Women taking low-dose oral contraceptives can prevent or reverse these symptoms by consuming a diet with generous amounts of vitamin B-6 or by taking a modest vitamin B-6 supplement.

Antacids People often take antacids to treat indigestion or stomach discomfort. Certain antacids contain aluminum or magnesium hydroxide, which combine with phosphorus and fluoride in the gut to form salts that cannot be absorbed. Chronic use of these antacids by some people may eventually result in the loss of phosphorus from bone, possibly hastening the course of bone disease.

Laxatives Because constipation becomes more common with age, many elderly people use laxatives frequently. This practice can have negative effects on nutrition. Repeated use of certain types of laxatives can cause calcium, potassium, and fat depletion. Mineral oil should not be used as a laxative, because it prevents the absorption of fat-soluble vitamins, including vitamin D. Losses of vitamin D and minerals could be especially damaging to people with osteoporosis.

Increasing the fiber and fluid content of your diet is a safer alternative. (However, remember that very high fiber intakes may reduce mineral absorption, as we discussed in Chapter 12.) Adequate exercise can also help.

Diuretics Diuretics cause the kidneys to excrete increased amounts of sodium and water. People who suffer from edema (accumulation of water in the tissues) or hypertension may become chronic users of diuretics.

Many diuretics cause potassium to be excreted along with the sodium and water, which can lead to severe electrolyte imbalance. For this reason, physicians advise people taking certain diuretics to eat several good sources of potassium daily or take potassium supplements. People who regularly use diuretics may also become depleted in other minerals; they should be sure to ask their doctor or druggist about possible nutrient–drug interactions.

Drugs to Lower Blood Cholesterol Some medications can lower blood cholesterol by reducing the usual absorption of cholesterol-containing bile acids from the GI tract, causing them to be excreted in the feces. The body is then forced to draw from internal cholesterol to make more bile acids; this, in turn, reduces the overall blood cholesterol level. Cholestyramine is a drug commonly used for this purpose.

Such drugs carry a possible unfortunate side effect: they may block the absorption of fat-soluble vitamins A, D, E, and K, which are normally carried into the body with the bile acids. For this reason, physicians may recommend supplements containing the fat-soluble vitamins and folic acid, which is also partially lost.

Anticoagulants Cardiovascular diseases that involve a high risk of clot formation are often treated with anticoagulants (other than aspirin) to reduce the likelihood of blood cells' sticking together and blocking the artery. Omega-3 fatty acids, found in deep-water fish oil capsules, also reduce clotting. A person who consumes both may tend to bleed too easily. The unsupervised use of fish oil capsules is not recommended for anyone, much less for a person already taking anticoagulants. Eating fish while on anticoagulant therapy, by contrast, is not likely to supply enough omega-3 fatty acids to cause a bleeding problem.

Anticonvulsants Anticonvulsants, which are taken by people prone to epileptic seizures, increase the liver's capacity to metabolize and then eliminate vitamin D. Because the body needs vitamin D to absorb calcium, a calcium deficiency can occur in a person taking anticonvulsants. Therefore, people using these medications need to be sure to consume enough vitamin D or have sufficient sun exposure to make up for the losses.

Some anticonvulsants, such as Dilantin, may also interfere with the absorption of folic acid. Patients should ask their doctors whether they need supplements of folic acid to avoid megaloblastic anemia.

How Nutrients Affect Drugs

Now let's consider how nutrients can affect drug utilization. The timing of meals and levels of certain food components, such as protein, alcohol, dietary fiber, and methlyxanthines, can have major effects on drug absorption and metabolism. The following sections provide some examples of these effects. This information certainly is not complete. Rather, it is designed to make the point that nutrients can interact even with commonly used drugs. In some situations, nutrient–drug interactions can have drastic consequences (Roe, 1988).

Effects on Absorption Foods and beverages that are present in the GI tract with a medication may affect the drug's absorption. Calcium from milk can block the antibiotic tetracycline; the drug and the calcium form a complex, preventing absorption of both substances. With aspirin, food both slows down the rate of absorption and reduces the amount absorbed.

In other cases, food increases the proportion of medicine absorbed or hastens the absorption rate; Darvon, lithium, Valium, and Inderal are examples. Because drugs taken with meals stay in your stomach longer, they have more time to dissolve and get into a readily absorbable form. Also, some drugs have an irritating effect on your stomach; doctors advise taking such drugs with food, because the presence of food may lessen the irritation.

Effects on Metabolism After a drug has been absorbed, nutrients present in the body can affect the drug's metabolism. Protein is more likely to be influential in this regard: high-protein diets generally enhance drug metabolism, and low-protein diets slow drug metabolism (Roe, 1988). Excessive consumption of foods high in vitamin K, such as liver and green vegetables, can hinder the effectiveness of some anticoagulant drugs. In one case, the anticoagulant drug dicumarol was rendered ineffective because the patient customarily ate almost a pound of broccoli per day. This makes another good argument for why it is better to eat a varied diet than to eat excessive amounts of few foods—even if they are very nutritious ones.

A group of antidepressant drugs called monoamine oxidase inhibitors (examples: Parnate, Marplan, and Nardil) can interact with certain components of fermented foods (such as aged cheese) to produce a sudden elevation in blood pressure. If people taking these drugs do not avoid cheese and other offending foods, they may experience a potentially fatal hypertensive crisis. Physicians who prescribe and pharmacists who dispense these drugs are careful to educate people about which foods to avoid.

Alcohol is a dietary substance that affects the metabolism of many medications. In some instances, alcohol exaggerates the effect of a drug; in some other cases, it diminishes it. The consequences can be extreme: alcohol and certain medications can be a fatal mix.

Guidelines for Taking Medications

To avoid undesirable food–drug interactions, consumers should carefully follow instructions for use. This applies to both prescription and over-the-

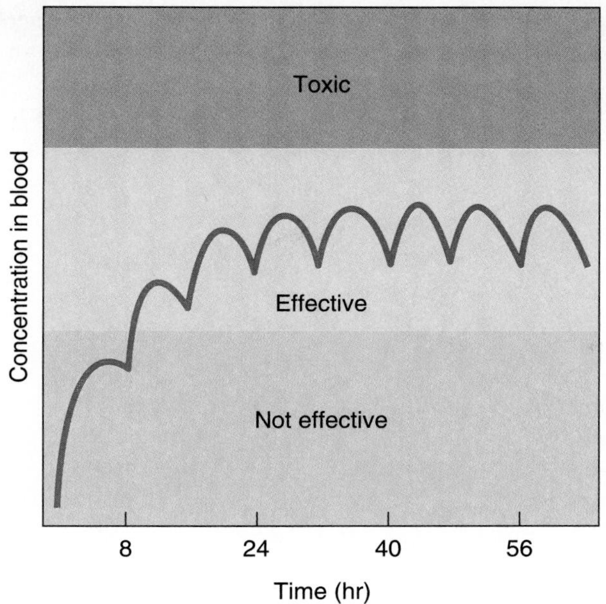

FIGURE 17.9
Medication, dose, and interval.

Medications can help only when they are in the effective range in your blood, a circumstance that depends on your taking them at the recommended amount and intervals of time. Other substances in your body—food, beverages, alcohol—can also affect whether an effective level is reached and how long it persists (see text).

counter drugs. Your doctor, a pharmacist, and product labels and package inserts are all good sources of information.

You should also adhere to the following general guidelines:

- Follow recommendations regarding dosage and timing for taking medications. This is necessary for reaching and maintaining an effective level in the body (Figure 17.9).
- Follow recommendations about whether to take the medication with meals or between meals. Taking a drug "between meals" means waiting at least 2 hours after your last meal before taking the drug and then waiting at least 1 hour before eating again.
- Find out whether any particular foods or beverages are contraindicated with particular medications you use.
- If a medication needs to be taken with a liquid, take it with a generous amount of water unless otherwise instructed. The drug will be absorbed more efficiently if it is dilute (Roe, 1988).
- If you are likely to consume alcoholic beverages during the course of drug therapy, find out whether your drug is one of the many that interacts negatively with alcohol.
- Tell your health care professionals about all medications and nutritional supplements, both prescription and over-the-counter, that you take. This is important not only for helping you avoid nutrient–drug interactions but also for avoiding drug–drug interactions.
- Eat a nutritionally balanced diet from a variety of foods. Medications cannot, by themselves, restore or maintain good health. Good nutrition is a necessary part of good health, and a balanced diet reduces the risk of drug–nutrient interactions.

Influences of Alcohol on Nutrition and Health

Alcoholic beverages have been part of human culture since ancient times. The Egyptians used wine in religious ceremonies and as a medicine; Aztec

TABLE 17.2 Alcohol and Kcalorie Content of Alcoholic Drinks[a]

Beverage	Alcohol (% by Volume)	Serving Size (Ounces)	Alcohol (Grams per Serving)	Kcalories per Serving
Beer	4.5	12	13	150
Light beer	3.7	12	11	100
Wine	11.5	5	14	110
Light wine	6–10	5	7–12	65
Wine cooler	3.5–6	12	10–17	220
Sherry	19	3	14	125
Gin, vodka, rum, rye, whiskey (80 proof)	40	1.5	14	100
Cordials, liqueurs (25–100 proof)	12.5–50	1	3–16	50–100
Martini		2.5	22	156
Bloody Mary		5	14	116
Tom Collins		7.5	16	121
Daiquiri		2	14	111

[a]All figures are for drinks without ice. One serving of any listed drink contains approximately one-half ounce of alcohol.
Source: Adapted from Tufts University Diet and Nutrition Letter, 1986

and Incan societies enjoyed an alcoholic beverage made from corn (Wotecki and Thomas, 1992). But the effects of alcohol intake are not always benign; as early as the ancient Roman civilization, the negative effects of alcohol on pregnant women were recognized. Since that time, many other effects of alcohol ingestion have been identified.

Problems with alcohol are significant in the United States, partly because of the number of people who consume alcoholic beverages. An estimated one-tenth of American adults drink heavily, one-fourth are moderate drinkers, one-third are light drinkers, and the remaining one-third abstain (National Research Council, 1989). This means that there are over 100 million adult drinkers in the United States. Consumption figures indicate that alcohol accounts for 4.5% of the energy value of the average American diet (Shaw and Lieber, 1988).

Many younger people also consume alcohol. Sixty-six percent of high school seniors interviewed by the National Institute on Alcohol Abuse and Alcoholism reported that they had consumed alcohol within the past month, and 5% said they drank daily. In another study, 37% said they had five or more drinks on at least one occasion in the previous 2 weeks (National Research Council, 1989).

Beer and ales, wines, and liquors are the common sources of alcohol. Although they differ in the percentage of alcohol they contain, a standard serving of any one of them puts approximately ½ ounce of alcohol into the consumer (Table 17.2).

The consumption of alcohol affects your body within minutes; and if ingested regularly in large amounts over a period of years, alcohol is likely to have serious long-term effects on health.

Short-Term Effects of Alcohol Consumption

Alcohol needs no digestion. It is a simple molecule that is readily absorbed and circulated through your body in the bloodstream. Like some other drugs, it can be absorbed from your stomach; whatever passes into the small intestine is readily absorbed from there. Although its own entry into your body is uncomplicated, alcohol can disturb your body's handling of foods and nutrients, and, particularly after heavy drinking, it can cause diarrhea.

Your Body's Rapid Response to Alcohol Because alcohol is a toxic substance, your body's normal reaction is to get rid of it or to metabolize it into harmless end-products. Enzymes in your stomach have the first opportunity to metabolize alcohol (Frezza et al., 1990). Your kidneys and lungs excrete predictable percentages of it, which explains why a breath test can provide a reliable measure of alcohol in the body. Your liver, which plays the major role in detoxification, begins to metabolize alcohol as quickly as it circulates through. In most people, it takes the liver anywhere from 1 to 2 hours to change ½ ounce of alcohol into harmless metabolites.

Alcohol has an anaesthetic (depressant) effect on the nervous system. First, it affects your forebrain, impairing your judgment, reducing your inhibitions, and making you feel euphoric and relaxed. If you drink more, your midbrain also becomes involved, and muscular coordination, reflexes, and speech are impaired. At even higher intakes, your hindbrain is affected: senses are dulled, and stupor results. If a person drinks so much that the part of the brain that controls vital functions is greatly depressed, a person can lose consciousness and die.

For any given person in a particular instance, the effects of alcohol depend on body size (a person with a larger body mass is less affected), the time frame within which the person drank the alcohol, other foods or beverages that were consumed, and drinking history (people who drink routinely tend to be less affected, unless they have liver damage). Over the years, various studies have shown that women are more severely affected than men (Mezey et al., 1988; Witteman et al., 1990). Recent research helps explain why: in women, enzymes in the stomach metabolize less alcohol than they do in men. Therefore, more alcohol reaches the bloodstream of a woman than of a man (Frezza et al., 1990). Because of these many variables, it is almost impossible to generalize about how many drinks it takes to reach a particular level of impairment.

Alcohol intake has an effect on food consumption. A small amount of alcohol usually stimulates your appetite and fosters social interaction. For this reason, an increasing number of hospitals and nursing homes in the United States serve a small amount of wine or beer before meals. By contrast, a large amount of alcohol depresses appetite. When alcoholic beverages displace food, nutrient intakes are likely to be low, because alcoholic beverages are poor sources of nutrients themselves. Some heavy consumers of alcohol get as much as half of their kcalories from alcohol. Alcohol can alter the metabolism of many nutrients, but moderate alcohol intake has little effect on nutritional status (Shaw and Lieber, 1988).

Strategies for Preventing Short-Term Problems from Alcohol People can *moderate*, but not eliminate, the effects of alcohol in a number of ways. If you expect to drink during a social event but do not want to experience effects beyond those of mild euphoria and elation, there are things you can do to help reduce the impact of alcohol.

First, eat something before you start drinking. The presence of any food in your stomach delays the absorption of alcohol. Second, pace your consumption so that you are not drinking faster than the rate at which your liver can detoxify the alcohol. If you limit your intake to approximately one drink per 1½ hours, you are not likely to become seriously impaired. If you are thirsty and want to drink more than that, alternate alcoholic beverages with nonalcoholic beverages; ask for just a mixer every other time. Or drink more dilute beverages, such as wine coolers (wine with sparkling water). However, be aware that "lite" beers and wines, although lower in kcalories, are not necessarily much lower in alcohol than the regular versions (Table 17.3). If you are the host or hostess, be sure that you provide an acceptable nonalcoholic alternative to your guests.

You Tell Me

At times when people have had too much to drink, they wish for a way to hurry up the rate at which their liver can detoxify alcohol. There is no such thing.

What does this say about the possibility of coffee "sobering up" a person who has drunk too much? What is the benefit of a cold shower? Exercise? Sleep?

The fact is that ounces of prevention are worth hours of cure. The best way to limit short-term consequences is to limit alcohol intake. The Dietary Guidelines recommend that a woman have no more than one drink per day; a man, no more than two. Of course, some people should have none at all: pregnant women, people intending to drive, people using certain medications, and people who are alcohol dependent. (Later in this chapter we'll offer more information about alcohol dependence.)

Long-Term Effects of Alcohol Consumption

Regular consumption of large amounts of alcohol over a period of years has damaging effects. Alcohol affects the function of many organs and systems. It can also cause nutritional deficiencies, especially in thiamin, riboflavin, niacin, folic acid, and vitamin B-6. In fact, alcohol consumption is probably the number-one cause of multinutrient deficiency in the United States (Wotecki and Thomas, 1992). Deficiencies occur because alcohol interrupts the body's normal processing of nutrients anywhere from ingestion through excretion (Watson and Watzl, 1992).

Chronic consumers of alcohol are at increased risk for the following:

- liver diseases (fatty liver, alcoholic hepatitis, cirrhosis)
- pancreatitis
- heart degeneration
- hypertension and stroke, perhaps in conjunction with job stress (Schnall et al., 1992)
- hyperlipidemia (with very high intakes)
- nervous system diseases
- cancer of the alimentary canal: mouth, pharynx, larynx, esophagus (National Research Council, 1989); colon and rectum (Henderson et al., 1991)

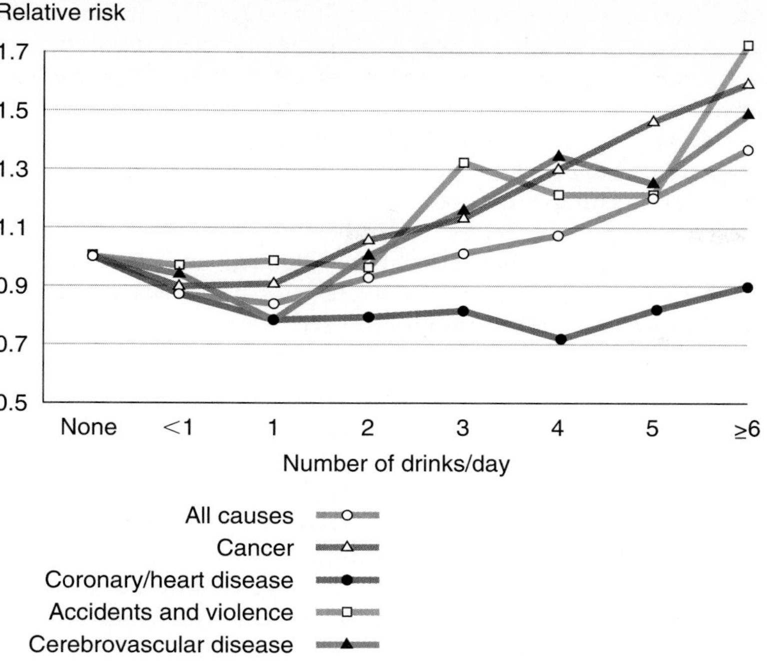

FIGURE 17.10 Relationship of habitual alcohol consumption to causes of death.

Several large studies show that at moderate levels of intake, alcohol consumption reduces risk of coronary heart disease. However, beyond two drinks per day, the risk of death from cancer, stroke, and other causes increases.

Source: Marmot and Brunner,

- osteoporosis in men (Spencer et al., 1986)
- fetal alcohol syndrome
- alcohol dependency

Some of these are discussed below.

Liver Diseases Chronic alcohol intake causes liver disease through direct toxic effects, but these effects do not totally account for the occurrence of liver disease; not everybody who regularly drinks gets liver disease. Nutrition also has an influence: the less food drinkers consume, the more likely they are to develop severe liver disease.

In the first phase of liver disease, called *fatty liver,* fat accumulates in the liver because of many alcohol-induced changes in the metabolism of energy nutrients and in fat mobilization. The second phase is *alcoholic hepatitis*—that is, inflammation of the liver. Both of these conditions can be reversed if the person avoids alcohol and follows sound health practices. **Cirrhosis,** an irreversible condition, occurs when fibrous deposits scar the liver, interfering with its function. Because the liver is the primary site for many metabolic reactions, its progressive destruction by cirrhosis can be fatal.

cirrhosis—scarring of the liver by fibrous deposits that interfere with its function; an irreversible condition

Cardiovascular Diseases Recently there has been a great deal of interest in the effect of alcohol on diseases of the cardiovascular system. Although alcohol in large amounts is known to have negative effects (see the list above), considerable recent research suggests that lesser amounts of alcohol could have beneficial effects on the cardiovascular system.

In general, scientists have found that people who drink one to four alcoholic drinks per day have lower rates of death from heart disease than those who do not consume any alcohol (Marmot and Brunner, 1991; Rimm et al., 1991; Steinberg et al., 1991; Renaud and de Lorgeril, 1992). Figure 17.10

shows drinkers' relative risk for heart disease. (Notice that the risk of various other causes of death goes up with increased drinking, however.)

What could explain this apparent effect of alcoholic beverages? The mechanisms are unclear. Several research teams suggest that alterations in blood lipids may be responsible, particularly elevations in HDL cholesterol (see Chapter 6) (Steinberg et al., 1991); but another group does not see a cardiovascular advantage in the blood lipid changes that occur (Seppa et al., 1992). Alcohol may reduce the likelihood of blood to clot, which other components of the diet may also affect (Renaud and de Lorgeril, 1992). Other substances in alcoholic beverages may be of benefit: *tannins* and *resveratrol* (a natural mold inhibitor) in red wines have been suggested as possibilities.

alcohol dependence—inability to limit the amount of alcohol consumed despite the problems it causes

Alcohol Dependence Another serious concern about alcohol intake is that some people develop **alcohol dependence** (become alcoholics). This condition does not necessarily involve the problems of physical health listed in the preceding section, although it can. The *Diagnostic and Statistical Manual of Mental Disorders (DSM-III-R)* (American Psychiatric Association, 1987) describes dependence as a condition in which a person cannot control his or her use of a psychoactive substance despite the adverse consequences it causes. It is estimated that one in ten Americans who drinks is an alcoholic.

Scientists believe that heredity as well as environment plays a role in the development of alcoholism. In 1990, a team of scientists claimed they had isolated a gene much more likely to be found in alcoholics: 78% of the alcoholic subjects in their study had this particular gene, and only 28% of those without the gene were alcoholic (Blum et al., 1990). Further work is needed to assess the relative importance of the environment and heredity in the development of alcoholism. However, knowing that there is a physical basis for alcoholism may help people who are alcoholic to accept treatment.

Once a person has a dependence, most experts believe that the only effective way to deal with the disease is for the dependent person to quit drinking. There are many drug treatment centers that help affected people and their families cope with this disease.

Live Well in the 1990s!

You create your own lifestyle, and it's up to you whether you include practices that are healthy. Public health agencies send out these messages loud and clear:

- *If you smoke, quit.* Smoking is the single most preventable cause of death in America, responsible for one death in six. Even if you gain weight when you quit (those who do usually gain less than 10 pounds), *the health benefits of not smoking* are much greater than the negative impact of the gain in weight.
- *Get regular exercise.* Get involved in activities that enhance strength, flexibility, and cardiorespiratory fitness.
- *Eat in a way that provides the nutrients you need, maintains your best weight, and reduces risk factors for disease.*
- *Get adequate sleep.* Scientists don't know exactly why we need sleep, but normal function and health deteriorate if we don't get enough.
- *Keep your psychologic stress level under control.* Although psychologists have found that a certain amount of stress is beneficial, too much is damaging.

TABLE 17.3 Nutrition Quacks Have a Familiar Sound

Their promises all sound appealing and genuine, but they are hollow. These are among the more common claims and practices of nutrition hucksters:

- Suggesting that most people are poorly nourished
- Claiming that most disease is due to faulty diet, which can be remedied by the product they sell
- Claiming that diseases for which medical science does not yet have highly effective treatment (such as AIDS and certain forms of cancer) can be cured through their nutrition program
- Claiming that emotional stress can be relieved by taking high doses of nutrients
- Recommending that everybody take vitamin and mineral supplements or eat "health" foods
- Claiming that natural vitamins are better than synthetic ones
- Claiming that megavitamins can improve the function of the immune system
- Claiming that modern processing methods and storage remove all nutritive value from our food
- Claiming that all additives and preservatives are poisons
- Warning that sugar is a deadly poison
- Telling you that it is easy to lose weight with their method
- Using anecdotes and testimonials as the only support for their claims
- Claiming that the medical establishment refuses to acknowledge their nutrition "cures" because doctors would lose business
- Displaying credentials not recognized by responsible scientists or educators

---

- *Avoid substance abuse, whether alcohol or other drugs.* If you find yourself hooked, get help. Many types of intervention programs are available as well as groups for continuing support.
- *Get medical help when you need it.*

Yearning for Easy Solutions to Difficult Problems

All of the preceding advice is undoubtedly familiar to you, but it may not seem easy to accomplish. After all, you have other things to do with your time—such as going to school, earning a living, or caring for a family—that may already make life as full as you think you can handle. You may think that you simply don't have the time for regular exercise or eating right; but the feelings of well-being you can gain from healthy living can more than make up for the time it takes.

There may be times when you will hear what seem to be easy ways to get around eating well. We remind you that there is a great deal of nutrition quackery targeted at people who hope for improvement in their lives and who are willing to spend money to get results easily when, in some cases, the results may not even be attainable. Major targets for quackery among the adult population are people who want to lose weight, people with arthritis, people with terminal illness, and healthy but fearful elderly. Table 17.3 identifies some of the popular claims of nutrition quacks and what they falsely promise nutrition can do. Knowledge is your best defense against this health fraud (Renner, 1989).

TABLE 17.4 Daily Food Intake Recommendations for Adults of All Ages

This table reemphasizes the recommendations of the Food Guide Pyramid.

Food Group	Recommended Servings	Comments
Bread, rice, cereal, and pasta	6–11	Most adults could benefit from more whole-grain breads, pastas, crackers, and cereals, because their fiber helps maintain normal intestinal function, which may diminish with age. Increase your fluid intake with an increase in fiber.
Vegetables	3–5	These are excellent sources of vitamins A and C; they also contain various anticarcinogens. When you want more to eat but do not want more fat, cholesterol, or sodium, eat more of these.
Fruits	2–4	Like vegetables, some fruits are good sources of vitamins.
Milk, yogurt, and cheese	*Through age 24 years:* 3 *Age 25 and older:* 2	If you have lactose intolerance, try cheese, low-fat yogurt, or low-lactose forms of milk.
Meat, poultry, fish, beans, eggs, and nuts	Equivalent of 5–7 oz. of meat	When you eat meat alternatives of plant origin, include a good source of vitamin C at the same meal to increase your absorption of iron.
Fats, oils, and sweets	Go easy!	Gradually reduce your intake of these, because energy needs diminish with the years. Consider some products with fat and sugar substitutes. Better yet, maintain a more active lifestyle, which has multiple benefits.

Whenever possible, eat your meals with somebody. When people share mealtime with others, they usually eat better than when they eat alone. The pleasure of someone's company at a meal adds another healthy dimension to nutrition for living.

Assuming Self-Responsibility for Nutrition

Good nutrition does not depend on eating a certain number of times per day or eating a particular amount at each meal. You might eat "three square meals" per day, or you might pick up smaller amounts more often, a practice that has been dubbed "grazing." You can nourish yourself well either way, provided your total intake follows the principles of variety, balance, and moderation that characterize a healthy diet. Table 17.4 reviews the Food Guide Pyramid recommendations for total daily intake for adults and emphasizes some points about the food groups that are especially relevant to adults.

The following sections suggest what to keep in mind in the various locations in which we make decisions about what to eat.

At the Food Store Most people still eat most meals at home, even though we eat an increasing number of meals away from home. This calls for food shopping.

According to market research, the average consumer goes to the grocery store 2.3 times per week and makes most decisions at the shelf (Opinion Research Corporation, 1989; Light et al., 1989). Knowing this, many processors use food product labels to attract consumers' attention, provide information about products, and make products seem more appealing. There also may be separate promotional/informational materials near products or at store information centers.

When considering the nutritional merits of items on the shelf, you can get the most specific information by going straight to the product's nutrition fact panel. Of less specific help are the descriptive terms printed elsewhere on the label, such as *light* or *low in cholesterol,* which now are defined by federal regulation (Congressional Federal Register, 1993). If you have medical restrictions—for example, a low-sodium diet—it may pay to learn what the descriptors *no, low, less,* and *light* mean in regard to the substance you're concerned about (see Chapters 6, 9, and 12).

An alternative to doing all of your thinking in the store is to do some planning before you go shopping. If you don't prepare food "from scratch," you may intend to do nothing more challenging than making a sandwich, pouring a glass of milk or bowl of cereal, or heating a prepared entree. If that describes you, here are some things to keep in mind when making food choices.

When looking for prepared main dishes, look for the lower fat and lower salt varieties. If these are not available where you shop, try to reduce your intake of fat and salt in your other choices for the day.

Don't bypass the fruit and vegetable section. If you do, you may be cheating yourself out of an adequate diet: it's hard to get enough vitamins A and C without these foods. Besides, fresh fruit is very easy to use; you don't even have to dirty a plate or fork to eat it. Many kinds require just washing, and others need just peeling before you eat them. If making salads is too much work for you, consider fixing frozen vegetables. Simply cook them for a few minutes on the stove top or in the microwave oven for a quick dish that may be even more nutritious than a "fresh" vegetable.

It may be that time pressure is partly responsible for how you deal with food. If that's the case, you could look for help in a book such as *Eating on the Run* (Tribole, 1992). It gives tips on how to nourish yourself well "from airline meals to microwave zapping."

If you have more time to cook, consider the ideas in the next section.

At Home Most people who cook regularly are interested in getting good-tasting, nourishing food to the table within a reasonable amount of time. They are probably also interested in the cost issue; even if you assign a cost to your time, home-cooked food usually costs less than buying a similarly prepared product. People may also prefer cooking their own food so that they can individualize the product, have control over the ingredients, and/or economize on the total energy used to produce the item (Gussow, 1988).

Some newer cookbooks incorporate many of these goals. Look for those that are designed to be compatible with the Dietary Guidelines. Such recipes will include good sources of nutrients and fiber; at the same time, they will be moderate in fat, cholesterol, salt, and sugar. Some of these cookbooks are written by nutrition professionals such as registered dietitians or nutritionists or are produced by their professional associations; others are published by health groups such as the American Heart Association.

The United States Department of Agriculture (USDA) has prepared a booklet called *Shopping for Food and Making Meals in Minutes* that offers some quick and good recipes (United States Department of Agriculture, Human Nutrition Information Service No. 232-10). In addition, magazines such as *Cooking Light* and *Eating Well* are dedicated to a nutritious eating style that provide you with more than enough new recipes; they often feature foods of interesting ethnic origins and take advantage of seasonal foods. Even some professional chefs have cooperated with health experts and produced a recipe booklet *Resetting the American Table,* "a new approach to eating that tastes good and is good for you" (The American Institute of Wine & Food, 1992).

If you have favorite recipes, you may now suspect that some do not fit well with the dietary principles for good health. Does this mean that you should throw away the whole lot? Not at all. Some recipes may be fine as they are (for example, ¼ cup of fat in a dessert recipe that serves 8 people is hardly a problem). Some recipes might be high in fat, sugar, and/or salt, but these foods may be important family traditions; if you don't have them often or eat much of them, they won't affect your overall nutrition significantly.

Finally, you may be able to modify some recipes that are staples for you. In casserole dishes, you can often cut down or eliminate added fat. In baked goods, you may be able to cut fat by one-fourth to one-third of the original amount; the same often can be done for sugar, and even larger cutbacks may be possible for salt. You can increase fiber by substituting whole-grain pasta, rice, and other grains and flour. If you plan to do much recipe modification, get a good set of guidelines for doing so; some products will tolerate change better than others (Stark, 1988).

The Slice of Life on page 589 describes a system two sisters developed for preparing good-tasting, healthy food for their own families and their parents—all in a way that was enjoyable, economical, and time-efficient.

In Your Briefcase or Backpack It would be very difficult to obtain a good diet for the whole day from foods that can be carried easily, can be eaten by hand, and can do without refrigeration for several hours; but some foods pack quite well. Fresh fruit, dried fruit, and juice boxes are very portable. So are crackers, bagels, and pretzels. Nuts, seeds, and cereals also qualify. You can combine a variety of dried fruit, cereal, pretzels, and smaller amounts of nuts and seeds into a mix.

At Your Worksite Employers are interested in enhancing the health of their employees. In a survey of private-sector employers with more than 50 employees, 66% had offered one or more of the following types of pro-

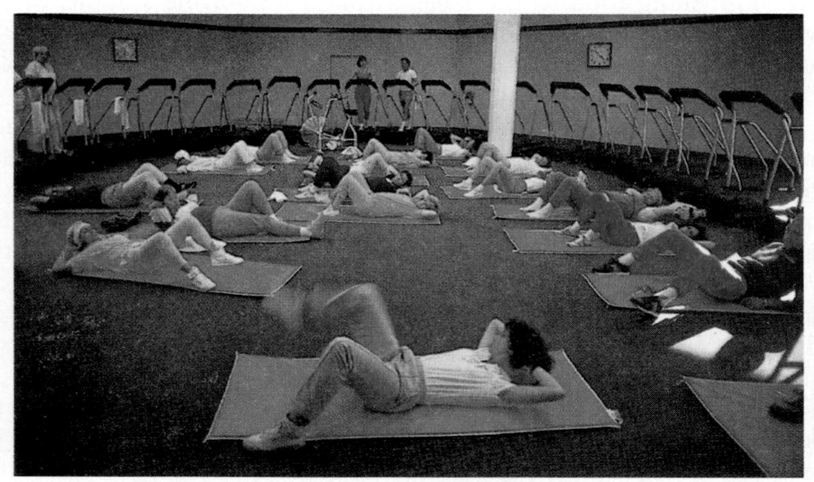

FIGURE 17.11
Lifestyle improvement in the workplace.

Increasing numbers of employers are providing facilities in which their workers can exercise, get nutritious meals, and learn about stress reduction. Such programs can benefit both employees and employers.

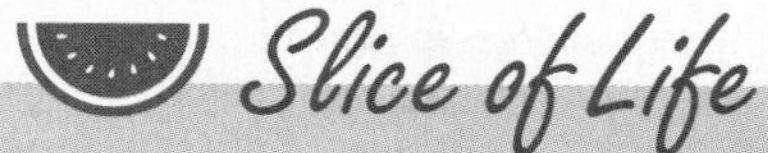

Benefits of a Family Food Factory

Paulette Smith and Patty Paulson are sisters; each is married and has children. They have found they can double both flavor and fun when they team up in the kitchen. Every Wednesday, they spend the day shopping, cooking, and planning menus for the following week. By the end of the day, they have packed four tasty and nutritious entrees, in quantities large enough to serve their families and their parents, into reusable food containers. Then the freezer-ready creations are labeled, dated, and delivered.

"With leftovers, we have enough food prepared to last all week," Patty said. "That's important to me because the reason I don't work (out of the home) is so I can be with my kids. I don't want to be intensely involved in the kitchen when they are home. But on the weekend we like to make something fresh, not from the freezer. That's when we grill hamburgers or cook a roast."

The Wednesday cooking project originated as a Christmas gift to their parents. "We were looking for something original, although neither one of us likes cooking that much." But their mother likes cooking even less, and their dad is supposed to be on a special diet, so they thought their idea could help. By choosing recipes carefully, they have found foods that fit their dad's diet and that everybody likes. This is quite an achievement, because they are feeding three generations.

Their recipes come from a variety of cookbooks and magazines that feature healthy cooking, such as *Living Fit* magazine and *Jane Brody's Good Food Book.* "We adapt all our recipes. We take a basic idea and make it simpler. We look for low-calorie, low-cholesterol recipes," Paulette said. "And we always double the vegetables." Each weekly menu includes beef, chicken, fish, and vegetarian entrees. (One of the children has chosen to be a vegetarian.)

Many of the entrees include vegetables such as beans, peppers, and tomatoes, which both sisters grow in their own gardens and freeze for year-round use. They supplement their own supply with produce from the Farmers' Market. Of course, there is more shopping to do.

"We meet at Woodman's Food Market, and we have our system down so well, we shoot through the store," Patty said. But the Wednesday cooking bees aren't all work. "We have fun, and we get a chance to catch up on the latest while we get our week's cooking out of the way," Patty said.

Adapted from *The Wisconsin State Journal,* May 27, 1990.

grams within the last 5 years: smoking cessation, general health risk assessment, care of the back, coping with stress, exercise, accident prevention, nutrition education, blood pressure control, and weight control (Fielding and Piserchia, 1989).

Having a positive attitude about health promotion, most employers are willing to listen to suggestions for improvement in their on-site food service, which could be anything from a vending machine to a full cafeteria line. If the available food does not provide for healthy choices, find out who makes decisions about the food service within your organization and talk with them. They are likely to listen, because employers know that sick employees cost them money.

Some employers actually seek employee opinion: one innovative program in the public sector involved having firefighters taste-test recipes that were lower in fat, cholesterol, and sodium than their usual fare. As a result, the men learned about the potential benefits of these changes in diet, and they began to use new recipes at the firehouse.

At Restaurants When ordering from a restaurant menu, select foods prepared by methods that retain nutrients and minimize fat, such as broiling, baking, poaching, grilling, stir-frying, and steaming. It is better to avoid frequent consumption of things that are described as deep-fried, creamed, battered, or rich, or served with gravy, cheese sauce, hollandaise sauce, or pastry. Sometimes a restaurant will accommodate special requests for people on modified diets; for example, omitting the salt on broiled meat or fish is an easy way to satisfy a customer.

TABLE 17.5 Making Healthy Choices in Ethnic Restaurants

Positive Choices	Cautions
Italian	
Minestrone soup	Antipasto plates
Breadsticks	Buttered garlic bread
Vinegar and oil dressing	Creamy Italian dressing
Pasta with red sauce such as marinara	Creamy white or butter sauce, such as Alfredo
Chicken cacciatore	Italian sausage
Cappuccino	Italian ice cream
Chinese	
Wonton soup	
Hot and sour soup	Fried wontons
Beef with broccoli	Egg rolls
Chicken, scallops, or shrimp with vegetables	Sweet and sour pork or shrimp
Steamed rice	Lemon chicken
	Peking duck
Mexican	
Black bean soup, menudo	Guacamole dip with taco chips
Salsa	Sour cream and cheese
Soft, plain tortillas	Crispy, fried tortillas
Burritos, soft tacos, enchiladas, tamales	Tacos, refried beans, tostadas, chile rellenos, quesadillas

Source: Adapted from The American Dietetic Association, 1990.

Soup and salad bars, healthy as they sound, call for careful selection as well. Enjoy all the fresh vegetables and fruit you want, but go easy on the fat. A low-fat or low-kcalorie salad dressing is a better choice. Broth-based soups are a better choice than creamed soups, but both are quite salty. If salt is of concern to you, have only a small portion of soup.

Ethnic restaurants can provide healthful and adventurous eating, but you still need to keep the principles of good nutrition in mind. There is no cuisine that gets a blanket recommendation for good nutrition: every cuisine seems to have some items that are stellar examples of healthy food but others that are higher in fat, cholesterol, or salt than is recommended. Table 17.5 gives examples of better choices from three cuisines.

A booklet published by the USDA, *Eating Better When Eating Out* (United States Department of Agriculture, Human Nutrition Information Service No. 232-11), provides many other suggestions for restaurant eating. Some restaurants have gained the privilege of using the seal of the American Heart Association (AHA) on menu items that are low in fat and cholesterol. You can call your local AHA office to find out which restaurants in your area provide that service.

From Carry-Out Places Carry-out foods are increasing in popularity faster than any other type of food service. More and more people want to eat at home but not cook. Of course, the same nutritional principles we have discussed above for selecting food in other settings apply here as well.

There is increasing variety in the foods available to carry out. Of course, there's the usual fast-food fare, but you might also find Asian or Cajun take-out. There are standard chilled delicatessen foods prepared on-site, as well as the newer commercially prepared *sous-vide* (chilled and vacuum-packed) items that might be held under refrigeration for a couple of weeks before they are consumed.

Food safety may be a special concern for some of these foods, because the opportunity for microbiologic contamination of mixed or cooked items is always greater and because these foods may be in and out of the temperature danger zone a number of times before they are eaten. Furthermore, because a few types of pathogenic microorganisms thrive even at refrigerator temperatures, items held under refrigeration for long periods (such as sous-vide products) could become sources of foodborne illness. A cautious approach when using such foods would be to buy only as much as you expect to eat at the upcoming meal. It is expected that future standards for production of these foods will provide greater confidence about microbiologic safety.

From the discussion above, you can see that there are healthy food options to suit a variety of lifestyles. By devoting a small amount of time to choosing your foods wisely, you can make sure the foods you eat meet your health goals.

Summary

- Nutrition, along with other lifestyle factors, affects health during the adult years; these practices assume greater importance as the likelihood of our living longer increases. Although genetic influences are also involved, lifelong habits of nutrition can modify health and longevity within inherited limits. Because of the cumulative effects of lifestyle practices, there are greater differences among the health conditions of elderly adults than among those of any other age peers.

- The changes of aging take place gradually, and their rate and sequence vary in different individuals. The nutrition-related effects include a decreased need for energy, and possible changes in digestion, absorption, and metabolism of nutrients. More research is needed to clarify these changes and the specific nutrient needs that result from them.

- Some of the health problems seen in some adults are atherosclerosis, cancer, constipation, diverticular disease, diabetes, obesity, hypertension, osteoporosis, **periodontal disease, arthritis,** and **dementia.** Infectious diseases are becoming greater problems, as the incidence of AIDS and tuberculosis increase. Nutrition is one of the factors that plays a role in the development and the course of many of these conditions.

- Every species of animals, including humans, has a **maximum life span,** which appears to be set genetically. **Life expectancy,** or **average life span,** is the statistical average length of life for a given group of animals, and **longevity** is the length of time an individual actually lives. Nutrition may play a role in determining life expectancy and longevity, although no scientifically valid studies have ever shown that supplements or special foods will prolong human life more than an ordinary well-balanced diet.

- Medications can influence nutrition by affecting appetite, the absorption of nutrients, their metabolism, and/or excretion. Individuals who use any drug for a long period of time, who use several drugs in combination, or who have marginal nutritional status are at greatest risk of drug-induced nutritional problems. Examples of commonly used drugs that can have consequences for nutrition are aspirin, oral contraceptives, antacids, laxatives, diuretics, cholesterol-lowering drugs, anticoagulants, and anticonvulsants. Nutrients can also affect drug utilization. Nutrient–drug interactions can be minimized by eating a balanced diet and carefully following the instructions for use of medications.

- Alcohol is a widely used drug that can influence short-term and long-term health both by affecting nutrition and by producing direct toxic effects on the body. People who use alcohol heavily over long periods of time are much more likely to suffer health problems, including liver diseases such as **cirrhosis,** heart problems, and alcoholism; genetics also plays a role. Treatment is available for people with indications of **alcohol dependence.**

- Research shows that adopting practices such as adequate exercise, good nutrition, and refraining from smoking pays you back in better health and possibly also longer life. There are no short-cuts to good health, although quacks are eager to exchange their empty promises for your money.
- No matter how many meals you eat per day or where you get your food, you can eat in a healthful way. Learning how to make better choices at the grocery store, at home, at work, at restaurants, and on the run can help equip you for doing what you want to do in life.

References

American Dietetic Association. 1990. *Healthful eating all around town.* Chicago, IL: The American Dietetic Association.

American Institute of Wine & Food. 1992. *Resetting the American table.* San Francisco, CA: The American Institute of Wine & Food.

American Psychiatric Association. 1987. *Diagnostic and statistical manual of mental disorders. Third edition-revised (DSM-III-R).* Washington, DC: The American Psychiatric Association.

Astrand, P.O. 1992. Physical activity and fitness. *American Journal of Clinical Nutrition* 55(Supplement): 1231S–1236S.

Balsam, A.L., J.M. Carlin, and B.L. Rogers. 1992. Weekend home-delivered meals in elderly nutrition programs. *Journal of the American Dietetic Association* 92: 1125–1127.

Blair, S.N., H.W. Kohl, R.S. Paffenbarger, D.G. Clark, K.H. Cooper, and L.W. Gibbons. 1989. Physical fitness and all-cause mortality: A prospective study of healthy men and women. *Journal of the American Medical Association* 262:2395–2401.

Blum, K., E.P. Noble, P.J. Sheridan, A. Montgomery, T. Ritchie, P. Jagadeeswaran, H. Nogami, A.H. Briggs, and J.B. Cohn. 1990. Allelic association of human dopamine D-2 receptor gene in alcoholism. *Journal of the American Medical Association* 263:2055–2060.

Blumberg, J.B. 1992. Dietary antioxidants and aging. *Contemporary Nutrition* 17(no.3). Minneapolis: General Mills.

Bollet, A.J. 1988. Nutrition and diet in rheumatic disorders. In *Modern nutrition in health and disease,* ed. M.E. Shils and V.R. Young. Philadelphia: Lea & Febiger.

Browner, W.S., J. Westenhouse, and J.A. Tice. 1991. What if Americans ate less fat? *Journal of the American Medical Association* 265:3285–3291.

Chandra, R.K. 1989. Nutritional regulation of immunity and risk of infection in old age. *Immunology* 67:141–147.

Chernoff, R. 1991. *Geriatric nutrition.* Gaithersburg, MD: Aspen Publishers.

Congressional Federal Register. 1993. Food labeling regulations. Washington, DC: *Congressional Federal Register,* January 6, 1993.

Dwyer, J.T., R.L. Bye, P.L. Holt, and S.R. Lauze. 1988. Unproven nutrition therapies for AIDS: What is the evidence? *Nutrition Today* 23(no.2):25–33.

Evans, W. and I.H. Rosenberg. 1991. *Biomarkers: The 10 determinants of aging you can control.* New York: Simon & Schuster.

Fielding, J.E. and P.V. Piserchia. 1989. Frequency of worksite health promotion activities. *American Journal of Public Health* 79:16–20.

Flieger, K. 1988. Why do we age? *FDA Consumer,* October, 1988:20–25.

Frezza, M., C. DiPadova, G. Pozzato, M. Terpin, E. Baraona, and C.S. Lieber. 1990. High blood alcohol levels in women. *New England Journal of Medicine* 322:95–99.

Good, R.A. and E. Lorenz. 1988. Nutrition, immunity, aging, and cancer. *Nutrition Reviews* 46(no.2):62–67.

Gray, G. 1989. Nutrition and dementia. *Journal of the American Dietetic Association* 89:1795–1802.

Greger, J.L. 1989. Potential for trace mineral toxicities and deficiencies in the elderly. *Current Topics in Nutrition and Disease* 21:171–199.

Greger, J.L. 1993. Aluminum metabolism. *Annual Review of Nutrition* 13:43–63.

Gussow, J.D. 1988. Does cooking pay? *Journal of Nutrition Education* 20:221–226.

Henderson, B.E., R.K. Ross, and M.C. Pike. 1991. Toward the primary prevention of cancer. *Science* 254: 1131–1138.

Heymsfield, S.B., J. Wang, S. Lichtman, Y. Kamen, J. Kehayias, and R.N. Pierson, Jr. 1989. Body composition in elderly subjects: A critical appraisal of clinical methodology. *American Journal of Clinical Nutrition* 50:1167–1175.

Hooper, C. 1992. Encircling a mechanism in Alzheimer's disease. *The Journal of NIH Research* 4:48–54.

Human Nutrition Information Service (HNIS). 1988. *Nationwide food consumption survey: Continuing survey of food intakes by individuals.* Washington, DC: United States Department of Agriculture.

Jarvis, W.T. 1990. Arthritis: Folk remedies and quackery. *Nutrition Forum* 7(no.1):1–8.

Kinsella, K.G. 1992. Changes in life expectancy 1900–1990. *American Journal of Clinical Nutrition* 55(Supplement):1196S–1202S.

Landesman, S.H. 1993. Commentary: Tuberculosis in New York City—the consequences and lessons of failure. *American Journal of Public Health* 83:766–767.

Leaf, A. 1988. The aging process: Lessons from observations in man. *Nutrition Reviews* 46(no.2):40–44.

Light, L., B. Portnoy, J.E. Blair, J.M. Smith, A.B. Rodgers, E. Tuckermanty, J. Tenney, and O. Mathews. 1989. Nutrition education in supermarkets. *Family and Community Health* 12(no.1):43–52.

Marmot, M. and E. Brunner. 1991. Alcohol and cardiovascular disease: The status of the U-shaped curve. *British Medical Journal* 303:565–567.

Marx, J. 1990. NGF and Alzheimer's: Hopes and fears. *Science* 247:408–410.

Masoro, E.J. 1992. Retardation of aging processes by food restriction: An experimental tool. *American Journal of Clinical Nutrition* 55(Supplement):1250S–1252S.

Mazess, R.B. and S.H. Forman. 1979. Longevity and age exaggeration in Vilcabamba, Ecuador. *Journal of Gerontology* 34:94–98.

McGandy, R.B., C.H. Barrows, A. Spanias, A. Meredith, J.L. Stone, and A.H. Norris. 1966. Nutrient intakes and energy expenditure in men of different ages. *Journal of Gerontology* 21:581–587.

Meydani, S.N., M. Meydani, and P.M. Barklund. 1989. Effect of vitamin E supplementation on immune responsiveness of the aged. *Annals of the New York Academy of Sciences* 510:283–290.

Mezey, E., C.J. Kolman, A.M. Diehl, M.C. Mitchell, and H.F. Herlong. 1988. Alcohol and dietary intake in the development of chronic pancreatitis and liver disease in alcoholism. *American Journal of Clinical Nutrition* 48:148–151.

Monti, D., L. Troiano, F. Tropea, E. Grassilli, A. Cossarizza, D. Barozzi, M.C. Pelloni, M.G. Tamassia, G. Bellomo, and C. Franceschi. 1992. Apoptosis—programmed cell death: A role in the aging process? *American Journal of Clinical Nutrition* 55(Supplement):1208S–1215S.

National Center for Health Statistics. 1977. *Dietary intake findings: United States, 1971–74.* Data from the National Health Survey, Series II, No. 202. DHEW Publications No. [HRA]77-1647. Hyattsville, MD: Public Health Service.

National Research Council. 1989. *Diet and health.* Washington, DC: National Academy Press.

Opinion Research Corporation. 1989. Trends: Consumer attitudes and the supermarket—1989. Washington, DC: Food Marketing Institute.

Paffenbarger, R.S., R.T. Hyde, A.L. Wing, and C.C. Hsieh. 1986. Physical activity, all-cause mortality, and longevity of college alumni. *New England Journal of Medicine* 314:605–613.

Pivonka, E.E. and K.K. Grunewald. 1990. Aspartame- or sugar-sweetened beverages: Effects on mood in young women. *Journal of the American Dietetic Association* 90:250–254.

RDA Subcommittee. 1989. *Recommended dietary allowances.* Washington, DC: National Academy of Sciences.

Renaud, S. and M. de Lorgeril. 1992. Wine, alcohol, platelets, and the French paradox for coronary heart disease. *Lancet* 339:1523–1526.

Renner, J.H. 1989. Knowledge best defense against health fraud. *Food and Nutrition News* 61(no.4):21–23.

Rimm, E.B., E.L. Giovannucci, W.C. Willett, G.A. Colditz, A. Ascherio, B. Rosner, and M.J. Stampfer. 1991. Prospective study of alcohol consumption and risk of coronary disease in men. *Lancet* 338:464–468.

Roe, D.A. 1988. Diet, nutrition and drug reactions. In *Modern nutrition in health and disease,* ed. M.E. Shils and V.R. Young. Philadelphia: Lea & Febiger.

Roe, D.A. 1989. Nutritional surveillance of the elderly: Methods to determine program impact and unmet need. *Nutrition Today* 24(no.5):24–29.

Roe, D.A. 1992. *Geriatric nutrition.* Englewood Cliffs, NJ: Prentice Hall.

Rosenberg, I. 1991. Nutrition and aging. In *Nutrition in the '90s,* ed. G.E. Gaull, F.N. Kotsonis, and M.A. Mackey. New York: Marcel Dekker, Inc.

Rosenberg, I.H. and J.W. Miller. 1992. Nutritional factors in physical and cognitive functions of elderly people. *American Journal of Clinical Nutrition* 55(Supplement):1237S–1243S.

Rowe, J.W. and R.L. Kahn. 1987. Human aging: Usual and successful. *Science* 237:143–149.

Russell, R.M. 1992. Changes in gastrointestinal function attributed to aging. *American Journal of Clinical Nutrition* 55(Supplement):1203S–1207S.

Ryan, A.S., G.A. Martinez, J.L. Wysong, and M.A. Davis. 1989. Dietary patterns of older adults in the United States, NHANES II 1976–1980. *American Journal of Human Biology* 1:321–330.

Schiffman, S.S. 1991. Taste and smell losses with age. *Contemporary Nutrition* 16(no.2). Minneapolis: General Mills.

Schnall, P.L., J.E. Schwartz, P.A. Landsbergis, K. Warren, and T.G. Pickering. 1992. Relation between job strain, alcohol, and ambulatory blood pressure. *Hypertension* 19:488–494.

Seppa, K., P. Sillanaukee, T. Pitkajarvi, M. Nikkila, and T. Koivula. 1992. Moderate and heavy alcohol consumption have no favorable effect on lipid values. *Archives of Internal Medicine* 152:297–300.

Shaw, S. and C.S. Lieber. 1988. Nutrition and diet in alcoholism. In *Modern nutrition in health and disease,* ed. M.E. Shils and V.R. Young. Philadelphia: Lea & Febiger.

Spencer, H., N. Rubio, E. Rubio, M. Indreika, and A. Seitam. 1986. Chronic alcoholism: Frequently overlooked cause of osteoporosis in men. *The American Journal of Medicine* 80:393–397.

Stark, C. 1988. Revitalize your recipes for better health. *Food for Health,* April 1988. Ithaca, NY: Cornell Cooperative Extension.

Steinberg, D., T.A. Pearson, and L.H. Kuller. 1991. Alcohol and atherosclerosis. *Annals of Internal Medicine* 114:967–976.

Stone, R. 1986. Aging in the eighties, age 65 years and over—use of community services. *Advancedata* 124:1–5.

Task Force on Nutrition Support in AIDS. 1989. Guidelines for nutrition support in AIDS. *Nutrition Today* 24(no.4):27–33.

Tribole, E. 1992. *Eating on the run.* Champaign, IL: Leisure Press.

Tufts University Diet and Nutrition Letter. 1986. To drink or not to drink? That's one of the questions. *Tufts University Diet and Nutrition Letter* 4(no.4):4.

United States Department of Agriculture, Human Nutrition Information Service. *Shopping for food & making meals in minutes.* Home and Garden Bulletin No. 232-10. Washington, DC: U.S. Government Printing Office.

United States Department of Agriculture, Human Nutrition Information Service. *Eating better when eating out.* Home and Garden Bulletin No. 121-11. Washington, DC: U.S. Government Printing Office.

Vaughan, L., F. Zurlo, and E. Ravussin. 1991. Aging and energy expenditure. *American Journal of Clinical Nutrition* 53:821–825.

Watson, R.R. and B. Watzl, eds. 1992. *Nutrition and alcohol.* Boca Raton, FL: CRC Press.

Weindruch, R. and R.L. Wilford. 1988. The retardation of aging and disease by dietary restriction. Springfield, IL: Charles C. Thomas.

White, J.V., J.T. Dwyer, B.M. Posner, R.J. Ham, D.A. Lipschitz, and N.S. Wellman. 1992. Nutrition Screening Initiative: Development and implementation of the public awareness checklist and screening tools. *Journal of the American Dietetic Association* 92:163–167.

Widdowson, E.M. 1992. Physiological processes of aging: Are there special nutritional requirements for elderly people? Do McCay's findings apply to humans? *American Journal of Clinical Nutrition* 55(Supplement): 1246S–1250S.

Witteman, J.C., W.C. Willett, M.J. Stampfer, G.A. Colditz, F.J. Kok, F.M. Sacks, F.E. Speizer, B. Rosner, and C.H. Hennekens. 1990. Relation of moderate alcohol consumption and risk of systemic hypertension in women. *American Journal of Cardiology* 65:633–637.

Wolman, P.G. 1987. Management of patients using unproven regimens for arthritis. *Journal of the American Dietetic Association* 87:1211–1214.

Work, J.A. 1989. Strength training: A bridge to independence for the elderly. *The physician and sports medicine* 17(no.11):135–138.

Wotecki, C.E. and P.R. Thomas. 1992. *Eat for life.* Washington, DC: The National Academy Press.

Zheng, J.J. and I.H. Rosenberg. 1989. What is the nutritional status of the elderly? *Geriatrics* 44(no.6):57–64.

IN THIS CHAPTER

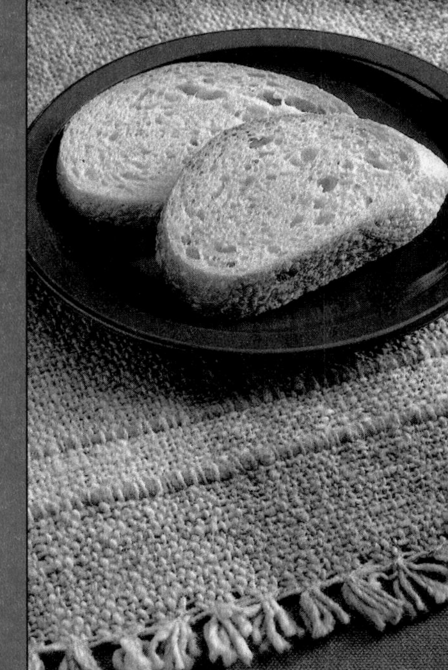

Chapter 18

Expanding Your Concerns

Throughout this book, the emphasis has been largely personal. We've discussed what nutrients do for *you* and which foods provide them. And we've urged you to consider whether you need to make some changes in *your* eating habits to improve *your* health. We've never questioned whether the right kinds and adequate amounts of food were available to you; we've simply assumed that you have access to a varied and plentiful supply.

Fortunately, most of you *do* have the food you need. But for many others, there is no guarantee that there will be enough to eat today, tomorrow, or the next day.

This situation causes some people constant concern about whether they will have the energy they need to carry out daily activities and whether their children will have enough food to grow, learn, and function well. For the most deprived of all, the amount of food available today will make the ultimate difference between life and death. You have seen their pictures on TV and in the print media, looking at you from places like Somalia and Bosnia . . . and from the rural areas and inner cities of America.

Now that you know the devastating effects of undernutrition, it's time to look beyond your own circumstances and focus on people who don't have enough to eat. The problem will not go away. It is the cause of incredible suffering, and we are losing valuable human resources because of it. Furthermore, we need to choose solutions wisely, because if our methods are short-sighted, they may irreparably damage the natural systems that affect the well-being—in fact, the very survival—of us all.

The challenge of adequately feeding the world's people involves not only agricultural issues but also environmental, political, economic, educational, and health care matters. The topic is so vast and multidimensional that this chapter can provide only a brief introduction to some of the major elements involved. Although the issues are intertwined, we will organize them into discussions of factors that affect food production, food demand, and food distribution.

But first, let's look at the extent of the problem.

How Many People Have Too Little Food?

It is very difficult to say with accuracy how many people in the world do not have enough to eat. There are many challenges in defining the condition and estimating how many are affected.

You also see different terms used. The word *hunger,* with a vague meaning, is in common use. *Undernutrition* can be defined in more precise, clinical terms, but it is also used in a very general way. Experts usually use the term **food insecurity,** which means not having enough food for normal health and physical activity (Unklesbay, 1992). When you see any of these terms in this chapter, think of the definition of food insecurity.

food insecurity—not having enough food for normal health and physical activity

Food insecurity may be ongoing or intermittent. An example of the intermittent condition is a poor farmer who has adequate food during much of the year but experiences serious shortage before the harvest. Intermittent food insecurity also occurs in developed countries, for example, when people receiving government food assistance run out of money before their next check arrives. To have **food security,** by contrast, you must have assurance of ongoing, safe, nutritionally adequate, and affordable food obtainable through ordinary channels.

food security—having enough to eat now and being assured of having enough in the future

Estimates of the number of people who don't have enough to eat are staggering. At the low end of the range, the World Bank estimates that about

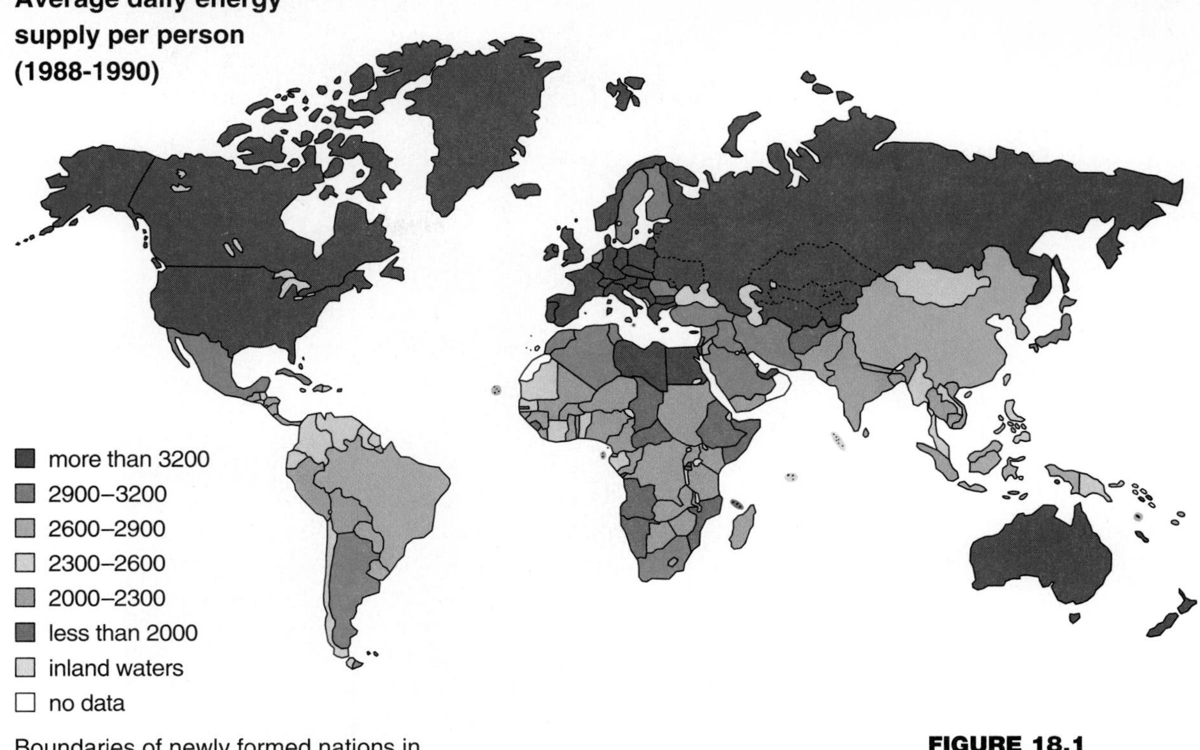

FIGURE 18.1
Hunger and glut.

The world's food supplies are very unevenly divided among countries. This map shows the difference between those countries in which people are likely to have largely enough to eat (blue, dark green, light green); those in which the average daily kcalorie supply is lower (yellow); and those in which hunger and malnutrition are most likely to be widespread (orange). The most seriously affected countries, in which the daily intake is less than 2000 kcalories per person, are colored red.

Source: Food and Agriculture Organization, 1992.

100 million of the world's 5.2 billion people are food insecure (Unklesbay, 1992). A (ten-fold higher!) estimate is that well over 1 billion of the world's people are malnourished (World Resources Institute, 1992). United Nations data put the number at approximately 800,000 (United Nations ACC/SCN, 1992).

Figure 18.1 shows where people experience food insecurity and where it is most severe. The United Nations Food and Agriculture Organization estimated in 1992 that 33% of the people in Africa are chronically undernourished, as are 19% in the Far East, 13% in Latin America, and 12% in the Near to Middle East.

Keep in mind that the map in Figure 18.1 refers to *average consumption data;* some people within a population get far less than the average to eat. The United States provides an example: although average consumption indicates that we are actually overfed as a nation, some Americans are hungry. How many Americans are affected? In the United States, the assumption is that all people living below the *official poverty line* are hungry. This means that in 1991, when the U.S. Census Bureau reported that 35.7 million Americans were living in poverty, 14.2% of us were hungry.

Some experts believe that this figure underrepresents hunger in America, because many people with incomes at or above the official poverty line seek emergency food aid (Clancy and Bowering, 1992). However, others point out that most people who are called "hungry" in the United States are not as nutritionally deprived as most "hungry" people in the developing countries (Foster, 1992). To get a better estimate, questions regarding how often and for how long people are without food will be added to future U.S. nutrition surveys (Briefel and Wotecki, 1992).

FIGURE 18.2
Hunger in the midst of plenty.

Even in the developed countries, where average intakes of food are more than adequate, some members of the population do not have enough to eat.

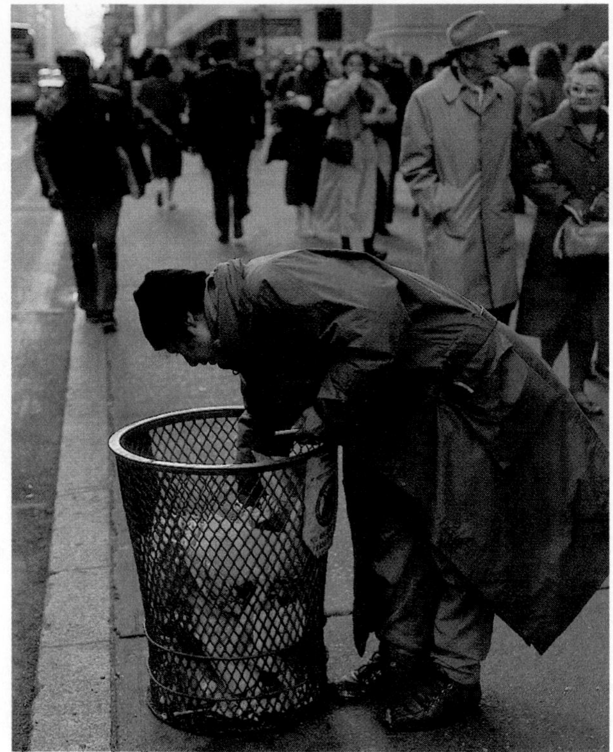

To summarize: despite many difficulties in quantifying the problem, both in the United States and around the world, it is clear that some degree of food insecurity affects large numbers of people. Worldwide, estimates suggest that as many as one in five of us do not have enough to eat.

Now let's look at factors that affect food production.

What It Takes to Produce Food

Our early ancestors were hunter-gatherers who relied on nature to supply their food. An environment with suitable natural resources was necessary for plant growth which, in turn, supported animal and human life.

Now, population pressures in most parts of the world call for farming that will yield more food than nature can provide unassisted. The basic production resources are still vital, but in addition, new agricultural technologies are needed to increase food production.

Basic Agricultural Production Resources

Four environmental resources are needed for producing food: land, water, climate, and energy. If any one of these is inadequate or unsuitable, less food can be grown.

arable land—soil fit for cultivation

Land For food production, land needs to be **arable;** that is, it must have sufficient topsoil containing the chemical substances that plants need.

There is a limited amount of arable land, and the great majority of high-quality land is already in use. Those areas that are now being brought into production are offset by other land going out of agricultural use (we discuss this topic further later in the chapter). Land that is only marginal for food production—such as steep hillsides—cannot provide much help; once

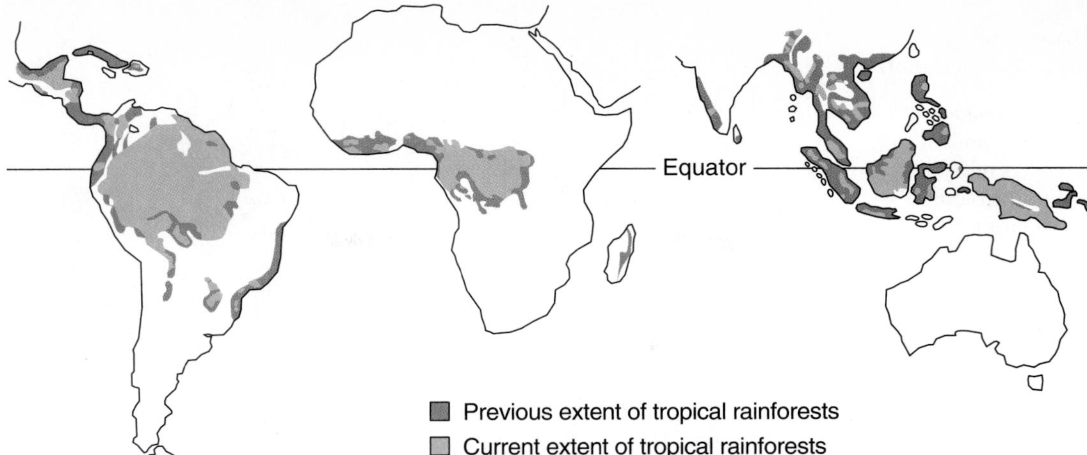

FIGURE 18.3
Tropical deforestation: so what if the trees disappear?

Although clearing the rainforest temporarily provides land for farming and ranching, it adds to the serious long-term problems of land depletion and erosion, global warming, and decrease in biologic diversity.
Source: Smithsonian Institution, 1988.

it is cleared, wind and water erosion quickly remove the topsoil, and the land soon becomes useless for farming.

The land of the tropical rainforest is marginal as well; nonetheless, poor farmers go there to clear land, establish homes, and eke out a living for their families. After just a few years of intense cultivation, the topsoil becomes so depleted and eroded that it is no longer sufficiently productive. Farmers then stake out another area of forest, clear it, and use it until it, too, fails to provide subsistence. Rainforest areas are also cleared for cattle ranching. Between 1961 and 1978, 39% of forests and woodlands in Brazil and Central America were slashed and burned for this reason (Brown et al., 1992).

Tropical deforestation impacts the entire globe. One effect, discussed in the section on climate, is that the burning and loss of trees results in an increase in carbon dioxide (CO_2) in the atmosphere. Deforestation also brings about a reduction in *biologic diversity;* that is, it causes the extinction of some plants and animals more rapidly than would occur naturally (Ryan, 1992). It has been found that many extinct forms of plants and animals played crucial roles in natural systems. This can have practical consequences to farmers, for example, if natural predators of crop pests are eliminated.

How extensive is rainforest destruction? The World Resources Institute estimates that each year, 17 million hectares—an area the size of the state of Washington—are cleared. Overall, tropical rainforests have been reduced by nearly half their original area (Ryan, 1992). Figure 18.3 shows where the losses have occurred.

You Tell Me

Figure 18.1 shows where hunger is most serious. Figure 18.3 shows where the rainforest has been lost. Note that hunger and environmental degradation are often seen together.

Which condition probably came first? How can each affect the other?

Because the use of marginal land cannot increase food production in the long term, emphasis must be put on sustaining the productivity of land of good quality. A major villain that destroys land is erosion of topsoil. Experts

FIGURE 18.4
Desertification in the Sahel.

In the sub-Saharan region of Africa, overgrazing and cutting down trees have resulted in losses of topsoil that could have supported crops.

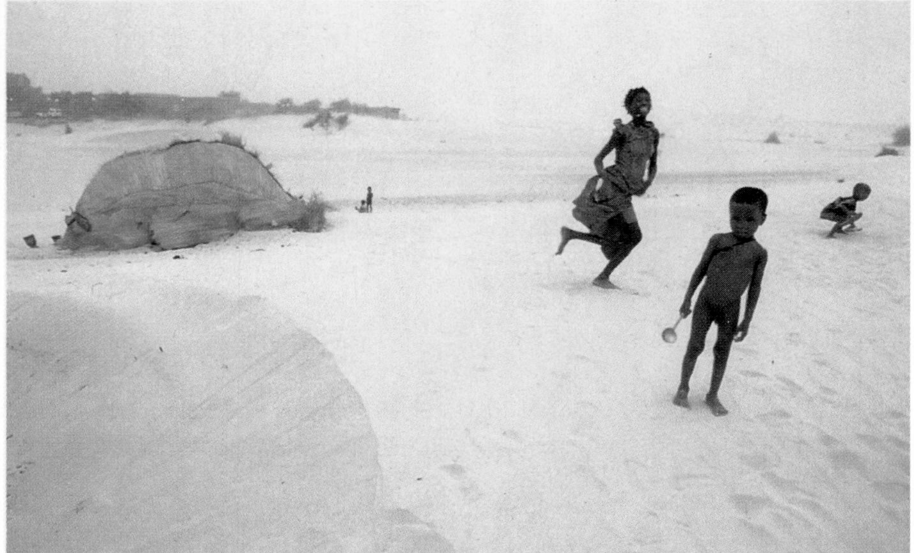

estimate that erosion is gradually stripping topsoil from almost one-third of the world's cropland (Brown et al., 1992). Substantial losses of cultivable land have occurred in India and in the sub-Saharan region of Africa, where denuding of the land and consequent loss of topsoil have allowed the deserts to advance (Figure 18.4).

Erosion occurs in the United States as well, but there is some relatively good news. Soil conservation legislation enacted in the 1985 Food Security Act is paying off: the amount of annual loss in this country has been reduced by one-third, thanks to two key provisions of the law. One provides payment to farmers who plant grass or trees on land that is at high risk of erosion; this helps because plants hold the topsoil. The other provision requires that farmers develop and implement a comprehensive soil-conservation plan by 1995 or lose all federal farm program benefits (Brown et al., 1992). So far, the United States is the only major food-producing country to respond legislatively to the erosion threat.

Even if erosion could be eliminated, though, some farmland would be lost by yet another means—conversion to nonfarm uses, such as building sites and highways. In China, for example, nearly 1% of the nation's cropland is given over annually to new homes and factories. Urban sprawl is claiming cropland in Bangkok, Thailand, and along the Nile River in Egypt. Other land is lost each year to unwise irrigation practices, as the next section describes.

Water Experts predict that water will become the most critically limiting natural resource for agriculture (Unklesbay, 1992). Water keeps topsoil from blowing away and provides the moisture plants need. The drought of the summer of 1988 in North America was a searing testimony to the critical nature of water: grain production in the United States and Canada was reduced by almost one-fourth. The drought in southern and eastern Africa in the early 1990s was partly responsible for one of the most severe famines ever experienced there (United Nations ACC/SCN, 1992).

In areas where rainfall is consistently inadequate, the use of surface water or groundwater for irrigation has enabled land to become more productive. Between 1950 and 1978, irrigated area in the world more than doubled; since then, the increase has slowed dramatically (Brown et al., 1992).

Part of the reason for the slowdown is that the extent to which these water supplies can be tapped is limited. In parts of China, which leads the world in irrigated land, irrigation is lowering the water table by more than 3 feet per year; parts of the United States have had a similar experience. In the Commonwealth of Independent States (formerly the USSR), irrigation has diminished the volume of some rivers. If these trends were to continue, irrigation would ultimately become impossible, as would providing adequate water for people in urban areas. Already, the use of water for irrigation has created competition for fresh water between farmers and city dwellers.

Poorly managed irrigation poses another risk: it can cause land to become infertile through waterlogging or through accumulation of mineral salts. If this accumulation reaches toxic levels, the condition is called *salinization*. Careful management can extend the land's productivity.

Water is also important as the natural habitat of certain animal foods: fish and shellfish from oceans, lakes, and rivers make important contributions to the diets of many people. We know, though, that food from these sources also has a limit: whereas the worldwide fish catch increased by 67% from 1969 to 1989, preliminary data show a decline of about 4% in 1990, the first decline in many years (World Resources Institute, 1992).

But fish taken from the wild is not the only possible source of seafood; both saltwater and freshwater fish are now produced by **fish farming,** or **aquaculture.** The expanding use of this technology currently accounts for about 13% of total fish harvested (World Resources Institute, 1992). Fish farming provides good conditions for the reproduction of finfish and shellfish and protects maturing fish from natural predators. As a result, the number of young that reach an appropriate size for food is hundreds of times what nature would have allowed.

fish farming, aquaculture—producing seafood in a protected environment

Shrimp and salmon are the two largest crops produced by aquaculture. China and Norway, respectively, produce the largest amounts of these seafoods (Unklesbay, 1992). Tilapia, perhaps the easiest fish to farm, is produced in large amounts in Asia and Africa each year. The United States produces catfish, white sturgeon, trout, salmon, oysters, mussels, and abalone by aquaculture.

This is an industry with clear opportunities for expansion. But as with any technology, scientists already have learned that aquaculture can be environmentally damaging if practiced unwisely. Rapid expansion of the prawn culture in Thailand has brought about destruction of mangrove forests along the country's southeast coast (World Resources Institute, 1992).

Climate Suitable climate is also necessary for plants to thrive. Plants need particular temperatures and amounts of sunlight, and they are affected by the concentration of various gases in the atmosphere. Although you might imagine that the tropics would be ideal for agriculture because of the region's year-round warmth and light, these conditions also foster weeds, pests, and diseases. The most productive areas are generally in the temperate zones, where winter serves as an effective herbicide and pesticide.

The climate of an area is not fixed for all time: scientists know that very gradual climatic changes have occurred over the millennia. Most scientists believe that human activities are accelerating and adding to these changes (World Resources Institute, 1992). Three major climatic concerns discussed in this section are global warming, acid rain, and the hole in the ozone layer.

Atmospheric temperature records indicate that temperatures since 1880 have been rising erratically, the situation known as **global warming** (Brown et al., 1992). Although there is circumstantial evidence that an increase in

global warming—increasing average world temperature

the levels of carbon dioxide, methane, and some other gases in the atmosphere act as a "greenhouse" to bring this about, this is difficult to prove conclusively, and it is a topic of serious scientific debate. Some scientists argue that by the time cause and effect could be established, the problem would no longer be correctable (Unklesbay, 1992); therefore, they urge immediate action to reduce the production of these gases.

fossil fuels—coal, natural gas, oil; energy sources naturally created from organic (carbon-containing) materials, which also usually contain sulfur and nitrogen compounds

The atmosphere's increase in carbon dioxide (CO_2), the predominant greenhouse gas, is primarily the result of two human activities. One is the burning of **fossil fuels,** which occurs mainly in the industrialized countries and produces nearly 6 billion tons of carbon annually. The other cause is the burning of forests, some of which occurs spontaneously, but most of which is deliberately set to clear tracts in the tropical rainforest. This produces 1–2 billion tons of carbon per year (Brown et al., 1992). The destruction of trees adds to the CO_2 burden of the atmosphere in another way: because trees are natural *users of* CO_2, deforestation reduces the ecosystem's own ability to deal with CO_2.

What's the harm in global warming? One likely problem is a public health concern: rising temperatures may extend the regions in which disease-causing organisms can thrive, because microorganisms tend to reproduce more rapidly in warmer environments (Doll, 1992).

Another problem concerns the food supply: experts anticipate a reduction in the amount of food that could be produced. Rising temperatures gradually melt the polar ice caps, causing the level of oceans to rise and submerge productive farmland. This is not a fantasy: many scientists believe this is already happening. Although other factors may contribute, one acre of land along the Louisiana coast is lost every 16 minutes to the rising water level of the Gulf of Mexico (Unklesbay, 1992). Other countries are thought to be much more affected. Global warming is also expected to result in lower rainfall, more hurricanes, and more pollution from increased use of air conditioners—all of which would reduce crop yields.

acid rain—acidic sulfur- and nitrogen-containing particles released into the atmosphere by burning fossil fuels; may settle in wet form (rain, snow) or as dry particles

Acid rain is another serious environmental problem that results from excessive combustion of fossil fuels. The sulfur- and nitrogen-containing by-products that industry, vehicles, and other fossil fuel users spew into the air damage both water and land resources. For example, as a result of the acidification of some trout streams in Norway, the fish populations have decreased by about three-fourths. On land, acid rain harms plant foliage. The rapid decline of European forests since 1970 offers persuasive evidence: 75% of commercial forests have suffered damage (World Resources Institute, 1992). Crops of all kinds are affected where acid rain falls.

ozone layer—the protective envelope of ozone gas that completely surrounds our planet, providing protection from most ultraviolet radiation

A hole in the **ozone layer** is the third major concern. The ozone layer shields the earth from most of the sun's harmful ultraviolet rays, which are capable of causing cancer, cataracts, and a reduction in the effectiveness of the immune system (Brown et al., 1992). Now that a hole has appeared over the Antarctic zone, we are losing protection against these rays.

There are harmful effects on food production as well. Ultraviolet rays can damage the simple organisms that are at the low end of the food chain, affecting the well-being of the whole chain (Doll, 1992). Basic agricultural crops, such as wheat and rice, are stunted by ultraviolet exposure. Research on soybeans, one of the more radiation-sensitive crops, has shown that each 1% increase in ultraviolet radiation results in a 1% decline in yield (Brown et al., 1992).

What are we doing to contribute to this problem? The ozone layer is being damaged primarily by *chlorofluorocarbons (CFCs),* a group of chemicals used in aerosol sprays, air conditioners, refrigerators, foamed plastics, and the manufacture of microchips. By a complicated process, one molecule

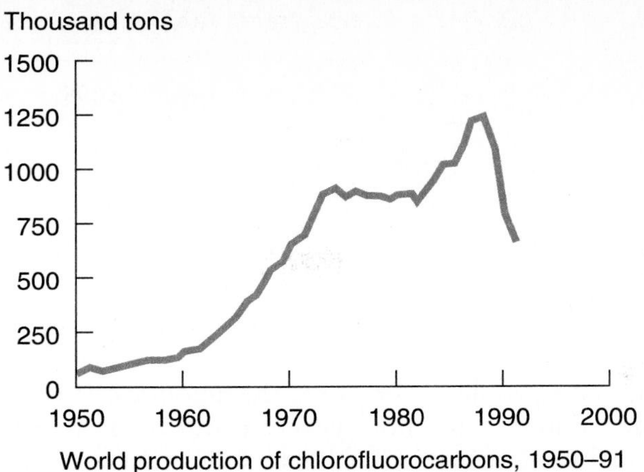

FIGURE 18.5
Chlorofluorocarbons (CFCs)—the cause of the hole in the ozone layer.

We have made progress in curtailing the use of CFCs, largely by eliminating their use in aerosol cans. Next, we need to recycle the CFCs existing in refrigerators and air conditioners to avoid their release into the atmosphere.
Source: Brown et al., 1992.

of chlorine can destroy as many as 100,000 molecules of ozone (Unklesbay, 1992). Some agreement about international phase-down of CFCs has been achieved. Although the United States led the way in 1978 by banning the use of CFCs as propellants in aerosol cans, much remains to be done (Figure 18.5).

Energy Energy is the last basic production resource. Cultivation of a crop from planting to harvest requires the investment of human, animal, and/or mechanical energy (Figure 18.6).

The developed countries use methods that are highly mechanized and rely heavily on fossil fuels. Such fuels are also ingredients of most herbicides, pesticides, and nitrogenous fertilizers (Unklesbay, 1992).

Nonetheless, the amount of commercially produced energy used for agriculture in any country is a relatively small proportion of total energy usage. In the United States, for example, only 1% of energy is used for agriculture; in Zimbabwe, the figure is 12% (World Resources Institute, 1992). Although you might think from these numbers that Zimbabwe uses more energy for agriculture than does the United States, the opposite is true. Zimbabwe uses much less energy for farming, but the percentage is higher because Zimbabwe uses *so little* energy for other purposes. The developing countries, in fact, want more energy for all purposes, such as household use, industry, and transportation, as well as agriculture.

FIGURE 18.6
Energy in agriculture.

Energy of various types is used for food production. Human labor, the first form used, is still the major source in many areas of the world. Although machines that use fossil fuels make it possible for a small number of farmers to produce food for large numbers of people, this contributes to the deterioration of the environment and depletes a finite resource.

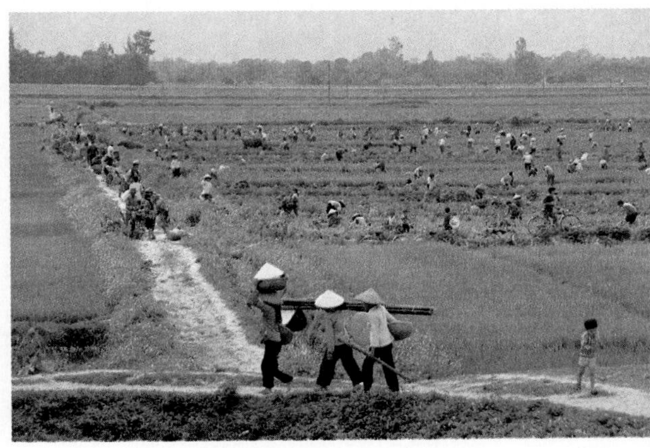

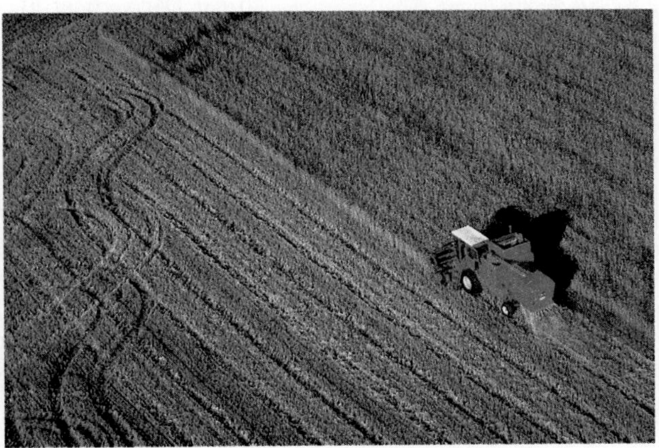

TABLE 18.1 Proven World Energy Reserves

Fuel Type	Years of Reserves Based on 1989 Production Rates
Oil	40
Natural gas	60
Coal	390

Data source: World Resources Institute, 1992.

This poses two problems. For one, the amount of fossil fuels is finite. Table 18.1 shows how many more years various fuels are estimated to last, based on annual usage figures of the late 1980s. Yet if countries use more fuel in the future, the fossil fuel supplies will be depleted even sooner. Therefore, on the world scene, countries compete with each other for fuel, and within each country, all economic sectors compete with each other for fuel.

The other major problem is that the burning of fossil fuels is environmentally detrimental, as you learned in the section on climate. Although coal, the dirtiest fuel, is not used for agricultural purposes, all other fossil fuels are damaging, too. Therefore, the concerns expressed about the burning of fossil fuels for industrial and transportation uses apply to agricultural uses as well.

Technologic Aids to Production

Technologic advancements, such as irrigation and fertilization, can help farmers produce food beyond the original capabilities of their basic production resources. Development of higher-yielding hybrids has also greatly increased food production.

Green Revolution—the surge in grain productivity occurring between 1960 and 1985 as the result of improved varieties, irrigation, and fertilization

The Green Revolution The effectiveness of using these three technologies together—irrigation, fertilization, and special hybrids—was well demonstrated in the 1960s, when the **Green Revolution** began. This agricultural movement enabled many Third World nations, especially those in Asia, to increase their food production many times over. A downside of the Green Revolution, however, was that these intensive farming methods led in some areas to environmental degradation from overuse of pesticides and fertilizers. Overall, though, the benefits of the Green Revolution were considerable, and they are still being realized—but they have probably reached their limit (Brown et al., 1992).

biotechnology—the use of living systems for the production of useful products

Biotechnology Biotechnology is at the leading edge of the agricultural and life sciences. **Biotechnology** involves the use of living systems—including plants, animals, microbes, and any part of these organisms—for the production of useful products. Although the term is modern, the practice itself has been going on for more than 8000 years. For example, the production of cheese, yogurt, alcoholic beverages, vinegar, and sourdough all depend on bacteria, so they fit the definition of biotechnologic processes. Recent examples include the extensive use of enzymes by the food processing industry to produce high-fructose corn syrups, beverage clarifiers, meat tenderizers, and texture modifiers.

The newest aspect of biotechnology involves making genetic changes in living systems. In a process known as **genetic engineering,** a gene that carries a desirable characteristic of a particular plant or animal is implanted into the genetic structure of a different plant or animal that lacks the trait. Genetic engineering has the potential to provide plants with resistance to insects, diseases, and herbicides; to improve nutritional quality; to reduce naturally occurring toxicants; and to reduce risk of damage from early frost. In animals produced for meat, genetic engineering can stimulate growth, promote more growth from a given amount of feed, and reduce fat content while increasing lean muscle mass.

genetic engineering—making changes in the genetic makeup of plants or animals by incorporating genes from other species

Some types of changes mentioned above have been accomplished in the past with selective breeding programs. Genetic engineering, however, can realize benefits far more rapidly and in a more controlled fashion than the earlier methods. The potential of biotechnology and genetic engineering for the food production and processing industries is enormous, but because they represent the unknown, these advances arouse many fears and anxieties—some justified, some not.

One application that has received wide publicity is the use of *bovine growth hormone (BGH),* also called *bovine somatotropin (BST)* produced by genetically engineered bacteria. Researchers have found that regularly injecting dairy cows with a small amount of this growth hormone, which is similar to that produced naturally in the cow's body, enhances milk production. But the future use of this technology is in question, because some opponents believe that it favors large agricultural operations rather than smaller family farms, which cannot afford the technology. Others believe that implementing the technology is unreasonable, because costly federal programs are already necessary to *limit* milk production and stabilize prices. Still others seem to fear the technology mainly because it is new. Taking legal opposition, legislatures in several states have limited or delayed the sale of milk produced with BGH.

Another application of current interest is increasing the disease resistance of plants through genetic engineering. This can be done by identifying bacteria that naturally produce pesticides, isolating the part of the bacterial genetic material responsible for the pesticide production, and introducing it into certain plants. Such *biopesticides* will be degradable and will not accumulate in the environment. Of course, the fact that biopesticides are natural does not automatically mean they're safe; their potential toxicity to humans will have to be evaluated carefully (Hall, 1991). This research investment can have a financial and environmental payback if it's found that new varieties of crops can be grown with less pesticide. Already, programs of *integrated pest management* that involve using pest-resistant varieties, applying pesticides only when significant damage occurs, introducing natural predators of pests, and/or using other nonchemical means have saved farmers millions of dollars (Greene, 1991).

Genetic engineering and biotechnology are not inherently good or bad; it all depends on how they are used. Early on, food scientists urged the government to develop clear and rational policies for regulating bioengineered products, and in June 1992, the Food and Drug Administration (FDA) announced food biotechnology guidelines for new plant varieties. The guidelines introduced six flow charts that identify the steps for the food industry to use in evaluating a bioengineered product, showing the points at which federal agencies need to be involved (Food Chemical News, 1992). Figure 18.7 shows one of these "decision trees."

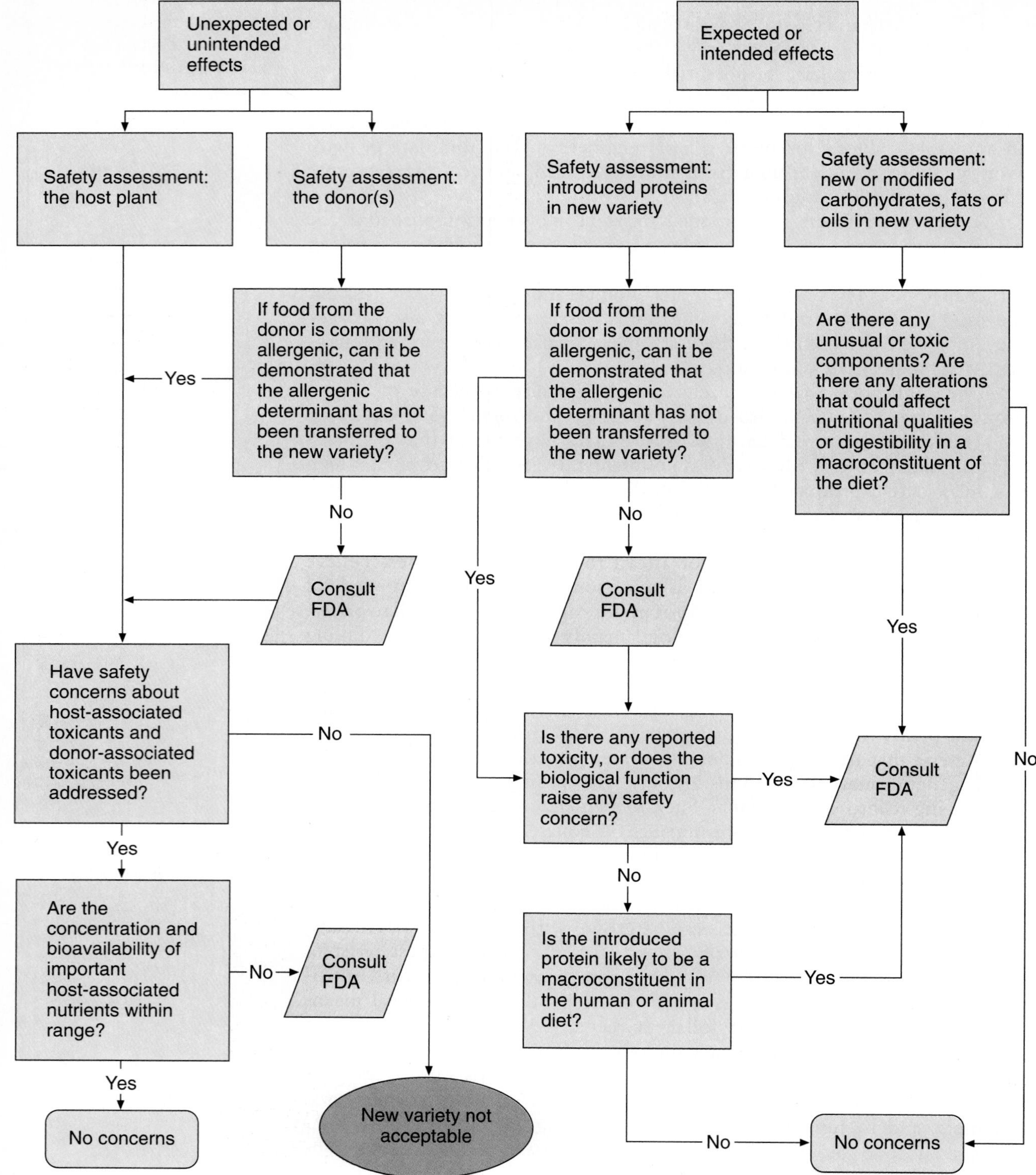

FIGURE 18.7
Evaluating the risks of genetically engineered plant varieties.

This "decision tree" summarizes the processes the FDA requires for developing new plant varieties. Both the plant being improved (the host) and the plant supplying genetic material (the donor) must be evaluated for safety.

Source: Adapted from *Food Chemical News,* June 1, 1992.

You Tell Me

"Nutriceuticals" (a term the popular press has coined) are foods that are designed to protect against illness. For example, one company has produced milk and eggs containing substantial amounts of antibodies that combat common pathogenic bacteria. The antibodies were produced by cows and chickens that had been repeatedly vaccinated with dead bacteria (New York Times, 1992).

Does this method meet the definition of a *biotechnologic process?* Would it be correct to call the products *genetically engineered?* Do you think that this is an appropriate use of this technology, or is it going too far for you? (These products have not been approved by the FDA, and they pose difficult regulatory issues.)

The Concept of Sustainability

In recent years, experts have become increasingly alarmed about the negative effects of agricultural practices on the resource base. What good is it to have a bigger harvest this year if your farming methods damage your soil so you can't produce as much next year? This concern has led to interest in **sustainable agriculture.**

sustainable agriculture—method of growing crops that fosters the maintenance and continued productivity of the soil

Sustainable agriculture, in its most idealistic sense, puts protection of the environment above everything else (Unklesbay, 1992). It sacrifices short-term production gains for long-term preservation of soil, water, climate, and energy supplies. Farmers could have difficulty making a living if they implemented these goals strictly.

Therefore, in the developed countries, variations of sustainable agriculture that *reduce* damage to the environment while still allowing for profitable operation are evolving. For example, *alternative agriculture* "reduces the use of chemicals and fertilizers with the greatest potential to harm the environment or the health of farmers or consumers" (World Resources Institute, 1992) without precluding the use of all farm chemicals; related terms are *ecologic agriculture, low input sustainable agriculture (LISA)* and *integrated pest management (IPM).* Such programs are beginning to get research and education support from the United States Department of Agriculture (USDA). To date, such systems involve only a small fraction of farmers; overall, our agricultural practices are still largely unsustainable (World Resources Institute, 1992).

The developed countries want to see developing countries take sustainability seriously, too, but conflict exists between the basic interests of these two factions. As we saw in discussions at the 1992 United Nations-sponsored "Earth Summit" in Rio de Janeiro, the developed countries' principal concern is environmental issues, whereas the developing countries are preoccupied with their poverty and need for economic development (Malone, 1992).

You Tell Me

The developing countries do not give the same high priority to concerns about the slashing and burning of the rainforest as do the developed countries. The developing countries, rather, focus on the fact that the developed countries, with only about one-fifth of the world's population, ►

produce and consume four-fifths of all the world's goods and services each year, creating far more environmental pollution than does the burning of the rainforest. At the same time, the *basic* needs of many people in the developing countries are not being met.

Taking these facts into account, what initiatives could provide some satisfaction for both sides? (Good luck—this question was difficult for the representatives to the 1992 World Summit to answer.)

The Extent of Demand for Food

Producing food is only one part of the world food equation; another important component is how much food is *needed and wanted.* Clearly, the demand for food is increasing.

Population One key element of demand is the size of the population. How many people need to be fed? World population is increasing at a rapid rate; after taking more than 100 years to double from 1.25 billion to 2.5 billion in 1950, population doubled again in only 37 years. In 1991, world population grew by a record 92 million, pushing the global total to 5.4 billion (Brown et al., 1992). The vast majority of these increases occurred in the developing countries.

Population trends are often described in terms of *rates* of population change. Keeping in mind that a growth rate of zero means that the size of the population is holding steady, you can see that even when the population growth rate declines from 2.06% to 1.73%, as it did during the 1970s, population is still increasing dramatically. In recent years, the rate has stalled at 1.73% (Horiuchi, 1992).

How is the world population likely to change from here on? The United Nations has made various projections, as shown in Figure 18.8; they differ widely, depending on assumptions about life expectancies and birth rates.

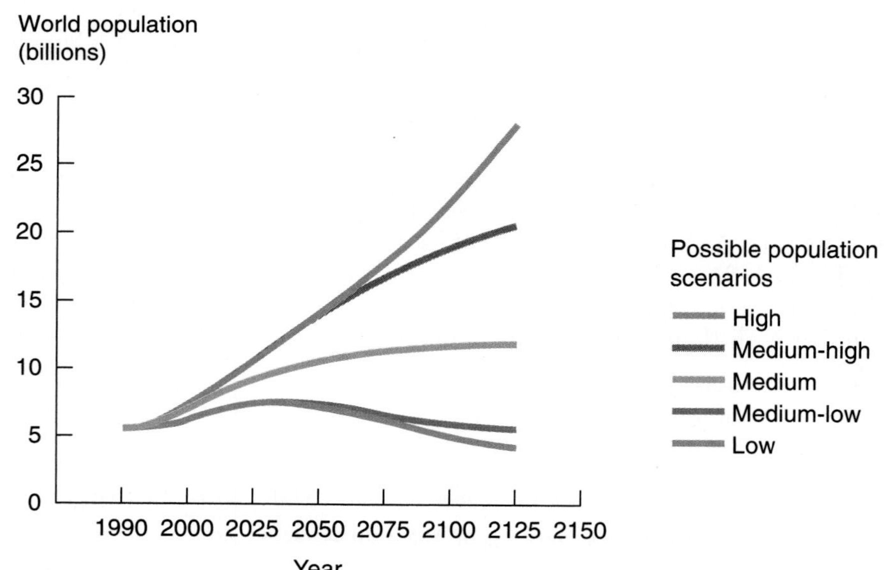

FIGURE 18.8
Population projections—United Nations style.

In 1992, the UN released a series of world population projections. They vary dramatically, depending on assumptions regarding life expectancy and fertility rates. For the near future, *all* projections predict large population increases.

Source: United Nations Population Division, 1992.

The UN's medium projection suggests that the world's population will reach 6 billion before the year 2000, reach 10 billion in 2050, and finally stabilize at 11.6 billion shortly after 2200 (World Resources Institute, 1992).

Attempts to decrease fertility have been faced with a "catch-22"; while high population levels decrease the amount of available food, the lack of available food fosters higher birth rates. Why is this?

There seem to be a variety of reasons (Bryant et al., 1985). In some of the world's most economically depressed countries, a person's only assurance of being cared for in old age is to have children to provide support. But if death rates of children are high, people must have many children to ensure that some will survive to adulthood. Therefore, social security is one reason that fertility rates tend to be kept high. Wanting extra help with agricultural and household labor and following religious beliefs that forbid birth control are other reasons.

Historically, one factor has been shown to lower a population's birth rate: achieving a reasonable quality of life, including an adequate standard of living, a sense of well-being, and assurance of economic and food security. These bring about a decline in the death rate, which is followed (usually decades later) by a decline in the birth rate. This is called the **demographic transition theory** (Foster, 1992). People who are committed to this theory believe that the way to reduce population growth is to address the causes of poverty.

demographic transition theory—pattern of population growth in which economic development brings about a drop in the death rate, which is followed later by a decline in the birth rate

Others look for more direct and rapid ways to bring down the birth rate—that is, family planning and birth control. Family planning programs, when strong and well-managed, have been highly effective: they reduce family size and lead to better health for mothers and children. The voluntary use of contraception in poor countries has risen from 10% of couples in the 1960s to 51% today, during which time the average number of births per woman dropped from 6 to 4 (World Resources Institute, 1992).

The Food People Need and Want Demand goes beyond the number of mouths there are to feed. It is also partly a matter of the amount of food people need to eat. Certainly, people who do not have enough to eat now want more in the future.

Another factor is the *type* of food people want. History shows that as people's incomes rise, their dietary preferences change. The classic illustration is shown in Figure 18.9: as incomes rise, people's consumption of sugar, animal protein, and fat increases, whereas consumption of starches and vegetable protein decreases (Foster, 1992). (These changes may not all be *desirable* from a health perspective, but they do occur.)

Demand for more animal products promotes an increase in the production of these products. This, in turn, affects the food supply. As we mentioned in Chapter 7 (on protein), when animals are fed grains that people could consume, a great deal of energy is lost in the process. But before you become too critical of the kinds of changes hungry people desire, read the Slice of Life on page 611.

Closer to home, here's another example of how economics can affect demand for food. The Soviets, after a bad harvest in 1973, bought substantial amounts of wheat on the world market. In response, grain prices went up around the world. In anticipation of high feed prices, beef prices in the United States also went up, and consumers cut back their consumption drastically. To stretch their beef purchases, many turned to pasta dishes—which caused tomato paste to became scarce, and its price to shoot up (Foster, 1992).

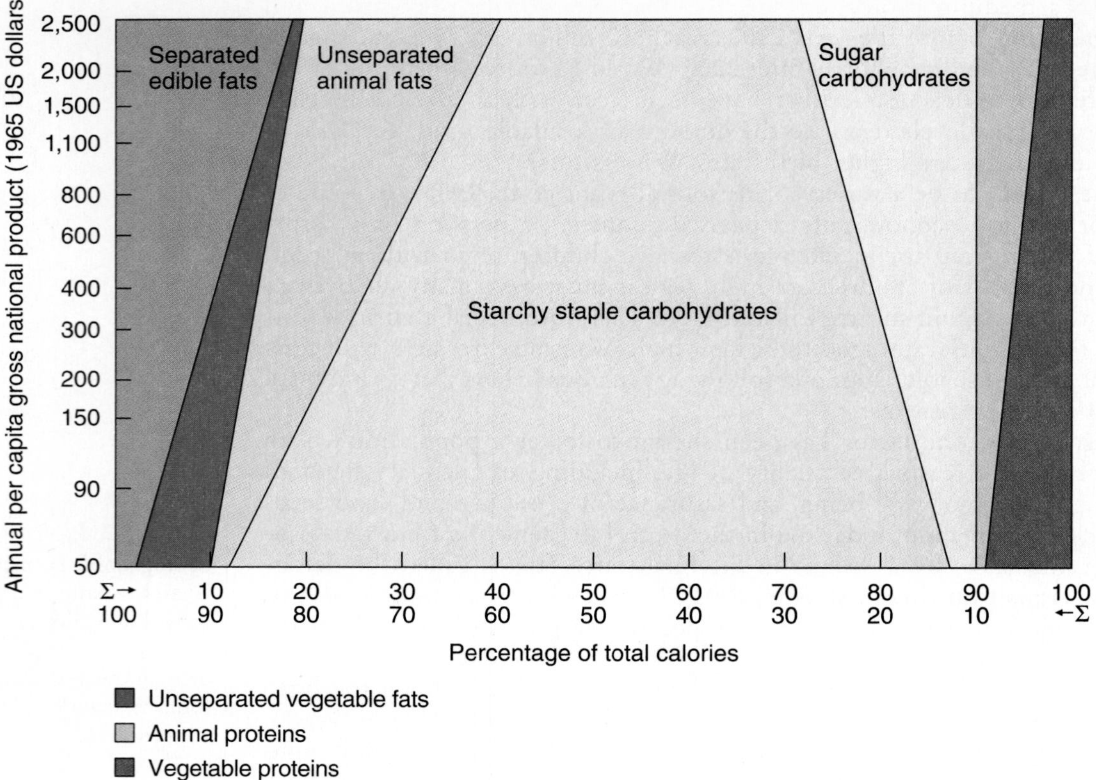

FIGURE 18.9
Changes in income causes changes in intake.

As peoples' incomes increase, they want to eat different kinds of foods—generally more meat products and refined sugar. At the same time, intake of plant foods decreases, as this classic illustration shows. Overall, fat intake increases and carbohydrate intake decreases (Perisse et al., 1969).

Distribution—Getting Food to People

Now that you have learned about factors that affect food production and demand, consider this fact: if all the food in the world were divided equally among the entire global population, each person's share would provide adequate nourishment. But as you learned at the start of the chapter, food is *not* distributed evenly: about one-fifth of the world's people have too little to eat.

What causes this?

In some countries, the food needs of the population have greatly outstripped the ability of their lands to yield it. The solution, it would seem, would be to purchase food from countries that produce more food than they need. However, poverty prevents much of this: poverty is the major cause of hunger.

Poverty is not an independent culprit, though; its effects are intertwined with many other factors, as you will read below.

Poverty

According to the World Watch Institute, a think tank concerned with issues of sustainability, approximately 60% of the world's people live in countries where the per capita annual income is below $2000. During the 1980s, per capita incomes declined dramatically in parts of Africa, and, to a lesser extent, in Latin America and parts of Asia (Brown et al., 1992). The gap between rich and poor is widening.

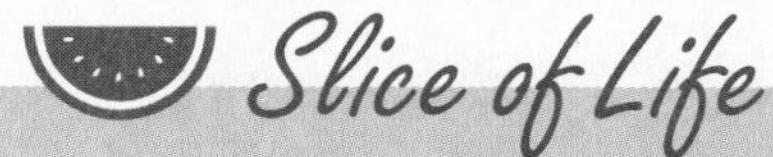

Food Choice and Income

In Chapter 1, you learned that our food choices are influenced by many factors—inborn, cultural, and individual. One individual factor is what you can afford. The poorer you are to begin with, the more dramatic are the changes you are likely to make when your circumstances improve.

The following describes the experience of Nicholas, a U.S. university student who became a Peace Corps volunteer in Zaire, and the local food customs he encountered there. We cannot know definitively to what extent the food choices of the people in this community were matters of cultural influence, sensory preference, or economic necessity, but if you put yourself in their place, what dietary changes would you make first if you had more money?

Here's an excerpt from a letter Nicholas wrote to his family after several months in Zaire:

> A few days ago, I ate palm grubs which, I have to admit, are rivaled in taste only by a certain bright green grasshopper which is around just once a year. They remind me of that chewing gum with liquid in the middle that squirts out when you bite it . . . what's it called?
>
> This is *makelele* season, named after a big ugly bug resembling a grasshopper. It burrows into the sand and makes a lot of noise at night. (*Makelele* means "noise" in Kikongo.) Kids particularly like to dig them up, leaving holes in the ground all over the place. They wrap them up in leaves and put them on wood coals. It is good to see the kids eating these bugs, since they contain more protein than they usually get. They eat caterpillars here, too, and I have got so I can eat them. It's been a lot easier to get used to some of the local fish and vegetables, though, which really are quite good . . . even with my cooking, Mom.
>
> Although there isn't much food, people are generous and invite me to dinner sometimes. They serve everything in covered dishes. Once the father set a dish in front of me, smiled politely, lifted the cover, and there was a little cooked mouse. It was on its back, feet up, hair charred off by the fire. The family was very polite, and so was I. Yes, I did have a little bit of the mouse.

You Tell Me

Some college students believe they are living "pretty close to the bone" at school. But if you think you are poor, compare your resources to those of people in the *poorest fifth* of the world's population: most of them have a per capita income of less than $275 *per year* (World Resources Institute, 1992).

For what period of time (days, weeks, or months) would $275 cover your expenses for rent, food, and clothing? (Don't even consider school-related expenses, such as tuition and books.) How could you modify your lifestyle to live within a budget of this amount?

You may think that because many of the world's poor are farmers, their ability to grow their own food should lessen their plight, but even most farmers expect to buy some of their food. Poor farmers have additional problems: they are likely to have marginal land and may not be able to afford adequate agricultural supplies, such as seed and fertilizers. In addition, their untrained farming practices often lead to further deterioration of their environment, resulting in a downward spiral of productivity (World Resources Institute, 1992).

FIGURE 18.10
The gender gap.

Women do 80% of the agricultural work in Africa, but they do not get equitable income or education. These women of Mali are processing rice for export.

Source: OXFAM America, Boston, Massachusetts.

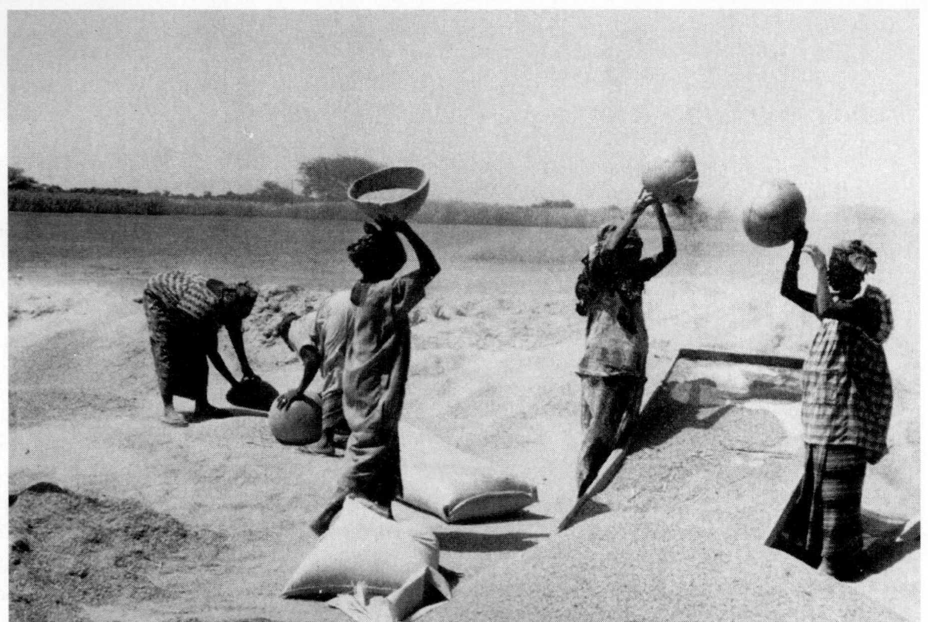

Another problem related to poverty is that people who don't have enough to eat become too physically weak to work. They are more susceptible to illness and cannot afford health care when they become sick. Illness increases the need for nutrients, resulting in a downward spiral for health, too. Death rates among infants and young children are high, and life expectancy is 20 years less in many low-income countries than it is in high-income countries (World Resources Institute, 1992).

Cultural Practices and the Gender Gap

Cultural practices can affect food distribution in many ways. A very direct effect in some cultures where there is not sufficient food to go around is that the men eat first, taking as much as they want at meals and leaving less than enough for the women and children.

Cultural patterns also affect education. Over 100 million children in the poorer countries receive no primary education at all, and the literacy rate of women is only three-fourths that of men (World Resources Institute, 1992). For example, only 57% of girls in Nepal are sent to primary school, whereas over 80% of boys attend. In terms of impact on the family, however, the education of women is estimated to be twice as important as education of men. Households in which the woman has had a primary education are likely to have higher incomes, better nutrition, healthier children, and less child mortality (World Resources Institute, 1992).

Another cultural mind-set ultimately has negative nutritional effects: women in many of the developing countries are viewed as "unproductive" in the eyes of society. Yet women do the majority of the work, working longer than their male relatives (Figure 18.10).

This cultural attitude plays out in grossly unequal allocation of resources—including food, credit, education, jobs, information, or training. Without these resources, women's ability to produce and earn are severely hampered. Since women's earnings are totally used for their families' needs—whereas men keep a portion of their earnings for their own purposes—these practices further impoverish families (Jacobson, 1992). Unfor-

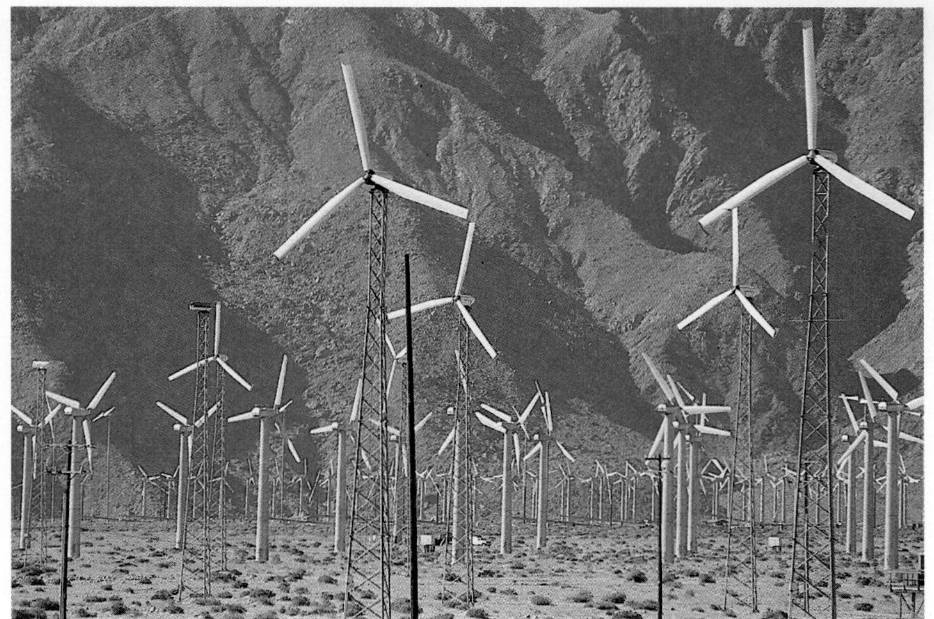

FIGURE 18.12
Power without pollution!

California supplies 1% of its electricity needs from "wind farms" such as this one near Palm Springs. Over the next decade, the state hopes to increase that share to 10%.

energy efficient; in Kenya, for example, an improved cooking stove more than doubled the efficiency of fuel. Another strategy is to switch fuel: natural gas puts out only half as much CO_2 as other fossil fuels. Third, alternative energy sources that do minimal environmental damage could be used to a greater extent; examples include hydroelectric power, wind turbines (Figure 18.12), and solar power collected in photovoltaic cells (Lenssen, 1992).

Nuclear power is another alternative to fossil fuels. This source of energy, of course, carries its own environmental risks (see Chapter 14). For nuclear energy to be feasible, there must be adequate research and development to ensure safe production, use, and waste disposal.

New Grain Varieties One international agricultural scientist ventures the educated guess that genetic engineering may provide the next surge of increased production (Chandler, 1992). Whereas varieties that brought about the Green Revolution required ideal conditions of fertilizer and irrigation, genetic engineering may bring about new varieties of grain that produce higher yields under less advantageous conditions.

Reducing Demand for Food—Access to Birth Control

Although many programs in family planning exist both in developed and in developing countries, they have not yet reached all who would use them. If family planning services were available to all women who say they want no more children, the number of births would drop by an estimated 27% in Africa, 33% in Asia, and 35% in Latin America (World Resources Institute, 1992).

Improving Distribution of Food

Initiatives to improve distribution of food are important for the future, because the gap between rich and poor has been widening. Below are two ideas that can help.

Forgiveness of Foreign Debt As we discussed earlier, developing countries that have large debts to developed nations sometimes feel trapped into making their payments in ways that are damaging to themselves and to their environment in the long term. Canceling part or all of the debt provides an opportunity for promoting sustainable development.

Debt relief can be granted on the condition, for example, that the developing country provide human development programs for its citizens. "Debt for nature" swaps are another helpful option—requiring the developing country to implement programs that protect natural resources in exchange for debt forgiveness (World Resources Institute, 1992).

Getting Away From the Livestock Economy Animals that eat table scraps or graze on land not suitable for cultivation have played largely beneficial roles in people's nutrition and in the human economy for thousands of years. Current high-volume methods used in production of animal products have led to environmental problems, however. Manure pollutes rivers and groundwater, and animals release significant amounts of methane, one of the "greenhouse gases," into the environment. Cattle ranching and other livestock operations are expensive in yet another way: animal products receive two-thirds of all agricultural subsidies (Durning and Brough, 1992).

New Zealand has taken a radical step. Formerly providing some of the world's highest price supports for sheep producers, the government eliminated most agricultural subsidies out of economic necessity. Unexpected environmental benefits emerged; and although farm earnings suffered, experts expect that in the long term, New Zealand's wool and dairy products will capture larger shares of the world market because of their lower costs (Durning and Brough, 1992).

How Can You Have an Impact?

The challenges involved in providing food security to the world's people are enormous. Even the efforts described above, each of which may have only a minor effect on improving prospects for the future, can seem daunting to an individual.

How can you—one person—have a positive impact on such a situation? Whether you want to provide help in your local community or beyond, there are opportunities to get involved. The Thinking for Yourself on page 619 gives you some options.

Now you've come to the end of this book. Throughout your study, you've learned about the benefits of good nutrition, as well as the damage that results from malnutrition. We hope you have also learned how to think critically about nutrition and health issues, because this skill will help you evaluate what you read and hear on these topics in the future. Nutrition will certainly continue to make news, as scientists uncover more information about how our diets can affect the quality and possibly even the length of our lives.

Further, we hope that your introduction to the interrelationships between feeding the world's people and sustaining our environment will have an impact on your political decisions and lifestyle, as you find your own way to help those who don't have enough to eat.

In every way, we wish you the best in using your nutrition for living.

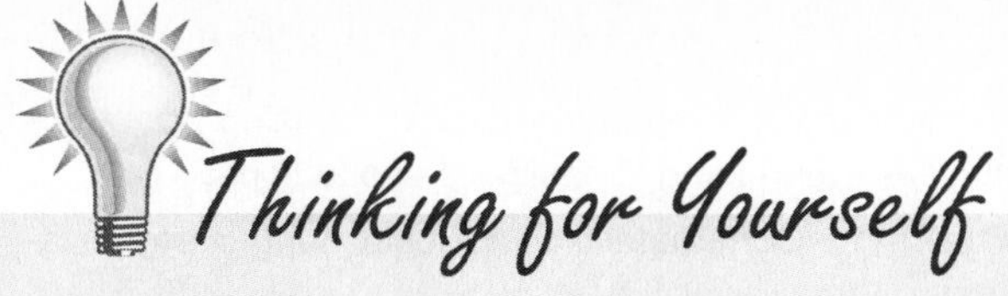

Food Security—Becoming Part of the Solution

The Situation

Having read this chapter, you are more aware of the extent of hunger, and you want to help. But what can you do that will make a difference?

You try to recall recent appeals for help. You remember a request for donations to stock a local emergency food bank, an appeal to help cook for an area homeless shelter, and solicitations by international hunger relief organizations. You remember hearing people say that "we should give up eating so much meat, because it takes food out of the mouths of people who are starving."

Is Your Information Accurate and Relevant?

- Food banks, homeless shelters, and hunger relief agencies can help people who need food (more about this below).
- Eating less meat will not necessarily help someone in a developing country. Who would buy, store, ship, and distribute the food you don't eat? You might think eating less meat would help because livestock consume grain that could be eaten by people. But experts say that this is not the problem: even with livestock eating approximately one-third of the world's grain, there is currently enough grain for everybody—but the hungry cannot afford to buy it (Dommen, 1992). However, there is one way that eating less meat *could* help others: if you spent less money on your new eating style, you could contribute the savings to a hunger relief agency.

What Else Should You Consider?

Let's go back to the first items on your list.

Food banks, homeless shelters, and similar emergency services can help unfortunate individuals through tough times, and they deserve your support. Consider volunteering some Saturday mornings at a food pantry or spending one evening per week serving meals at a homeless shelter. While providing help directly, you can further increase your awareness of hunger and whom it affects.

But even though these programs help, their existence represents failure—the failure of the government's social service system (especially the federal Food Stamp Program) adequately to meet the needs of America's hungry people. Some of the working poor need but cannot get food stamps. Part of the problem is that a person has to be extremely poor to qualify. Another problem is that an outdated formula is used to determine the allotment; therefore, grants often are not large enough, causing some recipients to seek supplemental emergency help (Clancy and Bowering, 1992). In the short run, increasing the allotments would help. In the long run, the best solution would be to help employable people get jobs at which they can earn a living wage, reserving food stamps for those who truly cannot work.

Solving these problems calls for major political change, which is another way you can help. Start by studying issues. Because hunger is a global concern, go beyond (but don't exclude) domestic concerns. Learn about such diverse matters as the social service network, the environment, sustainable agriculture, family planning, agricultural subsidies and tariffs, forgiveness of foreign debt, and development programs. Then, as a well-informed citizen, make your opinions known to your elected representatives . . . and also ask candidates running for office about their positions on these issues. Ask tough questions, and don't be satisfied with rhetoric for answers.

Another way to help is to modify your lifestyle. Because the world food situation is firmly linked with environmental issues, anything you do to safeguard land, water, or air helps. Reducing your use of fossil fuels by walking or riding a bicycle instead of driving a car helps. Not being wasteful when heating or cooling your living space helps. Recycling reusable materials helps.

Try to influence the environmental practices of the food industry as well. You could participate in citizen movements that pressure food companies to adopt more environmentally responsible production, processing, packaging, and distribution methods. Such groups also urge the general public to make food product choices based on these issues (Wittwer, 1992). Of course, often you cannot know the product's history, but you may be able to determine whether the packaging seems excessive or environmentally burdensome. You could press for the government to sanction the use of an "environmentally friendly" label logo to be used only on products that qualify.

Donating money is another way to provide assistance to hungry people, either in the United States or in a developing country. To be sure that as much as possible of the money you contribute will be spent for service, ask organizations for their annual reports. These reports will show you which organizations spend more on providing help and less on administering the programs. Also, you may want to specify whether your dollars should be used for temporary famine relief or for programs that focus on long-term development.

Going beyond any of the above ideas, you might even let your commitment direct your life after college. Consider volunteering for the Peace Corps, or consider a career that deals with problems of hunger and the environment. Such work will not put you at the top of the pay scale, but it will rate you high in your contributions to society.

Now What Do You Think?

The suggestions above do not exhaust the possibilities; they are ideas to stimulate your own thinking about opportunities around you. Consider these actions:

- Option 1 Contribute time to local hunger organizations.
- Option 2 Participate in meaningful political change.
- Option 3 Make lifestyle changes consistent with environmental sustainability.
- Option 4 Pressure the food industry to use environmentally responsible methods.
- Option 5 Contribute money to hunger relief organizations that have records of effectiveness.
- Option 6 Volunteer for a limited term with the Peace Corps or other international relief group.
- Option 7 Choose a career or position aimed at solving problems of hunger and the environment.

What other options do you see? Which do you choose?

Summary

- As many as one in five of the earth's people experiences **food insecurity. Food security** is the ongoing assurance of safe, nutritionally adequate, and affordable food obtainable through ordinary channels.
- One of the three major factors affecting food availability is the world's capacity for production. This, in turn, is affected by basic production resources. Most of the world's **arable land** is already used for agricultural purposes; the productivity of this land needs to be sustained. Water for irrigation is becoming depleted in some areas, whereas the use of water for **aquaculture** or **fish farming** is increasing. Three important climatic concerns are **global warming, acid rain,** and the hole in the **ozone layer.** Energy is needed to cultivate food; the most commonly used fuels are finite and originate as **fossil fuels.**
- The **Green Revolution** gives testimony to the food production benefits of technology. Now, **biotechnology,** including **genetic engineering,** is at the forefront of biologic research and offers possibilities for the future. Many technologies currently used do not contribute to **sustainable agriculture.**
- Demand for food is partly a function of population size. Because families in some cultures have many children as a form of social security, improving their overall economic status brings down the birth rate, a phenomenon described by the **demographic transition theory.** Demand is also reflected in people's wanting different types of food as their economic circumstances improve.
- At present, there is enough food in the world for everybody to have an adequate amount, but many do not; therefore, the problem is inequitable distribution. Poverty is the major cause of food insecurity. The gender gap, governmental policies (such as forcing farmers to raise a **cash crop**), international trade agreements, and appropriate **infrastructures** also affect distribution.
- To bring about food security in the future, we need to explore all factors that influence food production, demand, and distribution. Many creative initiatives are already under way, but many more are needed. There are many things you can do to help.

References

Borlaug, N.E. 1992. Lighting fires at the grass roots. *Food Technology* 46(no.7):84–85.

Briefel, R.R. and C.E. Wotecki. 1992. Development of food sufficiency questions for the Third National Health and Nutrition Examination Survey. *Journal of Nutrition Education* 24:24S–28S.

Brown, L.R., C. Flavin, and H. Kane. 1992. *Vital signs 1992.* New York: W.W. Norton & Company.

Bryant, C.A., A. Courtney, B.A. Markesbery, and K.M. DeWalt. 1985. *The cultural feast.* St. Paul: West Publishing Company.

Chandler, R.F. 1992. The role of the international agricultural research centers in increasing the world food supply. *Food Technology* 46(no.7):86–88.

Clancy, K.L. and J. Bowering. 1992. The need for emergency food: Poverty problems and policy responses. *Journal of Nutrition Education* 24:12S–17S.

Doll, R. 1992. Health and the environment in the 1990s. *American Journal of Public Health* 82:933–941.

Dommen, A. 1992. Can we solve the world food problem by giving up bacon and eggs? In *The world food problem,* by P. Foster. Boulder, CO: Lynne Rienner Publishers.

Durning, A.T. and H.B. Brough. 1992. Reforming the livestock economy. In *State of the world 1992,* ed. L. Starke. New York: W.W. Norton & Company.

Food and Agriculture Organization (FAO). 1992. *World food supplies and prevalence of chronic undernutrition in developing regions as assessed in 1992.* New York: The United Nations.

Food Chemical News. 1992. Plant biotech FDA decision trees to guide industry. *Food Chemical News,* June 1, 1992.

Foster, P. 1992. *The world food problem.* Boulder, CO: Lynne Rienner publishers.

Greene, C. 1991. Environmental concern sparks renewed interest in IPM. *Food Review* 14(no.2):8–11.

Hall, R.L. 1991. Food safety and biotechnology. *Nutrition Today* 45(no.3):15–20.

Horiuchi, S. 1992. Stagnation in the decline of the world population growth rate during the 1980s. *Science* 257:761–765.

Jacobson, J.L. 1992. *Gender bias: Roadblock to sustainable development.* Worldwatch paper 110. Washington, DC: Worldwatch Institute.

Jesse, E. and B. Cropp. 1987. Fluid milk reconstitution: Issues and impacts. Marketing and policy briefing paper, Department of Agricultural Economics, University of Wisconsin.

Lenssen, N. 1992. *Empowering development: The new energy equation.* Washington, DC: Worldwatch Institute.

Malone, T.F. 1992. The world after Rio. *American Scientist* 80:530–532.

Mellor, J.W. and S. Gavian. 1987. Famine: Causes, prevention, and relief. *Science* 235:539–545.

New York Times. 1992. Dairy items could fight illnesses. *San Jose Mercury News,* July 11, 1992.

Perisse, J., F. Sizaret, and P. Francoise. 1969. The effect of income on the structure of the diet. *FAO Newsletter 7* (July–September):2.

Postel, S. 1992. Denial in the decisive decade. In *State of the world 1992,* ed. L. Starke. New York: W.W. Norton & Company.

Renner, M. 1992. Creating sustainable jobs in industrial countries. In *State of the world 1992,* ed. L. Starke. New York: W.W. Norton & Company.

Ryan, J.C. 1992. *Life support: Conserving biological diversity.* Worldwatch paper 108. Washington, DC: The Worldwatch Institute.

Testin, R.F. and P.J. Vergano. 1991. Food packaging. *Food Review* 14(no.2):31–33.

UNICEF. 1991. *The state of the world's children, 1992.* New York: UNICEF.

United Nations ACC/SCN. 1992. *Second report on the world nutrition situation.* New York: The United Nations.

United Nations Population Division. 1992. *Long-range world population projections: Two centuries of population growth, 1950–2150.* New York: The United Nations.

Unklesbay, N. 1992. *World food and you.* New York: Food Products Press.

Uphoff, N. 1988. Assisted self-reliance: Working with, rather than for, the poor. In *Strengthening the poor: What have we learned?,* ed. J.P. Lewis. New Brunswick, N.J.: Transaction Books.

Wittwer, S.H. 1992. The "greening effect": Implications for consumer food choices. *Food & Nutrition News* 64:15–17.

World Resources Institute. 1992. *World resources 1992–1993: Toward sustainable development.* London: Oxford University Press.

Appendices

Reliable Sources of Nutrition Information

Semitechnical Periodicals

These materials contain reviews that are suitable for people without a strong science background. Most of them are available by subscription, except those indicated with an asterisk (*), which are available to health and education professionals on request.

***Contemporary Nutrition**
A monthly newsletter. Contains one referenced nutrition review topic by recognized expert per issue.

General Mills, Inc.
P.O. Box 5588
Stacy, MN 55079

Dairy Council Digest
A bimonthly newsletter. Contains one referenced nutrition review topic per issue.

National Dairy Council
6300 North River Road
Rosemont, IL 60018-4233

***Dietetic Currents**
A bimonthly newsletter. Contains one referenced nutrition review topic by recognized expert per issue.

Ross Laboratories
Director of Professional Services
625 Cleveland Avenue
Columbus, OH 43216

Environmental Nutrition
A newsletter published ten times per year. Contains reviews of current issues and books and a readers' forum.

2112 Broadway
New York, NY 10023

FDA Consumer
A monthly magazine. Contains articles on concerns and actions of the FDA.

Superintendent of Documents
Government Printing Office
Washington, DC 20402

***Food and Nutrition News**
A newsletter published five times per year. Contains one referenced article by recognized expert per issue; other features.

National Livestock and Meat Board
444 North Michigan Avenue
Chicago, IL 60611

Harvard Medical School Health Letter
A monthly newsletter. Contains information on a variety of health topics, including nutrition.

Department of Continuing Education
164 Longwood Avenue
Harvard Medical School
Boston, MA 02115

National Council Against Health Fraud Newsletter
A monthly newsletter. Contains information concerning health misinformation, faddism, and fraud.

NCAHF
P.O. Box 1276
Loma Linda, CA 92354

Tufts University Diet and Nutrition Letter
A monthly newsletter. Contains reviews of current issues and books; questions and answers.

Tufts Diet and Nutrition Letter
P.O. Box 57857
Boulder, CO 80322-7857

(continued)

Respected Professional Journals

Although this listing includes the journals that are most likely to carry original nutrition research, many other journals occasionally do also. Several of these journals feature technical review articles.

American Journal of Clinical Nutrition
American Society for Clinical Nutrition
9650 Rockville Pike
Bethesda, MD 20814

American Journal of Public Health
American Publich Health Association
1015 Fifteenth Street NW
Washington, DC 20005

Food and Chemical Toxicology
Pergamon Press Journals Division
660 White Plains Road
Tarrytown, NY 10591-5153

Food Technology
Institute of Food Technologists
221 North LaSalle Street
Chicago, IL 60601

Gastroenterology
W.B. Saunders Co.
The Curtiss Center
Independence Square West
Philadelphia, PA 19106-3399

International Journal of Sport Nutrition
Human Kinetics Publishers, Inc.
P.O. Box 5076
Champaign, IL 61825-5076

Journal of the American Dietetic Association
American Dietetic Association
216 West Jackson Boulevard, Suite 800
Chicago, IL 60606-6995

Journal of American Medical Association (JAMA)
American Medical Association
515 North State Street
Chicago, IL 60610

Journal of Applied Physiology
American Physiological Society
9650 Rockville Pike
Bethesda, MD 20814

Journal of Nutrition
American Institute of Nutrition
9650 Rockville Pike
Bethesda, MD 20814

Journal of Nutrition Education
Williams and Wilkins
428 East Preston Street
Baltimore, MD 21202-3993

Lancet (British)
Williams and Wilkins
428 East Preston Street
Baltimore, MD 21202-3993

Medicine and Science in Sports and Exercise
Williams and Wilkins
428 East Preston Street
Baltimore, MD 21202-3993

Nature (British)
Macmillan Magazines Ltd.
Subscription Department
P.O. Box 1733
Riverton, NJ 08077-7333

New England Journal of Medicine
Massachusetts Medical Society
10 Shattuck Street
Boston, MA 02115-6094

Nutrition Reviews
Springer-Verlag New York, Inc.
175 Fifth Avenue
New York, NY 10010

Nutrition Today
Williams and Wilkins
428 East Preston Street
Baltimore, MD 21202

Pediatric Research
International Pediatric Research Foundation, Inc.
428 East Preston Street
Baltimore, MD 21202

Pediatrics
American Academy of Pediatrics
P.O. Box 927
Elk Grove Village, IL 60009-0927

Science
American Association for the Advancement of Science
1333 H Street, NW
Washington, DC 20005

Professional and Service Organizations

These are organizations that publish various nutrition-related materials but do not publish any of the journals just listed.

American Cancer Society
1599 Clifton Road
Atlanta, GA 30329

American Council on Science and Health
1995 Broadway, 16th Fl.
New York, NY 10023

American Dental Association
211 East Chicago Avenue
Chicago, IL 60611

American Geriatrics Society
770 Lexington Avenue, Suite 400
New York, NY 10021

American Heart Association
7320 Greenville Avenue
Dallas, TX 75231

American Home Economics Association
1555 King Street
Alexandria, VA 22314

Food and Nutrition Board
Institute of Medicine, National Academy of Sciences
2101 Constitution Avenue NW
Washington, DC 20418

March of Dimes Birth Defects Foundation
1275 Mamaroneck Avenue
White Plains, NY 10605

Office of Cancer Communications
National Cancer Institute
Bldg. 31, Room 10A29
9000 Rockville Pike
Bethesda, MD 20892

Federal Government Resources

These agencies will furnish lists of their nutrition-related government publications.

Consumer Information Center
U.S. General Services Administration
Washington, DC 20405

Food and Nutrition Information
National Agricultural Library
10301 Baltimore Blvd., Room 304
Beltsville, MD 20705

Local Resources

These are people whom you can contact in your own geographical area who are familiar with science-based nutrition information.

Cooperative extension agents
in county extension offices

Dietitians
in clinical positions in local hospitals or nursing homes

Home economists
employed in business (supermarkets, utilities, food processing companies, and so on)

Nutrition faculty
affiliated with a reputable department of nutritional science

Nutritionists
in city, county, or state public health departments

Summary of Examples of Recommended Nutrients for Canadians Based on Energy, Expressed as Daily Rates

Age	Sex	Energy kcal	Thiamin mg	Riboflavin mg	Niacin NE[b]	n-3 PUFA[a] g	n-6 PUFA g
Months							
0–4	Both	600	0.3	0.3	4	0.5	3
5–12	Both	900	0.4	0.5	7	0.5	3
Years							
1	Both	1100	0.5	0.6	8	0.6	4
2–3	Both	1300	0.6	0.7	9	0.7	4
4–6	Both	1800	0.7	0.9	13	1.0	6
7–9	M	2200	0.9	1.1	16	1.2	7
	F	1900	0.8	1.0	14	1.0	6
10–12	M	2500	1.0	1.3	18	1.4	8
	F	2200	0.9	1.1	16	1.1	7
13–15	M	2800	1.1	1.4	20	1.4	9
	F	2200	0.9	1.1	16	1.2	7
16–18	M	3200	1.3	1.6	23	1.8	11
	F	2100	0.8	1.1	15	1.2	7
19–24	M	3000	1.2	1.5	22	1.6	10
	F	2100	0.8	1.1	15	1.2	7
25–49	M	2700	1.1	1.4	19	1.5	9
	F	2000	0.8	1.0	14	1.1	7
50–74	M	2300	0.9	1.3	16	1.3	8
	F	1800	0.8[c]	1.0[c]	14[c]	1.1[c]	7[c]
75+	M	2000	0.8	1.0	14	1.0	7
	F[d]	1700	0.8[c]	1.0[c]	14[c]	1.1[c]	7[c]
Pregnancy (additional)							
1st Trimester		100	0.1	0.1	0.1	0.05	0.3
2nd Trimester		300	0.1	0.3	0.2	0.16	0.9
3rd Trimester		300	0.1	0.3	0.2	0.16	0.9
Lactation (additional)		450	0.2	0.4	0.3	0.25	1.5

[a]PUFA, polyunsaturated fatty acids
[b]Niacin Equivalents
[c]Level below which intake should not fall
[d]Assumes moderate physical activity

Source: Scientific Review Committee. *Nutrition Recommendations,* Ottawa, Canada: Health and Welfare, 1990. Reproduced with permission of Supply and Services Canada.

(continued)

Summary Examples of Recommended Nutrient Intake for Canadians Based on Age and Body Weight, Expressed as Daily Rates

Age	Sex	Weight kg	Protein g	Vit. A RE[a]	Vit. D μg	Vit. E mg	Vit. C mg	Folate μg	Vit. B_{12} μg	Calcium mg	Phosphorus mg	Magnesium mg	Iron mg	Iodine μg	Zinc mg
Months															
0–4	Both	6.0	12[b]	400	10	3	20	50	0.3	250[c]	150	20	10.3[d]	30	2[d]
5–12	Both	9.0	12	400	10	3	20	50	0.3	400	200	32	7	40	3
Years															
1	Both	11	19	400	10	3	20	65	0.3	500	300	40	6	55	4
2–3	Both	14	22	400	5	4	20	80	0.4	550	350	50	6	65	4
4–6	Both	18	26	500	2.5	5	25	90	0.5	600	400	65	8	85	5
7–9	M	25	30	700	2.5	7	25	125	0.8	700	500	100	8	110	7
	F	25	30	700	2.5	6	25	125	0.8	700	500	100	8	95	7
10–12	M	34	38	800	5	8	25	170	1.0	900	700	130	8	125	9
	F	36	40	800	5	7	25	180	1.0	1100	800	135	8	110	9
13–15	M	50	50	900	5	9	30	150	1.5	1100	900	185	10	160	12
	F	48	42	800	5	7	30	145	1.5	1000	850	180	13	160	9
16–18	M	62	55	1000	5	10	40[e]	185	1.9	900	1000	230	10	160	12
	F	53	43	800	2.5	7	30[e]	160	1.9	700	850	200	12	160	9
19–24	M	71	58	1000	2.5	10	40[e]	210	2.0	800	1000	240	9	160	12
	F	58	43	800	2.5	7	30[e]	175	2.0	700	850	200	13	160	9
25–49	M	74	61	1000	2.5	9	40[e]	220	2.0	800	1000	250	9	160	12
	F	59	44	800	2.5	6	30[e]	175	2.0	700	850	200	13	160	9
50–74	M	73	60	1000	5	7	40[e]	220	2.0	800	1000	250	9	160	12
	F	63	47	800	5	6	30[e]	190	2.0	800	850	210	8	160	9
75+	M	69	57	1000	5	6	40[e]	205	2.0	800	1000	230	9	160	12
	F	64	47	800	5	5	30[e]	190	2.0	800	850	210	8	160	9
Pregnancy (additional)															
1st Trimester			5	100	2.5	2	0	300	1.0	500	200	15	0	25	6
2nd Trimester			20	100	2.5	2	10	300	1.0	500	200	45	5	25	6
3rd Trimester			24	100	2.5	2	10	300	1.0	500	200	45	10	25	6
Lactation (additional)			20	400	2.5	3	25	100	0.5	500	200	65	0	50	6

[a]Retinol Equivalents
[b]Protein is assumed to be from breast milk and must be adjusted for infant formula.
[c]Infant formula with high phosphorus should contain 375 mg calcium.
[d]Breast milk is assumed to be the source of the mineral.
[e]Smokers should increase vitamin C by 50%.

Source: Scientific Review Committee. *Nutrition Recommendations,* Ottawa, Canada: Health and Welfare, 1990. Reproduced with permission of Supply and Services Canada.

(continued)

Canada's Food Guide to Healthy Eating (1992)

For people four years and over

Different People Need Different Amounts of Food

The amount of food you need every day from the 4 food groups and other foods depends on your age, body size, activity level, whether you are male or female and if you are pregnant or breastfeeding. That's why the Food Guide gives a lower and higher number of servings for each food group. For example, young children can choose the lower number of servings, while male teenagers can go to the higher number. Most other people can choose servings somewhere in between.

Food Group	Servings per Day	Examples of One Serving	Examples of Two Servings
Grain Products	5–12	1 slice bread 30 g cold cereal 175 mL (3/4 cup) hot cereal	1 bagel, pita, or bun 250 mL (1 cup) pasta or rice
Vegetables & Fruit	5–10	1 medium size vegetable or fruit 125 mL (1/2 cup) fresh, frozen, or canned vegetables or fruit 250 mL (1 cup) salad 125 mL (1/2 cup) juice	
Milk Products	Children, 4–9: 2–3 Youth, 10–16: 3–4 Adults: 2–4 Pregnant & Breastfeeding Women: 3–4	250 mL (1 cup) milk 50 g (3" × 1" × 1") cheese 50 g (2 slices) cheese 175 g (3/4 cup) yogourt	
Meat & Alternatives	2–3	50–100 g meat, poultry, or fish 50–100 g (1/3–2/3 can) fish 1–2 eggs 125–250 mL beans 100 g (1/3 cup) tofu 30 mL (2 tbsp) peanut butter	

Other Foods

Taste and enjoyment can also come from other foods and beverages that are not part of the 4 food groups. Some of these foods are higher in fat or Calories, so use these foods in moderation.

Enjoy eating well, being active and feeling good about yourself. That's VITALITY®.

 ISBN 0–662–19648–1

APPENDIX C

Table of Food Composition

About the Database

This table of food composition is compiled by N-Squared Computing in Salem, Oregon. The table offers about 2000 selected foods, including baby foods, dietary products, brand names, alcoholic beverages, and mixed dishes, as well as a large variety of raw and cooked common foods.

The foods, listed alphabetically in common household units for easy use, provide an analysis for 21 nutritional components. The nutritional data is verified by recognized reputable sources, such as the USDA and scientific journal articles, as well as fast food and manufacturers' data where appropriate.

This food table is a scaled-down version of the N-Squared 9700-food database and is copyrighted data that may not be reprinted without permission from N-Squared Computing.

Appendix C Table of Food Composition

Item	Food Name	Portion	Weight (g)	Food Energy (kcal)	Protein (g)	Total Fat (g)	Saturated Fat (g)	Cholesterol (mg)	Carbohydrate (g)	Calcium (mg)	Phosphorus (mg)	Sodium (mg)	Potassium (mg)	Iron (mg)	Zinc (cm)	Vitamin A (RE)	Thiamin (mg)	Riboflavin (mg)	Niacin (mg)	Vitamin B6 (mg)	Vitamin B12 (ug)	Folic Acid (ug)	Vitamin C (mg)
1041	Alfalfa seeds-sprouted-raw	1 cup	33	10	1	0	0	0	1	11	23	2	26	0.32	0.30	5	0.03	0.04	0.16	0.01	0.00	12	3
807	Allspice-ground	1 tsp	2	5	0	0	0	0	1	13	2	1	20	0.13	0.02	1	0.00	0.00	0.05	—	0.00	—	1
1137	Almond butter-plain	1 tbsp	16	101	2	9	1	0	3	43	84	2	121	0.59	0.49	0	0.02	0.10	0.46	0.01	0.00	10	0
1043	Amaranth-boiled-drained	1 cup	132	28	3	0	0	0	5	276	95	28	846	2.98	1.16	366	0.03	0.18	0.74	0.23	0.00	75	54
1042	Amaranth-raw	1 cup	28	7	1	0	0	0	1	60	14	5	171	0.65	0.25	82	0.01	0.04	0.18	0.05	0.00	24	12
1761	Apple butter	1 tbsp	20	37	0	0	0	0	9	3	4	0	50	0.10	0.01	0	0.00	0.00	0.04	0.01	0.00	0	0
947	Apples-can-sweet-heated	1 cup	204	137	0	1	0	0	34	8	11	7	142	0.49	0.10	11	0.02	0.02	0.17	0.09	0.00	0	0
949	Apples-dried-cooked-unsweetened	1 cup	255	145	1	0	0	0	39	8	23	52	267	0.84	0.12	4	0.02	0.05	0.33	0.13	0.00	0	3
948	Apples-dried-uncooked	1 cup	86	209	1	0	0	0	57	12	33	75	387	1.21	0.17	0	0.00	0.14	0.80	0.11	0.00	0	3
951	Apples-frozen-unsweetened-heated	1 cup	206	97	1	1	0	0	25	9	16	5	156	0.39	0.09	4	0.03	0.02	0.09	0.07	0.00	1	1
950	Apples-frozen-unsweetened-unheated	1 cup	173	83	0	1	0	0	21	8	13	5	134	0.32	0.08	6	0.02	0.02	0.07	0.06	0.00	1	0
945	Apples-raw-peeled	1 item	128	73	0	0	0	0	19	5	9	0	144	0.09	0.05	6	0.02	0.01	0.12	0.06	0.00	1	5
946	Apples-raw-peeled-boiled	1 cup	171	91	0	1	0	0	23	9	13	2	150	0.32	0.07	8	0.03	0.02	0.16	0.08	0.00	1	0
224	Apples-raw-sliced-with skin	1 cup	110	65	0	0	0	0	17	8	8	0	126	0.20	0.04	6	0.02	0.02	0.09	0.05	0.00	3	6
223	Apples-raw-with skin-2¾ inch diameter	1 item	138	81	0	0	0	0	21	10	10	1	159	0.25	0.05	7	0.02	0.02	0.11	0.07	0.00	4	8
226	Applesauce-canned-sweetened	1 cup	255	194	0	0	0	0	51	9	17	8	156	0.89	0.10	3	0.03	0.07	0.48	0.07	0.00	2	4
227	Applesauce-canned-unsweetened	1 cup	244	105	0	0	0	0	28	7	17	5	183	0.29	0.07	7	0.03	0.06	0.46	0.06	0.00	1	3
228	Apricot-raw-without pit	1 item	35	17	0	0	0	0	4	5	7	0	104	0.19	0.09	92	0.01	0.01	0.21	0.02	0.00	3	4
229	Apricots-canned-heavy syrup-with skin	1 cup	258	214	1	0	0	0	55	22	32	10	361	0.77	0.27	317	0.05	0.06	0.97	0.14	0.00	4	8
954	Apricots-canned-juice pack	1 cup	248	119	2	0	0	0	31	30	50	9	409	0.74	0.27	420	0.05	0.05	0.85	0.13	0.00	4	12
955	Apricots-canned-light syrup pack	1 cup	253	159	1	0	0	0	42	28	34	10	349	0.99	0.27	334	0.04	0.05	0.77	0.14	0.00	4	7
953	Apricots-canned-water pack	1 cup	243	66	2	0	0	0	16	19	32	7	467	0.78	0.27	314	0.05	0.06	0.96	0.13	0.00	4	8
231	Apricots-dried-sulfured-cooked-no sugar	1 cup	250	213	3	0	0	0	55	40	104	9	1222	4.17	0.66	591	0.02	0.08	2.36	0.29	0.00	0	4
230	Apricots-dried-sulfured-uncooked	1 cup	130	309	5	1	0	0	80	59	152	13	1791	6.11	0.97	941	0.01	0.20	3.90	0.20	0.00	13	3
956	Apricots-frozen-sweetened	1 cup	242	237	2	0	0	0	61	24	46	10	554	2.18	0.24	407	0.05	0.10	1.94	0.15	0.00	4	22
125	Apricots-halves-with skin-canned-water	1 serving	28	6	0	0	0	0	2	5	5	3	44	0.15	0.03	51	0.01	0.01	0.12	0.02	0.00	0	1
751	Arby's-beef and cheese sandwich	1 item	176	402	32	18	9	77	27	183	401	1634	345	5.05	5.37	58	0.38	0.46	5.90	0.34	2.05	41	0
2008	Arby's-chicken breast sandwich	1 item	184	493	23	25	5	91	48	111	290	1019	330	3.45	1.66	15	0.45	0.39	14.80	0.65	0.34	32	0
754	Arby's-club sandwich	1 item	252	560	30	30	12	100	43	200	433	1610	466	3.60	3.13	127	0.68	0.43	7.00	0.40	0.94	44	28
752	Arby's-ham and cheese sandwich	1 item	146	353	21	16	6	58	33	130	152	772	290	3.25	1.38	96	0.31	0.49	2.69	0.20	0.54	71	3
750	Arby's-roast beef sandwich	1 item	139	346	22	14	4	52	34	54	239	792	316	4.23	3.39	63	0.38	0.31	5.86	0.27	1.22	40	2
2009	Arby's-super roast beef sandwich	1 item	234	501	25	22	9	40	50	115	402	798	503	6.38	10.70	0	0.53	0.60	9.44	0.48	4.29	41	0
753	Arby's-turkey deluxe	1 item	236	510	28	24	—	70	46	80	—	1220	—	2.70	—	—	0.45	0.34	8.00	—	—	—	—
1738	Arthur Treacher-chicken sandwich	1 item	156	413	16	19	—	—	44	59	147	708	279	1.70	—	37	0.17	0.24	8.10	—	—	—	19
1044	Artichokes-boiled-drained	1 item	120	60	4	0	0	0	13	54	103	114	425	1.55	0.59	22	0.08	0.08	1.20	0.13	0.00	61	12
1691	Asparagus-canned-dietary pack-low sodium	1 cup	244	34	4	0	0	0	5	34	93	849	373	1.42	1.15	115	0.13	0.22	2.08	0.24	0.00	208	40
568	Asparagus-canned-spears-drained solids	1 cup	242	46	5	2	0	0	6	39	104	944	416	4.43	0.97	128	0.15	0.24	2.31	0.27	0.00	231	45
567	Asparagus-frozen-boiled-drained-spears	1 cup	180	50	5	1	0	0	9	41	99	7	392	1.15	1.00	147	0.12	0.19	1.87	0.04	0.00	242	44
565	Asparagus-frozen-boiled-drained-tips	1 cup	180	50	5	1	0	0	9	41	99	7	392	1.15	1.01	148	0.12	0.19	1.87	0.04	0.00	242	44
566	Asparagus-raw-boiled-drained-spears	1 cup	180	45	5	1	0	0	8	43	110	7	558	1.19	0.86	149	0.18	0.22	1.89	0.25	0.00	177	49
564	Asparagus-raw-boiled-drained-tips	1 cup	180	45	5	1	0	0	8	43	110	7	558	1.19	0.86	149	0.18	0.22	1.89	0.25	0.00	177	49
233	Avocado-raw-california	1 item	173	306	4	30	4	0	12	19	73	21	1097	2.04	0.73	106	0.19	0.21	3.32	0.48	0.00	113	14
234	Avocado-raw-florida	1 item	304	340	5	27	5	0	27	33	119	15	1484	1.61	1.28	186	0.33	0.37	5.84	0.85	0.00	162	24
1366	Baby food-apple betty	1 ounce	28	20	0	0	0	0	6	5	1	3	14	0.05	0.00	0	0.00	0.01	0.01	0.00	0.01	0	10
777	Baby food-apple blueberry	1 ounce	28	17	0	0	0	0	5	1	2	0	20	0.06	0.01	1	0.01	0.01	0.03	0.01	0.00	1	8
787	Baby food-apple juice	1 fl oz	31	14	0	0	0	0	4	1	2	1	28	0.18	0.01	1	0.00	0.01	0.03	0.01	0.00	0	18
788	Baby food-apple peach juice	1 fl oz	31	13	0	0	0	0	3	1	1	0	30	0.17	0.01	2	0.00	0.00	0.07	0.01	0.00	0	18
789	Baby food-apple prune juice	1 fl oz	31	23	0	0	0	0	6	3	5	2	46	0.29	0.02	1	0.00	0.00	0.09	0.01	0.00	0	21
778	Baby food-applesauce	1 ounce	28	12	0	0	0	0	3	1	2	1	20	0.06	0.01	0	0.00	0.01	0.02	0.01	0.00	1	11
802	Baby food-arrowroot cookie	1 item	6	24	0	1	0	0	4	2	7	22	9	0.18	0.03	—	0.03	0.03	0.34	0.00	0.00	1	0
779	Baby food-bananas & tapioca	1 ounce	28	16	0	0	0	0	4	1	2	3	25	0.06	0.02	1	0.00	0.01	0.05	0.03	0.00	2	5
759	Baby food-barley cereal with milk	1 ounce	28	31	1	1	0	0	5	65	43	14	54	3.50	0.24	6	0.14	0.16	1.70	0.03	0.09	3	0
792	Baby food-beef	1 ounce	28	30	4	2	1	4	0	2	24	23	62	0.42	0.70	16	0.00	0.04	0.81	0.04	0.40	2	1
1370	Baby food-beef & egg noodles-strained	1 ounce	28	15	1	1	0	2	2	3	8	8	13	0.12	0.11	31	0.01	0.01	0.21	0.01	0.03	1	0
767	Baby food-beef lasagna	1 ounce	28	22	1	1	—	—	3	5	11	129	35	0.25	0.20	100	0.02	0.03	0.38	0.02	0.15	2	1
768	Baby food-beef stew	1 ounce	28	14	1	0	0	4	2	3	12	98	40	0.20	0.25	95	0.00	0.02	0.37	0.02	0.15	2	1
1377	Baby food-beets-strained	1 ounce	28	10	0	0	0	0	2	4	4	24	52	0.09	0.03	1	0.00	0.01	0.04	0.01	0.00	9	1
1376	Baby food-buttered green beans-strained	1 ounce	28	9	0	0	0	0	2	18	6	1	45	0.36	0.06	13	0.01	0.03	0.10	0.01	0.00	8	2
604	Baby food-carrots-strained	1 ounce	28	8	0	0	0	0	2	6	6	11	56	0.10	0.04	325	0.01	0.01	0.13	0.02	0.00	4	2
1365	Baby food-cereal & egg yolks-strained	1 ounce	28	15	1	1	0	18	2	7	11	9	11	0.13	0.08	11	0.00	0.01	0.01	0.01	0.02	1	0

793	Baby food-chicken	1 ounce	28	37	4	2	1	—	0	18	27	13	40	0.40	0.34	11	0.00	0.04	0.92	0.06	0.11	3	1
770	Baby food-chicken & noodles	1 ounce	28	15	1	0	1	24	2	6	7	5	11	0.13	0.09	32	0.01	0.02	0.13	0.01	0.04	2	0
1371	Baby food-chicken stew-strained	1 ounce	28	22	2	1	0	8	2	10	14	114	26	0.19	0.12	50	0.01	0.02	0.33	0.01	0.04	0	1
763	Baby food-chocolate custard pudding	1 ounce	28	24	1	1	0	0	5	17	14	7	24	0.11	0.09	1	0.00	0.03	0.03	0.00	0.00	1	0
1362	Baby food-cookies-enriched	1 item	7	28	1	1	0	0	4	7	12	12	33	0.27	0.07	0	0.10	0.21	1.04	0.38	0.30	1	1
764	Baby food-cottage cheese and pineapple	1 ounce	28	20	1	0	0	3	4	7	11	15	12	0.03	0.04	1	0.01	0.02	0.01	0.00	0.02	1	7
769	Baby food-cream of chicken soup	1 ounce	28	16	1	1	0	1	2	10	8	5	22	0.09	0.07	33	0.00	0.01	0.11	0.01	0.02	2	0
1378	Baby food-creamed corn-strained	1 ounce	28	16	0	0	0	0	4	6	9	12	26	0.08	0.05	2	0.00	0.01	0.15	0.01	0.01	3	1
1367	Baby food-dutch apple	1 ounce	28	19	0	0	0	0	5	1	1	5	9	0.06	0.00	1	0.00	0.00	0.01	0.00	0.00	0	6
794	Baby food-egg yolks	1 serving	28	58	3	5	1	223	0	22	81	11	22	0.78	0.54	107	0.02	0.08	0.01	0.05	0.44	26	0
1368	Baby food-fruit dessert-strained	1 ounce	28	17	0	0	0	0	5	2	2	4	27	0.06	0.01	7	0.01	0.00	0.04	0.01	0.00	1	1
803	Baby food-garden vegetables	1 ounce	28	11	1	0	0	0	2	8	8	10	48	0.24	0.07	172	0.02	0.02	0.22	0.03	0.00	11	2
801	Baby food-green beans	1 ounce	28	7	0	0	0	0	2	11	6	1	45	0.21	0.06	13	0.01	0.02	0.10	0.01	0.00	10	2
795	Baby food-ham	1 ounce	28	32	4	2	1	—	0	2	23	12	58	0.29	0.64	3	0.04	0.04	0.75	0.07	0.03	1	1
796	Baby food-lamb	1 ounce	28	29	4	1	1	0	0	2	27	18	58	0.42	0.78	7	0.01	0.06	0.83	0.04	0.62	1	0
797	Baby food-liver	1 ounce	28	29	4	1	0	52	0	1	58	21	64	1.50	0.84	3247	0.01	0.51	2.36	0.10	0.61	96	6
771	Baby food-macaroni & cheese	1 ounce	28	17	1	1	0	2	2	15	16	21	13	0.09	0.10	1	0.02	0.02	0.13	0.01	0.01	0	0
1372	Baby food-macaroni with tomato and beef	1 ounce	28	16	1	0	0	1	3	5	12	5	27	0.14	0.09	26	0.02	0.02	0.23	0.01	0.07	6	0
780	Baby food-mango & tapioca	1 serving	28	23	0	0	0	0	6	1	2	1	17	0.03	0.02	19	0.01	0.01	0.07	0.03	0.00	1	35
760	Baby food-mixed cereal with milk	1 ounce	28	32	1	1	—	0	5	62	40	13	56	2.96	0.20	6	0.12	0.17	1.64	0.02	0.09	3	0
790	Baby food-mixed fruit juice	1 fl oz	31	14	0	0	0	0	4	2	2	1	31	0.10	0.01	1	0.01	0.00	0.04	0.01	0.00	2	20
772	Baby food-mixed vegetables	1 ounce	28	11	0	0	0	0	3	6	—	2	34	0.09	0.05	77	0.00	0.01	0.14	0.02	0.00	2	1
761	Baby food-oatmeal cereal with milk	1 ounce	28	33	1	1	0	0	4	62	45	13	58	3.44	0.26	6	0.14	0.16	1.70	0.02	0.09	3	0
1373	Baby food-orange apple juice	1 fl oz	31	13	0	0	0	0	3	3	2	1	43	0.06	0.01	2	0.01	0.01	0.06	0.01	0.00	4	24
1374	Baby food-orange apricot juice	1 fl oz	31	14	0	0	0	0	3	2	4	2	62	0.12	0.01	7	0.02	0.01	0.08	0.02	0.00	6	27
791	Baby food-orange juice	1 fl oz	31	14	0	0	0	0	3	4	3	0	57	0.05	0.02	2	0.01	0.01	0.07	0.02	0.00	8	19
1375	Baby food-orange prune juice	1 fl oz	31	22	0	0	0	0	5	4	3	1	56	0.27	0.01	4	0.01	0.04	0.12	0.02	0.00	4	20
765	Baby food-orange pudding	1 ounce	28	23	0	0	0	0	5	9	8	6	24	0.03	0.05	3	0.01	0.02	0.03	0.01	0.00	2	3
781	Baby food-papaya/apple & tapioca	1 ounce	28	20	0	0	0	0	5	2	2	1	22	0.13	0.01	2	0.00	0.01	0.03	0.01	0.00	1	32
1369	Baby food-peach cobbler-strained	1 ounce	28	18	0	0	0	0	5	1	1	2	15	0.03	0.09	4	0.00	0.00	0.07	0.00	0.00	0	6
782	Baby food-peaches	1 ounce	28	20	0	0	0	0	5	2	3	2	46	0.07	0.02	5	0.00	0.01	0.17	0.00	0.00	1	9
783	Baby food-pears	1 ounce	28	12	0	0	0	0	3	2	3	1	37	0.07	0.02	1	0.00	0.01	0.05	0.00	0.00	1	7
784	Baby food-pears & pineapple	1 ounce	28	12	0	0	0	0	3	3	2	1	33	0.07	0.02	1	0.01	0.01	0.06	0.01	0.00	1	8
804	Baby food-peas	1 ounce	28	11	1	0	0	0	2	6	12	1	32	0.27	0.10	16	0.02	0.02	0.29	0.02	0.00	7	2
785	Baby food-plums & tapioca	1 ounce	28	20	0	0	0	0	6	2	2	2	24	0.06	0.02	3	0.00	0.01	0.06	0.01	0.00	0	0
798	Baby food-pork	1 ounce	28	35	4	2	1	14	0	1	27	12	63	0.28	0.64	3	0.04	0.06	0.64	0.06	0.28	1	1
1363	Baby food-pretzels-enriched	1 item	6	24	1	0	0	0	5	1	7	16	8	0.23	0.05	0	0.03	0.02	0.21	0.01	0.00	6	0
786	Baby food-prunes & tapioca	1 ounce	28	20	0	0	0	0	5	4	4	1	50	0.10	0.03	13	0.01	0.02	0.15	0.02	0.00	0	0
762	Baby food-rice cereal with milk	1 ounce	28	33	1	1	0	0	5	68	50	13	54	3.46	0.18	6	0.13	0.14	1.48	0.03	0.09	2	0
805	Baby food-squash	1 ounce	28	7	0	0	0	0	2	7	4	1	51	0.08	0.04	57	0.00	0.02	0.10	0.02	0.00	4	2
806	Baby food-sweet potatoes	1 ounce	28	16	0	0	0	0	4	4	7	6	75	0.10	0.06	183	0.01	0.01	0.10	0.03	0.00	3	3
758	Baby food-teething biscuits	1 item	11	43	1	1	0	0	8	29	18	40	35	0.39	0.10	1	0.03	0.06	0.48	0.01	0.01	2	1
799	Baby food-turkey	1 ounce	28	32	4	2	1	—	0	7	36	16	65	0.34	0.52	48	0.01	0.06	1.04	0.05	0.28	3	1
773	Baby food-turkey & rice	1 ounce	28	14	1	0	0	3	2	6	6	5	12	0.07	0.07	27	0.00	0.01	0.09	0.01	0.03	1	0
766	Baby food-vanilla custard pudding	1 ounce	28	24	0	1	0	0	5	16	13	8	19	0.07	0.08	2	0.00	0.02	0.01	0.01	0.00	2	0
800	Baby food-veal	1 ounce	28	29	4	1	1	11	0	2	28	18	61	0.36	0.57	4	0.01	0.05	1.01	0.04	0.37	2	1
776	Baby food-veal & vegetables	1 ounce	28	20	2	1	0	6	2	3	15	7	43	0.17	0.28	21	0.01	0.02	0.46	0.02	0.13	2	1
774	Baby food-vegetables & beef	1 ounce	28	15	1	1	0	3	2	3	12	6	29	0.11	0.09	49	0.01	0.01	0.14	0.02	0.07	1	0
775	Baby food-vegetables & liver	1 ounce	28	11	1	0	0	0	2	2	11	5	27	0.63	0.11	208	0.01	0.08	0.34	0.02	0.51	8	1
1364	Baby food-zwieback cookies	1 piece	7	30	1	1	0	1	5	1	4	16	21	0.04	0.04	0	0.02	0.02	0.09	0.01	0.00	1	0
1379	Baby food-creamed peas-strained	1 ounce	28	15	1	1	0	0	3	4	9	4	25	0.16	0.11	2	0.03	0.02	0.23	0.01	0.02	6	1
1380	Baby food-creamed spinach-strained	1 ounce	28	11	1	0	0	0	2	25	15	14	54	0.18	0.09	118	0.00	0.03	0.06	0.02	0.02	17	3
1408	Bacon bits	1 tbsp	6	27	2	2	0	0	2	8	18	165	9	0.30	0.11	0	0.03	0.02	0.14	0.01	0.07	8	0
161	Bacon-pork-broiled/pan-fried/roasted	1 slice	6	36	2	3	1	5	0	1	21	101	31	0.10	0.21	0	0.04	0.02	0.46	0.02	0.11	0	2
319	Bagel-egg-3 inch diameter	1 item	55	163	6	1	—	8	31	23	37	198	41	1.46	0.29	24	0.21	0.16	1.94	0.02	0.05	13	0
320	Bagel-water-3 inch diameter	1 item	55	163	6	1	0	0	31	23	37	198	41	1.46	0.29	0	0.21	0.16	1.94	0.02	0.00	13	0
684	Baking powder-low sodium	1 tsp	4	7	0	0	0	0	2	207	314	0	471	0.00	—	0	0.00	0.00	0.00	—	—	—	0
681	Baking powder-no calcium sulfate	1 tsp	3	4	0	0	0	0	1	58	87	329	5	0.00	—	0	0.00	0.00	0.00	—	—	—	0
683	Baking powder-straight phosphate	1 tsp	4	5	0	0	0	0	1	239	359	312	6	0.00	—	0	0.00	0.00	0.00	—	—	—	0
682	Baking powder-with calcium sulfate	1 tsp	3	3	0	0	0	0	1	183	45	290	4	0.00	—	0	0.00	0.00	0.00	—	—	—	0
1611	Baking soda	1 tsp	3	0	0	0	0	0	0	—	—	821	—	—	—	0	0.00	0.00	0.00	0.00	0.00	0	0
1045	Balsam pear-leafy tips-boiled-drained	1 cup	58	20	2	0	0	0	4	24	45	8	349	0.59	0.17	100	0.09	0.16	0.58	0.44	0.00	51	32
1046	Balsam pear-pods-boiled-drained	1 cup	124	24	1	0	0	0	5	11	45	7	396	0.47	0.96	14	0.06	0.07	0.35	0.05	0.00	63	41

Dashes (—) in data spaces indicate that no data were reported.

Appendix C Table of Food Composition

Item	Food Name	Portion	Weight (g)	Food Energy (kcal)	Protein (g)	Total Fat (g)	Saturated Fat (g)	Cholesterol (mg)	Carbohydrate (g)	Calcium (mg)	Phosphorus (mg)	Sodium (mg)	Potassium (mg)	Iron (mg)	Zinc (cm)	Vitamin A (RE)	Thiamin (mg)	Riboflavin (mg)	Niacin (mg)	Vitamin B6 (mg)	Vitamin B12 (ug)	Folic Acid (ug)	Vitamin C (mg)
1048	Bamboo shoots-boiled-drained	1 cup	120	14	2	0	0	0	2	14	24	5	640	0.29	0.56	0	0.02	0.06	0.36	0.12	0.00	3	0
1049	Bamboo shoots-canned-drained	1 cup	131	25	2	1	0	0	4	11	33	9	105	0.42	0.85	1	0.03	0.03	0.18	0.18	0.00	4	1
1047	Bamboo shoots-raw	1 cup	151	41	4	0	0	0	8	20	89	6	805	0.76	1.66	3	0.23	0.11	0.91	0.36	0.00	11	6
236	Banana flakes-dehydrated or powdered	1 tbsp	6	22	0	0	0	0	5	1	5	0	92	0.07	0.04	2	0.01	0.02	0.17	—	0.00	—	0
235	Bananas-raw-peeled	1 item	114	105	1	1	0	0	27	7	22	1	451	0.35	0.19	9	0.05	0.11	0.62	0.66	0.00	22	10
1326	Barbecue loaf-pork and beef	1 slice	23	40	4	2	1	9	1	13	30	307	76	0.27	0.57	2	0.08	0.06	0.52	0.06	0.39	2	4
1486	Barbecued chicken-light and elegant	1 item	227	300	26	6	3	97	35	22	896	900	450	1.50	2.90	189	0.19	0.15	6.90	0.57	0.36	40	5
1952	Barley-dry-uncooked	1 cup	184	651	23	4	1	0	135	61	485	22	831	6.63	5.10	4	1.19	0.53	8.47	0.59	0.00	35	0
1953	Barley-pearled-light-cooked	1 cup	157	193	4	1	0	0	44	17	85	5	145	2.09	1.29	2	0.13	0.10	3.24	0.18	0.00	26	0
321	Barley-pearled-light-uncooked	1 cup	200	704	20	2	0	0	155	57	442	18	560	5.00	4.25	4	0.38	0.23	9.21	0.52	0.00	46	0
808	Basil-ground	1 tsp	1	4	0	0	0	0	1	30	7	0	48	0.59	0.08	13	0.00	0.00	0.10	—	0.00	—	1
809	Bay leaf-crumbled	1 tsp	1	2	0	0	0	0	0	5	1	0	3	0.26	0.02	4	0.00	0.00	0.01	—	0.00	—	0
1801	Beans-adzuki-boiled	1 cup	230	294	17	0	0	0	57	63	385	18	1224	4.60	4.06	1	0.27	0.15	1.65	0.22	0.00	279	0
1802	Beans-adzuki-canned-sweetened	1 cup	296	702	11	0	0	0	163	66	220	646	353	3.34	4.62	3	0.30	0.17	1.87	0.25	0.00	316	0
1804	Beans-baked beans-canned	1 cup	254	236	12	1	0	0	52	127	264	1008	752	0.74	3.56	43	0.39	0.15	1.09	0.34	0.00	61	8
1803	Beans-baked beans-home recipe	1 cup	253	382	14	13	5	13	54	155	275	1068	907	5.04	1.84	0	0.34	0.12	1.03	0.23	0.03	122	3
1805	Beans-black-cooked-boiled	1 cup	172	227	15	1	0	0	41	47	241	1	611	3.60	1.92	1	0.42	0.10	0.87	0.12	0.00	256	0
1806	Beans-french-cooked-boiled	1 cup	177	228	13	1	0	0	43	111	181	11	655	1.92	1.13	1	0.23	0.11	0.97	0.19	0.00	132	2
123	Beans-garbanzo-canned-reconstituted	1 serving	28	28	1	1	0	0	5	11	30	113	55	0.71	0.26	1	0.00	0.01	0.09	—	0.00	—	1
1678	Beans-garbanzo-dry-raw	1 cup	200	720	41	10	—	0	122	300	662	52	1594	13.80	—	10	0.62	0.30	4.00	—	0.00	—	—
509	Beans-great northern-dry-cooked-drained	1 cup	180	210	14	1	4	0	38	90	266	12	749	4.90	1.80	0	0.25	0.13	1.30	1.01	0.00	63	0
1688	Beans-green-canned-dietary-low sodium	1 cup	136	26	2	0	0	0	6	32	26	3	148	1.22	0.40	—	0.02	0.08	0.27	—	0.00	43	6
573	Beans-green-frozen-boiled-french style	1 cup	135	35	2	0	0	0	8	61	32	18	151	1.11	0.84	72	0.07	0.10	0.56	0.08	0.00	11	11
1712	Beans-kidney-canned-dietary-low sodium	1 cup	255	230	15	1	0	0	42	74	278	10	673	4.60	1.91	1	0.13	0.10	1.50	1.12	0.00	36	8
570	Beans-lima-baby-frozen-boiled-drained	1 cup	180	189	12	1	0	0	35	50	202	52	740	3.53	0.99	31	0.13	0.10	1.39	0.21	0.00	28	10
1690	Beans-lima-canned-dietary-low sodium	1 cup	248	186	11	1	0	0	34	70	176	10	668	3.94	1.58	43	0.07	0.11	1.32	0.15	0.00	40	22
1050	Beans-lima-canned-solids & liquids	1 cup	248	186	11	1	0	0	34	70	176	618	668	3.94	1.58	43	0.07	0.11	1.32	0.15	0.00	40	22
569	Beans-lima-frozen-boiled-drained	1 cup	170	170	10	1	0	0	32	38	153	90	694	2.32	0.74	32	0.12	0.10	1.80	0.21	0.00	111	22
515	Beans-lima-raw-boiled-drained	1 cup	170	209	12	1	0	0	40	54	221	29	969	4.17	1.34	63	0.24	0.16	1.77	0.33	0.00	45	17
579	Beans-mung-sprouted-boiled	1 cup	125	26	3	0	0	0	5	15	35	13	126	0.81	0.59	1	0.06	0.13	1.01	0.07	0.00	37	14
578	Beans-mung-sprouted-raw	1 cup	104	31	3	0	0	0	6	14	56	6	155	0.95	0.43	2	0.09	0.13	0.78	0.09	0.00	63	14
510	Beans-navy pea-dry-cooked-drained	1 cup	190	225	15	1	0	0	40	95	281	13	790	5.10	1.80	0	0.27	0.13	1.30	1.06	0.00	67	0
1051	Beans-navy-sprouted-boiled	1 ounce	28	22	2	0	0	0	4	5	29	4	90	0.60	0.28	0	0.11	0.07	0.36	0.06	0.00	30	5
1052	Beans-pinto-frozen-boiled	1 ounce	28	46	3	0	0	0	9	15	28	24	183	0.77	0.20	0	0.08	0.03	0.18	0.06	0.00	10	0
514	Beans-red kidney-canned-solids & liquids	1 cup	255	230	15	1	1	0	42	74	278	833	673	4.60	1.91	1	0.13	0.10	1.50	1.12	0.00	36	8
1810	Beans-refried	1 cup	253	271	16	3	1	0	47	116	213	1073	994	4.48	3.47	0	0.12	0.14	1.23	0.25	0.00	211	15
1735	Beans-refried-canned-sausage-old el paso	1 cup	200	388	14	26	7	16	26	88	258	624	600	4.16	1.76	0	0.29	0.14	0.63	0.31	0.00	254	6
1053	Beans-shellie-canned	1 cup	245	74	4	0	0	0	15	71	74	818	267	2.43	0.66	56	0.08	0.13	0.50	0.12	0.00	44	8
1807	Beans-small white-boiled	1 cup	179	254	16	1	0	0	46	131	302	4	828	5.08	1.95	0	0.42	0.11	0.49	0.23	0.00	245	0
574	Beans-snap-green-canned-drained-cuts	1 cup	135	27	2	0	0	0	6	35	34	339	147	1.20	0.39	47	0.02	0.08	0.27	0.05	0.00	43	7
41	Beans-snap-green-dietetic-low sodium	1 ounce	28	4	0	0	0	0	1	7	6	0	24	0.17	0.06	10	0.01	0.01	0.09	—	0.00	—	1
572	Beans-snap-green-frozen-boiled-cuts	1 cup	135	35	2	0	0	0	8	61	32	18	151	1.11	0.84	72	0.07	0.10	0.56	0.08	0.00	11	11
571	Beans-snap-green-raw-boiled	1 cup	125	44	2	0	0	0	10	58	49	4	374	1.60	0.45	84	0.09	0.12	0.77	0.07	0.00	42	12
577	Beans-snap-yellow/wax-canned	1 cup	136	27	2	0	0	0	6	35	26	341	148	1.22	0.39	48	0.02	0.08	0.27	0.05	0.00	43	7
576	Beans-snap-yellow/wax-frozen-boiled	1 cup	135	35	2	0	0	0	8	61	32	18	151	1.11	0.84	72	0.07	0.10	0.56	0.08	0.00	11	11
575	Beans-snap-yellow/wax-raw-boiled	1 cup	125	44	2	0	0	0	10	58	48	4	374	1.60	0.45	84	0.09	0.12	0.77	0.07	0.00	42	12
463	Beef and green peppers-stouffer	1 item	220	225	10	11	—	—	18	0	—	960	420	2.33	—	136	0.08	0.16	3.88	—	—	—	0
1442	Beef and spinach pasta shells-stouffer	1 item	255	290	19	11	—	—	28	—	—	1315	485	—	—	—	—	—	—	—	—	—	—
79	Beef burgundy-frozen dinner	1 item	142	144	17	5	—	—	6	5	—	411	147	0.60	—	449	0.04	0.24	4.10	—	—	—	0
1482	Beef burgundy-light and elegant dinner	1 item	255	230	23	4	3	95	25	14	172	1235	200	3.10	8.07	181	0.15	0.23	1.70	0.49	4.12	25	1
1450	Beef cubes in wine sauce-hormel entree	1 ounce	28	52	4	4	2	15	1	3	23	106	71	0.47	1.27	—	0.77	0.05	0.50	0.02	0.41	4	0
162	Beef cuts-lean and fat-simmered/roasted	1 slice	85	297	21	23	9	78	0	8	164	50	244	2.21	4.67	0	0.07	0.18	2.94	0.26	2.03	6	0
163	Beef cuts-lean only-simmered/roasted	1 slice	85	347	19	30	12	78	0	8	147	55	186	1.85	4.51	0	0.05	0.15	2.43	0.20	1.91	5	0
1631	Beef dinner-swanson frozen dinner	1 item	326	320	25	9	10	84	34	36	283	1085	616	3.98	4.69	1140	0.14	0.27	4.88	0.52	2.10	24	6
1483	Beef julienne-light and elegant dinner	1 item	241	260	21	7	—	—	27	27	152	990	240	4.90	—	356	0.09	0.10	3.50	—	—	—	4
178	Beef potpie-home recipe-⅓ of 9″ "pie"	1 slice	210	515	21	30	8	44	39	29	149	596	334	3.80	—	344	0.30	0.30	5.50	—	—	—	6
1449	Beef short ribs in barbecue sauce-hormel	1 ounce	28	54	5	3	2	15	1	3	28	176	92	0.73	1.71	11	0.01	0.07	0.66	0.03	0.52	11	0
1616	Beef sirloin tips-le menu	1 item	326	400	29	19	—	—	27	—	—	1100	—	—	—	—	—	—	—	—	—	—	—
1453	Beef stew-hormel entree	1 ounce	28	29	2	1	0	7	2	4	15	106	51	0.21	0.49	—	0.01	0.02	0.29	0.01	0.15	6	0
177	Beef stew-with vegetables	1 cup	245	220	16	11	5	72	15	29	184	1006	613	2.90	—	480	0.15	0.17	4.70	—	0.00	—	17

81	Beef stroganoff-frozen dinner	1 item	170	192	20	8	—	—	8	23	—	785	316	2.90	—	68	0.05	0.32	2.90	—	—	—	2
1484	Beef stroganoff-light and elegant	1 item	255	260	24	6	11	84	27	45	79	785	230	3.00	4.85	189	0.20	0.26	2.20	0.28	2.58	19	2
1485	Beef teriyaki-light and elegant	1 item	227	240	18	3	—	—	37	30	152	625	215	5.60	—	24	0.40	0.10	2.50	—	—	—	2
176	Beef-dried-cured-chipped	1 serving	71	117	21	3	1	65	1	4	124	2464	315	3.20	3.72	—	0.05	0.23	2.70	—	1.31	—	0
181	Beef-heart-cooked-simmered	1 slice	85	149	25	5	1	164	0	5	213	54	198	6.38	2.66	0	0.12	1.31	3.46	0.18	12.20	2	1
188	Beef-liver-fried in margarine	1 slice	85	184	23	7	2	410	7	9	392	90	309	5.34	4.63	9216	0.18	3.52	12.30	1.22	95.00	187	19
1755	Beef-pot roast-chuck-arm cut-cooked	1 slice	100	231	33	10	4	101	0	9	268	66	289	3.79	8.66	0	0.08	0.29	3.72	0.33	3.40	11	0
1756	Beef-pot roast-chuck-blade cut-cooked	1 slice	100	270	31	15	6	106	0	13	235	71	263	3.68	10.30	0	0.08	0.28	2.67	0.29	2.47	6	0
77	Beef-raviolios-canned with meat sauce	1 ounce	28	28	1	1	0	—	4	5	—	131	46	0.31	—	50	0.03	0.02	0.40	—	—	—	0
1757	Beef-rib steak-cooked	1 item	100	221	28	11	5	80	0	13	208	69	394	2.57	6.99	0	0.11	0.22	4.80	0.40	3.32	8	0
1750	Beef-steak-chicken fried	1 item	100	389	18	30	7	97	12	11	110	815	126	2.30	4.85	8	0.11	0.14	2.70	0.50	3.27	11	0
1758	Beef-tenderloin steak-broiled	1 item	100	204	28	9	4	84	0	7	238	63	419	3.58	5.59	0	0.13	0.30	3.92	0.38	0.44	8	0
868	Beer-budweiser	12 fl oz	360	150	1	0	0	0	14	12	48	24	84	0.12	0.00	0	0.02	0.10	1.62	0.18	0.12	22	0
869	Beer-light	12 fl oz	354	99	1	0	0	0	5	18	42	11	64	0.14	0.11	0	0.04	0.11	1.39	0.12	0.04	14	0
870	Beer-michelob	12 fl oz	360	160	1	0	0	0	16	12	48	24	84	0.12	0.00	0	0.02	0.10	1.62	0.18	0.12	22	0
871	Beer-natural light	12 fl oz	360	100	0	0	0	0	6	12	48	24	60	0.12	0.12	0	0.04	0.11	1.39	0.12	0.00	14	0
686	Beer-regular	12 fl oz	356	146	1	0	0	0	13	18	43	18	89	0.11	0.07	0	0.02	0.10	1.62	0.18	0.07	21	0
1327	Beerwurst-beer salami-beef	1 slice	6	20	1	2	1	4	0	1	6	62	10	0.09	0.15	0	0.00	0.01	0.20	0.01	0.12	0	1
1311	Beerwurst-beer salami-pork	1 slice	6	14	1	1	0	4	0	0	6	74	15	0.05	0.10	0	0.03	0.01	0.20	0.02	0.05	0	2
584	Beet greens-boiled-drained	1 cup	145	39	4	0	0	0	8	165	60	349	1318	2.76	0.73	740	0.17	0.42	0.72	0.19	0.00	21	36
1689	Beets-canned-dietary pack-low sodium	1 cup	246	71	2	0	0	0	17	34	39	113	349	1.65	0.57	2	0.03	0.09	0.37	0.14	0.00	71	10
581	Beets-sliced-boiled-drained	1 cup	170	53	2	0	0	0	11	19	53	83	530	1.05	0.43	2	0.05	0.02	0.46	0.05	0.00	90	9
583	Beets-sliced-canned-drained	1 cup	170	53	2	0	0	0	12	26	29	466	252	3.09	0.36	2	0.02	0.07	0.27	0.10	0.00	51	7
580	Beets-whole-boiled-drained	1 item	50	16	1	0	0	0	3	6	12	25	156	0.31	0.13	1	0.02	0.01	0.14	0.02	0.00	27	3
582	Beets-whole-canned	1 cup	246	71	2	0	0	0	17	34	39	647	349	1.65	0.57	2	0.03	0.09	0.37	0.14	0.00	71	10
322	Biscuits-baking powder-home recipe	1 item	28	105	2	5	1	0	13	34	49	175	33	0.40	—	0	0.08	0.08	0.70	—	—	—	0
323	Biscuits-baking powder-from mix	1 item	28	104	2	5	3	1	13	34	99	221	33	0.62	0.11	37	0.10	0.07	1.75	0.01	0.04	2	0
1642	Bisquick mix-dry	1 cup	112	480	8	16	—	—	76	—	—	1400	—	—	—	—	—	—	—	—	—	—	—
957	Blackberries-canned-heavy syrup pack	1 cup	256	236	3	0	0	0	59	54	36	7	254	1.66	0.47	56	0.07	0.10	0.74	0.09	0.00	68	7
958	Blackberries-frozen-unsweetened	1 cup	151	97	2	1	0	0	24	44	45	2	211	1.21	0.38	17	0.04	0.07	1.82	0.09	0.00	51	5
237	Blackberries-raw	1 cup	144	75	1	1	0	0	18	46	30	0	282	0.82	0.39	24	0.04	0.06	0.58	0.08	0.00	49	30
959	Blueberries-canned-heavy syrup pack	1 cup	256	225	2	1	0	0	57	14	26	9	102	0.84	0.17	16	0.09	0.14	0.29	0.09	0.00	4	3
960	Blueberries-frozen-unsweetened	1 cup	155	79	1	1	0	0	19	12	17	2	84	0.28	0.11	13	0.05	0.06	0.81	0.09	0.00	10	4
238	Blueberries-raw	1 cup	145	81	1	1	0	0	21	9	15	9	129	0.25	0.16	15	0.07	0.07	0.52	0.05	0.00	9	19
1328	Bockwurst-raw-pork-link	1 item	65	200	9	18	7	38	0	10	95	718	176	0.42	1.01	4	0.27	0.11	2.68	0.15	0.53	4	0
198	Bologna-cured pork-4 by ⅛ inch slice	1 slice	23	57	4	5	2	14	0	3	32	272	65	0.18	0.47	0	0.12	0.04	0.90	0.06	0.21	1	8
961	Boysenberries-canned-heavy syrup pack	1 cup	256	225	3	0	—	0	57	46	25	9	230	1.10	0.48	10	0.07	0.07	0.59	0.10	0.00	88	16
962	Boysenberries-frozen-unsweetened	1 cup	132	66	1	0	0	0	16	36	36	2	183	1.12	0.29	9	0.07	0.05	1.01	0.07	0.00	84	4
853	Brandy-california	1 item	30	73	—	0	0	0	—	—	—	—	—	—	—	—	—	—	—	—	—	—	—
854	Brandy-cognac-pony	1 item	30	73	0	0	0	0	0	0	1	0	1	0.01	0.01	0	0.00	0.00	0.00	0.00	0.00	0	0
1304	Bratwurst-pork-cooked-link	1 item	85	256	12	22	8	51	2	38	126	473	180	1.09	1.96	0	0.43	0.16	2.72	0.18	0.81	2	1
199	Braunschweiger-liver sausage-cured pork	1 slice	18	65	2	6	2	28	1	2	30	206	36	1.68	0.51	759	0.05	0.28	1.51	0.06	3.62	8	2
1737	Bread sticks-vienna type	1 item	35	106	3	1	—	0	20	16	31	548	33	0.30	—	0	0.02	0.03	0.30	—	—	—	0
325	Bread-boston brown-canned	1 slice	45	95	2	1	0	0	21	41	72	112	131	0.90	—	0	0.06	0.04	0.70	—	—	—	0
327	Bread-cracked wheat-enriched	1 slice	25	66	2	1	0	0	13	16	32	108	33	0.67	—	0	0.10	0.10	0.84	0.02	0.00	—	0
1935	Bread-crisp-breakfast-wasa	1 slice	14	54	2	2	—	0	9	—	—	70	35	—	—	—	—	—	—	—	—	—	—
1931	Bread-crisp-whole grain-wasa	1 slice	6	22	1	0	0	0	5	1	6	4	6	0.29	0.05	0	0.03	0.02	0.32	0.00	0.00	1	0
329	Bread-french-enriched	1 slice	35	98	3	1	0	0	18	39	28	193	30	1.08	0.22	0	0.16	0.12	1.40	0.02	0.00	13	0
332	Bread-italian-enriched	1 slice	30	85	3	0	0	0	17	5	23	152	22	0.70	—	0	0.12	0.07	1.00	0.02	0.00	11	0
1934	Bread-melba toast-plain	1 slice	5	16	1	0	0	0	3	5	10	30	11	0.09	0.06	0	0.01	0.01	0.10	0.00	0.00	1	0
1933	Bread-melba toast-wheat	1 slice	5	16	1	0	0	0	3	5	10	30	11	0.10	0.07	0	0.01	0.01	0.10	0.01	0.00	1	0
1932	Bread-melba toast-wheat-unsalted	1 slice	5	16	1	0	0	0	3	5	10	5	11	0.10	0.07	0	0.01	0.01	0.10	0.01	0.00	1	0
1394	Bread-mixed grain-toasted	1 slice	22	66	3	1	—	0	12	27	54	105	56	0.83	0.31	0	0.08	0.10	1.06	0.03	0.00	17	0
1393	Bread-mixed grain-untoasted	1 slice	25	64	2	1	—	0	12	26	53	103	55	0.82	0.30	0	0.10	0.10	1.04	0.03	0.00	16	0
1940	Bread-oat bran-no cholesterol	1 slice	45	99	4	1	—	0	18	—	—	204	—	—	—	—	—	—	—	—	—	—	—
1945	Bread-oatmeal and bran	1 slice	36	90	4	2	0	0	15	40	50	140	64	1.08	0.38	0	0.15	0.10	1.60	0.02	0.02	11	0
1409	Bread-pita	1 item	38	105	4	1	0	0	21	31	38	215	45	0.92	0.26	0	0.17	0.08	1.40	0.04	0.00	22	0
338	Bread-pumpernickel	1 slice	32	82	3	1	—	0	15	23	70	173	139	0.88	0.37	0	0.11	0.17	1.06	0.05	0.00	—	0
334	Bread-raisin-enriched	1 slice	25	70	2	1	0	0	13	26	23	94	60	0.78	0.16	0	0.08	0.16	1.02	0.01	0.00	9	0
336	Bread-rye-american-light	1 slice	25	66	2	1	—	0	12	20	36	174	51	0.68	0.32	0	0.10	0.08	0.83	0.02	0.00	10	0
330	Bread-vienna-enriched	1 slice	25	70	2	1	0	0	13	28	20	138	22	0.77	0.16	0	0.12	0.09	1.00	0.01	0.00	9	0
362	Bread-wheat-firm-enriched-toasted	1 slice	21	59	2	1	0	0	11	17	63	153	42	0.82	0.40	0	0.07	0.05	0.92	0.05	0.00	13	0
359	Bread-wheat-soft-enriched-toasted	1 slice	24	67	3	1	—	0	13	20	72	175	49	0.94	0.46	0	0.08	0.06	1.05	0.05	0.00	15	0

Dashes (—) in data spaces indicate that no data were reported.

Appendix C Table of Food Composition

Item	Food Name	Portion	Weight (g)	Food Energy (kcal)	Protein (g)	Total Fat (g)	Saturated Fat (g)	Cholesterol (mg)	Carbohydrate (g)	Calcium (mg)	Phosphorus (mg)	Sodium (mg)	Potassium (mg)	Iron (mg)	Zinc (cm)	Vitamin A (RE)	Thiamin (mg)	Riboflavin (mg)	Niacin (mg)	Vitamin B6 (mg)	Vitamin B12 (ug)	Folic Acid (ug)	Vitamin C (mg)
1396	Bread-wheat-toasted-home recipe	1 slice	22	68	2	2	0	0	12	20	64	91	87	0.68	0.57	0	0.06	0.04	0.81	0.05	0.03	13	0
352	Bread-white-firm-enriched	1 slice	23	61	2	1	0	0	11	29	25	118	26	0.65	0.14	0	0.11	0.07	0.86	0.01	0.00	8	0
353	Bread-white-firm-enriched-toasted	1 slice	20	65	2	1	0	0	12	22	23	117	28	0.60	0.14	0	0.07	0.06	0.80	0.01	0.00	8	0
0	Bread-white-soft	1 slice	25	67	2	1	0	0	12	32	27	129	28	0.71	0.16	0	0.12	0.08	0.94	0.01	0.00	9	0
350	Bread-white-soft-enriched-crumbs	1 cup	45	120	4	2	0	0	22	57	49	231	50	1.28	0.28	0	0.21	0.14	1.69	0.02	0.00	16	0
349	Bread-white-soft-enriched-cubes	1 cup	30	80	2	1	0	0	15	38	32	154	34	0.85	0.19	0	0.14	0.09	1.13	0.01	0.00	11	0
341	Bread-white-soft-toasted	1 slice	22	67	2	1	0	0	12	32	27	129	28	0.72	0.16	0	0.10	0.08	0.94	0.01	0.00	9	0
361	Bread-whole wheat-firm-enriched	1 slice	25	61	2	1	0	0	11	18	65	159	44	0.86	0.42	0	0.09	0.05	0.96	0.05	0.00	14	0
1395	Bread-whole wheat-home recipe	1 slice	25	67	2	2	0	0	12	20	63	89	85	0.67	0.56	11	0.07	0.04	0.80	0.05	0.03	12	0
358	Bread-whole wheat-soft-enriched	1 slice	28	69	3	1	—	0	13	20	73	178	49	0.96	0.47	0	0.10	0.06	1.07	0.05	0.00	15	0
324	Breadcrumbs-dry-grated-enriched	1 cup	100	390	13	5	1	0	73	122	141	736	152	3.60	—	0	0.35	0.35	4.80	—	—	—	0
963	Breadfruit-raw	1 item	384	396	4	1	0	0	104	65	115	8	1882	2.07	0.46	15	0.42	0.12	3.46	0.36	0.00	39	111
1749	Brisket-lean-cooked	1 slice	100	241	29	13	5	93	0	6	239	72	287	2.77	6.88	0	0.07	0.22	3.75	0.30	2.55	8	0
590	Broccoli-frozen-boiled-drained	1 cup	185	52	6	0	0	0	10	94	102	44	333	1.13	0.56	350	0.10	0.15	0.84	0.24	0.00	104	74
587	Broccoli-raw	1 cup	88	25	3	0	0	0	5	42	58	24	286	0.77	0.35	136	0.06	0.11	0.56	0.14	0.00	63	82
588	Broccoli-raw-boiled-drained	1 cup	155	43	5	1	0	0	8	71	92	40	453	1.30	0.59	215	0.09	0.18	0.89	0.22	0.00	78	116
412	Brownies with nuts-home recipe	1 item	20	95	1	6	2	0	10	8	30	50	38	0.40	—	7	0.04	0.03	0.20	—	—	—	0
414	Brownies-chocolate icing-frozen	1 item	25	105	1	5	2	13	15	10	31	59	44	0.40	0.36	8	0.03	0.03	0.20	0.04	0.05	3	0
413	Brownies-commercially prepared	1 item	60	243	3	10	3	9	39	25	87	153	83	1.29	0.55	3	0.07	0.13	0.58	0.03	0.15	4	3
592	Brussels sprouts-frozen-boiled	1 cup	155	65	6	1	0	0	13	37	84	36	504	1.15	0.56	92	0.16	0.18	0.83	0.45	0.00	157	71
591	Brussels sprouts-raw-boiled	1 cup	156	61	4	1	0	0	14	56	87	33	495	1.87	0.52	112	0.17	0.12	0.95	0.28	0.00	94	97
1956	Buckwheat groats-roasted-cooked	1 cup	198	182	7	1	0	0	40	14	139	8	175	1.58	1.21	0	0.08	0.08	1.86	0.15	0.00	27	0
1955	Buckwheat groats-roasted-dry	1 cup	164	567	19	4	1	0	123	29	523	18	525	4.05	3.97	0	0.37	0.45	8.42	0.58	0.00	69	0
1954	Buckwheat-raw-whole	1 cup	170	583	23	6	1	0	122	31	590	2	782	3.74	4.08	0	0.17	0.72	11.90	0.36	0.00	51	0
384	Bulgur-canned-seasoned	1 cup	135	245	8	4	—	0	44	27	263	621	151	1.90	—	0	0.08	0.05	4.10	—	—	—	0
1957	Bulgur-cooked	1 cup	182	152	6	0	0	0	34	18	73	9	124	1.75	1.04	0	0.10	0.05	1.82	0.15	0.00	33	0
1674	Bulgur-dry-commercial	1 cup	140	479	17	2	0	0	106	49	419	23	573	3.44	2.70	0	0.33	0.16	7.16	0.48	0.00	37	0
1054	Burdock root-boiled-drained	1 item	166	146	3	0	—	0	35	82	154	7	597	1.28	0.63	0	0.07	0.10	0.53	0.46	0.00	32	4
1889	Burger King-croissant-egg and cheese	1 item	127	369	13	25	14	216	24	244	349	551	174	2.20	1.76	300	0.19	0.38	1.51	0.10	0.78	36	0
1890	Burger King-croissant-egg/cheese/ham	1 item	152	475	19	34	18	213	24	144	336	1080	272	2.13	2.17	135	0.52	0.30	3.19	0.23	1.01	36	11
1736	Burger King-whopper hamburger	1 item	261	630	26	36	17	104	50	104	312	990	520	6.00	5.25	192	0.02	0.03	5.20	0.31	2.81	31	13
1897	Burrito-beans and cheese	1 item	93	189	8	6	3	14	28	107	90	583	248	1.14	0.82	118	0.11	0.36	1.79	0.13	0.45	41	1
105	Butter-regular-pat	1 item	5	36	0	4	3	11	0	1	1	41	1	0.01	0.00	8	0.00	0.00	0.00	0.00	0.01	0	0
103	Butter-regular-stick	1 item	113	813	1	92	57	248	0	27	26	937	29	0.18	0.06	855	0.01	0.04	0.05	0.00	0.14	3	0
104	Butter-regular-tablespoon	1 tbsp	14	100	0	11	7	31	0	3	3	116	4	0.02	0.01	105	0.00	0.01	0.01	0.00	0.02	0	0
921	Butter-unsalted-pat	1 item	5	36	0	4	3	11	0	1	1	1	1	0.01	0.00	38	0.00	0.00	0.00	0.00	0.01	0	0
108	Butter-whipped-pat	1 item	4	27	0	3	2	8	0	1	1	31	1	0.01	0.00	29	0.00	0.00	0.00	0.00	0.01	0	0
106	Butter-whipped-stick	1 item	76	542	1	61	38	165	0	18	17	625	20	0.12	0.04	570	0.00	0.03	0.03	0.00	0.10	2	0
107	Butter-whipped-tablespoon	1 tbsp	9	65	0	7	5	20	0	2	2	74	2	0.01	0.01	68	0.00	0.00	0.00	0.00	0.01	0	0
944	Butter-whipped-unsalted-pat	1 item	4	27	0	3	2	8	0	1	1	0	1	0.01	0.00	29	0.00	0.00	0.00	0.00	0.01	0	0
1452	Cabbage rolls in tomato sauce-hormel	1 ounce	28	23	1	1	0	3	3	6	16	127	87	0.25	0.19	—	0.76	0.02	0.29	0.03	0.10	3	0
84	Cabbage rolls-frozen dinner	1 item	227	168	11	6	—	—	17	49	—	1026	290	1.40	—	136	0.09	0.16	2.70	—	—	—	0
598	Cabbage-celery-raw	1 cup	76	12	1	0	0	0	2	59	22	7	181	0.24	0.18	91	0.03	0.04	0.30	0.18	0.00	60	21
595	Cabbage-common-boiled-drained	1 cup	145	31	1	0	0	0	7	48	36	28	297	0.57	0.23	13	0.08	0.08	0.33	0.09	0.00	29	35
594	Cabbage-common-raw-shredded	1 cup	90	22	1	0	0	0	5	42	21	16	221	0.50	0.16	11	0.05	0.03	0.27	0.09	0.00	51	43
593	Cabbage-common-raw-sliced	1 cup	70	17	1	0	0	0	4	33	16	13	172	0.39	0.13	9	0.04	0.02	0.21	0.07	0.00	40	33
596	Cabbage-red-raw-shredded	1 cup	70	19	1	0	0	0	4	36	29	8	144	0.34	0.15	3	0.04	0.02	0.21	0.15	0.00	15	40
597	Cabbage-savoy-raw-shredded	1 cup	70	19	1	0	0	0	4	25	29	20	161	0.28	0.19	70	0.05	0.02	0.21	0.13	0.00	56	22
599	Cabbage-white mustard-boiled	1 cup	170	20	3	0	0	0	3	158	49	58	631	1.77	0.29	437	0.05	0.11	0.73	0.28	0.00	69	44
589	Cabbage-white mustard-raw	1 cup	70	9	1	0	0	0	2	74	26	46	176	0.56	0.13	210	0.03	0.05	0.35	0.14	0.00	46	32
386	Cake-angel food-prepared from mix	1 slice	53	142	4	0	—	0	32	50	63	142	52	0.45	0.11	0	0.06	0.12	0.59	0.01	0.02	5	0
1399	Cake-cheesecake-commercial	1 slice	85	257	5	16	7	57	24	48	75	189	83	0.41	0.36	43	0.03	0.11	0.39	0.05	0.42	15	4
1606	Cake-cheesecake-wt watchers	1 slice	113	180	6	6	5	23	25	60	106	366	192	1.80	0.61	90	0.05	0.31	1.14	0.05	0.25	13	0
388	Cake-coffee-prepared from mix	1 slice	72	230	5	7	2	—	38	44	125	310	78	1.20	—	24	0.14	0.15	1.30	—	—	—	0
392	Cake-devils food with icing-from mix	1 slice	69	235	3	8	3	33	40	41	72	180	90	1.00	—	20	0.07	0.10	0.60	—	—	4	0
403	Cake-fruitcake-dark-home recipe	1 slice	15	57	1	2	0	7	9	11	17	24	74	0.42	—	4	0.02	0.02	0.17	—	—	—	0
395	Cake-gingerbread-prepared from mix	1 slice	63	175	2	4	1	1	32	57	63	90	173	0.90	0.28	0	0.09	0.11	0.80	0.05	0.07	5	0
1397	Cake-pineapple upside down-home recipe	1 slice	70	221	2	9	2	20	35	50	44	167	119	1.11	0.38	54	0.11	0.08	0.74	0.04	0.06	8	4
409	Cake-pound-home recipe	1 slice	33	160	2	10	6	68	16	6	24	58	20	0.50	—	16	0.05	0.06	0.40	—	—	2	0
405	Cake-sheet-no icing-home recipe	1 slice	86	315	4	12	3	1	48	55	88	382	68	0.90	0.30	30	0.13	0.15	1.10	0.02	0.09	6	0

407	Cake-sheet-plain-uncooked white icing	1 slice	121	445	4	14	5	1	77	61	91	274	74	0.80	—	48	0.14	0.16	1.10	—	—	7	0
411	Cake-sponge-home recipe	1 slice	66	188	5	3	1	162	36	25	65	164	59	1.11	0.80	25	0.09	0.13	0.73	0.04	0.33	15	0
1746	Cake-strawberry shortcake	1 serving	175	344	5	9	—	—	61	73	84	—	—	2.00	—	86	0.17	0.21	1.30	—	—	—	89
1398	Cake-streusel type-with icing-from mix	1 slice	50	172	2	8	—	—	25	27	99	214	55	0.68	0.20	6	0.06	0.06	0.46	0.02	0.10	5	0
397	Cake-white/chocolate icing-home recipe	1 slice	71	271	3	11	3	3	42	70	127	200	77	0.68	0.26	4	0.07	0.11	0.68	0.02	0.06	4	0
399	Cake-yellow/chocolate icing-home recipe	1 slice	69	268	3	11	3	36	40	57	61	191	73	0.79	0.34	10	0.08	0.10	0.66	0.02	0.12	6	0
1312	Canadian bacon-pork-grilled	1 slice	23	43	6	2	1	14	0	3	69	360	91	0.19	0.40	0	0.19	0.05	1.61	0.11	0.18	1	5
1786	Candy-almond joy	1 ounce	28	151	2	8	2	1	19	60	68	22	114	0.25	0.41	3	0.02	0.10	0.18	0.02	0.18	4	0
1785	Candy-bit o honey	1 ounce	28	121	1	4	2	—	21	13	—	—	—	0.25	—	—	0.00	0.13	1.40	—	—	—	—
537	Candy-caramels-plain/chocolate	1 ounce	28	115	1	3	2	0	22	42	35	74	54	0.40	0.18	0	0.01	0.05	0.10	0.01	0.04	2	0
540	Candy-chocolate coated peanuts	1 ounce	28	160	5	12	4	0	11	33	84	16	143	0.40	—	0	0.10	0.05	2.10	—	—	—	0
539	Candy-chocolate-semisweet	1 cup	170	860	7	61	36	0	97	51	255	3	553	4.40	2.55	9	0.02	0.14	0.90	0.07	0.00	5	0
541	Candy-fondant-uncoated	1 ounce	28	105	0	1	0	0	25	4	2	60	1	0.30	0.00	0	0.00	0.00	0.00	0.00	0.00	0	0
542	Candy-fudge-chocolate-plain	1 ounce	28	115	1	3	1	0	21	22	24	54	42	0.30	0.08	0	0.01	0.03	0.10	0.01	0.06	1	0
543	Candy-gum drops	1 ounce	28	100	0	0	0	0	25	2	0	10	1	0.10	0.00	0	0.00	0.00	0.00	0.00	0.00	0	0
544	Candy-hard	1 ounce	28	110	0	0	0	0	28	6	2	9	1	0.50	—	0	0.00	0.00	0.00	—	—	—	0
1787	Candy-jelly beans	1 item	3	7	0	0	0	0	3	0	0	0	0	0.03	—	0	0.00	—	—	—	—	—	0
1784	Candy-kit kat bar	1 item	43	210	3	11	6	3	25	65	78	38	129	0.56	0.43	9	0.03	0.11	0.10	0.02	0.07	3	0
1780	Candy-life savers	1 item	2	8	0	0	0	0	2	0	0	1	0	0.04	—	0	0.00	0.00	0.00	—	—	—	0
1790	Candy-lollipop	1 item	28	108	0	0	0	0	28	0	0	—	—	0.00	—	0	0.00	0.00	0.00	—	—	—	0
1781	Candy-m & m-plain-package	1 item	45	220	3	10	—	—	31	—	—	—	—	—	—	—	—	—	—	—	—	—	—
1711	Candy-milk chocolate bar-no sugar	1 item	10	60	1	4	—	—	5	—	—	10	—	—	—	—	—	—	—	—	—	—	—
1676	Candy-milk chocolate with almonds	1 ounce	28	151	3	10	4	5	15	65	77	23	125	0.50	0.44	21	0.02	0.12	0.20	0.01	0.15	4	0
1675	Candy-milk chocolate with peanuts	1 ounce	28	154	4	11	5	—	13	49	83	19	138	0.40	—	15	0.07	0.07	1.40	—	—	—	0
538	Candy-milk chocolate-plain	1 ounce	28	145	2	9	6	0	16	65	65	28	109	0.30	—	24	0.02	0.10	0.10	—	—	2	0
1783	Candy-milky way bar	1 item	60	260	3	9	5	4	43	79	79	114	157	0.42	0.43	4	0.02	0.14	0.25	0.02	0.22	4	0
1788	Candy-peanut brittle	1 ounce	28	123	2	4	2	0	20	11	35	9	43	0.56	0.28	2	0.02	0.01	1.30	0.02	0.00	14	0
1789	Candy-peanut butter cup	1 piece	17	92	2	5	3	3	9	15	41	55	68	0.24	0.24	1	0.05	0.03	0.80	0.03	0.04	17	0
1782	Candy-snickers bar	1 item	57	270	6	13	5	9	33	66	102	145	189	0.46	0.63	3	0.03	0.10	1.68	0.06	0.17	29	0
964	Carambola-raw	1 item	127	42	1	0	0	0	10	6	20	2	207	0.33	0.14	63	0.04	0.03	0.52	0.13	0.00	11	27
692	Carbonated soda-club	12 fl oz	355	0	0	0	0	0	0	12	0	72	0	0.04	0.36	0	0.00	0.00	0.00	0.00	0.00	0	0
693	Carbonated soda-cola type	12 fl oz	370	151	0	0	0	0	38	11	44	15	4	0.11	0.04	0	0.00	0.00	0.00	0.00	0.00	0	0
1412	Carbonated soda-cream flavored	12 fl oz	371	190	0	0	0	0	49	19	0	45	4	0.18	0.26	0	0.00	0.00	0.00	0.00	0.00	0	0
1415	Carbonated soda-diet cola-nutrasweet	12 fl oz	355	4	0	0	0	0	0	14	32	21	0	0.11	0.29	0	0.01	0.08	0.00	0.00	0.00	0	0
1414	Carbonated soda-dr. pepper type cola	12 fl oz	370	151	0	0	0	0	38	11	41	37	4	0.14	0.02	0	0.00	0.00	0.00	0.00	0.00	0	0
695	Carbonated soda-ginger ale	12 fl oz	366	125	0	0	0	0	32	11	0	26	4	0.60	0.24	0	0.00	0.00	0.00	0.00	0.00	0	0
694	Carbonated soda-grape	12 fl oz	372	160	0	0	0	0	42	11	0	56	4	0.30	0.30	0	0.00	0.00	0.00	0.00	0.00	0	0
1876	Carbonated soda-lemon lime/7up	12 fl oz	368	148	0	0	0	0	38	7	0	41	4	0.25	0.18	0	0.00	0.00	0.06	0.00	0.00	0	0
696	Carbonated soda-root beer	12 fl oz	370	151	0	0	0	0	39	18	0	48	4	0.18	0.26	0	0.00	0.00	0.00	0.00	0.00	0	0
1460	Carbonated soda-tab-low calorie cola	12 fl oz	354	0	0	0	0	0	0	—	45	45	—	—	—	—	—	—	—	—	—	—	—
1879	Carbonated soda-tonic water/quinine	12 fl oz	366	125	0	0	0	0	32	4	0	15	0	0.04	0.37	0	0.00	0.00	0.00	0.00	0.00	0	0
965	Carissa-raw	1 item	20	12	0	0	—	0	3	2	1	1	52	0.26	—	1	0.01	0.01	0.04	—	0.00	—	8
345	Carnation instant breakfast-chocolate	1 item	36	130	7	1	—	—	23	100	150	136	422	4.50	3.00	525	0.30	0.07	5.00	0.40	0.60	0	27
344	Carnation instant breakfast-eggnog	1 item	34	130	7	0	0	0	23	100	150	196	266	4.50	3.00	525	0.30	0.07	5.00	0.40	0.60	0	27
343	Carnation instant breakfast-vanilla	1 item	35	130	7	0	0	0	24	100	150	145	382	4.50	3.00	525	0.30	0.07	5.00	0.40	0.60	0	27
1055	Carrot juice-canned	1 cup	246	98	2	0	0	0	23	59	103	71	718	1.13	0.44	6335	0.23	0.14	0.95	0.53	0.00	9	21
601	Carrot-raw-scraped-shredded	1 cup	110	47	1	0	0	0	11	30	48	39	355	0.55	0.22	3094	0.11	0.06	1.02	0.16	0.00	15	10
600	Carrot-raw-scraped-whole	1 item	72	31	1	0	0	0	7	19	32	25	233	0.36	0.14	2025	0.07	0.04	0.67	0.11	0.00	10	7
602	Carrots-boiled-drained-sliced	1 cup	156	70	2	0	0	0	16	48	47	103	354	0.97	0.47	3830	0.05	0.09	0.79	0.38	0.00	22	4
1692	Carrots-canned-dietary pack-low sodium	1 cup	246	57	2	0	0	0	12	62	49	96	426	1.50	0.71	3239	0.05	0.07	1.04	0.28	0.00	20	7
603	Carrots-canned-sliced-drained	1 cup	146	34	1	0	0	0	8	37	35	352	261	0.93	0.38	2010	0.03	0.04	0.81	0.16	0.00	13	4
634	Carrots-frozen-boiled-drained	1 cup	146	53	2	0	0	0	12	41	38	86	231	0.69	0.35	2584	0.04	0.05	0.64	0.19	0.00	16	4
35	Catsup-tomato-heinz lite	1 tbsp	15	8	0	0	0	0	2	7	8	110	54	0.10	—	21	0.01	0.01	0.20	—	—	—	2
37	Catsup-tomato-low sodium-heinz	1 tbsp	15	8	0	0	0	0	2	7	8	90	54	0.10	—	21	0.01	0.01	0.20	—	—	—	2
674	Catsup-tomato-regular	1 tbsp	15	15	0	0	0	0	4	3	8	156	54	0.10	0.03	21	0.01	0.01	0.20	0.02	0.00	1	2
607	Cauliflower-frozen-boiled	1 cup	180	34	3	0	0	0	7	31	43	32	250	0.74	0.23	4	0.07	0.10	0.56	0.16	0.00	74	56
606	Cauliflower-raw-boiled-drained	1 cup	124	30	2	0	0	0	6	34	44	8	400	0.52	0.30	2	0.08	0.06	0.68	0.25	0.00	63	69
605	Cauliflower-raw-chopped	1 cup	100	24	2	0	0	0	5	29	46	15	355	0.58	0.18	2	0.08	0.06	0.63	0.23	0.00	66	72
609	Celery-pascal-raw-diced	1 cup	120	19	1	0	0	0	4	48	30	104	344	0.48	0.16	16	0.06	0.05	0.39	0.10	0.00	34	8
608	Celery-pascal-raw-stalk	1 item	40	6	0	0	0	0	1	16	10	35	115	0.16	0.05	5	0.02	0.02	0.13	0.04	0.00	11	3
1239	Cereal-100% bran	1 cup	66	178	8	3	1	0	48	46	801	457	824	8.12	5.74	0	1.60	1.80	20.90	2.10	6.30	47	63
1240	Cereal-100% natural-plain	1 cup	104	489	12	22	15	0	65	181	383	45	514	3.07	2.35	6	0.31	0.56	2.37	0.19	0.13	31	0
1218	Cereal-40% bran flakes-kelloggs	1 cup	39	127	5	1	0	0	31	19	192	363	248	11.20	5.10	516	0.50	0.60	6.90	0.70	2.10	138	0

Dashes (—) in data spaces indicate that no data were reported.

Item	Food Name	Portion	Weight (g)	Food Energy (kcal)	Protein (g)	Total Fat (g)	Saturated Fat (g)	Cholesterol (mg)	Carbohydrate (g)	Calcium (mg)	Phosphorus (mg)	Sodium (mg)	Potassium (mg)	Iron (mg)	Zinc (cm)	Vitamin A (RE)	Thiamin (mg)	Riboflavin (mg)	Niacin (mg)	Vitamin B6 (mg)	Vitamin B12 (ug)	Folic Acid (ug)	Vitamin C (mg)
1219	Cereal-40% bran flakes-post	1 cup	47	152	5	1	0	0	37	21	296	431	251	7.50	2.50	622	0.60	0.70	8.30	0.80	2.50	166	0
1197	Cereal-all bran	1 cup	85	212	12	2	0	0	63	69	794	961	1051	13.50	11.20	1125	1.11	1.28	15.00	1.53	0.00	301	45
1198	Cereal-alpha bits	1 cup	28	111	2	1	0	0	25	8	51	219	110	1.80	1.50	375	0.40	0.40	5.00	0.50	1.50	100	0
1199	Cereal-apple jacks	1 cup	28	110	2	0	0	0	26	3	30	125	23	4.50	3.70	375	0.40	0.40	5.00	0.50	0.00	100	15
1200	Cereal-bran buds	1 cup	85	220	12	2	0	0	65	57	740	523	1425	13.50	11.20	1125	1.11	1.28	15.00	1.53	0.00	301	45
1201	Cereal-bran chex	1 cup	49	156	5	1	0	0	39	29	327	455	394	7.80	2.14	11	0.60	0.26	8.60	0.90	2.60	173	26
369	Cereal-bran flakes-ralston	1 cup	49	159	6	1	0	0	39	27	273	456	191	7.80	2.04	649	0.60	0.70	8.60	0.90	2.60	173	26
1202	Cereal-c.w. post-plain	1 cup	97	432	9	15	11	0	69	47	224	167	198	15.40	1.64	1284	1.30	1.50	17.10	1.70	5.10	342	0
1203	Cereal-c.w. post-with raisins	1 cup	103	446	9	15	11	0	74	51	232	160	260	16.40	1.64	1364	1.30	1.50	18.10	1.90	5.50	364	0
1204	Cereal-cap'n crunch	1 cup	37	156	2	3	2	0	30	6	47	278	48	9.83	4.01	5	0.66	0.71	8.64	1.00	2.34	238	0
1205	Cereal-cap'n crunch-crunchberries	1 cup	35	146	2	3	2	0	29	11	47	243	49	9.04	3.56	5	0.59	0.67	8.13	0.93	2.51	128	0
1206	Cereal-cheerios	1 cup	23	89	3	1	0	0	16	39	107	246	81	3.61	0.63	300	0.30	0.34	4.00	0.41	1.20	5	12
1207	Cereal-cocoa krispies	1 cup	36	139	2	1	0	0	32	6	47	275	53	2.30	1.90	477	0.50	0.50	6.30	0.60	0.02	127	19
1208	Cereal-cocoa pebbles	1 cup	33	133	2	2	1	0	28	6	25	155	54	2.05	1.72	430	0.42	0.49	5.72	0.59	1.72	115	0
1209	Cereal-corn bran	1 cup	36	125	2	1	—	0	30	41	52	310	70	12.20	4.00	8	0.37	0.70	10.90	0.86	1.39	232	0
1210	Cereal-corn chex	1 cup	28	111	2	0	0	0	25	3	11	271	23	1.80	0.10	14	0.40	0.07	5.00	0.50	1.50	100	15
1211	Cereal-corn flakes-kelloggs	1 cup	23	88	2	0	0	0	20	1	14	281	21	1.43	0.06	300	0.30	0.34	4.00	0.41	0.00	80	12
1212	Cereal-corn flakes-low sodium	1 cup	25	100	2	0	0	0	22	11	12	3	18	0.56	0.07	10	0.00	0.05	0.11	0.02	0.00	2	0
371	Cereal-corn flakes-ralston	1 cup	25	98	2	0	0	0	22	2	10	239	22	0.60	0.06	10	0.10	0.00	1.10	0.02	0.00	2	13
363	Cereal-corn grits-regular-enriched-hot	1 cup	242	145	3	0	0	0	32	0	29	0	53	1.55	0.17	—	0.24	0.15	1.96	0.06	0.00	2	—
364	Cereal-corn grits-regular-unenriched-hot	1 cup	242	145	3	0	0	0	32	0	29	0	53	1.55	0.17	—	0.24	0.15	1.96	0.06	0.00	2	—
374	Cereal-corn-shredded-added sugar	1 cup	25	95	2	0	0	0	22	1	10	247	—	0.60	0.09	0	0.33	0.05	4.40	0.45	1.33	88	13
1213	Cereal-cracklin bran	1 cup	60	229	6	9	6	0	41	40	241	487	355	3.80	3.20	794	0.80	0.90	10.60	1.10	0.00	212	32
1937	Cereal-cracklin oat bran-kelloggs	1 serving	28	110	3	4	1	0	20	20	150	140	160	1.80	1.50	180	0.38	0.43	5.00	0.50	1.50	100	15
1258	Cereal-cream of rice-cooked	1 cup	244	127	2	0	0	0	28	7	42	2	49	0.49	0.39	0	0.00	0.00	0.98	0.07	0.00	7	0
1260	Cereal-cream of wheat-instant	1 cup	241	153	4	1	0	0	32	59	43	6	48	12.00	0.41	0	0.20	0.10	1.80	0.03	0.00	11	0
1145	Cereal-cream of wheat-packet size	1 item	150	132	3	0	0	0	29	40	20	241	55	8.10	0.23	1250	0.40	0.20	5.00	0.50	0.00	100	0
1259	Cereal-cream of wheat-regular-hot	1 cup	251	133	4	1	0	0	28	50	42	2	43	10.30	0.33	0	0.25	0.00	1.51	0.04	0.00	10	0
1214	Cereal-crisp rice-low sodium	1 cup	26	105	1	0	0	0	24	17	27	3	20	0.80	0.39	0	0.00	0.05	0.36	0.04	0.00	3	0
1215	Cereal-crispy rice	1 cup	28	112	2	0	0	0	25	5	31	208	27	0.71	0.47	0	0.11	0.03	2.02	0.04	0.08	3	1
1216	Cereal-crispy wheats and raisins	1 cup	43	150	3	1	0	0	35	71	117	204	174	6.80	0.51	569	0.60	0.60	7.60	0.80	2.30	15	0
365	Cereal-farina-cooked-enriched-hot	1 cup	233	117	3	0	0	0	25	5	28	0	30	1.17	0.16	—	0.19	0.12	1.28	0.02	0.00	5	—
1217	Cereal-fortified oat flakes	1 cup	48	177	9	1	0	0	35	68	176	429	343	13.70	1.50	636	0.60	0.70	8.40	0.90	2.50	169	0
1220	Cereal-froot loops-general mills	1 cup	28	111	2	1	0	0	25	3	24	145	26	4.50	3.70	375	0.40	0.40	5.00	0.50	0.00	100	15
372	Cereal-frosted flakes-kellogg	1 cup	35	133	2	0	0	0	32	1	26	284	22	2.20	0.05	463	0.50	0.50	6.20	0.60	0.00	124	19
373	Cereal-frosted flakes-ralston	1 cup	38	149	2	1	0	0	34	4	9	247	24	1.00	0.82	503	0.50	0.60	6.70	0.70	2.00	3	20
1221	Cereal-frosted mini wheats-kelloggs	1 item	7	26	1	0	0	0	6	2	19	2	24	0.45	0.38	94	0.09	0.11	1.25	0.13	0.00	25	4
1222	Cereal-frosted rice krispies-kelloggs	1 cup	28	109	1	0	0	0	26	1	27	240	21	1.80	0.31	375	0.40	0.40	5.00	0.50	0.00	100	15
1223	Cereal-granola-homemade	1 cup	122	594	15	33	6	0	67	76	494	12	612	4.84	4.47	10	0.73	0.31	2.14	0.43	0.00	99	1
1234	Cereal-granola-nature valley	1 cup	113	503	12	20	13	0	76	71	354	232	389	3.78	2.19	8	0.39	0.19	0.83	0.09	0.00	85	0
1225	Cereal-grape nuts flakes-post	1 cup	33	116	3	0	0	0	27	13	97	250	113	5.17	0.65	430	0.42	0.49	5.72	0.59	1.72	115	0
1224	Cereal-grape nuts-post	1 cup	114	407	13	0	0	0	94	43	286	792	381	4.95	2.51	1500	1.48	1.71	20.10	2.05	6.04	402	0
1226	Cereal-heartland natural-plain	1 cup	115	499	12	18	10	0	79	75	416	294	385	4.33	3.04	7	0.36	0.16	1.61	0.19	0.00	64	1
1228	Cereal-honey bran	1 cup	35	119	3	1	0	0	29	16	132	202	151	5.60	0.90	463	0.50	0.50	6.20	0.60	1.90	23	19
1227	Cereal-honey nut cheerios-general mills	1 cup	33	125	4	1	0	0	27	23	122	299	115	5.20	0.87	437	0.40	0.50	5.80	0.60	1.70	22	17
1229	Cereal-honeycomb-post	1 cup	22	86	1	0	0	0	20	4	22	166	70	1.40	1.20	291	0.30	0.30	3.90	0.40	1.20	78	0
1230	Cereal-king vitaman	1 cup	21	85	1	1	1	0	18	2	27	161	26	12.70	0.16	717	0.92	1.06	12.90	1.18	4.13	286	33
1231	Cereal-kix	1 cup	19	74	2	0	0	0	16	24	26	226	30	5.41	0.16	250	0.25	0.28	3.33	0.34	1.00	67	10
1232	Cereal-life-plain/cinnamon	1 cup	44	162	8	1	0	0	32	154	238	229	197	11.60	1.45	3	0.95	1.00	11.60	0.08	0.00	37	1
1233	Cereal-lucky charms	1 cup	32	125	3	1	0	0	26	36	88	227	66	5.10	0.56	424	0.40	0.50	5.60	0.60	1.70	6	17
1261	Cereal-malt o meal-cooked	1 cup	240	122	4	0	0	0	26	5	23	2	31	9.50	0.17	0	0.40	0.30	5.90	0.02	0.00	6	0
1262	Cereal-maypo-cooked-hot	1 cup	240	170	6	2	—	0	32	125	248	9	211	8.40	1.49	702	0.70	0.80	9.40	0.90	2.80	9	28
1235	Cereal-nutri grain-barley	1 cup	41	153	5	0	0	0	34	11	126	277	108	1.45	5.40	543	0.50	0.60	7.20	0.70	2.20	145	22
1236	Cereal-nutri grain-corn	1 cup	42	160	3	1	0	0	36	1	120	276	98	0.89	5.50	556	0.50	0.60	7.40	0.80	2.20	148	22
1237	Cereal-nutri grain-rye	1 cup	40	144	4	0	0	0	34	8	104	272	72	1.13	5.30	530	0.50	0.60	7.00	0.70	2.10	141	21
1238	Cereal-nutri grain-wheat	1 cup	44	158	4	1	0	0	37	12	164	299	120	1.24	5.80	583	0.60	0.70	7.70	0.80	2.30	155	23
1970	Cereal-oat bran-cooked	1 cup	219	88	7	2	0	0	25	22	261	2	201	1.93	1.16	0	0.35	0.07	0.32	0.06	0.00	13	0
1936	Cereal-oat bran-kelloggs	1 serving	28	100	4	1	—	0	22	—	150	270	115	4.50	3.75	180	0.38	0.43	5.00	0.50	1.50	—	—
1901	Cereal-oat bran-quaker	1 cup	85	270	18	6	1	0	51	60	600	15	540	5.40	3.60	1028	0.90	0.31	15.00	1.49	5.18	48	0
1941	Cereal-oat bran-raisin/spice-hot	1 ounce	28	100	3	1	—	0	19	16	148	10	100	0.70	0.82	0	0.06	0.05	1.20	0.08	0.00	24	0

366	Cereal-oatmeal-cooked	1 cup	234	145	6	2	0	0	25	20	178	1	132	1.59	1.15	7	0.26	0.05	0.30	0.05	0.00	9	—
1871	Cereal-oatmeal-raw	1 cup	81	311	13	5	1	0	54	42	384	3	284	3.41	2.48	10	0.59	0.11	0.63	0.10	0.00	26	0
1147	Cereal-oats-apple/cinnamon-quaker-packet	1 item	149	135	4	2	0	0	26	158	117	222	107	6.07	0.70	435	0.48	0.28	5.13	0.70	0.00	137	0
1148	Cereal-oats-bran/raisin-quaker-packet	1 item	195	158	5	2	0	0	30	173	206	247	236	7.61	1.35	479	0.56	0.63	8.12	0.76	0.00	155	0
1149	Cereal-oats-cinnamon/spice-quaker-packet	1 item	161	177	5	2	0	0	35	172	146	280	104	6.65	0.97	475	0.56	0.34	5.66	0.77	0.00	153	0
1150	Cereal-oats-maple/sugar-quaker-packet	1 item	155	163	5	2	0	0	32	162	143	280	102	6.35	0.87	451	0.53	0.32	5.35	0.74	0.00	145	0
1146	Cereal-oats-plain-quaker-instant-packet	1 item	177	104	4	2	0	0	18	163	133	286	100	6.32	0.87	455	0.53	0.29	5.49	0.74	0.00	150	0
375	Cereal-oats-puffed-added sugar	1 cup	25	100	3	1	0	0	19	44	102	294	—	4.00	0.69	275	0.33	0.38	4.40	0.45	1.33	6	13
1241	Cereal-product 19-kelloggs	1 cup	33	126	3	0	0	0	27	4	47	378	51	21.00	0.50	1748	1.70	2.00	23.30	2.30	7.00	466	70
1242	Cereal-raisin bran-kelloggs	1 cup	49	154	5	1	0	0	37	17	183	359	256	6.00	5.02	500	0.49	0.59	6.69	0.69	2.02	133	0
1243	Cereal-raisin bran-post	1 cup	57	174	5	1	0	0	43	27	238	370	350	9.03	3.01	750	0.74	0.85	10.00	1.02	3.01	201	0
370	Cereal-raisin bran-ralston	1 cup	56	178	4	0	0	0	47	27	247	486	287	6.70	1.67	556	0.60	0.60	7.40	0.70	2.20	148	2
1151	Cereal-ralston-cooked-hot	1 cup	253	134	6	1	0	0	28	14	148	4	153	1.64	1.42	0	0.20	0.18	2.05	0.11	0.11	18	0
1244	Cereal-rice chex	1 cup	25	100	1	0	0	0	23	4	25	211	29	1.59	0.35	2	0.33	0.01	4.44	0.45	1.34	89	13
1245	Cereal-rice krispies-kelloggs	1 cup	28	112	2	0	0	0	25	4	34	340	30	1.80	0.48	375	0.40	0.40	5.00	0.50	0.00	100	15
377	Cereal-rice-puffed-added sugar	1 cup	28	115	1	0	0	0	26	3	14	21	43	0.00	1.48	300	0.00	0.00	0.00	0.50	1.48	99	15
376	Cereal-rice-puffed-plain	1 cup	14	56	1	0	0	0	13	1	14	0	16	0.15	0.14	0	0.02	0.01	0.42	0.01	0.00	3	0
1263	Cereal-roman meal-cooked	1 cup	241	147	7	1	—	0	33	30	215	3	302	2.12	1.78	0	0.24	0.12	3.08	0.11	0.00	24	0
1246	Cereal-special k-kelloggs	1 cup	21	83	4	0	0	0	16	6	41	199	37	3.39	2.81	280	0.28	0.32	3.75	0.38	0.01	75	11
1247	Cereal-sugar corn pops-kelloggs	1 cup	28	108	1	0	0	0	26	1	28	103	17	1.80	1.50	375	0.40	0.40	5.00	0.50	0.00	100	15
1248	Cereal-sugar smacks-kelloggs	1 cup	38	141	3	1	0	0	33	4	41	100	56	2.39	0.38	500	0.49	0.57	6.67	0.68	0.00	134	20
1249	Cereal-super sugar crisp-post	1 cup	33	123	2	0	0	0	30	7	60	29	123	2.10	1.70	437	0.40	0.50	5.80	0.60	1.70	116	0
1250	Cereal-tasteeos	1 cup	24	94	3	1	0	0	19	11	96	183	71	3.82	0.69	318	0.31	0.36	4.22	0.43	1.27	9	13
1251	Cereal-team	1 cup	42	164	3	1	0	0	36	6	65	259	71	2.57	0.58	556	0.50	0.60	7.40	0.80	2.20	7	22
1252	Cereal-toasties-post	1 cup	23	88	2	0	0	0	20	1	10	238	26	0.60	0.07	300	0.30	0.34	4.00	0.41	1.20	80	0
1253	Cereal-total-general mills	1 cup	33	116	3	1	0	0	26	56	137	409	123	21.00	0.78	1748	1.70	2.00	23.30	2.30	7.00	466	70
1254	Cereal-trix-general mills	1 cup	28	109	2	0	0	0	25	6	19	181	27	4.52	0.13	371	0.37	0.43	5.00	0.51	1.51	3	15
1255	Cereal-wheat chex	1 cup	46	169	5	1	1	0	38	18	182	308	174	7.30	1.23	0	0.60	0.17	8.10	0.80	2.40	162	24
378	Cereal-wheat flakes-added sugar	1 cup	30	105	3	0	0	0	24	12	83	368	81	4.80	0.67	330	0.40	0.45	5.30	0.54	1.59	9	16
1256	Cereal-wheat germ-brown sugar and honey	1 cup	113	426	25	9	2	0	69	38	971	3	803	7.71	14.10	0	1.41	0.70	4.73	0.83	0.00	298	0
382	Cereal-wheat germ-toasted	1 cup	113	432	33	12	2	0	56	51	1295	5	1070	10.30	18.80	50	1.89	0.93	6.31	1.11	0.00	398	7
380	Cereal-wheat-puffed-added sugar	1 serving	38	138	6	0	—	0	30	11	135	2	132	1.80	0.90	0	0.08	0.09	4.10	0.07	0.00	12	0
379	Cereal-wheat-puffed-plain	1 cup	12	44	2	0	0	0	10	3	43	0	42	0.57	0.28	0	0.02	0.03	1.30	0.02	0.00	4	0
367	Cereal-wheat-rolled-cooked-hot	1 cup	240	180	5	1	0	0	41	19	182	535	202	1.70	1.15	0	0.17	0.07	2.20	—	—	26	0
381	Cereal-wheat-shredded-biscuit	1 item	24	83	3	0	0	0	19	10	86	0	77	0.74	0.59	0	0.07	0.06	1.08	0.06	0.00	12	0
368	Cereal-wheat-whole meal-cooked-hot	1 cup	245	110	4	1	0	0	23	17	127	535	118	1.20	1.18	0	0.15	0.05	1.50	—	—	27	0
1264	Cereal-wheatena-cooked	1 cup	243	136	5	1	—	0	29	10	146	5	187	1.36	1.68	0	0.02	0.05	1.34	0.05	0.00	17	0
1257	Cereal-wheaties	1 cup	29	101	3	1	0	0	23	44	100	363	108	4.60	0.65	384	0.40	0.40	5.10	0.50	1.50	9	15
1265	Cereal-whole wheat natural	1 cup	242	150	5	1	0	0	33	17	167	1	171	1.50	1.16	0	0.17	0.12	2.15	0.18	0.00	27	0
858	Champagne-domestic-glassful	1 item	120	84	0	0	0	0	3	—	—	—	—	—	—	—	—	—	—	—	—	—	—
1057	Chard-swiss-boiled-drained	1 cup	175	35	3	0	0	0	7	102	58	313	961	3.96	0.57	549	0.06	0.15	0.63	0.15	0.00	15	32
1056	Chard-swiss-raw	1 cup	36	7	1	0	0	0	1	21	12	64	198	0.81	0.12	113	0.01	0.03	0.13	0.03	0.00	3	6
24	Cheese food-american-pasteurized process	1 ounce	28	93	6	7	4	18	2	163	130	337	79	0.24	0.85	78	0.01	0.13	0.04	0.04	0.32	2	0
1441	Cheese pasta shells/meat sauce-stouffer	1 item	255	320	19	14	8	169	30	146	238	1310	465	3.44	3.13	209	0.24	0.40	4.42	0.26	1.34	26	8
1677	Cheese souffle-home recipe	1 cup	95	207	9	16	7	137	6	191	185	346	115	1.00	1.03	152	0.05	0.23	0.20	0.06	0.35	14	0
25	Cheese spread-american-processed	1 ounce	28	82	5	6	4	16	2	159	202	381	69	0.09	0.73	67	0.01	0.12	0.04	0.03	0.11	2	0
22	Cheese-american-pasteurized process	1 ounce	28	106	6	9	6	27	0	174	211	406	46	0.11	0.85	103	0.01	0.10	0.02	0.02	0.20	2	0
1	Cheese-blue	1 ounce	28	100	6	8	5	21	1	150	110	396	73	0.09	0.75	61	0.01	0.11	0.29	0.05	0.35	10	0
1433	Cheese-blue-crumbled-unpacked	1 cup	135	477	29	39	25	102	3	712	523	1884	346	0.42	3.59	292	0.04	0.52	1.37	0.22	1.64	49	0
884	Cheese-brick	1 ounce	28	105	7	8	5	27	1	191	128	159	38	0.12	0.74	92	0.00	0.10	0.03	0.02	0.36	6	0
885	Cheese-brie	1 ounce	28	95	6	8	5	28	0	52	53	178	43	0.14	0.68	57	0.02	0.15	0.11	0.07	0.47	18	0
2	Cheese-camembert-wedge	1 item	38	114	8	9	6	27	0	147	132	320	71	0.12	0.90	105	0.01	0.19	0.24	0.09	0.49	24	0
886	Cheese-caraway	1 ounce	28	107	7	8	5	26	1	191	139	196	26	0.18	0.83	90	0.01	0.13	0.05	0.02	0.08	5	0
3	Cheese-cheddar-cut pieces	1 ounce	28	114	7	9	6	30	0	204	145	176	28	0.19	0.88	90	0.01	0.11	0.02	0.02	0.23	5	0
4	Cheese-cheddar-inch cubes	1 item	17	69	5	6	4	18	0	124	88	107	17	0.12	0.54	55	0.01	0.07	0.01	0.01	0.14	3	0
1929	Cheese-cheddar-lowfat-low sodium-pauly	1 ounce	28	83	9	5	1	14	1	200	137	68	32	0.20	0.88	18	0.01	0.01	0.03	0.02	0.24	5	0
5	Cheese-cheddar-shredded	1 cup	113	455	28	38	24	119	1	815	579	701	111	0.77	3.51	359	0.03	0.42	0.09	0.08	0.94	21	0
887	Cheese-cheshire	1 ounce	28	110	7	9	6	29	1	182	131	198	27	0.06	0.79	84	0.01	0.08	0.02	0.02	0.23	5	0
888	Cheese-colby	1 ounce	28	112	7	9	6	27	1	194	129	171	36	0.22	0.87	88	0.00	0.11	0.03	0.02	0.23	5	0
9	Cheese-cottage-1% lowfat-unpacked	1 cup	226	164	28	2	1	10	6	138	302	918	193	0.32	0.86	25	0.05	0.37	0.29	0.15	1.43	28	0
8	Cheese-cottage-2% lowfat-unpacked	1 cup	226	203	31	4	3	19	8	155	340	918	217	0.36	0.95	47	0.05	0.42	0.33	0.17	1.61	30	0
6	Cheese-cottage-4% fat-large curd-unpack	1 cup	225	232	28	10	6	34	6	135	297	911	189	0.32	0.83	110	0.05	0.37	0.28	0.15	1.40	27	0
7	Cheese-cottage-4% fat-small curd-unpack	1 cup	210	217	26	9	6	31	6	126	277	850	177	0.29	0.78	103	0.04	0.34	0.27	0.14	1.31	26	0

Dashes (—) in data spaces indicate that no data were reported.

Appendix C Table of Food Composition

Item	Food Name	Portion	Weight (g)	Food Energy (kcal)	Protein (g)	Total Fat (g)	Saturated Fat (g)	Cholesterol (mg)	Carbohydrate (g)	Calcium (mg)	Phosphorus (mg)	Sodium (mg)	Potassium (mg)	Iron (mg)	Zinc (cm)	Vitamin A (RE)	Thiamin (mg)	Riboflavin (mg)	Niacin (mg)	Vitamin B6 (mg)	Vitamin B12 (ug)	Folic Acid (ug)	Vitamin C (mg)
10	Cheese-cottage-dry curd-uncreamed	1 cup	145	123	25	1	0	10	3	46	151	19	47	0.33	0.68	13	0.04	0.21	0.23	0.12	1.20	21	0
16	Cheese-cottage-with fruit-unpacked	1 cup	226	279	22	8	5	25	30	108	236	915	151	0.25	0.66	84	0.04	0.29	0.23	0.12	1.12	22	0
11	Cheese-cream	1 ounce	28	100	2	10	6	31	1	23	30	85	34	0.34	0.15	122	0.01	0.06	0.03	0.01	0.12	4	0
889	Cheese-edam	1 ounce	28	101	7	8	5	25	0	207	152	274	53	0.12	1.06	78	0.01	0.11	0.02	0.02	0.44	5	0
890	Cheese-feta	1 ounce	28	75	4	6	4	25	1	140	96	316	18	0.18	0.82	36	0.04	0.24	0.28	0.12	0.48	9	0
891	Cheese-fontina	1 ounce	28	110	7	9	5	33	0	156	98	227	18	0.06	0.99	100	0.01	0.06	0.04	0.02	0.48	2	0
1928	Cheese-garlic-lowfat-low sodium-pauly	1 ounce	28	80	8	6	3	20	0	—	—	95	—	—	—	—	—	—	—	—	—	—	—
892	Cheese-gjetost	1 ounce	28	132	3	8	5	27	12	113	126	170	399	0.15	0.32	78	0.09	0.39	0.23	0.08	0.69	1	0
893	Cheese-gouda	1 ounce	28	101	7	8	5	32	1	198	155	232	34	0.07	1.11	55	0.01	0.10	0.02	0.02	0.44	6	0
894	Cheese-gruyere	1 ounce	28	117	8	9	5	31	0	287	172	95	23	0.05	1.11	104	0.02	0.08	0.03	0.02	0.45	3	0
895	Cheese-limburger	1 ounce	28	93	6	8	5	26	0	141	111	227	36	0.04	0.60	109	0.02	0.14	0.05	0.02	0.30	16	0
896	Cheese-monterey jack	1 ounce	28	106	7	9	5	25	0	212	126	152	23	0.20	0.85	81	0.00	0.11	0.03	0.02	0.23	5	0
1927	Cheese-monterey jack-lowfat-low sodium	1 ounce	28	80	8	6	3	20	0	—	—	95	—	—	—	—	—	—	—	—	—	—	—
13	Cheese-mozzarella-made from skim milk	1 ounce	28	72	7	5	3	16	1	183	131	132	24	0.06	0.78	50	0.01	0.09	0.03	0.02	0.23	2	0
12	Cheese-mozzarella-made from whole milk	1 ounce	28	80	6	6	4	22	1	147	105	106	19	0.05	0.63	68	0.00	0.07	0.02	0.02	0.19	2	0
897	Cheese-muenster	1 ounce	28	104	7	9	5	27	0	203	133	178	38	0.12	0.80	96	0.00	0.09	0.03	0.02	0.42	3	0
898	Cheese-neufchatel	1 ounce	28	74	3	7	4	22	1	21	39	113	32	0.08	0.15	96	0.00	0.06	0.04	0.01	0.08	3	0
14	Cheese-parmesan-grated	1 cup	100	456	42	30	19	79	4	1376	807	1862	107	0.95	3.19	211	0.05	0.39	0.32	0.11	1.40	8	0
902	Cheese-pimento-processed	1 ounce	28	106	6	9	6	27	0	174	211	405	46	0.12	0.84	108	0.01	0.10	0.02	0.02	0.20	2	1
899	Cheese-port du salut	1 ounce	28	100	7	8	5	35	0	184	102	151	39	0.12	0.74	114	0.00	0.07	0.02	0.02	0.43	5	0
17	Cheese-provolone	1 ounce	28	100	7	8	5	20	1	214	141	248	39	0.15	0.92	69	0.01	0.09	0.04	0.02	0.42	3	0
19	Cheese-ricotta-made with part skim milk	1 cup	246	340	28	20	12	76	13	669	449	307	308	1.08	3.30	319	0.05	0.46	0.19	0.05	0.72	32	0
18	Cheese-ricotta-made with whole milk	1 cup	246	428	28	32	20	124	7	509	389	207	257	0.94	2.85	362	0.03	0.48	0.26	0.11	0.83	30	0
20	Cheese-romano	1 ounce	28	110	9	8	5	29	1	302	215	340	25	0.22	0.73	49	0.01	0.11	0.02	0.02	0.32	2	0
900	Cheese-roquefort	1 ounce	28	105	6	9	5	26	1	188	111	513	26	0.16	0.59	89	0.01	0.17	0.21	0.04	0.18	14	0
21	Cheese-swiss	1 ounce	28	107	8	8	5	26	1	272	171	74	31	0.05	1.11	72	0.01	0.10	0.03	0.02	0.48	2	0
1930	Cheese-swiss-lowfat-low sodium-pauly	1 ounce	28	97	9	7	5	19	1	273	172	32	32	0.05	1.11	72	0.01	0.11	0.03	0.02	0.48	2	0
23	Cheese-swiss-pasteurized process	1 ounce	28	95	7	7	5	24	1	219	216	388	61	0.17	1.02	69	0.00	0.08	0.01	0.01	0.35	2	0
901	Cheese-tilsit	1 ounce	28	96	7	7	5	29	1	198	142	213	18	0.06	0.99	89	0.02	0.10	0.06	0.02	0.60	6	0
1329	Cheesefurter-pork and beef	1 item	43	141	6	13	5	29	1	25	76	465	89	0.46	0.97	16	0.11	0.07	1.25	0.05	0.74	1	8
966	Cherimoya-raw	1 item	547	514	7	2	—	0	131	126	219	—	—	2.74	—	6	0.55	0.60	7.11	—	0.00	—	49
967	Cherries-sour-canned-water pack	1 cup	244	88	2	0	0	0	22	27	24	17	239	3.34	0.17	184	0.04	0.10	0.43	0.11	0.00	20	5
968	Cherries-sour-frozen-unsweetened	1 cup	155	71	1	1	0	0	17	20	25	2	192	0.82	0.16	135	0.07	0.05	0.21	0.10	0.00	7	3
239	Cherries-sour-red-canned in heavy syrup	1 cup	256	233	2	0	0	0	60	26	26	18	238	3.33	0.15	183	0.04	0.10	0.43	0.11	0.00	20	5
970	Cherries-sweet-canned-juice pack	1 cup	250	135	2	0	0	0	35	35	55	8	328	1.45	0.25	31	0.05	0.06	1.02	0.08	0.00	11	6
969	Cherries-sweet-canned-water pack	1 cup	248	114	2	0	0	0	29	27	38	3	325	0.89	0.19	40	0.06	0.10	1.02	0.07	0.00	10	5
971	Cherries-sweet-frozen-sweetened	1 cup	259	231	3	0	0	0	58	31	41	3	515	0.91	0.10	49	0.07	0.12	0.46	0.09	0.00	11	3
240	Cherries-sweet-raw	1 item	7	5	0	0	0	0	1	1	1	0	15	0.03	0.00	1	0.00	0.00	0.03	0.00	0.00	0	0
1174	Chervil-dried	1 tsp	1	1	0	0	0	0	0	8	3	0	28	0.19	0.05	—	—	—	—	0.01	0.00	—	—
1701	Chewing gum-candy coated	1 item	2	5	0	0	0	0	2	0	0	0	0	0.00	0.00	0	0.00	0.00	0.00	0.00	0.00	0	0
1666	Chewing gum-wrigleys	1 item	3	10	0	0	0	0	2	3	0	0	0	0.00	0.00	0	0.00	0.00	0.00	0.00	0.00	0	0
214	Chicken a la king-cooked-home recipe	1 cup	245	470	27	34	13	186	12	127	358	759	404	2.50	—	226	0.10	0.42	5.40	—	—	—	12
1487	Chicken and broccoli-light and elegant	1 item	270	290	19	11	—	—	30	204	240	805	180	1.60	—	75	0.11	0.21	1.80	—	—	—	1
1458	Chicken and dumplings with gravy-hormel	1 ounce	28	31	3	1	0	9	2	5	29	116	45	0.15	0.19	65	0.01	0.03	0.62	0.04	0.06	11	0
215	Chicken and noodles-cooked-home recipe	1 cup	240	365	22	18	6	96	26	26	247	600	149	2.20	—	80	0.05	0.17	4.30	—	—	—	0
1628	Chicken burgundy-classic lite dinner	1 item	319	240	23	5	—	—	24	—	—	—	—	—	—	—	—	—	—	—	—	—	—
1439	Chicken cacciatore-stouffer dinner	1 item	319	310	25	11	8	166	29	75	398	1135	300	3.87	4.09	176	0.24	0.42	18.20	0.95	0.57	22	33
216	Chicken chow mein-canned	1 cup	250	95	7	0	0	98	18	45	85	722	418	1.30	—	30	0.05	0.10	1.00	—	—	—	13
217	Chicken chow mein-home recipe	1 cup	250	255	31	10	2	98	10	58	293	717	473	2.50	—	56	0.08	0.23	4.30	—	—	—	10
360	Chicken chow mein-lean cuisine dinner	1 item	319	250	14	5	—	25	36	—	—	1030	270	—	—	—	—	—	—	—	—	—	—
1438	Chicken crepes/mushroom sauce-stouffer	1 item	234	390	30	22	7	76	19	54	192	1040	420	2.62	1.13	910	0.15	0.19	7.99	0.46	0.19	28	33
1633	Chicken dinner-swanson frozen dinner	1 item	326	660	26	33	7	111	64	112	295	1610	602	2.70	2.63	323	0.33	0.39	10.30	0.45	0.36	30	12
1437	Chicken divan-stouffer frozen dinner	1 item	241	335	21	22	9	86	14	269	295	830	415	1.72	2.03	221	0.13	0.44	4.63	0.29	0.74	41	20
1617	Chicken florentine-le menu frozen dinner	1 item	354	510	28	28	8	121	35	122	320	985	653	2.93	2.85	351	0.36	0.42	11.20	0.49	0.39	33	13
1293	Chicken frankfurter	1 item	45	116	6	9	2	45	3	43	48	617	38	0.90	0.47	17	0.03	0.05	1.39	0.14	0.11	2	0
1614	Chicken kiev-le menu frozen dinner	1 item	234	500	21	30	5	80	35	80	212	745	432	1.94	1.89	232	0.24	0.28	7.37	0.33	0.26	22	9
1618	Chicken parmigiana-le menu	1 item	333	390	26	19	—	—	28	—	—	900	—	—	—	—	—	—	—	—	—	—	—
1488	Chicken parmigiana-light and elegant	1 item	227	260	28	6	7	172	23	73	394	685	310	2.80	2.89	128	0.33	0.20	6.60	0.45	0.53	22	7
1440	Chicken pasta shells-stouffer dinner	1 item	255	400	26	22	3	165	24	59	226	1060	350	3.71	2.16	177	0.30	0.43	7.46	0.35	0.39	28	28
218	Chicken potpie-baked-home recipe	1 slice	232	545	23	31	11	72	42	70	232	593	343	3.00	—	618	0.34	0.31	5.50	—	—	—	5

Item	Food	Amount	Col 1	Col 2	Col 3	Col 4	Col 5	Col 6	Col 7	Col 8	Col 9	Col 10	Col 11	Col 12	Col 13	Col 14	Col 15	Col 16	Col 17	Col 18	Col 19	Col 20	Col 21
1295	Chicken roll-light	1 slice	28	45	6	2	1	14	1	12	45	166	65	0.28	0.21	7	0.02	0.04	1.50	0.06	0.04	1	0
1296	Chicken spread-canned	1 tbsp	13	25	2	2	2	7	1	16	12	50	14	0.30	0.15	3	0.00	0.02	0.36	0.02	0.02	0	0
1271	Chicken-back-fried-flour coated	1 item	144	477	40	30	8	128	9	35	239	130	325	2.33	3.56	53	0.15	0.34	10.50	0.44	0.40	12	0
1272	Chicken-back-stewed	1 item	122	316	27	22	6	96	0	22	146	78	178	1.48	2.36	113	0.05	0.18	5.30	0.18	0.22	6	0
1875	Chicken-breast and wing-breaded-fried	1 serving	163	494	36	30	8	149	20	60	307	975	566	1.49	1.55	58	0.14	0.30	12.00	0.57	0.67	9	0
1275	Chicken-breast-no skin-fried	1 item	172	322	58	8	2	156	1	28	424	136	474	1.96	1.86	12	0.14	0.22	25.40	1.10	0.62	8	0
1276	Chicken-breast-no skin-roasted	1 item	172	284	53	6	2	146	0	26	392	126	440	1.78	1.72	11	0.12	0.20	23.60	1.02	0.58	6	0
1273	Chicken-breast-roasted	1 item	196	386	58	15	4	166	0	28	420	138	480	2.08	2.00	55	0.13	0.23	24.90	1.08	0.64	6	0
1274	Chicken-breast-stewed	1 item	220	404	60	16	5	166	0	28	344	136	390	2.02	2.12	54	0.09	0.25	17.20	0.64	0.46	6	0
212	Chicken-breast-with skin-fried in batter	1 item	280	728	70	37	10	238	25	56	516	770	564	3.50	2.66	57	0.32	0.41	29.50	1.20	0.82	16	0
210	Chicken-breast-with skin-fried in flour	1 item	196	436	62	17	5	176	3	32	456	150	506	2.34	2.14	29	0.16	0.26	26.90	1.14	0.68	8	0
213	Chicken-canned-boneless-with broth	1 item	142	234	31	11	3	78	0	20	350	714	196	2.25	2.00	100	0.02	0.18	8.99	0.50	0.42	6	3
1285	Chicken-capon-roasted	1 item	1274	2914	369	148	42	1098	0	182	3140	626	3252	18.90	22.10	260	0.89	2.17	114.00	5.50	4.14	70	0
1467	Chicken-drumstick & thigh-breaded-fried	1 serving	148	430	30	27	7	165	16	36	240	756	446	1.60	3.24	67	0.14	0.43	7.21	0.33	0.83	10	0
211	Chicken-drumstick-with skin-fried/flour	1 item	49	120	13	7	2	44	1	6	86	44	112	0.66	1.42	12	0.04	0.11	2.96	0.17	0.16	4	0
1266	Chicken-giblets-fried-flour coated	1 cup	145	402	47	20	6	647	6	26	414	164	478	15.00	9.09	5195	0.14	2.21	15.90	0.88	19.30	550	13
1267	Chicken-giblets-simmered	1 cup	145	228	38	7	2	570	1	18	331	85	229	9.34	6.63	3234	0.13	1.38	5.95	0.49	14.70	545	12
1268	Chicken-gizzard-simmered	1 cup	145	222	39	5	2	281	2	14	225	97	259	6.02	6.35	82	0.04	0.35	5.76	0.17	2.81	77	2
387	Chicken-glazed-with rice-lean cuisine	1 item	241	270	26	8	—	55	23	—	—	810	380	—	—	—	—	—	—	—	—	—	—
1269	Chicken-heart-simmered	1 cup	145	268	38	12	3	350	0	27	289	70	192	13.10	10.60	12	0.10	1.07	4.06	0.47	10.60	116	3
1278	Chicken-leg-no skin-roasted	1 item	95	182	26	8	2	89	0	12	174	87	230	1.24	2.71	18	0.07	0.22	6.00	0.35	0.31	8	0
1279	Chicken-leg-no skin-stewed	1 item	101	187	27	8	2	90	0	11	151	78	192	1.41	2.81	18	0.06	0.22	4.85	0.22	0.23	8	0
1277	Chicken-leg-roasted	1 item	114	265	30	15	4	105	0	14	199	99	256	1.52	2.96	46	0.08	0.24	7.06	0.37	0.35	8	0
1294	Chicken-liver pate-canned	1 tbsp	13	26	2	2	1	51	1	1	23	50	12	1.19	0.28	28	0.01	0.18	0.98	0.03	1.05	42	1
1270	Chicken-liver-simmered	1 cup	140	219	34	8	3	883	1	20	437	71	196	11.90	6.07	6886	0.21	2.45	6.23	0.82	27.10	1077	22
1920	Chicken-sweet and sour-budget gourmet	1 serving	284	350	18	7	1	40	53	60	163	640	429	0.72	1.44	80	0.12	0.34	3.00	0.38	0.17	13	2
1619	Chicken-sweet and sour-le menu dinner	1 item	298	450	20	22	1	53	42	37	171	1170	450	1.95	1.51	45	0.14	0.18	6.95	0.40	0.18	14	32
1280	Chicken-thigh-fried-flour coated	1 item	62	162	17	9	3	60	2	8	116	55	147	0.93	1.56	18	0.06	0.15	4.31	0.21	0.19	5	0
1281	Chicken-thigh-no skin-roasted	1 item	52	109	14	6	2	49	0	6	95	46	124	0.68	1.34	10	0.04	0.12	3.39	0.18	0.16	4	0
1950	Chicken-thin sliced-smoked-land o frost	1 serving	28	60	5	4	1	21	1	0	39	182	49	0.36	0.53	0	0.00	0.03	1.60	0.07	0.06	2	0
1282	Chicken-wing-fried-flour coated	1 item	32	103	8	7	2	26	1	5	48	25	57	0.40	0.56	12	0.02	0.04	2.14	0.13	0.09	1	0
1283	Chicken-wing-roasted	1 item	34	99	9	7	2	29	0	5	51	28	62	0.43	0.62	16	0.01	0.04	2.26	0.14	0.10	1	0
1284	Chicken-wing-stewed	1 item	40	100	9	7	2	28	0	5	48	27	56	0.45	0.65	16	0.02	0.04	1.85	0.09	0.07	1	0
1058	Chicory greens-raw-chopped	1 cup	180	41	3	1	0	0	8	180	85	81	756	1.62	0.76	720	0.11	0.18	0.90	0.19	0.00	197	43
1059	Chicory roots-raw	1 item	60	44	1	0	0	0	11	25	37	30	174	0.48	0.20	1	0.02	0.02	0.24	0.15	0.00	14	3
179	Chili con carne-with beans-canned	1 cup	255	340	19	16	8	38	31	82	321	1354	594	4.30	—	30	0.08	0.18	3.30	0.26	—	—	—
810	Chili powder	1 tsp	3	8	0	0	—	0	1	7	8	26	50	0.37	0.07	91	0.01	0.02	0.21	—	0.00	—	2
1809	Chili with beans-canned	1 cup	255	286	15	14	6	43	30	119	393	1330	932	8.75	5.10	86	0.12	0.27	0.91	0.34	0.03	58	4
1898	Chimichanga-beef	1 item	174	425	20	20	9	9	43	63	123	910	587	4.55	4.95	15	0.48	0.64	5.77	0.27	1.52	31	5
1306	Chitterlings-pork-simmered	1 ounce	28	86	3	8	3	41	0	8	13	11	2	1.05	1.44	0	0.00	0.02	0.03	0.00	0.29	1	0
1061	Chives-freeze dried	1 tbsp	0	1	0	0	0	0	0	2	1	0	6	0.04	0.01	14	0.00	0.00	0.01	0.00	0.00	0	1
1060	Chives-raw-chopped	1 tbsp	3	1	0	0	0	0	0	2	2	0	8	0.05	0.01	19	0.00	0.01	0.02	0.01	0.00	0	2
546	Chocolate beverage powder-dry milk	1 ounce	28	100	5	1	1	2	20	167	155	147	227	0.50	0.34	3	0.04	0.21	0.20	0.00	0.68	12	1
547	Chocolate beverage powder-no dry milk	1 ounce	28	99	1	1	1	0	26	11	36	60	168	0.89	0.44	1	0.01	0.04	0.14	0.00	0.00	2	0
697	Chocolate-bitter-for baking	1 ounce	28	145	3	15	9	0	8	22	109	1	235	1.90	0.30	6	0.01	0.07	0.40	0.01	0.00	3	0
180	Chop suey-with beef and pork-home recipe	1 cup	250	300	26	17	9	64	13	60	248	1052	425	4.80	—	120	0.28	0.38	5.00	—	—	—	33
1330	Chorizo-pork and beef-link	1 item	60	273	15	23	9	53	1	5	90	741	239	0.95	2.05	0	0.38	0.18	3.08	0.32	1.20	1	0
1739	Churchs chicken-white meat	1 item	100	327	21	23	—	—	10	94	—	498	186	1.00	—	48	0.10	0.18	7.20	—	—	—	1
855	Cider-fermented	1 fl oz	30	12	0	0	0	0	0	2	2	0	36	0.11	0.01	0	0.01	0.01	0.03	0.01	0.00	0	0
811	Cinnamon-ground	1 tsp	2	6	0	0	0	0	2	28	1	1	11	0.88	0.05	1	0.00	0.00	0.03	—	0.00	—	1
812	Cloves-ground	1 tsp	2	7	0	0	0	0	1	14	2	5	23	0.18	0.02	1	0.00	0.01	0.03	—	0.00	—	2
1607	Cobbler-weight watchers-frozen	1 slice	124	160	1	6	—	—	26	—	—	—	—	—	—	—	—	—	—	—	—	—	—
873	Cocktail-daiquiri	1 item	100	186	0	0	0	0	7	3	6	5	21	0.15	0.06	1	0.01	0.00	0.04	0.01	0.00	2	2
874	Cocktail-eggnog	1 item	123	335	4	16	2	94	18	44	74	75	178	0.70	0.61	25	0.04	0.11	0.00	0.07	0.57	15	0
875	Cocktail-gin rickey	1 item	120	150	0	0	0	0	1	2	1	19	12	0.00	0.10	0	0.01	0.00	0.00	0.00	0.00	1	4
876	Cocktail-highball	1 fl oz	29	26	0	0	0	0	0	1	1	4	1	0.01	0.02	0	0.00	0.00	0.01	0.00	0.00	0	0
877	Cocktail-manhattan	1 fl oz	29	64	0	0	0	0	1	1	2	1	7	0.03	0.01	0	0.00	0.00	0.03	0.00	0.00	0	0
878	Cocktail-martini	1 fl oz	28	63	0	0	0	0	0	1	1	1	5	0.03	0.01	0	0.00	0.00	0.00	0.00	0.00	0	0
879	Cocktail-mint julep	1 item	300	212	0	0	0	0	3	0	10	0	6	0.13	0.11	0	0.02	0.01	0.03	0.00	0.00	0	0
880	Cocktail-old fashioned	1 item	100	180	0	0	0	0	4	0	4	1	2	0.04	0.04	0	0.01	0.00	0.01	0.00	0.00	0	0
1880	Cocktail-pina colada-home recipe	1 fl oz	31	58	0	1	0	0	9	3	2	2	22	0.07	0.04	0	0.01	0.00	0.04	0.01	0.00	3	1
881	Cocktail-planters punch	1 item	100	175	0	0	0	0	8	4	3	—	—	0.10	—	0	0.10	0.00	0.00	—	—	—	8
882	Cocktail-rum sour	1 item	100	165	0	0	0	0	0	0	4	1	2	0.04	0.04	0	0.01	0.00	0.01	0.00	0.00	0	0

Dashes (—) in data spaces indicate that no data were reported.

Item	Food Name	Portion	Weight (g)	Food Energy (kcal)	Protein (g)	Total Fat (g)	Saturated Fat (g)	Cholesterol (mg)	Carbohydrate (g)	Calcium (mg)	Phosphorus (mg)	Sodium (mg)	Potassium (mg)	Iron (mg)	Zinc (cm)	Vitamin A (RE)	Thiamin (mg)	Riboflavin (mg)	Niacin (mg)	Vitamin B6 (mg)	Vitamin B12 (ug)	Folic Acid (ug)	Vitamin C (mg)
883	Cocktail-tom collins	1 fl oz	30	16	0	0	0	0	0	1	0	5	2	0.00	0.02	0	0.00	0.00	0.00	0.00	0.00	0	1
1154	Coconut cream-raw	1 cup	240	792	9	83	74	0	16	26	293	10	781	5.47	2.30	0	0.07	0.00	2.14	0.07	0.00	34	7
1155	Coconut milk-raw	1 cup	240	552	6	57	51	0	13	39	240	37	630	3.94	1.61	0	0.06	0.00	1.82	0.08	0.00	39	7
1418	Coffee substitute-prepared	8 fl oz	242	12	0	0	0	0	2	7	17	10	58	0.14	0.07	0	0.02	0.00	0.52	0.02	0.00	1	0
731	Coffee-brewed	8 fl oz	237	5	0	0	0	0	1	5	2	5	128	0.12	0.05	0	0.00	0.00	0.53	0.00	0.00	0	0
732	Coffee-instant-prepared	8 fl oz	239	5	0	0	0	0	1	7	7	7	86	0.12	0.07	0	0.00	0.00	0.68	0.00	0.00	0	0
611	Collards-frozen-boiled-drained	1 cup	170	61	5	1	—	0	12	357	46	85	427	1.90	0.46	1017	0.08	0.20	1.08	0.19	0.00	129	45
610	Collards-raw-boiled-drained	1 cup	128	35	2	0	0	0	8	29	10	21	168	0.21	0.14	349	0.03	0.07	0.37	0.07	0.00	8	16
415	Cookie-chocolate chip-baked from mix	1 item	11	50	1	2	1	6	7	3	7	38	14	0.23	0.05	6	0.01	0.02	0.20	0.00	—	1	0
416	Cookie-chocolate chip-from home recipe	1 item	10	46	1	3	1	5	6	3	8	21	21	0.25	0.04	1	0.02	0.02	0.15	0.00	0.01	1	0
1715	Cookie-chocolate chip-low sodium	1 item	5	25	1	1	0	5	3	2	6	5	7	0.15	0.04	2	0.01	0.01	0.08	0.00	0.01	0	0
417	Cookie-fig bar-commercial	1 item	14	53	1	1	0	0	11	10	8	45	41	0.34	0.09	3	0.02	0.02	0.18	0.02	0.00	1	0
1716	Cookie-fudge-low sodium	1 item	5	25	1	1	0	0	3	3	7	5	7	0.16	0.05	2	0.01	0.01	0.13	0.00	0.01	0	0
418	Cookie-gingersnap-from home recipe	1 item	7	34	0	2	—	0	5	3	4	20	14	0.16	0.03	1	0.01	0.01	0.12	0.00	0.01	1	0
419	Cookie-macaroon	1 item	19	90	1	5	—	0	13	5	16	6	88	0.15	—	0	0.01	0.03	0.10	—	—	—	0
420	Cookie-oatmeal/raisin-from mix	1 item	13	62	1	3	1	0	9	4	14	37	23	0.29	0.09	2	0.02	0.02	0.24	0.01	—	2	0
1656	Cookie-peanut butter-from mix	1 item	10	50	1	3	1	3	6	12	24	57	19	0.19	0.75	3	0.02	0.02	0.38	0.01	0.01	2	0
421	Cookie-plain-prepared from mix	1 item	12	60	1	3	1	0	8	4	9	65	6	0.15	0.03	8	0.03	0.02	0.23	0.01	—	1	0
422	Cookie-sandwich-chocolate/vanilla	1 item	10	50	1	2	1	0	7	3	24	63	4	0.18	0.09	0	0.02	0.03	0.18	0.00	0.00	0	0
1384	Cookie-sugar-from mix	1 item	20	99	1	5	—	—	13	21	38	109	14	0.39	0.05	3	0.04	0.02	0.47	0.01	—	2	0
423	Cookie-vanilla wafer	1 item	4	19	0	1	0	3	3	2	3	10	3	0.06	—	1	0.01	0.01	0.08	—	—	—	0
736	Cordials/liqueur-54 proof	1 fl oz	34	97	0	0	0	0	12	0	0	1	1	0.02	0.02	0	0.00	0.00	0.03	0.00	0.00	0	0
1175	Coriander leaf-dried	1 tsp	1	2	0	0	0	0	0	7	3	1	27	0.25	—	—	0.01	0.01	0.06	—	0.00	—	3
1959	Corn bran-crude	1 cup	76	170	6	1	0	0	65	32	55	5	33	2.12	1.18	5	0.01	0.08	2.08	0.12	0.00	3	0
1389	Corn chips	1 ounce	28	155	2	9	2	0	17	37	55	164	43	0.38	0.44	11	0.05	0.03	0.55	0.05	0.00	2	1
2025	Corn dog-plain	1 item	175	460	17	19	5	79	56	101	166	972	262	6.18	1.31	36	0.29	0.71	4.16	0.10	0.44	60	0
1680	Corn fritter	1 item	35	132	3	8	2	25	14	22	54	167	47	0.60	0.24	14	0.06	0.07	0.60	0.02	0.06	11	1
1734	Corn germ-toasted	1 ounce	28	130	5	7	—	0	12	3	444	—	—	2.18	2.97	2	0.47	0.21	0.60	0.39	—	26	1
1961	Corn grits-dry	1 cup	156	579	14	2	0	0	124	3	114	1	213	6.10	0.64	0	1.00	0.59	7.73	0.23	0.00	7	0
1958	Corn kernels-whole grain	1 cup	166	606	16	8	1	0	123	12	349	58	476	4.50	3.66	78	0.64	0.33	6.02	1.03	0.00	32	0
408	Corn souffle-stouffer frozen side dish	1 item	113	155	4	7	—	—	19	48	—	510	190	0.40	—	94	0.08	0.16	0.80	—	—	34	0
1693	Corn-creamed-canned-dietary-low sodium	1 cup	256	184	4	1	0	0	46	8	131	8	343	0.97	1.36	26	0.06	0.14	2.46	0.16	0.00	115	12
613	Corn-ear-frozen-boiled-drained	1 item	126	117	4	1	0	0	28	4	95	5	316	0.77	0.79	27	0.22	0.09	1.91	0.28	0.00	38	6
614	Corn-frozen-boiled-drained-kernels	1 cup	165	134	5	0	0	0	34	4	78	8	228	0.50	0.56	41	0.11	0.12	2.10	0.16	0.00	33	4
612	Corn-kernels from one ear-boiled-drained	1 item	77	83	3	1	0	0	19	2	79	13	192	0.47	0.37	17	0.17	0.06	1.24	0.05	0.00	36	5
617	Corn-sweet-canned-drained	1 cup	165	134	4	2	0	0	31	8	107	533	322	1.42	0.64	26	0.05	0.13	1.98	0.08	0.00	80	14
1679	Corn-sweet-canned-low sodium	1 cup	256	156	5	1	0	0	38	10	131	8	392	0.90	0.92	31	0.07	0.16	2.40	0.10	0.00	98	17
616	Corn-sweet-canned-vacuum packed	1 cup	210	166	5	1	0	0	41	10	134	572	390	0.88	0.96	51	0.09	0.15	2.45	0.12	0.00	104	17
615	Corn-sweet-cream style-canned	1 cup	256	184	4	1	0	0	46	8	131	730	343	0.97	1.36	26	0.06	0.14	2.46	0.16	0.00	115	12
1063	Corn-with red and green peppers-canned	1 cup	227	170	5	1	0	0	41	11	141	788	347	1.79	0.84	52	0.05	0.18	2.16	0.22	0.00	77	20
1385	Cornbread-home recipe	1 slice	45	108	2	4	1	0	16	49	44	126	42	0.67	0.21	7	0.08	0.08	0.68	0.03	0.08	5	0
175	Corned beef hash-canned	1 cup	220	400	19	25	12	50	24	29	147	1188	440	4.40	—	—	0.02	0.20	4.60	—	—	—	—
1331	Corned beef loaf-jellied	1 slice	28	44	7	2	1	13	0	3	21	270	29	0.58	1.16	0	0.00	0.03	0.50	0.03	0.36	2	2
174	Corned beef-canned	1 serving	85	213	23	13	5	73	1	17	94	855	116	1.77	3.03	0	0.02	0.20	2.90	0.11	1.38	3	0
427	Cornmeal-degermed-enriched-cooked	1 cup	240	878	20	4	1	0	186	12	202	7	389	9.91	1.73	98	1.72	0.98	12.10	0.62	0.00	115	0
426	Cornmeal-degermed-enriched-dry	1 cup	138	505	12	2	0	0	107	7	116	4	224	5.70	0.99	57	0.99	0.56	6.95	0.35	0.00	66	0
429	Cornmeal-degermed-unenriched-cooked	1 cup	240	878	20	4	1	0	186	12	202	7	389	2.64	1.73	98	0.34	0.12	5.60	0.62	0.00	115	0
428	Cornmeal-degermed-unenriched-dry	1 cup	138	505	12	2	0	0	107	7	116	4	224	1.52	0.99	57	0.19	0.07	1.38	0.35	0.00	66	7
1560	Cornmeal-self rising-degermed	1 cup	138	490	12	2	0	0	103	483	860	1860	235	6.53	1.38	57	0.94	0.53	6.30	0.54	0.00	43	0
425	Cornmeal-whole grain-bolted	1 cup	122	407	10	4	1	0	86	440	981	1521	311	7.03	2.44	57	0.81	0.49	6.46	0.66	0.00	70	0
424	Cornmeal-whole grain-dry	1 cup	122	442	10	4	1	0	94	7	294	43	350	4.21	2.21	57	0.47	0.25	4.43	0.37	0.00	31	0
1706	Cornstarch	1 cup	128	488	0	0	0	0	117	2	16	11	4	0.61	0.08	0	0.00	0.00	0.00	0.00	0.00	0	0
1963	Couscous-cooked	1 cup	179	200	7	0	0	0	42	14	39	9	104	0.68	0.47	0	0.11	0.05	1.76	0.09	0.00	27	0
1962	Couscous-dry	1 cup	184	692	24	1	0	0	142	44	313	18	305	1.99	1.52	0	0.30	0.14	6.42	0.20	0.00	37	0
1422	Crackers-animal-ralston	1 item	2	9	0	0	0	0	1	0	1	8	2	0.06	0.01	0	0.01	0.01	0.07	0.00	0.00	0	0
1423	Crackers-cheddar snacks-ralston	1 item	2	7	0	0	—	—	1	1	2	14	2	0.07	0.01	0	0.01	0.01	0.07	0.00	0.01	0	0
1386	Crackers-cheese	1 item	1	5	0	0	0	0	1	1	2	12	2	0.04	0.01	0	0.00	0.00	0.08	0.00	0.01	0	0
1430	Crackers-cheese and chives-ralston	1 item	2	7	0	0	—	—	1	1	2	14	2	0.07	0.01	0	0.01	0.01	0.08	0.00	0.01	0	0
1424	Crackers-cheese snacks-ralston	1 item	1	6	0	0	0	0	1	1	1	10	2	0.05	0.01	0	0.01	0.01	0.05	0.00	0.04	0	0
430	Crackers-graham-plain	1 item	7	28	1	1	0	0	5	3	11	33	28	0.25	0.05	0	0.01	0.04	0.25	0.01	0.00	1	0

1387	Crackers-graham-sugar-honey	1 item	7	30	1	1	0	0	5	3	8	33	12	0.18	0.05	0	0.02	0.02	0.22	0.01	0.00	1	0
1425	Crackers-oyster-ralston	1 item	0	2	0	0	0	0	0	0	0	5	1	0.02	0.00	0	0.00	0.00	0.02	0.00	0.00	0	0
1426	Crackers-rich and crisp-ralston	1 item	3	16	0	1	—	0	2	2	4	21	3	0.09	0.02	0	0.02	0.01	0.12	0.00	0.00	0	0
1869	Crackers-ritz	1 item	3	18	0	1	—	0	2	5	8	32	3	0.10	—	—	0.01	0.01	0.10	—	—	—	—
1419	Crackers-ry krisp-natural-ralston	1 item	2	8	0	0	0	0	2	1	7	19	10	0.09	0.06	—	0.01	0.01	0.03	0.01	—	1	—
1420	Crackers-ry krisp-seasoned-ralston	1 item	2	8	0	0	—	0	2	1	6	27	11	0.08	0.06	—	0.01	0.01	0.07	0.00	—	1	—
1421	Crackers-ry krisp-sesame-ralston	1 item	3	8	0	0	—	0	2	1	8	29	12	0.09	0.07	1	0.01	0.01	0.03	0.01	—	1	—
1427	Crackers-rye snacks-ralston	1 item	2	9	0	0	—	0	1	0	2	14	3	0.07	0.02	0	0.01	0.01	0.06	0.00	0.01	0	0
431	Crackers-rye wafers	1 item	7	23	1	0	0	0	5	4	25	57	39	0.25	—	0	0.02	0.02	0.10	—	—	—	0
432	Crackers-saltines	1 item	3	13	0	0	0	1	2	1	3	37	3	0.13	0.02	0	0.13	0.01	0.10	0.00	0.00	0	0
1431	Crackers-sesame and wheat-ralston	1 item	2	9	0	0	—	0	1	1	3	17	4	0.08	0.03	0	0.01	0.01	0.08	0.00	0.01	0	0
1428	Crackers-snackers-ralston	1 item	4	18	0	1	—	0	2	1	3	24	4	0.10	0.02	0	0.01	0.02	0.15	0.00	0.00	0	0
1650	Crackers-triscuits	1 item	5	21	0	1	0	0	3	1	9	24	6	0.15	0.07	0	0.02	0.01	0.21	0.01	0.04	1	0
1429	Crackers-wheat snacks	1 item	2	9	0	0	0	0	1	0	3	12	3	0.07	0.03	4	0.01	0.01	0.08	0.00	0.01	0	0
1651	Crackers-wheat thins	1 item	2	9	0	0	—	0	1	—	—	—	—	—	—	—	—	—	—	—	—	—	—
1925	Crackers-whole wheat-low sodium	1 serving	8	30	1	0	0	0	7	2	14	31	33	0.30	0.08	1	0.04	0.03	0.36	0.01	0.00	2	0
1926	Crackers-whole wheat-sodium free	1 serving	8	30	1	0	0	0	7	2	14	1	35	0.25	0.11	0	0.04	0.02	0.33	0.01	0.07	2	0
1637	Cranapple juice cocktail-ocean spray	1 fl oz	32	5	0	0	0	0	1	1	0	1	8	0.05	0.01	—	0.00	0.01	0.02	—	0.00	0	14
1717	Cranapple juice-canned	1 cup	253	170	0	0	0	0	43	18	8	5	68	0.15	0.10	0	0.01	0.05	0.15	0.05	0.00	1	81
241	Cranberry juice cocktail-bottled	1 cup	253	144	0	0	0	0	36	8	5	10	46	0.38	0.18	0	0.02	0.02	0.09	0.05	0.00	1	90
1638	Cranberry juice cocktail-ocean spray	1 fl oz	32	6	0	0	0	0	5	1	0	1	8	0.05	0.01	0	0.00	0.01	0.02	0.01	0.00	0	14
242	Cranberry sauce-canned-sweetened	1 cup	277	418	1	0	0	0	108	11	17	80	72	0.61	0.14	6	0.04	0.06	0.28	0.04	0.00	—	11
1436	Cream chipped beef-stouffer dinner	1 item	156	235	12	16	5	28	10	127	171	900	290	1.65	1.69	72	0.06	0.28	2.20	0.13	0.95	9	6
28	Cream-coffee-table-light-fluid	1 cup	240	469	6	46	29	159	9	231	192	95	292	0.10	0.65	519	0.08	0.36	0.14	0.08	0.53	6	2
26	Cream-half & half-milk and cream-fluid	1 cup	242	315	7	28	17	89	10	254	230	98	314	0.17	1.23	315	0.09	0.36	0.19	0.09	0.80	6	2
38	Cream-imitation-liquid-non dairy-frozen	1 cup	245	333	2	24	5	0	28	22	157	194	466	0.07	0.05	66	0.00	0.00	0.00	0.00	0.00	0	0
40	Cream-imitation-non dairy-powdered	1 cup	94	514	5	33	31	0	52	21	397	170	763	1.08	0.48	57	0.00	0.16	0.00	0.00	0.00	0	0
2019	Cream-mocha mix-non dairy	1 tbsp	15	20	1	2	1	0	1	—	—	5	20	—	—	—	—	—	—	—	—	—	—
36	Cream-sour-cultured	1 cup	230	493	7	48	30	102	10	268	195	123	331	0.14	0.62	546	0.08	0.34	0.15	0.04	0.69	25	2
903	Cream-sour-half & half	1 tbsp	15	20	0	2	1	6	1	16	14	6	19	0.01	0.08	20	0.01	0.02	0.01	0.00	0.05	2	0
904	Cream-sour-imitation	1 ounce	28	59	1	6	5	0	2	1	13	29	46	0.11	0.34	0	0.00	0.00	0.00	0.00	0.00	0	0
48	Cream-sour-imitation-nonfat dry milk	1 cup	235	415	8	39	31	0	11	266	205	240	380	0.10	—	6	0.09	0.38	0.20	—	—	—	2
42	Cream-whipped-imitation-non dairy-frozen	1 cup	75	239	1	19	16	0	17	5	6	19	14	0.09	0.02	194	0.00	0.00	0.00	0.00	0.00	0	0
44	Cream-whipped-imitation-non dairy-powder	1 cup	80	151	3	10	9	8	13	72	69	53	121	0.03	0.22	87	0.02	0.09	0.05	0.02	0.21	3	1
34	Cream-whipped-imitation-pressurized	1 cup	60	154	2	13	8	46	7	61	54	78	88	0.03	0.22	165	0.02	0.04	0.04	0.03	0.18	2	0
46	Cream-whipped-imitation-pressurized	1 cup	70	184	1	16	13	0	11	4	13	43	13	0.01	0.01	99	0.00	0.00	0.00	0.00	0.00	0	0
32	Cream-whipping-heavy-unwhipped-fluid	1 cup	238	821	5	88	55	326	7	154	149	89	179	0.07	0.55	1051	0.05	0.26	0.09	0.06	0.43	9	1
30	Cream-whipping-light-unwhipped-fluid	1 cup	239	699	5	74	46	265	7	166	146	82	231	0.07	0.60	809	0.06	0.30	0.10	0.07	0.47	9	1
410	Creamed spinach-stouffer side dish	1 item	128	190	4	15	—	—	9	—	—	855	585	—	—	—	—	—	—	—	—	—	—
1065	Cress-garden-raw	1 cup	50	16	1	0	0	0	3	40	38	8	304	0.66	0.12	465	0.04	0.13	0.50	0.12	0.00	40	35
1652	Croutons-herb seasoned	1 cup	30	100	4	0	0	0	20	29	42	372	39	1.54	0.30	0	0.13	0.20	1.72	0.00	0.00	0	0
619	Cucumber-raw-sliced	1 cup	104	14	1	0	0	0	3	15	18	2	155	0.29	0.24	5	0.03	0.02	0.31	0.05	0.00	15	5
618	Cucumber-raw-whole	1 item	301	39	2	0	0	0	9	42	51	6	448	0.84	0.69	15	0.09	0.06	0.90	0.16	0.00	42	14
390	Cupcake with chocolate icing	1 item	36	130	2	5	2	15	21	47	71	120	42	0.40	—	12	0.05	0.06	0.40	—	—	—	0
393	Cupcake-devils food with chocolate icing	1 item	35	120	2	4	2	40	20	21	37	91	46	0.50	—	10	0.03	0.05	0.30	—	—	2	0
389	Cupcake-no icing	1 item	25	90	1	3	1	0	14	40	59	113	21	0.30	—	8	0.05	0.05	0.40	—	—	—	0
1178	Curry powder	1 tsp	2	6	0	0	—	0	1	10	7	1	31	0.59	0.08	2	0.01	0.01	0.07	—	0.00	—	0
86	Custard-baked	1 cup	265	305	14	15	7	278	29	297	310	209	387	1.10	—	87	0.11	0.50	0.30	—	—	—	1
1466	Dairy queen-banana split	1 item	383	540	10	15	—	30	91	350	250	—	—	1.80	—	225	0.60	0.60	0.80	—	0.90	—	18
1462	Dairy queen-dip ice cream cone-regular	1 item	156	300	7	13	—	20	40	200	150	—	—	0.40	—	90	0.09	0.34	0.00	—	0.60	—	0
1465	Dairy queen-float	1 item	397	330	6	8	—	20	59	200	200	—	—	0.00	—	30	0.12	0.17	0.00	—	0.60	—	0
1461	Dairy queen-ice cream cone-regular	1 item	142	226	5	8	5	38	33	212	192	126	233	0.21	0.78	87	0.07	0.36	0.43	0.09	0.28	7	2
1463	Dairy queen-ice cream sundae-regular	1 item	177	319	6	10	6	23	53	232	255	204	443	0.66	1.06	75	0.07	0.34	1.20	0.14	0.73	11	3
1464	Dairy queen-malt-regular	1 item	418	600	15	20	—	50	89	500	400	—	—	3.60	—	225	0.12	0.60	0.80	—	1.80	—	4
620	Dandelion greens-boiled	1 cup	105	35	2	1	0	0	7	147	44	46	244	1.89	0.29	1229	0.14	0.18	0.54	0.17	0.00	13	19
1891	Danish pastry-cheese	1 item	91	353	6	25	5	20	29	70	80	320	116	1.85	0.63	43	0.27	0.21	2.55	0.06	0.23	15	3
1892	Danish pastry-cinnamon	1 item	88	349	5	17	3	28	47	37	74	326	96	1.80	0.49	5	0.26	0.19	2.20	0.06	0.22	14	3
1893	Danish pastry-fruit	1 item	94	335	5	16	3	19	45	22	69	333	110	1.40	0.48	24	0.29	0.21	1.79	0.06	0.23	15	2
434	Danish pastry-plain	1 item	65	250	4	14	5	0	29	69	66	249	61	1.20	0.55	11	0.16	0.15	1.47	—	—	—	0
244	Dates-domestic-natural and dry-chopped	1 cup	178	490	4	1	0	0	131	57	71	5	1161	2.05	0.52	9	0.16	0.18	3.92	0.34	0.00	22	0
243	Dates-domestic-natural and dry-whole	1 item	8	23	0	0	0	0	6	3	3	0	54	0.10	0.02	0	0.01	0.01	0.18	0.02	0.00	1	0
1180	Dill weed-dried	1 tsp	1	3	0	0	0	0	1	18	5	2	33	0.49	0.03	—	0.00	0.00	0.03	0.02	0.00	—	—
337	Dip-bacon and horseradish-kraft	1 tbsp	15	30	1	3	—	0	2	—	—	100	—	—	—	—	—	—	—	—	—	—	—

Dashes (—) in data spaces indicate that no data were reported.

Appendix C Table of Food Composition

Item	Food Name	Portion	Weight (g)	Food Energy (kcal)	Protein (g)	Total Fat (g)	Saturated Fat (g)	Cholesterol (mg)	Carbohydrate (g)	Calcium (mg)	Phosphorus (mg)	Sodium (mg)	Potassium (mg)	Iron (mg)	Zinc (cm)	Vitamin A (RE)	Thiamin (mg)	Riboflavin (mg)	Niacin (mg)	Vitamin B6 (mg)	Vitamin B12 (ug)	Folic Acid (ug)	Vitamin C (mg)
331	Dip-buttermilk-kraft	1 tbsp	15	40	1	4	—	3	1	—	—	135	—	—	—	—	—	—	—	—	—	—	—
339	Dip-clam-kraft	1 tbsp	15	30	1	2	—	5	2	—	—	115	—	—	—	—	—	—	—	—	—	—	—
333	Dip-french onion-kraft	1 tbsp	15	30	1	2	—	0	2	—	—	120	—	—	—	—	—	—	—	—	—	—	—
342	Dip-garlic-kraft	1 tbsp	15	30	1	2	—	0	2	—	—	80	—	—	—	—	—	—	—	—	—	—	—
335	Dip-green onion-kraft	1 tbsp	15	25	1	2	—	0	2	—	—	85	—	—	—	—	—	—	—	—	—	—	—
328	Dip-guacamole-kraft	1 tbsp	15	25	1	2	—	0	2	—	—	108	—	—	—	—	—	—	—	—	—	—	—
1751	Dip-jalapeno bean-fritos	1 ounce	28	33	2	1	0	1	3	7	23	163	77	0.39	0.10	4	0.02	0.03	1.10	0.03	0.00	20	0
326	Dip-jalapeno pepper-kraft	1 tbsp	15	25	1	2	—	0	2	—	—	80	—	—	—	—	—	—	—	—	—	—	—
436	Doughnuts-cake-plain	1 item	25	104	1	6	1	10	12	11	55	139	27	0.37	0.13	2	0.06	0.05	0.43	0.01	—	2	0
437	Doughnuts-yeast-glazed	1 item	50	205	3	11	3	13	22	16	33	117	34	0.60	—	5	0.10	0.10	0.80	—	—	11	0
1286	Duck-flesh & skin-roasted	1 item	764	2574	145	217	74	640	0	86	1190	454	1560	20.60	14.20	483	1.33	2.06	36.90	1.40	2.26	50	0
1287	Duck-no skin-roasted	1 item	442	890	104	50	18	396	0	52	898	286	1114	11.90	11.50	103	1.15	2.08	22.50	1.10	1.76	44	0
1681	Eclair-custard with chocolate icing	1 item	100	239	6	14	—	—	23	80	112	82	122	0.70	—	68	0.04	0.16	0.10	—	—	—	0
1647	Egg roll-beef and shrimp-frozen-la choy	1 item	12	27	1	1	0	2	4	2	5	81	15	0.13	0.07	12	0.01	0.01	0.14	0.01	0.02	1	2
920	Egg substitute-frozen	1 cup	240	384	27	27	5	5	8	175	172	479	512	4.75	2.35	324	0.29	0.93	0.34	0.32	0.81	39	1
918	Egg substitute-liquid	1 cup	251	211	30	8	2	3	2	133	304	444	828	5.27	3.26	542	0.28	0.75	0.28	0.01	0.75	37	0
919	Egg substitute-powder	1 serving	28	126	16	4	1	162	6	92	136	227	211	0.90	0.52	105	0.06	0.50	0.16	0.04	1.00	35	0
917	Egg-duck-whole-fresh-raw	1 item	70	130	9	10	3	619	1	45	154	102	156	2.70	0.99	279	0.11	0.28	0.14	0.18	3.78	56	0
99	Egg-fried in butter-whole-large-chicken	1 item	46	92	6	7	2	211	1	25	89	162	61	0.72	0.55	114	0.03	0.24	0.04	0.07	0.42	18	0
100	Egg-hard cooked-no shell-large-chicken	1 item	50	77	6	5	2	213	1	25	86	62	63	0.60	0.52	84	0.03	0.26	0.03	0.06	0.56	22	0
101	Egg-poached-whole-large-chicken	1 item	50	74	6	5	2	212	1	25	89	140	60	0.72	0.55	95	0.03	0.22	0.03	0.06	0.40	18	0
97	Egg-raw-white-large-chicken	1 item	33	17	4	0	0	0	0	2	4	55	48	0.01	0.00	0	0.00	0.15	0.03	0.00	0.07	1	0
96	Egg-raw-whole-large-chicken	1 item	50	75	6	5	2	213	1	25	89	63	60	0.72	0.55	95	0.03	0.25	0.04	0.07	0.50	23	0
98	Egg-raw-yolk-large-chicken	1 item	17	59	3	5	2	213	0	23	81	7	16	0.59	0.52	323	0.03	0.11	0.00	0.07	0.52	24	0
102	Egg-scrambled-with milk & butter-chicken	1 item	61	101	7	7	2	215	1	44	104	171	84	0.73	0.61	119	0.03	0.27	0.05	0.07	0.47	18	0
1066	Eggplant-boiled-drained	1 cup	96	27	1	0	0	0	6	6	21	3	238	0.34	0.14	6	0.07	0.02	0.58	0.08	0.00	14	1
972	Elderberries-raw	1 cup	145	106	1	1	0	0	27	55	57	9	406	2.32	0.16	87	0.10	0.09	0.73	0.33	0.00	9	52
1406	Enchilada-cheese	1 item	163	320	10	19	11	44	29	324	133	784	240	1.31	2.51	186	0.09	0.42	1.91	0.39	0.74	34	1
1904	Enchirito-cheese/beef/bean	1 item	193	344	18	16	8	49	34	217	224	1251	560	2.39	2.75	134	0.18	0.69	2.99	0.21	1.63	254	5
621	Endive-raw-chopped	1 cup	50	9	1	0	0	0	2	26	14	11	157	0.42	0.40	103	0.04	0.04	0.20	0.01	0.00	71	3
1964	Farina-enriched-dry	1 cup	176	649	19	1	0	0	137	25	154	5	165	6.54	0.94	—	1.01	0.63	7.12	0.10	0.00	42	—
922	Fat-animal-chicken-for cooking	1 tbsp	13	115	0	13	4	11	0	0	0	0	0	0.00	0.00	0	0.00	0.00	0.00	0.00	0.00	0	0
111	Fat-animal-lard (pork)	1 cup	205	1849	0	205	80	195	0	0	0	0	0	0.00	0.23	0	0.00	0.00	0.00	0.00	0.00	0	0
433	Fettucini alfredo-stouffer frozen dinner	1 item	142	270	8	18	—	—	19	—	—	1195	240	—	—	—	—	—	—	—	—	—	—
1915	Fettucini-chicken-budget gourmet	1 serving	284	400	23	21	—	100	29	200	—	740	—	1.80	—	350	0.15	0.43	6.00	—	—	—	2
975	Figs-canned-heavy syrup pack	1 cup	259	228	1	0	0	0	59	69	26	3	258	0.73	0.29	10	0.06	0.10	1.11	0.18	0.00	5	3
974	Figs-canned-water pack	1 cup	248	131	1	0	0	0	35	69	25	2	255	0.72	0.30	10	0.06	0.09	1.10	0.17	0.00	5	2
976	Figs-dried-uncooked	1 cup	199	507	6	2	0	0	130	287	135	22	1417	4.44	1.01	26	0.14	0.18	1.38	0.45	0.00	15	2
973	Figs-raw	1 item	50	37	0	0	0	0	10	18	7	1	116	0.18	0.07	7	0.03	0.03	0.20	0.06	0.00	3	1
391	Filet of fish divan-lean cuisine dinner	1 item	351	270	31	10	—	85	16	—	—	780	850	—	—	—	—	—	—	—	—	—	—
394	Filet of fish florentine-lean cuisine	1 item	255	240	26	9	—	100	13	—	—	700	540	—	—	—	—	—	—	—	—	—	—
1648	Fish and chips-van de kamps dinner	1 item	224	500	16	30	6	33	45	35	271	551	785	2.22	1.00	18	0.24	0.14	4.27	0.41	0.68	23	11
1593	Fish eggs-carp/cod/pike/shad-roe-raw	1 ounce	28	39	6	2	0	106	0	6	114	26	63	0.17	0.28	22	0.07	0.21	0.51	0.05	2.84	23	5
1572	Fish eggs-caviar-sturgeon-granular	1 tbsp	16	40	4	3	1	94	1	44	57	240	29	1.90	0.15	90	0.03	0.10	0.02	0.05	3.20	8	0
149	Fish sticks-breaded-frozen-cooked	1 ounce	28	77	4	3	1	32	7	6	51	165	74	0.21	0.19	9	0.04	0.05	0.60	0.02	0.51	5	0
1857	Fish-abalone-cooked-fried	1 serving	85	161	17	6	1	80	9	32	184	502	241	3.23	0.80	2	0.19	0.11	1.62	0.13	0.59	5	2
1856	Fish-abalone-raw	1 serving	85	89	15	1	0	72	5	26	162	256	213	2.71	0.70	2	0.16	0.09	1.28	0.13	0.62	4	2
1568	Fish-anchovy-fillet-canned	1 item	4	8	1	0	0	3	0	9	10	147	22	0.19	0.10	1	0.00	0.02	0.80	0.01	0.04	1	0
1569	Fish-bass-black-baked	1 ounce	28	32	5	1	0	19	0	23	57	20	101	0.42	0.19	—	—	—	—	—	—	—	—
1570	Fish-bass-striped-broiled	1 serving	159	154	28	4	1	127	0	22	373	110	501	1.33	0.64	170	0.19	0.22	2.91	0.69	6.07	10	3
1702	Fish-bass-striped-oven fried	1 item	200	392	43	17	—	—	13	—	—	—	—	—	—	—	—	—	—	—	—	—	—
145	Fish-bluefish-baked with butter	1 item	155	246	41	8	2	108	0	45	445	161	—	1.10	—	24	0.17	0.16	2.90	—	1.64	—	—
1571	Fish-bluefish-broiled	1 serving	150	186	30	6	1	88	0	10	341	90	558	0.72	1.21	179	0.09	0.12	8.93	0.60	8.09	2	0
1819	Fish-carp-cooked-dry heat	1 serving	85	138	19	6	1	72	0	44	451	54	363	1.35	1.62	8	0.12	0.06	1.79	0.19	1.25	15	1
1820	Fish-catfish-breaded-fried	1 serving	85	195	15	11	3	69	7	37	184	238	289	1.22	0.73	7	0.06	0.11	1.94	0.16	1.62	14	0
1859	Fish-clams-breaded-fried	1 serving	85	172	12	9	2	52	9	54	160	309	277	11.80	1.24	77	0.09	0.21	1.75	0.05	34.20	16	9
147	Fish-clams-canned-solids and liquids	1 ounce	28	13	2	0	0	18	1	16	39	15	40	1.17	0.35	—	0.00	0.03	0.30	—	5.40	—	—
1860	Fish-clams-cooked-moist heat	1 serving	85	126	22	2	0	57	4	78	287	95	534	23.80	2.32	145	0.13	0.36	2.85	0.09	84.10	16	19
146	Fish-clams-raw-meat only	1 serving	85	63	11	1	0	29	2	39	144	48	267	11.90	1.16	77	0.07	0.18	1.50	0.05	42.00	14	11
1573	Fish-cod-atlantic-cooked-dry heat	1 piece	180	189	41	2	0	99	0	25	248	141	440	0.88	1.04	25	0.16	0.14	4.52	0.51	1.89	15	2

1574	Fish-crab cake	1 item	60	93	12	5	1	90	0	63	128	198	195	0.65	2.46	49	0.05	0.05	1.74	0.10	3.56	25	2
148	Fish-crab meat-king-canned-unpacked	1 cup	135	135	24	3	1	135	1	61	246	675	149	1.10	5.83	—	0.11	0.11	2.60	—	13.50	—	—
1848	Fish-crab-alaska king-raw	1 serving	85	71	16	1	0	36	0	39	186	711	173	0.50	5.05	6	0.04	0.04	0.94	0.13	7.65	37	6
1851	Fish-crab-blue-canned	1 cup	135	134	28	2	0	120	0	136	351	450	505	1.13	5.42	3	0.11	0.11	1.85	0.20	0.62	57	4
1852	Fish-crab-blue-cooked-moist heat	1 cup	135	138	27	2	0	135	0	140	278	376	437	1.22	5.69	3	0.14	0.07	4.46	0.24	9.86	69	4
1703	Fish-crab-deviled	1 cup	240	451	27	23	5	223	32	113	329	2081	398	2.90	5.45	330	0.19	0.26	3.60	0.31	8.69	88	14
1850	Fish-crab-dungeness-raw	1 serving	85	73	15	1	0	50	1	39	155	251	301	0.32	3.63	23	0.04	0.14	2.67	0.13	7.65	37	3
1849	Fish-crab-imitation-surimi	1 serving	85	87	10	1	0	17	9	11	240	715	77	0.33	0.28	17	0.03	0.02	0.15	0.03	1.36	1	0
1704	Fish-crab-imperial	1 cup	220	323	32	17	4	275	9	132	365	1602	288	2.00	6.41	211	0.13	0.26	2.40	0.31	10.60	83	11
1576	Fish-crab-steamed-pieces	1 cup	155	150	30	2	0	82	0	92	434	1662	406	1.18	11.80	14	0.08	0.09	2.08	0.28	17.80	79	12
1853	Fish-crayfish-cooked-moist heat	1 serving	85	97	20	1	0	151	0	26	281	58	298	2.67	1.43	19	0.15	0.07	2.50	0.15	2.94	3	3
1822	Fish-croaker-breaded-fried	1 serving	85	188	16	11	3	71	6	27	184	296	289	0.73	0.44	19	0.08	0.11	3.66	0.22	1.79	15	0
1823	Fish-eel-cooked-dry heat	1 serving	85	201	20	13	3	137	0	22	235	55	297	0.54	1.77	966	0.16	0.04	3.81	0.07	2.45	15	2
1824	Fish-flatfish-cooked-dry heat	1 serving	85	100	21	1	0	58	0	15	246	89	292	0.29	0.54	9	0.07	0.10	1.85	0.20	2.13	8	0
1913	Fish-gefiltefish-commercial-with broth	1 piece	42	35	4	1	0	13	3	10	31	220	38	1.04	0.34	11	0.03	0.03	0.42	0.03	0.35	1	0
1825	Fish-grouper-cooked-dry heat	1 serving	85	100	21	1	0	40	0	18	121	45	403	0.96	0.43	43	0.07	0.01	0.32	0.30	0.59	9	0
150	Fish-haddock-breaded-fried	1 piece	85	140	17	5	1	42	5	34	210	150	296	1.00	—	—	0.03	0.06	2.70	—	1.10	—	2
1578	Fish-haddock-broiled	1 serving	85	95	21	1	0	63	0	36	205	74	339	1.15	0.41	16	0.03	0.04	3.94	0.29	1.18	11	0
1579	Fish-halibut-all types-broiled in butter	1 piece	125	214	32	9	—	75	0	20	310	168	656	1.00	—	255	0.06	0.09	10.40	—	—	—	—
1886	Fish-halibut-cooked-broiled	1 serving	85	119	23	2	0	35	0	51	242	59	490	0.91	0.45	46	0.06	0.08	6.06	0.34	1.16	12	0
1580	Fish-herring-atlantic-broiled	1 serving	85	173	20	10	2	66	0	63	258	98	356	1.20	1.08	26	0.10	0.25	3.50	0.30	11.20	10	1
1827	Fish-herring-atlantic-raw	1 serving	85	134	15	8	2	51	0	49	201	76	278	0.94	0.84	24	0.08	0.20	2.73	0.26	11.60	9	1
1581	Fish-herring-canned-solids and liquids	1 serving	100	208	20	14	—	98	0	147	297	—	—	1.80	—	—	0.18	—	—	—	—	—	—
1582	Fish-herring-pickled-bismarck type	1 item	50	131	7	9	1	7	5	39	45	435	35	0.61	0.27	129	0.02	0.07	1.65	0.09	2.14	1	0
1584	Fish-lobster newburg	1 cup	250	485	46	27	30	376	13	218	480	573	428	2.30	4.16	530	0.18	0.28	1.56	0.17	4.11	32	1
1585	Fish-lobster thermidor	1 serving	157	405	29	27	19	236	15	290	451	360	388	1.90	2.61	295	0.15	0.51	4.80	0.11	2.58	20	0
1854	Fish-lobster-cooked-moist heat	1 ounce	28	28	6	0	0	20	0	17	53	108	100	0.11	0.83	7	0.00	0.02	0.30	0.02	0.88	3	0
1583	Fish-lobster-northern-raw	1 ounce	28	26	5	0	0	27	0	14	41	84	78	0.09	0.86	6	0.00	0.01	0.41	0.02	0.26	3	0
1587	Fish-mackerel-atlantic-canned	1 cup	190	296	44	12	3	150	0	458	572	720	369	3.88	1.94	248	0.08	0.40	11.70	0.40	13.20	10	2
1586	Fish-mackerel-atlantic-raw	1 ounce	28	58	5	4	1	20	0	3	62	26	89	0.46	0.18	14	0.05	0.09	2.58	0.11	2.47	0	0
1828	Fish-mackerel-cooked-dry heat	1 serving	85	223	20	15	4	64	0	13	236	71	341	1.33	0.80	46	0.14	0.35	5.82	0.39	16.20	1	0
1829	Fish-mullet-cooked-dry heat	1 serving	85	128	21	4	1	54	0	26	207	60	389	1.20	0.75	36	0.09	0.09	5.36	0.42	0.21	8	1
1862	Fish-mussel-blue-cooked-moist heat	1 serving	85	147	20	4	1	48	6	28	242	313	228	5.71	2.27	77	0.26	0.36	2.55	0.09	20.40	64	12
1588	Fish-mussels-atlantic/pacific-meat only	1 ounce	28	27	4	1	—	16	1	25	67	81	90	0.97	—	—	0.05	0.06	—	—	—	—	—
1861	Fish-mussels-blue-raw	1 cup	150	129	18	3	1	42	6	39	296	429	479	5.92	2.40	72	0.24	0.32	2.40	0.08	18.00	63	12
151	Fish-ocean perch-breaded-fried	1 piece	85	195	16	11	3	32	6	28	192	128	242	1.10	—	—	0.10	0.10	1.60	—	0.85	—	—
1830	Fish-ocean perch-cooked-dry heat	1 serving	85	103	20	2	0	46	0	117	235	82	298	1.00	0.52	12	0.11	0.11	2.07	0.23	0.98	9	1
1590	Fish-octopus-raw	1 serving	85	70	13	1	0	41	2	45	158	196	298	4.51	1.43	38	0.03	0.03	1.79	0.31	17.00	14	4
1863	Fish-oyster-eastern-canned	1 cup	248	171	18	6	2	136	10	112	344	278	568	16.60	226.00	223	0.37	0.41	3.09	0.24	47.50	22	12
1864	Fish-oyster-eastern-cooked-moist heat	1 serving	85	117	12	4	1	93	7	76	236	190	389	11.40	155.00	145	0.25	0.28	2.12	0.08	32.50	15	7
1589	Fish-oysters-breaded-fried	1 serving	85	167	7	11	3	69	10	53	135	355	208	5.91	74.10	77	0.13	0.17	1.40	0.05	13.30	12	3
152	Fish-oysters-eastern-raw-meat only	1 cup	248	171	18	6	2	136	10	111	344	277	568	16.60	226.00	222	0.34	0.41	3.25	0.12	47.50	25	12
1865	Fish-oysters-pacific-raw	1 serving	85	69	8	2	0	43	4	7	138	90	143	4.34	14.10	69	0.06	0.20	1.71	0.04	13.60	9	7
1831	Fish-perch-cooked-dry heat	1 serving	85	100	21	1	0	98	0	87	218	67	292	0.99	1.21	9	0.07	0.10	1.62	0.12	1.87	5	1
1832	Fish-pike-cooked-dry heat	1 serving	85	96	21	1	0	43	0	62	239	42	281	0.60	0.73	20	0.06	0.07	2.38	0.12	1.96	15	3
1841	Fish-pollock-atlantic-raw	1 serving	85	78	17	1	0	60	0	51	188	73	303	0.39	0.40	9	0.04	0.16	2.78	0.24	2.71	3	0
1833	Fish-pollock-cooked-dry heat	1 serving	85	96	20	1	0	82	0	5	410	99	329	0.24	0.51	20	0.06	0.07	1.40	0.06	3.57	3	0
1834	Fish-pompano-cooked-dry heat	1 serving	85	179	20	10	4	54	0	36	290	65	541	0.57	0.59	31	0.58	0.13	3.23	0.20	1.02	15	0
1839	Fish-red snapper-cooked-dry heat	1 serving	85	109	22	1	0	40	0	34	171	48	444	0.20	0.37	30	0.05	0.00	0.29	0.39	2.98	5	1
1591	Fish-red snapper-raw	1 serving	85	85	17	1	0	31	0	27	169	54	355	0.15	0.30	26	0.04	0.00	0.24	0.34	2.55	4	1
1592	Fish-rockfish-cooked-dry heat	1 serving	100	121	24	2	0	44	0	12	228	77	520	0.53	0.53	66	0.04	0.08	3.92	0.27	1.20	10	1
1596	Fish-salmon patty	1 serving	100	239	16	12	3	64	16	78	104	96	89	1.24	0.84	20	0.12	0.22	4.00	0.07	3.00	13	4
1597	Fish-salmon rice loaf	1 serving	100	122	12	5	3	116	7	180	262	753	275	1.23	0.92	115	0.08	0.28	4.30	0.21	2.24	21	2
1594	Fish-salmon-broiled or baked-with butter	1 serving	100	182	27	7	1	47	0	18	418	116	443	1.20	0.66	48	0.16	0.06	9.80	0.22	2.71	5	2
1835	Fish-salmon-cooked-moist heat	1 serving	85	157	23	6	1	42	0	39	248	50	454	0.76	0.44	15	0.16	0.17	7.14	0.39	3.06	4	1
153	Fish-salmon-pink-canned-solids & liquids	1 serving	85	118	17	5	1	47	0	181	279	471	277	0.72	0.78	14	0.02	0.16	5.56	0.26	5.85	13	0
1595	Fish-salmon-smoked	1 serving	100	117	18	4	1	23	0	11	164	784	175	0.85	0.31	26	0.02	0.10	4.72	0.28	3.26	2	0
154	Fish-sardines-atlantic-canned in oil	1 item	12	25	3	1	0	17	0	46	59	61	48	0.35	0.16	8	0.01	0.03	0.63	0.02	1.07	1	0
1598	Fish-sardines-canned in tomato sauce	1 item	38	68	6	5	1	23	0	91	139	157	130	0.87	0.53	27	0.02	0.09	1.60	0.05	3.42	9	0
1599	Fish-scallops-bay and sea-steamed	1 ounce	28	32	7	0	—	15	1	33	96	75	135	0.85	—	—	—	—	—	—	—	—	—
155	Fish-scallops-frozen-breaded-fried	1 item	15	32	3	2	0	9	2	6	35	70	50	0.12	0.16	3	0.01	0.02	0.23	0.02	0.20	3	0
1866	Fish-scallops-raw	1 serving	85	75	14	1	0	28	2	20	186	137	274	0.25	0.81	13	0.01	0.06	0.98	0.13	1.30	14	3
1836	Fish-sea bass-cooked-dry heat	1 serving	85	105	20	2	1	45	0	11	211	74	279	0.32	0.44	54	0.11	0.13	1.62	0.39	0.26	5	0

Dashes (—) in data spaces indicate that no data were reported.

Appendix C Table of Food Composition

Item	Food Name	Portion	Weight (g)	Food Energy (kcal)	Protein (g)	Total Fat (g)	Saturated Fat (g)	Cholesterol (mg)	Carbohydrate (g)	Calcium (mg)	Phosphorus (mg)	Sodium (mg)	Potassium (mg)	Iron (mg)	Zinc (cm)	Vitamin A (RE)	Thiamin (mg)	Riboflavin (mg)	Niacin (mg)	Vitamin B6 (mg)	Vitamin B12 (ug)	Folic Acid (ug)	Vitamin C (mg)
156	Fish-shad-baked-butter/margarine & bacon	1 serving	100	201	23	11	2	69	0	24	313	79	377	0.60	—	9	0.13	0.26	8.60	—	—	—	—
1837	Fish-shark-raw	1 serving	85	111	18	4	1	43	0	29	179	67	136	0.71	0.36	60	0.04	0.05	2.50	0.34	1.27	3	0
157	Fish-shrimp-canned meat	1 cup	128	154	30	3	0	222	1	75	299	216	269	3.50	1.61	23	0.04	0.05	3.53	0.14	1.44	2	3
1855	Fish-shrimp-cooked-moist heat	1 serving	85	84	18	1	0	166	0	33	116	190	155	2.63	1.33	56	0.03	0.03	2.20	0.11	1.26	3	2
158	Fish-shrimp-french fried	1 serving	85	206	18	10	2	150	10	57	185	292	191	1.07	1.17	48	0.11	0.12	2.61	0.08	1.59	7	1
1600	Fish-smelt-atlantic-canned	1 item	20	40	4	3	—	—	0	72	74	—	—	0.34	—	—	—	—	—	—	—	—	—
1838	Fish-smelt-cooked-dry heat	1 serving	85	105	19	3	0	77	0	66	251	66	316	0.98	1.80	15	0.63	0.12	1.50	0.15	3.37	4	0
1577	Fish-sole/flounder-baked	1 serving	127	148	31	2	0	86	0	23	368	133	436	0.43	0.80	14	0.10	0.15	2.77	0.31	3.19	11	4
1868	Fish-squid-cooked-fried	1 serving	85	149	15	6	2	221	7	33	213	260	237	0.86	1.48	9	0.05	0.39	2.21	0.05	1.04	5	4
1867	Fish-squid-raw	1 serving	85	78	13	1	0	198	3	27	188	37	209	0.58	1.30	9	0.02	0.35	1.85	0.05	1.10	4	4
1601	Fish-sturgeon-steamed	1 serving	100	135	21	5	1	75	0	40	263	108	364	2.00	0.54	243	0.08	0.09	9.80	0.22	2.60	17	0
1840	Fish-surimi	1 serving	85	84	13	1	0	26	6	8	240	122	95	0.22	0.28	17	0.02	0.02	0.19	0.03	1.36	1	0
1602	Fish-swordfish-broiled-butter/margarine	1 serving	100	174	28	6	2	4	0	7	275	478	354	1.30	1.38	616	0.04	0.05	10.90	0.36	1.90	3	3
1842	Fish-swordfish-cooked-dry heat	1 serving	85	132	22	4	1	43	0	5	287	98	314	0.88	1.25	35	0.04	0.10	10.00	0.32	1.72	2	1
1843	Fish-tilefish-cooked-dry heat	1 serving	85	125	21	4	1	54	0	22	201	50	435	0.26	0.45	18	0.12	0.16	2.98	0.26	2.13	15	0
1603	Fish-trout-brook-cooked	1 serving	100	196	24	11	1	69	0	218	272	79	602	1.10	1.31	96	0.12	0.06	2.50	0.44	3.25	17	1
1844	Fish-trout-rainbow-cooked-dry heat	1 serving	85	128	22	4	1	62	0	73	273	29	539	2.07	1.18	19	0.07	0.19	5.87	0.39	2.98	15	3
1845	Fish-tuna-bluefin-cooked-dry heat	1 serving	85	156	25	5	1	42	0	9	277	43	275	1.11	0.65	643	0.24	0.26	8.96	0.45	9.25	2	0
159	Fish-tuna-canned in oil-drained solids	1 serving	85	168	25	7	1	15	0	11	264	301	176	1.18	0.77	20	0.03	0.10	10.50	0.09	1.87	5	0
354	Fish-tuna-dietetic-low sodium-drained	1 ounce	28	36	8	1	0	10	0	1	63	11	74	0.34	0.14	7	0.01	0.01	3.52	0.11	0.40	0	—
355	Fish-tuna-light-canned in water-drained	1 serving	85	111	25	0	0	15	0	10	158	303	267	2.72	0.37	20	0.03	0.10	10.50	0.32	1.87	4	0
351	Fish-tuna-white-albacore-canned in water	1 serving	85	116	23	2	1	35	0	3	227	333	241	0.51	0.40	20	0.00	0.04	4.93	0.37	1.87	4	0
1846	Fish-tuna-yellowfin-raw	1 serving	85	92	20	1	0	38	0	14	162	32	377	0.62	0.44	15	0.37	0.04	8.33	0.77	0.44	2	1
1605	Fish-white perch-fried filet	1 item	65	108	13	5	—	—	0	9	113	—	—	0.70	—	0	0.04	0.05	2.70	—	—	—	0
1604	Fish-whitefish-lake-baked-stuffed	1 serving	100	215	15	14	—	—	6	—	246	195	291	0.50	—	601	0.11	0.11	2.30	—	—	—	0
1847	Fish-whiting-cooked-dry heat	1 serving	85	98	20	1	0	71	0	53	242	113	369	0.36	0.45	29	0.06	0.05	1.42	0.15	2.21	13	0
1624	Flounder filet-le menu frozen dinner	1 item	298	350	22	17	—	—	27	—	—	1125	—	—	—	—	—	—	—	—	—	—	—
1951	Flour-arrowroot	1 cup	128	457	0	0	0	0	113	51	7	2	14	0.42	0.09	0	0.00	0.00	0.00	0.01	0.00	9	0
1643	Flour-barley	1 cup	112	401	11	2	0	0	86	46	417	3	179	4.82	2.77	0	0.62	0.13	4.82	0.36	0.00	54	0
383	Flour-buckwheat-whole groat	1 cup	120	402	15	4	1	0	85	49	404	0	692	4.88	3.75	0	0.50	0.23	7.38	0.70	0.00	64	0
1808	Flour-carob	1 cup	103	185	5	1	0	0	92	359	81	36	852	3.03	0.94	2	0.06	0.48	1.95	0.38	0.00	30	0
1644	Flour-corn-masa-sifted	1 cup	114	416	11	4	1	0	87	161	255	6	340	8.22	2.03	0	1.63	0.86	11.20	0.42	0.00	28	0
1960	Flour-corn-whole grain	1 cup	117	422	8	5	1	0	90	8	318	6	369	2.78	2.02	55	0.29	0.09	2.22	0.43	0.00	30	0
1095	Flour-potato	1 cup	179	628	14	1	0	0	143	59	319	61	2843	30.80	2.92	0	0.75	0.25	6.09	0.01	0.00	91	34
1976	Flour-rice-brown	1 cup	158	574	11	4	1	0	121	18	533	12	456	3.13	3.87	0	0.70	0.13	10.00	1.16	0.00	25	0
1645	Flour-rice-white	1 cup	158	578	9	2	1	0	127	16	155	1	120	0.55	1.26	0	0.22	0.03	4.09	0.69	0.00	6	0
1978	Flour-rye-dark	1 cup	128	415	18	3	0	0	88	72	809	2	934	8.26	7.19	0	0.40	0.32	5.47	0.57	0.00	77	0
1979	Flour-rye-light	1 cup	102	374	9	1	0	0	82	21	198	2	238	1.84	1.78	0	0.34	0.09	0.82	0.24	0.00	23	0
1658	Flour-sesame-lowfat	1 cup	100	333	50	2	0	0	36	149	757	39	397	14.20	10.00	6	2.52	0.27	12.50	0.14	0.00	29	0
1672	Flour-soybean-lowfat	1 cup	88	313	38	6	—	0	32	231	558	1	1636	8.00	—	7	0.73	0.32	2.30	—	—	—	0
1982	Flour-triticale-whole grain	1 cup	130	439	17	2	0	0	95	46	417	3	606	3.37	3.46	0	0.49	0.17	3.72	0.52	0.00	96	0
502	Flour-wheat-enriched-sifted	1 cup	115	419	12	1	0	0	88	17	124	2	123	5.34	0.81	0	0.90	0.57	6.79	0.05	0.00	30	0
503	Flour-wheat-enriched-unsifted	1 cup	125	455	13	1	0	0	95	18	135	2	134	5.80	0.88	0	0.98	0.62	7.38	0.06	0.00	33	0
504	Flour-wheat-white-cake/pastry-enriched	1 cup	109	395	9	1	0	0	85	16	93	2	115	7.98	0.67	0	0.97	0.47	7.40	0.04	0.00	21	0
1991	Flour-wheat-white-for bread	1 cup	137	495	16	2	0	0	99	21	133	2	136	6.04	1.17	0	1.11	0.70	10.40	0.05	0.00	40	0
505	Flour-wheat-white-self rising-enriched	1 cup	125	443	12	1	0	0	93	423	744	1588	155	5.84	0.78	0	0.84	0.52	7.29	0.06	0.00	53	0
1992	Flour-wheat-white-tortilla mix	1 cup	111	450	11	12	5	0	75	228	233	751	111	7.83	0.71	0	0.82	0.55	6.46	0.04	0.00	26	0
506	Flour-wheat-whole grain-stirred	1 cup	120	407	16	2	0	0	87	40	415	6	486	4.66	3.52	0	0.54	0.26	7.64	0.41	0.00	52	0
1511	Formula-similac-20 calorie-ross	1 fl oz	30	20	0	1	1	0	2	15	12	6	24	0.36	0.15	18	0.02	0.03	0.20	0.01	0.05	3	2
1521	Formula-SMA with iron-wyeth	1 fl oz	30	20	0	1	0	1	2	12	8	4	16	0.35	0.15	18	0.02	0.03	0.10	0.01	0.04	1	2
202	Frankfurter (hot dog)-no bun-beef & pork	1 item	57	183	6	17	6	29	1	6	49	639	95	0.66	1.05	0	0.11	0.07	1.50	0.08	0.74	2	15
1447	French toast-from frozen-campbells	1 slice	50	94	4	5	—	—	11	34	—	235	54	1.10	—	15	0.04	0.09	0.70	—	—	—	0
1388	French toast-from home recipe	1 slice	65	153	6	7	0	0	17	72	85	257	86	1.34	0.55	22	0.12	0.16	1.01	0.04	0.29	18	0
1894	French toast-with butter	1 slice	68	178	5	9	4	59	18	37	73	257	89	0.95	0.30	60	0.29	0.25	1.96	0.03	0.18	15	0
1905	Frijoles-beans with cheese	1 cup	167	226	11	8	4	36	29	188	175	882	605	2.24	1.73	46	0.14	0.33	1.48	0.19	0.68	111	2
1731	Frog legs-fried-flour coated	1 item	24	70	4	5	1	32	2	5	39	119	65	0.33	0.27	0	0.03	0.06	0.30	0.03	0.11	6	1
1747	Frozen yogurt-fruit varieties	1 cup	226	216	7	2	—	—	42	200	200	—	—	0.00	—	0	0.01	0.26	0.00	—	—	—	0
1944	Fruit bar-oat bran-nuts-health valley	1 item	43	150	4	4	—	0	28	25	134	5	230	1.40	0.80	0	0.19	0.06	0.70	0.06	0.00	19	10
245	Fruit cocktail-canned in heavy syrup	1 cup	255	186	1	0	0	0	48	16	28	15	224	0.73	0.21	52	0.05	0.05	0.95	0.13	0.00	7	5
978	Fruit cocktail-canned-juice pack	1 cup	248	114	1	0	0	0	29	20	35	10	236	0.52	0.22	76	0.03	0.04	1.00	0.13	0.00	6	7

977	Fruit cocktail-canned-water pack	1 cup	245	78	1	0	0	0	21	12	27	10	230	0.61	0.22	61	0.04	0.03	0.89	0.13	0.00	7	5
127	Fruit cocktail-canned-water-dietetic	1 ounce	28	9	0	0	0	0	2	2	3	1	26	0.14	0.02	7	0.01	0.06	0.17	0.02	0.00	1	1
1895	Fruit pie-fried	1 item	85	266	2	14	7	13	33	12	38	325	51	0.89	0.17	33	0.10	0.08	0.98	0.03	0.08	4	1
1718	Fruit punch drink-canned	8 fl oz	248	117	0	0	0	0	30	20	2	55	62	0.52	0.30	10	0.06	0.06	0.06	0.00	0.00	3	73
1475	Fruit punch-powdered-with water	1 cup	262	97	0	0	0	0	25	42	52	37	3	0.13	0.08	0	0.00	0.01	0.00	0.00	0.00	0	31
1721	Fruit roll up-cherry	1 item	14	50	0	1	—	0	12	—	—	5	45	—	—	—	—	—	—	—	0.00	—	—
813	Garlic powder	1 tsp	3	9	0	0	0	0	2	2	12	1	31	0.08	0.07	—	0.01	0.00	0.02	—	0.00	—	—
1752	Garlic salt-frenchs	1 tsp	6	4	0	0	0	0	1	—	—	2050	—	—	—	—	—	—	—	—	0.00	—	—
1067	Garlic-raw-clove	1 item	3	4	0	0	0	0	1	5	5	1	12	0.05	0.04	0	0.01	0.00	0.02	0.04	0.00	0	1
1878	Gatorade-thirst quenching drink	8 fl oz	241	60	0	0	0	0	15	0	22	96	26	0.12	0.05	0	0.02	0.00	0.00	0.00	0.00	0	0
699	Gelatin dessert-prepared	1 cup	240	140	4	0	0	0	34	5	46	0	0	0.00	0.00	0	0.00	0.00	0.00	0.00	0.00	0	0
1636	Gelatin-d zerta-low calorie-prepared	1 cup	240	16	4	0	0	0	0	6	0	20	3	0.02	0.07	0	0.00	0.00	0.00	0.00	0.00	0	0
698	Gelatin-dry-envelope	1 item	7	25	6	0	0	0	0	0	0	8	180	0.40	0.00	0	0.00	0.00	0.00	0.00	0.00	0	4
1635	Gelatin-jello-sugar free-prepared	1 cup	240	16	2	0	0	0	0	—	—	120	—	—	—	—	—	—	—	—	—	—	—
1068	Ginger root-raw-sliced	1 cup	96	66	2	1	0	0	15	17	26	13	398	0.48	0.33	0	0.02	0.03	0.67	0.15	0.00	11	5
1183	Ginger-ground	1 tsp	2	6	0	0	0	0	1	2	3	1	24	0.21	0.08	0	0.00	0.00	0.09	—	0.00	—	—
1489	Glazed chicken-light and elegant	1 item	227	230	24	4	—	—	25	18	348	655	300	4.80	—	31	0.21	0.07	7.70	—	—	—	—
1288	Goose-flesh & skin-roasted	1 item	1548	4721	389	339	106	1416	0	201	4180	1084	5092	43.80	40.60	325	1.19	5.00	64.50	5.73	6.35	31	0
1297	Goose-liver pate-smoked-canned	1 tbsp	13	60	1	6	—	20	1	9	26	91	18	0.72	0.12	130	0.01	0.04	0.33	0.01	1.22	8	0
1289	Goose-no skin-roasted	1 item	1182	2813	342	150	54	1138	0	165	3652	898	4586	33.90	499.00	142	1.09	4.61	48.20	5.50	5.56	142	0
982	Gooseberries-canned-heavy syrup pack	1 cup	252	184	2	1	0	0	47	40	18	5	194	0.83	0.28	35	0.05	0.13	0.39	0.03	0.00	8	25
981	Gooseberries-raw	1 cup	150	66	1	1	0	0	15	38	41	2	297	0.47	0.18	44	0.06	0.05	0.45	0.12	0.00	9	42
1069	Gourd-white flowered-boiled	1 cup	146	22	1	0	0	0	5	35	19	3	248	0.37	1.02	0	0.04	0.03	0.57	0.06	0.00	6	12
1383	Granola bar	1 item	24	109	2	4	—	—	16	14	67	67	78	0.76	—	—	0.07	0.03	—	—	0.00	—	—
673	Granola clusters-nature valley	1 item	34	150	2	3	5	0	28	24	96	115	126	0.85	0.71	6	0.10	0.03	0.00	0.00	0.00	26	0
260	Grape drink-canned	1 cup	253	154	1	0	0	0	38	23	28	8	334	0.61	0.13	2	0.07	0.09	0.66	0.16	0.00	7	0
248	Grapefruit-canned in light syrup	1 cup	254	152	1	0	0	0	39	36	25	4	328	1.02	0.21	0	0.10	0.05	0.62	0.05	0.00	22	54
984	Grapefruit-canned-juice pack	1 cup	249	92	2	0	0	0	23	37	30	19	420	0.52	0.20	0	0.07	0.05	0.62	0.05	0.00	22	84
983	Grapefruit-canned-water pack	1 cup	244	88	1	0	0	0	22	37	24	5	322	1.00	0.22	0	0.10	0.05	0.61	0.05	0.00	22	53
246	Grapefruit-pink & red-raw	1 item	246	74	1	0	0	0	19	36	22	0	312	0.30	0.18	64	0.10	0.05	0.49	0.10	0.00	23	91
247	Grapefruit-white-raw	1 item	236	78	2	0	0	0	20	28	18	0	350	0.14	0.17	2	0.09	0.05	0.63	0.10	0.00	24	79
256	Grapes-raw-adherent skin (european) type	1 serving	160	114	1	1	0	0	28	17	21	3	296	0.41	0.09	12	0.15	0.09	0.48	0.18	0.00	6	17
255	Grapes-raw-slip skin (american) type	1 cup	92	58	1	0	0	0	16	13	9	2	176	0.27	0.04	9	0.09	0.05	0.28	0.10	0.00	4	4
986	Grapes-thompson-canned-heavy syrup pack	1 cup	256	187	1	0	0	0	50	25	44	14	264	2.41	0.13	16	0.08	0.06	0.32	0.17	0.00	7	3
985	Grapes-thompson-canned-water pack	1 cup	245	98	1	0	0	0	25	25	44	15	262	2.40	0.12	16	0.08	0.06	0.32	0.16	0.00	6	2
842	Gravy-beef-canned	1 cup	233	123	9	5	3	7	11	14	70	1305	189	1.63	2.33	0	0.08	0.08	1.54	0.02	0.23	5	0
845	Gravy-brown-from dry-prepared with water	1 cup	258	75	2	2	1	3	13	66	44	1076	57	0.24	0.31	0	0.04	0.09	0.81	0.00	0.00	0	0
843	Gravy-chicken-canned	1 cup	238	188	5	14	3	5	13	48	69	1373	260	1.12	1.90	264	0.04	0.10	1.05	0.02	0.24	5	0
844	Gravy-mushroom-canned	1 cup	238	119	3	6	1	0	13	17	36	1357	252	1.57	1.67	0	0.08	0.15	1.60	0.05	0.00	29	0
847	Gravy-pork-from dry-prepared with water	1 cup	258	77	2	2	1	3	13	31	44	1235	57	0.26	0.26	0	0.05	0.06	0.77	0.03	0.16	3	2
846	Gravy-turkey-canned	1 cup	238	121	6	5	1	5	12	10	69	1373	259	1.67	1.90	0	0.05	0.19	3.10	0.02	0.00	5	0
987	Guavas-common-raw	1 item	90	46	1	1	0	0	11	18	23	3	256	0.28	0.21	71	0.05	0.05	1.08	0.13	0.00	13	165
988	Guavas-strawberry-raw	1 item	6	4	0	0	0	0	1	1	2	2	18	0.01	0.01	1	0.00	0.00	0.04	0.01	0.00	1	2
1314	Ham and cheese loaf/roll	1 slice	28	74	5	6	2	16	0	17	72	381	84	0.26	0.57	7	0.17	0.05	0.98	0.07	0.23	1	7
1315	Ham and cheese spread	1 tbsp	15	37	2	3	1	9	0	33	74	179	24	0.11	0.34	14	0.05	0.03	0.32	0.02	0.11	0	1
1435	Ham and swiss cheese crepes-stouffer	1 item	213	410	25	25	—	—	23	—	—	905	345	—	—	—	—	—	—	—	—	—	—
1318	Ham salad spread	1 tbsp	15	32	1	2	1	6	2	1	18	137	23	0.09	0.17	0	0.07	0.02	0.31	0.02	0.11	0	1
1742	Ham-banquet frozen dinner	1 item	284	369	17	12	2	36	48	151	278	1590	125	2.50	2.50	1311	0.57	0.23	3.40	0.48	0.45	21	57
190	Ham-boiled-regular-11% fat-luncheon meat	1 slice	28	52	5	3	1	16	1	2	70	373	94	0.28	0.61	0	0.24	0.07	1.49	0.10	0.24	1	8
191	Ham-canned-chopped-luncheon meat	1 slice	21	50	3	4	1	10	0	1	29	287	60	0.20	0.38	0	0.11	0.04	0.67	0.07	0.15	1	0
1317	Ham-canned-extra lean-4% fat	1 cup	140	190	30	7	2	42	1	8	293	1589	487	1.29	3.12	0	1.45	0.35	6.85	0.63	0.99	7	39
867	Ham-canned-pork-roasted-13% fat	1 cup	140	316	29	21	7	87	1	11	340	1317	500	1.92	3.50	0	1.15	0.36	7.42	0.42	1.48	7	20
201	Ham-deviled-canned-luncheon meat	1 tbsp	13	45	2	4	2	10	0	1	12	160	—	0.30	0.24	0	0.02	0.01	0.20	0.04	0.09	—	—
1316	Ham-extra lean-5% fat-roasted	1 cup	140	203	29	8	3	74	2	11	275	1684	402	2.07	4.03	0	1.06	0.28	5.63	0.56	0.91	5	29
1319	Ham-lean only-roasted	1 cup	140	220	35	8	3	77	0	10	318	1858	442	1.32	3.60	0	0.95	0.36	7.03	0.66	0.98	6	0
872	Ham-minced-pork	1 slice	21	55	3	4	2	15	0	2	33	261	65	0.17	0.40	0	0.15	0.04	0.87	0.06	0.20	0	6
189	Ham-roasted-regular-11% fat-boneless	1 cup	140	249	32	13	4	83	0	12	393	2100	573	1.88	3.46	0	1.02	0.46	8.61	0.43	0.98	4	32
164	Hamburger patty-broiled-extra lean beef	1 item	85	218	22	14	5	71	0	6	137	60	266	2.00	4.63	6	0.05	0.23	4.22	0.23	1.84	8	0
165	Hamburger patty-broiled-medium-lean beef	1 item	85	231	21	16	6	74	0	9	134	65	256	1.79	4.56	9	0.04	0.18	4.39	0.22	2.00	8	0
1410	Hamburger-bacon and cheese-generic	1 item	150	464	25	27	—	68	29	116	302	660	339	3.74	5.25	75	0.15	0.27	4.89	0.24	1.80	26	2
1882	Hamburger-ground-regular-baked	1 serving	85	244	20	18	7	74	0	8	117	51	188	2.05	4.16	0	0.03	0.14	4.04	0.20	1.99	7	0
1883	Hamburger-ground-regular-fried	1 serving	85	260	20	19	8	75	0	10	145	71	255	2.08	4.31	0	0.03	0.17	4.96	0.20	2.30	8	0
1320	Headcheese-pork	1 slice	28	60	5	4	1	23	0	5	17	357	9	0.33	0.37	—	0.01	0.05	0.32	0.05	0.30	1	6

Dashes (—) in data spaces indicate that no data were reported.

Appendix C Table of Food Composition

Item	Food Name	Portion	Weight (g)	Food Energy (kcal)	Protein (g)	Total Fat (g)	Saturated Fat (g)	Cholesterol (mg)	Carbohydrate (g)	Calcium (mg)	Phosphorus (mg)	Sodium (mg)	Potassium (mg)	Iron (mg)	Zinc (cm)	Vitamin A (RE)	Thiamin (mg)	Riboflavin (mg)	Niacin (mg)	Vitamin B6 (mg)	Vitamin B12 (ug)	Folic Acid (ug)	Vitamin C (mg)
1965	Hominy-canned	1 cup	160	115	2	1	0	0	23	15	56	336	14	1.00	1.68	0	0.00	0.01	0.05	0.01	0.00	1	0
548	Honey-strained/extracted	1 tbsp	21	65	0	0	0	0	17	1	1	1	11	0.10	0.02	0	0.00	0.01	0.10	0.00	0.00	0	0
1641	Horseradish-prepared	1 tbsp	15	6	0	0	0	0	1	9	5	165	44	0.10	0.11	0	0.00	0.00	0.05	0.01	0.00	0	3
908	Hot cocoa-with milk-home recipe	1 cup	250	218	9	9	6	33	26	298	270	123	480	0.78	1.22	96	0.10	0.44	0.37	0.11	0.87	12	2
1411	Hot dog-plain with bun-generic	1 item	98	242	10	15	5	44	18	24	97	671	143	2.31	1.98	0	0.24	0.27	3.65	0.05	0.51	30	0
1814	Hummus	1 cup	246	421	12	21	3	0	50	123	275	600	428	3.86	2.71	5	0.23	0.13	1.01	0.98	0.00	146	19
1400	Ice cream sundae-caramel	1 item	165	323	8	10	5	26	53	201	231	208	338	0.23	0.88	56	0.07	0.31	1.01	0.05	0.64	13	4
1401	Ice cream sundae-hot fudge	1 item	165	297	6	9	5	22	50	216	238	190	413	0.61	0.99	46	0.07	0.31	1.12	0.13	0.68	10	2
1402	Ice cream sundae-strawberry	1 item	165	289	7	8	4	23	48	173	167	99	292	0.35	0.71	48	0.07	0.30	0.97	0.08	0.69	20	2
78	Ice cream-french vanilla-soft serve	1 cup	173	377	7	23	14	153	38	236	199	153	338	0.43	1.99	199	0.08	0.45	0.18	0.10	1.00	9	1
76	Ice cream-vanilla-hardened-10% fat	1 cup	133	269	5	14	9	59	32	176	134	116	257	0.12	1.41	133	0.05	0.33	0.13	0.06	0.63	3	1
80	Ice cream-vanilla-rich-hardened-16% fat	1 cup	148	349	4	24	15	88	32	151	115	108	221	0.10	1.21	207	0.04	0.28	0.12	0.05	0.54	2	1
82	Ice milk-vanilla-hardened-4.3% fat	1 cup	131	184	5	6	4	18	29	176	129	105	265	0.18	0.55	52	0.08	0.35	0.12	0.09	0.88	3	1
83	Ice milk-vanilla-soft serve-2.6% fat	1 cup	175	223	8	5	3	13	38	274	202	163	412	0.28	0.86	44	0.12	0.54	0.18	0.13	1.37	5	1
534	Icing-cake-chocolate-prepared from mix	1 cup	275	1035	9	38	23	0	185	165	305	882	536	3.30	—	174	0.06	0.28	0.60	—	—	—	1
535	Icing-cake-fudge-prepared from mix/water	1 cup	245	830	7	16	5	0	183	96	218	568	238	2.70	—	0	0.05	0.20	0.70	—	—	—	0
532	Icing-cake-white-boiled	1 cup	94	295	1	0	0	0	75	2	2	134	17	0.00	—	0	0.00	0.03	0.00	—	—	—	0
536	Icing-cake-white-uncooked	1 cup	319	1200	2	21	13	0	260	48	38	156	57	0.00	—	258	0.00	0.06	0.00	—	—	—	0
533	Icing-cake-white/coconut-boiled	1 cup	166	605	3	13	11	0	124	10	50	195	277	0.80	—	0	0.02	0.07	0.30	—	—	—	0
1305	Italian sausage-pork-link	1 item	67	216	13	17	6	52	1	16	114	618	204	1.01	1.59	0	0.42	0.16	2.79	0.22	0.87	3	1
1740	Jack in the box-breakfast jack sandwich	1 item	121	301	18	13	—	182	28	177	310	1037	190	2.50	1.80	133	0.41	0.47	5.10	0.14	1.10	—	3
1469	Jack in the box-jumbo jack cheeseburger	1 item	272	628	32	35	15	110	45	273	411	1666	499	4.60	4.80	220	0.52	0.38	11.30	0.31	3.05	—	5
1468	Jack in the box-jumbo jack hamburger	1 item	246	551	28	29	11	80	45	134	261	1134	492	4.50	4.20	74	0.47	0.34	11.60	0.30	2.68	—	4
1858	Jack in the box-moby jack sandwich	1 item	141	455	17	26	—	56	38	167	263	837	246	1.70	1.10	72	0.30	0.21	4.50	0.12	1.10	—	1
1470	Jack in the box-onion rings-bag	1 item	83	275	4	16	7	14	31	73	86	430	129	0.85	0.35	2	0.09	0.10	0.92	0.06	0.12	11	1
562	Jam/preserves-strawberry-low calorie	1 tsp	6	8	0	0	0	0	2	1	0	6	5	0.04	0.00	0	0.00	0.00	0.01	0.00	0.00	1	1
549	Jams/preserves-regular	1 tbsp	20	55	0	0	0	0	14	4	2	2	18	0.20	0.01	0	0.00	0.01	0.00	0.00	0.00	2	0
550	Jams/preserves-regular-packet size	1 item	14	40	0	0	0	0	10	3	1	1	12	0.10	0.01	0	0.00	0.00	0.00	0.00	0.00	1	0
551	Jellies-regular	1 tbsp	18	50	0	0	0	0	13	4	1	3	14	0.30	0.01	0	0.00	0.01	0.00	0.00	0.00	0	1
552	Jellies-regular-packet size	1 item	14	40	0	0	0	0	10	3	1	2	11	0.20	0.01	0	0.00	0.00	0.00	0.00	0.00	0	1
1070	Jerusalem artichokes-raw	1 cup	150	114	3	0	0	0	26	21	117	6	644	5.10	0.18	3	0.30	0.09	1.95	0.12	0.00	20	6
225	Juice apple-canned or bottled	1 cup	248	116	0	0	0	0	29	16	18	7	296	0.92	0.07	0	0.05	0.04	0.25	0.07	0.00	0	2
952	Juice-apple-frozen-diluted	1 cup	239	112	0	0	0	0	28	14	17	17	301	0.62	0.09	—	0.01	0.04	0.09	0.08	0.00	1	1
232	Juice-apricot nectar-canned	1 cup	251	141	1	0	0	0	36	17	23	9	286	0.96	0.23	330	0.02	0.04	0.65	—	0.00	3	1
257	Juice-grape-canned & bottled	1 cup	253	154	1	0	0	0	38	23	28	8	334	0.61	0.13	2	0.07	0.09	0.66	0.16	0.00	7	0
258	Juice-grape-frozen concentrate	1 item	216	387	1	1	0	0	96	28	32	15	160	0.78	0.28	6	0.11	0.20	0.93	0.32	0.00	10	179
259	Juice-grape-frozen-diluted	1 cup	250	128	0	0	0	0	32	9	11	5	53	0.26	0.10	2	0.04	0.07	0.31	0.11	0.00	3	60
251	Juice-grapefruit-canned-sweetened	1 cup	250	115	1	0	0	0	28	20	28	5	405	0.90	0.15	0	0.10	0.06	0.80	0.05	0.00	26	67
250	Juice-grapefruit-canned-unsweetened	1 cup	247	94	1	0	0	0	22	17	27	2	378	0.49	0.22	2	0.10	0.05	0.57	0.05	0.00	26	72
254	Juice-grapefruit-dehydrated-prepared	1 cup	247	100	1	0	0	0	24	22	40	2	412	0.20	—	2	0.10	0.05	0.50	—	0.00	—	91
252	Juice-grapefruit-frozen concentrate	1 item	207	302	4	1	0	0	72	56	101	6	1002	1.02	0.38	7	0.30	0.16	1.60	0.32	0.00	26	248
253	Juice-grapefruit-frozen-diluted	1 cup	247	101	1	0	0	0	24	20	35	2	336	0.35	0.12	2	0.10	0.05	0.54	0.11	0.00	9	83
249	Juice-grapefruit-raw	1 cup	247	96	1	0	0	0	23	22	37	2	400	0.49	0.12	2	0.10	0.05	0.49	0.11	0.00	25	94
263	Juice-lemon-canned & bottled	1 cup	244	51	1	1	0	0	16	27	22	51	249	0.32	0.15	4	0.10	0.02	0.48	0.11	0.00	25	61
264	Juice-lemon-frozen-single strength	1 cup	244	54	1	1	0	0	16	20	20	2	217	0.29	0.12	3	0.14	0.03	0.33	0.15	0.00	23	77
262	Juice-lemon-raw	1 cup	244	61	1	0	0	0	21	17	15	2	303	0.07	0.12	5	0.07	0.02	0.24	0.12	0.00	32	112
270	Juice-lime-canned & bottled	1 cup	246	52	1	1	0	0	17	30	25	39	185	0.57	0.15	4	0.08	0.01	0.40	0.07	0.00	19	16
269	Juice-lime-raw	1 cup	246	66	1	0	0	0	22	22	17	2	268	0.07	0.15	3	0.05	0.03	0.25	0.11	0.00	20	72
280	Juice-orange grapefruit-canned	1 cup	247	106	1	0	0	0	25	20	35	7	390	1.14	0.17	29	0.14	0.07	0.83	0.06	0.00	35	72
281	Juice-orange grapefruit-frozen-diluted	1 cup	248	110	1	0	0	0	26	20	32	2	439	0.20	0.18	27	0.15	0.02	0.70	0.06	0.00	—	102
276	Juice-orange-canned	1 cup	249	104	1	0	0	0	25	21	36	6	436	1.10	0.17	44	0.15	0.07	0.78	0.22	0.00	136	86
277	Juice-orange-canned-frozen concentrate	1 item	213	339	5	0	0	0	81	67	122	7	1435	0.74	0.39	59	0.60	0.14	1.53	0.33	0.00	331	294
279	Juice-orange-dehydrated-prepared	1 cup	248	115	1	0	0	0	27	25	40	2	518	0.50	—	50	0.20	0.07	1.00	—	0.00	—	109
278	Juice-orange-frozen concentrate-diluted	1 cup	249	112	2	0	0	0	27	22	40	2	474	0.24	0.13	19	0.20	0.05	0.50	0.11	0.00	109	97
275	Juice-orange-raw	1 cup	248	111	2	1	0	0	26	27	42	2	496	0.50	0.13	50	0.22	0.07	0.99	0.10	0.00	136	124
1008	Juice-passion fruit-purple	1 cup	247	126	1	0	0	0	34	9	31	15	687	0.59	0.14	177	0.00	0.32	3.61	0.14	0.00	19	74
1009	Juice-passion fruit-yellow	1 cup	247	148	2	0	0	0	36	10	62	15	687	0.89	0.14	595	0.00	0.25	5.53	0.14	0.00	19	45
299	Juice-pineapple-canned	1 cup	250	140	1	0	0	0	35	43	20	3	335	0.65	0.28	1	0.14	0.06	0.64	0.24	0.00	58	27
1021	Juice-pineapple-frozen-diluted	1 cup	250	130	1	0	0	0	32	28	20	3	340	0.75	0.28	3	0.18	0.05	0.50	0.19	0.00	27	30
306	Juice-prune-canned & bottled	1 cup	256	182	2	0	0	0	45	31	64	10	707	3.02	0.54	1	0.04	0.18	2.01	0.56	0.00	1	11

317	Juice-tangerine-canned-sweetened	1 cup	249	125	1	1	0	0	30	45	35	2	443	0.50	0.06	105	0.15	0.05	0.25	0.08	0.00	12	55
1040	Juice-tangerine-raw	1 cup	247	106	1	0	0	0	25	44	35	2	440	0.49	0.06	104	0.15	0.05	0.25	0.10	0.00	11	77
623	Kale-frozen-boiled-drained	1 cup	130	39	4	1	0	0	7	179	36	20	417	1.22	0.23	826	0.06	0.15	0.87	0.11	0.00	19	33
622	Kale-raw-boiled-drained	1 cup	130	42	2	1	0	0	7	94	36	30	296	1.17	0.31	962	0.07	0.09	0.65	0.18	0.00	17	53
1332	Kielbasa-pork and beef	1 slice	26	81	3	7	3	17	1	11	39	280	71	0.38	0.52	0	0.06	0.06	0.75	0.05	0.42	1	5
990	Kiwifruit-raw	1 item	76	46	1	0	0	0	11	20	30	4	252	0.31	0.13	13	0.02	0.04	0.38	0.07	0.00	29	75
1333	Knockwurst-pork and beef-link	1 item	68	209	8	19	7	39	1	7	67	687	136	0.62	1.13	0	0.23	0.10	1.86	0.11	0.80	1	18
1072	Kohlrabi-boiled-drained	1 cup	165	48	3	0	0	0	11	41	74	35	561	0.66	0.51	7	0.07	0.03	0.64	0.25	0.00	20	89
1071	Kohlrabi-raw	1 cup	140	38	2	0	0	0	9	34	64	28	490	0.56	0.04	6	0.07	0.03	0.56	0.21	0.00	23	87
991	Kumquats-raw	1 item	19	12	0	0	0	0	3	8	4	1	37	0.07	0.02	6	0.02	0.02	0.10	0.01	0.00	3	7
182	Lamb chop-rib-broiled-lean and fat	1 serving	85	307	19	25	11	84	0	16	151	64	230	1.60	3.40	0	0.08	0.19	5.95	0.09	2.16	12	0
183	Lamb chop-rib-broiled-lean only	1 serving	57	134	16	7	3	52	0	9	121	49	178	1.26	3.00	0	0.06	0.14	3.73	0.09	1.50	12	0
184	Lamb-leg-roasted-lean and fat	1 slice	85	219	22	14	6	79	0	9	162	56	266	1.69	3.74	—	0.09	0.23	5.60	0.13	2.20	17	—
185	Lamb-leg-roasted-lean only	1 slice	71	136	20	6	2	63	0	6	146	48	240	1.51	3.50	—	0.08	0.21	4.50	0.12	1.87	16	—
186	Lamb-shoulder-roasted-lean and fat	1 slice	85	235	19	17	7	78	0	17	156	56	214	1.67	4.44	—	0.08	0.20	5.23	0.11	2.24	18	—
187	Lamb-shoulder-roasted-lean only	1 slice	64	131	16	7	3	56	0	12	128	44	170	1.36	3.87	—	0.06	0.17	3.69	0.10	1.73	16	—
1490	Lasagna florentine-light and elegant	1 item	319	280	24	5	—	—	34	280	387	975	720	3.60	—	814	0.39	0.38	1.70	—	—	—	22
1921	Lasagna-3 cheese-budget gourmet	1 serving	284	400	22	17	6	65	38	500	286	760	437	2.70	1.84	186	0.38	0.51	4.00	0.16	0.36	24	2
1916	Lasagna-sausage-budget gourmet	1 serving	284	284	20	20	9	80	38	400	348	950	591	2.70	3.74	183	0.45	0.43	4.00	0.28	0.91	23	18
471	Lasagna-stouffer frozen dinner	1 item	298	385	28	14	—	—	36	410	—	1200	580	3.15	—	248	0.21	0.42	4.20	—	—	—	0
1074	Leeks-boiled-drained	1 item	124	38	1	0	0	0	9	37	21	12	108	1.36	0.07	6	0.03	0.03	0.25	0.14	0.00	30	5
1073	Leeks-raw	1 item	124	76	2	0	0	0	18	73	43	25	223	2.60	0.15	12	0.07	0.04	0.50	0.29	0.00	80	15
993	Lemon peel-raw	1 tbsp	6	4	0	0	0	0	1	8	1	0	10	0.05	—	0	0.00	0.01	0.02	0.01	0.00	—	8
265	Lemonade-canned-frozen concentrate	1 item	219	425	0	0	0	0	112	9	13	4	153	0.40	—	4	0.05	0.06	0.70	—	0.00	—	66
266	Lemonade-frozen concentrate-diluted	1 cup	248	105	0	0	0	0	28	2	3	0	40	0.10	—	1	0.01	0.02	0.20	—	0.00	12	17
992	Lemons-raw-unpeeled	1 item	108	22	1	0	0	0	12	66	16	3	157	0.76	0.11	3	0.05	0.04	0.22	0.12	0.00	11	83
261	Lemons-raw-without peel	1 item	58	17	1	0	0	0	5	15	9	1	80	0.35	0.04	2	0.02	0.01	0.06	0.05	0.00	6	31
1075	Lentils-sprouted-raw	1 cup	77	82	7	0	0	0	17	19	133	8	248	2.47	1.16	4	0.18	0.10	0.87	0.15	0.00	77	13
522	Lentils-whole-cooked	1 cup	198	231	18	1	0	0	40	37	356	4	731	6.59	2.50	2	0.34	0.15	2.10	0.35	0.00	358	3
624	Lettuce-butterhead-head	1 item	163	21	2	0	0	0	4	52	38	8	419	0.49	0.28	158	0.10	0.10	0.49	0.08	0.00	119	13
625	Lettuce-butterhead-leaves	1 slice	15	2	0	0	0	0	0	5	3	1	39	0.05	0.03	15	0.01	0.01	0.05	0.01	0.00	11	1
628	Lettuce-iceberg-raw-chopped	1 cup	55	7	1	0	0	0	1	11	11	5	87	0.28	0.12	18	0.03	0.02	0.10	0.02	0.00	31	2
626	Lettuce-iceberg-raw-head	1 item	539	70	5	1	0	0	11	102	108	49	852	2.70	1.19	178	0.25	0.16	1.01	0.22	0.00	302	21
627	Lettuce-iceberg-raw-leaves	1 piece	20	3	0	0	0	0	0	4	4	2	32	0.10	0.04	7	0.01	0.01	0.04	0.01	0.00	11	1
629	Lettuce-looseleaf-raw	1 cup	55	10	1	0	0	0	2	37	14	5	145	0.77	0.16	105	0.03	0.04	0.22	0.03	0.00	27	10
1665	Lettuce-romaine-raw-shredded	1 cup	56	9	1	0	0	0	1	20	25	4	162	0.62	0.14	146	0.06	0.06	0.28	0.03	0.00	76	13
267	Limeade-canned-frozen concentrate	1 item	218	410	0	0	0	0	108	11	13	2	129	0.20	—	0	0.02	0.02	0.20	—	0.00	—	26
268	Limeade-frozen concentrate-diluted	1 cup	247	100	0	0	0	0	27	3	3	2	32	0.00	—	0	0.00	0.00	0.00	—	0.00	—	6
994	Limes-raw	1 item	67	20	0	0	0	0	7	22	12	1	68	0.40	0.07	1	0.02	0.01	0.13	0.03	0.00	5	20
469	Linguini with clam sauce-stouffer dinner	1 item	298	285	17	8	—	—	36	—	—	1010	115	—	—	—	—	—	—	—	—	—	—
848	Liqueurs-anisette	1 item	20	74	0	0	0	0	7	—	—	—	—	—	—	—	—	—	—	—	—	—	—
849	Liqueurs-apricot brandy	1 item	20	64	0	0	0	0	6	1	1	2	11	0.02	0.01	0	0.01	0.00	0.02	0.00	0.00	1	3
850	Liqueurs-benedictine	1 item	20	69	—	0	0	0	7	—	—	—	—	—	—	—	—	—	—	—	—	—	—
851	Liqueurs-creme de menthe	1 fl oz	34	125	0	0	0	0	14	0	0	2	0	0.02	0.01	0	0.00	0.00	0.00	0.00	0.00	0	0
852	Liqueurs-curacao	1 item	20	54	—	0	0	0	6	—	—	—	—	—	—	—	—	—	—	—	—	—	—
1321	Liver cheese-pork	1 slice	38	116	6	10	3	66	1	3	79	466	86	4.12	1.41	1996	0.08	0.85	4.47	0.18	9.33	40	1
1322	Liverwurst-liver sausage-pork	1 slice	18	59	3	5	2	28	0	5	41	215	36	1.15	0.51	760	0.05	0.19	1.51	0.03	2.42	5	2
467	Lobster newburg-stouffer frozen dinner	1 item	184	350	15	29	—	—	9	—	—	700	190	—	—	—	—	—	—	—	—	—	—
995	Loganberries-frozen	1 cup	147	81	2	0	0	0	19	38	38	1	213	0.94	0.50	5	0.07	0.05	1.24	0.10	0.00	38	23
996	Longans-raw	1 item	3	2	0	0	0	0	0	0	1	0	9	0.00	0.00	—	0.00	0.00	0.01	—	0.00	—	3
997	Loquats-raw	1 item	10	5	0	0	0	0	1	2	3	0	26	0.03	0.01	15	0.00	0.00	0.02	—	0.00	—	0
1077	Lotus root-boiled-drained	1 ounce	28	19	0	0	0	0	5	7	22	13	103	0.26	0.09	0	0.04	0.00	0.09	0.06	0.00	2	8
1076	Lotus root-raw	1 item	115	64	3	0	0	0	20	52	115	46	639	1.33	0.45	0	0.18	0.25	0.46	0.21	0.00	15	51
1500	Low methionine diet formula-mead johnson	1 fl oz	30	20	1	1	—	0	2	19	15	9	23	0.38	0.16	15	0.02	0.02	0.20	0.01	0.06	3	2
1501	Low phenylalanine/tyrosine diet formula	1 fl oz	30	20	1	1	—	—	3	19	14	9	20	0.37	0.13	15	0.02	0.02	0.26	0.01	0.06	3	2
998	Lychees-raw	1 item	10	6	0	0	0	0	2	0	3	0	16	0.03	0.01	0	0.00	0.01	0.06	0.01	0.00	1	7
441	Macaroni & cheese-enriched-canned	1 cup	240	230	9	10	4	42	26	199	182	729	139	1.00	—	52	0.12	0.24	1.00	—	—	—	0
442	Macaroni & cheese-enriched-home recipe	1 cup	200	430	17	22	9	42	40	362	322	1086	240	1.80	—	172	0.20	0.40	1.80	—	—	—	0
1491	Macaroni and cheese-light and elegant	1 item	255	300	15	9	—	—	37	238	334	1015	210	2.00	—	60	0.34	0.43	1.50	—	—	—	0
438	Macaroni-cooked-firm stage-hot	1 cup	130	183	6	1	0	0	37	1	71	1	41	1.82	0.69	0	0.27	0.13	2.18	0.05	0.00	1	0
439	Macaroni-cooked-tender stage-cold	1 cup	105	148	5	1	0	0	30	8	57	1	33	1.47	0.56	—	0.22	0.10	1.76	0.04	0.00	8	0
440	Macaroni-cooked-tender stage-hot	1 cup	140	197	7	1	0	0	40	10	76	1	44	1.96	0.74	0	0.29	0.14	2.34	0.05	0.00	10	0
2000	Macaroni-vegetable-cooked	1 cup	134	172	6	0	0	0	36	15	67	8	42	0.66	0.59	7	0.15	0.08	1.44	0.03	0.00	8	0

Dashes (—) in data spaces indicate that no data were reported.

Item	Food Name	Portion	Weight (g)	Food Energy (kcal)	Protein (g)	Total Fat (g)	Saturated Fat (g)	Cholesterol (mg)	Carbohydrate (g)	Calcium (mg)	Phosphorus (mg)	Sodium (mg)	Potassium (mg)	Iron (mg)	Zinc (cm)	Vitamin A (RE)	Thiamin (mg)	Riboflavin (mg)	Niacin (mg)	Vitamin B6 (mg)	Vitamin B12 (ug)	Folic Acid (ug)	Vitamin C (mg)
1565	Macaroni-whole wheat-cooked	1 cup	140	174	7	1	0	0	37	21	124	4	61	1.49	1.13	0	0.15	0.06	0.99	0.11	0.00	7	0
1184	Mace-ground	1 tsp	2	8	0	1	0	0	1	4	2	1	8	0.24	0.04	1	0.01	0.01	0.02	—	0.00	—	—
999	Mangos-raw	1 item	207	135	1	1	0	0	35	21	22	4	322	0.26	0.07	806	0.12	0.12	1.21	0.28	0.00	29	57
1623	Manicotti-cheese-le menu frozen dinner	1 item	241	310	18	13	10	146	29	348	328	840	434	2.99	2.68	223	0.23	0.46	3.26	0.22	1.03	26	8
1914	Manicotti-cheese/meat-budget gourmet	1 serving	284	450	20	26	11	50	33	450	376	920	484	2.70	2.29	280	0.45	0.51	4.00	0.23	0.72	31	10
924	Margarine-corn-regular-hydrogenated-hard	1 tsp	5	34	0	4	1	0	0	1	1	44	2	0.00	—	47	0.00	0.00	0.00	0.00	0.00	0	0
929	Margarine-corn-regular-soft	1 tsp	5	34	0	4	1	0	0	1	1	51	2	0.00	0.00	47	0.00	0.00	0.00	0.00	0.00	0	0
925	Margarine-corn/soybean-unsalted	1 tsp	5	34	0	4	1	0	0	1	1	0	1	0.00	0.00	47	0.00	0.00	0.00	0.00	0.00	0	0
110	Margarine-diet/low calorie-mazola	1 tbsp	14	50	0	6	1	0	0	0	0	130	1	0.00	0.02	130	0.00	0.00	0.00	0.00	0.00	0	0
934	Margarine-imitation-40% fat	1 tsp	5	17	0	2	0	0	0	1	1	46	1	0.00	0.00	48	0.00	0.00	0.00	0.00	0.00	0	0
935	Margarine-imitation-spread-60% fat	1 tsp	5	26	0	3	1	0	0	1	1	48	1	0.00	0.00	48	0.00	0.00	0.00	0.00	0.00	0	0
933	Margarine-liquid-regular-soybean	1 tsp	5	34	0	4	1	0	0	3	2	37	4	0.00	0.00	47	0.00	0.00	0.00	0.00	0.01	0	0
112	Margarine-no stick-spray-mazola	1 serving	1	6	0	1	0	0	0	0	0	0	—	0.00	—	0	0.00	0.00	0.00	—	—	—	0
928	Margarine-regular-hard-unsalted	1 tsp	5	34	0	4	1	0	0	1	1	0	1	0.00	0.00	47	0.00	0.00	0.00	0.00	0.00	0	0
932	Margarine-regular-soft-unsalted	1 tsp	5	34	0	4	1	0	0	1	1	1	2	0.00	0.00	47	0.00	0.00	0.00	0.00	0.00	0	0
115	Margarine-regular-unspecified oils-pat	1 item	5	36	0	4	1	0	0	2	1	47	2	0.00	0.00	15	0.00	0.00	0.00	0.00	0.01	0	0
113	Margarine-regular-unspecified oils-stick	1 item	113	812	1	91	18	0	1	34	26	1066	48	0.07	0.00	338	0.01	0.04	0.03	0.01	0.11	1	0
114	Margarine-regular-unspecified oils-tbsp	1 tbsp	14	101	0	11	2	0	0	4	3	132	6	0.01	0.00	139	0.00	0.01	0.00	0.00	0.01	0	0
930	Margarine-safflower-regular-soft-tub	1 tsp	5	34	0	4	0	0	0	1	1	51	2	0.00	0.00	47	0.00	0.00	0.00	0.00	0.00	0	0
926	Margarine-safflower/soybean-hydrogenated	1 tsp	5	34	0	4	1	0	0	1	1	44	2	0.00	0.00	47	0.00	0.00	0.00	0.00	0.00	0	0
931	Margarine-soybean-soft-tub-unsalted	1 tsp	5	34	0	4	1	0	0	1	1	1	2	0.00	0.00	47	0.00	0.00	0.00	0.00	0.00	0	0
117	Margarine-unspecified oils-soft-tbsp	1 tbsp	14	100	0	11	2	0	0	4	3	151	5	0.00	0.00	139	0.00	0.00	0.00	0.00	0.01	0	0
116	Margarine-unspecified oils-soft-tub	1 cup	227	1626	2	183	31	0	1	60	46	2449	86	0.40	0.00	675	0.02	0.07	0.05	0.02	0.19	2	0
119	Margarine-whipped	1 tbsp	9	70	0	8	1	0	0	2	2	97	2	0.00	0.00	310	0.00	0.00	0.00	0.00	0.01	0	0
1185	Marjoram-dried	1 tsp	1	2	0	0	0	0	0	12	2	0	9	0.50	0.02	5	0.00	0.00	0.03	—	0.00	—	0
545	Marshmallows	1 ounce	28	90	1	0	0	0	23	5	2	11	2	0.50	0.01	0	0.00	0.00	0.00	0.00	0.00	0	0
1947	Matzos-american crackers-manischewitz	1 serving	28	115	3	2	0	0	22	6	40	1	52	1.02	0.51	0	0.16	0.09	1.14	0.03	0.00	10	0
1946	Matzos-daily thin tea-manischewitz	1 piece	26	103	3	0	—	0	22	—	—	—	34	1.00	—	—	—	—	—	—	—	—	—
1948	Matzos-matzo meal-manischewitz	1 cup	135	514	13	1	8	0	109	37	101	3	149	4.10	0.67	87	0.10	0.29	0.90	0.08	0.37	24	0
936	Mayonnaise-imitation-milk cream	1 tbsp	15	15	0	1	0	6	2	11	9	76	15	0.08	0.04	0	0.00	0.02	0.01	0.00	0.04	0	0
937	Mayonnaise-imitation-soybean	1 tbsp	15	35	0	3	1	4	2	0	0	75	2	0.00	0.02	0	0.00	0.00	0.00	0.00	0.00	0	0
938	Mayonnaise-imitation-soybean-chol free	1 tbsp	14	68	0	7	1	0	2	0	0	49	1	0.00	0.02	0	0.00	0.00	0.00	0.00	0.00	0	0
1640	Mayonnaise-light-low calorie-kraft	1 tbsp	14	40	0	4	0	5	1	0	0	15	1	0.00	0.02	1	0.00	0.00	0.00	0.00	0.01	0	0
138	Mayonnaise-soybean-commercial	1 tbsp	14	99	0	11	2	8	0	2	4	78	5	0.10	0.02	12	0.00	0.00	0.00	0.08	0.04	1	0
2006	Mcdonalds-apple danish	1 slice	115	390	6	18	3	26	51	14	31	370	69	1.37	0.23	35	0.28	0.20	2.20	0.03	0.00	3	16
737	Mcdonalds-big mac hamburger	1 item	215	560	25	32	10	103	43	256	314	950	237	4.00	4.70	106	0.48	0.41	6.81	0.27	1.80	21	2
738	Mcdonalds-cheeseburger	1 item	116	310	15	14	5	53	31	199	177	750	223	2.30	2.09	118	0.29	0.21	3.86	0.12	0.94	18	2
1873	Mcdonalds-chicken mcnuggets-6 piece	1 serving	113	290	19	16	4	65	17	13	—	520	—	1.00	—	0	0.11	0.12	8.97	—	—	—	0
2020	Mcdonalds-cinnamon and raisin danish	1 item	110	440	6	21	4	35	58	35	—	430	—	1.81	—	33	0.32	0.24	2.80	—	—	—	3
743	Mcdonalds-egg mcmuffin	1 item	138	290	18	11	4	226	28	256	319	740	213	2.77	1.80	150	0.47	0.33	3.71	0.16	0.80	44	1
742	Mcdonalds-filet o fish	1 item	142	440	14	26	5	50	38	165	229	1030	150	1.83	0.90	44	0.30	0.15	2.68	0.10	0.82	20	0
1872	Mcdonalds-french fries-regular order	1 serving	68	220	3	12	5	9	26	10	90	110	484	0.52	0.35	0	0.14	0.00	1.84	0.18	0.08	22	8
739	Mcdonalds-hamburger	1 item	102	260	12	10	4	37	31	122	110	500	215	2.29	2.05	46	0.28	0.16	3.84	0.12	0.84	17	2
2003	Mcdonalds-hashbrown potato	1 serving	55	130	1	7	3	9	15	6	39	330	238	0.27	0.18	0	0.06	0.02	0.85	0.07	0.00	4	2
1874	Mcdonalds-hot cakes with syrup	1 serving	176	410	8	9	4	21	74	114	501	640	187	2.08	0.60	52	0.32	0.33	2.82	0.12	0.19	9	5
2001	Mcdonalds-mcdlt hamburger	1 item	234	580	26	37	12	109	36	225	—	990	—	3.91	—	226	0.39	0.36	6.87	—	—	—	7
741	Mcdonalds-quarter pound cheeseburger	1 item	194	520	29	29	11	118	35	295	382	1150	341	3.72	5.70	211	0.37	0.39	6.73	0.23	2.15	23	3
740	Mcdonalds-quarter pounder hamburger	1 item	166	410	23	21	8	86	34	142	249	660	322	3.68	5.10	67	0.36	0.29	6.70	0.27	1.88	23	3
2007	Mcdonalds-raspberry danish	1 item	117	410	6	16	3	26	62	14	—	310	—	1.47	—	35	0.33	0.21	2.10	—	—	—	3
1888	Mcdonalds-sausage and egg biscuit	1 item	180	520	20	35	11	275	33	116	490	1250	319	3.16	2.16	88	0.53	0.35	3.99	0.20	1.37	40	0
2004	Mcdonalds-sausage biscuit	1 item	123	440	13	29	9	49	32	83	443	1080	196	1.98	1.54	0	0.49	0.21	3.96	0.11	0.50	9	0
2010	Mcdonalds-sausage mcmuffin	1 item	117	370	17	22	8	64	27	235	273	830	179	2.30	1.67	72	0.60	0.29	4.80	0.13	0.50	48	1
2005	Mcdonalds-sausage mcmuffin with egg	1 item	167	440	23	27	9	263	28	263	390	980	255	3.34	2.39	150	0.64	0.42	4.82	0.19	0.72	68	0
2002	Mcdonalds-scrambled eggs	1 serving	98	140	12	10	3	399	1	57	136	290	102	2.08	1.09	156	0.07	0.26	0.05	0.08	1.68	27	1
1870	Meat loaf-with celery and onions	1 serving	88	213	16	14	5	107	5	23	112	103	182	1.91	3.08	12	0.05	0.15	3.16	0.16	1.52	11	1
396	Meatball stew-lean cuisine frozen dinner	1 item	284	240	22	7	—	65	21	—	—	1250	410	—	—	—	—	—	—	—	—	—	—
461	Meatballs and noodles-stouffer dinner	1 item	312	475	25	27	—	—	33	—	—	1620	395	—	—	—	—	—	—	—	—	—	—
1741	Meatloaf-banquet frozen dinner	1 item	312	412	21	24	7	79	29	84	243	1991	468	4.30	3.35	427	0.16	0.22	4.20	0.36	1.21	48	8
1001	Melon balls-frozen	1 cup	173	57	1	0	0	0	14	17	21	54	484	0.50	0.29	307	0.29	0.04	1.11	0.18	0.00	45	11
271	Melons-cantaloupe-raw-cubed pieces	1 cup	160	56	1	0	0	0	13	18	27	14	494	0.34	0.26	516	0.06	0.03	0.92	0.18	0.00	27	68

Code	Food	Amount	1	2	3	4	5	6	7	8	9	10	11	12	13	14	15	16	17	18	19	20	21
1000	Melons-casaba-raw	1 cup	170	44	2	0	0	0	11	9	12	20	357	0.68	0.27	5	0.10	0.03	0.68	0.20	0.00	29	27
272	Melons-honeydew-raw-cubed pieces	1 cup	170	60	1	0	0	0	16	10	17	17	461	0.12	—	7	0.13	0.03	1.02	0.10	0.00	—	42
1630	Mexican dinner-swanson frozen dinner	1 item	454	590	20	29	10	44	64	198	340	1865	603	5.13	3.62	93	0.35	0.30	3.83	0.30	0.83	135	7
57	Milk-0% fat-skim-fluid	1 cup	245	86	8	0	0	4	12	302	247	126	406	0.10	0.98	150	0.09	0.34	0.22	0.10	0.93	13	2
58	Milk-0%-skim-milk solids added	1 cup	245	90	9	1	0	5	12	316	255	130	418	0.12	1.00	150	0.10	0.43	0.22	0.11	0.95	13	2
54	Milk-1% fat-lowfat-fluid	1 cup	244	102	8	3	2	10	12	300	235	123	381	0.12	0.95	150	0.10	0.41	0.21	0.11	0.90	12	2
55	Milk-1% fat-nonfat milk solids added	1 cup	245	104	9	2	1	10	12	313	245	128	397	0.12	0.98	150	0.10	0.42	0.22	0.11	0.94	13	2
56	Milk-1% fat-protein fortified	1 cup	246	119	10	3	2	10	14	349	273	143	444	0.15	1.11	150	0.11	0.47	0.25	0.12	1.05	15	3
53	Milk-2% fat-fluid-protein fortified	1 cup	246	137	10	5	3	19	14	352	276	145	447	0.15	1.11	150	0.11	0.48	0.25	0.13	1.05	15	3
51	Milk-2% fat-lowfat-fluid	1 cup	244	121	8	5	3	18	12	297	232	122	377	0.12	0.95	150	0.10	0.40	0.21	0.11	0.89	12	2
52	Milk-2% fat-nonfat milk solids added	1 cup	245	125	9	5	3	18	12	313	245	128	397	0.12	0.98	150	0.10	0.42	0.22	0.11	0.94	13	2
50	Milk-3.3% fat-whole-fluid	1 cup	244	150	8	8	5	33	11	291	228	120	370	0.12	0.93	92	0.09	0.40	0.21	0.10	0.87	12	2
60	Milk-buttermilk-cultured-fluid	1 cup	245	99	8	2	1	9	12	285	219	257	371	0.12	1.03	24	0.08	0.38	0.14	0.08	0.54	12	2
64	Milk-buttermilk-dried-sweet cream	1 cup	120	464	41	7	4	83	59	1421	1119	621	1910	0.36	4.82	79	0.47	1.90	1.05	0.41	4.59	57	7
69	Milk-chocolate-1% fat-fluid	1 cup	250	158	8	3	2	7	26	287	256	152	426	0.60	1.02	150	0.10	0.42	0.32	0.10	0.86	12	2
68	Milk-chocolate-2% fat-fluid	1 cup	250	179	8	5	3	17	26	284	254	150	422	0.60	1.02	150	0.09	0.41	0.32	0.10	0.85	12	2
67	Milk-chocolate-whole-fluid	1 cup	250	208	8	8	5	30	26	280	251	149	417	0.60	1.02	91	0.09	0.41	0.31	0.10	0.84	12	2
63	Milk-condensed-sweetened-canned	1 cup	306	982	24	27	17	104	166	868	775	389	1136	0.58	2.88	302	0.28	1.27	0.64	0.16	1.36	34	8
70	Milk-eggnog-commercial	1 cup	254	342	10	19	11	149	34	330	278	138	420	0.51	1.17	268	0.09	0.48	0.27	0.13	1.14	2	4
62	Milk-evaporated-skim-canned	1 cup	255	199	19	1	0	10	29	740	497	293	847	0.74	2.30	300	0.12	0.79	0.44	0.14	0.61	23	3
61	Milk-evaporated-whole-canned	1 cup	252	338	17	19	12	73	25	658	509	267	764	0.48	1.94	184	0.12	0.80	0.49	0.13	0.41	20	5
909	Milk-goat-whole-fluid	1 cup	244	168	9	10	7	28	11	326	270	122	499	0.12	0.73	135	0.12	0.34	0.68	0.11	0.16	1	3
910	Milk-human-whole-mature	1 cup	246	171	3	11	5	34	17	79	34	42	126	0.07	0.42	178	0.03	0.09	0.44	0.03	0.11	13	12
905	Milk-imitation	1 cup	244	150	4	8	2	0	15	79	181	191	279	0.95	2.88	0	0.03	0.22	0.00	0.00	0.00	0	0
911	Milk-indian buffalo-whole	1 cup	244	236	9	17	11	46	13	412	286	127	434	0.29	0.54	130	0.13	0.33	0.22	0.06	0.89	14	5
71	Milk-malted-chocolate flavor-prepared	1 cup	265	229	9	9	6	34	30	304	265	172	499	0.50	1.09	80	0.13	0.44	0.63	0.14	0.91	16	3
72	Milk-malted-natural flavor-prepared	1 cup	265	237	10	10	6	37	27	354	303	223	529	0.29	1.13	94	0.20	0.59	1.31	0.19	1.03	22	3
66	Milk-nonfat/skim-instantized-dried	1 cup	68	244	24	0	0	12	36	837	670	373	1160	0.21	3.00	484	0.28	1.19	0.61	0.24	2.72	34	4
65	Milk-nonfat/skim-instantized-envelope	1 item	91	326	32	1	0	17	48	1120	896	499	1552	0.28	4.01	648	0.38	1.59	0.81	0.31	3.63	45	5
59	Milk-nonfat/skim-protein fortified	1 cup	246	100	10	1	0	5	14	352	275	144	446	0.15	1.11	150	0.11	0.48	0.25	0.12	1.05	15	3
912	Milk-sheep-whole-fluid	1 cup	245	264	15	17	11	66	13	474	387	108	334	0.24	1.32	108	0.16	0.87	1.02	0.15	1.74	17	10
1813	Milk-soy-fluid	1 cup	240	79	7	5	1	0	4	10	118	29	338	1.39	0.55	7	0.39	0.17	0.35	0.10	0.00	4	0
907	Milk-whole-dry	1 cup	128	635	34	34	21	124	49	1168	993	475	1702	0.60	4.28	354	0.36	1.54	0.83	0.39	4.16	47	11
906	Milk-whole-low sodium	1 cup	244	149	8	8	5	33	11	246	209	6	617	0.12	0.93	95	0.05	0.26	0.11	0.08	0.88	12	2
73	Milkshake-chocolate-thick	1 item	300	356	9	8	5	32	64	396	378	333	672	0.93	1.44	78	0.14	0.67	0.37	0.08	0.95	15	0
74	Milkshake-vanilla-thick	1 item	313	350	12	9	6	37	56	457	361	299	572	0.31	1.22	107	0.09	0.61	0.46	0.13	1.63	21	0
1967	Millet-cooked	1 cup	240	286	8	2	0	0	57	7	240	5	148	1.51	2.18	0	0.25	0.20	3.19	0.26	0.00	46	0
1966	Millet-raw	1 cup	200	756	22	8	1	0	146	17	569	10	390	6.02	3.37	0	0.84	0.58	9.44	0.77	0.00	170	0
1753	Miso-fermented soybeans	1 cup	275	567	33	17	2	0	77	182	421	10030	451	7.54	9.13	25	0.27	0.69	2.37	0.59	0.00	91	0
1002	Mixed fruit-canned-heavy syrup pack	1 cup	255	184	1	0	0	0	48	3	26	10	214	0.92	0.18	49	0.04	0.10	1.53	0.09	0.00	8	176
1003	Mixed fruit-frozen-sweetened	1 cup	250	245	4	0	0	0	61	18	30	8	327	0.70	0.12	81	0.04	0.09	0.99	0.06	0.00	19	188
556	Molasses-cane-blackstrap	1 tbsp	20	45	0	0	0	0	11	137	17	18	585	3.20	0.07	0	0.02	0.04	0.40	0.04	0.00	0	0
555	Molasses-cane-light	1 tbsp	20	50	0	0	0	0	13	33	9	3	183	0.90	0.07	0	0.01	0.01	0.00	0.04	0.00	0	0
1504	Mono/disaccharide free diet formula-mead	1 fl oz	30	20	1	1	—	—	3	19	12	9	22	0.38	0.12	23	0.02	0.02	0.26	0.01	0.06	3	2
1334	Mortadella-pork and beef	1 slice	15	47	2	4	1	8	0	3	15	187	25	0.21	0.32	0	0.02	0.02	0.40	0.02	0.22	0	4
1943	Muffin-blueberry oat bran-health valley	1 item	57	140	4	4	—	0	27	27	144	95	260	1.40	0.80	0	0.23	0.09	0.05	0.08	0.00	14	5
443	Muffin-blueberry-from home recipe	1 item	40	110	3	4	1	21	17	34	53	252	46	0.60	—	18	0.09	0.10	0.70	—	—	—	0
444	Muffin-bran-from home recipe	1 item	40	112	3	5	1	21	17	54	111	168	99	1.26	1.08	40	0.10	0.11	1.26	0.11	0.09	17	2
445	Muffin-corn-from home recipe	1 item	40	125	3	4	1	21	19	42	68	192	54	0.70	—	25	0.10	0.10	0.70	—	—	—	0
447	Muffin-corn-from mix-with egg and milk	1 item	40	130	3	4	1	21	20	96	152	191	44	0.60	—	20	0.08	0.09	0.70	—	—	—	0
1382	Muffin-english-plain-toasted	1 item	53	154	5	1	0	0	30	105	73	414	364	1.83	0.47	0	0.24	0.21	2.43	0.03	0.00	21	0
1381	Muffin-english-plain-untoasted	1 item	56	133	4	1	2	0	26	91	63	358	314	1.58	0.40	0	0.26	0.18	2.10	0.02	0.00	18	0
446	Muffin-plain-from home recipe	1 item	40	120	3	4	1	21	17	42	60	176	50	0.60	—	8	0.09	0.12	0.90	—	—	—	0
1942	Muffin-raisin oat bran-health valley	1 item	57	140	5	3	0	0	31	33	160	100	290	1.70	0.90	0	0.25	0.09	0.50	0.09	0.00	15	4
1730	Muffin-soy	1 item	40	119	4	4	—	0	17	35	56	—	—	0.90	—	40	0.08	0.10	0.50	—	—	—	0
1004	Mulberries-raw	1 cup	140	60	2	1	0	0	14	55	53	14	271	2.59	0.17	4	0.04	0.14	0.87	0.07	0.00	8	51
1079	Mushrooms-boiled-drained	1 item	12	3	0	0	0	0	1	1	10	0	43	0.21	0.10	0	0.01	0.04	0.54	0.01	0.00	2	0
1080	Mushrooms-canned-drained	1 item	12	3	0	0	0	0	1	1	8	51	16	0.10	0.09	0	0.01	0.00	0.19	0.01	0.00	1	0
630	Mushrooms-raw-chopped	1 cup	70	18	1	0	0	0	3	4	73	3	259	0.87	0.51	0	0.07	0.31	2.88	0.07	0.00	15	2
631	Mustard greens-boiled-drained	1 cup	140	21	3	0	0	0	3	103	58	22	283	0.98	0.15	424	0.06	0.09	0.61	0.00	0.00	103	35
1682	Mustard-brown-prepared	1 cup	250	228	15	16	8	0	13	310	335	3268	325	4.50	0.79	0	0.07	0.02	0.41	0.09	0.00	11	2
1713	Mustard-low sodium-featherweight	1 tsp	5	4	0	0	—	0	0	4	4	1	7	0.10	—	—	—	—	—	—	—	—	—
700	Mustard-yellow-prepared	1 tsp	5	5	0	0	0	0	0	4	4	65	7	0.10	—	—	—	—	—	—	—	—	—

Dashes (—) in data spaces indicate that no data were reported.

Appendix C Table of Food Composition

Item	Food Name	Portion	Weight (g)	Food Energy (kcal)	Protein (g)	Total Fat (g)	Saturated Fat (g)	Cholesterol (mg)	Carbohydrate (g)	Calcium (mg)	Phosphorus (mg)	Sodium (mg)	Potassium (mg)	Iron (mg)	Zinc (cm)	Vitamin A (RE)	Thiamin (mg)	Riboflavin (mg)	Niacin (mg)	Vitamin B6 (mg)	Vitamin B12 (ug)	Folic Acid (ug)	Vitamin C (mg)
1899	Nachos-cheese	1 serving	113	345	9	19	8	18	36	272	276	816	172	1.27	1.78	92	0.19	0.37	1.53	0.20	0.82	10	1
1754	Natto-fermented soybeans	1 cup	280	468	47	21	4	0	32	103	182	20	697	10.40	8.48	0	0.07	0.50	1.10	0.36	0.00	22	0
1005	Nectarines-raw	1 item	136	67	1	1	0	0	16	7	22	0	288	0.20	0.12	100	0.02	0.06	1.35	0.03	0.00	5	7
435	Noodles romanoff-stouffer frozen dinner	1 item	113	170	6	9	—	—	16	88	—	675	95	0.80	—	61	0.08	0.16	0.80	—	—	—	—
1562	Noodles-cellophane/long rice-dry	1 cup	140	491	0	0	0	0	121	35	45	14	14	3.04	0.57	0	0.21	0.00	0.28	0.07	0.00	3	0
449	Noodles-chow mein-enriched	1 cup	45	237	4	14	2	0	26	9	72	197	54	2.13	0.63	4	0.26	0.19	2.68	0.05	0.00	10	0
1564	Noodles-egg-cooked	1 cup	160	213	8	2	0	53	40	19	110	11	45	2.54	0.99	10	0.30	0.13	2.38	0.06	0.14	11	0
448	Noodles-egg-enriched-cooked	1 cup	160	200	7	2	—	50	37	16	94	3	70	1.40	—	11	0.22	0.13	1.90	0.14	0.00	19	0
1563	Noodles-egg-spinach-cooked	1 cup	160	211	8	3	1	52	39	30	91	20	59	1.74	1.01	17	0.39	0.20	2.36	0.18	0.22	34	0
1725	Noodles-ramen-oriental	1 cup	227	207	6	9	0	36	31	18	70	829	69	1.78	0.62	221	0.16	0.10	1.42	0.07	0.01	8	0
1727	Noodles-soba-buckwheat-dry	1 ounce	28	95	4	0	0	0	21	10	72	225	72	0.77	0.49	0	0.14	0.04	0.92	0.07	0.00	17	0
1726	Noodles-somen-wheat-dry	1 ounce	28	101	3	0	0	0	21	7	23	523	47	0.38	0.13	0	0.03	0.01	0.25	0.01	0.00	4	0
521	Nut-filbert/hazel-dried-chopped	1 cup	115	727	15	72	5	0	18	216	359	3	512	3.76	2.76	8	0.58	0.13	1.30	0.70	0.00	83	1
531	Nut-walnut-persian/english	1 cup	120	770	17	74	7	0	22	113	380	12	602	2.93	3.28	15	0.46	0.18	1.25	0.67	0.00	79	4
814	Nutmeg-ground	1 tsp	2	12	0	1	1	0	1	4	5	0	8	0.07	0.05	0	0.01	0.00	0.03	—	0.00	—	—
507	Nuts-almonds-unblanched-shelled-chopped	1 cup	130	766	26	68	6	0	27	346	676	14	952	4.76	3.80	0	0.27	1.01	4.37	0.15	0.00	76	1
508	Nuts-almonds-unblanched-shelled-slivered	1 cup	115	677	23	60	6	0	24	306	598	13	842	4.21	3.36	0	0.24	0.90	3.87	0.13	0.00	68	1
1138	Nuts-beechnuts-dried	1 ounce	28	164	2	14	2	0	10	0	0	11	289	0.70	0.10	0	0.09	0.11	0.25	0.19	0.00	32	4
517	Nuts-brazil-dried-shelled	1 cup	140	918	20	93	23	0	18	246	840	3	840	4.76	6.43	0	1.40	0.17	2.27	0.35	0.00	6	1
1139	Nuts-butternuts-dried	1 ounce	28	174	7	16	0	0	3	15	127	0	119	1.14	0.89	3	0.11	0.04	0.30	0.16	0.00	19	1
1140	Nuts-cashews-dry roasted	1 cup	137	786	21	64	13	0	45	62	671	22	774	8.22	7.67	0	0.27	0.27	1.92	0.35	0.00	95	0
518	Nuts-cashews-oil roasted	1 cup	130	749	21	63	12	0	37	53	554	22	689	5.33	6.18	0	0.55	0.23	2.34	0.33	0.00	88	0
1142	Nuts-chestnuts-chinese-dried	1 ounce	28	103	2	1	0	0	23	8	44	2	206	0.65	0.40	9	0.07	0.08	0.37	0.19	0.00	31	17
1141	Nuts-chestnuts-chinese-raw	1 ounce	28	64	1	0	0	0	14	5	27	1	127	0.40	0.25	6	0.05	0.05	0.23	0.12	0.00	19	10
1152	Nuts-chestnuts-roasted	1 ounce	28	68	1	0	0	0	15	5	29	1	135	0.43	0.26	0	0.04	0.03	0.43	0.12	0.00	21	11
519	Nuts-coconut-dried-flaked-canned	1 cup	77	341	3	24	22	0	32	11	79	15	249	1.42	1.23	0	0.02	0.02	0.24	0.18	0.00	5	0
1153	Nuts-coconut-dried-shredded	1 cup	93	466	3	33	29	0	44	14	99	244	313	1.78	1.69	0	0.03	0.02	0.44	0.25	0.00	8	1
520	Nuts-coconut-raw-shredded	1 cup	80	283	3	27	24	0	12	12	90	16	285	1.94	0.88	0	0.05	0.02	0.43	0.04	0.00	21	3
1156	Nuts-hickory-dried	1 ounce	28	187	4	18	2	0	5	17	95	0	124	0.60	1.22	4	0.25	0.04	0.26	0.06	0.00	11	1
1157	Nuts-macadamia-dried	1 cup	134	941	11	99	15	0	18	94	182	7	493	3.23	2.29	0	0.47	0.15	2.87	0.26	0.00	21	0
1158	Nuts-macadamia-oil roasted	1 cup	134	962	10	103	15	0	17	60	268	9	441	2.41	1.47	1	0.29	0.15	2.71	0.27	0.00	21	0
1159	Nuts-mixed-dry roasted	1 cup	137	814	24	71	9	0	35	96	596	16	817	5.07	5.21	2	0.27	0.27	6.44	0.41	0.00	69	1
1160	Nuts-mixed-oil roasted	1 cup	142	876	24	80	12	0	30	153	659	16	825	4.56	7.22	3	0.71	0.32	7.19	0.34	0.00	118	1
523	Nuts-peanuts-oil roasted	1 cup	144	837	38	71	10	0	27	127	744	8	982	2.64	9.55	0	0.36	0.16	20.60	0.37	0.00	181	0
1763	Nuts-peanuts-oil roasted-salted	1 cup	144	837	38	71	10	0	27	127	744	624	982	2.64	9.55	0	0.36	0.16	20.60	0.37	0.00	181	0
1161	Nuts-peanuts-spanish-dried	1 cup	146	828	38	72	10	0	24	134	549	26	1029	6.69	4.77	0	0.93	0.20	17.60	0.51	0.00	350	0
526	Nuts-pecans-dried-halves	1 cup	108	720	8	73	6	0	20	39	314	1	423	2.30	5.91	14	0.92	0.14	0.96	0.20	0.00	42	2
1162	Nuts-pecans-oil roasted	1 cup	110	754	8	78	6	0	18	37	324	1	395	2.33	6.05	—	0.34	0.11	0.98	0.21	0.00	43	2
1163	Nuts-pistachio-dried	1 cup	128	739	26	62	8	0	32	173	644	7	1399	8.67	1.71	30	1.05	0.22	1.38	0.32	0.00	74	9
1164	Nuts-pistachio-dry roasted	1 cup	128	776	19	68	9	0	35	90	609	8	1242	4.06	1.74	31	0.54	0.32	1.80	0.33	0.00	76	9
1165	Nuts-soybean kernels-roasted	1 cup	108	489	40	26	3	0	33	149	392	4	1588	4.81	3.91	22	0.11	0.16	1.90	0.32	0.00	244	2
529	Nuts-walnut-black-dried-chopped	1 cup	125	759	30	71	5	0	15	72	580	2	655	3.84	4.28	37	0.27	0.14	0.86	0.69	0.00	82	4
530	Nuts-walnuts-finely ground	1 cup	80	486	20	45	3	0	10	46	371	1	419	2.46	2.74	24	0.18	0.09	0.60	0.44	0.00	52	3
1969	Oat bran-raw	1 cup	94	231	16	7	1	0	62	55	690	4	532	5.09	2.92	0	1.10	0.21	0.88	0.16	0.00	49	0
1971	Oats-rolled or oatmeal-dry	1 cup	81	311	13	5	1	0	54	42	384	3	284	3.41	2.48	20	0.59	0.11	0.63	0.10	0.00	26	0
1968	Oats-whole grain-uncooked	1 cup	156	607	26	11	2	0	104	84	816	3	669	7.37	6.19	0	1.19	0.22	1.50	0.19	0.00	87	0
1444	Ocean fish almondine	1 item	113	236	16	17	—	—	3	22	—	388	229	0.70	—	0	0.19	0.25	3.10	—	—	—	0
1445	Ocean fish with lemon sauce	1 serving	113	262	14	21	2	16	3	15	93	370	224	0.70	0.54	0	0.17	0.18	2.80	0.13	0.22	18	0
120	Oil-vegetable-corn	1 cup	218	1927	0	218	28	0	0	0	0	0	0	0.00	0.00	0	0.00	0.00	0.00	0.00	0.00	0	0
122	Oil-vegetable-olive	1 cup	216	1909	0	216	31	0	0	0	3	0	0	0.83	0.13	0	0.00	0.00	0.00	0.00	0.00	0	0
124	Oil-vegetable-peanut	1 cup	216	1909	0	216	36	0	0	0	0	0	0	0.06	0.02	0	0.00	0.00	0.00	0.00	0.00	0	0
927	Oil-vegetable-rice bran	1 tbsp	14	120	0	14	3	0	0	0	0	0	0	0.01	0.00	0	0.00	0.00	0.00	0.00	0.00	0	0
126	Oil-vegetable-safflower	1 cup	218	1927	0	218	21	0	0	0	0	0	0	0.00	0.00	0	0.00	0.00	0.00	0.00	0.00	0	0
923	Oil-vegetable-sesame	1 tbsp	14	120	0	14	2	0	0	0	0	0	0	0.00	0.00	0	0.00	0.00	0.00	0.00	0.00	0	0
128	Oil-vegetable-soybean	1 cup	218	1927	0	218	32	0	0	0	0	0	0	0.00	0.00	0	0.00	0.00	0.00	0.00	0.00	0	0
130	Oil-vegetable-soybean/cottonseed	1 cup	218	1927	0	218	38	0	0	0	0	0	0	0.00	0.00	0	0.00	0.00	0.00	0.00	0.00	0	0
632	Okra-raw-boiled-drained	1 cup	160	51	3	0	0	0	12	101	90	8	515	0.72	0.88	92	0.21	0.09	1.39	0.30	0.00	73	26
1323	Olive loaf-pork	1 slice	28	67	3	5	2	11	3	31	36	421	84	0.15	0.39	6	0.08	0.07	0.52	0.07	0.36	1	3
701	Olives-green-pickled-canned	1 item	4	4	0	1	0	0	0	2	1	81	2	0.05	0.01	1	0.00	0.00	0.00	0.00	0.00	0	0
702	Olives-mission-ripe-canned	1 item	3	5	0	1	0	0	0	3	0	19	1	0.03	0.01	1	0.00	0.00	0.00	0.00	0.00	0	0

1407	Omelet-two egg-ham and cheese	1 item	120	266	19	20	7	445	2	153	286	598	182	1.67	1.84	273	0.18	0.57	0.83	0.19	1.08	38	4
1187	Onion powder	1 tsp	2	7	0	0	0	0	2	8	7	1	20	0.05	0.05	—	0.01	0.00	0.01	—	0.00	—	0
1081	Onion rings-frozen-prepared-heated	1 item	10	41	1	3	1	0	4	3	8	38	13	0.17	0.04	2	0.03	0.01	0.36	0.01	0.00	1	0
635	Onions-mature-boiled-drained	1 cup	210	92	3	0	0	0	21	46	74	6	349	0.50	0.44	0	0.09	0.05	0.35	0.27	0.00	32	11
633	Onions-mature-raw-chopped	1 cup	160	61	2	0	0	0	14	32	53	5	251	0.35	0.30	0	0.07	0.03	0.24	0.19	0.00	30	10
636	Onions-young green	1 item	5	1	0	0	0	0	0	3	2	0	13	0.10	0.02	25	0.00	0.01	0.00	0.00	0.00	1	2
273	Oranges-raw-all common varieties-whole	1 item	131	62	1	0	0	0	15	52	18	0	237	0.13	0.09	27	0.11	0.05	0.37	0.08	0.00	40	70
274	Oranges-raw-sections without membranes	1 cup	180	85	2	0	0	0	21	72	25	0	326	0.18	0.13	37	0.16	0.07	0.51	0.11	0.00	55	96
815	Oregano-ground	1 tsp	2	5	0	0	0	0	1	24	3	0	25	0.66	0.07	10	0.01	—	0.09	—	0.00	—	—
398	Oriental beef-lean cuisine frozen dinner	1 item	245	250	18	7	—	35	28	—	—	1150	270	—	—	—	—	—	—	—	—	—	—
1417	Ovaltine-chocolate flavor-prepared/milk	1 cup	265	227	10	9	5	34	29	392	302	228	600	4.77	1.13	700	0.63	0.97	12.70	0.77	0.87	29	29
1416	Ovaltine-malt flavor-prepared with milk	1 cup	265	228	10	8	5	37	29	371	308	201	576	4.49	1.08	770	0.67	1.16	11.90	0.75	0.87	29	30
450	Pancakes-buckwheat-from mix	1 item	27	55	2	2	1	20	6	59	91	160	66	0.40	0.19	12	0.04	0.05	0.20	0.06	0.36	3	0
451	Pancakes-plain-from home recipe	1 item	27	60	2	2	1	20	9	27	38	160	33	0.40	0.19	6	0.06	0.07	0.50	0.06	0.36	3	0
452	Pancakes-plain-from mix	1 item	27	59	2	2	1	20	8	36	71	160	43	0.27	0.19	8	0.04	0.06	0.25	0.06	0.36	3	0
1728	Pancakes-soybean-25% soy flour	1 item	45	68	3	2	—	0	10	26	42	—	—	0.60	—	18	0.07	0.07	0.40	—	—	—	0
1006	Papaya nectar-canned	1 cup	250	143	0	0	0	0	36	25	0	13	78	0.85	0.38	28	0.02	0.01	0.38	0.02	0.00	5	8
282	Papayas-raw	1 cup	140	55	1	0	0	0	14	34	7	4	359	0.14	0.10	282	0.04	0.05	0.47	0.03	0.00	53	87
816	Paprika	1 tsp	2	6	0	0	0	0	1	4	7	1	49	0.50	0.08	127	0.01	0.04	0.32	—	0.00	—	1
817	Parsley-dried	1 tsp	0	1	0	0	0	0	0	4	1	1	11	0.29	0.01	7	0.00	0.00	0.02	0.00	0.00	0	0
637	Parsley-raw-chopped	1 tbsp	4	1	0	0	0	0	0	5	2	2	21	0.25	0.03	21	0.00	0.00	0.05	0.00	0.00	7	4
638	Parsnips-sliced-boiled-drained	1 cup	156	126	2	0	0	0	31	58	108	16	574	0.90	0.41	0	0.13	0.08	1.13	0.15	0.00	91	20
1007	Passion fruit-purple-raw	1 item	18	18	0	0	0	0	4	2	12	5	63	0.29	0.02	13	0.00	0.02	0.27	0.02	0.00	3	5
1995	Pasta-corn-cooked	1 cup	140	176	4	1	0	0	39	2	106	1	43	0.34	0.88	8	0.07	0.03	0.78	0.08	0.00	9	0
1996	Pasta-fresh-plain-cooked	1 ounce	28	38	1	0	0	10	7	2	18	2	7	0.33	0.16	2	0.06	0.04	0.28	0.01	0.04	2	0
1997	Pasta-fresh-spinach-cooked	1 ounce	28	37	1	0	0	10	7	5	16	2	11	0.32	0.18	4	0.05	0.04	0.29	0.03	0.04	5	0
1998	Pasta-homemade-with egg-cooked	1 ounce	28	37	2	0	0	12	7	3	15	24	6	0.33	0.13	2	0.05	0.05	0.36	0.01	0.03	6	0
1999	Pasta-homemade-without egg-cooked	1 ounce	28	35	1	0	0	0	7	2	11	21	5	0.32	0.11	0	0.05	0.04	0.38	0.01	0.00	5	0
1010	Peach nectar-canned	1 cup	249	134	1	0	0	0	35	13	16	17	101	0.47	0.20	64	0.01	0.04	0.72	0.02	0.00	3	13
285	Peaches-canned-heavy syrup pack	1 cup	256	189	1	0	0	0	51	8	28	15	235	0.69	0.05	85	0.03	0.06	1.57	0.05	0.00	8	7
286	Peaches-canned-water pack	1 cup	244	59	1	0	0	0	15	5	24	7	242	0.78	0.22	130	0.02	0.05	1.27	0.05	0.00	8	7
288	Peaches-dried-cooked-sulfured-no sugar	1 cup	258	199	3	1	0	0	51	23	98	5	826	3.38	0.46	51	0.01	0.05	3.92	0.10	0.00	0	10
287	Peaches-dried-uncooked-sulfured	1 cup	160	382	6	1	0	0	98	45	190	11	1594	6.50	0.91	346	0.00	0.34	7.00	0.11	0.00	0	8
290	Peaches-frozen-sliced-sweetened	1 cup	250	235	2	0	0	0	60	6	28	16	325	0.93	0.13	71	0.03	0.09	1.63	0.05	0.00	8	235
49	Peaches-halved-canned in water-dietetic	1 serving	28	7	0	0	0	0	2	1	3	1	30	0.11	0.03	12	0.00	0.01	0.11	—	0.00	—	1
284	Peaches-raw-sliced	1 cup	170	73	1	0	0	0	19	9	20	0	335	0.19	0.24	91	0.03	0.07	1.68	0.03	0.00	6	11
283	Peaches-raw-whole	1 item	87	37	1	0	0	0	10	4	10	0	171	0.10	0.12	47	0.02	0.04	0.86	0.02	0.00	3	6
47	Peaches-sliced-canned in water-dietetic	1 ounce	28	7	0	0	0	0	2	1	3	1	30	0.11	0.03	12	0.00	0.01	0.11	—	0.00	—	1
289	Peaches-spiced-canned-heavy syrup pack	1 cup	242	182	1	0	0	0	49	15	22	10	206	0.68	0.19	77	0.03	0.09	1.30	0.05	0.00	8	13
1884	Peanut butter-chunk style	1 tbsp	16	95	4	8	2	0	3	7	51	78	121	0.31	0.45	0	0.02	0.02	2.21	0.07	0.00	15	0
1639	Peanut butter-low sodium-peter pan	1 tbsp	16	95	5	9	1	0	3	5	60	5	110	0.29	0.47	0	0.02	0.02	2.15	0.06	0.00	13	0
1885	Peanut butter-old fashioned	1 tbsp	16	95	4	8	2	0	3	5	60	75	110	0.30	0.50	0	0.01	0.01	2.30	0.06	0.00	13	0
524	Peanut butter-smooth type	1 tbsp	16	94	4	8	2	0	3	5	52	77	115	0.27	0.40	—	0.02	0.02	2.09	0.06	0.00	13	0
1014	Pear nectar-canned	1 cup	250	150	0	0	0	0	39	13	8	10	33	0.65	0.18	0	0.01	0.03	0.32	0.04	0.00	3	3
294	Pears-canned-heavy syrup pack	1 cup	255	189	1	0	0	0	49	13	18	13	166	0.56	0.20	0	0.03	0.06	0.62	0.04	0.00	3	3
1012	Pears-canned-juice pack	1 cup	248	124	1	0	0	0	32	22	30	10	238	0.72	0.22	1	0.03	0.03	0.50	0.04	0.00	3	4
1011	Pears-canned-water pack	1 cup	244	71	0	0	0	0	19	10	17	5	129	0.51	0.22	0	0.02	0.02	0.13	0.03	0.00	3	2
1013	Pears-dried-uncooked	1 cup	180	472	3	1	0	0	125	60	106	10	959	3.78	0.70	1	0.01	0.26	2.47	0.13	0.00	0	13
45	Pears-halved-canned in water-dietetic	1 ounce	28	9	0	0	0	0	2	1	2	1	17	0.14	0.02	—	0.00	0.01	0.09	—	0.00	—	1
291	Pears-raw-bartlett-with skin	1 item	166	98	1	1	0	0	25	18	18	0	208	0.42	0.20	3	0.03	0.07	0.17	0.03	0.00	12	7
292	Pears-raw-bosc-with skin	1 item	141	83	1	1	0	0	21	16	16	1	176	0.35	0.17	3	0.03	0.06	0.14	0.03	0.00	10	6
293	Pears-raw-d'anjou-with skin	1 item	200	118	1	1	0	0	30	22	22	1	250	0.50	0.24	4	0.04	0.08	0.20	0.04	0.00	15	8
1696	Peas & carrots-canned-dietary-low sodium	1 cup	255	96	6	1	0	0	22	58	116	10	256	1.92	1.47	1471	0.19	0.14	1.48	0.22	0.00	47	17
1082	Peas and carrots-canned	1 cup	255	97	6	1	0	0	22	59	117	663	255	1.91	1.48	1471	0.19	0.14	1.48	0.22	0.00	47	17
1083	Peas and carrots-frozen-boiled	1 cup	160	77	5	1	0	0	16	37	78	109	253	1.50	0.72	1242	0.36	0.10	1.85	0.14	0.00	42	13
1084	Peas and onions-canned	1 cup	120	61	4	0	0	0	10	20	61	530	115	1.04	0.70	19	0.12	0.08	1.54	0.23	0.00	32	4
1085	Peas and onions-frozen-boiled	1 cup	180	81	5	0	0	0	16	25	61	67	211	1.60	0.52	63	0.27	0.12	1.88	0.16	0.00	36	12
516	Peas-blackeye/cowpeas-boiled-drained	1 cup	165	179	13	1	0	0	30	46	197	7	693	2.36	1.30	105	0.11	0.18	1.77	0.08	0.00	173	3
586	Peas-blackeye/cowpeas-frozen-boiled	1 cup	170	224	14	1	0	0	40	40	208	9	638	3.60	2.42	13	0.44	0.11	1.24	0.16	0.00	240	5
585	Peas-blackeye/cowpeas-raw-boiled	1 cup	165	160	5	1	0	0	34	211	84	7	690	1.85	1.70	130	0.17	0.24	2.32	0.11	0.00	210	4
640	Peas-edible podded-raw	1 cup	145	61	4	0	0	0	11	62	77	6	290	3.02	0.39	20	0.22	0.12	0.87	0.23	0.00	61	87
1694	Peas-green-canned-dietary-low sodium	1 cup	170	117	8	1	0	0	21	34	114	3	294	1.62	1.21	131	0.21	0.13	1.24	0.11	0.00	75	16
639	Peas-green-canned-drained	1 cup	170	117	8	1	0	0	21	34	114	372	294	1.62	1.21	131	0.21	0.13	1.24	0.11	0.00	75	16

Dashes (—) in data spaces indicate that no data were reported.

Item	Food Name	Portion	Weight (g)	Food Energy (kcal)	Protein (g)	Total Fat (g)	Saturated Fat (g)	Cholesterol (mg)	Carbohydrate (g)	Calcium (mg)	Phosphorus (mg)	Sodium (mg)	Potassium (mg)	Iron (mg)	Zinc (cm)	Vitamin A (RE)	Thiamin (mg)	Riboflavin (mg)	Niacin (mg)	Vitamin B6 (mg)	Vitamin B12 (ug)	Folic Acid (ug)	Vitamin C (mg)
641	Peas-green-frozen-boiled-drained	1 cup	160	125	8	0	0	0	23	38	144	139	269	2.51	1.50	107	0.45	0.16	2.37	0.18	0.00	94	16
525	Peas-split-dry-cooked	1 cup	200	230	16	1	0	0	42	22	178	8	592	3.40	2.10	8	0.30	0.18	1.80	0.10	0.00	129	1
39	Peas-sweet-canned in water-dietetic	1 ounce	28	12	1	0	0	0	2	6	17	1	27	0.60	0.19	16	0.02	0.02	0.20	—	0.00	—	3
1917	Pepper steak with rice-budget gourmet	1 serving	284	300	15	9	6	25	39	40	350	800	729	0.72	5.99	60	0.15	0.17	3.00	0.59	3.90	22	2
1620	Pepper steak-le menu frozen dinner	1 item	326	360	26	13	—	—	34	—	—	1045	—	—	—	—	—	—	—	—	—	—	—
818	Pepper-black	1 tsp	2	5	0	0	0	0	1	9	4	1	26	0.61	0.03	0	0.00	0.01	0.02	0.00	0.00	0	3
819	Pepper-red or cayenne	1 tsp	2	6	0	0	0	0	1	3	5	1	36	0.14	0.05	75	0.01	0.02	0.16	0.00	0.00	0	1
1188	Pepper-white	1 tsp	2	7	0	0	0	0	2	6	4	0	2	0.34	0.03	—	0.00	0.00	0.01	—	0.00	—	—
1335	Pepperoni-pork and beef	1 slice	6	27	1	2	1	4	0	1	7	112	19	0.08	0.14	0	0.02	0.01	0.27	0.01	0.14	0	0
1663	Peppers-hot chili-canned	1 cup	136	34	1	0	0	0	8	10	24	1595	254	0.68	0.23	83	0.03	0.07	1.09	0.21	0.00	14	92
1664	Peppers-hot chili-raw	1 cup	150	60	3	0	0	0	14	26	68	10	510	1.80	0.46	116	0.14	0.14	1.43	0.42	0.00	35	364
642	Peppers-hot-red-dried	1 tsp	2	5	0	0	0	0	1	5	4	20	20	0.30	0.05	130	0.00	0.02	0.20	0.00	0.00	0	0
1086	Peppers-jalapeno-canned-chopped	1 cup	136	33	1	1	0	0	1	35	23	1990	185	3.81	0.26	231	0.04	0.07	0.68	0.28	0.00	18	18
644	Peppers-sweet-boiled-drained	1 item	73	20	1	0	0	0	5	7	13	1	121	0.34	0.09	43	0.04	0.02	0.35	0.17	0.00	11	54
643	Peppers-sweet-raw	1 item	74	20	1	0	0	0	5	7	14	1	131	0.34	0.09	47	0.05	0.02	0.38	0.18	0.00	16	66
1016	Persimmons-japanese-dried	1 item	34	93	0	0	0	0	25	9	28	1	273	0.25	0.14	19	0.01	0.01	0.06	0.03	0.00	3	0
1015	Persimmons-japanese-raw	1 item	168	118	1	0	0	0	31	13	28	3	270	0.26	0.18	364	0.05	0.03	0.17	0.17	0.00	13	13
1017	Persimmons-native-raw	1 item	25	32	0	0	0	0	8	7	7	78	78	0.63	0.03	54	0.01	0.01	0.03	0.03	0.00	2	17
33	Pickle relish-hamburger-heinz	1 ounce	28	30	0	0	0	0	7	6	4	325	—	0.19	—	—	—	—	—	—	—	—	—
31	Pickle relish-hot dog-heinz	1 ounce	28	35	0	0	0	0	8	6	4	200	—	0.19	—	—	—	—	—	—	—	—	—
706	Pickle relish-sweet-chopped	1 tbsp	15	20	0	0	0	0	5	3	2	124	30	0.10	0.01	2	0.00	0.00	0.00	0.00	0.00	1	1
703	Pickle-dill-cucumber-medium sized	1 item	65	5	0	0	0	0	1	17	14	928	130	0.70	0.18	7	0.00	0.01	0.00	0.01	0.00	1	4
704	Pickle-fresh pack-cucumber-sliced	1 item	8	5	0	0	0	0	2	3	2	50	15	0.15	0.02	1	0.00	0.00	0.00	0.00	0.00	0	1
705	Pickle-sweet/gherkin-small-whole	1 item	15	20	0	0	0	0	5	2	2	128	30	0.20	0.02	1	0.00	0.00	0.00	0.00	0.00	0	1
454	Pie-apple-from home recipe	1 slice	135	323	3	14	4	0	49	12	31	207	115	1.22	0.23	5	0.15	0.11	1.24	0.04	0.00	7	2
456	Pie-banana cream-from home recipe	1 slice	130	285	6	12	4	40	40	86	107	252	264	1.00	—	66	0.11	0.22	1.00	—	—	—	1
458	Pie-blueberry-from home recipe	1 slice	135	325	3	15	4	0	47	15	31	361	88	1.40	—	8	0.15	0.11	1.40	—	0.00	—	4
401	Pie-boston cream-home recipe	1 slice	69	210	3	6	2	0	34	46	70	128	61	0.70	—	28	0.09	0.11	0.80	—	—	—	0
460	Pie-cherry-from home recipe	1 slice	135	350	4	15	4	0	52	19	34	410	142	0.90	—	118	0.16	0.12	1.40	—	0.00	—	0
1657	Pie-chocolate cream-from home recipe	1 slice	100	264	5	15	5	55	30	84	109	273	142	1.08	0.66	53	0.10	0.17	0.72	0.05	0.37	9	0
462	Pie-custard-from home recipe	1 slice	130	285	8	14	5	—	30	125	147	373	178	1.20	—	60	0.11	0.27	0.80	—	—	—	0
464	Pie-lemon meringue-from home recipe	1 slice	120	300	4	11	4	0	47	16	48	223	53	0.90	0.34	33	0.10	0.12	0.72	0.03	0.19	11	4
466	Pie-mince-from home recipe	1 slice	135	365	3	16	4	0	56	38	51	604	240	1.90	—	0	0.14	0.12	1.40	—	—	—	1
468	Pie-peach-from home recipe	1 slice	135	345	3	14	4	0	52	14	39	361	21	1.20	—	198	0.15	0.14	2.00	—	0.00	—	4
470	Pie-pecan-from home recipe	1 slice	118	495	6	27	4	0	61	55	122	260	145	3.70	—	40	0.26	0.14	1.00	—	—	—	0
472	Pie-pumpkin-from home recipe	1 slice	130	275	5	15	5	0	32	66	90	278	208	1.00	—	320	0.11	0.18	1.00	—	—	—	0
473	Piecrust-baked-from home recipe	1 item	180	900	11	60	15	0	79	25	90	1099	89	3.10	—	0	0.47	0.40	5.00	—	—	—	0
474	Piecrust-baked-prepared from mix	1 item	160	743	10	47	11	0	71	66	136	1300	90	3.05	—	0	0.54	0.40	4.95	—	—	—	0
1324	Pimento/pickle loaf-pork	1 slice	28	74	3	6	2	11	2	27	40	394	97	0.29	0.40	2	0.08	0.07	0.58	0.05	0.34	1	4
1683	Pimientos-4 ounce can or jar	1 item	113	31	1	1	0	0	7	8	19	35	311	1.70	0.22	260	0.02	0.07	0.50	0.19	0.00	14	107
1719	Pineapple grapefruit drink	1 cup	253	129	1	0	0	0	32	15	10	56	139	0.81	0.13	0	0.05	0.05	0.61	2.02	0.00	25	68
1720	Pineapple orange drink	1 cup	253	134	1	0	0	0	32	13	10	8	121	0.68	0.15	134	0.08	0.05	0.53	0.12	0.00	28	63
296	Pineapple-bits-canned in syrup	1 cup	252	131	1	0	0	0	34	36	17	3	266	0.98	0.29	4	0.23	0.06	0.74	0.19	0.00	12	19
1018	Pineapple-bits-canned-water pack	1 cup	246	79	1	0	0	0	20	37	10	2	312	0.98	0.30	4	0.23	0.06	0.73	0.18	0.00	12	19
1019	Pineapple-canned-juice pack	1 cup	250	150	1	0	0	0	39	34	16	4	304	0.70	0.24	10	0.24	0.05	0.71	0.19	0.00	12	24
1020	Pineapple-frozen-sweetened	1 cup	245	208	1	0	0	0	54	22	10	5	245	0.98	0.28	7	0.25	0.07	0.74	0.18	0.00	26	20
295	Pineapple-raw-diced	1 cup	155	76	1	1	0	0	19	11	11	2	175	0.57	0.12	4	0.14	0.06	0.65	0.14	0.00	16	24
43	Pineapple-sliced-dietetic-canned/water	1 ounce	28	13	0	0	0	0	4	3	1	1	24	0.11	0.07	1	0.03	0.01	0.09	—	0.00	—	2
1022	Pitanga-raw	1 item	7	2	0	0	0	0	1	1	1	0	7	0.01	—	11	0.00	0.00	0.02	—	0.00	—	2
475	Pizza-cheese-baked	1 slice	63	140	8	3	2	9	21	116	113	336	110	0.58	0.82	74	0.18	0.16	2.48	0.04	0.33	59	1
1896	Pizza-cheese/meat/vegetable	1 slice	79	184	13	5	2	21	21	101	131	382	178	1.53	1.12	101	0.21	0.17	1.96	0.09	0.36	27	2
1608	Pizza-combination-weight watchers	1 item	205	340	20	12	—	—	38	—	—	—	—	—	—	—	—	—	—	—	—	—	—
1668	Pizza-pepperoni-baked	1 slice	71	181	10	7	2	14	20	65	75	267	153	0.94	0.52	54	0.14	0.23	3.05	0.05	0.19	53	2
1024	Plantains-cooked	1 cup	154	179	1	0	0	0	48	3	43	8	716	0.89	0.20	140	0.07	0.08	1.16	0.37	0.00	40	17
1023	Plantains-raw	1 item	179	218	2	1	0	0	57	5	61	7	893	1.07	0.25	202	0.09	0.10	1.23	0.54	0.00	39	33
302	Plums-purple-canned-heavy syrup pack	1 cup	258	230	1	0	0	0	60	24	33	50	234	2.17	0.19	67	0.04	0.10	0.75	0.07	0.00	7	1
1026	Plums-purple-canned-juice pack	1 cup	252	146	1	0	0	0	38	25	39	3	389	0.84	0.27	254	0.06	0.15	1.19	0.07	0.00	7	7
1025	Plums-purple-canned-water pack	1 cup	249	102	1	0	0	0	28	17	33	2	314	0.40	0.19	228	0.05	0.10	0.92	0.07	0.00	7	7
300	Plums-raw-japanese & hybrid	1 item	66	36	1	0	0	0	9	3	7	0	114	0.07	0.07	21	0.03	0.06	0.33	0.05	0.00	1	6
301	Plums-raw-prune type	1 item	28	20	0	0	0	0	6	3	5	0	48	0.10	0.03	8	0.01	0.01	0.10	0.02	0.00	1	1

1087	Poi-taro root product	1 cup	240	269	1	0	0	0	65	37	94	28	439	2.11	0.53	5	0.31	0.10	2.64	0.66	0.00	51	10
1325	Polish sausage-pork	1 item	227	740	32	65	23	159	4	27	309	1989	538	3.27	4.38	0	1.14	0.34	7.82	0.43	2.22	5	2
1027	Pomegranates-raw	1 item	154	105	1	0	0	0	26	5	12	5	399	0.46	0.19	0	0.05	0.05	0.46	0.16	0.00	9	9
477	Popcorn-popped-oil & salt	1 cup	9	40	1	2	2	0	5	1	19	174	—	0.20	0.40	—	—	0.01	0.20	—	—	—	0
476	Popcorn-popped-plain	1 cup	6	25	1	0	0	0	5	1	17	0	—	0.20	0.50	—	—	0.01	0.10	0.01	0.00	—	0
478	Popcorn-popped-sugar coated	1 cup	35	135	2	1	1	0	30	2	47	0	—	0.50	—	—	—	0.02	0.40	—	—	—	0
707	Popsicle	1 item	95	70	0	0	0	0	18	0	0	0	4	0.00	0.00	0	0.00	0.00	0.00	0.00	0.00	0	0
511	Pork and beans with frankfurters-canned	1 cup	257	365	17	17	6	15	40	123	267	1105	604	4.45	4.81	39	0.15	0.14	2.32	0.12	0.00	77	6
513	Pork and beans with sweet sauce-canned	1 cup	253	281	13	4	1	18	53	154	266	850	673	4.20	3.80	28	0.12	0.15	0.89	0.22	0.00	95	8
512	Pork and beans with tomato sauce-canned	1 cup	253	248	13	3	1	17	49	141	297	1113	759	8.30	14.80	62	0.13	0.12	1.26	0.18	0.00	57	8
192	Pork chop-loin-broiled-lean and fat	1 item	82	284	19	22	8	77	0	5	193	54	287	0.66	2.01	2	0.69	0.29	4.32	0.31	0.81	4	0
193	Pork chop-loin-broiled-lean only	1 item	66	169	18	10	3	63	0	5	184	49	276	0.61	1.93	2	0.64	0.28	3.93	0.30	0.71	4	0
1455	Pork loin and gravy-hormel entree	1 ounce	28	40	5	2	1	9	1	2	32	133	82	0.17	0.37	—	2.61	0.04	0.86	0.06	0.07	10	0
194	Pork-center loin-roasted-lean and fat	1 item	88	268	22	19	7	80	0	5	173	56	284	0.87	1.80	2	0.73	0.21	4.44	0.35	0.53	1	0
195	Pork-center loin-roasted-lean only	1 slice	72	173	21	9	3	66	0	4	158	50	261	0.79	1.64	2	0.65	0.19	3.93	0.32	0.43	1	0
1313	Pork-feet-pickled	1 ounce	28	58	4	5	2	26	0	9	10	262	67	0.18	0.35	0	0.00	0.01	0.10	0.11	0.18	1	0
1307	Pork-feet-simmered	1 ounce	28	55	5	4	1	28	0	13	14	9	42	0.13	0.31	0	0.00	0.02	0.15	0.03	0.05	0	0
1308	Pork-kidneys-braised	1 cup	140	211	36	7	2	673	0	18	337	111	200	7.41	5.81	109	0.55	2.22	8.10	0.65	10.90	57	15
1309	Pork-liver-braised	1 ounce	28	47	7	1	0	101	1	3	68	14	43	5.09	1.91	1531	0.07	0.62	2.39	0.16	5.30	46	7
197	Pork-shoulder-roasted-lean only	1 cup	140	342	36	21	7	136	0	11	323	106	493	2.13	5.94	3	0.82	0.51	6.03	0.56	1.23	7	0
1432	Pork-spareribs-braised	1 ounce	28	113	8	9	3	34	0	13	74	26	91	0.53	1.30	1	0.12	0.11	1.55	0.10	0.31	1	0
196	Pork-tenderloin-roasted-lean only	1 ounce	28	47	8	1	0	26	0	3	82	19	153	0.44	0.85	1	0.27	0.11	1.33	0.12	0.16	2	0
1310	Pork-tongue-braised	1 serving	85	230	21	16	5	124	0	16	148	93	201	4.24	3.85	0	0.27	0.43	4.54	0.20	2.03	3	1
1472	Postum-instant grain beverage-dry mix	1 ounce	28	103	2	0	0	0	24	77	189	28	896	1.87	—	0	0.17	0.08	6.76	—	—	—	0
654	Potato chips-salt added	1 ounce	28	149	2	10	3	0	15	7	44	133	369	0.34	0.30	0	0.04	0.00	1.19	0.14	0.00	13	12
1096	Potato pancakes-home recipe	1 item	76	495	5	13	3	93	26	21	78	388	538	1.21	0.68	9	0.10	0.10	1.61	0.29	0.22	22	0
1097	Potato puffs-frozen-heated	1 item	7	16	0	1	0	0	2	2	3	52	27	0.11	0.02	0	0.01	0.01	0.15	0.02	0.00	1	0
1088	Potato skin-baked	1 item	58	115	2	0	0	0	27	20	59	12	332	4.08	0.28	0	0.07	0.06	1.78	0.36	0.00	13	8
1089	Potato-au gratin-home recipe	1 cup	245	323	12	19	12	56	28	292	277	1061	970	1.57	1.69	93	0.16	0.28	2.43	0.43	0.49	20	24
1090	Potato-au gratin-prepared from mix	1 ounce	28	26	1	1	1	—	4	24	27	125	62	0.09	0.07	9	0.01	0.02	0.27	0.01	0.00	2	1
1144	Potato-baked-flesh & skin-whole	1 item	202	220	5	0	0	0	51	20	115	16	844	2.75	0.65	—	0.22	0.07	3.32	0.70	0.00	22	26
645	Potato-baked-peeled after baking	1 item	156	145	3	0	0	0	34	8	78	8	610	0.55	0.45	0	0.16	0.03	2.18	0.47	0.00	14	20
646	Potato-boiled-peeled after boiling	1 item	136	118	3	0	0	0	27	7	60	5	515	0.42	0.41	0	0.14	0.03	1.96	0.41	0.00	14	18
647	Potato-boiled-peeled before boiling	1 item	135	116	2	0	0	0	27	10	54	7	443	0.42	0.37	0	0.13	0.03	1.77	0.36	0.00	12	10
1143	Potato-canned-drained	1 item	35	21	0	0	0	0	5	2	10	91	80	0.44	0.10	0	0.02	0.01	0.32	0.07	0.00	2	2
649	Potato-french fried-prepared from frozen	1 item	5	11	0	0	0	0	2	0	4	2	23	0.07	0.02	0	0.01	0.00	0.12	0.01	0.00	1	1
648	Potato-french fried-prepared from raw	1 item	5	14	0	1	0	0	2	1	6	11	43	0.07	0.02	0	0.01	0.00	0.16	0.01	0.00	1	1
1091	Potato-hash brown-prepared from raw	1 cup	156	239	4	22	8	0	12	13	66	37	501	1.26	0.47	0	0.12	0.03	3.12	0.43	0.00	12	9
650	Potato-hashed brown-prepared from frozen	1 cup	156	340	5	18	7	0	44	24	112	54	680	2.34	0.50	0	0.17	0.03	3.78	0.20	0.00	39	10
1912	Potato-hush puppies	1 serving	78	256	5	12	3	135	35	69	190	965	188	1.43	0.43	9	0.00	0.02	2.03	0.10	0.18	21	0
653	Potato-mashed-from dehydrated-with milk	1 cup	210	166	4	5	1	4	28	65	92	491	704	1.26	0.53	19	0.06	0.11	1.68	0.42	0.00	15	6
651	Potato-mashed-from raw-with milk	1 cup	210	162	4	1	1	4	37	55	100	636	628	0.57	0.60	4	0.19	0.08	2.35	0.49	0.11	17	14
652	Potato-mashed-home recipe-milk/butter	1 cup	210	223	4	9	2	4	35	55	97	620	607	0.55	0.57	42	0.18	0.08	2.27	0.47	0.00	17	13
1092	Potato-o'brien-home recipe	1 cup	194	157	5	2	2	7	30	70	97	421	516	0.91	0.59	93	0.15	0.11	1.96	0.41	0.16	16	32
1093	Potato-scalloped-home recipe	1 cup	245	211	7	9	6	29	26	140	154	821	926	1.40	0.98	47	0.17	0.23	2.58	0.44	0.00	21	26
1094	Potato-scalloped-prepared from mix	1 ounce	28	26	1	1	1	—	4	10	16	97	58	0.11	0.07	6	0.01	0.02	0.29	0.01	0.00	0	1
203	Potted meat-canned-beef/chicken/turkey	1 tbsp	13	30	2	2	1	15	0	—	—	156	—	—	—	—	0.00	0.03	0.20	—	—	—	—
1190	Poultry seasoning	1 tsp	2	5	0	0	—	0	1	15	3	0	10	0.53	0.05	4	0.00	0.00	0.05	—	0.00	—	0
479	Pretzel-dutch-twisted	1 item	16	60	2	1	—	0	12	4	21	258	21	0.20	0.17	0	0.05	0.04	0.70	0.00	0.00	3	0
481	Pretzel-thin-stick	1 item	0	1	0	0	0	0	0	0	0	5	0	0.01	0.00	0	0.00	0.00	0.01	0.00	0.00	0	0
480	Pretzel-thin-twisted	1 item	6	24	1	0	—	0	5	2	5	97	6	0.12	0.07	0	0.02	0.02	0.26	0.00	0.00	1	0
1029	Pricklypears-raw	1 item	103	42	1	1	—	0	10	58	25	5	227	0.31	—	5	0.01	0.06	0.47	—	0.00	—	14
1028	Prunes-canned-heavy syrup pack	1 cup	234	246	2	0	0	0	65	40	61	7	529	0.96	0.45	187	0.08	0.29	2.03	0.48	0.00	0	7
297	Prunes-dried-cooked-with sugar	1 cup	238	295	3	1	0	0	78	51	78	4	741	2.48	0.53	68	0.05	0.22	1.61	0.48	0.00	0	6
305	Prunes-dried-cooked-without sugar	1 cup	212	227	2	0	0	0	60	48	75	4	708	2.35	0.50	65	0.05	0.21	1.53	0.46	0.00	0	6
304	Prunes-dried-uncooked	1 cup	161	385	4	1	0	0	101	82	127	6	1200	3.99	0.85	320	0.13	0.26	3.16	0.43	0.00	6	5
1476	Pudding-banana cream-instant mix-jello	1 ounce	28	106	0	0	0	0	27	1	111	190	1	0.03	—	0	0.00	0.00	0.00	—	—	—	0
1477	Pudding-butterscotch-instant mix-jello	1 ounce	28	105	0	0	0	0	27	1	102	244	1	0.03	—	0	0.00	0.00	0.00	—	—	—	0
90	Pudding-chocolate-cooked-from mix & milk	1 cup	260	320	9	8	4	32	59	265	247	335	354	0.80	—	68	0.05	0.39	0.30	—	—	—	2
87	Pudding-chocolate-home recipe-starch	1 cup	260	385	8	12	8	32	67	250	255	145	445	1.30	—	78	0.05	0.36	0.30	—	—	—	1
91	Pudding-chocolate-instant-from mix	1 cup	260	325	8	7	4	28	63	374	237	322	335	1.30	—	68	0.08	0.39	0.30	—	—	—	2
1923	Pudding-chocolate-sugar free-2% milk	1 serving	133	100	5	3	—	—	14	150	300	310	—	0.72	—	40	0.06	0.26	—	—	—	—	—
1479	Pudding-coconut cream-instant mix-jello	1 ounce	28	117	0	3	1	3	23	9	10	186	55	0.17	0.07	0	0.00	0.00	0.03	0.01	0.08	1	0

Dashes (—) in data spaces indicate that no data were reported.

Item	Food Name	Portion	Weight (g)	Food Energy (kcal)	Protein (g)	Total Fat (g)	Saturated Fat (g)	Cholesterol (mg)	Carbohydrate (g)	Calcium (mg)	Phosphorus (mg)	Sodium (mg)	Potassium (mg)	Iron (mg)	Zinc (cm)	Vitamin A (RE)	Thiamin (mg)	Riboflavin (mg)	Niacin (mg)	Vitamin B6 (mg)	Vitamin B12 (ug)	Folic Acid (ug)	Vitamin C (mg)
1064	Pudding-corn	1 cup	250	273	11	13	6	250	32	100	143	138	402	1.40	1.25	90	1.03	0.32	2.47	0.30	0.23	63	7
1478	Pudding-lemon-instant mix-jello	1 ounce	28	105	0	0	0	0	27	1	111	190	1	0.03	—	0	0.00	0.00	0.00	—	—	—	0
1722	Pudding-rice with raisins	1 cup	265	387	10	8	—	—	71	260	249	188	469	1.10	—	35	0.08	0.37	0.50	—	—	—	0
89	Pudding-tapioca cream-home recipe-starch	1 cup	165	220	8	8	4	80	28	173	180	257	223	0.70	—	60	0.07	0.30	0.20	—	—	—	2
88	Pudding-vanilla (blancmange)-home recipe	1 cup	255	285	9	10	6	36	41	298	232	165	352	0.00	—	82	0.08	0.41	0.30	—	—	—	2
1924	Pudding-vanilla-sugar free-with 2% milk	1 serving	133	90	4	2	—	—	12	150	200	380	—	—	—	40	0.03	0.17	—	—	—	—	—
1030	Pummelo-sections-raw	1 cup	190	72	1	0	0	0	18	8	32	2	410	0.21	0.15	0	0.07	0.05	0.42	0.07	0.00	—	116
1098	Pumpkin pie mix-canned	1 cup	270	281	3	0	0	0	71	100	122	562	373	2.86	0.73	2241	0.04	0.32	1.01	0.43	0.00	95	9
1191	Pumpkin pie spice	1 tsp	2	6	0	0	—	0	1	12	2	1	11	0.34	0.04	0	0.00	0.00	0.04	—	0.00	—	0
1773	Pumpkin-boiled-drained-mashed	1 cup	245	49	2	0	0	0	12	37	74	3	564	1.40	0.56	265	0.08	0.19	1.01	0.11	0.00	21	12
656	Pumpkin-canned	1 cup	245	83	3	1	0	0	20	64	86	12	505	3.41	0.42	5404	0.06	0.13	0.90	0.14	0.00	30	10
1705	Pumpkin-raw-cubed	1 cup	116	30	1	0	0	0	8	24	51	1	1	0.93	0.37	186	0.06	0.13	0.70	0.06	0.00	16	10
1649	Quiche lorraine-frozen dinner-mrs smiths	1 item	269	720	34	41	—	95	54	97	—	1965	610	2.70	—	67	0.33	1.01	6.00	—	—	—	0
1031	Quinces-raw	1 item	92	52	0	0	0	0	14	10	16	4	181	0.64	0.04	4	0.02	0.03	0.18	0.04	0.00	3	14
1972	Quinoa-whole or ground	1 cup	170	636	22	10	1	0	117	102	697	36	1258	15.70	5.61	0	0.34	0.67	4.98	0.38	0.00	83	0
1684	Rabbit-stewed-boneless-skinless	1 serving	85	175	26	7	2	73	0	17	192	32	255	2.01	2.01	0	0.05	0.15	6.09	0.29	5.53	8	0
1659	Radish-daikon-sliced-boiled-drained	1 cup	147	25	1	0	0	0	5	25	35	19	419	0.22	0.19	0	0.00	0.03	0.22	0.06	0.00	26	22
657	Radishes-raw	1 item	5	1	0	0	0	0	0	1	1	1	10	0.01	0.01	0	0.00	0.00	0.01	0.00	0.00	1	1
307	Raisins-seedless	1 cup	145	435	5	1	0	0	115	71	141	17	1089	3.02	0.39	1	0.23	0.13	1.19	0.36	0.00	5	5
308	Raisins-seedless-packet	1 item	14	42	0	0	0	0	11	7	14	2	105	0.29	0.04	0	0.02	0.01	0.12	0.04	0.00	0	0
1032	Raspberries-canned-heavy syrup pack	1 cup	256	234	2	0	0	0	60	27	23	9	241	1.08	0.40	9	0.05	0.08	1.13	0.11	0.00	27	22
310	Raspberries-frozen-sweetened	1 cup	250	258	2	0	0	0	65	38	43	3	285	1.63	0.45	15	0.05	0.11	0.58	0.09	0.00	65	41
309	Raspberries-raw	1 cup	123	60	1	1	0	0	14	27	15	0	187	0.70	0.57	16	0.04	0.11	1.11	0.07	0.00	32	31
453	Ratatouille-stouffer frozen side dish	1 item	142	60	1	3	—	—	9	—	—	1320	505	1.00	—	146	0.03	0.20	1.00	—	—	—	10
312	Rhubarb-cooked from frozen-added sugar	1 cup	240	278	1	0	0	0	75	348	19	2	230	0.50	0.19	17	0.04	0.06	0.48	0.05	0.00	13	8
311	Rhubarb-cooked from raw-added sugar	1 cup	270	380	1	0	0	0	97	211	41	5	548	1.60	0.22	22	0.05	0.14	0.80	0.05	0.00	14	16
1748	Rice bran	1 ounce	28	80	5	0	1	0	16	16	119	5	593	4.56	1.72	0	0.78	0.08	9.66	1.16	0.00	18	0
1975	Rice bran-crude	1 cup	83	262	11	17	3	0	41	47	1392	4	1232	15.40	5.02	0	2.29	0.24	28.20	3.38	0.00	52	0
1724	Rice cake-low sodium	1 item	9	35	1	0	1	0	8	7	10	0	26	0.17	0.08	0	0.00	0.00	0.09	0.01	0.00	1	0
1723	Rice cake-regular	1 item	9	35	1	0	1	0	8	7	10	11	27	0.17	0.08	0	0.00	0.00	0.09	0.01	0.00	1	0
129	Rice-brown-long grain-cooked	1 cup	195	216	5	2	0	0	45	20	161	9	83	0.82	1.23	0	0.19	0.05	2.98	0.28	0.00	8	0
131	Rice-brown-long grain-raw	1 cup	185	685	15	5	1	0	143	43	616	13	413	2.72	3.74	0	0.74	0.17	9.42	0.94	0.00	36	0
1459	Rice-brown-uncle ben's	1 cup	146	220	5	2	0	0	46	16	222	2	172	0.90	—	0	0.18	0.04	4.20	—	—	—	0
1685	Rice-spanish-home recipe	1 cup	245	213	4	4	8	0	41	34	96	774	566	1.50	2.85	162	0.10	0.07	1.70	0.33	2.12	11	37
482	Rice-white-instant-hot	1 cup	165	162	3	0	0	0	35	13	23	5	7	1.04	0.40	0	0.12	0.08	1.45	0.02	0.00	6	0
484	Rice-white-long grain-cooked	1 cup	205	264	6	1	0	0	57	23	95	4	80	2.25	0.94	0	0.33	0.03	3.03	0.19	0.00	7	0
483	Rice-white-long grain-raw	1 cup	185	675	13	1	0	0	148	52	213	9	213	7.97	2.02	0	1.07	0.09	7.76	0.30	0.00	16	0
486	Rice-white-parboiled-cooked	1 cup	175	199	4	0	0	0	43	33	73	6	66	1.97	0.53	0	0.44	0.03	2.45	0.03	0.00	6	0
485	Rice-white-parboiled-dry	1 cup	185	686	13	1	0	0	151	112	252	9	222	6.60	1.77	—	1.10	0.13	6.72	0.65	0.00	31	0
1973	Rice-white-short grain-cooked	1 cup	205	267	5	0	0	0	59	2	67	1	54	2.99	0.82	0	0.34	0.03	3.06	0.12	0.00	3	0
1974	Rice-white-with pasta-cooked	1 cup	202	246	5	6	1	1	43	16	75	1147	85	1.90	0.56	0	0.25	0.16	3.60	0.20	0.12	15	0
1994	Rice-wild-cooked	1 cup	164	166	7	1	0	0	35	5	134	6	166	0.99	2.20	0	0.09	0.14	2.11	0.22	0.00	43	0
169	Roast beef-bottom round-cooked-lean only	1 slice	78	173	25	8	3	75	0	4	212	40	240	2.70	4.27	0	0.06	0.20	3.18	0.28	1.93	9	0
168	Roast beef-bottom round-lean and fat	1 slice	85	222	25	13	5	81	0	5	217	43	248	2.76	4.36	0	0.06	0.21	3.29	0.29	2.04	9	0
166	Roast beef-rib-broiled-lean and fat	1 slice	85	308	18	26	11	73	0	10	140	52	257	1.77	4.27	0	0.07	0.15	2.65	0.25	2.37	5	0
167	Roast beef-rib-broiled-lean only	1 slice	51	122	14	7	3	41	0	5	109	38	192	1.33	3.54	0	0.04	0.11	2.10	0.15	1.49	4	0
487	Roll-brown & serve-enriched	1 item	26	85	2	2	0	0	14	20	23	144	25	0.80	0.19	0	0.10	0.06	0.90	0.02	—	10	0
1902	Roll-cinnamon	1 item	26	100	2	4	1	0	14	8	22	96	36	0.49	0.10	4	0.07	0.07	0.45	0.02	0.00	6	0
492	Roll-cloverleaf-from home recipe	1 item	35	120	3	3	1	0	20	16	36	193	41	0.70	0.26	6	0.12	0.12	1.20	0.02	—	13	0
488	Roll-cloverleaf/pan-commercial-enriched	1 item	28	85	2	2	0	0	15	21	24	155	27	0.80	0.20	0	0.11	0.07	0.90	0.02	—	11	0
1729	Roll-croissant-sara lee	1 item	26	109	2	6	3	29	11	12	32	140	40	1.04	0.18	8	0.28	0.10	1.20	0.02	0.05	9	0
489	Roll-hamburger/hotdog-commercial	1 item	40	114	3	2	1	0	20	54	33	241	37	1.19	0.25	0	0.20	0.13	1.58	0.01	—	15	0
490	Roll-hard-commercial-enriched	1 item	50	155	5	2	0	0	30	24	46	312	49	1.20	0.30	0	0.20	0.12	1.70	0.02	0.00	30	0
491	Roll-submarine/hoagie-enriched	1 item	135	390	12	4	1	0	75	58	115	761	122	3.00	—	0	0.54	0.32	4.50	0.05	—	—	0
1653	Roll-whole wheat-homemade	1 item	35	90	4	1	0	0	18	34	98	197	102	0.80	0.60	0	0.12	0.05	1.10	0.08	0.05	16	0
298	Roselle-raw	1 cup	57	28	1	0	—	0	6	123	21	3	119	0.84	—	16	0.01	0.02	0.18	—	0.00	—	7
1192	Rosemary-dried	1 tsp	1	4	0	0	—	0	1	15	1	1	11	0.35	0.04	4	0.01	—	0.01	—	0.00	—	1
1099	Rutabagas-boiled-drained	1 cup	170	58	2	0	0	0	13	71	83	31	488	0.80	0.51	0	0.12	0.06	1.07	0.15	0.00	26	37
1977	Rye-whole-dry	1 cup	169	566	25	4	0	0	118	56	632	10	446	4.51	6.30	0	0.53	0.42	7.22	0.50	0.00	101	0
1193	Sage-ground	1 tsp	1	2	0	0	0	0	0	12	1	0	7	0.20	0.03	4	0.01	0.00	0.04	—	0.00	—	0

132	Salad dressing-blue cheese	1 tbsp	15	77	1	8	2	9	1	12	11	167	6	0.00	0.00	10	0.00	0.02	0.00	0.01	0.04	1	0
133	Salad dressing-blue cheese-low calorie	1 tbsp	16	10	0	1	1	4	1	10	8	177	5	0.00	—	9	0.00	0.01	0.00	—	—	—	0
1764	Salad dressing-caesar	1 tbsp	15	70	0	7	—	—	1	—	—	—	—	—	—	—	—	—	—	—	—	—	—
134	Salad dressing-french	1 tbsp	16	67	0	6	2	2	3	2	2	214	12	0.10	0.01	3	0.00	0.00	0.00	0.00	0.02	1	0
135	Salad dressing-french-low calorie	1 tbsp	16	22	0	1	0	1	4	2	2	128	13	0.10	0.03	0	0.00	0.00	0.00	0.00	0.00	0	0
1767	Salad dressing-garlic-prepared from mix	1 tbsp	16	83	0	9	1	0	1	3	3	222	6	0.05	0.02	7	0.00	0.00	0.00	0.00	0.00	—	0
1766	Salad dressing-green goddess	1 tbsp	14	68	0	7	1	0	1	2	1	150	9	0.05	0.04	1	0.00	0.01	0.02	0.00	0.04	1	0
144	Salad dressing-home recipe-cooked	1 tbsp	16	25	1	2	1	8	2	13	14	117	19	0.10	0.00	20	0.01	0.02	0.04	0.00	0.00	0	0
136	Salad dressing-italian	1 tbsp	15	69	0	7	1	0	2	1	1	116	2	0.00	0.02	4	0.00	0.00	0.00	0.00	0.02	1	0
137	Salad dressing-italian-low calorie	1 tbsp	15	16	0	2	0	1	1	0	1	118	2	0.00	0.02	0	0.00	0.00	0.00	0.00	0.00	0	0
139	Salad dressing-mayonnaise type	1 tbsp	15	57	0	5	1	4	4	2	4	104	1	0.00	0.03	10	0.00	0.00	0.00	0.00	0.03	1	0
140	Salad dressing-mayonnaise-low calorie	1 tbsp	16	20	0	2	0	2	2	3	4	44	1	0.00	—	12	0.00	0.00	0.00	—	—	—	—
1709	Salad dressing-miracle whip light	1 tbsp	14	45	0	4	—	5	2	—	—	95	—	—	—	—	—	—	—	—	—	—	—
942	Salad dressing-oil/vinegar-home recipe	1 tbsp	16	70	0	8	1	0	0	2	1	0	1	0.00	0.00	0	0.00	0.00	0.00	0.00	0.00	0	0
1765	Salad dressing-ranch style	1 tbsp	15	54	0	6	1	4	1	2	4	97	1	0.03	0.03	13	0.00	0.00	0.00	0.00	0.03	1	0
940	Salad dressing-russian	1 tbsp	15	76	0	8	1	0	2	3	6	133	24	0.10	0.07	32	0.01	0.01	0.10	0.01	0.05	2	1
939	Salad dressing-russian-low calorie	1 tbsp	16	23	0	1	0	1	5	3	6	141	26	0.10	0.02	3	0.00	0.00	0.00	0.00	0.02	1	1
941	Salad dressing-sesame seed	1 tbsp	15	68	1	7	1	0	1	—	—	153	24	0.09	0.02	32	0.00	0.00	0.00	0.00	0.00	0	0
1772	Salad dressing-sweet and sour	1 tbsp	15	29	0	0	0	0	7	1	1	68	14	0.01	0.00	0	0.00	0.00	0.01	0.00	0.00	0	1
142	Salad dressing-thousand island	1 tbsp	16	59	0	6	1	5	2	2	3	109	18	0.10	0.02	15	0.00	0.00	0.00	0.00	0.03	1	0
143	Salad dressing-thousand-low calorie	1 tbsp	15	24	0	2	0	2	3	2	3	153	17	0.10	0.02	15	0.00	0.00	0.00	0.00	0.03	1	0
1775	Salad-carrot raisin-home recipe	1 cup	268	306	4	12	7	33	56	96	130	377	928	3.00	0.54	1100	0.16	0.16	1.00	0.68	0.14	28	12
1887	Salad-chef-with ham and cheese	1 serving	200	196	13	13	7	46	7	227	251	567	415	1.17	1.73	740	0.34	0.24	2.21	0.21	0.47	46	24
1778	Salad-chicken	1 cup	205	502	26	36	4	67	17	128	207	1395	521	3.69	1.95	30	0.47	0.42	7.71	0.34	0.20	39	2
1062	Salad-coleslaw	1 tbsp	8	6	0	0	0	1	1	4	3	2	15	0.05	0.02	7	0.01	0.01	0.02	0.01	0.00	2	3
1575	Salad-crab	1 serving	100	145	12	9	1	69	5	38	129	487	260	0.60	2.78	9	0.06	0.06	1.30	0.12	4.74	35	2
980	Salad-fruit-canned-juice pack	1 cup	249	125	1	0	0	0	33	28	36	13	288	0.62	0.36	149	0.03	0.04	0.89	0.07	0.00	6	8
979	Salad-fruit-canned-water pack	1 cup	245	74	1	0	0	0	19	17	22	7	191	0.74	0.20	108	0.04	0.05	0.92	0.08	0.00	6	5
1826	Salad-green salad-tossed	1 serving	207	32	3	0	0	0	7	26	80	53	356	1.30	0.43	235	0.06	0.10	1.15	0.16	0.00	77	48
1774	Salad-macaroni	1 serving	28	51	1	3	0	1	5	5	12	148	21	0.27	0.09	4	0.03	0.02	0.21	0.02	0.01	2	1
1777	Salad-mandarin orange gelatin	1 serving	28	23	0	0	0	0	6	—	—	14	9	—	—	—	—	—	—	—	—	—	—
655	Salad-potato	1 cup	250	358	7	21	4	171	28	48	130	1323	635	1.63	0.78	82	0.19	0.15	2.23	0.35	0.39	17	25
1900	Salad-taco	1 serving	198	279	13	15	7	44	24	192	143	763	416	2.28	2.68	78	0.10	0.35	2.46	0.21	0.64	40	4
1776	Salad-three bean-alex	1 serving	28	33	1	0	—	—	7	—	—	107	63	—	—	—	—	—	—	—	—	—	—
121	Salad-three bean-canned-del monte	1 ounce	28	22	1	0	0	0	5	10	16	101	38	0.28	0.09	8	0.01	0.01	0.09	0.01	0.01	10	1
1779	Salad-waldorf gelatin	1 serving	28	27	2	0	0	0	5	5	10	16	14	0.11	0.08	5	0.01	0.01	0.05	0.02	0.01	2	1
206	Salami-cooked-beef-4 by ⅛ inch slice	1 slice	23	60	3	5	2	15	1	2	26	270	52	0.50	0.50	0	0.02	0.04	0.75	0.05	1.11	0	4
205	Salami-dry or hard-pork-slice	1 slice	10	41	2	3	1	8	0	1	23	226	38	0.13	0.42	0	0.09	0.03	0.56	0.06	0.28	0	0
1743	Salisbury steak-banquet frozen dinner	1 item	312	390	18	25	7	86	24	90	206	2059	387	3.50	3.61	791	0.16	0.19	3.60	0.36	1.34	48	7
402	Salisbury steak-lean cuisine	1 item	269	280	25	15	—	95	11	—	—	800	650	—	—	—	—	—	—	—	—	—	—
822	Salt-table salt	1 tsp	6	0	0	0	0	0	0	14	—	2132	0	0.00	—	0	0.00	0.00	0.00	0.00	0.00	0	0
943	Sandwich spread-commercial	1 tbsp	15	60	0	5	1	12	3	0	0	153	5	0.00	0.00	0	0.00	0.00	0.00	0.00	0.00	0	0
1744	Sandwich-blt-with mayonnaise	1 item	148	282	7	16	7	44	29	53	89	1222	274	1.50	1.84	174	0.16	0.14	1.60	0.23	0.55	26	13
1745	Sandwich-club	1 item	315	590	36	21	15	93	42	103	394	2601	583	4.30	3.91	350	0.38	0.41	10.20	0.50	1.17	55	27
1906	Sandwich-ham and cheese	1 item	146	353	21	16	6	58	33	130	152	772	290	3.25	1.38	77	0.31	0.49	2.69	0.20	0.54	71	3
1910	Sandwich-roast beef-plain	1 item	139	346	22	14	4	52	34	54	239	792	316	4.23	3.39	21	0.38	0.31	5.86	0.27	1.22	40	2
1911	Sandwich-roast beef-with cheese	1 item	176	402	32	18	9	77	27	183	401	1634	345	5.05	5.37	46	0.38	0.46	5.90	0.34	2.05	41	0
1907	Sandwich-steak	1 item	204	459	30	14	4	73	52	91	297	798	525	5.17	4.54	44	0.40	0.37	7.30	0.37	1.57	89	6
1909	Sandwich-submarine-roast beef	1 item	216	411	29	13	7	73	44	41	193	845	330	2.81	4.39	50	0.42	0.42	5.97	0.32	1.82	45	6
1908	Sandwich-submarine-with coldcuts	1 item	228	456	22	19	7	35	51	189	287	1650	394	2.51	2.58	79	1.00	0.80	5.50	0.13	1.09	54	12
1480	Sanka-decaffeinated coffee-prepared	1 fl oz	30	0	0	0	0	0	0	1	1	0	10	0.01	0.01	0	0.00	0.00	0.05	0.00	0.00	0	0
1033	Sapodilla-raw	1 item	170	140	1	2	0	0	34	36	20	20	328	1.36	0.17	10	0.00	0.03	0.34	0.06	0.00	24	25
1034	Sapotes-raw	1 item	225	302	5	1	—	0	76	88	63	23	774	2.25	—	92	0.02	0.05	4.05	—	0.00	—	45
685	Sauce-barbecue-ready to serve	1 cup	250	188	5	5	1	0	32	48	50	2032	435	2.25	0.50	218	0.08	0.05	2.25	0.19	0.00	10	18
833	Sauce-bearnaise-from dry mix-milk/butter	1 cup	255	701	8	68	42	189	18	230	186	1265	298	0.26	0.77	757	0.08	0.26	0.26	0.08	0.51	10	2
834	Sauce-cheese-from dry mix-milk/butter	1 cup	279	307	16	17	9	53	23	570	437	1566	554	0.27	0.97	117	0.15	0.56	0.32	0.14	1.12	13	2
27	Sauce-chili-bottled	1 tbsp	15	16	0	0	0	0	4	3	8	201	56	0.10	—	21	0.01	0.01	0.20	—	—	—	2
1714	Sauce-chili-low sodium	1 tbsp	14	8	0	0	0	0	2	—	—	10	—	—	—	—	—	—	—	—	—	—	—
835	Sauce-curry-from dry mix-with milk	1 cup	272	269	11	15	6	35	26	484	280	1276	495	1.09	1.09	41	0.11	0.54	0.54	0.11	1.09	16	3
989	Sauce-guava-cooked	1 cup	238	86	1	0	0	0	23	17	26	10	536	0.43	0.41	67	0.06	0.03	1.00	—	0.00	—	348
836	Sauce-hollandaise-dry mix-with milk	1 cup	255	703	8	68	42	189	18	240	194	1134	309	0.23	0.77	696	0.08	0.33	0.23	0.08	0.51	10	2
1122	Sauce-marinara-canned	1 cup	250	170	4	8	1	0	26	45	88	1573	1060	2.00	0.68	240	0.11	0.15	3.98	0.62	0.00	34	32
837	Sauce-mushroom-dry mix-with milk	1 cup	267	227	11	10	5	34	24	302	166	1535	494	0.53	1.34	94	0.19	0.80	4.81	0.19	0.80	40	2

Dashes (—) in data spaces indicate that no data were reported.

Appendix C Table of Food Composition

Item	Food Name	Portion	Weight (g)	Food Energy (kcal)	Protein (g)	Total Fat (g)	Saturated Fat (g)	Cholesterol (mg)	Carbohydrate (g)	Calcium (mg)	Phosphorus (mg)	Sodium (mg)	Potassium (mg)	Iron (mg)	Zinc (cm)	Vitamin A (RE)	Thiamin (mg)	Riboflavin (mg)	Niacin (mg)	Vitamin B6 (mg)	Vitamin B12 (ug)	Folic Acid (ug)	Vitamin C (mg)
348	Sauce-picante-canned	1 fl oz	16	9	0	1	0	0	2	4	8	218	77	0.25	—	23	0.02	0.01	0.22	—	—	—	9
347	Sauce-salsa with green chilies-canned	1 fl oz	16	10	0	1	0	0	2	4	9	111	87	0.28	—	39	0.02	0.01	0.29	—	—	—	9
1360	Sauce-sour cream-from mix-with milk	1 cup	314	509	19	30	16	91	45	546	—	1007	733	0.61	1.37	144	0.13	0.70	0.56	0.13	0.94	16	3
841	Sauce-soy	1 tbsp	18	10	1	0	0	0	2	3	20	1029	32	0.36	0.07	0	0.01	0.02	0.61	0.03	0.00	3	0
1815	Sauce-soy-tamari	1 tbsp	18	11	2	0	0	0	1	4	23	1005	38	0.43	0.08	0	0.01	0.03	0.71	0.04	0.00	3	0
1130	Sauce-spaghetti-tomato based-canned	1 cup	249	271	5	12	2	0	40	70	90	1235	956	1.62	0.52	306	0.14	0.15	3.75	0.88	0.00	54	28
29	Sauce-steak-heinz 57	1 tbsp	15	15	0	0	0	0	3	—	—	265	—	—	—	—	—	—	—	—	—	—	—
838	Sauce-stroganoff-from mix-prepared	1 cup	296	272	12	11	7	39	34	521	302	1829	672	1.33	1.10	127	0.86	0.77	0.76	0.12	0.59	9	1
839	Sauce-sweet/sour-from mix-prepared	1 cup	313	294	1	0	0	0	73	41	188	779	66	1.62	0.09	0	0.01	0.10	0.94	0.31	0.00	2	0
1655	Sauce-tabasco	1 tsp	5	0	0	0	0	0	0	0	1	22	3	0.03	0.01	3	0.00	0.01	0.00	0.01	0.00	1	3
346	Sauce-taco-canned	1 fl oz	16	11	0	1	—	0	2	6	10	128	88	0.30	—	4	0.02	0.01	0.27	—	—	—	6
141	Sauce-tartar-regular	1 tbsp	14	75	0	8	2	9	1	3	4	98	11	0.10	—	3	0.00	0.00	0.00	—	—	—	0
1613	Sauce-teriyaki-bottled-ready to serve	1 tbsp	18	15	1	0	0	0	3	5	28	690	41	0.31	0.02	0	0.01	0.01	0.23	0.02	0.00	4	0
840	Sauce-teriyaki-from mix-prepared-water	1 cup	283	130	4	1	0	0	28	113	215	4791	216	2.80	0.14	0	0.03	0.09	1.30	0.14	0.00	28	0
1710	Sauce-tomato-canned-low sodium-s&w	1 cup	226	90	4	0	0	0	18	32	72	65	838	1.74	0.57	221	0.16	0.14	2.60	0.36	0.00	20	30
1125	Sauce-tomato-canned-salt added	1 cup	245	74	3	0	0	0	18	34	78	1482	908	1.89	0.61	240	0.16	0.14	2.82	0.38	0.00	23	32
1126	Sauce-tomato-spanish-canned	1 cup	244	81	4	1	0	0	18	42	117	1152	900	8.49	0.83	242	0.18	0.15	3.15	0.43	0.00	33	21
1127	Sauce-tomato-with herbs/cheese-canned	1 cup	244	144	5	5	2	—	25	90	132	1325	869	2.12	0.88	240	0.19	0.30	2.95	0.05	0.00	20	25
1128	Sauce-tomato-with mushrooms-canned	1 cup	245	86	4	0	0	0	21	32	78	1107	931	2.18	0.52	233	0.18	0.27	3.10	0.33	0.00	23	30
1129	Sauce-tomato-with onions-canned	1 cup	245	103	4	0	0	0	24	42	96	1350	1012	2.28	0.56	208	0.18	0.33	3.04	0.65	0.00	55	31
1612	Sauce-white-dehydrated-prepared-milk	1 cup	264	240	10	14	6	34	21	425	256	797	443	0.26	0.55	92	0.08	0.45	0.53	0.07	1.06	16	3
728	Sauce-white-medium-with enriched flour	1 cup	250	405	10	31	19	33	22	288	233	796	348	0.50	0.52	115	0.12	0.43	0.70	0.06	0.70	12	2
1654	Sauce-worcestershire	1 tbsp	15	12	0	0	0	0	3	15	9	147	120	0.90	0.03	5	0.00	0.03	0.00	0.00	0.00	0	27
658	Sauerkraut-canned	1 cup	236	45	2	0	0	0	10	71	47	1560	401	3.47	0.45	5	0.05	0.05	0.34	0.31	0.00	56	35
1456	Sausage and gravy-hormel entree	1 ounce	28	31	2	2	1	2	2	29	33	119	84	0.10	0.27	22	0.04	0.06	0.21	0.02	0.07	1	0
204	Sausage-link-cooked-pork	1 item	13	48	3	4	1	11	0	4	24	168	47	0.16	0.33	0	0.10	0.03	0.59	0.04	0.22	0	0
200	Sausage-patty-cooked-fresh pork	1 item	27	100	5	8	3	22	0	9	50	349	97	0.34	0.68	0	0.20	0.07	1.22	0.09	0.47	1	0
207	Sausage-vienna-canned-beef and pork	1 item	16	45	2	4	1	8	0	2	8	152	16	0.14	0.26	0	0.01	0.02	0.26	0.02	0.16	1	0
1194	Savory-ground	1 tsp	1	4	0	0	0	0	1	30	2	0	15	0.53	0.06	7	0.01	—	0.06	—	0.00	—	—
1454	Scalloped potatoes and ham-hormel entree	1 ounce	28	28	2	1	1	4	3	8	23	146	68	0.11	0.17	8	0.05	0.03	0.37	0.02	0.06	6	1
1443	Scallops and shrimp mariner-stouffer	1 item	291	400	23	16	—	—	40	—	—	1120	355	—	—	—	—	—	—	—	—	—	—
400	Scallops/vegetables/rice-lean cuisine	1 item	312	220	17	3	—	20	32	—	—	1200	360	—	—	—	—	—	—	—	—	—	—
1457	Seafood gumbo-hormel entree	1 ounce	28	10	1	0	0	6	1	8	16	146	82	0.20	0.13	—	0.01	0.02	0.22	0.03	0.09	6	0
1918	Seafood newberg-budget gourmet	1 serving	284	350	17	12	34	70	43	100	460	660	704	0.72	4.74	40	0.23	0.26	2.00	0.20	4.67	37	1
1100	Seaweed-agar-dried	1 serving	28	87	2	0	0	0	23	178	15	29	320	6.08	1.65	0	0.00	0.06	0.06	0.09	0.00	165	0
1101	Seaweed-irishmoss-raw	1 ounce	28	14	0	0	0	0	3	20	45	19	18	2.53	0.55	3	0.00	0.13	0.17	0.02	0.00	52	3
1102	Seaweed-kelp (kombu)-raw	1 ounce	28	12	0	0	0	0	3	48	12	66	25	0.81	0.35	3	0.01	0.04	0.13	0.00	0.00	51	1
1103	Seaweed-laver (nori)-raw	1 ounce	28	10	2	0	0	0	1	20	17	14	101	0.51	0.30	148	0.03	0.13	0.42	0.05	0.00	42	11
1104	Seaweed-spirulina-dried	1 ounce	28	82	16	2	1	0	7	34	34	298	387	8.09	0.57	16	0.68	1.04	3.64	0.10	0.00	27	3
1105	Seaweed-wakame-raw	1 ounce	28	13	1	0	0	0	3	43	23	248	14	0.62	0.11	10	0.02	0.07	0.45	0.00	0.00	56	1
1171	Seeds-anise	1 tsp	2	7	0	0	0	0	1	14	9	0	30	0.78	0.11	—	—	—	—	—	0.00	—	—
1166	Seeds-breadfruit-roasted	1 ounce	28	59	2	1	0	0	11	24	50	8	307	0.26	0.29	8	0.12	0.07	2.10	0.12	0.00	17	2
1172	Seeds-caraway	1 tsp	2	7	0	0	0	0	1	14	12	0	28	0.34	0.12	1	0.01	0.01	0.08	—	0.00	—	—
1173	Seeds-celery	1 tsp	2	8	0	1	0	0	1	35	11	3	28	0.90	0.14	0	0.00	0.00	0.01	0.00	0.00	0	0
1176	Seeds-coriander	1 tsp	2	5	0	0	0	0	1	13	7	1	23	0.29	0.08	0	0.00	0.01	0.04	0.00	0.00	0	0
1177	Seeds-cumin	1 tsp	2	8	0	0	—	0	1	20	10	4	38	1.39	0.10	3	0.01	0.01	0.10	—	0.00	—	0
1179	Seeds-dill	1 tsp	2	6	0	0	0	0	1	32	6	0	25	0.34	0.11	0	0.01	0.01	0.06	—	0.00	—	—
1181	Seeds-fennel	1 tsp	2	7	0	0	0	0	1	24	10	2	34	0.37	0.07	0	0.01	0.01	0.12	—	0.00	—	—
1182	Seeds-fenugreek	1 tsp	4	12	1	0	—	0	2	6	11	2	28	1.24	0.09	—	0.01	0.01	0.06	—	0.00	2	0
1186	Seeds-mustard-yellow	1 tsp	3	15	1	1	0	0	1	17	28	0	23	0.33	0.19	0	0.02	0.01	0.26	—	0.00	—	—
1189	Seeds-poppy	1 tsp	3	15	1	1	0	0	1	41	24	1	20	0.26	0.29	0	0.02	0.01	0.03	0.01	0.00	0	0
527	Seeds-pumpkin/squash-dried	1 cup	138	747	34	63	12	0	25	59	1620	24	1114	20.70	10.30	53	0.29	0.44	2.41	0.12	0.00	79	3
1167	Seeds-pumpkin/squash-roasted	1 cup	64	285	12	12	2	0	34	35	59	12	588	2.12	6.59	4	0.02	0.03	0.18	0.02	0.00	6	0
1168	Seeds-sesame-dried-whole	1 cup	144	825	26	72	10	0	34	1404	906	16	674	21.00	11.20	1	1.14	0.36	6.50	1.14	0.00	139	0
1169	Seeds-sesame-roasted-whole	1 ounce	28	161	5	14	2	0	7	281	181	3	135	4.19	2.03	0	0.23	0.07	1.30	0.23	0.00	28	0
528	Seeds-sunflower-dried	1 cup	144	821	33	71	7	0	27	168	1015	4	992	9.75	7.29	7	3.29	0.36	6.48	1.81	0.00	327	2
1170	Seeds-sunflower-oil roasted	1 cup	135	830	29	78	8	0	20	76	1538	4	652	9.05	7.04	7	0.43	0.38	5.58	1.07	0.00	316	2
1980	Semolina	1 cup	167	601	21	2	0	0	122	28	227	2	311	7.28	1.75	0	1.35	0.95	10.00	0.17	0.00	120	0
820	Sesame seed-decorticated	1 tsp	3	16	1	1	0	0	0	4	21	1	11	0.21	0.28	0	0.02	0.00	0.13	0.00	0.00	0	0
1473	Shake 'n bake-package-general foods	1 ounce	28	116	2	4	—	—	18	14	44	984	57	0.71	—	62	0.16	0.18	2.19	—	—	—	0

1107	Shallots-freeze dried	1 tbsp	1	3	0	0	0	0	1	2	3	1	15	0.05	0.02	51	0.00	0.00	0.01	0.02	0.00	1	0
1106	Shallots-raw	1 tbsp	10	7	0	0	0	0	2	4	6	1	33	0.12	0.04	125	0.01	0.00	0.02	0.04	0.00	3	1
85	Sherbet-orange-2% fat	1 cup	193	270	2	4	2	14	59	103	74	88	198	0.31	1.33	39	0.03	0.09	0.13	0.03	0.16	14	4
109	Shortening-vegetable-soybean/cottonseed	1 cup	205	1812	0	205	51	0	0	0	0	0	0	0.00	0.00	0	0.00	0.00	0.00	0.00	0.00	0	0
1492	Shrimp creole-light and elegant	1 item	283	200	11	2	3	293	31	54	225	1045	200	2.50	2.40	889	0.22	0.03	3.26	0.32	1.91	14	1
1919	Sirloin tip/vegetables-budget gourmet	1 serving	284	310	16	18	2	40	21	60	195	570	504	0.36	4.39	150	0.15	0.17	4.00	0.44	1.87	16	2
1626	Sole-light-van de kamp's frozen dinner	1 item	142	293	16	18	0	45	17	39	200	412	453	0.93	0.56	10	0.13	0.13	3.27	0.25	1.35	36	21
557	Sorghum	1 tbsp	21	55	0	0	0	0	14	35	5	2	37	2.60	0.00	0	0.03	0.02	0.00	0.00	0.00	0	0
1981	Sorghum-whole-dry	1 cup	192	651	22	6	1	0	143	54	551	12	672	8.45	—	0	0.46	0.27	5.62	—	0.00	—	0
711	Soup-bean with bacon-canned-with water	1 cup	253	173	8	6	2	3	23	81	132	952	403	2.05	1.03	89	0.09	0.03	0.57	0.04	0.05	32	2
712	Soup-beef broth-canned-ready to eat	1 cup	240	17	3	1	0	0	0	14	31	782	130	0.41	0.00	0	0.01	0.05	1.87	0.02	0.17	5	0
722	Soup-beef broth-dehydrated-cubed	1 item	4	6	1	0	0	0	1	2	8	864	15	0.08	0.01	1	0.01	0.01	0.12	0.01	0.04	1	0
713	Soup-beef noodle-canned-prepared-water	1 cup	244	84	5	3	1	5	9	15	46	952	99	1.10	1.54	63	0.07	0.06	1.07	0.04	0.20	4	0
1338	Soup-beef-chunky-canned-ready to serve	1 cup	240	170	12	5	3	14	20	31	120	866	336	2.33	2.64	261	0.06	0.15	2.71	0.13	0.61	13	7
1337	Soup-black bean-canned-prepared-water	1 cup	247	116	6	2	0	0	20	45	107	1198	273	2.16	1.41	49	0.08	0.05	0.53	0.09	0.02	25	1
825	Soup-cheese-canned-prepared with milk	1 cup	251	230	9	15	9	48	16	288	250	1020	340	0.81	0.69	147	0.06	0.33	0.50	0.08	0.44	10	1
1339	Soup-chicken and dumplings-canned-milk	1 cup	241	96	6	6	1	34	6	15	60	860	116	0.63	0.37	52	0.02	0.07	1.75	0.04	0.16	2	0
826	Soup-chicken broth-canned-prepared-water	1 cup	244	39	5	1	0	1	1	9	73	776	210	0.51	0.25	0	0.01	0.07	3.35	0.02	0.24	5	0
827	Soup-chicken noodle-canned-with water	1 cup	241	75	4	2	1	7	9	17	36	1106	55	0.77	0.40	72	0.05	0.06	1.39	0.03	0.15	2	0
1769	Soup-chicken noodle-low sodium	1 cup	240	91	5	2	1	7	10	17	36	36	106	1.20	0.40	109	0.17	0.14	2.64	0.03	0.14	2	0
724	Soup-chicken noodle-prepared from dry	1 cup	252	53	3	1	0	3	7	33	33	1283	30	0.50	0.20	6	0.07	0.06	0.88	0.01	0.00	2	0
1340	Soup-chicken-chunky-canned-ready to eat	1 cup	251	178	13	7	2	30	17	24	113	887	176	1.73	1.00	130	0.09	0.17	4.42	0.05	0.25	5	1
1770	Soup-chicken-chunky-low sodium	1 cup	251	173	13	5	—	—	15	28	—	78	264	1.76	—	94	0.13	0.25	4.77	—	—	—	2
1341	Soup-chicken/rice-canned-ready to serve	1 cup	240	127	12	3	1	12	13	35	72	888	108	1.87	0.96	586	0.02	0.10	4.10	0.05	0.31	4	4
1342	Soup-chili-beef-canned-prepared-water	1 cup	250	170	7	7	3	13	22	43	148	1035	525	2.13	1.40	151	0.06	0.08	1.07	0.16	0.32	18	4
714	Soup-clam chowder-manhattan style-water	1 cup	244	78	2	2	0	2	12	27	42	578	188	1.63	0.98	96	0.03	0.04	0.82	0.10	4.05	10	4
828	Soup-clam chowder-new england-with milk	1 cup	248	163	9	7	3	22	17	187	157	992	300	1.48	0.80	40	0.07	0.24	1.03	0.13	10.30	10	4
1343	Soup-clam chowder-new england-with water	1 cup	244	95	5	3	0	5	12	44	54	915	146	1.49	0.75	1	0.02	0.04	0.96	0.08	8.00	4	2
1344	Soup-consomme-canned-prepared with water	1 cup	241	29	5	0	0	0	2	10	31	636	154	0.53	0.37	0	0.02	0.03	0.71	0.02	0.00	3	1
1771	Soup-corn-canned-low sodium-campbells	1 serving	305	191	3	5	—	—	31	28	—	33	164	0.80	—	93	0.10	0.15	1.90	—	—	—	6
1345	Soup-crab-canned-ready to serve	1 cup	244	76	5	2	0	10	10	66	88	1234	326	1.22	1.46	50	0.20	0.07	1.34	0.12	0.20	15	0
823	Soup-cream of asparagus-canned-with milk	1 cup	248	161	6	8	3	22	16	175	153	1041	359	0.87	0.93	83	0.10	0.28	0.88	0.06	0.50	30	4
824	Soup-cream of celery-canned-with milk	1 cup	248	164	6	10	4	32	15	186	151	1009	310	0.69	0.20	68	0.07	0.25	0.44	0.06	0.50	9	1
708	Soup-cream of chicken-canned-with milk	1 cup	248	191	7	12	5	27	15	180	152	1046	273	0.67	0.68	94	0.07	0.26	0.92	0.07	0.55	8	1
715	Soup-cream of chicken-canned-with water	1 cup	244	117	3	7	2	10	9	34	37	986	88	0.61	0.63	56	0.03	0.06	0.82	0.02	0.10	2	0
709	Soup-cream of mushroom-canned-milk	1 cup	248	203	6	14	5	20	15	178	156	1076	270	0.59	0.64	38	0.08	0.28	0.91	0.06	0.50	10	2
716	Soup-cream of mushroom-canned-with water	1 cup	244	129	2	9	2	2	9	46	50	1031	101	0.51	0.59	0	0.05	0.09	0.73	0.02	0.05	5	1
831	Soup-cream of potato-canned-with milk	1 cup	248	148	6	6	4	22	17	166	160	1060	323	0.54	0.68	67	0.08	0.24	0.64	0.09	0.50	9	1
832	Soup-cream of shrimp-canned-with milk	1 cup	248	164	7	9	6	35	14	164	337	1036	248	0.59	0.80	54	0.06	0.23	0.53	0.45	1.04	10	1
1346	Soup-escarole-canned-ready to serve	1 cup	248	27	2	2	1	2	2	32	79	3864	265	0.74	2.23	217	0.07	0.05	2.31	0.22	0.50	35	4
829	Soup-gazpacho-canned-ready to serve	1 cup	244	57	9	2	0	0	1	24	37	1183	224	0.98	0.24	20	0.05	0.02	0.93	0.15	0.00	10	3
1347	Soup-lentil with ham-canned-ready to eat	1 cup	248	139	9	3	1	7	20	42	184	1319	357	2.65	0.74	36	0.17	0.11	1.35	0.22	0.30	50	4
717	Soup-minestrone-canned-prepared-water	1 cup	241	82	4	3	1	2	11	34	55	911	313	0.92	0.74	234	0.05	0.04	0.94	0.10	0.00	16	1
1348	Soup-onion-canned-prepared with water	1 cup	241	58	4	2	0	0	8	27	12	1053	68	0.68	0.61	0	0.03	0.02	0.60	0.05	0.00	15	1
723	Soup-onion-dehydrated-packet	1 serving	39	115	5	2	1	2	21	55	126	3493	260	0.58	0.23	1	0.11	0.24	1.99	0.04	0.00	6	1
725	Soup-onion-dehydrated-prepared-water	1 cup	246	27	1	1	0	0	5	12	30	849	64	0.15	0.06	0	0.03	0.06	0.48	0.00	0.00	1	0
830	Soup-oyster stew-canned-prepared-milk	1 cup	245	134	6	8	5	32	10	167	162	1040	235	1.04	10.30	45	0.07	0.23	0.34	0.06	2.63	10	4
1349	Soup-oyster stew-canned-prepared-water	1 cup	241	58	2	4	3	15	4	22	48	981	48	0.99	10.30	7	0.02	0.04	0.23	0.01	2.19	2	3
1350	Soup-pea green-canned-prepared-milk	1 cup	254	239	13	7	4	18	32	173	238	1048	377	2.01	1.76	58	0.16	0.27	1.34	0.10	0.44	8	3
1351	Soup-pea green-canned-prepared/water	1 cup	250	165	9	3	1	0	27	28	124	988	190	1.95	1.71	20	0.11	0.07	1.24	0.05	0.00	2	2
1361	Soup-pea green-low sodium-canned-water	1 cup	250	165	9	3	1	0	27	28	124	33	190	1.95	1.71	20	0.11	0.07	1.24	0.05	0.00	2	2
718	Soup-pea-split-canned-prepared-water	1 cup	253	189	10	4	2	8	28	22	213	1008	399	2.28	1.32	44	0.15	0.08	1.48	0.07	0.00	3	1
1352	Soup-pepperpot-canned-prepared-water	1 cup	241	103	6	5	2	10	9	23	42	970	152	0.89	1.22	87	0.05	0.05	1.22	0.06	0.17	10	1
1354	Soup-tomato beef & noodle-canned-water	1 cup	244	139	4	4	2	5	21	17	56	917	221	1.12	0.75	53	0.08	0.09	1.87	0.09	0.19	7	0
1355	Soup-tomato bisque-canned-prepared-milk	1 cup	251	198	6	7	3	22	29	186	174	1108	604	0.88	0.63	110	0.11	0.27	1.25	0.14	0.44	21	7
1609	Soup-tomato bisque-low sodium-with water	1 cup	247	123	2	3	1	4	24	40	60	30	417	0.82	0.59	72	0.07	0.07	1.15	0.09	0.00	15	6
1356	Soup-tomato rice-canned-prepared/water	1 cup	247	119	2	3	1	2	22	22	33	815	330	0.79	0.51	76	0.06	0.05	1.06	0.08	0.00	14	15
726	Soup-tomato vegetable-prepared-dry	1 cup	253	56	2	1	0	0	10	8	29	1146	103	0.63	0.17	20	0.06	0.05	0.79	0.05	0.00	10	6
710	Soup-tomato-canned-prepared-milk	1 cup	248	161	6	6	3	17	22	159	149	932	449	1.81	0.29	108	0.13	0.25	1.52	0.16	0.44	21	68
719	Soup-tomato-canned-prepared-water	1 cup	244	85	2	2	0	0	17	12	34	871	263	1.76	0.24	69	0.09	0.05	1.42	0.11	0.00	15	66
1358	Soup-turkey noodle-canned-prepared-water	1 cup	244	68	4	2	1	5	9	12	48	815	75	0.94	0.58	29	0.07	0.06	1.40	0.04	0.15	2	0
1610	Soup-turkey noodle-low sodium-with water	1 cup	244	68	4	2	1	5	9	12	48	42	75	0.94	0.58	29	0.07	0.06	1.40	0.04	0.15	2	0
1359	Soup-turkey vegetable-canned-water	1 cup	241	72	3	3	1	2	9	17	40	905	175	0.77	0.61	244	0.03	0.04	1.01	0.05	0.17	5	0

Dashes (—) in data spaces indicate that no data were reported.

Appendix C Table of Food Composition

Item	Food Name	Portion	Weight (g)	Food Energy (kcal)	Protein (g)	Total Fat (g)	Saturated Fat (g)	Cholesterol (mg)	Carbohydrate (g)	Calcium (mg)	Phosphorus (mg)	Sodium (mg)	Potassium (mg)	Iron (mg)	Zinc (cm)	Vitamin A (RE)	Thiamin (mg)	Riboflavin (mg)	Niacin (mg)	Vitamin B6 (mg)	Vitamin B12 (ug)	Folic Acid (ug)	Vitamin C (mg)
1357	Soup-turkey-chunky-canned	1 cup	236	135	10	4	1	9	14	50	104	923	361	1.91	2.12	716	0.04	0.11	3.59	0.31	2.12	11	6
1768	Soup-vegetable beef-canned-low sodium	1 serving	305	165	12	4	1	6	18	49	50	57	455	1.39	1.94	553	0.24	0.33	4.20	0.10	0.39	13	11
720	Soup-vegetable beef-canned-with water	1 cup	245	78	6	2	1	5	10	17	42	960	174	1.13	1.55	189	0.04	0.05	1.03	0.08	0.31	11	2
1687	Soup-vegetable-canned-low sodium	1 cup	240	98	2	0	0	0	14	19	35	38	185	0.96	0.46	371	0.05	0.05	1.20	0.06	0.00	11	3
721	Soup-vegetarian-canned-prepared-water	1 cup	241	72	2	2	0	0	12	21	35	823	209	1.08	0.46	300	0.05	0.05	0.92	0.06	0.00	11	1
1353	Soup-vichyssoise-canned-prepared-milk	1 cup	248	148	6	6	4	22	17	166	160	1060	323	0.54	0.68	67	0.08	0.24	0.64	0.09	0.50	9	1
303	Soursop-raw-pulp	1 cup	225	149	2	1	—	0	38	32	61	32	626	1.35	—	1	0.16	0.11	2.03	0.13	0.00	—	46
1670	Soybeans-dry-cooked	1 cup	180	234	20	10	—	0	19	131	322	4	972	4.90	—	5	0.38	0.16	1.10	—	0.00	—	0
1108	Soybeans-green-boiled-drained	1 cup	180	254	22	12	1	0	20	261	284	25	970	4.50	1.64	29	0.47	0.28	2.25	0.11	0.00	201	31
1109	Soybeans-sprouted-steamed	1 cup	94	76	8	4	0	0	6	56	127	9	334	1.23	0.98	1	0.19	0.05	1.03	0.10	0.00	75	8
404	Spaghetti-beef and mushroom-lean cuisine	1 item	326	280	15	7	—	20	38	—	—	1450	580	—	—	—	—	—	—	—	—	—	—
493	Spaghetti-cooked-firm stage-al dente-hot	1 cup	130	190	7	1	—	0	39	14	85	1	103	1.40	0.70	0	0.23	0.13	1.80	0.08	0.00	16	0
494	Spaghetti-cooked-tender stage-hot	1 cup	140	155	5	1	—	0	32	11	70	1	85	1.30	0.70	0	0.20	0.11	1.50	0.09	0.00	17	0
1494	Spaghetti-light and elegant	1 item	290	290	16	8	—	—	40	100	252	700	273	6.00	—	157	0.25	0.15	3.36	—	—	—	10
496	Spaghetti/tomato/cheese-canned	1 cup	250	190	6	2	1	4	39	40	88	955	303	2.80	—	186	0.35	0.28	4.50	—	—	—	10
495	Spaghetti/tomato/cheese-home recipe	1 cup	250	260	9	9	2	4	37	80	135	955	408	2.30	—	216	0.25	0.18	2.30	—	—	—	13
498	Spaghetti/tomato/meat-canned	1 cup	250	260	12	10	2	39	29	53	113	1220	245	3.30	—	200	0.15	0.18	2.30	—	—	—	5
497	Spaghetti/tomato/meat-home recipe	1 cup	248	330	19	12	3	75	39	124	236	1009	665	3.70	—	1590	0.25	0.30	4.00	—	—	—	22
465	Spinach crepes/cheese sauce-stouffer	1 item	269	415	16	25	—	—	30	—	—	995	440	—	—	—	—	—	—	—	—	—	—
1110	Spinach souffle	1 cup	136	219	11	18	7	184	3	230	231	763	201	1.34	1.29	675	0.09	0.31	0.48	0.12	1.36	62	3
1698	Spinach-canned-dietary pack-low sodium	1 cup	234	45	5	1	0	0	7	194	75	746	538	3.70	0.98	1505	0.04	0.25	0.63	0.19	0.00	136	32
663	Spinach-canned-drained	1 cup	214	50	6	1	0	0	7	271	94	57	740	4.92	0.99	1878	0.03	0.30	0.83	0.21	0.00	209	31
1697	Spinach-canned-solids and liquids	1 cup	234	45	5	1	0	0	7	194	75	746	538	3.70	0.98	1505	0.04	0.25	0.63	0.19	0.00	136	32
661	Spinach-frozen-boiled-chopped	1 cup	205	57	6	0	0	0	11	299	98	176	611	3.12	1.44	1596	0.12	0.34	0.86	0.30	0.00	220	25
662	Spinach-leaf-frozen-boiled-drained	1 cup	190	53	6	0	0	0	10	277	91	164	566	2.89	1.33	1479	0.11	0.32	0.80	0.28	0.00	204	23
660	Spinach-raw-boiled-drained	1 cup	180	41	5	0	0	0	7	245	101	126	839	6.43	1.37	1474	0.17	0.43	0.88	0.44	0.00	262	18
659	Spinach-raw-chopped	1 cup	56	12	2	0	0	0	2	55	27	44	312	1.52	0.30	376	0.04	0.11	0.41	0.11	0.00	108	16
1662	Squash-acorn-baked	1 cup	205	115	2	0	0	0	30	90	93	9	896	1.91	0.35	88	0.34	0.03	1.81	0.40	0.00	38	22
1661	Squash-butternut-baked	1 cup	205	82	2	0	0	0	22	84	55	8	582	1.23	0.27	1435	0.15	0.04	1.99	0.25	0.00	39	31
1660	Squash-hubbard-boiled-mashed	1 cup	236	71	3	1	0	0	15	24	33	12	505	0.67	0.24	946	0.10	0.07	0.79	0.24	0.00	23	15
664	Squash-summer-boiled-sliced	1 cup	180	36	2	1	0	0	8	48	69	2	346	0.64	0.71	52	0.08	0.07	0.92	0.12	0.00	36	10
665	Squash-winter-bake-mashed	1 cup	205	80	2	1	0	0	18	29	41	2	896	0.68	0.53	730	0.17	0.05	1.44	0.15	0.00	57	20
1113	Squash-zucchini-froz-boiled	1 cup	223	38	3	0	0	0	8	38	56	4	433	1.07	0.45	96	0.09	0.09	0.86	0.10	0.00	17	8
1114	Squash-zucchini-italia-canned	1 cup	227	66	2	0	0	0	16	39	66	850	622	1.54	0.59	123	0.10	0.09	1.20	0.35	0.00	69	5
1112	Squash-zucchini-raw-boiled	1 cup	180	29	1	0	0	0	7	23	72	5	455	0.63	0.32	43	0.07	0.07	0.77	0.14	0.00	30	8
1111	Squash-zucchini-raw-sliced	1 cup	130	18	2	0	0	0	4	20	42	4	322	0.55	0.26	44	0.09	0.04	0.52	0.12	0.00	29	12
170	Steak-sirloin-broiled-lean and fat	1 item	85	238	23	15	6	77	0	9	185	54	306	2.56	4.89	15	0.10	0.22	3.29	0.34	2.26	8	0
171	Steak-sirloin-broiled-lean only	1 item	56	116	17	5	2	50	0	6	137	37	226	1.88	3.65	3	0.07	0.17	2.40	0.25	1.60	6	0
172	Steak-top round-broiled-lean and fat	1 slice	85	179	26	7	3	72	0	5	203	51	365	2.39	4.59	0	0.10	0.22	4.98	0.46	2.08	10	0
173	Steak-top round-broiled-lean only	1 slice	68	130	22	4	1	57	0	4	167	42	301	1.96	3.79	0	0.08	0.18	4.11	0.38	1.69	8	0
1035	Strawberries-canned-heavy syrup pack	1 cup	254	234	1	1	0	0	60	33	29	9	218	1.24	0.24	7	0.05	0.09	0.15	0.12	0.00	71	80
314	Strawberries-frozen-sweetened-sliced	1 cup	255	245	1	0	0	0	66	28	32	8	249	1.49	0.14	6	0.04	0.13	1.02	0.08	0.00	38	106
315	Strawberries-frozen-sweetened-whole	1 cup	255	199	1	0	0	0	54	28	31	3	250	1.20	0.13	7	0.04	0.20	0.75	0.07	0.00	10	101
1036	Strawberries-frozen-unsweetened	1 cup	149	52	1	0	0	0	14	24	19	3	221	1.12	0.19	7	0.03	0.06	0.69	0.04	0.00	25	61
313	Strawberries-raw-whole	1 cup	149	45	1	1	0	0	11	21	28	1	247	0.57	0.19	4	0.03	0.10	0.34	0.09	0.00	26	85
1471	Stuffing mix-chicken-general foods	1 ounce	28	107	4	1	0	15	21	29	37	488	77	1.08	0.35	5	0.15	0.09	1.28	0.06	0.05	3	0
1707	Stuffing mix-dry form	1 cup	30	111	4	1	—	—	22	37	57	399	52	1.00	—	0	0.07	0.08	1.00	—	—	—	0
1708	Stuffing mix-prepared	1 cup	140	501	9	31	—	—	50	92	136	1254	126	2.20	—	91	0.13	0.17	2.10	—	—	—	0
385	Subway sandwich-ham and cheese-on wheat	1 item	194	673	39	22	7	73	86	—	—	2508	918	—	—	—	—	—	—	—	—	—	—
1115	Succotash-boiled-drained	1 cup	192	221	10	2	0	0	47	33	225	33	787	2.92	1.22	56	0.32	0.18	2.55	0.22	0.00	63	16
559	Sugar-brown-pressed down	1 cup	220	820	0	0	0	0	212	187	42	66	757	7.50	0.59	0	0.02	0.07	0.40	0.09	0.00	0	0
1760	Sugar-equal-packet size	1 item	1	4	0	0	0	0	1	0	0	0	0	0.00	0.00	0	0.00	0.00	0.00	0.00	0.00	0	0
1759	Sugar-sweet & low-packet size	1 item	1	4	0	0	0	0	1	0	0	4	3	0.00	0.00	0	0.00	0.00	0.00	0.00	0.00	0	0
561	Sugar-white-granulated	1 tbsp	12	45	0	0	0	0	12	0	0	0	0	0.00	0.01	0	0.00	0.00	0.00	0.00	0.00	0	0
563	Sugar-white-powdered-sifted	1 cup	100	385	0	0	0	0	100	0	0	1	3	0.10	0.00	0	0.00	0.00	0.00	0.00	0.00	0	0
1451	Swedish meatballs in sauce-hormel entree	1 serving	28	44	3	3	2	8	2	15	39	165	87	0.49	0.39	11	1.07	0.06	0.53	0.03	0.18	9	0
666	Sweet potato-baked-peeled	1 item	114	117	2	0	0	0	28	32	63	11	397	0.51	0.33	2487	0.08	0.15	0.69	0.28	0.00	26	28
667	Sweet potato-boiled-mashed	1 cup	328	344	5	1	0	0	80	70	88	42	602	1.83	0.87	5594	0.17	0.46	2.10	0.80	0.00	36	56
668	Sweet potato-candied	1 piece	105	144	1	3	1	0	29	27	27	73	198	1.19	0.16	440	0.02	0.04	0.41	0.04	0.03	12	7
669	Sweet potato-canned-mashed	1 cup	255	258	5	1	0	0	59	76	133	191	536	3.39	0.54	3857	0.07	0.23	2.44	0.17	0.00	27	13

670	Sweet potato-canned-vacuum pack	1 cup	200	182	3	0	0	0	42	44	98	106	624	1.78	0.36	1596	0.07	0.11	1.48	0.38	0.00	33	53
1686	Sweetbreads-calf-braised	1 serving	85	143	28	3	—	—	0	—	—	—	—	—	—	—	0.05	0.14	2.50	—	—	—	—
1448	Swiss steak in gravy-hormel entree	1 ounce	28	34	4	2	1	8	1	5	15	110	86	0.46	0.57	76	0.02	0.05	0.91	0.04	0.32	27	0
554	Syrup-chocolate flavored-fudge-thick	1 fl oz	38	125	2	5	3	0	20	48	60	27	107	0.50	0.30	18	0.02	0.08	0.20	—	—	—	0
553	Syrup-chocolate flavored-thin	1 fl oz	38	83	1	0	0	0	22	6	35	20	106	0.60	0.30	0	0.01	0.03	0.20	0.00	0.00	2	0
558	Syrup-corn-table blends-light and dark	1 tbsp	21	60	0	0	0	0	15	9	3	15	1	0.80	0.01	0	0.00	0.00	0.00	0.00	0.00	0	0
560	Syrup-pancake-karo	1 tbsp	21	60	0	0	0	0	15	9	3	35	1	0.80	0.00	0	0.00	0.00	0.00	0.00	0.00	0	0
1634	Syrup-pancake-light-aunt jemima	1 fl oz	39	60	0	0	0	0	15	1	4	18	7	0.05	0.01	0	0.00	0.01	0.00	0.00	0.00	0	0
1667	Taco	1 item	171	370	21	21	11	57	27	221	203	802	473	2.42	3.93	147	0.15	0.45	3.22	0.24	1.04	23	2
744	Taco bell-bean burrito	1 item	168	332	17	12	6	79	43	144	143	1030	405	3.84	3.04	240	0.28	0.60	3.86	0.21	1.00	73	3
745	Taco bell-beef burrito	1 item	110	262	13	10	5	33	29	42	88	746	370	3.05	2.37	42	0.12	0.46	3.23	0.16	0.99	20	1
746	Taco bell-beefy tostada	1 item	225	334	16	17	12	75	30	190	173	870	490	2.45	3.18	383	0.09	0.50	2.85	0.26	1.13	0	4
749	Taco bell-burrito supreme	1 item	225	457	21	22	8	126	43	146	245	367	350	3.80	5.85	216	0.45	0.92	6.17	0.27	1.53	43	8
2018	Taco bell-double beef burrito supreme	1 item	255	457	24	22	10	57	42	145	548	1053	431	3.95	5.93	286	0.43	2.19	3.68	0.35	2.18	132	9
2024	Taco bell-enchirito	1 item	213	382	20	20	9	54	31	269	—	1243	—	2.84	—	290	0.26	0.42	2.32	—	—	—	28
2021	Taco bell-mexican pizza	1 serving	223	575	21	37	11	52	40	257	360	1031	408	3.74	2.32	295	0.32	0.33	2.96	0.27	0.20	113	31
2011	Taco bell-nachos	1 serving	106	346	7	19	6	9	38	191	439	399	159	0.93	2.58	169	0.01	0.16	0.68	0.12	0.62	16	2
2012	Taco bell-nachos bellgrande	1 serving	287	649	22	35	12	36	61	297	—	997	674	3.48	—	341	0.10	0.34	2.17	—	—	—	58
2023	Taco bell-pintos & cheese	1 serving	128	190	9	9	4	16	19	156	175	642	399	1.42	1.08	132	0.05	0.15	0.40	0.19	0.08	98	51
2014	Taco bell-soft taco	1 item	92	228	12	12	5	32	18	116	132	516	178	2.27	1.36	64	0.39	0.22	2.74	0.16	0.31	40	1
2013	Taco bell-taco bellgrande	1 item	163	355	18	23	11	56	18	182	234	472	334	1.92	2.40	254	0.11	0.29	2.02	0.28	0.55	71	5
2022	Taco bell-taco light	1 item	170	410	19	29	12	56	18	155	—	594	316	2.44	—	199	0.20	0.33	2.51	—	—	—	5
2016	Taco bell-taco salad with salsa/no shell	1 serving	530	520	31	31	14	80	30	367	567	1431	1151	5.14	9.14	908	0.26	0.64	3.17	0.78	4.29	99	76
2015	Taco bell-taco salad with salsa/shell	1 serving	595	941	36	61	19	80	63	398	637	1662	1212	7.10	10.30	888	0.51	0.75	4.78	0.88	4.82	111	77
2017	Taco bell-taco salad-no salsa-no shell	1 serving	530	502	30	31	14	80	26	331	567	1056	988	4.54	9.14	572	0.25	0.50	3.17	0.78	4.29	99	74
747	Taco bell-taco-regular	1 item	171	370	21	21	11	57	27	221	203	802	473	2.42	3.93	257	0.15	0.45	3.22	0.24	1.04	23	2
748	Taco bell-tostada-regular	1 item	144	223	10	10	5	30	27	211	116	543	403	1.88	1.90	187	0.10	0.33	1.33	0.17	0.68	75	1
1390	Taco shells	1 item	11	50	1	2	0	0	7	16	25	20	27	0.29	0.14	5	0.03	0.02	0.19	0.04	0.00	3	0
1037	Tamarinds-raw	1 item	2	5	0	0	0	0	1	1	2	1	13	0.06	0.00	0	0.01	0.00	0.04	0.00	0.00	0	0
1474	Tang-instant breakfast drink-orange-dry	1 ounce	28	104	0	0	0	0	26	71	76	13	81	0.03	—	535	0.00	0.00	0.00	—	—	—	107
1038	Tangerines-canned-juice pack	1 cup	249	92	2	0	0	0	24	27	25	13	331	0.67	1.27	212	0.20	0.07	1.11	0.11	0.00	12	85
1039	Tangerines-canned-light syrup pack	1 cup	252	154	1	0	0	0	41	18	25	15	197	0.93	0.61	212	0.13	0.11	1.12	0.11	0.00	12	50
316	Tangerines-raw-peeled	1 item	84	37	1	0	0	0	9	12	8	1	132	0.09	0.20	77	0.09	0.02	0.13	0.06	0.00	17	26
1117	Taro root-cooked-sliced	1 cup	132	187	1	0	0	0	46	24	100	20	638	0.95	0.36	0	0.14	0.04	0.67	0.44	0.00	25	7
1116	Taro root-raw-sliced	1 cup	104	111	2	0	0	0	28	45	87	11	615	0.57	0.24	0	0.10	0.03	0.62	0.29	0.00	23	5
1195	Tarragon-ground	1 tsp	2	5	0	0	—	0	1	18	48	1	48	0.52	0.06	7	0.00	0.02	0.14	—	0.00	—	—
733	Tea-brewed	8 fl oz	237	2	0	0	0	0	1	0	2	7	88	0.05	0.05	0	0.00	0.03	0.00	0.00	0.00	12	0
1877	Tea-herbal-brewed	8 fl oz	237	2	0	0	0	0	0	5	0	2	21	0.19	0.10	0	0.02	0.01	0.00	0.00	0.00	1	0
735	Tea-instant-prepared-sweetened	8 fl oz	259	88	0	0	0	0	22	5	3	8	49	0.05	0.08	0	0.00	0.05	0.09	0.01	0.00	10	0
734	Tea-instant-prepared-unsweetened	8 fl oz	237	2	0	0	0	0	0	5	2	7	47	0.04	0.07	0	0.00	0.01	0.09	0.01	0.00	1	0
1812	Tempeh-soybean product	1 cup	166	330	32	13	2	0	28	154	342	10	609	3.75	3.00	114	0.22	0.18	7.69	0.50	1.66	86	0
1336	Thuringer/cervelat-pork	1 slice	23	77	4	7	3	17	0	3	26	286	62	0.58	0.59	0	0.04	0.08	0.99	0.06	1.27	0	5
821	Thyme-ground	1 tsp	1	4	0	0	0	0	1	26	3	1	11	1.73	0.09	5	0.01	0.01	0.07	—	0.00	—	—
499	Toaster pastries/pop tarts	1 item	50	196	2	6	—	0	35	97	97	230	85	2.00	0.29	96	0.16	0.17	2.10	0.19	0.00	40	0
1817	Tofu-fried	1 piece	13	35	2	3	0	0	1	48	37	2	19	0.63	0.26	0	0.02	0.01	0.01	0.01	0.00	3	0
1818	Tofu-okara	1 cup	122	94	4	2	0	0	15	98	73	11	259	1.59	0.68	0	0.02	0.02	0.12	0.14	0.00	32	0
1816	Tofu-raw-firm	1 cup	252	365	40	22	3	0	11	517	479	35	597	26.40	3.96	43	0.40	0.26	0.96	0.23	0.00	74	1
1671	Tofu-soybean curd	1 piece	120	86	9	5	3	0	3	154	151	8	50	2.30	1.00	0	0.07	0.04	0.10	0.06	0.05	21	0
675	Tomato juice-canned	1 cup	244	42	2	0	0	0	10	22	46	881	537	1.42	0.34	137	0.11	0.08	1.64	0.27	0.00	49	45
75	Tomato juice-low sodium	1 cup	244	42	2	0	0	0	10	22	46	24	537	1.42	0.34	137	0.11	0.08	1.64	0.27	0.00	49	45
1123	Tomato paste-canned-low sodium	1 cup	262	220	10	2	0	0	49	92	207	172	2442	7.83	2.10	647	0.41	0.50	8.44	1.00	0.00	59	111
1699	Tomato paste-canned-salt added	1 cup	262	220	10	2	0	0	49	92	207	2070	2442	7.83	2.10	647	0.41	0.50	8.44	1.00	0.00	59	111
676	Tomato powder	1 ounce	28	86	4	0	0	0	21	47	84	38	547	1.30	0.49	490	0.26	0.22	2.59	0.13	0.00	34	33
1124	Tomato puree-canned-low sodium	1 cup	250	103	4	0	0	0	25	38	100	50	1050	2.33	0.55	340	0.18	0.14	4.29	0.38	0.00	28	88
1700	Tomato puree-canned-salt added	1 cup	250	103	4	0	0	0	25	38	100	998	1050	2.33	0.55	340	0.18	0.14	4.29	0.38	0.00	28	88
1695	Tomato-canned-dietary pack-low sodium	1 cup	240	48	2	1	0	0	10	62	46	31	530	1.46	0.38	144	0.11	0.07	1.76	0.22	0.00	19	36
1119	Tomato-cooked-stewed-home recipe	1 cup	101	80	2	3	1	0	13	26	38	460	249	1.07	0.18	68	0.11	0.08	1.12	0.09	0.00	11	18
1120	Tomato-red-canned-stewed	1 cup	255	66	2	0	0	0	17	84	51	648	609	1.86	0.43	140	0.12	0.09	1.82	0.04	0.00	14	34
672	Tomato-red-canned-whole	1 cup	240	48	2	1	0	0	10	62	46	391	530	1.46	0.38	144	0.11	0.07	1.76	0.22	0.00	19	36
1121	Tomato-red-canned-with green chilies	1 cup	241	36	2	0	0	0	9	48	34	966	258	0.63	0.31	94	0.08	0.05	1.54	0.25	0.00	22	15
1118	Tomato-red-raw-boiled	1 cup	240	65	3	1	0	0	14	14	74	26	670	1.34	0.26	178	0.17	0.14	1.80	0.23	0.00	31	55
671	Tomato-red-ripe-raw	1 item	123	26	1	0	0	0	6	6	30	11	273	0.55	0.11	76	0.07	0.06	0.77	0.10	0.00	19	24
1561	Tomatoes-green-raw	1 item	123	30	1	0	0	0	6	16	34	16	251	0.63	0.09	79	0.07	0.05	0.62	0.10	0.00	11	29

Dashes (—) in data spaces indicate that no data were reported.

Appendix C Table of Food Composition

Item	Food Name	Portion	Weight (g)	Food Energy (kcal)	Protein (g)	Total Fat (g)	Saturated Fat (g)	Cholesterol (mg)	Carbohydrate (g)	Calcium (mg)	Phosphorus (mg)	Sodium (mg)	Potassium (mg)	Iron (mg)	Zinc (cm)	Vitamin A (RE)	Thiamin (mg)	Riboflavin (mg)	Niacin (mg)	Vitamin B6 (mg)	Vitamin B12 (ug)	Folic Acid (ug)	Vitamin C (mg)
1646	Tortilla chips-doritos	1 ounce	28	139	2	7	1	0	19	30	59	180	51	0.50	0.24	5	0.03	0.03	0.04	0.10	0.00	4	0
1391	Tortilla-corn	1 item	30	67	2	1	0	0	13	42	55	53	52	0.57	0.43	5	0.05	0.03	0.38	0.09	0.00	6	0
1669	Tortilla-flour	1 item	30	95	3	2	1	0	17	46	25	113	30	1.10	0.23	0	0.01	0.08	1.00	0.01	0.00	4	0
459	Tuna noodle casserole-stouffer dinner	1 item	163	200	10	9	—	—	18	98	—	670	210	1.15	—	54	0.17	0.23	3.45	—	—	—	—
160	Tuna-salad-celery/mayonnaise/pickle/egg	1 cup	205	350	30	22	4	68	7	41	291	434	—	2.70	—	118	0.08	0.23	10.30	—	—	—	2
1627	Turf and surf-classic lite frozen dinner	1 item	283	250	29	8	—	—	15	—	—	—	—	—	—	—	—	—	—	—	—	—	—
1298	Turkey & gravy-frozen	1 cup	240	160	14	6	2	43	11	33	194	1328	146	2.22	1.68	20	0.06	0.31	4.32	0.23	0.58	10	0
1922	Turkey a la king/rice-budget gourmet	1 serving	284	390	20	18	4	75	36	150	212	740	451	1.08	1.92	100	0.15	4.00	5.00	0.56	0.30	41	2
1622	Turkey breast-le menu frozen dinner	1 item	319	470	27	24	—	—	36	—	—	1165	—	—	—	—	—	—	—	—	—	—	—
1632	Turkey dinner-swanson frozen dinner	1 item	326	340	20	10	6	74	42	84	305	1295	635	2.67	2.64	771	0.26	0.27	7.91	0.56	0.42	42	13
1299	Turkey ham-cured thigh meat	1 slice	28	37	5	1	0	16	0	3	54	283	92	0.79	0.84	0	0.02	0.07	1.00	0.07	0.07	2	0
1300	Turkey loaf-breast	1 serving	28	31	6	0	0	12	0	2	65	406	79	0.11	0.32	0	0.01	0.03	2.36	0.10	0.57	1	0
1301	Turkey pastrami	1 slice	28	40	5	2	1	15	0	3	57	297	74	0.47	0.61	0	0.02	0.07	1.00	0.08	0.07	1	0
457	Turkey pie-stouffer frozen dinner	1 item	284	460	20	26	—	—	35	—	—	1735	270	—	—	—	—	—	—	—	—	—	—
1302	Turkey roll-light	1 ounce	28	42	5	2	1	12	0	11	52	139	71	0.36	0.44	0	0.03	0.06	1.99	0.09	0.07	1	0
1303	Turkey roll-light and dark	1 ounce	28	42	5	2	1	16	1	9	48	166	77	0.38	0.57	0	0.03	0.08	1.36	0.08	0.07	1	0
455	Turkey tetrazzini-stouffer frozen dinner	1 item	170	240	12	14	—	—	17	72	—	620	200	0.60	—	41	0.12	0.24	2.40	—	—	—	—
222	Turkey-breast-no skin-roasted	1 item	612	826	184	5	1	510	0	76	1370	318	1784	9.36	10.60	0	0.26	0.80	45.90	3.42	2.36	38	0
219	Turkey-dark meat-no skin-roasted	1 cup	140	262	40	10	3	119	0	45	286	110	406	3.27	6.25	0	0.09	0.35	5.11	0.50	0.52	13	0
1290	Turkey-giblets-simmered	1 cup	145	242	39	7	2	606	3	19	296	86	290	9.72	5.34	2629	0.07	1.31	6.53	0.47	34.80	501	3
1291	Turkey-gizzard-simmered	1 cup	145	236	43	6	2	336	1	22	186	79	306	7.88	6.03	81	0.05	0.47	4.45	0.17	2.76	75	2
220	Turkey-light meat-no skin-roasted	1 cup	140	219	42	5	1	97	0	27	307	89	426	1.88	2.85	0	0.09	0.18	9.57	0.75	0.52	8	0
221	Turkey-light/dark meat-no skin-roasted	1 cup	140	238	41	7	2	107	0	35	298	99	418	2.49	4.34	0	0.09	0.26	7.62	0.64	0.52	10	0
1292	Turkey-liver-simmered	1 cup	140	237	34	8	3	876	5	15	381	89	272	10.90	4.33	5288	0.07	1.99	8.32	0.73	66.50	932	3
1493	Turkey-sliced-light and elegant	1 item	227	230	20	5	—	—	25	18	121	1020	280	1.00	—	171	0.12	0.14	4.60	—	—	—	1
1949	Turkey-thin sliced-smoked-land o frost	1 serving	28	50	5	3	1	23	1	40	58	283	80	0.36	0.84	0	0.00	0.03	1.20	0.12	0.10	2	0
1196	Turmeric-ground	1 tsp	2	8	0	0	—	0	1	4	6	1	56	0.91	0.10	—	0.00	0.01	0.11	—	0.00	0	1
679	Turnip greens-frozen-boiled	1 cup	164	49	5	1	0	0	8	249	56	25	367	3.18	0.67	1309	0.09	0.12	0.77	0.11	0.00	65	36
678	Turnip greens-raw-boiled	1 cup	144	29	2	0	0	0	6	197	42	42	292	1.15	0.20	792	0.07	0.10	0.59	0.26	0.00	171	40
677	Turnips-boiled-drained-diced	1 cup	156	28	1	0	0	0	8	34	30	78	211	0.34	0.31	0	0.04	0.04	0.47	0.11	0.00	14	18
1403	Turnover-apple	1 ounce	28	85	1	5	1	1	11	4	11	109	14	0.31	0.05	2	0.03	0.02	0.33	0.01	0.03	1	0
1404	Turnover-cherry	1 ounce	28	84	1	5	1	4	11	4	14	124	20	0.23	0.06	12	0.02	0.02	0.21	0.01	0.00	1	0
1405	Turnover-lemon	1 ounce	28	93	1	5	1	7	12	4	18	95	14	0.39	0.08	12	0.06	0.03	0.57	0.01	0.06	1	0
1762	Twinkie-hostess	1 item	42	143	1	4	—	21	26	19	—	189	—	0.55	—	8	0.06	0.06	0.50	—	—	—	0
1903	Vanilla-pure	1 tsp	5	14	0	0	0	0	1	0	—	0	0	0.00	—	0	0.00	0.00	0.00	—	0.00	—	0
1446	Veal parmigiana	1 item	213	296	24	14	9	162	17	97	401	973	466	2.30	3.63	123	0.30	0.38	6.80	0.43	1.21	25	6
1629	Veal steak-classic lite frozen dinner	1 item	312	280	25	8	6	60	27	171	299	1738	932	3.58	4.18	241	0.36	0.43	6.51	0.53	0.85	62	33
208	Veal-leg-top round-pan fried	1 serving	85	179	27	7	3	89	0	5	237	64	362	0.75	2.75	0	0.06	0.30	1.00	0.41	1.23	13	0
209	Veal-rib-separable lean only-braised	1 serving	85	185	29	7	2	123	0	20	186	84	270	1.23	5.08	0	0.05	0.26	6.72	0.29	1.30	14	0
1505	Veal-shoulder-arm-lean only-roasted	1 serving	85	139	22	5	2	93	0	23	192	77	302	0.98	3.67	0	0.06	0.28	7.00	0.25	1.33	15	0
1131	Vegetable juice-canned	1 cup	242	46	2	0	0	0	11	27	41	883	467	1.02	0.48	283	0.10	0.07	1.76	0.34	0.00	51	67
118	Vegetable juice-snap e tom-tomato	1 cup	243	46	2	0	0	0	9	37	41	1298	688	1.94	0.49	103	0.10	0.07	2.43	0.34	0.00	51	10
15	Vegetable juice-v-8 cocktail-low sodium	1 cup	243	51	0	0	0	0	10	39	—	58	571	1.46	—	437	0.05	0.07	1.94	—	0.00	—	53
1434	Vegetable juice-v8-regular	1 cup	243	49	0	0	0	0	10	29	41	819	513	1.46	0.49	342	0.05	0.05	1.70	0.34	0.00	51	49
1615	Vegetable lasagna-le menu frozen dinner	1 item	312	400	15	24	9	39	30	296	274	1135	519	3.18	1.45	723	0.23	0.47	3.27	0.34	0.20	78	62
356	Vegetable spray-pam-butter flavored	1 serving	1	7	0	1	0	0	0	0	0	0	0	0.00	—	0	—	—	—	—	—	—	0
357	Vegetable spray-pam-unflavored	1 serving	1	7	0	1	0	0	0	0	0	0	0	0.00	—	0	—	—	—	—	—	—	0
1132	Vegetables-mixed-canned-drained	1 cup	163	77	4	0	0	0	15	44	69	243	474	1.71	0.67	1899	0.08	0.08	0.94	0.13	0.00	39	8
680	Vegetables-mixed-frozen-boiled	1 cup	182	107	5	0	0	0	24	46	93	64	308	1.49	0.89	778	0.13	0.22	1.55	0.14	0.00	35	6
1733	Venison-dried-salted	1 serving	100	142	31	1	—	—	0	60	298	—	—	1.90	—	—	0.09	0.34	10.00	—	—	—	—
1732	Venison-roasted	1 slice	100	146	30	2	2	82	0	20	264	70	336	3.50	4.52	0	0.37	0.28	7.40	0.26	6.22	7	0
727	Vinegar-cider	1 tbsp	15	0	0	0	0	0	1	1	1	0	15	0.10	0.02	0	0.00	0.00	0.00	0.00	0.00	0	0
1673	Vinegar-distilled	1 cup	240	29	0	0	0	0	12	14	22	2	36	1.44	0.00	0	0.00	0.00	0.00	0.00	0.00	0	0
500	Waffles-enriched-from home recipe	1 item	75	245	7	13	2	45	26	154	135	445	129	1.48	0.65	28	0.18	0.24	1.46	0.05	0.37	14	0
501	Waffles-enriched-from mix-egg & milk	1 item	75	205	7	8	3	45	27	179	257	514	146	1.00	—	34	0.14	0.22	0.90	—	—	—	0
1392	Waffles-frozen	1 item	37	103	2	4	—	0	16	30	141	256	78	1.80	0.30	95	0.17	0.20	1.93	0.10	—	1	0
1939	Waffles-oat bran-no cholesterol-eggo	1 item	39	110	3	4	1	0	16	20	135	220	194	1.80	0.67	100	0.15	0.17	0.78	0.20	0.60	16	0
1413	Water-mineral-perrier	1 cup	237	0	0	0	0	0	0	32	0	3	0	0.00	0.00	0	0.00	0.00	0.00	0.00	0.00	0	0
1821	Water-municipal tap	1 cup	237	0	0	0	0	0	0	5	0	7	1	0.01	0.06	0	0.00	0.00	0.00	0.00	0.00	0	0
1134	Waterchestnuts-chinese-canned	1 cup	140	70	1	0	0	0	17	6	28	12	164	1.22	0.54	1	0.02	0.03	0.50	0.22	0.00	8	2

1133	Waterchestnuts-chinese-raw	1 cup	124	131	2	0	0	0	30	14	78	17	724	0.07	0.62	0	0.17	0.25	1.24	0.41	0.00	20	5
1135	Watercress-raw	1 cup	34	4	1	0	0	0	0	40	20	14	112	0.06	0.04	160	0.03	0.04	0.07	0.04	0.00	3	15
318	Watermelon-raw	1 cup	160	51	1	1	—	0	12	13	14	3	186	0.27	0.11	59	0.13	0.03	0.32	0.23	0.00	4	15
756	Wendys-double hamburger	1 item	226	540	34	27	11	122	40	102	314	791	569	5.95	5.68	31	0.36	0.39	7.57	0.54	4.07	27	1
755	Wendys-single hamburger	1 item	218	511	26	27	10	86	40	96	233	825	479	4.92	4.87	93	0.42	0.38	7.28	0.33	2.38	36	3
757	Wendys-triple hamburger	1 item	259	693	50	42	16	142	29	65	393	713	785	8.33	10.80	47	0.31	0.56	11.00	0.62	4.92	31	1
1989	Wheat bran-crude	1 cup	60	130	9	3	0	0	39	44	608	2	710	6.34	4.36	0	0.31	0.35	8.15	0.78	0.00	48	0
1990	Wheat germ-crude	1 cup	115	414	27	11	2	0	60	44	968	14	1026	7.20	14.10	0	2.17	0.57	7.84	1.50	0.00	324	0
1988	Wheat-durum	1 cup	192	651	26	5	1	0	137	65	975	3	827	6.76	7.98	0	0.80	0.23	12.90	0.80	0.00	83	0
1983	Wheat-hard red-spring	1 cup	192	632	30	4	1	0	131	48	637	4	653	6.92	5.34	0	0.97	0.21	11.00	0.65	0.00	83	0
1984	Wheat-hard red-winter	1 cup	192	628	24	3	1	0	137	56	552	4	697	6.12	5.08	0	0.74	0.22	10.50	0.58	0.00	72	0
1986	Wheat-hard white	1 cup	192	657	22	3	1	0	146	61	682	4	829	8.76	6.39	0	0.74	0.21	8.41	0.71	0.00	72	0
1985	Wheat-soft red-winter	1 cup	168	556	17	3	0	0	125	46	828	4	667	5.39	4.41	0	0.66	0.16	8.06	0.46	0.00	68	0
1987	Wheat-soft white	1 cup	168	571	18	3	1	0	127	57	675	3	730	9.02	5.82	0	0.69	0.18	8.01	0.63	0.00	68	0
1993	Wheat-sprouted	1 cup	108	214	8	1	0	0	46	30	216	18	182	2.32	1.79	0	0.24	0.17	3.33	0.29	0.00	41	3
915	Whey-acid-dry	1 tbsp	3	10	0	0	0	0	2	59	39	28	66	0.04	0.18	1	0.02	0.06	0.03	0.02	0.07	1	0
913	Whey-acid-fluid	1 cup	246	59	2	0	0	1	13	253	191	118	352	0.20	1.06	5	0.10	0.34	0.19	0.10	0.44	5	0
916	Whey-sweet-dry	1 tbsp	8	26	1	0	0	0	6	59	70	80	155	0.07	0.15	1	0.04	0.17	0.09	0.04	0.18	1	0
914	Whey-sweet-fluid	1 cup	246	66	2	1	1	5	13	115	112	132	396	0.15	0.32	12	0.09	0.39	0.18	0.08	0.68	2	0
857	Whiskey/gin/rum/vodka-100 proof	1 fl oz	28	82	0	0	0	0	0	0	1	0	0	0.01	0.01	0	0.00	0.00	0.00	0.00	0.00	0	0
687	Whiskey/gin/rum/vodka-80 proof	1 fl oz	28	64	0	0	0	0	0	0	1	0	1	0.03	0.02	0	0.00	0.00	0.00	0.00	0.00	0	0
688	Whiskey/gin/rum/vodka-86 proof	1 fl oz	28	70	0	0	0	0	0	0	1	0	1	0.01	0.01	0	0.00	0.00	0.01	0.00	0.00	0	0
689	Whiskey/gin/rum/vodka-90 proof	1 fl oz	28	73	0	0	0	0	0	0	0	1	0	0.00	0.00	0	0.00	0.00	0.00	0.00	0.00	0	0
856	Whiskey/gin/rum/vodka-94 proof	1 fl oz	28	77	0	0	0	0	0	0	1	0	0	0.01	0.01	0	0.00	0.00	0.00	0.00	0.00	0	0
1811	Wine cooler-white wine and 7up	1 serving	102	55	0	0	0	0	6	6	7	7	41	0.19	0.06	0	0.00	0.00	0.04	0.01	0.00	0	2
861	Wine-california/red-glassful	1 item	102	85	0	0	0	0	3	8	13	10	116	0.97	0.10	0	0.01	0.03	0.08	0.04	0.01	1	0
690	Wine-dessert	1 fl oz	30	46	0	0	0	0	4	2	3	3	28	0.07	0.02	0	0.01	0.01	0.06	0.00	0.00	0	0
859	Wine-madeira-glassful	1 item	100	105	0	0	0	0	1	8	9	5	92	0.24	0.07	0	0.02	0.02	0.21	0.00	0.00	0	0
860	Wine-muscatel/port-glassful	1 item	100	158	0	0	0	0	14	8	9	4	75	1.61	0.06	0	0.01	0.01	0.20	0.05	0.00	2	0
691	Wine-red-table	1 fl oz	30	21	0	0	0	0	1	2	4	19	41	0.13	0.03	0	0.00	0.01	0.02	0.01	0.00	1	0
1881	Wine-rose-table	1 fl oz	30	21	0	0	0	0	0	2	4	1	29	0.11	0.02	0	0.00	0.01	0.02	0.01	0.00	0	0
862	Wine-sauterne-glassful	1 item	100	84	0	0	0	0	4	8	14	2	89	0.41	0.07	0	0.00	0.02	0.07	0.02	0.01	1	0
863	Wine-sherry-dry-glassful	1 item	60	84	0	0	0	0	5	5	8	2	45	0.25	0.04	0	0.01	0.01	0.10	0.01	0.01	1	0
864	Wine-vermouth-dry-glassful	1 item	100	105	0	0	0	0	1	8	14	4	75	0.41	0.07	0	0.01	0.01	0.20	0.02	0.01	1	0
865	Wine-vermouth-sweet-glassful	1 item	100	167	0	0	0	0	12	8	9	9	92	0.24	0.07	0	0.02	0.02	0.21	0.00	0.00	0	0
1481	Wine-white-table	1 fl oz	30	20	0	0	0	0	0	3	4	1	24	0.09	0.02	0	0.00	0.00	0.02	0.00	0.00	0	0
1078	Yam-mountain-hawaii-steamed	1 cup	145	119	3	0	0	0	29	11	57	18	717	0.62	0.46	0	0.13	0.02	0.19	0.30	0.00	18	0
1136	Yams-boiled or baked-drained	1 cup	136	158	2	0	0	0	38	19	66	11	911	0.70	0.27	0	0.13	0.04	0.75	0.31	0.00	22	17
1621	Yankee pot roast-le menu frozen dinner	1 item	312	360	27	15	—	—	29	—	—	830	—	—	—	—	—	—	—	—	—	—	—
729	Yeast-baker's-dry-active-package	1 serving	7	20	3	0	0	0	3	3	90	1	140	1.10	—	0	0.16	0.38	2.60	0.14	0.00	286	0
730	Yeast-brewer's-dry	1 tbsp	8	25	3	0	0	0	3	17	140	9	152	1.40	0.64	0	1.25	0.34	3.00	0.20	0.00	313	0
92	Yogurt-fruit flavors-lowfat-added solids	1 cup	227	231	10	2	2	10	43	345	271	133	442	0.16	1.68	31	0.08	0.40	0.22	0.09	1.06	21	2
1938	Yogurt-original coffee-lowfat-dannon	1 serving	227	200	10	3	2	11	34	389	306	140	498	0.16	1.88	30	0.10	0.46	0.24	0.10	1.20	24	2
93	Yogurt-plain-lowfat-milk solids added	1 cup	227	144	12	4	2	14	16	415	326	159	531	0.18	2.02	45	0.10	0.49	0.26	0.11	1.28	25	2
94	Yogurt-plain-nonfat-milk solids added	1 cup	227	127	13	0	0	4	17	452	355	174	579	0.20	2.20	5	0.11	0.53	0.28	0.12	1.39	28	2
95	Yogurt-plain-whole milk-no solids	1 cup	227	139	8	7	5	29	11	274	215	105	351	0.11	1.34	84	0.07	0.32	0.17	0.07	0.84	17	1
406	Zucchini lasagna-lean cuisine	1 item	312	260	20	7	—	20	28	—	—	1050	570	—	—	—	—	—	—	—	—	—	—
1625	Zucchini romano-le menu frozen dinner	1 item	234	350	17	19	—	—	27	—	—	680	—	—	—	—	—	—	—	—	—	—	—

Dashes (—) in data spaces indicate that no data were reported.

Fiber Content of Foods

Food	Serving Size	Weight (g)	Dietary Fiber (g/serving) Insoluble	Soluble	Total
Bread, cereal, rice, and pasta					
Biscuits, baking powder	1	28	0.5	0.2	0.7
Bread, French	1 slice	35	0.7	0.3	1.0
Bread, white wheat, regular slice	1 slice	28	0.5	0.2	0.7
Bun, hamburger	1 bun	40	0.7	0.3	1.0
Cake, yellow, 1⁄16 of round cake	1 piece	75	0.8	0.2	1.0
Cereal, All Bran	1⁄3 cup	28	7.8	0.6	8.4
Cereal, 40% bran flakes	1 cup	39	6.8	0.8	7.6
Cereal, cornflakes	1 cup	25	1.0	0.1	1.1
Cereal, Cream of Wheat, quick, cooked	1 cup	245	1.5	0.4	1.9
Cereal, Frosted Miniwheats	1 cup	55	4.1	0.4	4.5
Cereal, Honey Smacks	3⁄4 cup	28	0.5	0.1	0.6
Cereal, oat bran, uncooked	1⁄3 cup	28	3.0	1.8	4.8
Cereal, oatmeal, old fashion, cooked	1 cup	240	2.7	1.7	4.4
Cereal, Product 19	3⁄4 cup	28	1.4	0.1	1.5
Cereal, Rice Krispies	1 cup	28	0.4	0.1	0.5
Cereal, shredded wheat	1 biscuit	25	2.5	0.3	2.8
Cereal, Special K	1 1⁄3 cup	28	0.7	0.1	0.8
Cereal, Total	1 cup	33	1.0	tr	1.0
Cereal, Wheaties	1 cup	28	2.7	0.5	3.2
Cookies, ginger snaps	10 cookies	70	0.9	0.4	1.3
Cookies, plain sugar, medium size	2 cookies	16	0.1	0.1	0.2
Corn bread	1 piece	55	1.5	0.1	1.6
Cracker, graham, plain	2 squares	14	0.3	0.1	0.4
Cracker, saltine	4 crackers	11	0.2	0.1	0.3
Flour, all-purpose white wheat	1 cup	115	2.2	1.1	3.3
Ice cream cone	1 cone	12	0.3	0.1	0.4
Macaroni, cooked	1 cup	130	2.2	0.3	2.5
Muffin, English	1	57	1.3	0.4	1.7
Muffin, plain	1	40	0.5	0.1	0.6
Noodles, egg, cooked	1 cup	160	2.2	0.5	2.7
Pie crust	1 pie shell	180	3.2	1.0	4.2
Rice, medium grain, regular, cooked	1 cup	175	1.1	0.1	1.2
Spaghetti, cooked, tender stage	1 cup	140	1.5	0.6	2.1
Sweet roll, cinnamon	1 rectangle	75	1.2	0.5	1.7
Taco shell	1	11	0.7	0.1	0.8
Tortilla, flour	1	28	0.3	0.1	0.4
Wheat germ	1 tbsp	6	0.7	0.1	0.8

Food	Serving Size	Weight (g)	Dietary Fiber (g/serving) Insoluble	Soluble	Total
Vegetables					
Asparagus, whole spears, canned	1 cup	244	3.0	0.9	3.9
Avocado	½ avocado	120	3.1	1.6	4.7
Bean sprouts, canned	½ cup	62	0.6	0.1	0.7
Beans, green, whole cut, canned	1 cup	135	1.8	0.6	2.4
Beets, cut, canned	1 cup	170	2.2	0.7	2.9
Broccoli, fresh, cooked, ½ in. pieces	1 cup	155	4.8	0.6	5.4
Brussels sprouts, frozen, cooked	1 cup	155	5.5	0.8	6.3
Cabbage, raw, shredded	1 cup	80	1.3	0.1	1.4
Carrots, raw, peeled	1 carrot	81	1.9	0.2	2.1
Cauliflower, fresh, cooked, drained	1 cup	125	2.3	0.4	2.7
Celery, raw, chopped	1 cup	120	2.0	0.1	2.1
Corn, whole kernel, frozen, cooked	1 cup	165	3.3	0.1	3.4
Cucumber, raw, unpeeled	9 slices	28	0.2	tr	0.3
Cucumber, raw, peeled	9 slices	28	0.2	tr	0.2
Mushrooms, canned	½ cup	78	1.8	0.2	2.0
Onion, yellow, raw, chopped	1 tbsp	10	0.2	tr	0.2
Peas, green, canned	1 cup	170	5.0	0.6	5.6
Green pepper, raw, chopped	1 cup	150	2.3	0.3	2.6
Potato, baked, with skin	1	202	3.7	1.2	4.9
Potato, boiled, cubed, without skin	1 cup	155	1.5	0.4	1.9
Potato, french fries, 2 to 3½ in.	10 strips	50	0.9	0.2	1.1
Pumpkin, canned	1 cup	245	5.8	1.3	7.1
Radish, red, raw	10 radishes	50	0.7	tr	0.7
Squash, zucchini, raw	1 cup	130	1.1	0.1	1.2
Sweet potato, cut, canned	1 cup	200	2.6	0.7	3.3
Tomatoes, canned	1 cup	241	1.4	0.4	1.8
Turnip greens, frozen, cooked	1 cup	165	3.9	0.3	4.2
Vegetarian vegetable soup, canned	1 cup	245	1.6	0.6	2.2
Fruits					
Apple, unpeeled, large (2½ per pound)	1	180	3.3	0.3	3.6
Apple, peeled, large (2½ per pound)	1	180	2.3	0.3	2.6
Apricots, canned in syrup	1 cup	258	3.4	1.3	4.7
Banana	1	175	2.1	0.8	2.9
Blueberries, fresh	1 cup	145	3.6	0.4	4.0
Cantaloupe, raw, cubed	1 cup	160	1.0	0.2	1.2
Cherries, tart, canned	1 cup	244	1.8	0.4	2.2
Grapefruit, with membrane	½	184	2.0	0.5	2.5
Grapefruit, sections	1 cup	200	0.7	0.2	0.9
Grapes, Thompson green, seedless	10 grapes	50	0.4	0.1	0.5
Nectarine, unpeeled	1	150	1.2	0.6	1.8

Food	Serving Size	Weight (g)	Dietary Fiber (g/serving)		
			Insoluble	Soluble	Total
Fruits					
Orange, large	1	200	2.7	1.1	3.8
Pear, canned	1 cup	244	3.5	0.8	4.3
Pear, Barlett, fresh, unpeeled	1	180	4.2	0.8	5.0
Pineapple, canned	1 cup	246	1.5	0.2	1.7
Plum, Friar, fresh, unpeeled	1	66	0.6	0.2	0.8
Strawberries, fresh	1 cup	149	2.1	0.6	2.7
Tangerine	1	135	1.9	0.5	2.4
Watermelon, raw, cubed	1 cup	160	0.5	0.1	0.6
Beans and Nuts					
Almonds, with skin	15 nuts	15	5.0	0.6	5.6
Kidney beans, canned	1 cup	255	10.2	2.9	13.1
Lima beans, green, canned	1 cup	170	6.4	0.7	7.1
Peanuts, roasted in shell	10 nuts	27	1.8	0.1	1.9
Peanut butter	1 tbsp	16	1.0	0.1	1.1
Pork and beans, canned in tomato sauce	1 cup	255	7.7	3.4	11.1
Walnuts, English, chopped	1 cup	120	4.5	0.1	4.6
Fats, oils, and sweets					
Catsup	1 tbsp	15	0.1	0.1	0.2
Olives, green, with pimento	4 olives	26	0.5	0.1	0.6
Olives, black	10 olives	40	0.9	tr	0.9
Pickle, dill	1 pickle	65	0.7	tr	0.8

Data source: Marlett, J.A. 1992. Content and composition of 117 frequently consumed foods. *Journal of the American Dietetic Association* 92:175–186.

APPENDIX E

Chemical Structures of the Vitamins

The fat-soluble vitamins

Vitamin E

(all- *trans* retinoids)
Vitamin A

Vitamin D

(menadione)

(phylloquinone)
Vitamin K

The water-soluble vitamins

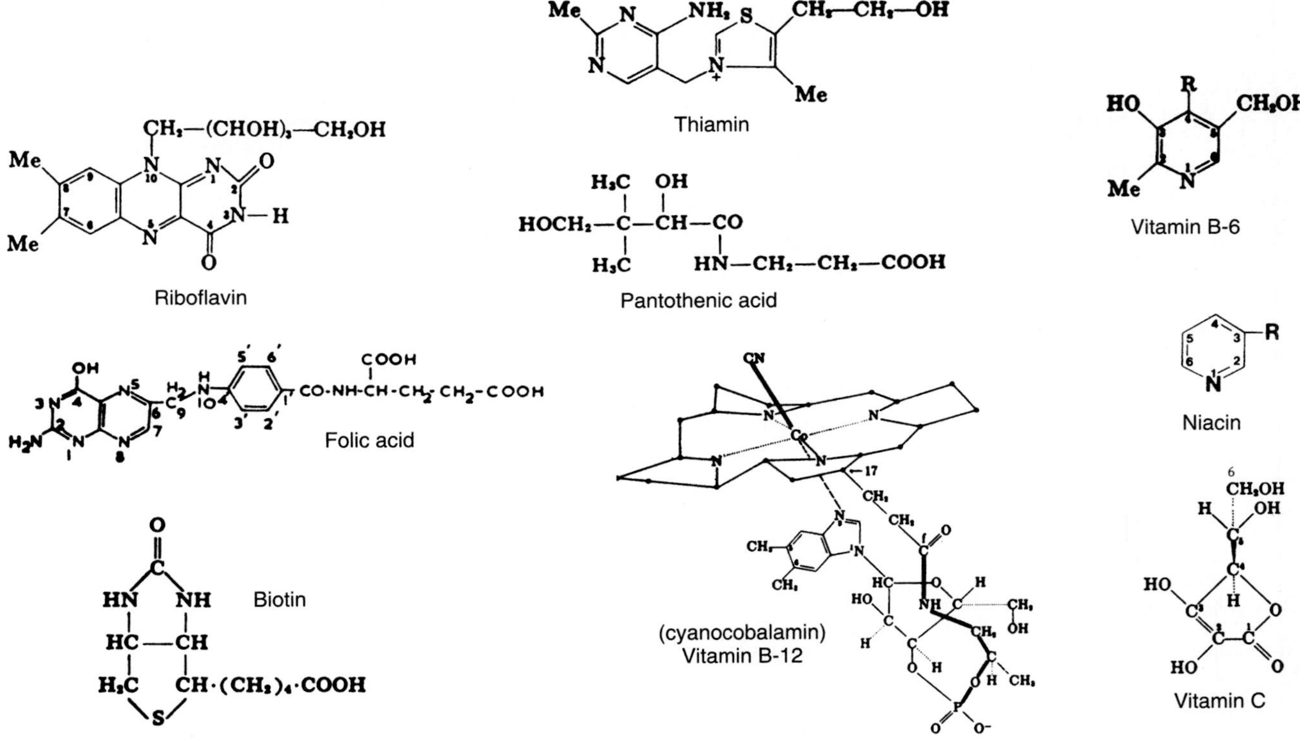

Me = methyl group (CH_3) R = group that can vary

Reprinted from Journal of Nutrition. 1990. Nomenclature policy: generic descriptors and trivial names for vitamins and related compounds.

Credits

Text and Art Credits

Chapter 1
Slice of Life from Ron Paquin, Robert Doherty, *Not First in Nobody's Heart: The Life Story of a Contemporary Chippewa.* 1992. Iowa State U. Press, Ames, IA
Fig. 1.12: Adapted from Mertz, W. 1983. "The Significance of trace elements for health. *Nutrition Today* 18(no.5):27. Reproduced with permission of *Nutrition Today Magazine*, P.O. Box 1829, Annapolis, MD 21404.
Fig. 1.14: Adapted from Olson, R.E. 1978. Clinical nutrition - where human ecology and internal medicine meet. *Nutrition Today* 13(no.4):18-28. Reproduced with permission of *Nutrition Today Magazine*, P.O. Box 1829, Annapolis, MD 21404.

Chapter 2
Table 2.1: McLaren, D.S. 1988. *Modern Nutrition in Health and Disease*, eds. M.E. Shils, V.R. Young, Lea & Febiger, Philadelphia; Heymsfield, S.B. and P.J. Williams, 1988, *Modern Nutrition in Health and Disease*, as above; some data from Weinsier, R.L. and C.E. Butterworth, 1981. *Handbook of Clinical Nutrition*, C.V. Mosby Co., St. Louis and Mayo Clinic health Letter, October 1991. Your fingernails: What do they reveal about your health.
Sample Act on Fact 2.1, 2.2: Adapted with permission from *Recommended Dietary Allowances: 10th Edition*. Copyright ©1989 by the National Academy of Sciences. Courtesy of the National Academy Press, Washington, D.C.
Table 2.3: Some data from Zeman, F. and D.M. Ney, 1988. *Applications of Clinical Nutrition*, Prentice-Hall, Englewood Cliffs, NJ and from USDA Consumer Nutrition Division, 1983. The thrifty food plan, 1983. Hyattsville, MD: Human Nutrition Information Service, USDA.
Table 2.4: "The Exchange Lists are the basis of a meal planning system designed by a committee of the American Diabetes Association and The American Dietetic Association. While designed primarily for people with diabetes and others who must follow special diets, the Exchange Lists are based on principles of good nutrition that apply to everyone. Exchange Lists for Meal Planning ©1986 American Diabetes Association.

Chapter 3
Fig. 3.7: Elaine N. Marieb, *Human Anatomy & Physiology*, 2nd Edition, fig. 24.2, p. 769, Redwood City, CA: Benjamin/Cummings, 1992. Copyright ©1992 Benjamin/Cummings Publishing Co., Inc.

Chapter 4
Table 4.1: Greenleaf, J.E. 1982. The body's need for fluids. NASA Ames Research Center.
Fig. 4.7: Elaine N. Marieb, *Human Anatomy & Physiology*, 2nd Ed., fig. 27.7, p. 910, Redwood City, CA: Benjamin/Cummings, 1992. Copyright ©1992 Benjamin/Cummings Publishing Co., Inc.

Chapter 5
Table 5.2: Institute of Food Technologists, (IFT) 1989. Ingredients for sweet success. *Food Technology* 43:94-116. IFT. 1987. Sweeteners: Nutritive and non-nutritive. *Contemporary Nutrition* 12(no. 9); Jain, N.K., V.P. Patel, C.S. Pitchumone. 1987. Sorbitol intolerance in adults. *Journal of Clinical Gastroenterology* 9:317-319.
Table 5.3: Matthews, R.H., P.R. Pehrsson, M. Farhat-Sabet. 1987. *Sugar Content of Selected Foods*. Washington, D.C.: US Dept. of Agriculture; Pennington, J.A. 1989. *Food Values of Portions Commonly Used*. NY: Harper & Row.
Table 5.7: Reprinted from Applegate, L., *Power Foods*. Copyright ©1991 by Rodale Press, Inc. Permission granted by Rodale Press, Inc., Emmaus, PA 18098.
Table 5.8: Data from Marlett, J.A. 1992. Content and composition of dietary fiber in 117 frequently consumed foods. *Journal of the American Dietetic Association* 92:175-186.
Fig. 5.5: Elaine N. Marieb, *Human Anatomy & Physiology*, 2nd Ed., Redwood City, CA: Benjamin/Cummings, 1992. Copyright ©1992 Benjamin/Cummings Publishing Co., Inc. Fig. 17-16, p. 566.
Fig. 5.7: Adapted from Bergstrom, J. et al., Diet, Muscle, Glycogen and Physical Performance. *Acta Physiologica Scandinavica* 71:140, 1967.

Chapter 6
Table 6.2: Anon. 1989. Fats, oils, and fat substitutes. *Food Technology* 43:66-74; Anon. 1990. Fat substitute update. *Food Technology* 44:92-97.; Waring, S. 1988. Shortening replacement in cakes. *Food Technology* 42:114-117; Nutrifat. 1988. The Nutrasweet Ca, Consumer Affairs Div., personal communication, 1992.
Table 6.6: Adapted from Linscheer, W.G. & A.J. Vergroesen, 1988. Lipids. In *Modern Nutrition in Health and Disease*, M.E. Shils & V.R. Young, eds. Lea & Febiger,Philadelphia.
Table 6.7: Report of the National Cholesterol Education Program, 1988. Expert Panel on Detection, Evaluation, and Treatment of High Blood Cholesterol in Adults. *Archives of Internal Medicine* 148:36-69.
Table 6.8: Hepburn, R.N, J. Exler, J.L. Weibrauch, 1986. Provisional tables on the content of omega-3 fatty acids and other fat components of selected foods. *Journal of the American Dietetic Association* 86:788-793.
Fig. 6.2: Neil Campbell, *Biology*, 3rd Edition, Copyright ©1993 Benjamin/Cummings Publishing Co., Redwood City, CA: Benjamin/Cummings Publishing Co. fig. 8.7, p. 156.
Fig. 6.7: McNamara, D.J. 1987. Effects of fat modified diets on cholesterol and lipoprotein metabolism. Reproduced with permission from the *Annual Review of Nutrition*, Vol. 7,273-290, ©1987 by Annual Reviews, Inc.
Fig. 6.9: McNamara, D.J. 1987. Effects of fat modified diets on cholesterol and lipoprotein metabolism. Reproduced with permission from the *Annual Review of Nutrition*, Vol. 7,273-290, ©1987 by Annual Reviews, Inc.
Fig. 6.17: Adapted from American Cancer Society, 1992. Cancer Facts and Figures - 1992. Atlanta, GA: American Cancer Society.
Fig. 6.12: Modified from Zilversmit, D.B. and C. Stark, 1984. Diet and cardiovascular disease. *Professional Perspectives*. June, 1984, Ithaca, NY: Cornell University Extension. With permission of the author.
Fig. 6.13: Adapted from Farrand, M.E., and L. Mojonnier. 1980. Nutrition in the multiple risk factor intervention trial [MRFIT]. *Journal of the American Dietetic Association* 76:347-351.
Fig. 6.14: National Research Council, 1989. *Diet and Health*. Washington, D.C.: National Academy Press.
Fig. 6.19: Carroll, K.K. 1991. "Nutrition and cancer: Fat." *Nutrition, Toxicity, and Cancer*, I.R. Rowland, ed. Boca Raton, FL, CRC Press.

Chapter 7
Fig. 7.7: A.P. Spence and E.B. Mason, *Human Anatomy & Physiology*, ©1983 Benjamin/Cummings Publishing Co., Redwood City, CA: Benjamin/Cummings Publishing Co. fig. 11.8, p. 299.

Chapter 8
Act on Fact 8.1: Table A adapted with permission from *Recommended Dietary Allowances: 10th Edition*. Copyright © 1989 by the National Academy of Sciences. Courtesy of the National Academy Press, Washington, D.C.
Table 8.1: Data from Taylor, C.M. & G. McLeod, 1949. *Rose's laboratory handbook for dietetics*, 5th Ed., p. 18, Macmillan; Durnin, J.V.G.A. & R. Passmore. 1967. Energy, work, and leisure. In *Energy and protein requirements*. FAO/WHO McArdle, W.D., F.I. Katch, V.L. Katch, 1981. Exercise physiology. Lea & Febiger; Passmore, R., J.V.G.A., Durnin. 1955. Human energy expenditure. *Physiological Reviews* 35:801-840.
Table 8.2: Adapted from *Recommended Dietary Allowances, 10th Ed.*, 1989, with permission of the National Academy Press, Washington, D.C.
Table 8.3: Data from Kolasa, K., A.C. Jobe, C. Dunn, 1991. "Consult a physician before starting any weight loss..." *Nutrition Today* 26(no. 6):25-31.
Table 8.5: Some data from Ganong, W.F., 1991. *Review of medical physiology*, p. 273. E. Norwalk, CT: Lange Medical Publications.

Fig. 8.3: Adapted from Poehlman, E.T., 1989. "A review: Exercise and its influence on resting energy metabolism in man." *Medicine and Science in Sports and Exercise* 21:515-525. Copyright ©1989 The American College of Sports Medicine.

Chapter 9

Table 9.1: Data from Bray, G.A. 1992. Pathophysiology of obesity. *American Journal of Clinical Nutrition* 55:488S-494S.
Table 9.2: Adapted from National Institutes of Health, 1992.
Table 9.3: McArdle, W.D., F.I. Katch, V.L.Katch, *Exercise Physiology*, 3rd Ed., Philadelphia: Lea & Febiger.
Table 9.5: Copyright ©1992 Green Mountain at Fox Run, Ludlow, VT 05149. A residentially-based weight and health management center for women only.
Ch. 9 You Tell Me p. 275: *Cases from Weighty Issues: Dangers and Deceptions of the Weight Loss Industry*. NY: Communications Division, NYC Department of Consumer Affairs.
Act on Fact 9.2: Adapted from "Finding the Fat in Food," 1991. University of Wisconsin-Madison: Nutrition Education Program. Data from the 1989 Recommended Dietary Allowances for average energy allowances.
Fig. 9.2: G.A. Bray, Pathophysiology of obesity. 1992 *American Journal of Clinical Nutrition*, 55:488S-494S.
Fig. 9.3: Adapted from Taylor et al., Performance capacity and effects of caloric restriction with hard physical work on young men. 1957. *Journal of Applied Physiology* 10:421-429.
Fig. 9.5: Bray, G.A. and S.D. Gray, 1988. Obesity: Part I: Pathogenesis. *Western Journal of Medicine* 149:429-441.
Fig. 9.6: Bray, G.A. and S.D. Gray, 1988. Obesity: Part I: Pathogenesis. *Western Journal of Medicine* 149:429-441.
Fig. 9.11: S.L. Gortmaker, W.H. Dietz, L.W. Cheung. 1990. Inactivity, diet, and the fattening of America. *Journal of the American Dietetic Association* 90:1247-1252, 1255. Copyright ©The American Dietetic Association. Reprinted by permission from *Journal of The American Dietetic Association*.
Fig. 9.12: S.M. Garn, 1985. Continuities and changes in fatness from infancy through adulthood. *Current Problems in Pediatrics* 15:1-47. By permission of Mosby-Year Book, Inc.
Fig. 9.15: W.D. McArdle, F.I. Katch, V.L. Katch. 1991. *Exercise Physiology*, 3rd Ed. Philadelphia: Lea & Febiger.
Fig. 9.18: R.B. Stuart, C. Mitchell, J.A. Jensen. 1981. Therapeutic options in the management of obesity. *Medical Psychology: Contributions to Behavioral Medicine*. NY: Academic Press.

Chapter 10

Table 10.1: American Psychiatric Association: *Diagnostic and Statistical Manual of Mental Disorders, Third Edition, Revised*, Washington, D.C., American Psychiatric Association, 1987.
Table 10.2: American Psychiatric Association: Diagnostic and Statistical Manual of Mental Disorders, Third Edition, Revised, Washington, D.C., American Psychiatric Association, 7.
Table 10.3: Adapted from Adams, L.B. and M.B. Shafer, 1988. Early manifestations of eating disorders in adolescents: Defining those at risk. *Journal of Nutrition Education* 20:307-312.
Slice of Life p. 320: L.Hall and L. Cohn. 1992. *Bulimia: A Guide to Recovery*, Carlsbad, CA: Gurze Books.
Slice of Life p. 316-317: Crisp, A.H. 1980. *Anorexia Nervosa: Let Me Be*. London: Academic Press.
Table 10.4: B.T. Walsh, Pharmacotherapy of eating disorders. In *The Eating Disorders*, ed. B.J. Blinder, F.F. Chaitin, R.S. Goldstein. 1988. NY: PMA Publishing Corporation.
Table 10.5: J. Rodin and L. Larson. 1992. Social Factors and the Ideal Body Shape. In *Eating, Body Weight, and Performance in Athletes*, ed. J.D. Brownell, J. Rodin, J.H. Wilmore. Philadelphia: Lea & Febiger.
Slice of Life p. 322: Stein and B.C. Unell. 1986. *Anorexia Nervosa: Finding the Life Line*. Minneapolis: CompCare Publications. Reprinted with permission.

Chapter 11

Table 11.1: RDA Subcommittee, 1989. *Recommended Dietary Allowances*. Washington, D.C. National Academy Press; Shils, M.E. and V.R. Young, 1988. *Modern Nutrition in Health and Disease*. Philadelphia: Lea & Febiger.
Table 11.2: HNIS: *Agricultural handbook 8 series on composition of foods*. Washington, D.C.: U.S. Department of Agriculture; ESHA Research - Nutrition Systems.
Table 11.3: Data adapted from Pennington, J.A. 1989. *Food values of portions commonly used*. Philadelphia: J.B. Lippincott. By permission of Dr. Pennington.
Table 11.4: Data adapted from Pennington, J.A. 1989. *Food values of portions commonly used*. Philadelphia: J.B. Lippincott. By permission of Dr. Pennington.
Table 11.5: Data from Suttie, J.W. 1992. Vitamin K and human nutrition. Journal of American Dietetic Association 92:585-590.
Fig. 11.3: Bauerfeind, J.C. 1988. Vitamin A deficiency: A staggering problem of health and sight. *Nutrition Today* 23:34-36.(March/April)
Fig. 11.4: Bauerfeind, J.C. 1988. Vitamin A deficiency: A staggering problem of health and sight. *Nutrition Today* 23:34-36. (March/April)

Chapter 12

Table 12.1: Nielsen, F.H. 1988. Ultra trace minerals, *Modern Nutrition in Health and Disease*, eds. M.E. Shils and V.R. Young, Philadelphia: Lea & Febiger.
Table 12.2: 1)Shils, M.E. 1988. Magnesium. In *Modern Nutrition in Health & Disease*, eds. M.E. Shils, V.R. Young. Philadelphia: Lea & Febiger; 2)Fairbanks, V.F., E. Beutler. Iron. [from same as 1); 3)Solomons, N.W. Zinc and copper. (from same as 1);4) RDA Subcommittee. 1989. *Recommended dietary allowances*. Washington, D.C. National Academy Press; 5)Underwood, E.J. 1977. *Trace elements in human and animal nutrition*. NY: Academic Press.
Table 12.4: Data from Leveille, G.A., M.E. Zabik, K.J. Morgan. 1983. *Nutrients in foods*. Cambridge, MA: The Nutrition Guild.
Slice of Life p. 394: Marshall, C.W. 1983. *Vitamins and minerals: Help or harm?* Philadelphia: George F. Stickley Company.
Fig. 12.3: *Nutrition Review*. 1991. 49:24-25. Springer-Verlag.
Fig. 12.9: Sweeney, E.A. and J.A. Shaw. 1988. Nutrition in relation to dental medicine, in *Modern Nutrition in Health and Disease*, eds. M.E. Shils and V.R. Young, Lea & Febiger.

Chapter 13

Table 13.1: Data from American Dietetic Association 1991; Food Marketing Institute Survey, 1992.
Table 13.3: Data from Pennington, J.A., 1989, *Food values of portions commonly used*. NY: Harper & Row; Science and Education Administration, 1985. *Nutritive value of foods*. Home and Garden Bulletin No. 72. Washington, D.C.: U.S. Department of Agriculture.
Fig. 13.6: Tannenbaum, Young, Archer, fig. 14.6, p. 488, "Vitamins and Minerals." In *Food Chemistry*, 3rd Ed., O.R. Fennema, ed., Marcel Dekker, Inc., New York, 1985. Reprinted by courtesy of Marcel Dekker, Inc.
Table 13.2: Karmas, E. and R.S. Harris, eds. 1988. *Nutritional Evaluation of Food Processing*. NY: Chapman and Hall

Chapter 14

Ch. 14 Thinking for Yourself: From Carol Sugarman, "FDA Approves Irradiation of Poultry," *The Washington Post*, May 2, 1990. Copyright ©1990 The Washington Post. Reprinted with permission.
Table 14.1: Adapted from Annest, J.L., K.R. Mahaffey, D.H. Cox, J.Roberts, 1982. Blood lead levels for persons 6 months to 74 years of age: United States, 1976-80. *National Center for Health Statistics Advance Data* 79:1-24.
Table 14.2: Gold et al., 1987. Ranking possible carcinogenic hazards. *SCIENCE* 236: 271-280 and Ames & Gold, 1987. Pesticides, risk and applesauce. *SCIENCE* 236:755-757. Copyright ©1987 by the American Association for the Advancement of Science.
Table 14.3: Wilson, R. & E.A.C. Crouch, 1987. Risk assessment and comparisons: An introduction. *SCIENCE* 236:267-70. Copyright ©1987 by the American Association for the Advancement of Science.
Table 14.4: Adapted from Roberts, H.R. and J.J. Barone, 1983. Caffeine content of food products. *Reprinted from Food Technology*. 1983. 37(9):32-39. Copyright © Institute of Food Technologists.
Table 14.5: Adapted from the Committee on Nitrite and Alternative Curing Agents in Food, 1981, with the permission of the National Academy Press, Washington, D.C.

Fig. 14.1: Adapted from Murphy, S.D. Toxicological assessment of food residues. Reprinted from *Food Technology*. 1979. 33(6):35-42. Copyright © Institute of Food Technologists.

Fig. 14.2: Glass, R.I., M. Libel, A.D. Brandling-Bennett. 1992. *SCIENCE* 256:1254-55. American Association for the Advancement of Science and Centers for Diseases Control.

Fig. 14.3: Adapted from Leveille, G.A., M.A. Uebersax. 1979. Fundamentals of food science for the dietitian: Thermal processing. *Dietetic Currents* 6(no.3). Columbus, OH: Ross Laboratories.

Fig. 14.5: Adapted from Food Safety and Inspection Service. 1984. *The Safe Food Book*. Home and Garden Bulletin No. 24. Washington, D.C. United States Department of Agriculture, 1984.

Fig. 14.6: Reprinted from U.S. Department of Agriculture, 1990. *Chartbook Agriculture Handbook no. 689*, Washington, D.C.

Chapter 15

Slice of Life 15.1: Satter, E. 1986. *Child of Mine*. Palo Alto, CA: Bull Publishing Co.

Table 15.1: Adapted from Williams, S.R. 1988. Nutrition for high risk populations. In *Nutrition Throughout the Life Cycle*, Eds. S.R. Williams, B.S. Worthington Roberts. St.Louis, MO: Times Mirror/Mosby College Publishing.

Table 15.3: Adapted from Mutch, P.B., 1988. *Food Journal of Clinical Nutrition* 48:913-919. and RDA Subcommittee 1989. *Recommended dietary allowances*. Washington, D.C. National Academy Press.

Table 15.4: Jensen, R.G., A.M. Ferris, C.J. Lammi-Keefe. 1992. Lipids in human milk and infant formulas. Reproduced with permission from the *Annual Review of Nutrition*, Vol. 12, pp. 417-441. Copyright ©1992 by Annual Reviews, Inc.

Fig. 15.1: Adapted from Committee on Nutritional Status During Pregnancy and Lactation, 1990. *Nutrition During Pregnancy, Appendix B*. Washington, D.C.: National Academy Press.

Fig. 15.3: Adapted from Moore, K.L., *The Developing Human*, 4th Ed. Philadelphia: W.B. Saunders Co.1988. With permission.

Fig. 15.4: Data from RDA Subcommittee, National Resarch Council, 1989. *Recommended dietary allowances*. Washington, D.C.: National Academy Press.

Fig. 15.10: Adapted from National Center for Health Statistics, NCHS Growth Charts, 1976. *Monthly Vital Statistics Report* Vol. 25, No. 3, Supp. (HRA)76-1120. Health Resources Administration, Rockville, MD, June 1976. Data from the Fels Research Institute, Yellow Springs, OH 1976 Ross Laboratories, Columbus, OH 43216.

Chapter 16

Slice of Life 16: Satter, E., *How To Get Your Kid To Eat But Not Too Much*, Bull Publishing, Palo Alto, CA. Used with permission.

Table 16.1: Adapted from Hertzler, A.A. 1989. *Journal of Nutrition Education*. 21:100 B-C.; Sigman-Grant, M. 1992. *Nutrition Today* 27(no. 4):13-17. Williams & Wilkins.

Table 16.2: Sigman-Grant, M. 1992. Feeding pre-schoolers: Balancing nutritional and developmental needs. *Nutrition Today* 27(no.4):13-17. Williams & Wilkins.

Table 16.4: Adapted from Gillespie, A. 1983. Asessing snacking behavior in children. *Ecology of Food and Nutrition* 13:167-172.

Table 16.5: American School Health Assn., Assn. for the Advancement of Health Education, Society for Public Health Education,Inc. 1989. *The National Adolescent Student Health Survey: A Report on the Health of America's Youth*. A cooperative project of U.S.D.H.H.S., P.H.S., Office of Disease Prevention and Health Promotion, Centers for Disease Control, National Institute on Drug Abuse.

Table 16.6: American College of Sports Medicine. 1976. Position stand on weight loss in wrestlers. *Medicine and Science in Sports and Exercise* 8(no.2):xi-xiii.

Fig. 16.1: Data from National Research Council,1989. *Recommended dietary allowances*. Washington, D.C.: National Academy of Sciences.

Fig. 16.2: Adapted from J.A. Harris, C.M.Jackson, R.E. Scammon, *The Measurement of Man*, 1927, University of Minnesota Press.

Fig. 16.5: Data from National Research Council,1989. *Recommended dietary allowances*. Washington, D.C.: National Academy of Sciences; RDA Subcommittee, 1989.

Fig. 16.7: Adapted from Valadian, I. and D. Porter, 1977. *Physical growth and development from conception to maturity: A programmed text*. Boston: Little, Brown & Co.

Fig. 16.8: Courtesy: National Dairy Council.

Chapter 17

Slice of Life p. 589: From Jackie Bradley, "Organization Is A Key Ingredient for Two Sisters," *The Wisconsin State Journal*, May 27, 1990.

Slice of Life p. 566: Adapted from The Milwaukee Journal, Monday, Dec. 8, 1986. Reprinted with permission of The Milwaukee Journal.

Fig 17.5: White, J.V., J.T. Dwyer, B.M. Posner, R.J. Ham, D.A. Lipschitz, N.S. Wellman. 1992. Nutrition Screening Initiative: Development and implementation of the public awareness checklist and screening tools. *Journal of the American Dietetic Association* 92:163-167. ©American Dietetic Association. By permission of the *Journal of the American Dietetic Association*.

Table 17.1: Evans, W. and I.H. Rosenberg. 1991. *Biomarkers: The 10 Determinants of Aging You Can Control*. NY: Simon & Schuster.

Table 17.2: Adapted from *Tufts University Diet and Nutrition Letter*, 1986. To drink or not to drink? That's one of the questions. *Tufts University Diet and Nutrition Letter* 4(no. 1):4.

Table 17.4: Adapted from USDA Consumer Nutrition Division, 1983. *The Thrifty Food Plan*, 1983. Hyattsville, MD: Human Nutrition Information Service. US Department of Agriculture.

Table 17.5: American Dietetic Association, *Healthful Eating All Around Town*, 1990. Copyright ©American Dietetic Association. Reprinted by permission.

Fig. 17.1: Flieger, K. 1988. Why do we age? *FDA Consumer*, October 1988:20-25. U.S. Bureau of the Census.

Fig. 17.3: From Alexander Leaf, *Growing Old*. Copyright ©1973 by Scientific American, Inc. All rights reserved.

Fig. 17.4: Data from National Center for Health Statistics, 1977. Dietary Intake Findings: United States, 1971-74; *National Health Survey*, Series 11, No. 202. DHEW Publications No.[HRA] 77-1647. Hyattsville, MD: Public Health Service.

Fig. 17.10: Marmot, M. and E. Brunner. 1991. Alcohol and cardiovascular disease: The Status of the U-Shaped Curve. *British Medical Journal* 303:565-567.

Chapter 18

Table 18.1: World Resources Institute. 1992. *World Resources 1992-1993: Toward Sustainable Development*. London: Oxford University Press.

Fig. 18.1: Information Division, FAO of the United Nations.

Fig. 18.3: Smithsonian Institution, *Tropical Rainforests: Disappearing Treasure*, Traveling Ext. Service, 1988.

Fig. 18.5: Brown, L.R., C. Flavin, H. Kane. 1992. *Vital Signs 1992*. W.W. Norton.

Fig. 18.7: Plant biotech FDA decision trees to guide industry, *Food Chemical News*, June 1, 1992.

Slice of Life p. 613: From Introduction to J.L. Jacobsen, *Gender Bias: Roadblock to Sustainable Development*, 1992, Worldwatch paper 110. Washington, D.C., Worldwatch Institute.

Fig. 18.8: United Nations Population Division, *Long Range Population Projections: Two Centuries of Population Growth, 1950-2150*, executive summary.

Fig. 18.9: Adapted from Perisse, J., F. Sizaret, P. Francoise. 1969. The effect of income on the structure of the diet. *FAO Newsletter* 7(July-Sept.):2

Fig. 18.11: Brown, L.R., C. Flavin, H. Kane. 1992. *Vital Signs 1992*. W.W. Norton.

Appendix B (first page): Scientific Review Committee. 1990. *Nutrition Recommendations*. Ottawa, Canada: Health and Welfare. (second page): Adapted from "Canada's Food Guide," Health and Welfare Canada, 1983, Minister of Supply and Services Canada. (third page): From *Canada's Food Guide to Health Eating 1992*. Minister of Supply and Services Canada 1992. Cat. No. H39-252/1992E.

Appendix C: Reprinted with permission from N-Squared Computing, 3040 Commercial St. SE, Suite 240, Salem, OR 97302. Developer of the Diet Simple Plus/Fitness Evaluator Software.

Inside Back Cover: Adapted from *Recommended Dietary Allowances, 10th Edition*, ©1989 National Academy of Sciences, National Academy Press, Washington, D.C.

Page Opposite Inside Back Cover: Adapted from *Recommended Dietary Allowances, 10th Edition*, ©1989 National Academy of Sciences, National Academy Press, Washington, D.C.

Photograph Credits

Chapter 1
Part 1 Opener: Richard Tauber; Chapter Opener: Richard Tauber
1.1a: Matt Meadows/Peter Arnold, Inc. 1.1b: Peter Gridley/FPG International. 1.2: Ron Chapple/FPG International. 1.3a: Lawrence Migdale/Stock Boston. 1.3b: John Coletti/Stock Boston. 1.6: Richard Hutchings/Photo Researchers. 1.7: Laura Dwight/Peter Arnold, Inc. 1.8: Richard Hutchings/Photo Researchers. 1.9a: Jeff Persons/Stock Boston. 1.9b: Richard Tauber. 1.11: Milton Potts/Photo Researchers. 1.13: Doug Plummer/Photo Researchers.

Chapter 2
Chapter Opener: Richard Tauber
2.1a: Suzanne Arms. 2.1b: Richard Tauber. 2.4: Richard Tauber. "Pieces of the Pyramid"; pp. 45-52: Richard Tauber.

Chapter 3
Chapter Opener: Richard Tauber
3.3: Shaffer/Smith Photography. 3.4: Suzanne Arms. 3.6b: Peter Arnold, Inc. 3.9a: Ed Reschke/Peter Arnold, Inc. 3.9b: Ed Reschke/Peter Arnold, Inc. 3.9c: Ed Reschke/Peter Arnold, Inc. 3.16: Gary Haynes/The Image Works.

Chapter 4
Part 2 Opener: Richard Tauber; Chapter Opener: Richard Tauber
4.8: Olaf Kallstran/Jeroboam. Box, p. 111: Kent Reno/Jeroboam.

Chapter 5
Chapter Opener: Richard Tauber
5.6: Hattie Young/Photo Researchers; Science Photo Library. 5.8: Ted Kerasote/Photo Researchers.

Chapter 6
Chapter Opener: Richard Tauber
6.1b: Alfred Owczarzak/Biological Photo Service. 6.10b: Martin M. Rotker/Photo Researchers. 6.15: Bob Daemmrich/Stock Boston. 6.16: Brock May/Photo Researchers.

Chapter 7
Chapter Opener: Richard Tauber
7.5a: CNRI/SPL/Photo Researchers. 7.5b: Bill Longcore/Photo Researchers. 7.9: Richard Tauber. 7.10: Photo Researchers/Omikron. 7.11: Teri Stratford/Photo Researchers.

Chapter 8
Part 3 Opener: Richard Tauber; Chapter Opener: Richard Tauber
8.2a: Comstock Inc./M+C Werner. 8.2b: Edward Lettau/Photo Researchers. 8.2c: Jan Lukas/Photo Researchers. 8.2d: David Ryan/Photo 20-20. 8.2e: Gerard Vandystadt/Photo Researchers.

Chapter 9
Chapter Opener: Richard Tauber
9.1: Bettmann Archive. 9.4, Left to right: Art Resource, Bettmann Archive, Cooper Hewitt Museum Picture Library, Reuters/Bettmann. 9.7: Peter Menzel/Stock Boston. 9.10: John Running. 9.13: Erika Stone/ Peter Arnold, Inc. 9.14a: Peter Arnold/Peter Arnold, Inc. 9.14b: Bruce Byers/FPG International. 9.19: Bob Daemmrich/Image Works. Box, p. 304: Bettmann Archive.

Chapter 10
Chapter Opener: Richard Tauber
10.2: UPI/Bettmann Newsphotos. 10.3: Bob Daemmrich/Image Works. 10.4: W Hill/Image Works.

Chapter 11
Part 4 Opener: Terry Heffernan, Inc.; Chapter Opener: Terry Heffernan, Inc.
11.3a: J. Christopher Bauernfeind/Nutrition Today. 11.7a: Biophoto Associates, Science Source/Photo Researchers. 11.7b: Dr. F.C. Skvara/Peter Arnold, Inc. 11.8: Richard Tauber.

Chapter 12
Chapter Opener: Terry Heffernan, Inc.
12.2: Michael Klein/Peter Arnold, Inc. 12.6: Stephen L. Feldman/Photo Researchers. 12.7a: Biophoto Associates, Science Source/Photo Researchers. 12.7b: Biophoto Associates/Photo Researchers. 12.8: John Paul Kay/Peter Arnold, Inc. 12.10: K.M. Hambidge, P.A. Walravens, and K.H. Neldner. In Zinc and Copper Clinical Medicine, eds. K.M. Hambidge and B.L. Nichols. New York: Spectrum Publishers, 1978.

Chapter 13
Part 5 Opener: Richard Tauber; Chapter Opener: Richard Tauber
13.1: Larry Lefever/Grant Heilman Photography, Inc. 13.2: National Livestock and Meat Board. 13.3: Larry Lefever/Grant Heilman Photography, Inc. 13.4: Martin J. Heade/Bettmann Archive. 13.8: Richard Tauber.

Chapter 14
Chapter Opener: Richard Tauber
14.4: Andrew Syred/Photo Researchers.

Chapter 15
Part 6 Opener: Richard Tauber; Chapter Opener: Richard Tauber
15.2 left: Lennart Nilsson/Boehringer Ingelheim International. 15.2 middle and right: Lennart Nilsson. 15.5: Streissguth, A.P., Clarren, S.K., and K.L. Jones, Natural History of the Fetal Alcohol Syndrome: A ten-year follow-up of eleven patients. Lancet 2 (July 1985):85-92. 15.6: Suzanne Arms. 15.7: Suzanne Arms. 15.8: David Johnsen, Case Western Reserve University. 15.9: C. Seghers/Photo Researchers.

Chapter 16
Chapter Opener: Richard Tauber
16.3a: Bob Daemmrich/Image Works. 16.3b: Laura Dwight/Peter Arnold, Inc. 16.4a: Kosti Ruohomaa/Black Star. 16.4b: John Troha/Black Star. 16.6: Mike Douglas/Image Works.

Chapter 17
Chapter Opener: Richard Tauber
17.6: Catherine Ursillo/Photo Researchers. 17.7: Suzanne Arms. 17.8: AP/Wide World Photos. 17.11: Spencer Grant/Photo Researchers.

Chapter 18
Chapter Opener: Richard Tauber
18.2: Andrew Holbrooke/Black Star. 18.4: Steve McCurry/Magnum. 18.6a: Paul Miller/Black Star. 18.6b: Bob Krist/Black Star. 18.10: OXFAM America. 18.12: M. Granitsas/Image Works.

Index

NOTE: Page numbers on which tables appear are followed by *t*.

Estimated Safe and Adequate Daily Dietary Intakes of Selected Vitamins and Minerals[a]

Category	Age (years)	Vitamins: Biotin (μg)	Vitamins: Pantothenic Acid (mg)
Infants	0-0.5	10	2
	0.5-1	15	3
Children and adolescents	1-3	20	3
	4-6	25	3-4
	7-10	30	4-5
	11+	30-100	4-7
Adults		30-100	4-7

Category	Age (years)	Trace Elements[b]: Copper (mg)	Manganese (mg)	Fluoride (mg)	Chromium (μg)	Molybdenum (μg)
Infants	0-0.5	0.4-0.6	0.3-0.6	0.1-0.5	10-40	15-30
	0.5-1	0.6-0.7	0.6-1.0	0.2-1.0	20-60	20-40
Children and adolescents	1-3	0.7-1.0	1.0-1.5	0.5-1.5	20-80	25-50
	4-6	1.0-1.5	1.5-2.0	1.0-2.5	30-120	30-75
	7-10	1.0-2.0	2.0-3.0	1.5-2.5	50-200	50-150
	11+	1.5-2.5	2.0-5.0	1.5-2.5	50-200	75-250
Adults		1.5-3.0	2.0-5.0	1.5-4.0	50-200	75-250

[a] Because there is less information on which to base allowances, these figures are not given in the main table of RDA and are provided here in the form of ranges of recommended intakes.
[b] Since the toxic levels for many trace elements may be only several times usual intakes, the upper levels for the trace elements given in this table should not be habitually exceeded.

Estimated Sodium, Chloride, and Potassium Minimum Requirements for Healthy Persons[a]

Age	Weight (kg)[a]	Sodium (mg)[a,b]	Chloride (mg)[a,b]	Potassium (mg)[c]
Months				
0-5	4.5	120	180	500
6-11	8.9	200	300	700
Years				
1	11.0	225	350	1,000
2-5	16.0	300	500	1,400
6-9	25.0	400	600	1,600
10-18	50.0	500	750	2,000
> 18[d]	70.0	500	750	2,000

[a] No allowance has been included for large, prolonged losses from the skin through sweat.
[b] There is no evidence that higher intakes confer any health benefit.
[c] Desirable intakes of potassium may considerably exceed these values (~3,500 mg for adults).
[d] No allowance included for growth, pregnancy, or lactation.